TOURO COLLEGE LIBRARY
Kings Hwy

WITHDRAWN

Treatment of Childhood Disorders

Third Edition

Treatment of Childhood Disorders

Third Edition

TOURO COLLEGE LIBRARY
Kings Hwy

edited by
Eric J. Mash
Russell A. Barkley

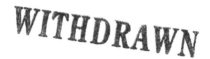

THE GUILFORD PRESS
New York   London

KH

© 2006 The Guilford Press
A Division of Guilford Publications, Inc.
72 Spring Street, New York, NY 10012
www.guilford.com

All rights reserved

No part of this book may be reproduced, translated, stored in a retrieval system, or
transmitted, in any form or by any means, electronic, mechanical, photocopying,
microfilming, recording, or otherwise, without written permission from the Publisher.

Printed in the United States of America

This book is printed on acid-free paper.

Last digit is print number: 9   8   7   6   5   4   3   2   1

Library of Congress Cataloging-in-Publication Data
Treatment of childhood disorders / edited by Eric J. Mash, Russell A. Barkley.—3rd ed.
    p. cm.
    Includes bibliographical references and index.
    ISBN-10 1-57230-921-0   ISBN-13 978-1-57230-921-0 (hardcover)
    1. Behavior disorders in children—Treatment.   2. Affective disorders in children—
Treatment.   3. Behavior therapy for children.   4. Child psychopathology.   5. Child
psychotherapy.   6. Behavioral assessment of children.   I. Mash, Eric J.   II. Barkley, Russell
A., 1949– .
    [DNLM: 1. Child Behavior Disorders—therapy.   2. Developmental Disabilities—
therapy.   3. Mood Disorders—Infant.   4. Mood Disorders—Child.   5. Behavior Therapy—
Infant.   6. Behavior Therapy—Child.
WS 350.6 T784 2006]
RJ506.B44T73 2006
618.92′8914—dc22

                                                                          2005019901

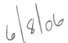
6\8\06

To my wife, Heather,
and to the memory of three special girlfriends—
Annie, Tootie, and Sadie

—E. J. M.

To Steve, Ken, and Pat

—R. A. B.

About the Editors

Eric J. Mash, PhD, is Professor of Psychology in the Department of Psychology and Program in Clinical Psychology at the University of Calgary. He is a fellow of the American and Canadian Psychological Associations; has served as an editor, editorial board member, and editorial consultant for many scientific and professional journals; and has written or edited numerous books and journal articles related to children's mental health, child and adolescent psychopathology, child and adolescent psychotherapy, and child and family assessment. Dr. Mash's research has focused on family relationships across a variety of child and family disorders, including attention-deficit/hyperactivity disorder, conduct problems, internalizing disorders, and maltreatment. He is a recipient of the Leadership Education in Neurodevelopmental Disabilities Distinguished Alumnus Award from the Oregon Health & Science University.

Russell A. Barkley, PhD, is Research Professor of Psychiatry at the State University of New York (SUNY) Upstate Medical University at Syracuse. In 1978, he founded the Neuropsychology Service at the Medical College of Wisconsin and Milwaukee Children's Hospital, and served as its Chief until 1985. He then moved to the University of Massachusetts Medical School, where he served as Director of Psychology from 1985 to 2000 and established the research clinics for both child and adult attention-deficit/hyperactivity disorder (ADHD). In 2003, he relocated to a position as Professor in the Department of Psychiatry at the Medical University of South Carolina. He joined the faculty of the SUNY Upstate Medical University in 2005. Dr. Barkley has published 15 books, more than 200 scientific articles and book chapters, and 7 videos on ADHD and related disorders, including childhood defiance, and is editor of the newsletter *The ADHD Report*. A frequent conference presenter and speaker who is widely cited in the national media, he is past president of the Section on Clinical Child Psychology, Division 12 of the American Psychological Association, and of the International Society for Research in Child and Adolescent Psychopathology. His distinguished research contributions have been recognized with awards from the American Association of Applied and Preventive Psychology, the American Academy of Pediatrics, the Section on Clinical Child Psychology of the American Psychological Association, and the Society for a Science of Clinical Psychology.

Contributors

Sandra T. Azar, PhD, Department of Psychology, Pennsylvania State University, University Park, Pennsylvania

Russell A. Barkley, PhD, Department of Psychiatry, State University of New York Upstate Medical University at Syracuse, Syracuse, New York

Sandra A. Brown, PhD, Departments of Psychiatry and Psychology, University of California at San Diego, La Jolla, California; Psychology Service, Veterans Affairs San Diego HealthCare System, San Diego, California

Vinita Chhabra, MEd, Child Development and Behavior Branch, National Institute of Child Health and Human Development, National Institutes of Health, Bethesda, Maryland

Bruce F. Chorpita, PhD, Department of Psychology, University of Hawaii at Manoa, Honolulu, Hawaii

Jack M. Fletcher, PhD, Department of Pediatrics, University of Texas Health Sciences Center, Houston, Texas

John P. Foreyt, PhD, Behavioral Medicine Research Center, Baylor College of Medicine, Houston, Texas

Kevin Frissell, MS, Department of Psychiatry and Human Behavior, Brown University, Providence, Rhode Island

Lynn S. Fuchs, PhD, Department of Special Education, Vanderbilt University, Nashville, Tennessee

Richard H. Gilchrist, MD, Akron Children's Hospital, Akron, Ohio

Rand Glenn, MA, Department of Educational Psychology, University of Texas, Austin, Texas

Benjamin L. Handen, PhD, Departments of Psychiatry and Pediatrics, University of Pittsburgh School of Medicine, Pittsburgh, Pennsylvania; John Merck Child Outpatient Program, Western Psychiatric Institute and Clinic, Pittsburgh, Pennsylvania

Michele Hauser, MD, Department of Educational Psychology, University of Texas, Austin, Texas

Christine A. Hovanitz, PhD, Department of Psychology, University of Cincinnati, Cincinnati, Ohio

Julie S. Kotler, MS, Department of Psychology, University of Washington, Seattle, Washington

G. Reid Lyon, PhD, Child Development and Behavior Branch, National Institute of Child Health and Human Development, National Institutes of Health, Bethesda, Maryland

Laura MacPherson, PhD, Alcohol and Addiction Studies, Department of Biology and Medicine, Brown University, Providence, Rhode Island

Eric J. Mash, PhD, Department of Psychology, University of Calgary, Calgary, Alberta, Canada

Robert J. McMahon, PhD, Department of Psychology, University of Washington, Seattle, Washington

Johanna Molnar, MS, Department of Educational Psychology, University of Texas, Austin, Texas

Mark G. Myers, PhD, Department of Psychiatry, University of California at San Diego, La Jolla, California

Crighton Newsom, PhD, Southwest Ohio Developmental Center, Batavia, Ohio

Walker S. Carlos Poston II, PhD, Department of Psychology, University of Missouri, Kansas City, Missouri

Janay Sander, PhD, Department of Educational Psychology, University of Texas, Austin, Texas

Sarah Schnoebelen, PhD, Department of Educational Psychology, University of Texas, Austin, Texas

Cheri J. Shapiro, PhD, Department of Psychology, University of South Carolina, Columbia, South Carolina

Jane Simpson, PhD, Department of Educational Psychology, University of Texas, Austin, Texas

Bradley H. Smith, PhD, Department of Psychology, University of South Carolina, Columbia, South Carolina

Michael A. Southam-Gerow, PhD, Department of Psychology, Virginia Commonwealth University, Richmond, Virginia

Kevin D. Stark, PhD, Department of Educational Psychology, University of Texas, Austin, Texas

Lisa Terre, PhD, Department of Psychology, University of Missouri, Kansas City, Missouri

Karen C. Wells, PhD, Family Studies Program and Clinic, Department of Psychiatry, Duke University, Durham, North Carolina

David A. Wolfe, PhD, Centre for Prevention Science, Centre for Addiction and Mental Health, London, Ontario, Canada; Departments of Psychology and Psychiatry, University of Toronto, Toronto, Ontario, Canada; Faculty of Education, University of Western Ontario, London, Ontario, Canada

Vicky Veitch Wolfe, PhD, Child and Adolescent Centre, London Health Sciences Centre, London, Ontario, Canada

Preface

Our goal for this volume has remained largely unchanged from the two previous editions—that is, to construct a resource of both scholarly and practical information on evidence-based, scientifically established treatments for childhood psychological disorders. Its companion volumes, Mash and Terdal's *Assessment of Childhood Disorders* (New York: Guilford Press, 1997) and our own *Child Psychopathology* (New York: Guilford Press, 2003), complete the set by providing similar scientifically based information on the nature and evaluation of those disorders. As in our past editions, we have been fortunate to be joined by highly regarded experts on each disorder and its treatment, so as to provide our readers with the state of both the science and art of treatment. We wish to express our gratitude here to all of them for the substantial investment of time and effort they have put into bringing their respective chapters up to date. With more than 8 years having elapsed since the second edition, hundreds of research publications on the treatments for each disorder needed to be consulted for their implications in revising this volume. Eschewing once again the typical fads, fashions, guru-based clinical dogmas, and "alternative" (a/k/a unscientific) approaches to treatment, our experts instead review the scientifically based options for treatment and use what can be extrapolated from that empirical basis to educate readers on the best approaches currently recognized for each disorder. We were especially interested in information not only on the efficacy of interventions as demonstrated in clinical trials conducted by experts and often in university settings, but also on the effectiveness of these same treatments as they are likely to be instituted in more naturalistic, typical clinical settings where such information may be available. We believe that the authors have successfully attained this goal. The result is not simply a compendium of treatment options, but a set of thoughtful and well-reasoned reviews and critiques of the rationales or conceptual bases for the treatments available, the factors that may moderate or mediate their effectiveness with various client populations, and the available evidence for their efficacy and effectiveness.

Whereas in the earlier volumes we likened our text to a family snapshot, capturing the dynamic field of treatment at a single point in time, this third edition comes with a more historical basis. It is therefore more akin to a family video, for it retains the richness of the past two decades and what was known over that span of time, while appreciating the ebb and flow of more recent findings and indicating future directions (to the extent that these can be discerned). It is evident that we know far more now about the treatment of childhood disorders than ever before, and that the self-correcting nature of this clinical–scientific enterprise has succeeded in paring away those approaches that seemed initially promising but proved not to be so, while retaining and enhancing the evidentiary basis of those having greater utility. New approaches to treatment have also been identified, and, as one would expect from a maturing clinical science, more is known about the combinations of therapies than was heretofore the case. We believe our authors have done an exceptional job of capturing this dynamic, self-correcting, yet advancing state of knowledge of the treatment scene, and we hope that you will agree with our assessment.

Besides our obvious appreciation to this volume's many contributors, we are also grateful for the exceptional assistance of Marie Sprayberry, Judith Grauman, Laura Specht Patchkofsky, Carolyn Graham, and others at The Guilford Press for shepherding this project to its fruition. They have made us and our contributors appear to be far better writers than we have a right to claim. We are also indebted to Seymour Weingarten, Editor in Chief, and Bob Matloff, President, of The Guilford Press—longstanding friends who have repeatedly supported this and other works of ours for more than 25 years. And, of course, this work would not have been possible without the love, encouragement, and support of our families—Heather Mash, and Pat, Steve, and Ken Barkley—to whom we once again express our deep appreciation. Learn and enjoy. *Bon appétit!*

ERIC J. MASH, PhD
RUSSELL A. BARKLEY, PhD

Contents

I. INTRODUCTION

1. Treatment of Child and Family Disturbance: 3
A Cognitive-Behavioral Systems Perspective
Eric J. Mash

II. BEHAVIOR DISORDERS

2. Attention-Deficit/Hyperactivity Disorder   65
Bradley H. Smith, Russell A. Barkley, and Cheri J. Shapiro

3. Conduct Problems   137
Robert J. McMahon, Karen C. Wells, and Julie S. Kotler

III. EMOTIONAL AND SOCIAL DISORDERS

4. Fears and Anxieties   271
Bruce F. Chorpita and Michael A. Southam-Gerow

5. Depressive Disorders during Childhood and Adolescence   336
*Kevin D. Stark, Janay Sander, Michele Hauser, Jane Simpson,
Sarah Schnoebelen, Rand Glenn, and Johanna Molnar*

IV. DEVELOPMENTAL DISORDERS

6. Mental Retardation   411
Benjamin L. Handen and Richard H. Gilchrist

7. Autistic Spectrum Disorders   455
Crighton Newsom and Christine A. Hovanitz

8. Learning Disabilities   512
G. Reid Lyon, Jack M. Fletcher, Lynn S. Fuchs, and Vinita Chhabra

Contents

V. CHILDREN AT RISK

9. Child Physical Abuse and Neglect 595
Sandra T. Azar and David A. Wolfe

10. Child Sexual Abuse 647
Vicky Veitch Wolfe

VI. PROBLEMS OF ADOLESCENCE

11. Adolescent Substance Use Problems 731
*Laura MacPherson, Kevin Frissell, Sandra A. Brown,
and Mark G. Myers*

12. Eating Disorders 778
Lisa Terre, Walker S. Carlos Poston II, and John P. Foreyt

Author Index 831
Subject Index 866

I

INTRODUCTION

1

Treatment of Child and Family Disturbance

A COGNITIVE-BEHAVIORAL SYSTEMS PERSPECTIVE

Eric J. Mash

About 20% of children and adolescents[1] in the United States suffer from some type of mental health problem during the course of a year (U.S. Department of Health and Human Services, 1999), and about 50% of all mental disorders in adults have an onset prior to age 14 (Kessler, Bergland, Demler, Jin, & Walters, 2005). Thus mental illnesses begin early in life and are both common and protracted (Insel & Fenton, 2005). Furthermore, the number of children experiencing mental health problems may be on the rise (Achenbach, Dumenci, & Rescorla, 2003). For example, the World Health Organization (WHO) estimates that by 2020, neuropsychiatric disorders in children will increase internationally by 50% compared with other health-related problems, making them one of the top five causes of childhood illness, disability, and death (U.S. Public Health Service, 2001). These disorders and related problems are associated with enormous distress and impairment in young people, including substance abuse, school failure, criminal activity, lack of vocational success, work problems, and suicide (Mash & Barkley, 2003).

In addition to personal suffering, the financial costs to society of childhood disorders are large. Each year about 6–12% of children in the United States alone receive some form of mental health service, at an estimated cost of $12 billion or more (Achenbach et al., 2003; Ringel & Sturm, 2001). These costs are actually likely to be underestimates of the problem's magnitude, since as many as three-quarters of children who are in need of help do not receive it (Katoaka, Zhang, & Wells, 2002). Although the costs of mental health care are considerable, the direct and indirect long-term costs to society of not providing appropriate services to youths are much greater. Such costs include the loss in productivity associated with a failure to complete high school, criminal justice costs, lost tax and employment insurance premium revenues, increased income support costs, and lost work due to mental illness and associated medical conditions. Thus the economic logic of providing effective treatments for children with mental health problems is compelling: Treating such problems is costly, but not treating them is even more costly, and a luxury that society can ill afford (WHO, 2005).

Great strides have been made over the past decade in developing effective intervention and prevention programs for children who are experiencing or at risk for a broad array of mental health problems (Hibbs & Jensen, 2005; Kazdin & Weisz, 2003). These advances are evident for most childhood disorders and particularly so for previously neglected ones, such as childhood depression (Compton, March, et al., 2004; Hammen & Rudolph, 2003; Rudolph, Hammen, & Daley, 2006). However, as discussed throughout this volume, much work remains to be done, particularly with respect to developing coordinated services and supports that can be effectively delivered across a variety of

3

real-life settings to those children who most need them (Chorpita, Daleiden, & Weisz, 2005; President's New Freedom Commission on Mental Health, 2003; Weisz, Jensen, & McLeod, 2005).

The term "psychotherapy" has been used to describe "an array of nonmedical interventions designed to alleviate nonnormative psychological distress, reduce maladaptive behavior, or increase deficient adaptive behavior through counseling, interaction, a training program, or a predetermined treatment plan" (Weisz, Doss, & Hawley, 2005, p. 338). Current psychotherapeutic interventions for children are extremely diverse and include cognitive-behavioral therapy, parent training, family-focused treatments, community-based treatments, home–school programs, multisystemic therapy, interpersonal therapy, stress management procedures, pivotal response training, anger management training, and social skills training, to name a few. In light of this diversity (and following Barlow, 2004), I use the term "psychological treatment(s)" in this chapter rather than the more generic term "psychotherapy," to differentiate these approaches from the more traditional forms of intervention (e.g., play therapy) that have been used with children.

The behavioral, psychological, interpersonal, physical, and learning problems for which children are referred to professionals for help are numerous and varied (Herbert, 2005; Hersen & Ammerman, 1999; Mash & Barkley, 2003; Mash & Wolfe, 2005). Adaptation difficulties that lead to referral for services frequently reflect developmentally and/or situationally inappropriate or exaggerated expressions of behavior that may at times also occur in children who are not referred (Achenbach, Howell, Quay, & Conners, 1991; Achenbach & Rescorla, 2001; Mash & Dozois, 2003). As a result, decisions regarding the referral, evaluation, and treatment of any child are embedded within the child's social and cultural milieu, and are always the result of ongoing judgments that are made or not made by significant individuals in the child's environment, usually parents and teachers (Mash & Terdal, 1997b). The professionals who evaluate and treat disturbed children and their families come from numerous disciplines and backgrounds. They include psychologists, educators, pediatricians, child psychiatrists, nurses, social workers, speech and language pathologists, physical and occupational therapists, day care specialists, recreational therapists, and others. It is not surprising, therefore, that a tremendous number and diversity of treatments for children and families exist (see Barrett & Ollendick, 2004; Christopherson & Mortweet, 2001; Hibbs & Jensen, 2005; Johnson, Rasbury, & Siegel, 1997; Kazdin & Weisz, 2003; Kratochwill & Morris, 1993; Mash & Barkley, 1998; Walker & Roberts, 2001; Weisz, 2004), with some conservative estimates listing well over 550 different varieties of psychosocial interventions alone (Kazdin, 2000). The actual number is much higher when joint forms of psychosocial treatment and combined psychosocial and psychopharmacological treatments for children are included.

In light of the heterogeneity of circumstances leading up to and surrounding the identification, referral, evaluation, and treatment of children with problems, it is believed that these activities are best depicted as ongoing decision-making/problem-solving processes (e.g., Evans & Meyer, 1985; Herbert, 1987; Kanfer & Schefft, 1988; Mash, 1998; Nezu, Nezu, & Lombardo, 2004; Schroeder & Gordon, 2002). These processes are directed at providing answers to such questions as these:

- Should this child's difficulties be treated?
- What are the projected outcomes in the absence of treatment?
- What types of treatment are likely to be most effective?
- Who is (are) the best person(s) to provide treatment?
- What are the most appropriate settings in which to carry out treatment (e.g., clinic, home, school, community)?
- What types of treatments are likely to be the most feasible, efficient, and cost-effective in the setting(s) in which they are typically provided?
- Which types of interventions are likely to be the most acceptable to the child, parents, and other family and community members?
- What is the motivation of the child and caregivers to implement these interventions (i.e., readiness for change)?
- When should treatment be initiated, and when should it be terminated?
- What changes or adjustments in treatment are needed as intervention progresses?
- Is the intervention having the desired impact, and are these effects maintained over time?
- Has the treatment resulted in clinically meaningful changes for the child and family?

Since a number of people are typically involved in decision making, it is also crucial that the process of answering these questions is a collaborative one that encourages shared decision making among parents, youngsters, and professionals; reduces disagreements; builds consensus; and helps to promote realistic expectations throughout assessment and treatment (Hamilton, 2004). Such collaboration is important, because parents, children, and professionals frequently do not agree on the nature of the children's problems (Hawley & Weisz, 2003). For example, in one study of outpatient-clinic-referred children and their parents, it was found that 63% of parent–child pairs failed to agree on even a single problem at the outset of treatment (Yeh & Weisz, 2001). The ultimate goals of a collaborative and iterative decision-making process should be to achieve effective solutions to the problems being faced by children and their families, and to promote and enhance long-term adjustments and quality of life.

It is my view, and that of the authors represented in this book, that decisions concerning the questions above and related issues are best made when they are based on a consistently applied theoretical framework, well-established research findings relevant to both typical and atypical child and family functioning, evidence-based treatment procedures, and operational rules that are sensitive to the realities and changing demands of clinical practice and to the broader sociocultural context in which treatments are carried out. Kazdin (1997) has provided a useful framework that is consistent with the general cognitive-behavioral systems orientation of this volume, in which the steps needed to advance the development of effective treatments for children and families are specified (see Table 1.1). This model emphasizes the importance of theory and data about specific childhood disorders, as well as the need for carefully specified evidence-based treatment strategies with known boundary conditions. Although such an amalgamation of theory, research, and practice is more an ideal than a fact at the present time, current cognitive-behavioral systems perspectives approximate this integration most closely, and this volume is based on these approaches.

Although many practicing child and family therapists continue to identify their approach as "eclectic," therapists' use of cognitive-behavioral, behavioral, and (to a lesser degree)

TABLE 1.1. A Model for Developing Effective Treatments: Steps toward Progress

1. Conceptualization of the dysfunction: Propose key areas, processes, and mechanisms that relate to the development, onset, and escalation of dysfunction.
2. Research on processes related to dysfunction: Test proposed processes in relation to the dysfunction.
3. Conceptualization of treatment: Propose key areas, processes, and mechanisms through which treatment may achieve its effects, and describe how the procedures relate to these processes.
4. Specification of treatment: Operationalize the procedures, preferably in manual form, that identify how one changes the key processes. Provide material to codify the procedures, to evaluate treatment integrity, and to replicate the treatment in research and practice.
5. Tests of treatment outcome: Test the impact of treatment, drawing on diverse designs (e.g., open [uncontrolled] studies, single-case designs, and full-fledged clinical trials) and types of studies (e.g., dismantling, parametric studies, and comparative outcome studies) as relevant.
6. Tests of treatment processes: Identify whether the intervention techniques, methods, and procedures within treatment actually affect those processes that are critical to the model.
7. Tests of the boundary conditions and moderators: Examine the child, parent, family, and contextual factors with which treatment interacts. The boundary conditions or limits of application are identified through interactions of treatment and diverse attributes within empirical tests.

Note. From Kazdin (1997, p. 117). Copyright 1997 by Erlbaum. Adapted by permission.

family systems approaches has become increasingly predominant, with 60–75% of all clinical child and pediatric psychologists identifying with these orientations (Mullins, Hartman, Chaney, Balderson, & Hoff, 2003; Weersing, Weisz, & Donenberg, 2002). Nevertheless, we believe that the complexity of childhood disorders, the diversity of circumstances under which they occur and are treated, the evolving nature of cognitive-behavioral treatments, efforts to integrate different therapy orientations (e.g., Fauber & Kendall, 1992; Goldfried, 1995; Kaslow & Lebow, 2002; Kendall, 1982; Norcross & Goldfried, 1992), the widespread use of combined and multimodal treatments (e.g., Kazdin, 1996a), and the uncertainties regarding the clinical significance and long-term effectiveness of current treatments for children (Chorpita et al., 2002; Chorpita & Nakamura, 2004; Weisz, 2004; Weisz, Han, & Valeri, 1997) would contraindicate a rigid adherence to *any* narrowly defined therapeutic perspective.

It is the purpose of this initial chapter to provide an overview of historical and recent developments, conceptual issues, and practical concerns associated with the treatment of child and family disturbances from a cognitive-behavioral systems perspective, and also to describe some of the common features of this approach. The general themes raised in this introductory chapter are elaborated in the chapter discussions of specific child and family disorders that follow.

HISTORICAL ANTECEDENTS AND EARLY DEVELOPMENTS

There have been several descriptions of the early development of behavioral and cognitive-behavioral approaches to the treatment of children and families (e.g., Kazdin, 1978; O'Leary & Wilson, 1987; Ollendick, 1986; Ollendick & Cerny, 1981; Ross, 1981). This development is briefly highlighted here. Although it is possible to find examples of the application of behavioral principles with children throughout the history of humankind (Lasure & Mikulas, 1996), systematic applications are usually identified as beginning with the rise of behaviorism in the early 1900s, as reflected in the classic studies on the conditioning and elimination of children's fears (Jones, 1924; Watson & Rayner, 1920), and in Pavlov's experimental research that established the foundations for classical conditioning. The time from 1930 to 1950 represented child behavior therapy's latency period, with a few reports in the 1930s describing the treatment of isolated problems such as bedwetting (Mowrer & Mowrer, 1938), stuttering (Dunlap, 1932), and fears (Holmes, 1936; Weber, 1936).

It was not until the 1950s and early 1960s that behavior therapy began to emerge as a systematic approach to the treatment of child and family disorders. The classic works of Wolpe (1958), Salter (1949), Lazarus (1958; Lazarus & Abramovitz, 1962), Skinner (1953), Eysenck (1960), and Bijou (Bijou & Baer, 1961) all contributed to behavior therapy's early development. The behavioral approaches that emerged during the 1950s and early 1960s

were counterreactions to the then-dominant psychodynamic perspective. Most behavioral work with children was carried out with developmentally delayed or severely disturbed youngsters, for whom psychoanalytic practices were perceived as not being very appropriate or effective. Much of this work took place in institutions or classrooms—settings that were thought to provide the kind of environmental control needed to "modify" behavior effectively. Early case studies were designed primarily to demonstrate the applicability of one learning principle or another, and showed relatively little attention to the clinical significance of treatment or its long-term impact on the child and family. As Wachtel (1977) pointed out, many of the most prominent figures in the early behavior therapy movement were psychologists who were almost exclusively experimental researchers, with little or no clinical experience. In retrospect, early case reports underestimated the complexity of clinical phenomena and failed to communicate the subtleties needed to understand and mediate the gap between laboratory-based principles of behavior change and clinical practice (Kazdin, 1988a). As I discuss later, this gap—which is currently seen as a "disconnect" between clinical investigators who evaluate the effectiveness of treatments under controlled conditions, and practitioners who are on the front line of services for children—continues to present major challenges for the field (Chorpita et al., 2005; Weisz, Jensen, et al., 2005).

The case study phase of child behavior therapy is perhaps most clearly illustrated in the 1965 volume edited by Ullmann and Krasner, entitled *Case Studies in Behavior Modification*. The childhood behaviors treated in these case reports included phobias, thumb sucking, eliminative disturbances, tantrums, isolate behavior, crying, crawling, vomiting, hyperactivity, and noncompliance. Most of these reports devoted little attention to the larger social or cultural networks in which these specific behavior problems occurred, or to issues such as generalization, long-term follow-up, the possible negative effects of treatment, or the clinical significance of change. With few exceptions, they also ignored or minimized diagnostic considerations, comorbid conditions, developmental factors, cognitive processes, possible biological determinants, the use of medications, and therapeutic processes (such as the therapeutic alliance or resistance).

Early behavioral work with children and families was derived primarily from an operant/reinforcement tradition. A major development in the field was the establishment of the *Journal of Applied Behavior Analysis* in 1968, which provided an outlet for treatment studies with children and also served to define, shape, and reshape the field of applied behavior analysis (Baer, Wolf, & Risley, 1968, 1987). The establishment of journals such as *Behaviour Research and Therapy* and *Behavior Therapy*, and later *Child and Family Behavior Therapy, Behavior Modification, Journal of Behavior Therapy and Experimental Psychiatry, Behavioral Assessment, Cognitive Therapy and Research*, and *Cognitive and Behavioral Practice*, further legitimized and promoted behavioral and cognitive-behavioral applications in clinical child psychology.

Work during the late 1960s foreshadowed developments of the 1970s, as reflected in several noteworthy clinical research programs and publications. Tharp and Wetzel's (1969) *Behavior Modification in the Natural Environment* provided a model that redirected intervention into the community and provided a beginning systems framework for treatment. Mischel's (1968) *Personality and Assessment* focused attention on the importance of examining behavior in relation to context and established the conceptual foundations upon which behavioral assessment was built. Bandura's *Principles of Behavior Modification* (1969) and Kanfer and Phillips's *Learning Foundations of Behavior Therapy* (1970) placed behavioral approaches more squarely within a clinical context, broadened the range of principles upon which behavioral procedures were based, and laid the groundwork for the many cognitive approaches that were to develop in the 1970s and beyond. Kanfer and Saslow's (1965, 1969) model for "behavioral diagnosis" established the complex network of factors that needed to be considered in treatment, and by doing so provided an early decision-making approach to treatment. Patterson's (Patterson, Ray, & Shaw, 1968) work with antisocial children extended the locus of behavioral intervention from the child to the family, and from the clinic to the home and classroom. The work of operant psychologists such as Lindsley, Bijou, Baer, Wolf, Risley, Hopkins, and many others refined many of the behavioral procedures and extended them across a range of settings, especially the classroom. Finally, Lovaas's early work with children with autism helped to establish the range of procedures used in working with children with developmental disabilities; it also provided the needed impetus for addressing such important issues as generalization of treatment effects, the appropriateness/acceptability of using aversive procedures in a clinical context, and ethical issues in behavior therapy more generally (Lovaas, Freitag, Gold, & Kasorla, 1965). Although there were undoubtedly many other important developments during the late 1960s, the aforementioned seem especially noteworthy in retrospect.

It is difficult to place the events of the 1970s and beyond into a neat temporal perspective, partly due to the enormous change and growth in cognitive-behavioral concepts and applications that have taken place. However, the continuing work of several investigators firmly established the new conceptual and technological base for child and family cognitive-behavioral therapy. Patterson's (Patterson, 2005; Patterson, Reid, Jones, & Conger, 1975) program for antisocial children and adolescents; Forehand and McMahon's (1981; McMahon & Forehand, 2003) child management training program for parents of oppositional children; Lovaas's continuing work with young children with autism (Lovaas, 2002; Lovaas, Koegel, Simmons, & Long, 1973); O'Leary's classroom interventions (O'Leary, Becker, Evans, & Saudargas, 1969); Barkley's (1987, 1997b) program for teaching child management skills to parents of children with what is now known as attention-deficit/hyperactivity disorder (ADHD) or with defiant behavior, and later to parents of defiant teens (Barkley, Edwards, & Robin, 1999); Meichenbaum's (1977) promotion of cognitive-behavioral therapy; Kendall's cognitive-behavioral strategies for impulsive children and for children with anxiety disorders (Kendall, 2005; Kendall & Braswell, 1985); Lewinsohn, Clarke, and colleagues' cognitive-behavioral treatment for adolescent depression (Lewinsohn, Clarke, Hops, & Andrews, 1990); Henggeler's multisystemic family- and community-based treatment for high-risk adolescents (Curtis, Ronan, & Borduin, 2004; Henggeler & Lee, 2003; Swenson, Henggeler, Taylor, & Addison, 2005); and the systematic interventions and ecological applications by operant psychologists in classroom, day care, group home, and work environments all served to shape the field.

As described in the sections that follow, further expansion and later extensions of this body of work continued to move behavioral applications into cognitive and affective processes, family intervention, health psychology, behavioral pediatrics, community intervention, environmental engineering, and early intervention and prevention. The cumulative impact of Alan Kazdin's writings and research over the past 35 years has been monumental. His work has helped to bring cognitive-behavioral approaches into mainstream clinical child psychology; to bridge the gaps among work in clinical child psychology, child psychiatry, and developmental psychopathology; and to provide the impetus for the current emphasis on evidence-based child and family interventions. All of the aforementioned developments have resulted in most practicing child behavior therapists' identifying with a cognitive-behavioral orientation (Elliott, Miltenberger, Kaster-Bundgaard, & Lumley, 1996), and in an integration of cognitive-behavioral assessment and treatment approaches within the mainstream practice of clinical child psychology (Mash & Hunsley, 2004).

DEVELOPMENTS FROM THE 1980s ONWARD

Beginning with the 1980s, many conceptual, methodological, and societal developments have shaped, and continue to shape, current cognitive-behavioral approaches to the treatment of child and family disturbance. These include the following:

1. A growing recognition of the need for a systems perspective to guide cognitive-behavioral assessment and treatment (e.g., Dishion & Snyder, 2004; Emery, Fincham, & Cummings, 1992; Henggeler & Lee, 2003; Kanfer & Schefft, 1988).
2. An increased developmental emphasis in the design and implementation of cognitive-behavioral treatments (e.g., Harris & Ferrari, 1983; Holmbeck, Greenley, & Franks, 2003, 2004; Kendall, Lerner, & Craighead, 1984; Meyers & Cohen, 1990).
3. An increased sensitivity to the role of individual differences, including personality, gender, ethnic, cultural, and biological factors, in moderating the effectiveness of treatment (e.g., Bell, Foster, & Mash, 2005; Haynes & Uchigakiuchi, 1993b; Iwamasa, 1996; Neal-Barnett & Smith, 1996; Russo & Budd, 1987; Sonderegger & Barrett, 2004; Strayhorn, 1987).
4. A heightened interest in the potential utility of clinical diagnosis and empirical classification as decision aids in formulating effective treatments (e.g., Achenbach, 1993, 2001a; Achenbach & McConaughy, 1997; Harris & Powers, 1984; Mash & Hunsley, 2005; Mash & Terdal, 1997b; Silverman & Saavedra, 2004).
5. A growing view of cognitive-behavioral intervention as a collaborative clinical decision-making process (e.g., Evans & Meyer, 1985; Greene & Ablon, 2005; Herbert, 1987; Kanfer & Busemeyer, 1982; Nezu & Nezu, 1989, 1993; Webster-Stratton & Herbert, 1994).
6. An increased emphasis on prevention, and the development of early intervention programs for high-risk children, youths, and families (e.g., Clarke et al., 1995; Conduct Problems Prevention Research Group, 1992; Dunst, Trivette, & Deal, 1988; McEachin, Smith, & Lovaas, 1993; Peters & McMahon, 1996; Peterson & Mori, 1985; Peterson, Zink, & Downing, 1993; Roberts & Peterson, 1984).
7. A focus on the interrelated influences of child cognitions and affects on behavior, as assessed and treated within the context of ongoing social interactions (e.g., Finch, Nelson, & Ott, 1993; Gottman & Katz, 1996; Kendall, 2005; Lochman, 1987; Schwebel & Fine, 1992).
8. An increased emphasis on the treatment of childhood disorders in the context of the family (Alexander & Sexton, 2002; Henggeler et al., 1997; Henggeler & Borduin, 1990; Mash & Johnston, 1996; Schwebel & Fine, 1994), including efforts to integrate individual and family therapy approaches (Fauber & Kendall, 1992; Fauber & Long, 1991), and the extensive involvement of family members in treatment programs for a wide range of childhood disorders.
9. The proliferation of cognitive-behavioral practices in child health care settings and their application to a growing number of health-related problems (e.g., Gross & Drabman, 1990; Koetting, Peterson, & Saldana, 1997; Roberts, 2003).
10. A growing acceptance of the notion that

individualized treatments should also be population-specific, focusing on parameters that are relevant to particular types of childhood disorders (Kazdin, 1997; Lee & Mash, 1990; Mash & Barkley, 1998, 2003; Mash & Terdal, 1997b).

11. An increased emphasis on the use of multimodal and combined (e.g., behavior therapy and medication) intervention strategies (Compton, McKnight, & March, 2004; Kazdin, 1996a; MTA Cooperative Group, 2004; Ollendick, 2004; Treatment for Adolescents with Depression Study [TADS] Team, 2004).

12. An increasing awareness that effective cognitive-behavioral treatments, like medications, can produce side effects (unwanted or undesirable changes in behavior or family systems) in a minority of those in treatment. These side effects can include deviancy training (increased aggression) as a byproduct of social skills groups that include aggressive children (Antshel & Remer, 2003; Dishion, McCord, & Poulin, 1999); increased family conflict secondary to training in problem-solving and communication training for families with defiant teens or teens with ADHD (Barkley, Edwards, Laneri, Fletcher, & Metevia, 2001; Barkley, Guevremont, Anastopoulos, & Fletcher 1992); and the potential at least for misuse of coercive punishment tactics by abusive parents undergoing behavioral parent training programs (DuCharme, Atkinson, & Poulton, 2000)—just to name a few. All of these suggest the need for greater attention to preexisting characteristics of children and their families, and to their potential impact on treatment-emergent side effects.

13. An increasing emphasis on the detailed specification of treatment strategies and procedures, as reflected in a growing number of treatment manuals for such child and adolescent disorders as oppositional defiant disorder and ADHD (Barkley, 1997b; Barkley et al., 1999); conduct problems (Dishion & Kavanagh, 2003; Greene & Ablon, 2005; Henggeler, Schoenwald, Borduin, Rowland, & Cunningham, 1998; McMahon & Forehand, 2003), anxiety disorders (Kendall, Hudson, Choudhury, Webb, & Pimentel, 2005; Kendall, Kane, Howard, & Siqueland, 1992), mood disorders (Clarke &

Lewinsohn, 1995; Mufson, Dorta, Moreau, & Weissman, 2004; Stark & Kendall, 1996), separation anxiety (Eisen & Schaefer, 2005), obsessive–compulsive disorder (Knox, Albano, & Barlow, 1993; March, Franklin, & Foa, 2005), posttraumatic stress disorder (Amaya-Jackson et al., 2003), and relationship violence (Wolfe et al., 1996; Wolfe, Scott, & Crooks, 2005).

14. Increased attention to models of child and family intervention that are sensitive to changing sociocultural demographics and needs (American Psychological Association, 1996), the realities and constraints of present-day health care delivery systems (Mash & Hunsley, 1993; Norcross, Karg, & Prochaska, 1997; Roberts & Hurley, 1997; Strosahl, 1994, 1996; WHO, 2005), and the everyday demands of clinical practice (Adelman, 1995; Clement, 1996; Kazdin, 1997).

15. A growing recognition of the general importance of accountability in treatment, with a concomitant emphasis on the need for evidence-based treatments (Hibbs, 2001; Hibbs & Jensen, 2005; Hoagwood, Hibbs, Brent, & Jensen, 1995; Kazdin & Weisz, 2003; Ollendick & King, 2004; Weisz, 2004) and cost-effective interventions such as group treatments (Barrett, Healy-Farrell, & March, 2004; Flannery-Schroeder, Choudhury, & Kendall, 2005; Hoag & Burlingame, 1997; Niec, Hemme, Yopp, & Brestan, 2005; Stoiber & Kratochwill, 1998) and behavioral consultations (Sheridan, Kratochwill, & Bergan, 1996). The recent emphasis on evidence-based treatments for children and adolescents has had a particularly large impact on clinical child research and practice.

Cognitive-Behavioral Systems Perspective

A key development in child and family cognitive-behavioral therapy has been the growing tendency to design and implement treatments based on a systems perspective of child and family functioning (Chronis, Chacko, Fabiano, Wymbs, & Pelham, 2004; Henggeler et al., 1998; Mash, 1998; Miller & Prinz, 1990; Stormshak & Dishion, 2002). This approach is consistent with a more general trend toward the use of systems models in related fields, such as developmental psychology (e.g.,

Bronfenbrenner, 1986; Cowan, 1997; Fogel & Thelen, 1987), developmental psychopathology (Davies & Cicchetti, 2004; Dishion & Snyder, 2004: Sameroff, 1995), and couple and family therapy (Birchler, Doumas, & Fals-Stewart, 1999; Gurman & Kniskern, 1991; Sexton & Weeks, 2003). Many of the other developments that have occurred in child and family cognitive-behavioral therapy appear to be either directly or indirectly related to the adoption of a systems perspective. Although a thorough presentation of contemporary systems models for child and family treatment is beyond the scope of this chapter (see Steinglass, 1987, for an overview), concepts that are particularly relevant for cognitive-behavioral clinical child practice include (1) the view of child and family disorders as constellations of interrelated response systems and subsystems; (2) the need to consider the child and family's entire situation in assessing the impact of any single variable; (3) the ideas that similar behaviors can result from different sets of initiating factors (referred to as "equifinality"), and that different behaviors can result from similar sets of initiating factors (referred to as "multifinality"); (4) a recognition that intervention is likely to lead to multiple outcomes, including readjustments of relationships within the family system (e.g., Brunk, Henggeler, & Whelan, 1987); and (5) the notion that family systems and subsystems possess dynamic properties and are constantly changing over time (Hollandsworth, 1986). As will be illustrated throughout this volume, all of these concepts have important implications for the manner in which treatments for children and families are selected, implemented, and evaluated.

Isolated elements of a systems formulation have characterized behavioral and cognitive-behavioral approaches to child and family treatment throughout their inception and development. For example, concepts such as situationism (Mischel, 1968), social learning (Bandura, 1969, 1986), reciprocity (Patterson, 1976, 1982), behavioral ecology (Willems, 1974), intervention in the natural environment (Tharp & Wetzel, 1969), response classes (Voeltz & Evans, 1982), triple-response system assessment (Eifert & Wilson, 1991), keystone behaviors (Wahler, 1975), setting events (Wahler & Fox, 1981; Wahler & Graves, 1983), stimulus generalization (Stokes & Baer, 1977), and response generalization (Kazdin, 1982b) all suggest the complex interplay of variables associated with a systems orientation. However, explicit systems formulations have only fairly recently been brought to bear in child and family cognitive-behavioral therapy, both as a general therapeutic orientation (e.g., Robin & Foster, 1989; Sexton & Alexander, 2003) and in specific areas such as conduct disorder (Henggeler et al., 1998), autism (Harris, 1984), school and learning problems (Evans & Meyer, 1985; Kratochwill, Albers, & Shernoff, 2004), anxiety disorders (Dadds & Barrett, 2001), and child abuse (Azar & Wolfe, Chapter 9, this volume).

Progression toward a systems perspective has resulted in a number of related developments in the cognitive-behavioral treatment of child and family disorders, including (1) continued extension of cognitive-behavioral practices into new areas; (2) a greater awareness both of the need for testable theories of disorders, and of how such theories may affect treatment designs; (3) an emphasis on the use of combined and multimodal treatments; (4) increasing specialization; (5) a broadening of treatment goals; (6) a growing recognition of the need for multidisciplinary approaches to treatment; and (7) an expanded concept of treatment to include a range of treatment delivery models and a broader public health perspective.

Extension into New Areas

The range of individual response systems (e.g., behavioral, cognitive, emotional, physical), family subsystems (e.g., mother–child, father–child, adult couple, sibling), and settings (e.g., home, school, day care, neighborhood, outpatient clinic, hospital, summer camp, workplace) encompassed by a systems perspective has promoted the extension of cognitive-behavioral practices into new problem areas, with different populations, and in new settings. Perhaps the most visible extension has been in the area of pediatric and health psychology (e.g., Gross & Drabman, 1990; Roberts, 2003). The range of problems treated also continues to grow, as interventions have become increasingly sensitive to the interrelationships among the behavioral, emotional, cognitive, and physical manifestations of child and family disorders (e.g., Crick & Dodge, 1994; Kendall, 1987). Applications in the areas of social competence (e.g., Lochman, 1988; Lochman & Wells, 1996), sexual abuse (e.g., Wolfe, Chapter 10, this volume; Wolfe & Birt, 1997), child and adolescent depression (e.g., Stark et al., Chapter 11, this volume), teenage drinking and substance abuse (e.g., MacPherson, Frissell, Brown, & Myers, Chapter 5, this volume), accident prevention (e.g., Peterson & Mori, 1985), and childhood anxiety disorders (e.g., Chorpita & Southam-Gerow, Chapter 4, this volume; Davis & Ollendick, 2005) illustrate this growth.

Use of Combined and Multimodal Treatments

The multidimensional nature of the causes and contexts of child and family disorders; the limited therapeutic effects of single-modality treatments; and the desire for more powerful treatments to produce clinically significant, generalizable, and long-lasting effects have led to an increased use of combined and multimodal treatments (Kazdin, 1996a). The term "combined treatments" generally refers to the use of two of more interventions, each of which can stand on its own as a treatment strategy. In some instances, combinations of stand-alone interventions may cross conceptual approaches—for example, when cognitive-behavioral and pharmacological treatments are used for children with ADHD (Arnold, Abikoff, & Wells, 1997; Barkley, 2006; MTA Cooperative Group, 2004) or children with obsessive–compulsive disorder (Piacentini & Graae, 1997), or when cognitive-behavioral treatment and family therapy are combined (Fauber & Kendall, 1992). In other instances, combined treatments may be derived from the same overall conceptual approach—for example, the use of social skills training and cognitive restructuring in a group treatment program for adolescents with depression or social phobia (Clarke, Lewinsohn, & Hops, 1990; King, Muris, & Ollendick, 2005), or the use of individual behavior management and family behavior therapy in the treatment of children with oppositional defiant disorder or ADHD (Chronis et al., 2004; Fauber & Long, 1991).

There are numerous theoretical, practical, and evaluation-related issues associated with the use of combined treatments. Paramount among these are (1) the need for models to guide decision making with respect to when, how, and under what circumstances combined treatments are required; and (2) the need for a variety of research strategies to determine the

incremental gains, synergistic effects, and conditions associated with the effective use of combined treatments. Clearly, more treatment is not synonymous with more *effective* treatment—and in the absence of decision rules and research to guide when combined treatments are to be used, there is the potential danger of using cost-inefficient, time-consuming, and potentially detrimental treatments in an effort to introduce the most "powerful" intervention possible, using an "everything but the kitchen sink" model of service delivery. Experience and research have both shown that providing more and more integrated services for children do not necessarily produce better outcomes (Bickman, 1996, 1997, 2002; Bickman, Smith, Lambert, & Andrade, 2003). Kazdin (1996a) has presented a detailed and thought-provoking discussion of these and many other issues related to the use of combined treatments.

Increasing Specialization

Extension of cognitive-behavioral practice into new areas has also been accompanied by increasing specialization. Such specialization indicates a recognition of the unique developmental demands, setting events, controlling variables, and intervention requirements associated with particular age groups, problems, ethnic and cultural groups, and settings. In referring to developments in child behavior therapy, Hersen and Van Hasselt (1987) noted that "the field has become more differentiated, with many of our colleagues specializing in the treatment of certain age groups and particular disorders. As time goes on we see fewer generalists in behavior therapy with children and adolescents" (p. xi). The chapters in this volume bear witness to the fact that the conceptual formulations, clinical procedures, and operational rules associated with various childhood disorders are quite different, and that effective intervention requires a thorough understanding of the specific parameters and empirical findings associated with particular clusters of problems, situations, and risk factors. This is reflected in the rapidly growing number of evidence-based treatment guidelines that focus on *specific* childhood disorders and problems (e.g., www.aacap.org/clinical/parameters; www.nice.org.uk/page.aspx?o=guidelines.completed; www.effectivechildtherapy.com; www.aap.org/policy/paramtoc.html).

Broadening of Treatment Goals

The systems perspective in child and family cognitive-behavioral therapy also has implications for the manner in which treatment goals are defined and the range of treatment outcomes is evaluated. Although early behavioral interventions were criticized for their overemphasis on management, compliance, and the short-term reduction of symptomatic distress (e.g., Winett & Winkler, 1972), recent applications have shown an increasing sensitivity to the need to develop skills and competencies in both the child and his or her social environment, and to minimize adverse outcomes through the use of maintenance and prevention strategies. As Blechman (1985) has stated, "Children with behavior problems deserve more in the way of treatment than training to conform quietly to the demands of poorly functioning homes and schools. Contemporary behavior therapy aspires to reshape the social environment, so that family and classroom foster children's social, emotional, and intellectual competence" (p. ix). The focus of treatment needs to be on changes that make a meaningful difference in a child's life, and producing changes that are statistically significant may not be sufficient in achieving this objective.

Current cognitive-behavioral treatments are directed at the family and/or peer group, not just the child (e.g., Dishion & Kavanagh, 2003; Howard & Kendall, 1996; March & Mulle, 1998). An increasing number of studies support the notion that more effective treatment outcomes are achieved when treatment focuses on the child *and* on relevant family subsystems. For example, in treating children with conduct disorder, Dadds, Schwartz, and Sanders (1987) compared child management training alone with a combination of child management training plus partner support training, which focused on reducing marital conflict and improving communication and problem solving. Although there were no group differences immediately following treatment, the partner support condition was associated with better child and family outcomes at a 6-month follow-up for families in which there was marital discord. Other studies have found that the addition of a family component to treatment that focused on interactions, managing emotion, communication, and problem solving significantly enhanced short-term outcome and long-term maintenance in children with

anxiety disorders (Barrett, Dadds, & Rapee, 1996).

These findings, and those from many other investigations to be discussed in this volume, all reinforce the notion that treatment goals should focus on building skills in the child and his or her social environment that will reduce impairment and facilitate long-term adjustment, not just on the elimination of problem behaviors and/or the short-term reduction of subjective distress. In some instances, impairment in functioning may be a more sensitive indicator of later outcomes for the child than specific symptoms may be (Vander Stoep, Weiss, McKnight, Beresford, & Cohen, 2002). Although symptom reduction is one important goal of therapy, other treatment goals and outcomes are also of crucial importance to the child, family, and society at large. These include (1) outcomes related to child functioning, such as degree of impairment in functioning, prosocial competence, and academic performance; (2) outcomes related to family functioning, such as level of family dysfunction, marital/couple and sibling relationships, stress, quality of life, burden of care, and family support; and (3) outcomes of societal importance, such as the child's participation in school-related activities (increased attendance, reduced truancy, reduction in school dropout), decreased involvement in the juvenile justice system, reduced need for special services, reduction in accidental injuries or substance abuse, and enhancement of physical and mental health (Kazdin, 1997).

Cognitive-behavioral therapies have typically emphasized the goal of helping children and families to achieve control over their thoughts and feelings as a vehicle for behavior change. A recent trend in work with adults is toward helping some clients *accept* rather than *control* their thoughts and feelings as a key element for behavior change (e.g., Hayes, Follette, & Linehan, 2004; Jacobson & Christensen, 1996). Although experiential acceptance and its relationship to behavior change in interventions with children and families have not received systematic attention to date, there has been an implicit emphasis on this goal in several applications of work with children and families. For example, treatments for children with ADHD or with developmental disabilities are often directed at helping parents accept their reactions to their children's condition, while providing them with alternative strategies for coping with their own reactions and their children's behavior (Barkley, 1997b). Some treatments for adolescents with social phobia help the youths understand and accept the adaptive nature of anxiety as a reaction to perceived threat as one element of treatment. And some treatments for depression teach children secondary control strategies (e.g., adjusting their beliefs, expectations, or interpretations of events) for dealing with distressing conditions that may not be modifiable (Weisz, Southam-Gerow, Gordis, & Connor-Smith, 2003).

The goal of acceptance in the context of the rapid developmental change and malleability that characterize childhood is likely to be controversial and in some ways antagonistic with the current emphasis on prevention. On the other hand, an accumulating body of evidence suggesting the importance of early dispositions and styles of information processing and emotion regulation for a number of childhood disorders (e.g., ADHD, early-onset conduct disorder, social phobia, autism, and learning disabilities) suggests that a recognition and acceptance of these "basic" tendencies by children and families may be an important element for teaching coping strategies and achieving effective behavior change. This hypothesis is worthy of further exploration.

Multidisciplinary Perspective

The adoption of a systems viewpoint has also reinforced the need for a multidisciplinary perspective on the cognitive-behavioral treatment of child and family disorders. As stated by Kanfer and Schefft (1988), "The systems approach implies the relevance of different knowledge bases, particularly the social and biological sciences. It is multidisciplinary, and effective treatment often requires familiarity with information that cuts across disciplines" (p. 19). The interlocking network of physical, behavioral, social, and learning difficulties that characterizes most childhood disorders necessitates a multidisciplinary approach to both treatment and prevention (e.g., Jason, Felner, Hess, & Moritsugo, 1987). The coordinated use of medication and psychosocial interventions for children with a variety of disorders (see Pappadopulos, Guelzow, Wong, Ortega, & Jensen, 2004)—for example, ADHD (e.g., Smith, Barkley, & Shapiro, Chapter 2, this volume), conduct disorder and aggression

(McMahon, Wells, & Kotler, Chapter 3, this volume), autism (e.g., Schroeder, Gualtieri, & Van Bourgondien, 1986), anxiety disorders (Piacentini & Graae, 1997), depression (e.g., TADS Team, 2004), mental retardation (Handen & Gilchrist, Chapter 6, this volume), and child and adolescent schizophrenia (Asarnow, Tompson, & McGrath, 2004)—illustrates this point. So too does the integration of cognitive-behavioral procedures with effective teaching strategies for learning disabilities (e.g., Lyon, Fletcher, Fuchs, & Chhabra, Chapter 8, this volume), or with required medical procedures for childhood chronic illnesses (e.g., Johnson & Rodrigue, 1997).

Expanded Concept of Treatment and Range of Treatment Delivery Models

The complexity of a systems framework underscores the notion that different child and family problems and circumstances require different solutions. Conventional models of cognitive-behavioral treatment have consisted of brief time-limited interventions focusing on already identified problems. Treatment is carried out for several weeks or months until the problem is eliminated, at which time the treatment is withdrawn. Even within this model, it has been recognized that concerted efforts must be made both during treatment and, to a lesser extent, after treatment is terminated (e.g., booster sessions), if gains are to be maintained (Mash & Terdal, 1980). Although conventional models of treatment may be appropriate for many acute or focal problems of mild severity, it is clear that other treatment delivery models may be needed for more complex, severe, or chronic difficulties.

As possible alternatives to the conventional care model of treatment, Kazdin (1997) has highlighted two types of continuing care models. The first is a "chronic care model," in which treatment is maintained and adjusted in the same way that it would be for children with a chronic illness such as diabetes mellitus or asthma. Ongoing treatment is needed to ensure that the benefits of treatment are maintained. ADHD and early-onset conduct disorder are two long-term and persistent problems in which a chronic care model of treatment may be needed. The second approach to continuing care is a "dental care model," in which ongoing follow-ups are carried out on a regular basis following initial treatment, in much the same way that regular dental checkups are recommended at 6-month intervals. Follow-up visits may be conducted on a periodic basis at prescribed intervals involving key transitions (e.g., a change in school), or on an "as-needed" basis related to emergent issues in development and adjustment.

Conventional models of treatment, in which a child is seen individually by a therapist for a limited number of treatment sessions in the clinic, fail to recognize the many other options for helping children with problems that are available and that are currently being used. These options include many different treatment agents (e.g., parents, teachers, siblings, peers, foster parents), settings (e.g., home, school, community, residential, day care, summer camps, foster homes, Web-based treatments), and formats (e.g., group therapy; Clarke et al., 1990; Malekoff, 2004). Current cognitive-behavioral systems approaches to child and family treatment recognize the need for a continuum of intervention activities and treatment delivery models—ranging from primary prevention programs, to targeted preschool and early school interventions, to focused intensive treatments for severe and chronic problems. An illustration of one such intervention continuum, showing the wide range of intervention and prevention activities encompassed under the concept of "treatment" with children and families, is presented in Figure 1.1 (Adelman & Taylor, 1993).

Developmental Emphasis

Early behavioral applications were decidedly insensitive to the need for incorporating developmental information into their assessments and treatments. This was due in part to their almost exclusive reliance on such principles of learning as positive reinforcement, negative reinforcement, extinction, and punishment, which were presumed to apply universally across all age groups and populations without regard for developmental status. Cognitive-behavioral treatments have become increasingly sensitive to the developmental issues surrounding diagnosis (e.g., Peterson, Burbach, & Chaney, 1989), assessment (e.g., Mash & Terdal, 1997b; Yule, 1993), and treatment (e.g., Harris & Ferrari, 1983; Holmbeck et al., 2003, 2004; Kendall et al., 1984; McMahon & Peters, 1985; Meyers & Cohen, 1990; Weisz &

Hawley, 2002). Also, behavioral conceptualizations of child and family disturbance have increasingly attempted to conceptualize, describe, predict, and suggest ways to alter the developmental progression of child and family disorders—for example, in the cases of antisocial children (Dishion & Kavanagh, 2003; Patterson, 2005), children with autism (e.g., Lovaas, 1987, 2002; Newsom & Hovanitz, Chapter 7, this volume), children with ADHD (Barkley et al., 1997), or children who have been abused or neglected (e.g., Azar & Wolfe, Chapter 9, this volume). Although this increased developmental emphasis continues to be an exciting and needed direction in the field, the incorporation of developmental findings and principles into cognitive-behavioral practice is a complex affair, and the degree to which it has been accomplished to date remains rudimentary at best.

Part of the difficulty in achieving a clinical–developmental integration is in specifying precisely what such an integration would require. At its simplest level (the one that has characterized cognitive-behavioral approaches to date), a developmental emphasis involves some recognition that the child's age, developmental level, and gender play a significant role in determining the methods of treatment that are likely to be most effective, and that normative information about development may facilitate clinical decision making by suggesting such things as what the boundaries for typical development are, when intervention is or is not required, and what constitute appropriate treatment goals. Normative information may also provide a basis for evaluating the clinical significance of change (Sheldrick, Kendall, & Heimberg, 2001). For example, Kazdin, Esveldt-Dawson, French, and Unis (1987) found that even though a problem-solving skills training program was more effective than a relationship-oriented approach in treating children with conduct disorder, the adjustment of these children was still outside the norms for a nonclinical population at a 1-year follow-up. Similarly, Barkley and colleagues (1992) found that although adolescents with ADHD improved following treatment, the functioning of most did not show clinically significant improvements when compared with the functioning of control adolescents.

At a more complex level, a developmental emphasis would require the incorporation of

Intervention Continuum	***Types of Activities*** (directed at system changes and individual needs)

Primary prevention ("public health")

1. Programs designed to promote and maintain
   - safety (at home and at school)
   - physical and mental health (including healthy start initiatives, immunizations, substance abuse prevention, violence prevention, health/mental health education, sex education and family planning, and so forth)

2. Preschool programs (encompassing a focus on health and psychosocial development)
   - parent education and support
   - day care
   - early education
   - identification and amelioration of physical and mental health and psychosocial problems

Early-age targeted intervention

3. Early school adjustment programs
   - welcoming and transition support into school life for students and their families (especially immigrants)
   - personalized instruction in the primary grades
   - additional support in class for identified students
   - parent involvement in problem solving
   - comprehensive and accessible psychosocial and physical and mental health programs (primary grades)

Early-after-onset correction

4. Improvement and augmentation of ongoing regular support
   - preparation and support for school and life transitions
   - teaching "basics" of remediation to regular teachers (including use of available resource personnel, peer and volunteer support)
   - parent involvement in problem solving
   - providing support for parents in need
   - comprehensive and accessible psychosocial and physical and mental health programs (including interventions for students and families targeted as high risks—all grades)
   - emergency and crisis prevention and response mechanisms

5. Interventions prior to referral for intensive treatments
   - staff development (including consultation)
   - short-term specialized interventions (including resource teacher instruction and family mobilization; programs for pregnant minors, substance abusers, gang members, and other potential dropouts)

Treatment for severe/chronic problems

6. Intensive treatments—referral to and coordination with
   - special education
   - dropout recovery and follow-up support
   - services for severe/chronic psychosocial/mental/physical health problems

FIGURE 1.1. From prevention to treatment: A continuum of programs for amelioration of learning, behavior, and socioemotional problems. From Adelman and Taylor (1993, p. 279). Copyright 1993 by Wadsworth, Inc. Reprinted by permission of Brooks/Cole Publishing Company.

developmental principles and findings into our conceptualizations of child and family psychopathology—such that treatments are sensitive not only to a child's age and sex, but also to ongoing developmental *processes* as they unfold and interact with and within one or more dynamic and changing social systems. At this level, our treatments not only would be sensitive to developmental parameters, but would be *derived from* our knowledge of relevant developmental processes, including neurodevelopmental processes (Courchesne, Townsend, & Chase, 1995), cognition (Noam, Chandler, & LaLonde, 1995), attachment (Rutter, 1997), self-control (Barkley, 1997a), and emotion regulation (Izard, Fine, Mostow, Trentacosta, & Campbell, 2002). However, the principles and processes that are deemed to be most important vary across developmental theories; the empirical base describing these processes is just beginning to emerge from recent longitudinal investigations; and the decision rules by which developmental knowledge can be translated into clinical practice are not well developed at this time. In light of this, there is likely to be continued exploration of the boundaries for developmental applications of cognitive-behavioral treatments with children and families. Research in the field of developmental psychopathology has provided a growing empirical base to guide these new interventions (Cicchetti & Cohen, 1995a, 1995b; Cicchetti & Hinshaw, 2002).

Within the field of developmental psychopathology, organizational–developmental approaches that consider development as involving progressive reorganizations in response to changing environmental demands (e.g., Cicchetti & Cohen, 1995c), and models that conceptualize early development in terms of child and family coping responses (e.g., Emery & Kitzmann, 1995; Tronick & Gianino, 1986), seem especially consistent with a cognitive-behavioral perspective. Within these views, the origins of child and family disorders are seen as breakdowns in adaptational processes. For a variety of reasons, both the child and family fail to cope adequately with either normative or non-normative events. These models consider adaptational outcomes in relation to the complex interaction between and among external events, perceptual and cognitive appraisals of such events, internal conditions (e.g., values, physical status, personality traits), external resources for coping (e.g., social support), decision-making processes, and preferred coping strategies.

Age

Therapists report using different treatment approaches for children of different ages—for example, using more behavioral (vs. cognitive or psychodynamic) techniques with younger children displaying externalizing (vs. internalizing) problems (Weersing et al., 2002). A common assumption in the treatment of children has been that interventions directed at younger children are likely to be more effective. In part, this is because younger children are presumed to be more malleable than older children, and because maladaptive patterns of behavior have had less time to become well established. Some indirect support for this assumption comes from a meta-analysis carried out by Weisz, Weiss, Alicke, and Klotz (1987), who found a mean effect size of 0.92 for treatment studies with children ages 4–12, compared with a mean effect size of 0.58 for children ages 13–18. However, findings of interactions between age and outcome are inconsistent, with one meta-analysis reporting the largest effect size for adolescents (Weisz, Weiss, Han, Granger, & Morton, 1995).

Age effects in treatment are also likely to interact with the type of treatment under consideration. For example, in one meta-analysis of studies using just cognitive-behavioral therapy, it was predicted that effect sizes would be larger for adolescents than for younger children, because adolescents function at a higher cognitive level and thus are more likely to learn the cognitive skills needed in treatment. This prediction was supported, with an effect size of 0.92 for 11- to 13-year-old adolescents, compared with effect sizes of 0.55 in children ages 7–11 years and 0.57 in children ages 5–7 years (Durlak, Fuhrman, & Lampman, 1991). Although both common sense and clinical sensitivity would indicate that different approaches are required for children of different ages, few empirical studies have demonstrated specific cognitive-behavioral strategies to be more or less effective with children of different ages.

More importantly, the issue is not so much the differential effectiveness of the same treatment procedure at different ages, but rather the extent to which we can identify specific age-related developmental processes and capacities and incorporate them into treatment in order to produce more effective outcomes. At best, age is a summary measure of many diverse developmental influences—biological, social, cognitive, and contextual—each of which is deserving of attention in its own right. For example, at what ages can mental imagery be used in reducing fears, or can cognitive self-instruction be employed in regulating impulsive behavior? How might the application of a time-out procedure be different for 3- to 5-year-olds versus school-age children? How might explanations of procedures be adjusted to take into account a child's cognitive capabilities? In one study, Wurtele, Marrs, and Miller-Perrin (1987) found that participant modeling procedures were more effective than symbolic modeling procedures in teaching personal safety skills to kindergarten children, although this difference was not significant at a 6-week follow-up. These authors emphasized the importance of including active rehearsal in programs for young children, and noted that some prevention studies have found that young children may have difficulty understanding the abstract concepts involved in a cognitive approach.

Gender

Few studies have examined the general effectiveness of treatment as a function of children's gender, and findings in this area are variable. In one meta-analysis of treatment outcome studies, Casey and Berman (1985) found that the percentage of boys in the sample was negatively correlated with treatment outcome. Weisz, Weiss, Alicke, and colleagues (1987) found no difference in mean effect size for treatment studies with males versus females. And Weisz, Weiss, and colleagues (1995) found mean effect sizes for adolescent girls that were approximately twice as large as those for adolescent boys and for younger children of both genders. As with age, a critical question related to gender differences is how information regarding these differences might suggest different treatment strategies. To date, few cognitive-behavioral treatment studies have directly addressed this question. However, numerous studies have reported sex differences in the expression of childhood disorders (Bell et al., 2005; Crick & Zahn-Waxler, 2003; Zoccolillo, 1993), which may suggest different intervention protocols for boys versus girls. To illustrate, a few of these studies are described below.

Moran and Eckenrode (1988) examined the relationship between social stress and depression in adolescent males and females. It was found that female early adolescents were significantly more affected by social stress than male age-mates, but that older males and females were similarly affected. Other studies (e.g., Nolen-Hoeksema, Girgus, & Seligman, 1988) have shown peer popularity or rejection to be more highly correlated with depression in girls than in boys. Such findings suggest that interventions directed at enhancing peer relationships may be especially critical for young adolescent females.

Block and Gjerde (1990) found that the predictors at age 14 of depressive symptomatology at age 18 were quite different for boys versus girls. Fourteen-year-old girls subsequently expressing depressive tendencies were described as vulnerable, anxious, somaticizing, and showing generally low esteem. In contrast, 14-year-old boys who later showed high depressive symptomatology tended to show an early lack of concern for satisfying interpersonal relationships, and subsequent antisocial and hostile characteristics. Introspective concern with self-adequacy seemed to be a less salient issue for boys. Early intellective incompetence predicted later depressive symptoms for boys, whereas early intellective competence predicted depressive symptomatology for girls.

Block, Block, and Keyes (1988) found that the personality concomitants and antecedents of drug use differed somewhat as a function of gender and the drug used. At age 14, the use of marijuana was related to ego undercontrol, while the use of harder drugs reflected an absence of ego resiliency, with undercontrol also being a contributing factor. For girls, adolescent drug use was related to both undercontrol and lower ego resiliency at 3–4 years of age; for boys, preschool undercontrol was a strong predictor of adolescent drug use, but there was no impact of ego resiliency. Early family environments that were characterized by an unstructured and laissez-faire atmosphere, with little pressure to achieve, were related to adolescent drug use in girls but not in boys. For boys only, drug use was related to an IQ decline from ages 11 to 18.

Studies of the psychophysiology of disruptive behavior in boys versus girls suggest that girls' disruptive behavior may be more closely connected to experiences of anxiety than such behavior in boys is (Zahn-Waxler, Cole, Welsh,

& Fox, 1995), and that although rates of disruptive behavior are lower in girls than boys, girls show a higher incidence of comorbid disorders (Zahn-Waxler, 1993). Such findings would suggest that different interventions may be needed for girls and boys with disruptive behavior disorders. For example, combined interventions that focus on conduct problems and anxiety and mood disorders may be especially important in treating the comorbid conditions observed in females with disruptive behavior disorders.

Research has also found that girls are more likely to be emotionally upset by aggressive social exchanges than boys (Crick, 1995), and when angry are more likely than boys to use indirect and relational forms of aggression, such as verbal insults, gossip, tattling, ostracism, threatening to withdraw their friendship, getting even, or third-party retaliation (Crick, Bigbee, & Howes, 1996). As girls move into adolescence, the function of their aggressive behavior centers increasingly around group acceptance and affiliation, whereas for boys aggression remains confrontational in nature. These and other findings suggest different avenues for the treatment of aggression in girls versus boys (Ehrensaft, 2005).

There also may be gender differences in children's preferences for treatment agents. For example, Winter, Hicks, McVey, and Fox (1988) found that children's choices regarding the people (i.e., peers, parents, experts) they would consult for different types of problems varied as a function of the children's age and sex. Furthermore, in choosing consultants, females valued familiarity, whereas males valued expertise. Although a number of the studies just described do not address treatment concerns directly, their findings do suggest that the focus of both treatment and prevention efforts needs to be different for boys and girls of different ages (Kavanagh & Hops, 1994).

Despite these findings and substantial interest in gender differences in treatment needs and responsiveness, very little research has examined this issue. In relation to conduct problems, Chamberlain and Reid (1994) found that delinquent boys and girls referred for treatment foster care responded to treatment differently, and recommended that treatment with antisocial girls focus on stabilizing the daily environment and behavior problems, preventing additional changes in placement, developing planful competency, and learning skills to replace relational

aggression. However, other studies using multisystemic treatment (MST) have not reported sex differences in the effectiveness of treatment (Borduin et al., 1995). Some possible reasons for these differences across studies may be the number of girls in each sample, as well as the types of outcome measures used. For example, some studies assess outcomes such as crime rates, aggression, and delinquency, but do not include sex-specific outcomes such as pregnancy, suicide attempts, and early childbearing. Girls with conduct problems are less likely to receive services for their problems (Offord, Boyle, & Racine, 1991), perhaps as a result of their displaying fewer disruptive behaviors than boys.

Norms

The uses of normative information in cognitive-behavioral assessment have received extensive discussion (e.g., Edelbrock, 1984; Hartmann, Roper, & Bradford, 1979), and many of these uses parallel those for treatment. Briefly, normative information is important in identifying problems; increasing diagnostic sensitivity to age, gender, ethnic, and other differences; evaluating parent and teacher expectations; identifying difficulties that are likely to be chronic versus those that are common and transient; deciding when treatment is indicated; establishing treatment goals; suggesting different forms of treatment; and evaluating the clinical significance of change (Achenbach, 2001b; Mash & Terdal, 1997b).

Normative information may also suggest possible goals for prevention studies. For example, Kline, Canter, and Robin (1987) reported that 15–40% of junior and senior high school students may experience problems related to alcohol use, and found that measures of family functioning such as disengagement, poor communication, and family approval of alcohol were highly predictive of teenage drinking. Rubenstein, Heeren, Houssman, Rubin, and Stechler (1988) reported not only that 20% of the adolescents in their high school sample were suicidal, but that they were virtually indistinguishable on all measures from their hospitalized suicidal sample. Of the high school sample of adolescents, 75% had received no therapeutic intervention in the year of their suicide attempt. Carlson, Asarnow, and Orbach (1987) reported that although rates of completed suicide were low prior to the age of 14 years, suicidal ideation and nonfatal suicide attempts were not uncommon in preadolescent children. Such ideation and nonfatal attempts have been noted prior to completed suicides, and they sometimes occur in the context of depression. The normative information derived from the Rubenstein and colleagues (1988) and Carlson and colleagues (1987) studies suggests that there are significant numbers of unidentified and/or untreated suicidal adolescents in the public schools, and that there is a need for early intervention and prevention programs in this area.

Recognition of Individual Differences

Cognitive-behavioral approaches have shown a growing concern for how individual differences in inborn and/or acquired characteristics of both children and parents moderate and mediate treatment outcomes. Characteristics such as child temperament, personality disorders, parental anxiety and depression, and the generalized expectations and attributions of parents have all been identified as possible moderators or mediators of treatment outcome. In addition to basic biological differences (e.g., child temperament, social inhibition, arousability, threshold to novel events, emotion regulation, sensitivity to aversive stimuli), background characteristics (e.g., intelligence, social status, or family configuration) may influence the child's and family's style of social problem solving, their attributional processes, and their reactions to specific types of treatment. For example, in the case of parents, generalized expectancies concerning what the future holds—referred to as "dispositional optimism or pessimism" (Scheier & Carver, 1985)—could determine the success of behavioral parent training programs, to the extent that they influence the coping mechanisms invoked by the parents. Optimists focus on active problem solving in coping with stress, whereas pessimists focus on their feelings of distress, disengage from goal-directed activities, and give up their goals when obstacles intervene (Carver & Scheier, 1986).

Maternal depression and anxiety, parental psychopathy, parental substance abuse, marital/couple conflict, parental attributional styles, and parenting self-esteem are examples of other parent characteristics that may be related to treatment outcomes. It has also been found that family members of children with a wide range of childhood disorders (e.g.,

ADHD, anxiety, depression) have an elevated risk for psychopathology—often for disorders that are the same as or similar to those of the children. This possibility needs to be carefully considered in treatment, since many cognitive-behavioral interventions with children rely extensively on the involvement of family members in treatment, and the presence of the disorder in the parents may interfere with treatment efficacy if not also addressed. Sonuga-Barke, Daley, and Thompson (2002), for example, found that children with ADHD whose mothers had high levels of adult ADHD showed limited improvements following a parent training program, in contrast to those children with ADHD whose mothers displayed lower levels of adult ADHD. These investigators concluded that the treatment of maternal ADHD might be a prerequisite step for successful psychosocial treatment of children with ADHD. Consistent with this conclusion, Evans, Vallano, and Pelham (1994) found that a mother with ADHD did better in parent training when her own ADHD was treated with medication.

One child characteristic that seems especially important for both treatment and prevention is intelligence, which appears to be an attenuating factor for many different kinds of problems (e.g., Lynam, Moffitt, & Stouthamer-Loeber, 1993). For example, Kandel and colleagues (1988) reported that in a group at high risk for criminality, cohort members who have committed serious crimes evidenced lower IQ scores than cohort members with no criminal records. Their interpretation was that within the high-risk group higher IQ led to school success and greater rewards, which in turn led to greater attachment to school and bonding to the conventional social order. Also, Schonfeld, Shaffer, O'Conner, and Portnoy (1988) have reported a direct link between deficiencies in cognitive functioning and conduct disorder in boys, and argue that the nature of this deficiency is one of acculturational learning broadly defined, rather than a narrowly focused social-cognitive deficit.

Recent research has found that cognitive-behavioral interventions with community-based samples of parents and children may not be as effective as interventions with parents and children who are referred to clinics for treatment, and that community-identified samples may be less likely to participate fully in treatment and more likely to terminate treatment prematurely (Smith et al., Chapter 2, this volume). Understanding the individual differences that may contribute to such differential participation and treatment outcomes in community samples seems especially important in the context of current prevention efforts directed at children and families whose problems have not yet resulted in referral. In this regard, one characteristic that may be especially important is a parent's (and child's) "readiness for change," and there is a need to understand the structural stages and processes of change that support or impede such a readiness (e.g., Littell & Girvin, 2005; Prochaska, 1994).

Clinical Diagnosis and Empirical Classification

Early cognitive-behavioral treatments minimized the need for formal clinical diagnosis and/or assignment to groups based on empirical classification procedures, and emphasized the importance of individualized behavioral assessments. However, current research and practice have increasingly acknowledged the potential benefits to be derived from the use of standardized diagnostic systems, such as the *Diagnostic and Statistical Manual of Mental Disorders*, fourth edition, text revision (DSM-IV-TR; American Psychiatric Association, 2000) or the *International Classification of Diseases*, 10th revision (ICD-10; WHO, 1992); multivariate classification strategies (e.g., Achenbach, 1993, 1995; Reynolds & Kamphaus, 2004); and classification models based on a developmental perspective (e.g., Garber, 1984; Zero to Three/National Center for Clinical Infant Programs, 1994). Such approaches are intended to supplement rather than replace the individualized and contextually grounded assessments characteristic of an individualized and ongoing behavioral/functional analysis (Carr, 1994; Hayes & Follette, 1992; Haynes & Heiby, 2004; Haynes & Uchigakiuchi, 1993a; Mash & Terdal, 1997b).

Many treatment programs have been instituted with poorly or globally defined groups of children and little regard for comorbidity or family and cultural context (Jensen, 2003). Although some studies suggest that the presence of comorbid externalizing disorders or other anxiety disorders may not make a difference in treatment effectiveness for children with a primary diagnosis of an anxiety disorder (Flannery-Schroeder, Suveg, Safford, Kendall, & Webb, 2004; Kendall, Brady, & Verduin, 2001), other research suggests differential outcomes for children with ADHD with comorbid conduct disorder versus those with ADHD alone.

Classification efforts focusing on the refinement and development of subtypes of child and family disorders have potential for determining the kinds of treatments that are likely to be most effective for individuals and families showing particular constellations of characteristics (i.e., client–treatment matching). Categorization efforts to date have attempted to subtype disturbed children on the basis of dimensions such as social withdrawal (Rubin & Stewart, 1996), styles of social information processing (Milich & Dodge, 1984), peer social status (Lochman & Lampron, 1986), comorbid disorders (Caron & Rutter, 1991), and types of violence (Tolan & Guerra, 1994) and aggression (Crick & Dodge, 1996), to name a few. To illustrate in the case of aggression, "reactive" aggression occurs in response to actions by others, whereas "proactive" aggression involves taking the offensive without provocation through domination, bullying, or threats. Reactive aggression is associated with deficits and distortions in children's taking in and interpreting information in social situations, including a limited use of social information in reaching interpersonal decisions and a tendency to think that others have bad intentions. In contrast, proactive aggression is associated with a restricted and mostly aggressive behavioral repertoire (Crick & Dodge, 1996). Subgrouping children based on the dimension of proactive versus reactive aggression may lead to a relative difference in emphasis on the use of cognitive strategies (in the case of children who display reactive aggression) versus the use of skill-based or problem-solving strategies (in the case of the latter).

The importance of differential diagnosis is also evident in the work on children who have conduct disorder with and without comorbid disorders such as ADHD or anxiety disorders (Hinshaw & Lee, 2003; Lynam, 1996, 1997). Children with diagnoses of conduct disorder *and* ADHD show a more diverse and serious pattern of antisocial behavior than children with a diagnosis of conduct disorder alone. When ADHD is present, the onset of conduct disorder is earlier, the developmental progression from less serious to more serious antisocial behavior may be more rapid, and the risk for psychopathy may be greater than for a child with conduct disorder alone. In other instances, when conduct disorder is accompanied by anxiety, the conduct problem symptoms may be less severe. These differences in behavior and outcomes related to comorbid conditions and developmental history in the case of children with conduct disorder suggest the need for different treatment recommendations based on these factors.

Therapy as a Collaborative Decision-Making Process

A number of writers have emphasized the need for a collaborative clinical decision-making approach to cognitive-behavioral interventions with disturbed children and families (Herbert, 1987; Kanfer & Busemeyer, 1982; Nezu & Nezu, 1989, 1993; Webster-Stratton & Herbert, 1994). In many ways, this approach extends and formalizes the everyday decision-making/problem-solving processes used by parents (e.g., Holden, 1985), teachers (Evans & Meyer, 1985), children (Urbain & Kendall, 1980), and adolescents (Tisdelle & St. Lawrence, 1988). The models presented by Kanfer (Kanfer & Busemeyer, 1982; Kanfer & Schefft, 1988), Evans and Meyer (1985), Herbert (1981, 1987), Webster-Stratton and Herbert (1994), and Henggeler and colleagues (1994) provide excellent descriptions of a collaborative decision-making perspective. In contrast to earlier cognitive-behavioral approaches, which were concerned with the use of specific techniques derived from principles of learning, decision-making approaches emphasize the collaborative and flexible application and reapplication of various treatment strategies over time as needed. Decisions concerning the utilization of specific procedures are made within a broader clinical context that takes into account the phase of treatment (Kanfer & Schefft, 1988), the cognitive activities and potential decision-making biases of the clinician (e.g., Kanfer, 1985; Tabachnik & Alloy, 1988), and the social context and values surrounding treatment. Some of the more common features of collaborative decision-making approaches include an emphasis on the use of flexible and ongoing decisional strategies (Kanfer & Busemeyer, 1982); a systems orientation (Evans, 1985); the development of generic strategies intended to optimize the effectiveness of more specific target-oriented tactics (Kanfer & Schefft, 1988); creation of a favorable therapeutic environment; identification and elabora-

tion of decision points in treatment (e.g., seeking help, terminating treatment); client participation in decision making; and a sensitivity to the varying needs of different treatment phases.

An emphasis on the flexible use of strategies as a medium in which specific cognitive-behavioral techniques are applied is perhaps the major distinguishing feature of these approaches. As reflected in the following quotations, the concern is with process and not just with techniques. In describing their model of educational decision making, Evans and Meyer (1985) state:

> Our approach involves an extension and elaboration of standard behavior modification methods. It is a "second generation" of behavior modification in which the focus is no longer simply on the derivation of techniques from learning principles, but on how these principles may be most effectively adapted to the instructional situation and extended to deal with the total educational needs of the child. This volume is about educational programming, not just the design of isolated behavioral interventions; about clinical strategies and the values that influence clinical decisions, not just techniques that produce behavior change. (p. 2)

And Herbert (1987), in a practical manual for treating children's problems, states: "There is no one way of carrying out assessments and behavioural programmes. There is nothing preordained about the ordering of the steps suggested" (p. v).

Although the flexibility inherent in the approach being described here has some appeal, there is a need for specific guidelines concerning how clinical *strategies* are to be implemented from a cognitive-behavioral perspective with children and families. As Kanfer and Schefft (1988) note, there are many descriptions of therapy methods (e.g., biofeedback, modeling, parent training, cognitive change methods, relationship enhancement methods), but "there are only a few books that offer clinicians a conceptually consistent framework for structuring each step of the change process, regardless of the specific treatment used" (p. xvi). Implicit in a probabilistic decision-making approach is the notion that there are many different ways to achieve the same treatment objective, and that it is possible to identify alternative treatment goals and choices for the same client, depending on the circumstances. No proposed solution can be rigidly adhered to, since each step in treatment is presumed to generate new information that requires ongoing adjustments in the program. In light of the many possible choices that are involved, further elaboration and empirical validation of the decision rules to be used in treatment are clearly needed, in much the same way that specific techniques have been described and validated. Although the desirability of such validation has been acknowledged, it remains to be seen whether systematic quantification of the complex judgmental process involved in treatments for children and families is even possible (Kanfer & Schefft, 1988).

Any decision rules in treatment are likely to be contextually specific, and there is a need to identify the parameters under which specific rules may or may not apply. I believe that the accumulated knowledge concerning *specific* childhood disorders represents a critical dimension for clinical decision making, and this view is reflected in the organization of the current volume. A host of other factors also contribute to the selection and sequencing of treatments for children and families, including characteristics of the family subsystems that are involved (e.g., child, parent–child, adult couple, sibling) and their cultural context; the overt versus covert nature of the problem; characteristics of the primary agent of treatment (e.g., therapist, parent, teacher, child); the treatment setting (e.g., home, classroom); applicable psychological principles and techniques; empirical support for the efficacy and effectiveness of specific treatments for particular problems; and the therapist's orientation (Wolfe & Goldfried, 1988). Collaborative therapeutic decision making is an interactive process that incorporates information from each of these areas and more in formulating an overall intervention strategy.

Decision-making frameworks also emphasize the importance of adapting decision-making rules to the various phases of treatment (e.g., the therapist's response to a missed first vs. a missed ninth treatment session), and several writers have delineated such phases. For example, Kanfer and Schefft (1988) describe seven phases of treatment: (1) role structuring and the creation of a therapeutic alliance; (2) developing a commitment for change; (3) the behavioral analysis; (4) negotiating treatment objectives and methods; (5) implementing treatment and maintaining motivation; (6) monitoring and evaluating progress; and (7) maintenance, generalization, and termination of treatment.

Herbert (1987) has presented three general phases. The first initial screening involves explaining the therapist's role, identifying problems, identifying the child's and family's assets, specifying the desired outcomes, constructing a problem profile, teaching clients to think in antecedent–behavior–consequence (A-B-C) terms, and establishing problem priorities. The second phase, moving from data collection to problem formulation, includes specifying relevant situations, assessing the extent and severity of the problem, providing the clients with appropriate materials, and determining the frequency and intensity of the problem. The third phase, intervention, involves planning treatment, formulating objectives, selecting procedures and methods, developing a treatment plan, working out practicalities of implementation, evaluating the plan, initiating the program, phasing out intervention, and conducting follow-up.

Conceptual models and decision guides to therapeutic choices within each of these phases for specific problems are just beginning to emerge in cognitive-behavioral child and family interventions, and it is not possible to do justice to the many complexities involved in this brief introductory discussion. The interested reader may wish to consult Evans and Meyer (1985), Herbert (1987), and Kanfer and Schefft (1988) for particularly detailed accounts of how collaborative decisional models can be implemented in different types of therapeutic contexts.

Emphasis on Prevention

In general, the costs of mental health services for children have been found to increase with the children's age. For example, Ringel and Sturm (2001) reported the yearly costs of mental health care to be $35 per preschool-age child, $163 per child age 6–11, and $293 per adolescent. The reasons for these higher costs for older children may relate to the nature of their acts (e.g., implications of actions, seriousness of problems), resistance to treatment (requiring more intensive interventions for older children), or other factors. Whatever the reason(s) for the higher costs, the benefits of heading off problems before they develop seem self-evident for both personal and economic reasons. Cognitive-behavioral approaches have shown a growing concern for both primary and secondary prevention programs for children and families (e.g., Conduct Problems Prevention Research Group, 1997; Lochman & Wells, 2004; Rickel & Allen, 1987; Roberts & Peterson, 1984; Spence, Sheffield, & Donovan, 2005). These programs have included interventions with high-risk populations directed at minimizing the likelihood of several known adverse outcomes (e.g., the sequelae associated with abusive family situations); interventions directed at reducing the future risk of specific problems, such as depression or the abuse of alcohol or drugs; interventions designed to facilitate transitions and to minimize their negative impact (e.g., new school, foster placement); interventions intended to increase children's and families' general adaptive competencies (e.g., early social skills training); and, interventions designed to increase children's and families' overall health, safety, and physical well-being (Jason, 1980).

Some examples of areas in which prevention efforts have been carried out include accident prevention (e.g., Christopherson, 1986; Mori & Peterson, 1986; Wright, Flagler, & Friedman, 1988), child abduction (e.g., Flanagan, 1986), sexual abuse (e.g., Harvey, Forehand, Brown, & Holmes, 1988; Wurtele, Kast, & Kondrick, 1988; Wurtele et al., 1987), practicing safer sex (e.g., Gordon & Craver, 1988), seat belt use (Malenfant, Wells, Van Houten, & Williams, 1996), teaching emergency fire safety skills to blind children and adolescents (e.g., Jones, Sisson, & Van Hasselt, 1984), and reducing relationship violence in teens (Wolfe et al., 1996).

In one prevention study, Markman, Floyd, Stanley, and Storaasli (1988) provided premarital intervention via a cognitive-behavioral approach that included communication and problem-solving skills training, clarifying and sharing expectations, and sensual/sexual enhancement. Although there were no differences in self-reported relational quality at posttreatment, there were differences 1½ years later that were maintained at 3 years. Markman and colleagues (1988) suggest that their premarital intervention served to reduce the declines in relationship quality that occur in most marriages over time. Similar longitudinal studies involving premarital or prenatal interventions that focus on parent–child relationships and the prevention of possible child and family disorders are needed.

Although investigations of child and parent behaviors have typically employed causal models in which single factors are hypothesized to uniquely determine outcomes, a number of studies across a wide variety of domains, such as IQ (e.g., Sameroff, Seifer, Barocas, Zax, & Greenspan, 1987), behavior disorders (e.g., Rutter, Tizard, Yule, Graham, & Whitmore, 1976), and child abuse (e.g., Egeland, Jacobvitz, & Sroufe, 1988), have shown that combinations of risk factors provide the best predictions of outcome (Mash & Dozois, 2003). In light of this, it follows that early prevention strategies should encompass multiple areas of child and family functioning. However, in considering various factors that have been shown to relate to child competence (e.g., maternal mental health, maternal anxiety, parental perspectives, maternal interactive behavior, maternal education, occupation of head of household, minority group status, family social support, family size, and stressful life events), Sameroff and colleagues (1987) noted that there is a large difference between the number of variables affecting a child's competence and the number that can be changed by our interventions. Only stress is likely to change by itself (for better or for worse), and psychological interventions for the individual often come down to altering maternal interactive behavior and maternal anxiety.

The fact that early circumstances and early personality characteristics seem to foreshadow so many later childhood disorders reinforces the need for early intervention. For example, in a study by Block and colleagues (1988), personality dimensions such as undercontrol and ego resiliency at 3 and 4 years were predictive of adolescent drug use 10 or 11 years later. Lerner, Hertzog, Hooker, Hassibi, and Thomas (1988) analyzed data from the New York Longitudinal Study and found two separate dimensions of negative emotional behavior—aggression (aggression, undercompliance, disobedience) and affect (anxiety, dissatisfaction, depression)—both at ages 1–6 and at ages 7–12. There was a substantial amount of developmental stability in individual differences on these dimensions, with autoregressive coefficients of .97 and .91 for aggression and affect, respectively. Aggression at age 7–12 was the best predictor of adolescent adjustment problems. Affect did not predict social maladjustment independent of aggression. These and many other findings suggest that it is especially critical for interventions to alter the course of early aggressive behavior, if later child maladjustment is to be prevented.

Cognition and Affect

Current cognitive-behavioral interventions with children and families have given increased attention to cognitive and affective processes in treatment. The growth of cognitive-behavioral therapy with children has continued unabated since the early 1970s, and this period has also witnessed a greater concern for the affective components of child and family disorders (including child and maternal anxiety and depression) and the interactions between children and parents, peers, and adult partners during emotionally charged social situations.

Cognitive-Behavioral Therapy

There are now many descriptions of behavioral interventions that take both child (Harris, Wong, & Keogh, 1985; Kendall, 2005) and family (Foster & Robin, 1998) cognitions into account. Although the long-term effectiveness of cognitive-behavioral interventions with children has yet to be determined (Lochman, 1988), and the concordance between cognitive-behavioral theory and therapy is not always clear (see Beidel & Turner, 1986, for a critique), a number of shared assumptions characterize current approaches:

1. Psychological disturbances are in part the results of faulty thought patterns, which include deficiencies in cognitive mediators and distortions in both cognitive content (e.g., erroneous beliefs) and cognitive process (e.g., irrational thinking and faulty problem solving). Various cognitive distortions and attributional biases have been identified in studies of children with depression (e.g., Asarnow, Carlson, & Guthrie, 1987), aggression (McMahon, Wells, & Kotler, Chapter 3, this volume), ADHD (Hoza, Pelham, Dobbs, Owens, & Pillow, 2002), and anxiety (e.g., Bell-Dolan, 1995; Bell-Dolan & Wessler, 1994). For example, Lochman (1987) found that during social interaction, aggressive boys tended to minimize perceptions of their own aggressiveness and to perceive their partners as more aggressive than they were. There is also some evidence of the specificity of cognitive distortions across different child psychiatric populations (e.g.,

Siqueland, Kendall, Stoff, & Pollack, 1987). The presence of cognitive distortions in disturbed populations is suggestive, but there is a need for longitudinal studies that would establish causal relationships between early cognitive distortions and later childhood psychopathology.

2. A goal of treatment is to identify maladaptive cognitions and to replace them with more adaptive ones.

3. The manner in which children and parents think about their environment determines their reactions to it (Meichenbaum, 1977).

4. Cognitive appraisals need to be evaluated in the context of ongoing social interaction (Gottman & Levenson, 1986). For example, Lochman (1987) found that nonaggressive boys in the early stages of conflict tended to assume greater responsibility for aggression, and suggested that this attribution of greater self-blame might motivate their efforts to modulate the expression of hostility. In contrast, if aggressive boys blamed others, they might begin to justify their subsequent peer aggression and to engage in conflict escalation.

5. Interventions need to take into account both the developmental continuities and changes in children's cognitive appraisals over time (e.g., Lochman, 1988; Mahoney & Nezworski, 1985).

If cognitive approaches to treatment are to be systematically evaluated, it will also be important to improve our methodologies for assessing those cognitions that are being targeted for change—for example, attributional styles, cognitive errors, and irrational beliefs (e.g., Robins & Hinkley, 1989)—and also to establish the relationship between cognitive changes and long-term behavioral outcomes.

Emotional Factors in Relationships

The progression in emphasis of cognitive-behavioral treatments has been from behaviors, to cognitions, to emotions, to strategies that attempt to integrate information from all three areas. The more recent interest in affect has included the following:

1. The development and refinement of interventions for disturbances that are predominantly affective in nature, such as childhood and adolescent depression (e.g., Stark et al., Chapter 5, this volume) and anxiety disor-

ders (e.g., Chorpita & Southam-Gerow, Chapter 4, this volume).

2. A concern for the ways in which emotional processes (e.g., arousal) moderate the expression of other types of behavior, such as social aggression (e.g., Lochman, 1988).

3. A concern for the ways in which a child's emotional status affects social-cognitive processes, such as attributions of causality.

4. A concern for the manner in which the emotional environment of a child's larger social system—for example, maternal depression (Goodman & Gotlib, 2002), maternal anxiety (Wood, McLeod, Sigman, Hwang, & Chu, 2003), maternal arousability (Wolfe & Bourdeau, 1987), marital/couple conflict (Gottman & Levenson, 1986), or family communication (Gottman, Katz, & Hooven, 1997)—affects the child's functioning.

The interest in affective processes has led to the development of such interventions as anger management and stress management training for both children and parents. It should be recognized that training (e.g., in child management) that occurs under safe, sterile conditions may not simulate the real-life context in which these skills must be exercised. Parenting in relatively unhurried and unstressful circumstances may require very different skills from parenting in situations where the child or parent is stressed, irritable, or rushed. Interventions must be generalizable to the emotionally charged situations that often set the stage for family conflict (Foster & Robin, 1998).

Population Specificity

Although cognitive-behavioral interventions have maintained their idiographic focus on individuals, individual behaviors, and treatment individualization as the "categorical imperative" in therapy (Wolpe, 1986), there is an increasing sensitivity to the unique characteristics and treatment needs associated with particular populations of children and families (Mash & Terdal, 1997b). For example, Ollendick and Cerny (1981) stated that "although basic concepts of behavior therapy may not change across populations, the manner in which those concepts are applied to particular populations may vary considerably" (p. 3). Whereas the latter part of this statement is undoubtedly true, it may well be that the basic concepts of

cognitive-behavioral therapy (e.g., relevant principles, conceptual framework for treatment, model of childhood disorder) also vary from population to population. As will be illustrated throughout this volume, intervention models need to be directed at the specific child and family characteristics that have been shown to be important for different disorders. Training protocols for parents of children with mental retardation (e.g., Baker, 1980), parents of defiant children (e.g., Barkley, 1997b), or abusive parents (e.g., Azar & Wolfe, Chapter 9, this volume) are likely to be quite different, as are the social skills training programs employed with children who have conduct disorder (e.g., McMahon et al., Chapter 3, this volume) versus autism (e.g., Newsom & Hovanitz, Chapter 7, this volume). An emphasis on populations rather than techniques in cognitive-behavioral therapy seems especially relevant for clinical practice, because, as noted by Kazdin (1988b, p. 3), "clinically, the major concern is not what the effects are of a particular treatment across a host of problem areas, but rather what the options are and what 'works' for a specific clinical problem."

CHILDHOOD DISORDERS

Consistent with a population-specific treatment focus, current cognitive-behavioral approaches acknowledge the importance of considering specific clinical problems as representing constellations of child–environment symptoms that commonly occur together (Mash & Terdal, 1997b). Such an approach capitalizes on established bodies of knowledge concerning the expression, prevalence, etiology, associated characteristics, prognosis, and prescribed treatments for specific problems, and attempts to use this information in order to design individualized programs of evidence-based intervention. The types of childhood problems that have most often been identified in clinical and empirical classification efforts are reflected in the major headings and subheadings of DSM-IV-TR (American Psychiatric Association, 2000). Although there are many unresolved conceptual and empirical issues surrounding all of the currently available classification systems for childhood disorders (Achenbach, 1985; Jablensky & Kendell, 2002; Lahey et al., 2004; Mash & Terdal, 1997b), the DSM-IV-TR categories are useful in orienting the reader to the types of childhood disorders discussed throughout this text. The disorders presented in Tables 1.2 through 1.5 are not intended to be exhaustive of all DSM diagnoses or combinations of diagnoses that apply to children. Rather, they are intended to provide an overview of the range and variety of disorders and problems that typically occur during childhood and for which children are most commonly referred for treatment. Further details concerning the characteristics of children with these problems are included in each of the chapters that follow and in Mash and Barkley (2003).

Table 1.2 lists DSM-IV-TR developmental and learning disorders, including mental retardation, pervasive developmental disorders (e.g., autistic disorder), specific problems related to reading and mathematics, and language and communication difficulties. A number of these disorders constitute chronic conditions that often reflect deficits in capacity rather than performance difficulties per se.

Table 1.3 lists the DSM-IV-TR categories for other disorders (besides those listed in Table 1.2) that are usually first diagnosed in infancy, childhood, or adolescence. These disorders

have traditionally been thought of not only as first occurring in childhood or as exclusive to childhood, but as requiring operational criteria different from those used to define disorders in adults.

Table 1.4 lists disorders that can be diagnosed in children (e.g., mood disorders, anxiety disorders, schizophrenia), but that are not listed in DSM-IV-TR as distinct disorders first occurring during childhood, or requiring operational criteria different from those used for adults. In many ways the DSM-IV-TR distinction between child and adult categories is arbitrary; it reflects our current lack of knowledge concerning the continuities between child and adult disorders more than it does the existence of qualitatively distinct conditions. Recent efforts to diagnose ADHD in adults illustrate this

---

TABLE 1.2. DSM-IV-TR Categories for Developmental and Learning Disorders, Usually First Diagnosed in Infancy, Childhood, or Adolescence

Mental retardation
  Mild, moderate, severe, profound, severity
    unspecified

Learning disorders
  Reading disorder
  Mathematics disorder
  Disorder of written expression
  Learning disorder not otherwise specified

Motor skills disorder
  Developmental coordination disorder

Communication disorders
  Expressive language disorder
  Mixed receptive–expressive language disorder
  Phonological disorder
  Stuttering
  Communication disorder not otherwise specified

Pervasive developmental disorders
  Autistic disorder
  Rett's disorder
  Childhood disintegrative disorder
  Asperger's disorder
  Pervasive developmental disorder not otherwise
    specified

TABLE 1.3. DSM-IV-TR Categories for Additional Disorders Usually First Diagnosed in Infancy, Childhood, or Adolescence

Attention-deficit and disruptive behavior disorders
  Attention-deficit/hyperactivity disorder
    Predominantly inattentive type
    Predominantly hyperactive–impulsive type
    Combined type
    Attention-deficit/hyperactivity disorder not
      otherwise specified
  Disruptive behavior disorders
    Conduct disorder
    Oppositional defiant disorder
    Disruptive behavior disorder not otherwise
      specified

Feeding and eating disorders of infancy or early childhood
  Pica
  Rumination disorder
  Feeding disorder of infancy or early childhood

Tic disorders
  Tourette's disorder
  Chronic motor or vocal tic disorder
  Transient tic disorder
  Tic disorder not otherwise specified

Elimination disorders
  Encopresis
  Enuresis

Other disorders of infancy, childhood, or adolescence
  Separation anxiety disorder
  Selective mutism
  Reactive attachment disorder of infancy or early
    childhood
  Stereotypic movement disorder
  Disorder of infancy, childhood, or adolescence
    not otherwise specified

TABLE 1.4. Selected Categories for Disorders of Childhood or Adolescence That Are Not Listed Separately in DSM-IV-TR as Ones Usually First Diagnosed in Infancy, Childhood, or Adolescence

Mood disorders
  Depressive disorders
    Major depressive disorder
    Dysthymic disorder
  Bipolar disorders

Anxiety disorders

Specific phobia, social phobia (social anxiety disorder), obsessive–compulsive disorder, posttraumatic stress disorder, panic disorder, generalized anxiety disorder, acute stress disorder, anxiety disorder due to . . . [indicate the general medical condition]

Somatoform disorders

Factitious disorders

Dissociative disorders

Sexual and gender identity disorders

Eating disorders

Sleep disorders

Schizophrenia and other psychotic disorders

Substance-related disorders

Impulse-control disorders not elsewhere classified

Adjustment disorders

Personality disorders

TABLE 1.5. Selected DSM-IV-TR Categories for Other Conditions That May Be a Focus of Clinical Attention during Childhood but Are Not Defined as Mental Disorders

Relational problems
  Relational problem related to a general mental disorder or general medical condition
  Parent–child relational problem
  Sibling relational problem
  Relational problem not otherwise specified

Problems related to abuse or neglect
  Physical abuse of child
  Sexual abuse of child
  Neglect of child

Bereavement

Borderline intellectual functioning

Academic problem

Child or adolescent antisocial behavior

Identity problem

---

problem. Although the criteria for ADHD were derived from work with children, and the disorder is included in the section of DSM-IV-TR on disorders that are usually first diagnosed in infancy, childhood, or adolescence, these criteria are also used to diagnose adults even though they do not fit the expression of the disorder in adults very well (Barkley, 2006). The more general issue here is whether there is a need for separate diagnostic criteria for children versus adults, or whether we can use the same criteria for both groups by adjusting them to take into account differences in developmental status—for example, by requiring fewer symptoms, different symptoms, or a shorter duration of impaired functioning.

Finally, Table 1.5 lists DSM-IV-TR categories for other conditions that are not defined as mental disorders, but that may be a focus of clinical attention during childhood. The categories included in this table are the ones that seem especially relevant to children, in that they emphasize relational problems, maltreatment, and academic and adjustment difficulties.

Since the criteria for judging "abnormality" in children are to a large extent social in nature, the determination of what constitutes a problem, and the likelihood of referral for treatment, will depend greatly upon the norms and expectations of key individuals in the child's environment. Children may not be accurate reporters of their own distress, especially when describing externalizing difficulties such as social aggression. The discrepancy in what constitutes "normal" for different individuals is illustrated in the following extreme example reported by Donnellan (1988):

> For two years the mother of a young man with autism would correct her son by saying, "Don't do that. It doesn't look normal." The son would stop the inappropriate behavior. Then she would add, "You want to look normal, don't you?" The son would say, "Yes." Then one day, it occurred to the mother to ask her son, "Do you know what normal means?" "Yes," he said, and the mother was impressed. She pushed for his definition. He said, "It's the second button from the left on the washing machine."

NEED FOR EFFECTIVE INTERVENTIONS

In spite of frequently acknowledged inconsistencies in the manner in which childhood disorders are conceptualized, defined, diagnosed, and assessed (Mash & Terdal, 1997a), epidemiological studies have been surprisingly consistent in their overall findings, reporting that between 5% and 15% of children and adolescents exhibit some type of mental health problem (Mash & Dozois, 2003; Mash & Wolfe, 2005; Roberts, Atkisson, & Rosenblatt, 1998). Although prevalence estimates vary as a function of the child's age, type of disorder, gender, socioeconomic status, ethnicity, and geographical region, they do indicate a rather substantial need for effective child mental health services (Kazdin, 1988b). If preventive psychological and health-related services for high-risk populations—such as children who have been physically or sexually abused (e.g., Wekerle & Wolfe, 2003), infants with interactional disturbances (e.g., Lyons-Ruth, Zeanah, & Benoit, 2003), children with learning disabilities (e.g., Lyon, Fletcher, & Barnes, 2003), chronically ill children (e.g., Peterson, Reach, & Grabe, 2003), children and adolescents with HIV/AIDS (Kalichman, 1997; Thomason, Bachanas, & Campos, 1996), or potential accident victims (e.g., Peterson & Brown, 1994)—are also taken into account, this need would be considerably greater (e.g., Rickel & Allen, 1987).

As noted at the outset of this chapter, most children who are in need of psychological services do not receive them (Kazdin, 1988b). Estimates indicate that only 20–33% of children with clinically significant disturbances actually receive treatment (Katoaka et al., 2002; Knitzer, 1982), and that children with more severe dysfunctions and those of Hispanic and African American origin are less likely to receive help (Katoaka et al., 2002; Sowder, 1975). On the other hand, the transient nature of many types of psychological disturbances during childhood would suggest that not all children exhibiting disorders or problems are best served through the provision of specialized psychological services. For many children, community, school, and other health care services may adequately address the personal and social adjustment difficulties they are experiencing.

EFFECTIVENESS OF COGNITIVE-BEHAVIORAL TREATMENTS FOR CHILDREN

The effectiveness of cognitive-behavioral treatments for children needs to be considered in relation to empirical evidence regarding the efficacy and effectiveness of psychotherapy with children more broadly (e.g., Weisz, Doss, et al., 2005; Weisz, Hawley, & Doss, 2004). The current emphasis on evidence-based treatments initially focused on criteria for empirically supported treatments with adults, and this focus rapidly extended to interventions for children (Chorpita et al., 2002; Lonigan, Elbert, & Bennett-Johnson, 1998). However, it was not too long ago that several researchers called attention to the scarcity of well-controlled outcome research on any form of therapy for children (e.g., Kendall & Koehler, 1985). For example, Kazdin (1988b) stated that "progress in the area of child treatment has been slow. There are many different treatments. . . . The great majority of these have not been shown to be effective. Even more regrettably, most of these techniques have never been carefully evaluated" (p. 9).

This state of affairs has been steadily changing, though, and the number of controlled outcome investigations for a wide range of childhood disorders has increased dramatically (Weisz, Hawley, et al., 2004). Nevertheless, the proportion of controlled outcome studies with children and families still pales in comparison to studies of psychotherapy with adults (Hibbs & Jensen, 2005). Even scarcer are controlled studies of treatment processes, such as the therapeutic relationship, treatment noncompliance, treatment involvement, or reasons for dropout in child treatment (DiGiuseppe, Linscott, & Jilton, 1996; Shelton, Levy, & Contributors, 1981). However, this situation also seems to be changing (e.g., Bickman et al., 2004; Chu & Kendall, 2004; Garcia & Weisz, 2002; Harwood & Eyberg, 2004; Hawley & Weisz, 2005; McLeod & Weisz, 2005; Shirk & Karver, 2003;

Several broad-based meta-analytic reviews ("meta-analysis" is a technique for pooling research findings across studies for statistical analysis) of treatment outcome studies with children have been conducted (Casey & Berman, 1985; Kazdin, Bass, Ayers, & Rodgers, 1990; Weisz, Weiss, Alicke, et al., 1987; Weisz, Weiss, et al., 1995), as well as more focused meta-analytic reviews of cognitive-behavioral therapy (Durlak et al., 1991). The main findings from these reviews have been presented by Weisz and colleagues (McLeod & Weisz, 2004; Weisz, Doss, et al., 2005; Weisz, Hawley, et al., 2004; Weisz, Jensen, et al., 2005) and Kazdin (1996b, p. 11) and may be summarized as follows:

1. The changes achieved by children receiving psychotherapy are greater than those for children not receiving therapy. This finding has been consistent across reviews.

2. The sizes of the mean treatment effects for treatment versus no treatment in published clinical trials are on the order of 0.5 to 0.8 across a broad range of treatment techniques, problems, and ages. These effect sizes are comparable to those reported for adults and fall in the range typically considered to be "medium" to "large."

3. Mean treatment effects reported in unpublished doctoral dissertations are significant and positive, but smaller than those reported in published clinical trials, with average effect sizes on the order of 0.23 to 0.27. These fall into the range typically considered "small" to "moderate."

4. The effects of treatment have not been shown to be reliably different for internalizing disorders (e.g., depression, anxiety, social withdrawal) versus externalizing disorders (e.g., ADHD, conduct disorder). Findings in this area have been inconsistent, with some reviews suggesting larger effect sizes for internalizing than for externalizing disorders, and others suggesting the opposite.

5. Treatment effects tend to be durable, with effects measured at follow-up being similar to those found immediately following treatment. In general, follow-up intervals average about 6 months.

6. Treatment effect sizes are about twice as large for problems that are specifically targeted in treatment as they are for changes in nonspecific areas of functioning. This suggests that treatments are producing focused effects (e.g., anxiety reduction) rather than nonspecific or global effects (e.g., feeling good).

Types of treatments—for example, behavioral versus nonbehavioral, or individual techniques within a given class of treatments—do not vary consistently in their relative effectiveness. Where differences have been found, they have favored cognitive and behavioral treatments over nonbehavioral treatments such as client-centered counseling or insight-oriented therapy (Weisz, Weiss, et al., 1995), albeit that these findings have been challenged on both conceptual and methodological grounds. For example, Weisz, Weiss, Alicke, and colleagues (1987) employed meta-analysis to investigate the effectiveness of psychotherapy with children and adolescents. They examined 108 well-designed outcome studies with participants ages 4–18. Findings showed that the average treated youngster was better adjusted than 79% of those not treated. These authors also found that behavioral treatments proved to be more effective than nonbehavioral treatments, regardless of the client's age, therapist's experience, or type of problem treated. The mean effect size for behavioral treatments was 0.88, compared with a mean effect size of 0.42 for nonbehavioral approaches. However, when comparisons were excluded in which the outcome measure was similar to the treatment procedure, this difference was nonsignificant. Weisz, Weiss, Alicke, and colleagues then reintroduced into their analysis those studies where inclusion of such outcome measures was deemed to be a fair test, and again found the behavioral procedures to be superior. These authors concluded that, overall, their findings make a case for the superiority of behavioral over nonbehavioral approaches in the treatment of children (Weiss & Weisz, 1995).

When the findings of the meta-analyses that have compared behavioral and nonbehavioral approaches are considered, it is important to note that these meta-analyses have included mostly studies involving group comparisons. This selection criterion probably underestimates the documented successes of behavioral and cognitive-behavioral procedures with children in studies employing single-subject research designs (e.g., Barlow & Hersen, 1984; Kazdin, 1982a). Although suggestions have been presented for using meta-analysis with within-subject designs (White, Rusch, Kazdin, & Hartmann, 1989), such analyses have received minimal attention. One exception is a meta-analysis of school interventions for children with ADHD that included between-subject, within-subject, and single-case studies (DuPaul & Eckert, 1997). The overall mean effect size for contingency management procedures was 0.6 for between-subject designs, nearly 1.0 for within-subject designs, and approximately 1.4 for single-case experimental designs. To date, other forms of therapy have not received the rigorous empirical evaluations characteristic of the cognitive-behavioral strategies used in many single-case studies, so direct comparisons across approaches cannot be made.

Although the meta-analytic findings present a generally positive picture of psychotherapy with children, and of behavioral and cognitive-behavioral approaches in particular, there are a number of important caveats. Weisz and colleagues (see Weisz & Weiss, 1993) have noted the important distinction between "research therapy" (i.e., therapy as carried out in laboratory outcome studies) and "clinic therapy" (i.e., therapy as carried out in clinics). Relative to research therapy, clinic therapy is typically conducted more often with children who have severe disorders (some of whom are coerced into treatment) and with ethnic minorities, is directed at a heterogeneous set of problems and children, focuses on multiple problems and goals, and is carried out in clinic or hospital settings by professional career therapists with large caseloads (Southam-Gerow, Weisz, & Kendall, 2003). In general, clinic therapy is generally less structured and more flexible, and it uses proportionately more nonbehavioral methods such as psychodynamic and eclectic approaches. In stark contrast to the meta-analytic findings for research therapy, as described above, similar analyses for nine studies of clinic therapy produced minimal effect sizes ranging from –0.40 to +0.29, with a mean effect size across studies of near 0 (Weisz, Donenberg, Han, & Weiss, 1995). Although the number of studies carried out in real-life clinical settings ("usual care") is small, this finding suggests multiple differences between the conditions in which usual care is provided and those found in clinical trials, with the latter being more favorable for producing change. To illustrate, parent training has been shown to be an effective treatment for preschool-age children with ADHD when delivered in specialized settings, but these benefits do not generalize to parent training that is delivered as part of routine primary care by nonspecialist health professionals (Barkley et al., 2000; Sonuga-Barke, Thompson, Daley, & Laver-Bradbury, 2004).

Similarly, other community-based mental health delivery systems for children have not found incremental improvement in outcomes related to the availability of comprehensive services. For example, in one large-scale study, the Fort Bragg Project, an integrated continuum of services was successfully implemented that provided good access, greater continuity of care, more client satisfaction, and treatment of children in less restrictive environments. However, costs were higher, and clinical outcomes were no better than those at a comparison site that provided services in a conventional manner (Bickman, 1996, 1997). These and other findings suggest that conventional services for children may be of limited effectiveness, and that integrating these interventions into more coordinated systems of care also shows minimal support for the beneficial effects of treatment. However, it is generally recognized that studies of child therapy outcomes in settings where it is typically conducted are few in number, and that it would be premature to draw any conclusions from the findings from clinic and community studies until more empirical data about therapy in practice are available (Shadish et al., 1997).

There is a clear need for additional information on the effectiveness of conventional forms of treatment for children. However, as Kazdin (2004) and Weisz, Jensen, and colleagues (2005) note, it is not just that more research is needed, but also that a different kind of research is needed—research that focuses on the conditions under which therapy for children is typically provided and on the therapies used most often in clinic settings. If systematic investigations of conventional treatments continue to provide weak results, further attention to the *reasons* for the large discrepancy between research therapy and clinic therapy will be needed. Since research therapy generally includes more behavioral and cognitive-behavioral treatments (Weisz, Doss, et al., 2005), and since these approaches are often not the first choice of treatment for most practitioners, one possible conclusion is that clinic therapy with children might be enhanced if cognitive-behavioral therapies were used more often. However, the exportability of these therapies may be premature when we consider that the conditions under which cognitive-behavioral therapies have been evaluated are quite different from those in which therapy is typically conducted in clinics. Evidence-based treatments need to be taken out of the laboratory, disseminated, and developed and evaluated in clinic practice before their generalizability can be assessed (Weisz, 2004; Weisz, Chu, & Polo, 2004). In order to achieve this goal, however, a number of obstacles will need to be overcome. These include practical constraints on practitioners' ability to use research; the acceptability of research products to clinicians, administrators, and clients; and the tendency to view dissemination as the one-way transmission of research to clinical practice, rather than as a two-way process (Addis, 2002; Herschell, McNeil, & McNeil, 2004: Hoagwood, 2002).

The evaluation of cognitive-behavioral treatments for children is compounded by the fact that comprehensive, multifaceted cognitive-behavioral programs are generally used, and it is difficult to evaluate the specific elements within such multimodal packages. Also, different aspects of a child's environment (e.g., with different family members, in different settings) are involved in treatment, and changes may occur not only in the child, but also in other systems in which the child functions (i.e., spillover effects). For example, as children come to view themselves as more competent and less avoidant, parents' perceptions about what their children can and can't do change as well. As a result, parents may begin to respond differently to their children, and their own feelings and functioning are improved (Kendall & Flannery-Schroeder, 1998). These more general spillover effects of treatment have not received sufficient attention in research to date. Moreover, in light of the rapid changes that take place during childhood, treatments that produce short-term effects are probably less meaningful in relation to childhood disorders than they might be with adults (Kazdin, 1988b). Consequently, more studies of long-term adjustment following treatment are needed, although such studies are difficult to conduct (e.g., Mash & Terdal, 1980).

Finally, and perhaps most importantly, blanket claims concerning the general effectiveness of cognitive-behavioral therapies for children and families make little sense. As Bornstein, Kazdin, and McIntyre (1985) noted more than 20 years ago, "Behavior therapy is not a monolithic, monomethodological approach. The area incorporates widely diverse methods and techniques with differential efficacy. To draw reasonable conclusions, we must examine the individual literatures for each technique as it is applied to specific problems" (p. 837).

Future work on the effectiveness of cognitive-behavioral treatment will probably require greater attention to the following: a wider range of child problems and disorders; the co-occurrence and interrelationships of childhood disorders and problems; a wider range of treatment models; identification of the necessary and sufficient components of treatment; understanding the moderators of treatment outcome; identification of the change processes that mediate treatment outcome; understanding the role of clinical processes such as the therapeutic relationship and alliance building (Shirk & Saiz, 1992); and evidence-based treatments that can be effectively delivered in real-world practice settings (Connor-Smith & Weisz, 2003; Kazdin, 2003a, 2003b, 2004; Weisz, Chu, et al., 2004; Weisz, Jensen, et al., 2005, pp. 14–19).

GENERAL FEATURES OF A COGNITIVE-BEHAVIORAL SYSTEMS PERSPECTIVE

A cognitive-behavioral systems perspective to the treatment of child and family disorders involves a collaborative problem-solving approach to treatment—one that is guided by a particular conceptual viewpoint and certain assumptions about child and family functioning; adheres to certain methodologies; and utilizes techniques that have empirical support and are evaluative, in the sense that they are self-correcting and constantly changing. Cognitive-behavioral therapy is therefore part of the larger armentarium of scientifically based treatments for childhood disorders, but by no means is the only such treatment. In a review two decades ago of input from several major figures in the field of child behavior therapy and elsewhere, Ollendick (1986) concluded that the major points emphasized in definitions of a behavioral perspective on child treatment were these: "(1) principles of behavioral psychology, most notably principles of learning; (2) use of strategies or procedures that are methodologically sound and empirically validated; and (3) application of such principles and procedures to adjustment problems of children and adolescents" (p. 527).

It is now even more apparent that the principles upon which cognitive-behavioral applications with children and families are based have become increasingly heterogeneous; they encompass elements derived from the areas of learning, cognitive psychology, developmental psychology, developmental psychopathology, social psychology, behavioral genetics, and the neurosciences. The appropriateness of such a conceptual expansion has not gone uncontested (e.g., Levis, 1988), but the current state of affairs seems to be the result of a gradual evolution in behavior therapy away from an ideological emphasis on principles of learning to a pragmatic search for effective scientifically based treatments, regardless of their theoretical origins (e.g., London, 1972). Although the development of a consistent conceptual framework is important for organizing cognitive-behavioral research and practice with children and families, a framework that is based exclusively on the extrapolation of laboratory principles of learning to the clinical context seems far too narrow, and the current commitment in cognitive-behavioral therapy is as much to empirical as to conceptual ties, if not more so (e.g., Kazdin, 1988a; Mash, 1998). As noted by Ross (1981), "The touchstone of a behavioral technique is whether it has objective, observable referents that permit one to put its validity to empirical test—not whether it fits neatly into the procrustean bed of one theory or another" (p. 2).

Given that cognitive-behavioral approaches are so thoroughly committed to a foundation of empiricism, the persistent contradictions between the vagaries and complexities of clinical practice and the rigor of laboratory-clinical research have been a continuing struggle. Clinical realities often require research-based treatment protocols to be altered or set aside in the interests of responsible practice. Some have suggested that the resolution of this paradox involves constructing a knowledge base for the therapeutic enterprise from *both* sources, although experience over the past half century tells us that this is more easily said than done (Goldfried & Wolfe, 1996; Weisz, Chu, et al., 2004).

Interestingly, the epistemological alliance between clinic and laboratory, as reflected in a scientific orientation to clinical practice, has been a double-edged sword for cognitive-behavioral approaches to child and family behavior therapy. This alliance has embraced two premises, each of which has been criticized as not providing a suitable model for practice.

Laboratory Research and Clinical Practice

The first premise is that cognitive-behavioral clinical practice is based on methods derived from empirically supported psychological principles, including, but not restricted to, those derived from studies of learning and cognition. The validity of this premise has been challenged both from within and from outside the field. For example, in his text on child behavior therapy, Ross (1981) stated, "It would be folly to assert that everything a behavior therapist does in the course of a treatment program, let alone in an individual treatment session, is explicitly and directly derived from empirically supported psychological principles" (p. 2). Similarly, Wachtel (1977), a psychoanalyst, noted:

> The more sophisticated among behavior therapists recognize that there is often only a loose, analogic connection between the methods they use and the learning experiments on which the methods are purportedly based. The various models of learning derived from experimental research serve only as stimulating guiding metaphors for much of the clinical work in the behavioral tradition . . . but they can be mischievous when the connection between clinic and laboratory is exaggerated or misconstrued for purposes of polemic or myth. (p. 8)

Wachtel went on:

> Behavior therapists are often effective precisely because they are not behavioristic in any narrowly construed way. In their clinical work they find it necessary to make inferences and to concern themselves with what their patients want and feel as well as what they do. Most of the practicing behavior therapists with whom I have discussed this issue have acknowledged privately that what they actually do looks quite different from what one would expect from reading the literature. (p. 8)

In support of this general view, findings from a survey two decades ago by Morrow-Bradley and Elliot (1986) indicated that only a very small proportion of practicing clinicians reported using research findings as a basis for their practice. However, later reports suggest that this situation is changing, with substantial numbers of clinicians indicating that research findings are useful in guiding their clinical practice (Beutler, Williams, Wakefield, & Entwistle, 1995). Apparently the road from clinical practice to the laboratory is less well traveled, however, with researchers being less likely to attempt to understand the problems that face clinical practitioners.

Empiricism and Clinical Practice

The second premise is that cognitive-behavioral clinical practice is closely wedded to empiricism, involving the collection of objective data prior to, during, and following treatment. However, guidelines for the uses of data collection in clinical practice are not readily available, and the extent to which such data collection facilitates meaningful outcomes in therapy has not been empirically documented. For example, Herbert (1987), in discussing his treatment manual for working with children and families, has stated:

> It [the manual] fails if it leads to some facile 'cookbook' application of techniques, or a mechanical insistence on numbers and measurement. The virtues of operationism can turn into quantiphrenia, which acts to the detriment of warm empathic interactions with parents and children. The emphasis on rigorous thinking and scientific assessment in this book is not meant to be at the expense of clinical art and sensitivity. 'Scientism,' a Pharasaical adherence to the letter rather than the spirit of the scientific method is to be avoided at all costs. (pp. 6–7)

The current emphasis on treatment accountability in mental health services for children and families has led to a renewed interest in data collection in clinical practice, and to the development of meaningful and workable assessment and evaluation protocols for assessing treatment outcomes in the clinical context (Mash & Hunsley, 2005; Ogles, Lambert, & Masters, 1996). The long-standing recognition by cognitive-behavioral therapists of the importance of evidence-guided clinical practice makes them especially sensitive to and well equipped for meeting current health care system requirements for greater accountability in practice.

PROTOTYPE FOR A COGNITIVE-BEHAVIORAL SYSTEMS APPROACH

The basic model for the treatment of childhood disorders from a cognitive-behavioral systems perspective involves a blend of epistemological assumptions; psychological principles; research findings; specific techniques (literally hundreds); operational rules for the selection and implementation of these techniques in relation to specific problems, concerns, and settings; and the continual evaluation of short- and long-term outcomes. Given the complexity of conditions and processes encompassed by this perspective, any single model that attempts to capture the processes of therapeutic intervention must be an oversimplification. Although there are no necessary or defining characteristics of a cognitive-behavioral systems approach to intervention with children and families, the

following conceptual, strategic, and procedural points, taken together, provide a general prototype for some of its more commonly occurring features.

Consistent Theoretical Framework

Cognitive-behavioral perspectives adhere to the general belief that good theory generates good practice, and that a consistent but flexible theoretical framework regarding behavior change principles and the nature and development of childhood disorders is needed to guide our intervention efforts (Bornstein & van den Pol, 1985; Herbert, 1987; Kazdin, 1997). For the reasons mentioned earlier, the epistemological framework for cognitive-behavioral interventions has been changing and evolving. Although a general commitment to a variety of cognitive-behavioral theories and models continues (e.g., instrumental, operant, respondent, drive reduction, mediational, observational/social learning, cognitive-behavior modification, applied behavior analysis), current approaches are perhaps best represented by a systems point of view. As noted by Kanfer and Schefft (1988), systems models provide the clinician with a perspective that will help to "guide decisions concerning what observations to make, what empirical data to select from various sciences, and at what systems level effective interventions should be conducted" (p. 19).

Within a general systems framework, the theoretical models being used to guide our treatments for disturbed children and families are becoming increasingly population-specific. For example, Patterson's (1986) performance model for social aggression suggests the importance of several molar and micro-level variables that are important to address in interventions with families of antisocial children. These include the extent to which a child is rejected or perceived as antisocial by others; the likelihood of the child's unprovoked negative behavior toward parents and siblings, and its duration; the extent to which the parents monitor their children and spend time with them; and the parents' inept discipline, as reflected in their use of explosive forms of punishment, negative actions and reactions, and inconsistent/erratic behavior.

As will be illustrated throughout this volume, the theoretical models underlying various child and family problems suggest very different sets of variables that are important in treatment (Mash & Barkley, 2003). The conceptual frameworks that guide our interventions for children with ADHD, anxiety, depression, abuse sequelae, mental retardation, or learning disabilities are likely to be quite different from one population to another. Models of service delivery for children with developmental disabilities are typically based on teaching long-term management and coping strategies, whereas intervention models for many other childhood disorders are based on a curative or corrective view that we can go in, fix the problem, and then terminate treatment. However, as I have noted, it is becoming more apparent that many childhood disorders that were previously treated from a curative perspective (e.g., early-onset conduct disorder, ADHD) may be more appropriately considered from a chronic illness model of coping and long-term management (Smith et al., Chapter 2, this volume; Kazdin, 1988b).

Conceptualization of Childhood Disorders

Although the number of child and family dysfunctions is large, a broad conceptualization of how such dysfunctions develop is needed in order to gather and organize information for assessment and treatment (Mash & Dozois, 2003). What is observed and emphasized during assessment and treatment will depend on the therapist's assumptions concerning child and family development, including the importance ascribed to social context, sociocultural norms, and biological factors. In light of the multiple etiologies underlying any child or family problem, all of these determinants will be involved (although their relative emphasis may vary, depending on the particular condition). Childhood disorders have been viewed as learned maladaptive habits, as physical defects and deficits, as failures in the adaptational process, and as system breakdowns. All of these views have some validity.

Most childhood disorders are best conceptualized as representing failures in adaptation on the part of the child and his or her social environment, and therapy is directed at corrective actions that will permit successful adaptation (or, in a preventive model, that will prevent or decrease the likelihood of future breakdowns). From a cognitive-behavioral systems perspective, childhood disorders are viewed as representing exaggerations, insufficiencies,

handicapping combinations, situationally inappropriate behaviors, or developmentally atypical expressions of behavior that are common to all children at certain ages. Although some childhood disorders (e.g., autism or childhood psychosis) may represent qualitatively distinct conditions (Kazdin & Kagan, 1994), for the most part, dysfunction is a matter of quantitative rather than qualitative variation in the expression of behavior, and the principles underlying the development and modification of typical and atypical behaviors are presumed to be similar. As I have noted, there is also an increasing acceptance of the view of childhood problems as constellations of behaviors, cognitions, and emotions, not simply as isolated responses (Mash & Dozois, 2003).

Importance of Reciprocal Influences

A cognitive-behavioral systems perspective recognizes the importance of the reciprocal influences that occur both within and between individuals (Bandura, 1986). Numerous studies have demonstrated reciprocity in parent–child and adult couple interactions across a wide range of disorders (e.g., Houts, Shutty, & Emery, 1985; Patterson, 1982; Patterson, Reid, & Dishion, 1992). At a more molar level, adult reactions to a child are affected by the age, gender, physical attractiveness, and temperament of the child (Bell & Harper, 1977; Mash, 1984). Child characteristics will also influence parental disciplinary practices. For example, a mother may exhibit more helping, rewarding, and overprotective behavior toward an anxious child, and more controlling and restrictive behavior toward a child with conduct problems or ADHD. Unidirectional models of intervention that fail to recognize the ongoing reciprocal social influences characterizing most child and family disorders are not likely to be very effective.

Evidence-Based Treatment and Clinical Sensitivity

In a relative sense, treatment from a cognitive-behavioral perspective is based on empirical data and well-documented theories, rather than on an accumulation of clinical folklore and experience. As much as possible, the description and treatment of child and family disorders from this perspective employ objectively defined terms and measurable operations, and are based on a quantitative analysis of actual performance (e.g., behavioral, cognitive, physiological), including a description of proximal and distal antecedent and consequent events. Many writers have adopted the view that the analytic approach and empirical methodologies characterizing cognitive-behavioral interventions are far more important dimensions than the model of behavior change a therapist subscribes to.

In spite of the acknowledged importance of an empirical perspective, there is a growing appreciation of some of the difficulties inherent in such an approach. For example, in describing their systems-oriented approach, Kanfer and Schefft (1988) state:

> While parameters and details may vary across clients and treatment settings, the approach presented here has wide applicability. It presumes that an empirical knowledge base is indispensable. But there is simply not sufficient scientific knowledge available at present (or may never be) to guide a therapist's action in all detail. Therefore, the empirical knowledge base has to be supplemented by extrapolations from personal experience, subjective judgments, and the realities of the present situation. But whenever strategies and tactics derived from scientific principles *are* available, intuition and subjectivity should never be substituted for them. (pp. xvii–xviii)

Thus empirically grounded cognitive-behavioral intervention with children and families also constitutes a craft—one that involves "a subtle amalgam of art and applied science," and that requires careful study and supervised practice (Herbert, 1987, p. 6).

Combined Emphasis on Proximal and Distal Controlling Events

From a cognitive-behavioral systems perspective, the controlling variables that are contemporaneous and present in the immediate situation have been given special emphasis in assessment and treatment. This is in contrast to orientations that focus on historical or temporally remote events. This emphasis on contemporaneous influences reflects the view that such events are likely to be more accessible and therefore more easily incorporated into our change efforts. This is especially so when a primary emphasis is placed on external environ-

mental events, as was the case with many of the early behavioral approaches. However, with the integration of the role of cognitive mediators into behavior therapy, symbolic processes give historical events contemporaneous representation, and any designation of what is considered contemporaneous and what is not becomes arbitrary and difficult to make.

In addition, numerous studies have established the important influence of extrasituational and temporally remote events on child and family functioning. External stressors such as marital/couple discord (e.g., O'Leary, 1984), negative interactions with neighbors or friends (e.g., Wahler, 1980), or neighborhood social disorganization (e.g., Caspi & Moffitt, 1995) may have direct effects on a mother's immediate reactions to her child's behavior. Cognitive-behavioral intervention programs that do not take these and other such events within the child's larger social system into account have not proved to be very effective (Patterson, 1982, 1996). The combined emphasis on proximal and distal, micro-level and molar controlling events is evident in the multimodal evidence-based intervention strategies presented throughout this volume.

Important Role of Assessment

Cognitive-behavioral assessment and cognitive-behavioral intervention are viewed as complementary and interactive. In fact, the use of systematic and user-friendly assessments in clinical practice has the potential to improve clinical care as much as the use of evidence-based treatments does (Kazdin, 2004). Initial intervention follows from a systematic behavioral or functional analysis, which considers the different system parameters and levels that are likely to be important for a particular child or family (Cone, 1997). Cognitive-behavioral analyses have often involved a single-level and linear consideration of antecedents, behaviors, and consequences (the A-B-C model). Although this approach continues to have enormous heuristic value in organizing information for intervention, it is limited in describing complex system relationships and the possible organizing role of cognitions and plans. Grawe and his coworkers (as described in Kanfer & Schefft, 1988, pp. 181–182) have presented an adaptation of the A-B-C model, referred to as "vertical" or "hierarchical" behavioral analysis. In this model, behavior is seen as being organized at hierarchical levels; the top of the hierarchy consists of themes, or beliefs and motives, that are related to specific responses in a situation. Hierarchical behavioral analysis appears to be a promising approach to organizing assessment information within a cognitive-behavioral systems perspective.

Terdal and I (Mash & Terdal, 1997b) have described child and family behavior assessment as involving a range of deliberate problem-solving strategies for understanding both disturbed and nondisturbed children and their social systems, including their families and peer groups. These strategies employ a flexible and ongoing process of hypothesis testing regarding the nature of the problem, its causes, the likely outcomes in the absence of intervention, and the anticipated effects of various treatments. Such hypothesis testing should be based on an understanding of the general theories, principles, and techniques of psychological assessment (e.g., Anastasi & Urbina, 1997; Cronbach, 1990; Sattler, 1992, 1997); information concerning typical child and family development (e.g., Mussen, 1983); and knowledge of populations of children and families showing similar types of problems, including information about incidence, prevalence, developmental characteristics, biological factors, and system parameters (e.g., Lewis & Miller, 1990; Mash & Barkley, 2003).

We (Mash & Hunsley, 2004; Mash & Terdal, 1997b) have described a number of commonly occurring conceptual, strategic, and procedural features of cognitive-behavioral assessments that, for the most part, parallel those associated with cognitive-behavioral treatment. These include the following:

1. An emphasis on conceptualizations of personality and atypical behavior that give greater relative emphasis to the child's thoughts, feelings, and behaviors as they occur in specific situations than to global underlying traits or dispositions.
2. An approach that is predominantly idiographic and individualized. Greater relative emphasis is given to understanding the individual child and family than to nomothetic comparisons that describe individuals primarily in relation to group norms.
3. An emphasis on the role of situational influences on behavior and the need to assess them in formulating effective treatments.
4. A recognition of the changes over time and reorganizations that often characterize child and family behavior, cognitions, and emotions.
5. A systems-oriented approach directed at describing and understanding the characteristics of children and families; the contexts in which these characteristics are expressed; and the structural organizations and functional relationships that exist between situations and behaviors, thoughts, and emotions.
6. An emphasis on contemporary controlling variables, in addition to the role of historical and more distal setting events.
7. A view of behaviors, cognitions, and affects as direct samples of the domains of interest, rather than as signs of some underlying or remote causes.
8. A focus on assessment information that is directly relevant to treatment, including such activities as pinpointing goals; selecting targets for intervention; choosing, designing, or implementing interventions; and evaluating therapy outcomes.
9. A reliance on a multimethod approach involving the flexible use of different informants and a variety of procedures, including observations, interviews, and questionnaires.
10. The use of a relatively low level of inference in interpreting assessment findings.
11. An ongoing and self-evaluating approach to assessment, with the need for further assessment being dictated in part by the efficacy of methods in facilitating desired treatment outcomes.
12. Assessment strategies—in particular, decisions regarding which variables to assess—that are guided by (a) knowledge concerning the characteristics of the child and family being assessed, and (b) the research literature on specific disorders (Mash & Barkley, 2003). Where assessments are theoretically driven, theories should be closely tied to the data.

The interested reader may wish to consult a number of comprehensive books and book chapters that review the underlying conceptual models and methods characteristic of behavioral assessment in general (e.g., Ciminero,

Calhoun, & Adams, 1986; Haynes & Heiby, 2004; Mash & Hunsley, 1990; Nelson & Hayes, 1986), and child and family behavioral assessment in particular (e.g., Bornstein & van den Pol, 1985; Mash & Hunsley, 2004; Mash & Terdal, 1997a, 1997b).

Ongoing Evaluation of Outcomes

Although it is recognized that clinical practice dictates placing higher priority on the discovery of solutions than on the demonstration of a functional relation between treatment and performance, accountability has and continues to be a central characteristic of cognitive-behavioral interventions with children and families. Single-subject designs, which are presumed to be more applicable in the clinical context than comparison group designs, have been developed to document the relation between treatment and outcome (e.g., Barlow & Hersen, 1984; Kazdin, 2003).

Idiographic Emphasis

A cognitive-behavioral systems perspective recognizes that within groups of children showing common symptom clusters, variation among individuals is the norm. Children and families with the same disorder may have different etiologies that are represented both in past events and in current controlling conditions. For example, with conduct disorder, the etiology may involve early ADHD, family interaction, or cultural influences. One major implication for intervention is that different treatments may be required for the same phenotypic expression of a disorder. Idiographic analyses permit this type of individualization of treatments for children within particular diagnostic categories.

Importance of Contextual Events

Cognitive-behavioral approaches are especially sensitive to the impact of situational context on behavior and the need to incorporate contextual information into treatment. Many studies have shown how context moderates the expression of behaviors, cognitions, and affects. For example, Asarnow and colleagues (1987) found that the negative biases of children ages 8–13 were not generalized across all situational contexts. Similarly, with aggressive boys, Lochman (1987) found that attributional pro-

cesses were distorted only when a child was interacting with another boy who had a different behavioral status (e.g., nonaggressive with aggressive vs. aggressive with aggressive or nonaggressive with nonaggressive), and who was typically much more aggressive or nonaggressive than himself. Interventions need to be sensitive to these types of situational variations.

Within a cognitive-behavioral systems framework for intervention, it is also important to identify the complex interrelationships among settings. For example, Pettit, Dodge, and Brown (1988) found that several dimensions of family experience were predictive of classroom social competence and problem solving. However, although early family experience with peers had a direct impact on peer outcomes, the impact of exposure to maternal values and expectations on social competence with peers was mediated by a child's social problem-solving skills. Such findings suggest the need to consider family relationship factors when preventive interventions in the area of classroom social competence are being designed.

Context also moderates the effectiveness of treatment, as, for example, when intervention takes place in the home versus the classroom. Expectations and responses of family members, teachers, and the child's peers all interact in determining the expression of childhood disorders, as well as the impact of various treatment strategies.

Family Involvement in Treatment

The cognitive-behavioral systems view often means that the child, family members, and other significant individuals will be actively involved in all phases of treatment. Koocher and Pedulla (1977) found that 94% of therapists reported seeing at least one parent and a child, and 23% reported teacher involvement as well. Early behavioral views promoted the idea that the most effective change agents would be individuals in the child's natural environment, such as parents and teachers (Tharp & Wetzel, 1969). Although the "child as target" focus of this viewpoint is somewhat antagonistic to current systems formulations, it was seen as both conceptually relevant and economical, and it spawned a rich and continuing tradition in child cognitive-behavioral therapy of involving parents (e.g., Dangel & Polster, 1984), teachers (e.g., Alberto & Troutman, 1982), peers (e.g., Strain, 1981), and siblings as change agents for children with a wide range of disorders.

The assumption that individuals in a child's natural environment are likely to be the most effective change agents has not been systematically tested. However, the meta-analysis by Weisz, Weiss, Alicke, and colleagues (1987) suggested an interaction between the agent of intervention and the nature of the child's problem. It was found that paraprofessionals and graduate students were equally effective as therapists in the treatment of undercontrolled types of problems, such as aggression and impulsivity, but that professionals were more effective in treating disorders of overcontrol, such as phobias and shyness. Also, graduate students and paraprofessionals were more effective with younger than with older children, whereas this was not the case for professionals. These findings suggest that the applicability of cognitive-behavioral models of parent training may depend on the nature of the disorder and the age of the child, although many other factors would also need to be considered in determining the primary agent of change.

A number of additional concerns must be addressed when parents are involved as therapists for their own children. For example, the relationships among family resources, well-being, and adherence to prescribed regimens would suggest that before parents are asked to carry out child-level interventions, efforts to meet more basic family needs must be made in order for parents to have the time, energy, and personal investment to work with their own children in a therapeutic or educational capacity (Dunst et al., 1988).

Importance of Cognitive Processes

Current practices emphasize that understanding the cognitive processes of both the child and significant others is essential to understanding and treating childhood disorders (Finch et al., 1993; Kendall, 2005; Schwebel & Fine, 1994). Cognitive-behavioral systems interventions are based on developing new behaviors, response strategies, and coping skills, and these types of learning are mediated in part by the beliefs, perceptions, expectations, and attributions of children and their families (Herbert, 1987).

Since the 1980s, there has been an increasing emphasis on the role of social cognition in both the developmental and clinical literatures (e.g., Miller, 1988). For example, in examining the link among family experience, social problem-solving skills, and children's social competence, Pettit and colleagues (1988) found that the strongest predictors of social competence were mothers' biased expectations (attributions of hostile intent). These authors suggest a developmental path running from maternal attitudes, values, and expectations to child social cognition to child social competence with peers. There seems to be a covert but pervasive influence of maternal attitudes, values, and expectations, and mothers may exert a more subtle influence on their children through verbal means than through other direct forms of control, such as harsh discipline. Pettit and colleagues hypothesize that through exposure to deviant maternal values, a child may learn to process social information in a deviant way when interacting with peers, and then comes to be perceived by teachers and peers as socially incompetent. Putallaz (1987) reported that mothers' social values, as expressed in their advised solutions to a hypothetical situation involving their children being teased, were predictive of children's social status in the classroom. However, solutions involving other social situations, such as entry into a new group, were not predictive. Such findings reinforce the need for a contextually specific approach to cognitive as well as behavioral interventions.

The Important Role of Genetic and Neurobiological Processes

The role of genetic, neurobiological, and neurodevelopmental processes, including basic maturational changes, has received increasing attention in cognitive-behavioral approaches to the treatment of childhood disorders. Studies of the effects of endocrine products, metabolites, neurotransmitters, and genetic structures on behavioral predispositions (e.g., Cicchetti & Cohen, 1995a, 1995b; Cicchetti & Walker, 2003) have necessitated a reappraisal of several learning-based theories and treatment approaches (Kanfer & Schefft, 1988; O'Leary & Wilson, 1987). Genetically influenced constitutional factors provide the medium in which psychological principles operate to produce both adaptive and maladaptive behavior. Biological determinants, biochemical disorders, or physical diseases frequently set limits on the skills a given child or family can learn; in turn, these limits influence decisions concerning the type of treatment that is likely to be most effective (Mash & Dozois, 2003; Ross, 1981).

The possible involvement of organic illness in many forms of childhood disorder necessitates an active collaboration with medical specialists. Strayhorn (1987) has presented several general guidelines in assessing the possibility of organic illness (e.g., toxic, traumatic, infectious, idiopathic, neoplastic, nutritional, collagen vascular/autoimmune, congenital/hereditary, endocrine, vascular, metabolic, or degenerative). An organic contribution is seen as more likely when functioning is grossly impaired, when there is a loss of previous ability in intellectual functioning, when explanations based on other grounds are not readily available, and when there are physical complaints and symptoms in addition to psychological ones (though physical symptoms need not be present at all for biological compromises or genetic factors to have played a role).

Beyond the psychological factors we have discussed, it is increasingly evident that virtually every disorder represented in this volume (ADHD, aggression, autism, depression, anxiety, etc.) has some genetic contribution to its variation within the population; in some cases, the genetic contribution accounts for the substantial majority of such variation (Mash & Barkley, 2003). Genes can and do make contributions to behavioral expressions and their variations and do so across the life span; indeed, learning as well as family environments would be impossible without such genetically mediated regulation of the underlying neuronal changes that permit us to learn and socialize at all (Pinker, 2002; Plomin, 1995; Ridley, 2002). The current focus on molecular genetics and the identification of candidate genes for many disorders discussed in this book are signs of this broadening conceptual shift, as are recent demonstrations that particular allele polymorphisms (gene variations) are associated with particular psychophysiological (electroencephalographic, evoked response) and neuropsychological variations and deficits. Neurological compromises may also make some contribution to etiology and variation (e.g., maternal smoking or perinatal brain hemorrhages to ADHD; intrauterine infections to autism; maternal drug abuse to childhood lan-

guage, learning, and broad cognitive disorders; etc.). These and other etiological factors are incorporated into the unique (unshared) environmental contributions that have likewise been revealed in behavioral genetic studies to influence the variation of nearly every disorder discussed here, often significantly more so than common (shared) or within-family environment. These genetic and neurological nongenetic contributions to behavioral variations are also historical events of some significance, raising additional challenges to a focus on immediate social events as the most functionally significant contributions to disordered behavior. Again, more important than a myopic adherence to some conceptually driven emphasis on immediate over distal or social-cognitive over biological events as having primacy in behavioral expressions is the greater commitment of the cognitive-behavioral systems approach to a scientific/empirical foundation to elucidating causal and contributory mechanisms, no matter where they originate.

Current cognitive-behavioral practices are based on a wide net of research findings, including those emanating from the biological sciences. This has led to the identification of important organismic variables and to information concerning the manner in which such variables interact with environmental factors in determining behavioral outcomes. For example, the relationship between child temperament and the quality of early parent–child relationships may be mediated by socioeconomic status, suggesting that early intervention with difficult infants may be more critical for low-socioeconomic-status families. Some longitudinal studies (e.g., Cohen, Velez, Brook, & Smith, 1989), have found that pre- and perinatal problems, as well as illnesses, accidents, and hospitalizations in early childhood, pose a biological risk for future psychopathology in children. Interestingly, these studies have tended to find that biological risk factors such as perinatal and early somatic problems are nonspecific; that is, they place a child at increased risk for all kinds of problems, including both externalizing and internalizing disorders, as well as substance abuse. Implicit in such findings is the notion that experiential factors both within and outside the family may mediate the expression of the disorder and should therefore be a high priority for intervention.

Development of Operational Rules for Implementing Treatment

The availability of operational rules for interpreting principles, in formulating assessment and treatment strategies, is limited. However, several investigators have suggested the form that such rules might take (Kazdin, 1997). For example, in the context of early intervention, Dunst and colleagues (1988, pp. 48–49) presented four general operating rules, each specifying a pragmatic relationship between an outcome and the action that has the greatest probability of achieving a desired goal:

1. To promote positive child, parent, and family functioning, base intervention efforts on family-identified needs, aspirations, and personal projects.
2. To enhance successful efforts toward meeting needs, use existing family functioning style (strengths and capabilities) as a basis for promoting the family's ability to mobilize resources.
3. To insure the availability and adequacy of resources for meeting needs, place major emphasis on strengthening the family's personal social network as well as promoting utilization of untapped but potential sources of informal aid and assistance.
4. To enhance a family's ability to become more self-sustaining with respect to meeting its needs, employ helping behaviors that promote the family's acquisition and use of competencies and skills necessary to mobilize and secure resources.

In the context of educational interventions for handicapped learners, Evans, Meyer, Derer, and Hanashiro (1985) suggest that because of the limited availability of educational programming time in proportion to the learning needs of children with disabilities, and because most excess behaviors can be effectively decreased by meeting educational needs rather than by behavior reduction procedures, "direct programming to modify a behavior should be considered a priority *only when unavoidable*" (p. 45; emphasis in original).

Concern for Treatment Generalization

Within a cognitive-behavioral systems framework, choices concerning the target of intervention, the agent of intervention, the setting in which intervention occurs, and the nature of the intervention should be based on the therapist's predictions concerning the generalizability of effects that can be achieved by intervening in one aspect of the family system versus another. The intent is to make choices that will maximize the impact of treatment throughout the relevant systems in which the child functions. Treatment generalization has been conceptualized as occurring across settings (e.g., clinic to home), across responses and response systems (e.g., from targeted to untargeted behaviors), over time (e.g., durable effects), and among family members (e.g., from target child to sibling). Findings from numerous investigations indicate that unless systematic steps are taken in treatment to promote generalization, it will not occur, and several writers have offered suggestions as to how generalization might be enhanced (e.g., Stokes & Baer, 1977). These suggestions have included the use of cognitive-behavioral therapy procedures, the enlistment of mediators in the child's natural environment, the use of multicomponent treatment strategies that focus on several family subsystems (e.g., parent–child and adult couple), the employment of self-management programs, and the use of specific procedures such as fading. The emphasis on cognitive processes and self-control in treatment has been viewed as one way of increasing generalization, by providing the child with internal self-regulators that will continue to operate across settings and time in the absence of external controls. This hypothesis has not been systematically tested, however, and studies are needed to determine whether cognitive therapies do in fact produce more generalized or more durable treatment effects with children and families, relative to other forms of treatment that do not include cognitive components.

Although follow-up studies have become increasingly common in the cognitive-behavioral literature (Barrett, Duffy, Dadds, & Rapee, 2001; Kendall, Safford, Flannery-Schroeder, & Webb, 2004), there is still a great need for studies that evaluate the long-term impact of child and family interventions. Complex issues surrounding the choice of follow-up intervals remain (e.g., Mash & Terdal, 1980), and the rapid developmental changes that characterize child and adolescent development make the assessment of long-term outcomes that much more difficult. A few investigators have suggested the possibility of "sleeper effects" in treatment; that is, performance at follow-up may actually be better than that immediately following treatment. This improvement has been hypothesized to be a function of the cumulative benefits derived from the continuing use of skills that were learned during treatment and the positive impact that such skills might have on the child's social system. Further investigations of possible "sleeper effects" are needed, and in these, it will be important to consider such posttreatment improvements against a baseline of growing maturity.

Several studies have found that treatments focusing on multiple family and school subsystems tend to produce more durable outcomes. For example, Dadds and colleagues (1987) found that child management training alone resulted in 6-month relapses in child problems, parent reports of difficulties, and marital dissatisfaction in families with marital discord. However, such relapses were less prevalent in families where child management training had been supplemented with partner support training in conflict resolution, communication, and problem solving. Epstein, Wing, Koeske, and Valoski (1987) found that at a 5-year follow-up of their diet management program, the children who had received combined parent and child training showed significantly greater weight reduction when compared to children who had been trained without their parents, or to controls. One-third of the children in the parent and child training group were within 20% of average weight, in comparison with only 5% of the controls.

Interest in Treatment Processes

A growing recognition of the importance of the general therapeutic milieu in moderating the effectiveness of cognitive-behavioral techniques has resulted in a greater interest in understanding treatment processes (e.g., resistance, treatment termination, treatment dropout). Although most forms of cognitive-behavioral intervention require a cooperative therapeutic relationship with children, parents, and teachers, these individuals are not always motivated for change (e.g., Chamberlain, Patterson, Reid, Kavanagh, & Forgatch, 1984). Consequently, there may be a need for special strategies designed to increase client involvement, in order to reduce the likelihood that premature intervention will lead to resistance and premature treatment termination (e.g., Ellis, 1985).

Kanfer and Schefft (1988) have described resistance and treatment noncompliance as representing a discrepancy between the client's behavior and the therapist's expectations. They also note that many possible sources of noncompliance need to be examined, including such things as client anxieties and self-doubts (e.g., fear of the future, giving up a known life pattern for a new and possibly worse state); client skill deficits; insufficient therapeutic structure or guidance; no motivation for change, due to secondary gain from symptoms; a countertherapeutic support network; and the client's lack of confidence in his or her ability to carry out therapeutic assignments. Understanding the different sources of therapeutic noncompliance will lead to different strategies for dealing with it in treatment.

Premature treatment termination has also been a concern in cognitive-behavioral work with children and families. The fact that as many as 40–60% of cases receiving outpatient care drop out of treatment makes this a significant concern (Kazdin, 1996c). In the review of child treatment outcome studies conducted by Weisz, Weiss, Alicke, and colleagues (1987), the mean number of therapy sessions was 9.5. However, this review also supported the idea that more intensive forms of treatment may produce more beneficial effects. In light of this, understanding the factors surrounding treatment dropout and developing methods to minimize them are priorities in cognitive-behavioral intervention. In a study by Weisz, Weiss, and Langmeyer (1987), dropouts and continuers in child psychotherapy were compared on a variety of child and family characteristics; these included child demographic variables, therapist variables, child problems, and parent perception variables. Surprisingly, the two groups were virtually indistinguishable on the basis of these characteristics. Weisz, Weiss, and Langmeyer suggested that source of referral and caretaker symptomatology factors (which were not included in their study) may be more important factors in determining whether or not families drop out of treatment.

In a study that focused on children with conduct problems, Kazdin (1996c) identified a number of factors associated with a greater risk of dropping out of treatment. Among these were lower income, dangerous neighborhood, younger mothers, one-parent families, greater perceived stress, maternal history of antisocial behavior, greater severity and duration of child conduct problem symptoms, greater number of parent-reported symptoms, below-average intelligence, poor school functioning, harsh parenting practices, and contacts with deviant peers. Kazdin (pp. 146–147) summarized his findings as follows:

1. Several factors increase the risk of families' dropping out of treatment; although many of these are related, they make separate contributions to predicting early termination from treatment.
2. The factors that predict early termination are much the same as those that predict poor long-term prognosis in children with conduct problems.
3. Reliable prediction of early treatment termination from the identified risk factors is possible.
4. Current parental psychopathology does not seem to predict early treatment termination.
5. Those high-risk families that continue in treatment do not profit very much from seeing treatment to the end of its course.

These findings suggest the need for decision models that view dropping out of treatment in the larger context of service delivery and utilization, and that focus on a wide variety of barriers to service utilization and their interaction (Kazdin, 1996c). Such decision models will need to be developed in the context of different childhood disorders; although there is likely to be some overlap, the barriers for children with conduct problems (e.g., socioeconomic disadvantage) are likely to differ from those for children with anxiety disorders (e.g., reluctance of parents to seek treatment) or children with autism (e.g., high burden of care).

Mechanisms of Change

As I have discussed, a large amount of research supports the efficacy of a variety of different treatment approaches for most childhood disorders and problems (Chorpita et al., 2002; Nock, 2003; Weisz, Hawley, & Doss, 2004). However, information regarding which treatment components are responsible for change, which mechanisms are involved, and which factors influence change is lacking for most treatments and disorders (Hudson, 2005; Kazdin, 2004, 2005; Kazdin & Nock, 2003; Nock, 2003; Weersing & Weisz, 2002). There is a need for more integrated theoretical models of how relevant mechanisms affect child out-

comes, both directly and indirectly (Patterson, 2005).

Emphasis on Self-Regulation, Self-Management, and Self-Control

A number of cognitive-behavioral models for intervention have emphasized the importance of examining self-regulatory systems as the basis for treatment (e.g., Kanfer & Schefft, 1988; Karoly, 1981). Self-initiated, self-maintained, and self-corrective internal processes—including self-observation, self-monitoring, self-reinforcement, imaging, planning, and decision making—have the potential for maintaining behavior over protracted periods of time, and by doing so can decrease the individual's dependence on environmental and biological factors. A self-management approach seems especially relevant for children and families, given that many of the disorders to be discussed in this volume represent a failure to develop (or a breakdown in) self-regulatory skills. Recent models of early intervention that have emphasized family needs assessment and concepts such as empowerment are consistent with the self-regulatory approach.

Self-management and self-regulation therapies are directed at teaching such processes as setting goals, evaluating norms and standards, monitoring and evaluating problem situations, planning, solving problems, examining choices, anticipating outcomes, employing self-reward and self-punishment, and understanding the relationships between cognitions and behavior. Appropriate use of these strategies assists children and family members in developing control over their behavior; over certain physiological reactions, such as anxiety, anger, and the experience of pain; and over cognitive or imaginally mediated reactions, such as intrusive thoughts, negative self-appraisals, or undesirable urges (Kanfer & Schefft, 1988). Achieving such control is intended to make the children and family members more proactive in their behavior, so that they are able to anticipate potentially conflictual situations, and have available a variety of mechanisms permitting them to cope effectively.

Concern for Ethical Standards

Criticism of some of the early behavior therapy practices, especially the use of aversive controls, has led to a special concern for the development of ethical standards for cognitive-behavioral intervention with children and families. Minimum ethical standards for practice include such things as selecting treatment goals and procedures that are in the best interests of the client; making sure that client participation is active and voluntary; keeping records that document the effectiveness of treatments in achieving its objectives; protecting the confidentiality of the therapeutic relationship; and ensuring the qualifications and competencies of the therapist (e.g., MacDonald, 1986). Guidelines for the responsible use of aversive procedures in behavioral intervention have also been developed (Favell et al., 1982), although the use of such procedures with children continues to decline.

Use of Specific Techniques and Technologies

The specific techniques that have been used in behavioral interventions for children and families are numerous; they are described in great detail throughout the chapters of this volume in relation to specific disorders. Some of the more commonly utilized general techniques are parent management training; modeling and role playing; relaxation procedures; desensitization and its many variants; exposure and response prevention; self-control and self-management methods; basic operant techniques, such as differential reinforcement, shaping, fading, punishment, and time out; cognitive change procedures, such as cognitive restructuring, stress inoculation, and cognitive coping strategies; social skills training; token systems; behavioral contracting; and environmental engineering.

Although, as noted earlier, flexibility is required in the clinical context, efforts to describe behavioral programs in as precise and replicable a fashion as possible have resulted in the availability of many useful assessment and intervention technologies. These include many detailed therapists' manuals for the assessment and treatment of a variety of child and family disorders (e.g., Barkley, 1997b; Blechman, 1985; Clarke & Lewinsohn, 1995; Evans & Meyer, 1985; Fleischman, Horne, & Arthur, 1983; Henggeler, 1991; Herbert, 1987; Kendall & Braswell, 1985; Kendall et al., 1992; Knox et al., 1993; McMahon & Forehand, 2003; Stark & Kendall, 1996); training materials and handouts for parents (e.g., Bernal & North, 1978); videotaped sequences of parent–child interaction (e.g., Wolfe & LaRose, 1986); computer simulations for training (e.g., Lambert, 1987); programs for data collection and treatment implementation utilizing microprocessors (e.g., Romancyzk, 1986); filmed presentations of treatment programs (e.g., Houts, Whelan, & Peterson, 1987); virtual-reality-assisted exposure for the treatment of fear (Rothbaum, 2004); an Internet intervention as an adjunctive therapy for pediatric encopresis (Ritterband, Cox, et al., 2003); and self-administered parent management training using a CD-ROM interactive program for delinquent children from low-income families (Gordon & Stanar, 2003) and children with health problems such as cystic fibrosis (Davis, Quittner, Stack, & Yang, 2004; Wade, 2004). Such technology is not intended to be a substitute for sound clinical decision making, but it does permit the training, transmission, and further evaluation of empirically well-documented techniques and procedures (Chorpita, Daleiden, & Burns, 2004; Ritterband, Gonder-Frederick, et al., 2003; Weingardt, 2004). These technologies and procedural specifications are viewed as key characteristics of evidence-based treatment, but will require further development and testing if they are to be effectively integrated into clinical practice (Carroll & Nuro, 2002; Henggeler & Schoenwald, 2002).

Use of Multiple Indicators to Assess Treatment Outcomes

A cognitive-behavioral systems perspective recognizes the need to use multiple indicators to assess the impact of treatment. Such indicators include reduction in symptoms; improvements in adjustment at home, at school, or in the community; increases in self-reported happiness and well-being; evaluations of relatives and friends that things are better; and prevention of possible further deterioration in a child's and family's adjustment. A concern for the clinical significance of therapeutic change has increased, and various methods have been presented to measure such change (Kazdin, 2001). Not only is it important to demonstrate that behavioral changes have occurred; it is essential that the magnitude and quality of these changes place the child and family within the boundaries of developmental, sociocultural, and personal norms for adjustment, and that they make a meaningful difference in the quality of their lives.

Concern for Consumer Satisfaction and the Acceptability of Treatments

A number of studies have examined the acceptability to consumers of various cognitive-behavioral interventions, and the possible factors mediating such acceptance (e.g., Elliott, 1988; Kazdin, 1981, 1984; LeBow, 1982; McMahon & Forehand, 1983; Witt & Elliott, 1986). For example, Tarnowski, Kelly, and Mendlowitz (1987) examined pediatric nurses' acceptability ratings of six behavioral interventions. Interventions directed at increasing desired behaviors were rated as more acceptable than reductive treatments, and treatment acceptability varied as a function of behavior problem severity. The medical severity of the child's condition did not significantly influence ratings. Furey and Basili (1988) attempted to predict consumer satisfaction in parent training for noncompliant children, and noted the importance of predicting what consumer satisfaction is going to be in advance, rather than determining what satisfaction is after the fact. Although clients' rights to self-determination, ethical and legal considerations, and common sense would certainly dictate the use of client-preferred treatment procedures, it has also been assumed that procedures perceived as objectionable or offensive by children and families will not be very effective, and that procedures clients prefer over others are likely to be more effective. However, the relationships between acceptability and outcome are just beginning to be empirically investigated.

The assessment of the social validity of interventions includes an expanded definition of "consumers," to acknowledge the range of community members and health care delivery personnel who are likely to influence the survival and effectiveness of an intervention program; the assessment of underrepresented populations, particularly lower-socioeconomic-status and minority group members; and increasing the involvement of consumers in the planning and evaluation of cognitive-behavioral programs, so as to educate consumers to make better-informed decisions about intervention (Schwartz & Baer, 1991).

Need to Consider Ethnic and Cultural Factors in Assessment and Treatment

In light of the family's central importance as a social unit and transmitter of sociocultural values, it is especially critical that interventions concerned with child behavior, child rearing, and other family issues establish some degree of congruence between the cognitive-behavioral therapy program and the sociocultural milieu in which it is carried out (Canino & Spurlock, 2000; Tharp, 1991). Often the rules that govern behavior and expectations for children are more explicit than those describing social intercourse among adults. The need to give greater attention to the cultural context of children and families participating in cognitive-behavioral interventions has received increased attention. This is evidenced in a recent call to consider parenting values and behaviors of specific ethnic minority groups (African, Asian, Hispanic, and Native Americans) in parent management training (Forehand & Kotchick, 1996), and in a special journal series devoted to ethnic and cultural diversity in cognitive and behavioral practice (Iwamasa, 1996). A consideration of treatment in relation to specific values, norms, expectations, and prescribed behaviors for different socioeconomic levels within cultures, across families that vary in their religious belief systems, for new immigrants, and across cultures is essential. Although cognitive-behavioral procedures have been applied across many different ethnic groups and cultures, cross-cultural assessment and treatment have received only minimal attention to date, particularly in the context of evidence-based treatments (Jackson, 2002; Verhulst et al., 2003).

There is some evidence to suggest that different practice elements may be used in treating children from different ethnic backgrounds as a function of the disorder of the child being treated. For example, Chorpita and colleagues (2005) reported differences in the practice elements used in treating specific phobias in Hispanic versus those used in treating Asian, African, and European American children. Relaxation, problem solving, tangible rewards, and self-monitoring procedures were not used in treating Hispanic children with specific phobias, but were used with other ethnic groups. Such differences between ethnic groups in practice elements were not found for other anxiety disorders, depression, or disruptive behavior disorders. These findings do not explain the differences, but they suggest that ethnicity is being used to guide choice of treatment for some problems and that further study of the reasons for this is warranted.

SUMMARY AND CONCLUSIONS

In this chapter, I have presented some of the major characteristics of a cognitive-behavioral systems perspective on the treatment of child and family disorders. The cognitive-behavioral systems perspective is depicted as a decision-making approach to treatment and prevention; it is based on a consistently applied theoretical framework, well-established research findings relevant to both typical and atypical child and family functioning, evidence-based treatment procedures, and operational rules that conform to the realities and changing demands of clinical practice. Recent developments in the field have included a growing systems emphasis; greater sensitivity to developmental factors; and an increased recognition of the importance of individual differences, biological determinants, and emotional, cognitive, and cultural factors in treatment. The need for further development of cognitive-behavioral treatment strategies that are sensitive to specific clinical problems is emphasized. The population-specific chapter presentations that follow provide detailed discussions of many of the issues that have been highlighted in this introductory presentation.

NOTE

1. Throughout the chapter I use the term "children" to denote children and adolescents. The focus of the chapter is on youths approximately 18 years of age and younger. Where the distinction between children and adolescents is relevant, this is noted.

REFERENCES

Achenbach, T. M. (1985). *Assessment and taxonomy of child and adolescent psychopathology.* Beverly Hills, CA: Sage.

Achenbach, T. M. (1993). *Empirically based taxonomy: How to use syndromes and profile types derived from the CBCL/4-18, TRF, and YSF.* Burlington: University of Vermont, Department of Psychiatry.

Achenbach, T. M. (1995). Diagnosis, assessment, and comorbidity in psychosocial treatment research. *Journal of Abnormal Child Psychology, 23,* 45–65.

Achenbach, T. M. (2001a). Challenges and benefits of assessment, diagnosis, and taxonomy for clinical practice and research. *Australian and New Zealand Journal of Psychiatry, 35,* 263–271.

Achenbach, T. M. (2001b). What are norms and why do we need valid ones? *Clinical Psychology: Science and Practice, 8,* 446–450.

Achenbach, T. M., Dumenci, L., & Rescorla, L. A. (2003). Are American children's problems still getting worse?: A 23-year comparison. *Journal of Abnormal Child Psychology, 31,* 1–11.

Achenbach, T. M., Howell, C. T., Quay, H. C., & Conners, C. K. (1991). National survey of problems and competencies among four- to sixteen-year-olds. *Monographs of the Society for Research in Child Development, 56*(3, Serial No. 225).

Achenbach, T. M., & McConaughy, S. H. (1997). *Empirically based assessment of child and adolescent psychopathology: Practical applications* (2nd ed.). Thousand Oaks, CA: Sage.

Achenbach, T. M., & Rescorla, L. A. (2001). *Manual for the ASEBA school-age forms and profiles: An integrated system of multi-informant assessment.* Burlington: University of Vermont, Research Center for Children, Youth, and Families.

Addis, M. E. (2002). Methods for disseminating research products and increasing evidence-based practice: Promises, obstacles, and future directions. *Clinical Psychology: Science and Practice, 9,* 367–378.

Adelman, H. S. (1995). Clinical psychology: Beyond psychopathology and clinical interventions. *Clinical Psychology: Science and Practice, 2,* 28–44.

Adelman, H. S., & Taylor, L. L. (1993). *Learning problems and learning disabilities: Moving forward.* Belmont, CA: Brooks/Cole.

Alberto, P. A., & Troutman, A. C. (1982). *Applied behavior analysis for teachers: Influencing student performance.* Columbus, OH: Merrill.

Alexander, J. F., & Sexton, T. L. (2002). Functional family therapy: A model for treating high-risk, acting-out youth. In F. Kaslow & J. L. Lebow (Eds.), *Comprehensive handbook of psychotherapy: Vol. 4. Integrative/eclectic* (pp. 111–132). New York: Wiley.

Amaya-Jackson, L., Reynolds, V., Murray, M. C., McCarthy, G., Nelson, A., Cherney, M. S., et al. (2003). Cognitive-behavioral treatment for pediatric posttraumatic stress disorder: Protocol and application in school and community settings. *Cognitive and Behavioral Practice, 10,* 204–213.

American Psychiatric Association. (2000). *Diagnostic and statistical manual of mental disorders* (4th ed., text rev.). Washington, DC: Author

American Psychological Association. (1996). *Violence and the family: Report of the American Psychological Association Presidential Task Force on Violence and the Family.* Washington, DC: Author.

Anastasi, A., & Urbina, S. (1997). *Psychological testing* (7th ed.). Upper Saddle River, NJ: Prentice Hall.

Antshel, K. M., & Remer, R. (2003). Social skills training in children with attention deficit hyperactivity disorder: A randomized-controlled clinical trial. *Journal of Clinical Child and Adolescent Psychology, 32,* 153–165.

Arnold, L. E., Abikoff, H. B., & Wells, K. C. (1997). National Institute of Mental Health Collaborative Multimodal Treatment Study of Children with ADHD (the MTA): Design challenges and choices. *Archives of General Psychiatry, 54,* 865–868.

Asarnow, J., Carlson, G. A., & Guthrie, D. (1987). Coping strategies, self-perceptions, hopelessness, and perceived family environments in depressed and suicidal children. *Journal of Consulting and Clinical Psychology, 55,* 361–366.

Asarnow, J. R., Tompson, M. C., & McGrath, E. P. (2004). Annotation: Childhood-onset schizophrenia: Clinical and treatment issues. *Journal of Child Psychology and Psychiatry, 45,* 180–194.

Baer, D. M., Wolf, M. M., & Risley, T. R. (1968). Some current dimensions of applied behavior analysis. *Journal of Applied Behavior Analysis, 1,* 91–97.

Baer, D. M., Wolf, M. M., & Risley, T. R. (1987). Some still-current dimensions of applied behavior analysis. *Journal of Applied Behavior Analysis, 20,* 313–327.

Baker, B. L. (1980). Training parents as teachers of their developmentally disabled children. In S. Saizinger, J. Antrobus, & J. Glick (Eds.), *The ecosystem of the sick child* (pp. 201–216). New York: Academic Press.

Bandura, A. (1969). *Principles of behavior modification.* New York: Holt, Rinehart & Winston.

Bandura, A. (1986). *Social foundations of thought and action: A social cognitive theory.* Englewood Cliffs, NJ: Prentice-Hall.

Barkley, R. A. (1987). *Defiant children: A clinician's manual for parent training.* New York: Guilford Press.

Barkley, R. A. (1997a). *ADHD and the nature of self-control.* New York: Guilford Press.

Barkley, R. A. (1997b). *Defiant children: A clinician's manual for assessment and parent training* (2nd ed.). New York: Guilford Press.

Barkley, R. A. (2006). *Attention-deficit hyperactivity disorder: A handbook for diagnosis and treatment* (3rd ed.). New York: Guilford Press.

Barkley, R. A., Edwards, G., Laneri, M., Fletcher, K., & Metevia, L. (2001). The efficacy of problem-solving training alone, behavior management training alone, and their combination for parent–adolescent conflict in teenagers with ADHD and ODD. *Journal of Consulting and Clinical Psychology, 69,* 926–941.

Barkley, R. A., Edwards, G., & Robin, A. R. (1999). *Defiant teens: A clinician's manual for family training.* New York: Guilford Press.

Barkley, R. A., Guevremont, D. C., Anastopoulos, A. D., & Fletcher, K. E. (1992). A comparison of three family therapy programs for treating family conflicts in adolescents with attention-deficit hyperactivity disorder. *Journal of Consulting and Clinical Psychology, 60,* 450–462.

Barkley, R. A., Shelton, T. L., Crosswait, C., Moorehouse, M., Fletcher, K., Barrett, S., et al. (1997). Preliminary findings of an early intervention program with aggressive hyperactive children. In C. F. Ferris & T. Grisso (Eds.), *Understanding aggressive behavior in children* (pp. 277–289). New York: New York Academy of Sciences.

Barkley, R. A., Shelton, T. L., Crosswait, C., Moorehouse, M., Fletcher, K., Barrett, S., et al. (2000). Early psycho-educational intervention for children with disruptive behavior: Preliminary post-treatment outcome. *Journal of Child Psychology and Psychiatry, 41,* 319–332.

Barlow, D. H. (2004). Psychological treatments. *American Psychologist, 59,* 869–878.

Barlow, D. H., & Hersen, M. (1984). *Single case experimental designs: Strategies for studying behavior change* (2nd ed.). New York: Pergamon Press.

Barrett, P. M., Dadds, M. R., & Rapee, R. M. (1996). Family treatment of childhood anxiety: A controlled trial. *Journal of Consulting and Clinical Psychology, 64,* 333–342.

Barrett, P. M., Duffy, A. L., Dadds, M. R., & Rapee, R. M. (2001). Cognitive-behavioral treatment of anxiety disorders in children: Long-term (6-year) follow-up. *Journal of Consulting and Clinical Psychology, 69,* 135–141.

Barrett, P. M., Healy-Farrell, L., & March, J. S. (2004). Cognitive-behavioral family treatment of childhood obsessive-compulsive disorder: A controlled trial. *Journal of the American Academy of Child and Adolescent Psychiatry, 43,* 46–62.

Barrett, P. M., & Ollendick, T. H. (2004). *Handbook of interventions that work with children and adolescents: Prevention and treatment.* New York: Wiley.

Beidel, D. C., & Turner, S. M. (1986). A critique of the theoretical bases of cognitive-behavior theories and therapy. *Clinical Psychology Review, 6,* 177–197.

Bell, D. J., Foster, S. L., & Mash, E. J. (Eds.). (2005). *Handbook of behavioral and emotional problems in girls.* New York: Kluwer Academic/Plenum Press.

Bell-Dolan, D. J. (1995). Social cue interpretation of anxious children. *Journal of Clinical Child Psychology, 24,* 1–10.

Bell-Dolan, D. J., & Wessler, A. E. (1994). Attributional style of anxious children: Extensions from cognitive theory and research on adult anxiety. *Journal of Anxiety Disorders, 8,* 79–96.

Bell, R. Q., & Harper, L. V. (1977). *Child effects on adults.* Hillsdale, NJ: Erlbaum.

Bernal, M. E., & North, J. (1978). A survey of parent training manuals. *Journal of Applied Behavior Analysis, 11,* 533–544.

Beutler, L. E., Williams, R. E., Wakefield, P. J., & Entwistle, S. R. (1995). Bridging scientist and practitioner perspectives in clinical psychology. *American Psychologist, 50,* 984–994.

Bickman, L. (1996). A continuum of care: More is

not always better. *American Psychologist, 51*, 689–701.

Bickman, L. (1997). Resolving issues raised by the Fort Bragg evaluation: New directions for mental health services research. *American Psychologist, 52*, 562–565.

Bickman, L. (2002). The death of treatment as usual: An excellent first step on a long road. *Clinical Psychology Science and Practice, 9*, 195–198.

Bickman, L., Andrade, A. R., Lambert, E. W., Doucette, A., Sapyta, J., Boyd, A. S., et al. (2004). Youth therapeutic alliance in intensive treatment settings. *Journal of Behavioral Health Services and Research, 31*, 134–148.

Bickman, L., Smith, C. M., Lambert, E. W., & Andrade, A. R. (2003). Evaluation of a congressionally mandated wraparound demonstration. *Journal of Child and Family Studies, 12*, 135–156.

Bijou, S. W., & Baer, D. M. (1961). *Child development: Systematic and empirical theory*. New York: Appleton-Century-Crofts.

Birchler, G. R., Doumas, D. M., & Fals-Stewart, W. S. (1999). The seven Cs: A behavioral systems framework for evaluating marital distress. *The Family Journal: Counseling and Therapy for Couples and Families, 7*, 253–264.

Blechman, E. A. (1985). *Solving child behavior problems at home and school*. Champaign, IL: Research Press.

Block, J., Block, J. H., & Keyes, S. (1988). Longitudinally foretelling drug usage in adolescence: Early childhood personality and environmental precursors. *Child Development, 59*, 336–355.

Block, J., & Gjerde, P. F. (1990). Depressive symptoms in late adolescence: A longitudinal perspective on personality antecedents. In J. E. Rolf, A. Masten, D. Cicchetti, K. Neuchterlein, & S. Weintraub (Eds.), *Risk and protective factors in the development of psychopathology* (pp. 334–360). New York: Cambridge University Press.

Borduin, C. M., Mann, B. J., Cone, L. T., Henggeler, S. W., Fucci, B. R., Blaske, D. M., et al. (1995). Multisystemic treatment of serious juvenile offenders: Long-term prevention of criminality and violence. *Journal of Consulting and Clinical Psychology, 63*, 569–578.

Bornstein, P. H., Kazdin, A. E., & McIntyre, T. J. (1985). Characteristics, trends, and future directions in child behavior therapy. In P. H. Bornstein & A. E. Kazdin (Eds.), *Handbook of clinical behavior therapy with children* (pp. 833–850). Homewood, IL: Dorsey Press.

Bornstein, P. H., & van den Pol, R. A. (1985). Models of assessment and treatment in child behavior therapy. In P. H. Bornstein & A. E. Kazdin (Eds.), *Handbook of clinical behavior therapy with children* (pp. 44–74). Homewood, IL: Dorsey Press.

Bronfenbrenner, U. (1986). Ecology of the family as a context for human development: Research perspectives. *Developmental Psychology, 22*, 723–742.

Brunk, M., Henggeler, S. W., & Whelan, J. P. (1987). Comparison of multisystemic therapy and parent training in the brief treatment of child abuse and neglect. *Journal of Consulting and Clinical Psychology, 55*, 171–178.

Canino, I. A., & Spurlock, J. (2000). *Culturally diverse children and adolescents: Assessment, diagnosis, and treatment* (2nd ed.). New York: Guilford Press.

Carlson, G., Asarnow, J. R., & Orbach, I. (1987). Developmental aspects of suicidal behavior in children. *Journal of the American Academy of Child and Adolescent Psychiatry, 26*, 186–192.

Caron, C., & Rutter, M. (1991). Comorbidity in child psychopathology: Concepts, issues, and research strategies. *Journal of Child Psychology and Psychiatry, 32*, 1063–1080.

Carr, E. G. (1994). Emerging themes in the functional analysis of problem behavior. *Journal of Applied Behavior Analysis, 27*, 393–399.

Carroll, K. M., & Nuro, K. F. (2002). One size cannot fit all: A stage model for psychotherapy manual development. *Clinical Psychology: Science and Practice, 9*, 396–406.

Carver, C. S., & Scheier, M. F. (1986, August). *Dispositional optimism: A theoretical analysis and implications for the self-regulation of behavior*. Paper presented at the annual meeting of the American Psychological Association, Washington, DC.

Casey, R. J., & Berman, J. S. (1985). The outcome of psychotherapy with children. *Psychological Bulletin, 98*, 388–400.

Caspi, A., & Moffitt, T. E. (1995). The continuity of maladaptive behavior: From description to understanding in the study of antisocial behavior. In D. Cicchetti & D. J. Cohen (Eds.), *Developmental psychopathology: Vol. 2. Risk, disorder, and adaptation* (pp. 472–511). New York: Wiley.

Chamberlain, P., Patterson, G. R., Reid, J. B., Kavanagh, K., & Forgatch, M. (1984). Observation of client resistance. *Behavior Therapy, 15*, 144–155.

Chamberlain, P., & Reid, J. B. (1994). Differences in risk factors and adjustment for male and female delinquents in treatment foster care. *Journal of Child and Family Studies, 3*, 23–39.

Chorpita, B. F., Daleiden, E. L., & Burns, J. A. (2004). Designs for instruction, designs for change: Distributing knowledge of evidence-based practice. *Clinical Psychology: Science and Practice, 11*, 332–335.

Chorpita, B. F., Daleiden, E. L., & Weisz, J. R. (2005). Identifying and selecting the common elements of evidence based interventions: A distillation and matching model. *Mental Health Services Research, 7*, 5–20.

Chorpita, B. F., & Nakamura, B. J. (2004). Four considerations for dissemination of intervention innovations. *Clinical Psychology: Science and Practice, 11*, 364–367.

Chorpita, B. F., Yim, L., Donkervoet, J. C., Aresdorf, A., Amundsen, M. J., McGee, C., et al. (2002). Toward large-scale implementation of empirically supported treatments for children: A review and observations by the Hawaii Empirical Basis to Services Task Force. *Clinical Psychology: Science and Practice, 9,* 165–190.

Christopherson, E. R. (1986). Accident prevention in primary care. *Pediatric Clinics of North America, 33,* 925–933.

Christopherson, E. R., & Mortweet, S. I. (2001). *Treatments that work with children: Empirically supported strategies for managing childhood problems.* Washington, DC: American Psychological Association.

Chronis, A. M., Chacko, A., Fabiano, G. A., Wymbs, B. T., & Pelham, W. E., Jr. (2004). Enhancements to the behavioral parent training paradigm for families of children with ADHD: Review and future directions. *Clinical Child and Family Psychology Review, 7,* 1–27.

Chu, B. C., & Kendall, P. C. (2004). Positive association of child involvement and treatment outcome within a manual-based cognitive-behavioral treatment for children with anxiety. *Journal of Consulting and Clinical Psychology, 72,* 821–829.

Cicchetti, D., & Cohen, D. J. (Eds.). (1995a). *Developmental psychopathology: Vol. 1. Theory and methods.* New York: Wiley.

Cicchetti, D., & Cohen, D. J. (Eds.). (1995b). *Developmental psychopathology: Vol. 2. Risk, disorder, and adaptation.* New York: Wiley.

Cicchetti, D., & Cohen, D. J. (1995c). Perspectives on developmental psychopathology. In D. Cicchetti & D. J. Cohen (Eds.), *Developmental psychopathology: Vol. 1. Theory and methods* (pp. 3–20). New York: Wiley.

Cicchetti, D., & Hinshaw, S. P. (2002). Editorial: Prevention and intervention science: Contributions to developmental theory. *Development and Psychopathology, 14,* 667–671.

Cicchetti, D., & Walker, E. F. (Eds.). (2003). *Neurodevelopmental mechanisms in psychopathology.* New York: Cambridge University Press.

Ciminero, A. R., Calhoun, K. S., & Adams, H. E. (Eds.). (1986). *Handbook of behavioral assessment* (2nd ed.). New York: Wiley-Interscience.

Clarke, G. N., Hawkins, W., Murphy, M., Sheeber, L. B., Lewinsohn, P. M., & Seeley, M. S. (1995). Targeted prevention of unipolar depressive disorder in an at-risk sample of high school adolescents: A randomized trial of a group cognitive intervention. *Journal of the American Academy of Child and Adolescent Psychiatry, 34,* 312–321.

Clarke, G. N., & Lewinsohn, P. M. (1995). *The adolescent coping with stress class: Leader manual.* Unpublished manual, Oregon Health Sciences University.

Clarke, G. N., Lewinsohn, P. M., & Hops, H. (1990). *Leader's manual for adolescent groups: Adolescent coping with depression course.* Retrieved from www.kpchr.org/public/acwd/acwd.html

Clement, P. W. (1996). Evaluation in private practice. *Clinical Psychology: Science and Practice, 3,* 146–159.

Cohen, P., Velez, C. N., Brook, J. S., & Smith, J. (1989). Mechanisms of the relation between perinatal problems, early childhood illness, and psychopathology in late childhood and adolescence. *Child Development, 60,* 701–709.

Compton, S. N., March, J. S., Brent, D., Albano, A. M., Weersing, V. R., & Curry, J. (2004). Cognitive-behavioral psychotherapy for anxiety and depressive disorders in children and adolescents: An evidence-based medicine review. *Journal of the American Academy of Child and Adolescent Psychiatry, 43,* 930–959.

Compton, S. N., McKnight, C. D., & March, J. S. (2004). Combining medication and psychosocial treatments: An evidence-based medicine approach. In T. L Morris & J. S. March (Eds.), *Anxiety disorders in children and adolescents* (2nd ed., pp. 355–370). New York: Guilford Press.

Conduct Problems Prevention Research Group. (1992). A developmental and clinical model for the prevention of conduct disorder: The FAST Track Program. *Development and Psychopathology, 4,* 509–527.

Conduct Problems Prevention Research Group. (1997, April). *Prevention of antisocial behavior: Initial findings from the Fast Track project.* Symposium presented at the biennial meeting of the Society for Research in Child Development, Washington, DC.

Cone, J. D. (1997). Issues in functional analysis in behavioral assessment. *Behaviour Research and Therapy, 35,* 259–275.

Connor-Smith, J. K., & Weisz, J. R. (2003). Applying treatment outcome research in clinical practice: Techniques of adapting interventions to the real world. *Child and Adolescent Mental Health, 8,* 3–10.

Courchesne, E., Townsend, J., & Chase, C. (1995). Neurodevelopmental principles guide research on developmental psychopathologies. In D. Cicchetti & D. J. Cohen (Eds.), *Developmental psychopathology: Vol. 1. Theory and methods* (pp. 195–226). New York: Wiley.

Cowan, P. A. (1997). Beyond meta-analysis: A plea for a family systems view of attachment. *Child Development, 68,* 601–603.

Crick, N. R. (1995). Relational aggression: The role of intent attributions, feelings of distress, and provocation type. *Development and Psychopathology, 7,* 313–322.

Crick, N. R., Bigbee, M. A., & Howes, C. (1996). Gender differences in children's normative beliefs about aggression: How do I hurt thee? Let me count the ways. *Child Development, 67,* 1003–1014.

Crick, N. R., & Dodge, K. A. (1994). A review and reformulation of social information processing mechanisms in children's social adjustment. *Psychological Bulletin, 115,* 74–101.

Crick, N. R., & Dodge, K. A. (1996). Social information-processing mechanisms in reactive and proactive aggression. *Child Development, 67,* 993–1002.

Crick, N. R., & Zahn-Waxler, C. (2003). The development of psychopathology in females and males: Current progress and future challenges. *Development and Psychopathology, 15*, 719–742.

Cronbach, L. J. (1990). *Essentials of psychological testing* (5th ed.). New York: Harper & Row.

Curtis, N. M., Ronan, K. R., & Borduin, C. M. (2004). Multisystemic treatment: A meta-analysis of outcome studies. *Journal of Family Psychology, 18*, 411–419.

Dadds, M. R., & Barrett, P. M. (2001). Practitioner review: Psychological management of anxiety disorders in childhood. *Journal of Child Psychology and Psychiatry, 42*, 999–1011.

Dadds, M. R., Schwartz, S., & Sanders, M. R. (1987). Marital discord and treatment outcome in behavioral treatment of child conduct disorders. *Journal of Consulting and Clinical Psychology, 55*, 396–403.

Dangel, R. F., & Polster, R. A. (Eds.). (1984). *Parent training: Foundations of research and practice*. New York: Guilford Press.

Davies, P. T., & Cicchetti, D. (2004). Editorial: Toward an integration of family systems and developmental psychopathology approaches. *Development and Psychopathology, 16*, 477–481.

Davis, M. A., Quittner, A. L., Stack, C. M., & Yang, M. C. K. (2004). Controlled evaluation of the STARBRIGHT CD-ROM program for children and adolescents with cystic fibrosis. *Journal of Pediatric Psychology, 29*, 259–267.

Davis, T. E., III, & Ollendick, T. H. (2005). Empirically supported treatments for specific phobia in children: Do efficacious treatments address the components of a phobic response? *Clinical Psychology: Science and Practice, 12*, 144–160.

DiGiuseppe, R., Linscott, J., & Jilton, R. (1996). Developing the therapeutic alliance in child-adolescent psychotherapy. *Applied and Preventive Psychology, 5*, 85–100.

Dishion, T. J., & Kavanagh, K. (2003). *Intervening in adolescent problem behavior: A family-centered approach*. New York: Guilford Press.

Dishion, T. J., McCord, J., & Poulin, F. (1999). When interventions harm: Peer groups and problem behavior. *American Psychologist, 54*, 755–764.

Dishion, T. J., & Snyder, J. (2004). An introduction to the special issue on advances in process and dynamic system analysis of social interaction and the development of antisocial behavior. *Journal of Abnormal Child Psychology, 32*, 575–578.

Donnellan, A. M. (1988, February). Our old ways just aren't working. *Dialect* [Newsletter of the Saskatchewan Association for the Mentally Retarded].

DuCharme, J., Atkinson, L., & Poulton, L. (2000). Success based, noncoercive treatment of oppositional behavior in children from violent homes. *Journal of the American Academy of Child and Adolescent Psychiatry, 39*, 995–1004.

Dunlap, K. (1932). *Habits: Their making and unmaking*. New York: Liveright.

Dunst, C., Trivette, C., & Deal, A. (1988). *Enabling and empowering families: Principles and guidelines for practice*. Cambridge, MA: Brookline Books.

DuPaul, G. J., & Eckert, T. L. (1997). The effects of school-based interventions for attention deficit hyperactivity disorder: A meta-analysis. *School Psychology Digest, 26*, 5–27.

Durlak, J. A., Fuhrman, T., & Lampman, C. (1991). Effectiveness of cognitive-behavior therapy for maladapting children: A meta-analysis. *Psychological Bulletin, 110*, 204–214.

Edelbrock, C. (1984). Developmental considerations. In T. H. Ollendick & M. Hersen (Eds.), *Child behavioral assessment: Principles and procedures* (pp. 20–37). New York: Pergamon Press.

Egeland, B., Jacobvitz, D., & Sroufe, L. A. (1988). Breaking the cycle of abuse. *Child Development, 59*, 1080–1088.

Ehrensaft, M. K. (2005). Interpersonal relationships and sex differences in the development of conduct problems. *Clinical Child and Family Psychology Review, 8*, 39–63.

Eifert, G. H., & Wilson, P. H. (1991). The triple response approach to assessment: A conceptual and methodological reappraisal. *Behaviour Research and Therapy, 29*, 283–292.

Eisen, A. R., & Schaefer, C. E. (2005). *Separation anxiety in children and adolescents: An individualized approach to assessment and treatment*. New York: Guilford Press.

Elliott, A. J., Miltenberger, R. G., Kaster-Bundgaard, J., & Lumley, V. (1996). A national survey of assessment and therapy techniques used by behavior therapists. *Cognitive and Behavioral Practice, 3*, 107–125.

Elliott, S. N. (1988). Acceptability of behavioral treatments: Review of variables that influence treatment selection. *Professional Psychology: Research and Practice, 19*, 68–80.

Ellis, A. (1985). *Overcoming resistance: Rational–emotive therapy with difficult clients*. New York: Springer.

Emery, R. E., Fincham, F. D., & Cummings, E. M. (1992). Parenting in context: Systemic thinking about parental conflict and its influence on children. *Journal of Consulting and Clinical Psychology, 60*, 909–912.

Emery, R. E., & Kitzmann, K. M. (1995). The child in the family: Disruptions in family functioning. In D. Cicchetti & D. J. Cohen (Eds.), *Developmental psychopathology: Vol. 2. Risk, disorder, and adaptation* (pp. 3–31). New York: Wiley.

Epstein, L. H., Wing, R. R., Koeske, R., & Valoski, A. (1987). Long-term effects of family based treatment of childhood obesity. *Journal of Consulting and Clinical Psychology, 55*, 91–95.

Evans, I. M. (1985). Building systems models as a strategy for target behavior selection in clinical assessment. *Behavioral Assessment, 7*, 21–32.

Evans, I. M., & Meyer, L. H. (1985). *An educative approach to behavior problems: A practical decision model for interventions with severely handicapped learners.* Baltimore: Brookes.

Evans, I. M., Meyer, L. H., Derer, K. R., & Hanashiro, R. Y. (1985). An overview of the decision model. In I. M. Evans & L. H. Meyer, *An educative approach to behavior problems: A practical decision model for interventions with severely handicapped learners* (pp. 43–61). Baltimore: Brookes.

Evans, S. W., Vallano, G., & Pelham, W. (1994). Treatment of parenting behavior with a psychostimulant: A case study of an adult with attention-deficit hyperactivity disorder. *Journal of Child and Adolescent Psychopharmacology, 4,* 63–69.

Eysenck, H. J. (Ed.). (1960). *Behavior therapy and the neuroses.* New York: Pergamon Press.

Fauber, R. L., & Kendall, P. C. (1992). Children and families: Integrating the focus of interventions. *Journal of Psychotherapy Integration, 2,* 107–123.

Fauber, R. L., & Long, N. (1991). Children in context: The role of the family in child psychotherapy. *Journal of Consulting and Clinical Psychology, 59,* 813–820.

Favell, J. E., Azrin, N. H., Baumeister, A. A., Carr, E. G., Dorsey, M. F., Forehand, R., et al. (1982). The treatment of self-injurious behavior (AABT Task Force Report, Winter, 1982). *Behavior Therapy, 13,* 529–554.

Finch, A. J., Jr., Nelson, W. M., III, & Ott, E. S. (Eds.). (1993). *Cognitive-behavioral procedures with children and adolescents: A practical guide.* Needham Heights, MA: Allyn & Bacon.

Flanagan, R. (1986). Teaching young children responses to inappropriate approaches by strangers in public places. *Child and Family Behavior Therapy, 8,* 27–43.

Flannery-Schroeder, E., Choudhury, M. S., & Kendall, P. C. (2005). Group and individual cognitive-behavioral treatments for youth with anxiety disorders: 1-year follow-up. *Cognitive Therapy and Research, 29,* 253–259.

Flannery-Schroeder, E., Suveg, C., Safford, S., Kendall, P. C., & Webb, A. (2004). Comorbid externalizing disorders and child anxiety treatment outcomes. *Behaviour Change, 21,* 14–25.

Fleischman, M. J., Horne, A. M., & Arthur, J. L. (1983). *Troubled families: A treatment program.* Champaign, IL: Research Press.

Fogel, A., & Thelen, E. (1987). Development of early expressive and communicative action: Reinterpreting the evidence from a dynamic systems perspective. *Developmental Psychology, 23,* 747–761.

Forehand, R. L., & Kotchick, B. A. (1996). Cultural diversity: A wake-up call for parent training. *Behavior Therapy, 27,* 187–206.

Forehand, R. L., & McMahon, R. J. (1981). *Helping the noncompliant child: A clinician's guide to parent training.* New York: Guilford Press.

Foster, S. L., & Robin, A. L. (1998). Parent–adolescent conflict and relationship discord. In E. J. Mash & R. A. Barkley (Eds.), *Treatment of childhood disorders* (2nd ed., pp. 647–691). New York: Guilford Press.

Furey, W. M., & Basili, L. (1988). Predicting consumer satisfaction in parent training for noncompliant children. *Behavior Therapy, 19,* 555–564.

Garber, J. (1984). Classification of child psychopathology: A developmental perspective. *Child Development, 55,* 30–48.

Garcia, J. A., & Weisz, J. R. (2002). When youth mental health care stops: Therapeutic relationship problems and other reasons for ending youth outpatient treatment. *Journal of Consulting and Clinical Psychology, 70,* 439–443.

Goldfried, M. R. (1995). *From cognitive-behavior therapy to psychotherapy integration: An evolving view.* New York: Springer.

Goldfried, M. R., & Wolfe, B. E. (1996). Psychotherapy practice and research: Repairing a strained relationship. *American Psychologist, 51,* 1007–1016.

Goodman, S. H., & Gotlib, I. H. (Eds.). (2002). *Children of depressed parents: Mechanisms of risk and implications for treatment.* Washington, DC: American Psychological Association.

Gordon, D. A., & Stanar, C. R. (2003). Lessons learned from the dissemination of parenting wisely: A parent training CD-ROM. *Cognitive and Behavioral Practice, 10,* 312–323.

Gordon, J. R., & Craver, J. N. (1988, January). *Safer sex: A self help manual.* Unpublished manual, University of Washington School of Social Work.

Gottman, J. M., & Katz, L. F. (1996). Parental meta-emotion philosophy and the emotional life of families: Theoretical models and preliminary data. *Journal of Family Psychology, 10,* 243–268.

Gottman, J. M., Katz, L. F., & Hooven, C. (1997). *Meta-emotion: How families communicate emotionally.* Mahwah, NJ: Erlbaum.

Gottman, J. M., & Levenson, R. W. (1986). Assessing the role of emotion in marriage. *Behavioral Assessment, 8,* 31–48.

Greene, R. W., & Ablon, J. S. (2005). *Treating explosive kids: The collaborative problem-solving approach.* New York: Guilford Press.

Gross, A. M., & Drabman, R. S. (Eds.). (1990). *Handbook of clinical behavioral pediatrics.* New York: Plenum Press.

Gurman, A. S., & Kniskern, D. P. (Eds.). (1991). *Handbook of family therapy* (Vol. 2). New York: Brunner/Mazel.

Hamilton, J. D. (2004). Evidence-based thinking and the alliance with parents. *Journal of the American Academy of Child and Adolescent Psychiatry, 43,* 105–108.

Hammen, C., & Rudolph, K. D. (2003). Childhood mood disorders. In E. J. Mash & R. A. Barkley (Eds.), *Child psychopathology* (2nd ed., pp. 233–278). New York: Guilford Press.

Harris, K. R., Wong, B. L., & Keogh, B. K. (Eds.). (1985). Cognitive-behavior modification with children: A critical review of the state of the art [Special issue]. *Journal of Abnormal Child Psychology, 3,* 329–476.

Harris, S. L. (1984). The family of the autistic child: A behavioral systems view. *Clinical Psychology Review, 4*, 227–239.

Harris, S. L., & Ferrari, M. (1983). Developmental factors in child behavior therapy. *Behavior Therapy, 14*, 54–72.

Harris, S. L., & Powers, M. D. (1984). Diagnostic issues. In T. H. Ollendick & M. Hersen (Eds.), *Child behavioral assessment: Principles and procedures* (pp. 38–57). New York: Pergamon Press.

Hartmann, D. P., Roper, B. L., & Bradford, D. C. (1979). Some relationships between behavioral and traditional assessment. *Journal of Behavioral Assessment, 1*, 3–21.

Harvey, P., Forehand, R., Brown, C., & Holmes, T. (1988). The prevention of sexual abuse: Examination of the effectiveness of a program with kindergarten-age children. *Behavior Therapy, 19*, 429–435.

Harwood, M. D., & Eyberg, S. M. (2004). Therapist verbal behavior early in treatment: Relation to successful completion of parent–child interaction therapy. *Journal of Clinical Child and Adolescent Psychology, 33*, 601–612.

Hawley, K. M., & Weisz, J. R. (2003). Child, parent, and therapist (dis)agreement on target problems in outpatient therapy: The therapist's dilemma and its implications. *Journal of Consulting and Clinical Psychology, 71*, 62–70.

Hawley, K. M., & Weisz, J. R. (2005). Youth versus parent working alliance in usual clinical care: Distinctive associations with retention, satisfaction, and treatment outcome. *Journal of Clinical Child and Adolescent Psychology, 34*, 117–128.

Hayes, S. C., Follette, V. M., & Linehan, M. M. (Eds.). (2004). *Mindfulness and acceptance: Expanding the cognitive-behavioral tradition.* New York: Guilford Press.

Hayes, S. C., & Follette, W. C. (1992). Can functional analysis provide a substitute for syndromal classification? *Behavioral Assessment, 14*, 345–365.

Haynes, S. N., & Heiby, E. M. (2004). *Comprehensive handbook of psychological assessment: Vol. 3. Behavioral assessment.* New York: Wiley.

Haynes, S. N., & Uchigakiuchi, P. (1993a). Functional analytic causal models and the design of treatment programs: Concepts and clinical applications with childhood behavior problems. *European Journal of Psychological Assessment, 9*, 189–205.

Haynes, S. N., & Uchigakiuchi, P. (1993b). Incorporating personality trait measures in behavioral assessment: Nuts in a fruitcake or raisins in a Mai Tai? *Behavior Modification, 17*, 72–92.

Henggeler, S. W. (1991, April). *Treating conduct problems in children and adolescents: An overview of the multisystemic approach with guidelines for intervention design and implementation.* Charleston: Division of Children, Adolescents and Their Families, South Carolina Department of Mental Health.

Henggeler, S. W., & Borduin, C. M. (1990). *Family therapy and beyond: A multisystemic approach to treating the behavior problems of children and adolescents.* Pacific Grove, CA: Brooks/Cole.

Henggeler, S. W., & Lee, T. (2003). Multisystemic treatment of serious clinical problems. In A. E. Kazdin & J. R. Weisz (Eds.), *Evidence-based therapies for children and adolescents* (pp. 301–322). New York: Guilford Press.

Henggeler, S. W., Rowland, M. D., Pickrel, S. G., Miller, S. L., Cunningham, P. B., Santos, A. B., et al. (1997). Investigating family-based alternatives to institution-based mental health services for youth: Lessons learned from the pilot study of a randomized field trial. *Journal of Clinical Child Psychology, 26*, 226–233.

Henggeler, S. W., & Schoenwald, S. K. (2002). Treatment manuals: Necessary, but far from sufficient. *Clinical Psychology: Research and Practice, 9*, 419–420.

Henggeler, S. W., Schoenwald, S. K., Borduin, C. M., Rowland, M. D., & Cunningham, P. B. (1998). *Multisystemic treatment of antisocial behavior in children and adolescents.* New York: Guilford Press.

Henggeler, S. W., Schoenwald, S. K., Pickrel, S. G., Brondino, S. J., Borduin, C. M., & Hall, J. A. (1994). *Treatment manual for family preservation using multisystemic therapy.* Charleston: South Carolina Health and Human Services Finance Commission.

Herbert, M. (1981). *Behavioural treatment of problem children: A practice manual.* London: Academic Press.

Herbert, M. (1987). *Behavioural treatment of children with problems: A practice manual* (2nd ed.). London: Academic Press.

Herbert, M. (2005). *Developmental problems of childhood and adolescence: Prevention, treatment, and training.* Malden, MA: Blackwell.

Herschell, A. D., McNeil, C. B., & McNeil, D. W. (2004). Clinical child psychology's progress in disseminating empirically supported treatments. *Clinical Psychology: Science and Practice, 11*, 267–288.

Hersen, M., & Ammerman, R. T. (Eds.). (1999). *Advanced abnormal child psychology* (2nd ed.). Hillsdale, NJ: Erlbaum.

Hersen, M., & Van Hasselt, V. B. (Eds.). (1987). *Behavior therapy with children and adolescents: A clinical approach.* New York: Wiley.

Hibbs, E. D. (2001). Evaluating empirically based psychotherapy research for children and adolescents. *European Child and Adolescent Psychiatry, 10*, 1–11.

Hibbs, E. D., & Jensen, P. S. (Eds.). (2005). *Psychosocial treatments for child and adolescent disorders: Empirically based strategies for clinical practice* (2nd ed.). Washington, DC: American Psychological Association.

Hinshaw, S. P., & Lee, S. S. (2003). Conduct and oppositional defiant disorders. In E. J. Mash & R. A. Barkley (Eds.), *Child psychopathology* (2nd ed., pp. 144–198). New York: Guilford Press.

Hoag, M. J., & Burlingame, G. M. (1997). Evaluating

the effectiveness of child and adolescent group treatment: A meta-analytic review. *Journal of Clinical Child Psychology, 26*, 234–246.

Hoagwood, K. (2002). Making the translation from research to its application. The *je ne sais pas* of evidence-based practices. *Clinical Psychology: Science and Practice, 9*, 210–213.

Hoagwood, K., Hibbs, E., Brent, D., & Jensen, P. (1995). Introduction to the special section: Efficacy and effectiveness in studies of child and adolescent psychotherapy. *Journal of Consulting and Clinical Psychology, 63*, 683–687.

Holden, G. W. (1985). Analyzing parental reasoning with microcomputer-presented problems. *Simulation and Games, 16*, 203–210.

Hollandsworth, J. G., Jr. (1986). *Physiology and behavior therapy.* New York: Plenum Press.

Holmbeck, G. N., Greenley, R. N., & Franks, E. A. (2003). Developmental issues and considerations in research and practice. In A. E. Kazdin & J. R. Weisz (Eds.), *Evidence-based psychotherapies for children and adolescents* (pp. 21–40). New York: Guilford Press.

Holmbeck, G. N., Greenley, R. N., & Franks, E. A. (2004). Developmental issues in evidence based practice. In P. M. Barrett & T. H. Ollendick (Eds.), *Interventions that work with children and adolescents: Prevention and treatment* (pp. 27–48). New York: Wiley.

Holmes, F. B. (1936). An experimental investigation of a method of overcoming children's fears. *Child Development, 7*, 6–30.

Houts, A. C., Shutty, M. S., & Emery, R. E. (1985). The impact of children on adults. In B. B. Lahey & A. E. Kazdin (Eds.), *Advances in clinical child psychology* (Vol. 8, pp. 267–307). New York: Plenum Press.

Houts, A. C., Whelan, J. P., & Peterson, K. (1987). Filmed versus live delivery of full-spectrum home training for primary enuresis: Presenting the information is not enough. *Journal of Consulting and Clinical Psychology, 55*, 902–906.

Howard, B., & Kendall, P. C. (1996). *Cognitive-behavioral family therapy for anxious children: Therapist manual.* Ardmore, PA: Workbook.

Hoza, B., Pelham, W. E., Jr., Dobbs, J., Owens, J. S., & Pillow, D. R. (2002). Do boys with attention-deficit/hyperactivity disorder have positive illusory self-concepts? *Journal of Abnormal Psychology, 111*, 268–278.

Hudson, J. L. (2005). Mechanisms of change in cognitive behavioral therapy for anxious youth. *Clinical Psychology: Science and Practice, 12*, 161–165.

Insel, T. R., & Fenton, W. S. (2005). Psychiatric Epidemiology: It's not just about counting anymore. *Archives of General Psychiatry, 62*, 590–592.

Iwamasa, G. Y. (1996). Introduction to the special series: Ethnic and cultural diversity in cognitive and behavioral practice. *Cognitive and Behavioral Practice, 3*, 209–213.

Izard, C. E., Fine, S., Mostow, A., Trentacosta, C., &

Campbell, J. (2002). Emotional processes in normal and abnormal development and preventive intervention. *Development and Psychopathology, 14*, 761–787.

Jablensky, A., & Kendell, R. E. (2002). Criteria for assessing a classification in psychiatry. In M. Maj & W. Gaebel (Eds.), *Psychiatric diagnosis and classification* (pp. 1–24). New York: Wiley.

Jackson, Y. (2002). Exploring empirically supported treatment options for children: Making the case for the next generation of cultural research. *Clinical Psychology: Research and Practice, 9*, 220–222.

Jacobson, N. S., & Christensen, A. (1996). *Integrative couple therapy: Promoting acceptance and change.* New York: Norton.

Jason, L. A. (1980). Prevention in the schools. In R. H. Price, R. F. Ketterer, B. C. Bader, & J. Morahan (Eds.), *Prevention in mental health: Research, policies, and practices* (pp. 109–134). Beverly Hills, CA: Sage.

Jason, L. A., Felner, R. D., Hess, R., & Moritsugo, J. N. (1987). *Prevention: Toward a multidisciplinary approach.* New York: Haworth Press.

Jensen, P. S. (2003). Comorbidity and child psychopathology: Recommendations for the next decade. *Journal of Abnormal Child Psychology, 31*, 293–300.

Johnson, J. H., Rasbury, W. C., & Siegel, L. J. (1997). *Approaches to child treatment: Introduction to theory, research, and practice* (2nd ed.). Needham Heights, MA: Allyn & Bacon.

Johnson, S. B., & Rodrigue, J. R. (1997). Health-related disorders. In E. J. Mash & L. G. Terdal (Eds.), *Assessment of childhood disorders* (3rd ed., pp. 481–519). New York: Guilford Press.

Jones, M. C. (1924). A laboratory study of fear: The case of Peter. *Journal of Genetic Psychology, 31*, 308–315.

Jones, R. T., Sisson, L. A., & Van Hasselt, V. B. (1984). Emergency fire-safety skills for blind children and adolescents: Group training and generalization. *Behavior Modification, 8*, 267–286.

Kalichman, S. C. (1997). HIV prevention for youth. *Child, Youth, and Family Services Quarterly, 20*(1), 1–3.

Kandel, E., Mednick. S. A., Kirkegaard-Sorensen, L., Hutchings, B., Knop, J. Rosenberg, R., et al. (1988). IQ as a protective factor for subjects at high risk for antisocial behavior. *Journal of Consulting and Clinical Psychology, 56*, 224–226.

Kanfer, F. H. (1985). Target selection for clinical change programs. *Behavioral Assessment, 7*, 7–20.

Kanfer, F. H., & Busemeyer, J. R. (1982). The use of problem-solving and decision-making in behavior therapy. *Clinical Psychology Review, 2*, 239–266.

Kanfer, F. H., & Phillips, J. S. (1970). *Learning foundations of behavior therapy.* New York: Wiley.

Kanfer, F. H., & Saslow, G. (1965). Behavioral analysis: An alternative to diagnostic classification. *Archives of General Psychiatry, 12*, 529–538.

Kanfer, F. H., & Saslow, G. (1969). Behavioral diagnosis. In C. M. Franks (Ed.), *Behavior therapy:*

Appraisal and status (pp. 417–444). New York: McGraw-Hill.

Kanfer, F. H., & Schefft, B. K. (1988). *Guiding the process of therapeutic change.* Champaign, IL: Research Press.

Karoly, P. (1981). Self-management problems in children. In E. J. Mash & L. G. Terdal (Eds.), *Behavioral assessment of childhood disorders* (pp. 79–126). New York: Guilford Press.

Kaslow, F., & Lebow, J. L. (Eds.). (2002). *Comprehensive handbook of psychotherapy: Vol. 4. Integrative/eclectic* (pp. 111–132). New York: Wiley.

Katoaka, S. H., Zhang, L., & Wells, K. B. (2002). Unmet need for mental health care among U.S. children: Variation by ethnicity and insurance status. *American Journal of Psychiatry, 159,* 1548–1555.

Kavanagh, K., & Hops, H. (1994). Good girls? Bad boys?: Gender and development as contexts for diagnosis and treatment. In T. H. Ollendick & R. J. Prinz (Eds.), *Advances in clinical child psychology* (Vol. 16, pp. 45–79). New York: Plenum Press.

Kazdin, A. E. (1978). *History of behavior modification.* Baltimore: University Park Press.

Kazdin, A. E. (1981). Acceptability of child treatment techniques: The influence of treatment efficacy and adverse side effects. *Behavior Therapy, 12,* 493–506.

Kazdin, A. E. (1982a). *Single-case research designs: Methods for clinical and applied settings.* New York: Oxford University Press.

Kazdin, A. E. (1982b). Symptom substitution, generalization, and response covariation: Implications for psychotherapy outcome. *Psychological Bulletin, 91,* 349–365.

Kazdin, A. E. (1984). Acceptability of aversive procedures and medication as treatment alternatives for deviant child behavior. *Journal of Abnormal Child Psychology, 12,* 289–302.

Kazdin, A. E. (1988a). Behavior therapy and the treatment of clinical dysfunction. *Contemporary Psychology, 33,* 686–687.

Kazdin, A. E. (1988b). *Child psychotherapy: Developing and identifying effective treatments.* New York: Pergamon Press.

Kazdin, A. E. (1996a). Combined and multimodal treatments in child and adolescent psychotherapy: Issues, challenges, and research directions. *Clinical Psychology: Science and Practice, 3,* 69–100.

Kazdin, A. E. (1996b). Developing effective treatments for children and adolescents. In E. D. Hibbs & P. S. Jensen (Eds.), *Psychosocial treatments for child and adolescent disorders: Empirically-based strategies for clinical practice* (pp. 9–18). Washington, DC: American Psychological Association.

Kazdin, A. E. (1996c). Dropping out of child psychotherapy: Issues for research and practice. *Clinical Child Psychology and Psychiatry, 1,* 133–156.

Kazdin, A. E. (1997). A model for developing effective treatments: Progression and interplay of theory, research, and practice. *Journal of Clinical Child Psychology, 26,* 114–129.

Kazdin, A. E. (2000). *Psychotherapy for children and adolescents: Directions for research and practice.* New York: Oxford University Press.

Kazdin, A. E. (2001). Almost clinically significant (*p* < .10): Current measures may only approach clinical significance. *Clinical Psychology: Science and Practice, 8,* 455–462.

Kazdin, A. E. (2003a). Psychotherapy for children and adolescents. *Annual Review of Psychology, 54,* 253–276.

Kazdin, A. E. (2003b). Psychotherapy for children and adolescents. In M. J. Lambert (Ed.), *Bergin and Garfield's handbook of psychotherapy and behavior change* (5th ed., pp. 543–589). New York: Wiley.

Kazdin, A. E. (2004). Evidence-based treatments: Challenges and priorities for practice and research. *Child and Adolescent Psychiatric Clinics of North America, 13,* 923–941.

Kazdin, A. E. (2005). Treatment outcomes, common factors, and continued neglect of mechanisms of change. *Clinical Psychology: Science and Practice, 12,* 184–188.

Kazdin, A. E., Bass, D., Ayers, W. A., & Rodgers, A. (1990). Empirical and clinical focus of child and adolescent psychotherapy research. *Journal of Consulting and Clinical Psychology, 62,* 100–110.

Kazdin, A. E., Esveldt-Dawson, K., French, N. H., & Unis, A. S. (1987). Problem-solving skills training and relationship therapy in the treatment of antisocial child behavior. *Journal of Consulting and Clinical Psychology, 55,* 76–85.

Kazdin, A. E., & Kagan, J. (1994). Models of dysfunction in developmental psychopathology. *Clinical Psychology: Science and Practice, 1,* 35–52.

Kazdin, A. E., & Nock, M. K. (2003). Delineating mechanisms of change in child and adolescent therapy: Methodological issues and research recommendations. *Journal of Child Psychology and Psychiatry, 44,* 1116–1129.

Kazdin, A. E., & Weisz, J. R. (Eds.). (2003). *Evidence-based psychotherapies for children and adolescents.* New York: Guilford Press.

Kendall, P. C. (1982). Integration: Behavior therapy and other schools of thought. *Behavior Therapy, 13,* 550–571.

Kendall, P. C. (1987). Ahead to basics: Assessments with children and families. *Behavioral Assessment, 9,* 321–332.

Kendall, P. C. (Ed.). (2005). *Child and adolescent therapy: Cognitive-behavioral procedures* (3rd ed.). New York: Guilford Press.

Kendall, P. C., Brady, E. U., & Verduin, T. L. (2001). Comorbidity in childhood anxiety disorders and treatment outcome. *Journal of the American Academy of Child and Adolescent Psychiatry, 40,* 787–794.

Kendall, P. C., & Braswell, L. (1985). *Cognitive-behavioral therapy for impulsive children.* New York: Guilford Press.

Kendall, P. C., & Flannery-Schroeder, E. C. (1998).

Methodological issues in treatment research for anxiety disorders in youth. *Journal of Abnormal Child Psychology, 26,* 27–38.

Kendall, P. C., Hudson, J. L., Choudhury, M., Webb, A., & Pimentel, S. (2005). Cognitive-behavioral treatment for childhood anxiety disorders. In E. D. Hibbs & P. S. Jensen (Eds.), *Psychosocial treatments for child and adolescent disorders: Empirically based strategies for clinical practice* (2nd ed., pp. 47–73). Washington, DC: American Psychological Association.

Kendall, P. C., Kane, M., Howard, B., & Siqueland, L. (1992). *Cognitive-behavioral therapy for anxious children.* Ardmore, PA: Workbook.

Kendall, P. C., & Koehler, C. (1985). Outcome evaluation in child behavior therapy: Methodological and conceptual issues. In P. H. Bornstein & A. E. Kazdin (Eds.), *Handbook of clinical behavior therapy with children* (pp. 75–122). Homewood, IL: Dorsey Press.

Kendall, P. C., Lerner, R. M., & Craighead, W. E. (1984). Human development and intervention in child psychopathology. *Child Development, 55,* 71–82.

Kendall, P. C., Safford, S., Flannery-Schroeder, E., & Webb, A. (2004). Child anxiety treatment: Outcomes in adolescence and impact on substance use and depression at 7.4 year follow-up. *Journal of Consulting and Clinical Psychology, 72,* 276–287.

Kessler, R. C., Berglund, P., Demler, O., Jin, R., & Walters, M. S. (2005). Lifetime prevalence and age-of-onset distributions of DSM-IV disorders in the National Comorbidity Survey replication. *Archives of General Psychiatry, 62,* 593–602.

King, N. J., Muris, P., & Ollendick, T. H. (2005). Childhood fears and phobias: Assessment and treatment. *Child and Adolescent Mental Health, 10,* 50–56.

Kline, R. B., Canter, W. A., & Robin, A. (1987). Parameters of teenage alcohol use: A path analytic conceptual model. *Journal of Consulting and Clinical Psychology, 55,* 521–528.

Knitzer, J. (1982). *Unclaimed children: The failure of public responsibility to children and adolescents in need of mental health services.* Washington, DC: Children's Defense Fund.

Knox, L. S., Albano, A. M., & Barlow, D. H. (1993). *Treatment of OCD in children: Exposure and response prevention.* Unpublished manuscript, Anxiety Disorders Clinic, University of Louisville.

Koetting, K., Peterson, L., & Saldana, L. (1997). Survey of pediatric hospitals' preparation programs: Evidence of the impact of health psychology research. *Health Psychology, 16,* 147–154.

Koocher, G. P., & Pedulla, B. M. (1977). Current practices in child psychotherapy. *Professional Psychology: Research and Practice, 8,* 275–287.

Kratochwill, T. R., Albers, C. A., & Shernoff, E. S. (2004). School-based interventions. *Child and Adolescent Psychiatric Clinics of North America, 13,* 885–904.

Kratochwill, T. R., & Morris, R. J. (Eds.). (1993).

Handbook of psychotherapy with children and adolescents. Needham Heights, MA: Allyn & Bacon.

Lahey, B. B., Applegate, B., Waldman, I. D., Loft, J. D., Hankin, B. L., & Rick, J. (2004). The structure of child and adolescent psychopathology: Generating new hypotheses. *Psychological Bulletin, 113,* 358–385.

Lambert, M. E. (1987). A computer simulation for behavior therapy training. *Journal of Behavior Therapy and Experimental Psychiatry, 18,* 245–248.

Lasure, L. C., & Mikulas, W. L. (1996). Biblical behavior modification. *Behaviour Research and Therapy, 34,* 563–566.

Lazarus, A. A. (1958). New methods in psychotherapy: A case study. *South African Medical Journal, 32,* 660–664.

Lazarus, A. A., & Abramovitz, A. (1962). The use of "emotive imagery" in the treatment of children's phobias. *Journal of Mental Science, 108,* 191–195.

LeBow, J. (1982). Consumer satisfaction with mental health treatment. *Psychological Bulletin, 91,* 244–259.

Lee, C. M., & Mash, E. J. (1990). Behaviour therapy. In B. Tonge, G. D. Burrows, & J. Werry (Eds.), *Handbook of studies on child psychiatry* (pp. 415–430). Amsterdam: Elsevier.

Lerner, J. V., Hertzog, C., Hooker, K. A., Hassibi, M., & Thomas, A. (1988). A longitudinal study of negative emotional states and adjustment from early childhood through adolescence. *Child Development, 59,* 356–366.

Levis, D. J. (1988). Integration of behavioral theory and practice. *The Behavior Therapist, 11,* 75.

Lewinsohn, P. M., Clarke, G. N., Hops, H., & Andrews, J. (1990). Cognitive-behavioral group treatment of depression in adolescents. *Behavior Therapy, 21,* 385–401.

Lewis, M., & Miller, S. M. (Eds.). (1990). *Handbook of developmental psychopathology: Perspectives in developmental psychology* (pp. 475–485). New York: Plenum Press.

Littell, J. H., & Girvin, H. (2005). Caregivers' readiness for change: Predictive validity in a child welfare sample. *Child Abuse and Neglect, 29,* 59–80.

Lochman, J. E. (1987). Self- and peer perceptions and attributional biases of aggressive and nonaggressive boys in dyadic interactions. *Journal of Consulting and Clinical Psychology, 55,* 404–410.

Lochman, J. E. (1988). *Effectiveness of a cognitive-behavioral intervention with aggressive boys.* Unpublished manuscript, Duke University Medical Center.

Lochman, J. E., & Lampron, L. B. (1986). Situational social problem-solving skills and self esteem of aggressive and nonaggressive boys. *Journal of Abnormal Child Psychology, 14,* 605–617.

Lochman, J. E., & Wells, K. C. (1996). A social-cognitive intervention with aggressive children: Prevention effects and contextual implementation issues. In R. DeV. Peters & R. J. McMahon (Eds.), *Preventing childhood disorders, substance abuse, and delinquency* (pp. 111–143). Thousand Oaks, CA: Sage.

Lochman, J. E., & Wells, K. C. (2004). The Coping Power Program for preadolescent boys and their parents: Outcome effects at the 1-year follow up. *Journal of Consulting and Clinical Psychology, 72,* 571–578.

London, P. (1972). The end of ideology in behavior modification. *American Psychologist, 27,* 913–920.

Lonigan, C. J., Elbert, J. C., & Bennett-Johnson, S. (1998). Empirically supported psychosocial interventions for children: An overview. *Journal of Clinical Child Psychology, 27,* 138–145.

Lovaas, O. I. (1987). Behavioral treatment and normal educational and intellectual functioning in young autistic children. *Journal of Consulting and Clinical Psychology, 55,* 3–9.

Lovaas, O. I. (2002). *Teaching individuals with developmental delays : Basic intervention techniques.* Austin, TX: PRO-ED.

Lovaas, O. I., Freitag, G., Gold, V. J., & Kasorla, I. C. (1965). Experimental studies in childhood schizophrenia: Analysis of self-destructive behavior. *Journal of Experimental Child Psychology, 2,* 67–84.

Lovaas, O.I., Koegel, R., Simmons. J. Q., & Long, J. S. (1973). Some generalization and follow-up measures on autistic children in behavior therapy. *Journal of Applied Behavior Analysis, 6,* 131–166.

Lynam, D. R. (1996). Early identification of chronic offenders: Who is the fledgling psychopath? *Psychological Bulletin, 120,* 209–234.

Lynam, D. R. (1997). Pursuing the psychopath: Capturing the fledgling psychopath in a nomological net. *Journal of Abnormal Psychology, 106,* 425–438.

Lynam, D. R., Moffitt, T. E., & Stouthamer-Loeber, M. (1993). Explaining the relation between IQ and delinquency: Race, class, test motivation, school failure, or self-control. *Journal of Abnormal Psychology, 102,* 187–196.

Lyon, R., Fletcher, J., & Barnes, M. C. (2003). Learning disabilities. In E. J. Mash & R. A. Barkley (Eds.), *Child psychopathology* (2nd ed., pp. 390–435). Guilford Press.

Lyons-Ruth, K., Zeanah, C. H., & Benoit, D. (2003). Disorder and risk for disorder during infancy and toddlerhood. In E. J. Mash & R. A. Barkley (Eds.), *Child psychopathology* (2nd ed., pp. 589–631). New York: Guilford Press.

MacDonald, L. (1986). Ethical standards for therapeutic programs in human services: An evaluation model. *The Behavior Therapist, 9,* 213–215.

Mahoney, M. J., & Nezworski, M. T. (1985). Cognitive-behavioral approaches to children's problems. *Journal of Abnormal Child Psychology, 13,* 467–476.

Malekoff, A. (2004). *Group work with adolescents: Principles and practice* (2nd ed.). New York: Guilford Press.

Malenfant, L., Wells, J. K., Van Houten, R., & Williams, A. F. (1996). The use of feedback signs to increase observed daytime seat belt use in two cities in North Carolina. *Accident Analysis and Prevention, 28,* 771–777.

March, J. S., Franklin, M., & Foa, E. (2005). Cognitive-behavioral psychotherapy for pediatric obsessive-compulsive disorder. In E. D. Hibbs & P. S. Jensen (Eds.), *Psychosocial treatments for child and adolescent disorders: Empirically based strategies for clinical practice* (2nd ed., pp. 121–142). Washington, DC: American Psychological Association.

March, J. S., & Mulle, K. (1998). *OCD in children and adolescents: A cognitive-behavioral treatment manual.* New York: Guilford Press.

Markman, H. J., Floyd, F. J., Stanley, S. M., & Storaasli, R. D. (1988). Prevention of marital distress: A longitudinal investigation. *Journal of Consulting and Clinical Psychology, 56,* 210–217.

Mash, E. J. (1984). Families with problem children. In A. Doyle, D. Gold, & D. Moskowitz (Eds.), *Children in families under stress* (pp. 65–84). San Francisco: Jossey-Bass.

Mash, E. J. (1998). Treatment of child and family disturbance: A behavioral–systems perspective. In E. J. Mash & R. A. Barkley (Eds.), *Treatment of childhood disorders* (2nd ed., pp. 3–51). New York: Guilford Press.

Mash, E. J., & Barkley, R. A. (Eds.). (1998). *Treatment of childhood disorders* (2nd ed.). New York: Guilford Press.

Mash, E. J., & Barkley, R. A. (Eds.). (2003). *Child psychopathology* (2nd ed.). New York: Guilford Press.

Mash, E. J., & Dozois, D. J. A. (2003). Child psychopathology: A developmental–systems perspective. In E. J. Mash & R. A. Barkley (Eds.), *Child psychopathology* (2nd ed., pp. 3–71). New York: Guilford Press.

Mash, E. J., & Hunsley, J. (1990). Behavioral assessment: A contemporary approach. In A. S. Bellack, M. Hersen, & A. E. Kazdin (Eds.), *International handbook of behavior modification and therapy* (2nd ed., pp. 87–106). New York: Plenum Press.

Mash, E. J., & Hunsley, J. (1993). Behavior therapy and managed mental health care: Integrating effectiveness and economics in managed mental health care. *Behavior Therapy, 24,* 67–90.

Mash, E. J., & Hunsley, J. (2004). Behavioral assessment: Sometimes you get what you need. In M. Hersen, S. Haynes, & E. Heiby (Eds.), *The comprehensive handbook of psychological assessment: Vol. 3. Behavioral assessment* (pp. 489–501). New York: Wiley.

Mash, E. J., & Hunsley, J. (2005). Evidence-based assessment of child and adolescent disorders: Issues and challenges. *Journal of Clinical Child and Adolescent Psychology, 34,* 362–379.

Mash, E. J., & Johnston, C. (1996). Family relational problems: Their place in the study of psychopathology. *Journal of Emotional and Behavioral Disorders, 4,* 240–254.

Mash, E. J., & Terdal, L. G. (1980). Follow-up assessments in behavior therapy. In P. Karoly & J. J. Steffan (Eds.), *The long-range effects of psychotherapy:*

Models of durable outcome (pp. 99–147). New York: Gardner Press.

Mash, E. J., & Terdal, L. G. (Eds.). (1997a). *Assessment of childhood disorders* (3rd ed.). New York: Guilford Press.

Mash, E. J., & Terdal, L. G. (1997b). Assessment of child and family disturbance: A behavioral systems approach. In E. J. Mash & L. G. Terdal (Eds.), *Assessment of childhood disorders* (3rd ed., pp. 3–68). New York: Guilford Press.

Mash, E. J., & Wolfe, D. A. (2005). *Abnormal child psychology* (3rd ed.). Belmont, CA: Wadsworth/Thomson.

McEachin, J. J., Smith, T., & Lovaas, I. O. (1993). Long-term outcome for children with autism who received early intensive behavioral treatment. *American Journal on Mental Retardation, 97,* 359–372.

McLeod, B. D., & Weisz, J. R. (2004). Using dissertations to examine potential bias in child and adolescent clinical trials. *Journal of Consulting and Clinical Psychology, 72,* 235–251.

McLeod, B. D., & Weisz, J. R. (2005). The Therapy Process Observational Coding System—Alliance Scale: Measure characteristics and prediction of outcome in usual clinical practice. *Journal of Consulting and Clinical Psychology, 73,* 323–333.

McMahon, R. J., & Forehand, R. L. (1983). Consumer satisfaction in behavioral treatment of children: Types, issues, and recommendations. *Behavior Therapy, 14,* 209–225.

McMahon, R. J., & Forehand, R. L. (2003). *Helping the noncompliant child: Family-based treatment for oppositional behavior* (2nd ed.). New York: Guilford Press.

McMahon, R. J., & Peters, R. D. (Eds.). (1985). *Childhood disorders: Behavioral–developmental approaches.* New York: Brunner/Mazel.

Meichenbaum, D. (1977). *Cognitive behavior modification.* New York: Plenum Press.

Meyers, A. W., & Cohen, R. (1990). Cognitive-behavioral approaches to child psychopathology: Present status and future directions. In M. Lewis & S. M. Miller (Eds.), *Handbook of developmental psychopathology: Perspectives in developmental psychology* (pp. 475–485). New York: Plenum Press.

Milich, R., & Dodge, K. A. (1984). Social information processing in child psychiatric populations. *Journal of Abnormal Child Psychology, 13,* 471–490.

Miller, G. E., & Prinz, R. J. (1990). Enhancement of social learning family interventions for childhood conduct disorder. *Psychological Bulletin, 108,* 291–307.

Miller, S. A. (1988). Parents' beliefs about children's cognitive development. *Child Development, 59,* 259–285.

Mischel, W. (1968). *Personality and assessment.* New York: Wiley.

Moran, P., & Eckenrode, J. (1988). *Social stress and depression during adolescence: Gender and age differences.* Unpublished manuscript, Department of Human Development and Family Studies, Cornell University.

Mori, L., & Peterson, L. (1986). Training preschoolers in home safety skills to prevent inadvertent injury. *Journal of Clinical Child Psychology, 15,* 106–114.

Morrow-Bradley, C., & Elliot, R. (1986). Utilization of psychotherapy research by practicing psychotherapists. *American Psychologist, 41,* 188–197.

Mowrer, O. H., & Mowrer, W. M. (1938). Enuresis: A method for its study and treatment. *American Journal of Orthopsychiatry, 8,* 436–459.

MTA Cooperative Group. (2004). National Institute of Mental Health Multimodal Treatment Study of ADHD follow-up: 24–month outcomes of treatment strategies for attention-deficit/hyperactivity disorder (ADHD). *Pediatrics, 113,* 754–761.

Mufson, L., Dorta, K. P., Moreau, D., & Weissman, M. M. (2004). *Interpersonal psychotherapy for depressed adolescents* (2nd ed.). New York: Guilford Press.

Mullins, L. L., Hartman, V. L., Chaney, J. M., Balderson, B. H. K., & Hoff, A. L. (2003). Training experiences and theoretical orientations of pediatric psychologists. *Journal of Pediatric Psychology, 28,* 115–122.

Mussen, P. H. (Series Ed.). (1983). *Handbook of child psychology* (4th ed., 4 vols.). New York: Wiley.

Neal-Barnett, A. M., & Smith, J. M., Sr. (1996). African American children and behavior therapy: Considering the Afrocentric approach. *Cognitive and Behavioral Practice, 3,* 351–369.

Nelson, R. O., & Hayes, S. C. (Eds.). (1986). *Conceptual foundations of behavioral assessment.* New York: Guilford Press.

Nezu, A. M., & Nezu, C. M. (1989). *Clinical decision making in behavior therapy: A problem-solving perspective.* Champaign, IL: Research Press.

Nezu, A. M., & Nezu, C. M. (1993). Identifying and selecting target problems for clinical interventions: A problem-solving model. *Psychological Assessment, 5,* 254–263.

Nezu, A. M., Nezu, C. M., & Lombardo, E. (2004). *Cognitive-behavioral case formulation to treatment design: A problem-solving approach.* New York: Springer.

Niec, L. N., Hemme, J. M., Yopp, J. M., & Brestan, E. V. (2005). Parent child interaction therapy: The rewards and challenges of a group format. *Cognitive and Behavioral Practice, 12,* 113–125.

Noam, G. G., Chandler, M., & LaLonde, C. (1995). Clinical–developmental psychology: Constructivism and social cognition in the study of psychological dysfunctions. In D. Cicchetti & D. J. Cohen (Eds.), *Developmental psychopathology: Vol. 1. Theory and methods* (pp. 424–464). New York: Wiley.

Nock, M. K. (2003). Progress review of the psychosocial treatment of child conduct problems. *Clinical Psychology: Science and Practice, 10,* 1–28.

Nolen-Hoeksema, S., Girgus, J. S., & Seligman, M. E. P. (1988, March). *A longitudinal study of depression in pre-adolescents: Sex differences in depression and related factors.* Paper presented at the meeting of the Society for Research on Adolescence, Alexandria, VA.

Norcross, J. C., & Goldfried, M. R. (Eds.). (1992). *Handbook of psychotherapy integration.* New York: Basic Books.

Norcross, J. C., Karg, R. S., & Prochaska, J. O. (1997). Clinical psychologists in the 1990s: II. *The Clinical Psychologist, 50*(3), 4–11.

Offord, D. R., Boyle, M. C., & Racine, Y. A. (1991). The epidemiology of antisocial behavior in childhood and adolescence. In D. J. Pepler & K. H. Rubin (Eds.), *The development and treatment of childhood aggression* (pp. 31–54). Hillsdale, NJ: Erlbaum.

Ogles, B. M., Lambert, M. J., & Masters, K. S. (1996). *Assessing outcome in clinical practice.* Needham Heights, MA: Allyn & Bacon.

O'Leary, K. D. (1984). Marital discord and children: Problems, strategies, methodologies and results. In A. Doyle, D. Gold, & D. S. Moskowitz (Eds.), *Children in families under stress* (pp. 35–36). San Francisco: Jossey-Bass.

O'Leary, K. D., Becker, W. C., Evans, M. B., & Saudargas, R. A. (1969). A token reinforcement program in a public school: A replication and systematic analysis. *Journal of Applied Behavior Analysis, 2,* 3–13.

O'Leary, K. D., & Wilson, G. T. (1987). *Behavior therapy: Application and outcome* (2nd ed.). Englewood Cliffs, NJ: Prentice-Hall.

Ollendick, T. H. (1986). Behavior therapy with children and adolescents. In S L. Garfield & A. E. Bergin (Eds.), *Handbook of psychotherapy and behavior change* (3rd ed., pp. 565–624). New York: Wiley.

Ollendick, T. H. (Ed.). (2004). *Phobic and anxiety disorders in children and adolescents: A clinician's guide to effective psychosocial and pharmacological interventions.* London: Oxford University Press.

Ollendick, T. H., & Cerny, J. A. (1981). *Clinical behavior therapy with children.* New York: Plenum Press.

Ollendick, T. H., & King, N. J. (2004). Empirically supported treatments for children and adolescents: Advances toward evidence-based practice. In P. M. Barrett & T. H. Ollendick (Eds.), *Handbook of interventions that work with children and adolescents: Prevention and treatment* (pp. 3–25). New York: Wiley.

Pappadopulos, E. A., Guelzow, B. T., Wong, C., Ortega, M., & Jensen, P. S. (2004). A review of the growing evidence base for pediatric psychopharmacology. *Child and Adolescent Psychiatric Clinics of North America, 13,* 817–856.

Patterson, G. R. (1976). The aggressive child: Victim and architect of a coercive system. In E. J. Mash, L. A. Hamerlynck, & L. C. Handy (Eds.), *Behavior modification and families* (pp. 267–316). New York: Brunner/Mazel.

Patterson, G. R. (1982). *Coercive family process.* Eugene, OR: Castalia.

Patterson, G. R. (1986). Performance models for antisocial boys. *American Psychologist, 41,* 432–444.

Patterson, G. R. (1996). Some characteristics of a developmental theory for early-onset delinquency. In M. F. Lenzenweger & J. J. Haugaard (Eds.), *Frontiers of developmental psychopathology* (pp. 81–124). New York: Oxford University Press.

Patterson, G. R. (2005). The next generation of PMTO models. *The Behavior Therapist, 28 (2),* 27–33.

Patterson, G. R., Ray, R. S., & Shaw, D. A. (Eds.). (1968). Direct intervention in families of deviant children [Special issue]. *Oregon Research Institute Research Bulletin, 8.*

Patterson, G. R., Reid, J. B., & Dishion, T. J. (1992). *Antisocial boys.* Eugene, OR: Castalia.

Patterson, G. R., Reid, J. B., Jones, R. R., & Conger, R. E. (1975). *A social learning approach to family intervention: Families with aggressive children* (Vol. 1). Eugene, OR: Castalia.

Peters, R. DeV., & McMahon, R. J. (Eds.). (1996). *Preventing childhood disorders, substance abuse, and delinquency.* Thousand Oaks, CA: Sage.

Peterson, L., & Brown, D. (1994). Integrating child injury and abuse–neglect research: Common histories, etiologies, and solutions. *Psychological Bulletin, 116,* 293–315.

Peterson, L., Burbach, D. J., & Chaney. J. (1989). Developmental issues. In C. G. Last & M. Hersen (Eds.), *Handbook of child psychiatric diagnosis* (pp. 463–482). New York: Wiley.

Peterson, L., & Mori, L. (1985). Prevention of child injury: An overview of targets, methods, and tactics for psychologists. *Journal of Consulting and Clinical Psychology, 53,* 58–595.

Peterson, L., Reach, K., & Grabe, S. (2003). Health-related disorders. In E. J. Mash & R. A. Barkley (Eds.), *Child psychopathology* (2nd ed., pp. 716–749). New York: Guilford Press.

Peterson, L., Zink, M., & Downing, J. (1993). Childhood injury prevention. In D. S. Glenwick & L. A. Jason (Eds.), *Promoting health and mental health in children, youth, and families* (pp. 51–73). New York: Springer.

Pettit, G. S., Dodge, K. A., & Brown, M. M. (1988). Early family experience, social problem solving patterns, and children's social competence. *Child Development, 59,* 107–120.

Piacentini, J., & Graae, F. (1997). Childhood OCD. In E. Hollander & D. Stein (Eds.), *Obsessive-compulsive disorders: Diagnosis, etiology, treatment* (pp. 23–46). New York: Marcel Dekker.

Pinker, S. (2002). *The blank slate: The modern denial of human nature.* Philadelphia: Viking.

Plomin, R. (1995). Genetics and children's experiences in the family. *Journal of Child Psychology and Psychiatry, 36,* 33–68.

President's New Freedom Commission on Mental Health. (2003). *Achieving the promise: Transforming mental health care in America.* Retrieved from www.mentalhealthcommission.gov

Prochaska, J. O. (1994). Strong and weak principles for progressing from precontemplation to action on the basis of twelve problem behaviors. *Health Psychology, 13,* 47–51.

Putallaz, M. (1987). Maternal behavior and children's sociometric status. *Child Development, 58,* 324–340.

Reynolds, C. R., & Kamphaus, R. W. (2004). *BASC-2: Behavior Assessment System for Children, Second Edition*. Circle Pines, MN: American Guidance Service.

Rickel, A. U., & Allen, L. (1987). *Preventing maladjustment from infancy through adolescence*. Newbury Park, CA: Sage.

Ridley, M. (2002). *Nature via nurture*. New York: HarperCollins.

Ringel, J. S., & Sturm, R. (2001). National estimates of mental health utilization and expenditures for children in 1998. *Journal of Behavioral Health Services and Research, 28*, 319–333.

Ritterband, L. M., Cox, D. J., Walker, L., Kovatchev, B., McKnight, L., Patel, K., et al. (2003). An Internet intervention as adjunctive therapy for pediatric encopresis. *Journal of Consulting and Clinical Psychology, 71*, 910–917.

Ritterband, L. M., Gonder-Frederick, L. A., Cox, D. J., Clifton, A. D., West, R. W., & Borowitz, S. M. (2003). Internet interventions: In review, in use, and into the future. *Professional Psychology: Research and Practice, 34*, 527–534.

Roberts, M. C. (Ed.). (2003). *Handbook of pediatric psychology* (3rd ed.). New York: Guilford Press.

Roberts, M. C., & Hurley, L. K. (1997). *Managing managed care*. New York: Plenum Press.

Roberts, M. C., & Peterson, L. (Eds.). (1984). *Prevention of problems in childhood: Psychological research and applications*. New York: Wiley.

Roberts, R., Attkisson, C., & Rosenblatt, A. (1998). Prevalence of psychopathology among children and adolescents. *American Journal of Psychiatry, 155*, 715–725.

Robin, A. L., & Foster, S. L. (1989). *Negotiating parent–adolescent conflict: A behavioral–family systems approach*. New York: Guilford Press.

Robins, C. J., & Hinkley, K. (1989). Social-cognitive processing and depressive symptoms in children: A comparison of measures. *Journal of Abnormal Child Psychology, 17*, 29–36.

Romancyzk, R. G. (1986). *Clinical utilization of microcomputer technology*. New York: Pergamon Press.

Ross, A. (1981). *Child behavior therapy: Principles, procedures and empirical basis*. New York: Wiley.

Rothbaum, B. O. (2004). Technology and manual-based therapies. *Clinical Psychology: Science and Practice, 11*, 339–341.

Rubenstein, J. L., Heeren, T., Houssman, D., Rubin, C., & Stechler, G. (1988, March). *Suicidal behavior in "normal" adolescents: Risk and protective factors*. Paper presented at the biennial meeting of the Society for Research in Adolescence, Alexandria, VA.

Rubin, K. H., & Stewart, S. L. (1996). Social withdrawal. In E. J. Mash & R. A. Barkley (Eds.), *Child psychopathology* (pp. 277–307). New York: Guilford Press.

Rudolph, K. D., Hammen, C., & Daley, S. E. (2006). Mood disorders. In D. A. Wolfe & E. J. Mash (Eds.), *Behavioral and emotional disorders in adolescents:*

Nature, assessment, and treatment (pp. 300–342). New York: Guilford Press.

Russo, D. C., & Budd, K. S. (1987). Limitations of operant practice in the study of disease. *Behavior Modification, 11*, 264–285.

Rutter, M. (1997). Clinical implications of attachment concepts: Retrospect and prospect. In L. A. Atkinson & K. J. Zucker (Eds.), *Attachment and psychopathology* (pp. 17–46). New York: Guilford Press

Rutter, M., Tizard, J., Yule, W., Graham, P., & Whitmore, K. (1976). Research report: Isle of Wight studies, 1964–1974. *Psychological Medicine, 6*, 313–332.

Salter, A. (1949). *Conditioned reflex therapy*. New York: Capricorn.

Sameroff, A. J. (1995). General systems theories and developmental psychopathology. In D. Cicchetti & D. J. Cohen (Eds.), *Developmental psychopathology: Vol. 1. Theory and methods* (pp. 659–695). New York: Wiley.

Sameroff, A. J., Seifer, R., Barocas, R., Zax, M., & Greenspan, S. (1987). Intelligence quotient scores of 4-year-old children: Social–environmental risk factors. *Pediatrics, 79*, 343–350.

Sattler, J. M. (1992). *Assessment of children: Revised and updated third edition*. San Diego, CA: Jerome M. Sattler.

Sattler, J. M. (1997). *Clinical and forensic interviewing of children and families: Guidelines for the mental health, education, pediatric, and child maltreatment fields*. San Diego, CA: Jerome M. Sattler.

Scheier, M. F., & Carver, C. S. (1985). Optimism, coping and health: Assessment and implications of generalized outcome expectancies. *Health Psychology, 4*, 219–247.

Schonfeld, I. S., Shaffer, D., O'Conner, P., & Portnoy, S. (1988). Conduct disorder and cognitive functioning: Testing three causal hypotheses. *Child Development, 59*, 993–1007.

Schroeder, C. S., & Gordon, B. N. (2002). *Assessment and treatment of childhood problems: A clinician's guide* (2nd ed.). New York: Guilford Press.

Schroeder, S. R., Gualtieri, C. T., & Van Bourgondien, M. E. (1986). Autism. In M. Hersen (Ed.), *Pharmacological and behavioral treatment: An integrative approach* (pp. 89–107). New York: Wiley.

Schwartz, I. S., & Baer, D. M. (1991). Social validity assessments: Is current practice state of the art? *Journal of Applied Behavior Analysis, 24*, 189–204.

Schwebel, A. I., & Fine, M. A. (1992). Cognitive-behavioral family therapy. *Journal of Family Psychotherapy, 3*, 73–91.

Schwebel, A. I., & Fine, M. A. (1994). *Understanding and helping families: A cognitive-behavioral approach*. Hillsdale, NJ: Erlbaum.

Sexton, T. L., & Alexander, J. F. (2003). Functional family therapy: A mature clinical model for working with at-risk adolescents and their families. In T. L. Sexton & G. R. Weeks (Eds.), *Handbook of family therapy:*

The science and practice of working with families and couples (pp. 323–348). New York: Brunner-Routledge.

Sexton, T. L., & Weeks, G. R. (Eds.). (2003). *Handbook of family therapy: The science and practice of working with families and couples*. New York: Brunner-Routledge.

Shadish, W. R., Matt, G. E., Navarro, A. M., Siegle, G., Crits-Christoph, P., Hazelrigg, M. D., et al. (1997). Evidence that therapy works in clinically representative conditions. *Journal of Consulting and Clinical Psychology, 65*, 355–365.

Sheldrick, R. C., Kendall, P. C., & Heimberg, R. G. (2001). The clinical significance of treatments: A comparison of three treatments for conduct disordered children. *Clinical Psychology: Science and Practice, 8*, 418–430.

Shelton, J. L., Levy, R. L., & Contributors. (1981). *Behavioral assignments and treatment compliance: A handbook of clinical strategies*. Champaign, IL: Research Press.

Sheridan, S. M., Kratochwill, T. R., & Bergan, J. R. (1996). *Conjoint behavioral consultation: A procedural manual*. New York: Plenum Press.

Shirk, S. R., & Karver, M. (2003). Prediction of treatment outcome from relationship variables in child and adolescent therapy: A meta-analytic review. *Journal of Consulting and Clinical Psychology, 71*, 452–464.

Shirk, S. R., & Saiz, C. S. (1992). Clinical, empirical, and developmental perspectives on the therapeutic relationship in child psychotherapy. *Development and Psychopathology, 4*, 713–728.

Silverman, W. K., & Saavedra, L. M. (2004). Assessment and diagnosis in evidence-based practice. In P. M. Barrett & T. H. Ollendick (Eds.), *Handbook of interventions that work with children and adolescents: Prevention and treatment* (pp. 49–70). New York: Wiley.

Siqueland, L., Kendall, P. C., Stoff, D., & Pollack, L. (1987). *Cognitive distortions and deficiencies in child psychiatric populations*. Unpublished manuscript, Department of Psychology, Temple University.

Skinner, B. F. (1953). *Science and human behavior*. New York: Macmillan.

Sonderegger, R., & Barrett, P. M. (2004). Assessment and treatment of ethnically diverse children and adolescents. In P. M. Barrett & T. H. Ollendick (Eds.), *Handbook of interventions that work with children and adolescents: Prevention and treatment* (pp. 89–111). New York: Wiley.

Sonuga-Barke, E. J. S., Daley, D., & Thompson, M. (2002). Does maternal ADHD reduce the effectiveness of parent training for preschool children's ADHD? *Journal of the American Academy of Child and Adolescent Psychiatry, 41*, 696–702.

Sonuga-Barke, E. J. S., Thompson, M., Daley, D., & Laver-Bradbury, C. (2004). Parent training for attention deficit/hyperactivity disorder: Is it as effective when delivered as routine rather than as specialist

care? *British Journal of Clinical Psychology, 43*, 449–457.

Southam-Gerow, M. A., Weisz, J. R., & Kendall, P. C. (2003). Youth with anxiety disorders in research and service clinics: Examining client differences and similarities. *Journal of Clinical Child and Adolescent Psychology, 32*, 375–385.

Sowder, B. J. (1975). *Assessment of child mental health needs* (Vols. 1–8). McLean, VA: General Research Corporation.

Spence, S. H., Sheffield, J. K., & Donovan, C. L. (2005). Long-term outcome of a school-based, universal approach to prevention of depression in adolescents. *Journal of Consulting and Clinical Psychology, 73*, 160–167.

Stark, K., & Kendall, P. C. (1996). *Treating depressed children: Therapist manual for "taking action."* Ardmore, PA: Workbook.

Steinglass, P. (1987). A systems view of family interaction and psychopathology. In T. Jacob (Ed.), *Family interaction and psychopathology: Theories, methods, and findings* (pp. 25–65). New York: Plenum Press.

Stoiber, K. C., & Kratochwill, T. R. (Eds.). (1998). *Handbook of group intervention for children and families*. Boston: Allyn & Bacon.

Stokes, T. F., & Baer, D. M. (1977). An implicit technology of generalization. *Journal of Applied Behavior Analysis, 10*, 349–367.

Stormshak, E. A., & Dishion, T. J. (2002). An ecological approach to child and family clinical and counseling psychology. *Clinical Child and Family Psychology Review, 5*, 197–215.

Strain, P. S. (Ed.). (1981). *The utilization of peers as behavior change agents*. New York: Plenum Press.

Strayhorn, J. M., Jr. (1987). Medical assessment of children with behavioral problems. In M. Hersen & V. B. Van Hasselt (Eds.), *Behavior therapy with children and adolescents: A clinical approach* (pp. 50–74). New York: Wiley.

Strosahl, K. D. (1994). Entering the new frontier of managed mental health care: Gold mines and land mines. *Cognitive and Behavioral Practice, 1*, 5–23.

Strosahl, K. D. (1996). Confessions of a behavior therapist in primary care: The odyssey and the ecstasy. *Cognitive and Behavioral Practice, 3*, 1–28.

Swenson, C. C., Henggeler, S. W., Taylor, I. S., & Addison, O. W. (2005). *Multisystemic therapy and neighborhood partnerships: Reducing adolescent violence and substance abuse*. New York: Guilford Press.

Tabachnik, N., & Alloy, L. B. (1988). Clinician and patient as aberrant actuaries: Expectation-based distortions in assessment of covariation. In L. Y. Abramson (Ed.), *Social cognition and clinical psychology* (pp. 295–365). New York: Guilford Press.

Tarnowski, K. J., Kelly, P. A., & Mendlowitz, D. R. (1987). Acceptability of behavioral pediatric interventions. *Journal of Consulting and Clinical Psychology, 55*, 435–436.

Tharp, R. G. (1991). Cultural diversity and treatment of

children. *Journal of Consulting and Clinical Psychology, 59,* 799–812.

Tharp, R. G., & Wetzel, R. J. (1969). *Behavior modification in the natural environment.* New York: Academic Press.

Thomason, B. T., Bachanas, P. J., & Campos, P. E. (1996). Cognitive behavioral interventions with persons affected by HIV/AIDS. *Cognitive and Behavioral Practice, 3,* 417–442.

Tisdelle, D. A., & St. Lawrence, J. S. (1988). Adolescent interpersonal problem-solving skills training: Social validation and generalization. *Behavior Therapy, 19,* 171–182.

Tolan, P. H., & Guerra, N. (1994, July). *What works in reducing adolescent violence: An empirical review of the field.* Boulder, CO: Center for the Study and Prevention of Violence.

Treatment for Adolescents with Depression Study (TADS) Team. (2004). Fluoxetine, cognitive-behavioral therapy, and their combination for adolescents with depression: Treatment for Adolescents with Depression Study (TADS) randomized controlled trial. *Journal of the American Medical Association, 292,* 807–820.

Tronick, E., & Gianino, A. (1986). Interactive mismatch and repair: Challenges to the coping infant. *Zero to Three, 6,* 1–6.

U.S. Department of Health and Human Services. (1999). *Mental health: A report of the Surgeon General.* Rockville, MD: National Institutes of Health, National Institute of Mental Health.

U.S. Public Health Service. (2001). *Report of the Surgeon General's Conference on Children's Mental Health: A national action agenda.* Washington, DC: U.S. Department of Health and Human Services.

Ullmann, L. P., & Krasner, L. (Eds.). (1965). *Case studies in behavior modification.* New York: Holt, Rinehart & Winston.

Urbain, E. S., & Kendall, P. C. (1980). Review of social-cognitive problem-solving interventions with children. *Psychological Bulletin, 88,* 109–143.

Vander Stoep, A., Weiss, N. S., McKnight, B., Beresford, S. A. A., & Cohen, P. (2002). Which measure of adolescent psychiatric disorder—diagnosis, number of symptoms, or adaptive functioning—best predicts adverse young adult outcomes? *Journal of Epidemiology and Community Health, 56,* 56–65.

Verhulst, F. C., Achenbach, T. M., van der Ende, J., Erol, N., Lambert, M. C., Leung, P. W. L., et al. (2003). Comparisons of problems reported by youths from seven countries. *American Journal of Psychiatry, 160,* 1479–1485.

Voeltz, L. M., & Evans, I. M. (1982). The assessment of behavioral interrelationships in child behavior therapy. *Behavioral Assessment, 4,* 131–165.

Wachtel, P. L. (1977). *Psychoanalysis and behavior therapy.* New York: Basic Books.

Wade, S. L. (2004). Commentary: Computer-based interventions in pediatric psychology. *Journal of Pediatric Psychology, 29,* 269–272.

Wahler, R. G. (1975). Some structural aspects of deviant child behavior. *Journal of Applied Behavior Analysis, 8,* 27–42.

Wahler, R. G. (1980). The insular mother: Her problems in parent–child treatment. *Journal of Applied Behavior Analysis, 13,* 207–219.

Wahler, R. G., & Fox, J. J. (1981). Setting events in applied behavior analysis: Toward a conceptual and methodological expansion. *Journal of Applied Behavior Analysis, 14,* 327–338.

Wahler, R. G., & Graves, M. G. (1983). Setting events in social networks: Ally or enemy in child behavior therapy? *Behavior Therapy, 14,* 19–36.

Walker, C. E., & Roberts, M. C. (Eds.). (2001). *Handbook of clinical child psychology* (3rd ed.). New York: Wiley.

Watson, J. B., & Rayner, R. (1920). Conditioned emotional reactions. *Journal of Experimental Psychology, 3,* 1–14.

Weber, J. (1936). An approach to the problem of fear in children. *Journal of Mental Science, 82,* 136–147.

Webster-Stratton, C., & Herbert, M. (1994). *Troubled families—problem children: Working with parents: A collaborative process.* Chichester, UK: Wiley.

Weersing, V. R., & Weisz, J. R. (2002). Mechanisms of action in youth psychotherapy. *Journal of Child Psychology and Psychiatry, 43,* 3–29.

Weersing, V. R., Weisz, J. R., & Donenberg, G. R. (2002). Development of the therapy procedures checklist: A therapist-report measure of technique use in child and adolescent treatment. *Journal of Clinical Child Psychology, 31,* 168–180.

Weingardt, K. R. (2004). The role of instructional design and technology in the dissemination of empirically supported, manual-based therapies. *Clinical Psychology: Science and Practice, 11,* 313–331.

Weiss, B., & Weisz, J. R. (1995). Relative effectiveness of behavioral versus nonbehavioral child psychotherapy. *Journal of Consulting and Clinical Psychology, 63,* 317–320.

Weisz, J. R. (2004). *Psychotherapy for children and adolescents: Evidence-based treatments and case examples.* Cambridge, UK: Cambridge University Press.

Weisz, J. R., Chu, B. C., & Polo, A. J. (2004). Treatment dissemination and evidence-based practice: Strengthening intervention through clinician–researcher collaboration. *Clinical Psychology: Science and Practice, 11,* 300–307.

Weisz, J. R., Donenberg, G. R., Han, S. S., & Weiss, B. (1995). Bridging the gap between laboratory and clinic in child and adolescent psychotherapy. *Journal of Consulting and Clinical Psychology, 63,* 688–701.

Weisz, J. R., Doss, A. J., & Hawley, K. M. (2005). Youth psychotherapy outcome research: A review and critique of the evidence base. *Annual Review of Psychology, 56,* 337–363.

Weisz, J. R., Han, S. S., & Valeri, S. M. (1997). More of what?: Issues raised by the Fort Bragg study. *American Psychologist, 52,* 541–545.

Weisz, J. R., & Hawley, K. M. (2002). Developmental

factors in the treatment of adolescents. *Journal of Consulting and Clinical Psychology, 70,* 21–43.

Weisz, J. R., Hawley, K. M., & Doss, A. J. (2004). Empirically tested psychotherapies for youth internalizing and externalizing problems and disorders. *Child and Adolescent Psychiatric Clinics of North America, 13,* 729–815.

Weisz, J. R., Jensen, A. L., & McLeod, B. D. (2005). Development and dissemination of child and adolescent psychotherapies: Milestones, methods, and a new deployment-focused model. In E. D. Hibbs & P. S. Jensen (Eds.), *Psychosocial treatments for child and adolescent disorders: Empirically based strategies for clinical practice* (2nd ed., pp. 9–39). Washington, DC: American Psychological Association.

Weisz, J. R., Southam-Gerow, M. A., Gordis, E. B., & Connor-Smith, J. (2003). Primary and secondary control enhancement training for your depression: Applying the deployment focused model of treatment development and testing. In A. E. Kazdin & J. R. Weisz (Eds.), *Evidence-based psychotherapies for children and adolescents* (pp. 165–183). New York: Guilford Press.

Weisz, J. R., & Weiss, B. (1993). *Effects of psychotherapy with children and adolescents.* Newbury Park, CA: Sage.

Weisz, J. R., Weiss, B., Alicke, M. D., & Klotz, M. L. (1987). Effectiveness of psychotherapy with children and adolescents: A meta-analysis for clinicians. *Journal of Consulting and Clinical Psychology, 55,* 542–549.

Weisz, J. R., Weiss, B., Han, S. S., Granger, D. A., & Morton, T. (1995). Effects of psychotherapy with children and adolescents revisited: A meta-analysis of treatment outcome studies. *Psychological Bulletin, 117,* 450–468.

Weisz, J. R., Weiss, B., & Langmeyer, D. B. (1987). Giving up on child psychotherapy: Who drops out? *Journal of Consulting and Clinical Psychology, 55,* 916–918.

Wekerle, C., & Wolfe, D. A. (2003). Child maltreatment. In E. J. Mash & R. A. Barkley (Eds.), *Child psychopathology* (2nd ed., pp. 632–684). New York: Guilford Press.

White, D. M., Rusch, F. R., Kazdin, A. E., & Hartmann, D. P. (1989). Applications of meta analysis in individual-subject research. *Behavioral Assessment, 11,* 281–296.

Willems, E. P. (1974). Behavioral technology and behavioral ecology. *Journal of Applied Behavior Analysis, 7,* 151–165.

Winett, R. A., & Winkler, R. C. (1972). Current behavior modification in the classroom: Be still, be quiet, be docile. *Journal of Applied Behavior Analysis, 5,* 499–504.

Winter, M. G., Hicks, R., McVey, G., & Fox, J. (1988). Age and sex differences in choice of consultant for various types of problems. *Child Development, 59,* 1046–1055.

Witt, J. C., & Elliott, S. N. (1986). Acceptability of classroom management procedures. In T. R. Kratochwill (Ed.), *Advances in school psychology* (pp. 251–288). Hillsdale, NJ: Erlbaum.

Wolfe, B. E., & Goldfried, M. R. (1988). Research on psychotherapy integration: Recommendations and conclusions from an NIMH workshop. *Journal of Consulting and Clinical Psychology, 56,* 448–451.

Wolfe, D. A., & Bourdeau, P. A. (1987). Current issues in the assessment of abusive and neglectful parent–child relationships. *Behavioral Assessment, 9,* 271–290.

Wolfe, D. A., & LaRose, L. (1986). *Child videotape series* [Videotape]. London, ON, Canada: University of Western Ontario.

Wolfe, D. A., Scott, K. S., & Crooks, C. (2005). Abuse and violence in adolescent girls' dating relationships. In D. J. Bell, S. L. Foster, & E. J. Mash (Eds.), *Handbook of behavioral and emotional problems in girls* (pp. 381–414). New York: Kluwer Academic/Plenum.

Wolfe, D. A., Wekerle, C., Gough, R., Reitzel-Jaffe, D., Grasley, C., Pittman, A., et al. (1996). *The youth relationships manual: A group approach with adolescents for the prevention of woman abuse and the promotion of healthy relationships.* Thousand Oaks, CA: Sage.

Wolfe, V. V., & Birt, J. (1997). Child sexual abuse. In E. J. Mash & L. G. Terdal (Eds.), *Assessment of childhood disorders* (3rd ed., pp. 569–623). New York: Guilford Press.

Wolpe, J. (1958). *Psychotherapy by reciprocal inhibition.* Stanford, CA: Stanford University Press.

Wolpe, J. (1986). Individualization: The categorical imperative of behavior therapy practice. *Journal of Behavior Therapy and Experimental Psychiatry, 17,* 145–153.

Wood, J. J., McLeod, B. D., Sigman, M., Hwang, W., & Chu, B. C. (2003). Parenting and child anxiety: Theory, empirical findings, and future directions. *Journal of Child Psychology and Psychiatry, 44,* 134–151.

World Health Organization (WHO). (1992). *The ICD-10 classification of mental and behavioural disorders: Clinical descriptions and diagnostic guidelines.* Geneva: Author.

World Health Organization (WHO). (2005). *Mental health policy and service guidance package: Child and adolescent mental health policies and plans.* Geneva: Author.

Wright, L., Flagler, S., & Friedman, A. G. (1988). Assessment for accident prevention. In P. Karoly (Ed.), *Handbook of child health assessment: Biopsychosocial perspectives* (pp. 491–518). New York: Wiley-Interscience.

Wurtele, S. K., Kast, L. C., & Kondrick, P. A. (1988). *Measuring young children's responses to sexual abuse prevention programs: The what-if situations test.* Unpublished manuscript, Department of Psychology, Washington State University.

Wurtele, S. K., Marrs, S. R., & Miller-Perrin, C. L. (1987). Practice makes perfect?: The role of participant modeling in sexual abuse prevention programs. *Journal of Consulting and Clinical Psychology, 55,* 599–602.

Yeh, M., & Weisz, J. R. (2001). Why are we here at the clinic?: Parent–child (dis)agreement on referral problems at outpatient treatment entry. *Journal of Consulting and Clinical Psychology, 69,* 1018–1025.

Yule, W. (1993). Developmental considerations in child assessment. In T. H. Ollendick & M. Hersen (Eds.), *Handbook of child and adolescent assessment* (pp. 15–25). Boston: Allyn & Bacon.

Zahn-Waxler, C. (1993). Warriors and worriers: Gender and psychopathology. *Development and Psychopathology, 5,* 79–89.

Zahn-Waxler, C., Cole, C. M., Welsh, J. D., & Fox, N. A. (1995). Psychophysiological correlates of empathy and prosocial behaviors in preschool children with behavior problems. *Development and Psychopathology, 7,* 27–48.

Zero to Three/National Center for Clinical Infant Programs. (1994). *Diagnostic classification of mental health and developmental disorders of infancy and early childhood (Diagnostic Classification: 0–3).* Washington, DC: Author.

Zoccolillo, M. (1993). Gender and the development of conduct disorder. *Development and Psychopathology, 5,* 65–78.

II

BEHAVIOR DISORDERS

2

Attention-Deficit/Hyperactivity Disorder

Bradley H. Smith, Russell A. Barkley, and Cheri J. Shapiro

Over the past century, numerous diagnostic labels have been given to clinically referred children who have significant deficiencies in behavioral inhibition, sustained attention, resistance to distraction, and the regulation of activity level. At present, "attention-deficit/ hyperactivity disorder" (ADHD) as defined by the *Diagnostic and Statistical Manual of Mental Disorders*, fourth edition, text revision (DSM-IV-TR; American Psychiatric Association, 2000) is the term used to describe this developmental disorder. Previously employed terms have been "brain-injured child syndrome," "hyperkinesis," "hyperactive child syndrome," "minimal brain dysfunction," and "attention deficit disorder (with or without hyperactivity)." Such periodic relabeling reflects a shifting emphasis in the primacy accorded certain symptom clusters within the disorder, based in part on the substantial research conducted each year on ADHD and on investigators' and theorists' interpretations of those findings.

This chapter provides a critical overview of the treatments that have been shown through scientific research to have some efficacy for the management of ADHD. This literature is voluminous, however, and so space here permits only a brief discussion and critique of each of the major treatments. More detailed discussions of these treatments can be found in the texts by Barkley (2006) and DuPaul and Stoner (2003). In addition to this chapter, perspectives on state-of-the-art treatment for ADHD are provided in published practice guidelines from the American Academy of Child and Adoles-

cent Psychiatry (McClellan & Werry, 2003), the American Academy of Pediatrics (2001), the American Medical Association (Goldman, Genel, Bezman, & Slanetz, 1998), and the Task Force on Empirically Validated Treatments commissioned by the American Psychological Association (Pelham, Wheeler, & Chronis, 1998). Our perspective on diagnosis and treatment is highly congruent with these authoritative sources, but adds the important considerations of practicality and safety of treatments to guide overall intervention planning for children and adolescents with ADHD.

The chapter begins with a brief overview of the nature of the disorder, its prevalence, its developmental course, and its etiologies. More detailed examinations of these topics can be found in the text by Barkley (2006). Subsequently, the main purpose of this chapter is addressed through a critical overview of various treatments for the disorder. Minimal information on the assessment of ADHD is provided here, due to both space limitations and the availability of more detailed information on this topic elsewhere (Barkley, 1997b, 2006; DuPaul & Stoner, 2003).

RECENT DEVELOPMENTS

Over the past decade, there have been several important developments related to the treatment of ADHD. These developments include (1) consensus statements from major professional and scientific organizations about appropriate treatment of ADHD; (2) proliferation in the variety of medications used to treat ADHD; (3) some major additions to the research literature on treatment of adolescents with ADHD; (4) unique insights about treatment from the Multimodal Treatment Study of ADHD, or MTA (MTA Cooperative Group, 1999a, 1999b, 2004a, 2004b); and (5) increased attention to alternative approaches to treatment development and evaluation, which emphasize treatment effectiveness as opposed to just treatment efficacy.

A noteworthy change from the preceding edition of this chapter is systematic consideration of the effectiveness and practicality of treatments. In that earlier edition, the primary emphasis was on the efficacy of treatments as determined in controlled clinical trials. The current chapter places equal or greater emphasis on the practicality of treatment.

"Practicality," as we use the term, is distinct from both "efficacy" and "effectiveness." "Efficacy" refers to demonstrated treatment success in controlled research studies, which often take place in clinical laboratories or university settings and are typically designed, supervised, and executed by experts and their students and staffs. "Effectiveness" refers to demonstrated treatment success in naturalistic settings more typical of those clinics, hospitals, and private practices in which patients are likely to seek treatment; the demonstration of effectiveness involves controlled scientific studies supervised or instituted by the clinicians typically practicing in those settings. "Practicality" here refers to the ease or convenience of carrying out the treatment, and hence the likelihood of its adoption in ordinary clinical practice. Classroom management or intensive all-day summer treatment approaches to ADHD may be both efficacious and effective; yet they may not necessarily be adopted in typical classroom or community settings if the labor they require for implementation is too great, or if the financial cost of doing so is disproportionate within the total school or community budget. This focus on practical considerations stems from a growing concern that empirically supported treatments are being underutilized—not only for children with ADHD, but in all of children's mental health. The consequence of this situation is that there is a two-tiered pattern of outcomes in the extant research literature. Specifically, meta-analytic reviews of the literature have found substantial evidence for beneficial effects of interventions studied in research set-

tings, but little or no evidence for beneficial effects of interventions delivered in typical clinical settings (Weisz, 2004).

This two-tiered system of outcomes seems to persist, despite some vigorous and well-planned efforts to disseminate the empirically validated treatments (e.g., Henggeler, Melton, Brondino, Scherer, & Hanley, 1997). The bad news is that, for a variety of reasons, clinicians in naturalistic settings did not implement empirically validated treatments with sufficient fidelity to get effective outcomes (Biglan, Mrazek, Carnine, & Flay, 2003). The good news is that several studies have found that fidelity of treatment implementation is positively correlated with beneficial outcomes (Biglan et al., 2003). Therefore, efforts to overcome barriers to effective implementation and promote treatment fidelity should result in better treatment outcomes. Consequently, this chapter pays close attention to barriers to dissemination of empirically supported treatments for ADHD; overcoming such barriers is an issue we call the "practicality" of treatment.

To help summarize issues of effectiveness, safety, and practicality, and to facilitate comparisons between treatments, we use a grading system for each of these three considerations. Our grades for empirical support of effectiveness are very similar to the ranking system proposed by Biglan and colleagues (2003), which is a refinement of a consensus system adopted by the American Psychological Association's Task Force on Empirically Validated Treatments. Specifically, in this chapter a treatment receives a grade of F if claims of effectiveness are based solely on clinical experience or weak quasi-experimental designs (e.g., single-group pre- to posttest studies). The grade of D is given to treatments possessing evidence of effectiveness from one well-designed, randomized clinical trial, or from an interrupted time series that was replicated across at least three cases. The grade of C is given when there has been replication of well-designed, randomized clinical trials or interrupted time series studies, but the replication has been conducted by the same group of researchers. Treatments receive a grade of B when there has been replication of well-designed, randomized clinical trials or interrupted time series studies by independent teams of researchers. Finally, a grade of A is assigned when the efficacy criteria to earn a B are met, *and* when there is evidence of effectiveness for the intervention as implemented in its intended setting.

PRIMARY SYMPTOMS

Children having ADHD, by definition, display difficulties with attention and/or impulse control relative to typical children of the same age and sex (American Psychiatric Association, 2000; Barkley, Cook, et al., 2002). "Attention" is a multidimensional construct that can refer to problems with alertness, arousal, selective or focused attention, sustained attention, distractibility, or span of apprehension, among others (Barkley, 1988; Mirsky, 1996). Research to date suggests that, among these elements, children with ADHD are likely to have their greatest difficulties with sustaining attention to tasks (persistence of responding), resisting distractions, and reengaging in initial tasks once disrupted (Barkley, 1997a, 1997c; Douglas, 1983). These difficulties are sometimes apparent in free-play settings, but are much more evident in situations requiring sustained attention to dull, boring, and/or repetitive tasks (Danforth, Barkley, & Stokes, 1991; Luk, 1985). However, even when those children are presented with apparently intrinsically interesting stimuli (such as a television program), attractive distracting stimuli (such as toys) may significantly impair their attention to and comprehension of events, relative to those of children who do not have ADHD (Lorch, Sanchez, van den Broek, Baer, & Hooks, 2000). More recent research is suggesting that the attention problems evident in ADHD are part of a larger domain of cognitive activities known as "executive functioning," and especially "working memory" (i.e., holding information in mind that is being used to guide performance) (Barkley, 1997a, 1997c). Specifically, evidence from the development of rating scales indicates that the DSM items used to define the attention deficits in ADHD load on a larger dimension containing items reflecting executive functioning and specifically working memory (Conners, 1998; Gioia, Isquith, Guy, & Kenworthy, 2000).

Often coupled with this difficulty in sustained attention is a deficiency in inhibiting behavior, or "impulsivity." Like attention, impulsivity is multidimensional in nature (Nigg, 1999, 2000, 2001). The deficit in ADHD is not so much in cognitive reflectiveness as mainly in the capacity to inhibit or delay prepotent responses, particularly in settings where those responses compete with rules (Barkley, 1997d). A "prepotent response" is one that would gain the immediate reinforcement (reward or escape) available in a given context, or that has a strong history of such reinforcement in the past. Those with ADHD have difficulties with sustained inhibition of such dominant responses over time (Nigg, 1999), as well as with poor delay of gratification (Rapport, Tucker, DuPaul, Merlo, & Stoner, 1986), a steeper discounting of the value of delayed over immediate rewards (Barkley, Edwards, Lanieri, Fletcher, & Metevia, 2001b), and impaired adherence to commands to inhibit behavior in social contexts (Danforth et al., 1991). This inhibitory deficit may also include a difficulty with interrupting an already ongoing response pattern (Schachar, Tannock, & Logan, 1993), particularly when given feedback about performance and errors. In the latter case, perseverative responding may be evident despite negative feedback concerning such responding, which may reflect an insensitivity to errors (Sergeant & van der Meere, 1988). Overall, individuals with ADHD have poorer inhibitory control and slower inhibitory processing than nondisabled controls do (Nigg, 2001).

Numerous studies have shown that children with ADHD tend to be more active, restless, and fidgety than typical children (Porrino et al., 1983; Teicher, Ito, Glod, & Barber, 1996). As with the other symptoms, there are significant situational fluctuations in this symptom (Luk, 1985; Porrino et al., 1983). It has not always been convincingly shown that hyperactivity distinguishes children with ADHD from other clinic-referred groups of children (Werry, Elkind, & Reeves, 1987; Werry, Reeves, & Elkind, 1987). It may be the pervasiveness of the hyperactivity across settings that separates ADHD from other diagnostic categories (Taylor, 1986).

ADHD symptoms of hyperactivity have been shown to decline significantly across the elementary school years, while problems with attention persist at relatively stable levels during this same period of development (Hart, Lahey, Loeber, Applegate, & Frick, 1995). One explanation that may account for such a state of affairs is that the hyperactivity reflects an early developmental manifestation of a more central deficit in behavioral inhibition. Studies that factor-analyze behavior ratings certainly show that hyperactivity and poor impulse control form a single dimension of behavior, as shown in the DSM-IV and DSM-IV-TR (Achenbach, 2001; DuPaul, 1991). This deficit in inhibition, of which early hyperactivity is a part, may become increasingly reflected in poor self-regulation over various developmental stages, even though the difficulties with excessive activity level may wane with maturation.

Difficulties with adherence to rules and instructions are also evident in children with ADHD (American Psychiatric Association, 2000; Barkley, 1997a). Care is taken here to exclude poor rule-governed behavior that may stem from sensory disabilities (e.g., deafness), impaired language development, or defiance or oppositional behavior. Nevertheless, children with ADHD typically show significant problems in complying with parental and teacher commands (Danforth et al., 1991), following experimental instructions in the absence of the experimenter (Draeger, Prior, & Sanson, 1986), and adhering to directives to defer gratification or resist temptations (Rapport, Tucker, et al., 1986). Like the other symptoms, rule-governed behavior is a multidimensional construct (Hayes, 1989). It remains to be shown which aspects of this construct are specifically impaired in ADHD.

DIAGNOSTIC CRITERIA

Between 1980 and the present, efforts have been made to develop more specific guidelines for the classification of children as having ADHD. These efforts have been increasingly based on an empirical approach to developing a taxonomy of child psychopathology. Although guidelines appeared in the DSM-II (American Psychiatric Association, 1968), these comprised merely a single sentence, along with the admonition not to grant the diagnosis if demonstrable brain injury were present. A more concerted effort at developing criteria appeared in the DSM-III (American Psychiatric Association, 1980), though it was still unempirical. These criteria were not examined in any field trial, but were developed primarily from expert opinion. In the subsequent revision of the DSM-III (DSM-III-R; American Psychiatric Association, 1987), an attempt was made to draw upon the results of factor-analytic studies of child behavior rating scales to aid in the selection of symptoms that might be included for ADHD (Spitzer, Davies, & Barkley, 1990). A small-scale field trial employing 500 children from multiple clinical sites was conducted to narrow down the potential list of symptoms, and a cutoff score on this list was chosen that best differentiated children with ADHD from other diagnostic groups.

The current diagnostic criteria codified in the DSM-IV and DSM-IV-TR (these are unchanged from the original to the text revision) are based on a better field trial and more thorough analysis of the results than the DSM-III-R (Applegate et al., 1997; Lahey et al., 1994). The DSM-IV-TR criteria appear in Table 2.1. Despite the increasingly empirical foundation of the DSM, there remain a few problems with these criteria; these include developmental sensitivity to the disorder, possible gender discrimination in diagnosis, an empirically unjustified age of onset of 7 years, and a vexing requirement for cross-setting impairment that is confounded with the problem of poor parent–teacher agreement (Barkley, 2006). Particularly problematic for the generality of these criteria is the fact that the field trial used primarily male children, ages 4–16 years, who were largely of European American background. Consequently, adjustments or allowances must be made when clinicians wish to apply the DSM criteria to females, young adults, and non-European ethnic groups. For example, the symptom of "often leaves seat" is irrelevant to adults with ADHD. Moreover, children whose onset of symptoms was sometime during the childhood years (prior to 13) should be considered as having a valid disorder because the DSM criterion for diagnosis that requires documentation of onset prior to age 7 has not been empirically validated and presumably may lead to an unacceptably high false negative rate when diagnosing ADHD (Barkley & Biederman, 1997).

Where sex differences exist, they indicate that girls with ADHD show less severe symptoms of both inattention and hyperactive–impulsive behavior, especially in school; fewer symptoms of oppositional defiant disorder (ODD) and conduct disorder (CD); greater intellectual deficits; and more symptoms of anxiety and depression than do boys with ADHD (Abikoff et al., 2002; Gershon, 2002; Hartung et al., 2002). Some recent studies indicate that girls with ADHD may employ more relational aggression than their peers without ADHD (Zalecki & Hinshaw, 2004).

TABLE 2.1. DSM-IV-TR Criteria for ADHD

A. Either (1) or (2):

(1) six (or more) of the following symptoms of **inattention** have persisted for at least 6 months to a degree that is maladaptive and inconsistent with developmental level:

Inattention
(a) often fails to give close attention to details or makes careless mistakes in schoolwork, work, or other activities
(b) often has difficulty sustaining attention in tasks or play activities
(c) often does not seem to listen when spoken to directly
(d) often does not follow through on instructions and fails to finish schoolwork, chores, or duties in the workplace (not due to oppositional behavior or failure to understand instructions)
(e) often has difficulty organizing tasks and activities
(f) often avoids, dislikes, or is reluctant to engage in tasks that require sustained mental effort (such as schoolwork or homework)
(g) often loses things necessary for tasks or activities (e.g., toys, school assignments, pencils, books, or tools)
(h) is often easily distracted by extraneous stimuli
(i) is often forgetful in daily activities

(2) six (or more) of the following symptoms of **hyperactivity–impulsivity** have persisted for at least 6 months to a degree that is maladaptive and inconsistent with developmental level:

Hyperactivity
(a) often fidgets with hands or feet or squirms in seat
(b) often leaves seat in classroom or in other situations in which remaining seated is expected
(c) often runs about or climbs excessively in situations in which it is inappropriate (in adolescents or adults, may be limited to subjective feelings of restlessness)
(d) often has difficulty playing or engaging in leisure activities quietly
(e) is often "on the go" or often acts as if "driven by a motor"
(f) often talks excessively

Impulsivity
(g) often blurts out answers before the questions have been completed
(h) often has difficulty awaiting turn
(i) often interrupts or intrudes on others (e.g., butts into conversations or games)

B. Some hyperactive–impulsive or inattentive symptoms that caused impairment were present before age 7 years.

C. Some impairment from the symptoms is present in two or more settings (e.g., at school [or work] and at home).

D. There must be clear evidence of clinically significant impairment in social, academic, or occupational functioning.

E. The symptoms do not occur exclusively during the course of a Pervasive Developmental Disorder, Schizophrenia, or other Psychotic Disorder and are not better accounted for by another mental disorder (e.g., Mood Disorder, Anxiety Disorder, Dissociative Disorder, or a Personality Disorder).

Code based on type:
314.01 Attention-Deficit/Hyperactivity Disorder, Combined Type: if both Criteria A1 and A2 are met for the past 6 months
314.00 Attention-Deficit/Hyperactivity Disorder, Predominantly Inattentive Type: if Criterion A1 is met but Criterion A2 is not met for the past 6 months
314.01 Attention-Deficit/Hyperactivity Disorder, Predominantly Hyperactive–Impulsive Type: if Criterion A2 is met but Criterion A1 is not met for the past 6 months

Coding note: For individuals (especially adolescents and adults) who currently have symptoms that no longer meet full criteria, "In Partial Remission" should be specified.

Note. From American Psychiatric Association (2000, pp. 92–93). Copyright 2000 by the American Psychiatric Association. Reprinted by permission.

PREVALENCE AND SEX RATIO

The DSM-IV-TR cites a prevalence of 3–7% of school-age children as probably having ADHD (American Psychiatric Association, 2000). In his review, Szatmari (1992) found that the prevalence varied from a low of 2% to a high of 6.3%. Most fell within the range of 4.2–6.3%. Another review found prevalence rates ranging from 1.6% to 16% (Goldman et al., 1998). Similar prevalence rates (4–8%) in elementary school–age children have been reported in several studies (Breton et al., 1999; Briggs-Gowan, Horwitz, Schwab-Stone, Leventhal, & Leaf, 2000). Some of the studies that have found lower rates of ADHD (i.e., in the 2–6% range) were likely affected by methodological issues such as rigid adherence to DSM criteria, use of earlier versions of the DSM in which the inattentive type of ADHD did not exist, and the fact that many studies relied exclusively on parent reports (Brenton et al., 1999). Higher prevalence rates occur if just a cutoff on teacher ratings is used (DuPaul, Power, Anastopoulos, & Reid, 1998 [up to 23%]; Nolan, Gadow, & Sprafkin, 2001 [15.8%]).

Sex and age differences in prevalence are routinely found in research. For instance, prevalence rates may be 4% in girls and 8% in boys in the preschool age group (Gadow, Sprafkin, & Nolan, 2001), but may fall to 2–4% in girls and 6–9% in boys during the 6- to 12-year-old age period, based on parent reports (Breton et al., 1999; Szatmari, Offord, & Boyle, 1989). The prevalence may decrease again, to 0.9–2% in girls and 1–5.6% in boys, by adolescence (Breton et al., 1999; Lewinsohn, Hops, Roberts, Seeley, & Andrews, 1993; Romano, Tremblay, Vitaro, Zoccolillo, & Pagani, 2001). Importantly, if (as specified in the DSM) both a symptom threshold and the requirement for impairment are used, the prevalence may decrease by 20–60% from the figure based on symptom thresholds alone (Breton et al., 1999; Romano et al., 2001; Wolraich, Hannah, Baumgaertel, & Feurer, 1998).

In large part, differences in prevalence rates across studies are due to different methods of selecting samples, differences in the nature of the populations themselves (urban vs. rural, etc.), differing definitions of the disorder, and certainly the variation in ages of the samples. Males are approximately three times more likely than females to have ADHD. The disorder decreases in both sexes across development. Despite all the factors affecting the prevalence of the disorder, there is a clear consensus that ADHD is a valid, diagnosable disorder (Barkley, Cook, et al., 2002).

ONSET, COURSE, AND OUTCOME

Studies of the developmental course and outcome of children with ADHD have been numerous and can only be briefly summarized here (for reviews, see Barkley, 2006; Weiss & Hechtman, 1993). Although some children with ADHD are reported to have been difficult in their temperament since birth or early infancy (Barkley, DuPaul, & McMurray, 1990; Ross & Ross, 1982), the majority appear to be identifiable by their caregivers as deviating from typical development at between 3 and 4 years of age (Barkley, Fischer, Newby, & Breen, 1988; Loeber, Green, Lahey, Christ, & Frick, 1992). However, it may be several years later before such children are brought to the attention of professionals. Although the diagnosis of ADHD among preschoolers may be more difficult, due to higher rates of disruptive behavior among the general population at this age, a few recent studies suggest that reliable and valid diagnosis can be made for children as young as 3 years and 7 months old (Hartung et al., 2002).

During their preschool years, children with ADHD are often excessively active, mischievous, noncompliant with parental requests, and difficult to toilet-train (Campbell, 2002; Hartsough & Lambert, 1985; Mash & Johnston, 1982). They may also already be manifesting some delays in academic readiness skills (Mariani & Barkley, 1997). Parental distress over child care and management is likely to reach its zenith between 3 and 6 years of age, declining thereafter as the deficits in attention and rule following improve (Barkley, Karlsson, & Pollard, 1985; Mash & Johnston, 1983). Yet, even into the elementary school years, the stress parents report in raising children with ADHD remains considerably higher than that for parents of children in control groups (Anastopoulos, Guevremont, Shelton, & DuPaul, 1992; Bussing et al., 2003; Fischer, 1990). Likewise, parents of teenagers with ADHD report high levels of stress and family conflict with these youths, particularly if the teens also carry a comorbid diagnosis of ODD (Barkley, Anastopoulos, Guevremont, &

Fletcher, 1992; Barkley, Fischer, Edelbrock, & Smallish, 1991; Edwards, Barkley, Laneri, Fletcher, & Metevia, 2001).

By entry into formal schooling (6 years of age), most children with ADHD have become recognizably deviant from their nondisabled peers in their poor sustained attention, impulsivity, and restlessness. Difficulties with aggression, defiance, or oppositional behavior may now emerge, if they did not earlier in development (Barkley, Fischer, Edelbrock, & Smallish, 1990; Barkley et al., 1991). Children with ADHD who develop these conduct problems or antisocial behaviors are likely to veer into a more severe path of maladjustment in later years than are those children with ADHD who do not develop aggressive/defiant behaviors or do so only to a limited degree (Barkley, Fischer, Smallish, & Fletcher, 2004a). During these elementary school years, the majority of children with ADHD have varying degrees of poor school performance, usually related to failure to finish assigned tasks in school or as homework, disruptive behavior during class activities, and poor peer relations with schoolmates. Learning disabilities in areas of reading, spelling, math, handwriting, and language, however, may also become manifest in a significant minority of children with ADHD, requiring additional special educational assistance beyond that typically needed to manage the ADHD symptoms (Barkley, 2006; Tannock, 2000b).

As teenagers, a small percentage of children with ADHD will have "outgrown" their symptoms, in that they now place within the broadly defined "normal" range in their symptom deviance. However, those who have subclinical levels of ADHD as adolescents or young adults may still be significantly impaired and might be considered to have ADHD if more developmentally appropriate diagnostic criteria were employed. Moreover, even when DSM criteria are used, the odds generally favor the continuation of the disorder, as studies have estimated that 43–80% continue to have the disorder into adolescence (Barkley, Fischer, et al., 1990; Biederman, Faraone, Milberger, et al., 1996; Mannuzza et al., 1993; Weiss & Hechtman, 1993).

For adolescents with ADHD, family conflicts may continue or even increase (Barkley, Anastopoulos, et al., 1992; Fletcher, Fischer, Barkley, & Smallish, 1996). These may now center around the teens' failure to accept responsibility for performing routine tasks, their

difficulties with being trusted to obey rules when away from home, and general difficulties in the problem-solving approaches that parents and adolescents with ADHD attempt to use in resolving conflicts (e.g., authoritarian, highly emotional, excessive use of ultimatums, etc.) (Robin, 1998). Among that subset of teens with ADHD who have had significant earlier problems with aggressive and oppositional behavior, delinquency and CD are more likely to emerge (if they have not done so already), as these adolescents spend greater amounts of unsupervised time in the community (Barkley, Fischer, et al., 1990; Mannuzza et al., 1991; Satterfield, Swanson, Schell, & Lee, 1994; Weiss & Hechtman, 1993). Greater-than-usual substance experimentation and abuse is likely to occur within the adolescent years, mainly among youths diagnosed with ADHD and comorbid CD (Barkley, Fischer, et al., 1990; Barkley et al., 2004a; Thompson, Riggs, Mikulich, & Crowley, 1996) or bipolar disorder (Biederman, Faraone, Mick, Wozniak, et al., 1996). An increasing number of studies have replicated and extended the original report of Weiss and Hechtman (1993) suggesting that both children with ADHD followed into adolescence and clinically referred teenagers (and adults) with ADHD have more automobile accidents and speeding citations than typical teens do (see Barkley, 2004b, for a review; see also Fischer, Barkley, Smallish, & Fletcher, in press). Research also suggests that up to 32% may fail to complete high school, and that most fail to pursue college programs after high school (Barkley, Fischer, Smallish, & Fletcher, 2004b; Weiss & Hechtman, 1993). A greater risk of teenage pregnancy has also been noted in a recent follow-up study (Barkley et al., 2004b). Certainly, the outcome of childhood ADHD in the adolescent years is far more negative than previous clinical lore had postulated.

Less research exists on the adult outcome of children with ADHD. What does exist suggests that from 8% to 66% may continue to have the disorder or are continuing to have symptoms of ADHD that significantly affect their lives (Barkley, Fischer, Smallish, & Fletcher, 2002). More recent studies using more modern diagnostic criteria for ADHD appear to demonstrate higher rates of persistence of the disorder than do earlier follow-up studies. Interpersonal problems continue to plague as many as 75% (Weiss & Hechtman, 1993). Juvenile convictions and symptoms of adult antisocial personality may occur in 23–45% (Barkley et al., 2004a; Fischer et al., in press), while 20–27% or more may have substance use disorders (Fischer, Barkley, Smallish, & Fletcher, 2002).

RELATED CHARACTERISTICS

Children with ADHD have a higher likelihood of having other medical, developmental, adaptive, behavioral, emotional, and academic difficulties than do peers who do not have ADHD. Delays in intelligence, academic achievement, and motor coordination are more prevalent in children with ADHD than in matched samples of nondisabled children or even in siblings (Barkley, 2006), as are delays in adaptive functioning more generally (Greene et al., 1996; Roizen, Blondis, Irwin, & Stein, 1994; Stein, Szumowski, Blondis, & Roizen, 1995). Problems with peer acceptance and in peer interactions are commonly documented in children with ADHD (Bagwell, Molina, Pelham, & Hoza, 2001; Erhardt & Hinshaw, 1994; Stroes, Alberts, & van der Meere, 2003).

As many as 87% of children with clinically diagnosed ADHD may have at least one other disorder, and 67% have at least two other disorders (Kadesjo & Gillberg, 2001). As noted earlier, children with ADHD are more likely to have coexisting symptoms of ODD and CD than are children without ADHD (Angold, Costello, & Erkanli, 1999). Depression and juvenile-onset bipolar disorder also appear to be more common in children with ADHD than would be expected in the general population (Biederman, Faraone, Mick, Moore, & Lelon, 1996; Jensen, Shervette, Xenakis, & Richters, 1993), especially when CD is present with ADHD (Angold et al., 1999). There is a modest increase in risk for anxiety disorders as well (Angold et al., 1999; Tannock, 2000a). The severity of the ADHD symptoms may in part predict the severity of and risk for these comorbid conditions (Gabel, Schmidtz, & Fulker, 1996).

Children with ADHD appear to have more minor physical anomalies than typically developing children (Quinn & Rapoport, 1974) and may be physically smaller than such children, at least during childhood (Spencer et al., 1996). They may also have more sleep difficulties than typical children (Ball & Koloian, 1995). However, prior beliefs that ADHD may have a higher-than-usual association with either allergies or asthma have not been corroborated by research (Biederman, Milberger, Faraone, Guite, & Warburton, 1994; McGee, Stanton, & Sears, 1993).

Research on the family interactions of children with ADHD suggests that their symptoms produce significant alterations in family functioning, particularly when these children are also manifesting problems with oppositional and defiant behavior (Johnston & Mash, 2001). Children with ADHD have been shown to be less compliant, more negative, and less able to sustain compliance than typical children during task completion with their mothers (see Danforth et al., 1991, for a review). Their mothers are more directive and negative, are more lax in their discipline, are less rewarding and responsive to their children's behavior, and show lower levels of maternal coping than mothers of typical children (Cunningham & Boyle, 2002; Keown & Woodward, 2002; McKee, Harvey, Danforth, Ulaszek, & Friedman, 2004); however, these problems are more closely aligned with level of child conduct problems than with severity of ADHD symptoms (Johnston, Murray, Hinshaw, Pelham, & Hoza, 2002; Kashdan et al., 2004). There appears to be less conflict in the task-related interactions of older children with ADHD than in those of younger children (Danforth et al., 1991). However, older children with ADHD remain deviant from same-age children in their noncompliance and parent–child conflicts, even into adolescence (Barkley et al., 1991; Edwards et al., 2001; Fletcher et al., 1996). Not surprisingly, these interaction problems are significantly greater in those teens with both ADHD and ODD than in those without comorbid ODD, as was evident in childhood ADHD.

It is also not surprising, then, that parents of children with ADHD report significantly greater stress in their parental roles than do parents of typical children (DuPaul, McGoey, Eckert, & VanBrakle, 2001; Harrison & Sofronoff, 2002; Johnston & Mash, 2001). Conflicts between parents and children with ADHD may also spill over into increased conflicts between the parents and their nondisabled children (Smith, Brown, Bunke, Blount, & Christophersen, 2002). Mothers of children with ADHD routinely manifest higher levels of depression as well (Cunningham & Boyle, 2002); this depression is associated with even greater parenting problems, as well as biased maternal reporting of children's severity of

ADHD symptoms as a function of depression-related distortions (Chi & Hinshaw, 2002). Childhood ADHD is also associated with higher levels of parental ADHD, and if children also manifest ODD or CD, parents may also manifest greater rates of mood, anxiety, and substance use disorders (Chronis et al., 2003).

Studies evaluating the impact of stimulant medication on these interactions suggest that the greater directive and negative behavior of the mothers of children with ADHD may be in part a reaction to their children's noncompliance and poor self-control, rather than a cause of it (Danforth et al., 1991). Moreover, these conflicts in social interactions appear to exist in the relations of children with ADHD with their fathers (Edwards et al., 2001; Tallmadge & Barkley, 1983) and teachers (Cunningham & Boyle, 2002; Whalen, Henker, & Dotemoto, 1980). Yet both children and teens with ADHD do not perceive their relations with parents as being more problematic than do control children (Edwards et al., 2001; Gerdes, Hoza, & Pelham, 2003; Hoza et al., 2004). These results and others on the perceptions of children with ADHD concerning their task performance indicate a positive illusory bias in their self-perceptions. That is, children with ADHD do not typically suffer from low self-esteem; rather, these children may have problems related to overly high self-esteem, or at least inflated self-perceptions of their performance abilities.

The peer relations of children and teens with ADHD are also more problematic than usual (Bagwell et al., 2001; Cunningham & Siegel, 1987); these youths experience more rejection and fewer close friendships. This is especially so for the subset having ODD/CD (Bagwell et al., 2001; DuPaul et al., 2001; Mikami & Hinshaw, 2003). Children with ADHD exhibit more negative behavior (DuPaul et al., 2001) and are less socially involved with playmates without ADHD during conversations; however, the children with ADHD may direct attention to their typical peers during play activities, receiving more structure in the form of praise and questioning from peers during the latter activities (Stroes et al., 2003). When children who have ADHD are presented with stories involving social problems, they have difficulty focusing on main story events, provide less relevant predictions about future outcomes, have more problems maintaining a positive outlook on future events, and do not generate as many socially acceptable solutions as peers without ADHD do (Zentall, Cassady, & Javorsky, 2001). Children with ADHD also encode fewer social cues and generate fewer responses than typical children, while those with comorbid ODD/CD demonstrate a greater propensity for aggressive responses than control children (Matthys, Cuperus, & van Engeland, 1999).

ETIOLOGIES

The various proposed etiologies for ADHD are too numerous to review here in any detail. Therefore, we concentrate on those for which there is substantial empirical support, but even they can only receive brief mention. More detailed information is available elsewhere (Accardo, Blondis, Whitman, & Stein, 2006; Barkley, 2006; Spencer, 2004). Although the definitive specific and most proximal causes of ADHD have not been established, the larger domains in which these precise causes are likely to exist have been much better clarified over the past decade. Substantial evidence points to both neurological and genetic contributions to this disorder, and even specific brain regions and specific genes are now being implicated as contributors. So, while the exact neurochemical or neuromechanical mechanisms remain to be established for ADHD, and the suites of genes contributing to its striking heritability have yet to be completely catalogued, there is little doubt that these etiological directions hold the greatest promise for understanding the causes of the disorder.

As we discuss below, purely social causes of ADHD can be largely ruled out as likely contributors to most forms of ADHD, and this is a major advance in itself. Social factors surely moderate types and degrees of impairments resulting from the disorder, and even risk for comorbid ODD or CD, as well as social prejudices against those having ADHD—not to mention access to services for its management. And they may even moderate severity of symptoms as perceived by caregivers. But as causes of disorder in and of themselves, social factors appear to have little research support.

Neurological Factors

A large number of studies have used neuropsychological tests of frontal lobe functions and have detected deficits in children and adults with ADHD (Barkley, 1997a; Barkley, Edwards, et al., 2001b; Murphy, Barkley, & Bush, 2001; Seidman et al., 1997, 2004), especially in response or "executive" inhibition (Nigg, 2001). The greatest support in meta-analyses of the burgeoning neuropsychological literature on ADHD is for difficulties not only with the cardinal domains of inattention and inhibition, but also with working memory (Frazier, Demaree, & Youngstrom, 2004; Hervey, Epstein, & Curry, 2004). Less evidence exists for difficulties in other executive abilities, such as planning and verbal fluency, response perseveration, and emotional self-regulation, but this is largely because there have been far fewer studies of these domains. Difficulties with sense of time have also been convincingly established (Barkley, Edwards, et al., 2001b; Barkley, Murphy, & Bush, 2001). Moreover, research shows that not only do siblings of children with ADHD who also have ADHD show similar executive function deficits; even those siblings who do not actually manifest ADHD appear to have mild yet significant impairments in these same executive functions (Seidman et al., 1995). Such findings imply a phenotypic dimension to ADHD that is present, albeit in milder form, among individuals who are genetically related to those with the disorder. Executive deficits in ADHD appear to arise from the same substantial shared genetic liability as do the ADHD symptoms themselves (Coolidge, Thede, & Young, 2000).

These inhibitory and executive deficits are not the results of comorbid disorders, such as ODD, CD, anxiety, or depression; these findings give investigators greater confidence in their affiliation with ADHD itself (Barkley, Edwards, et al., 2001b; Barkley, Murphy, et al., 2001; Bayliss & Roodenrys, 2000; Murphy et al., 2001; Nigg, Blaskey, Huang-Pollock, & Rappley, 2002). This is not to say that some other disorders (such as learning disabilities or autism) do not affect some executive function tasks (such as those of verbal working memory), perhaps owing to their associated deficits in language development. But it is to say that the pattern of deficits associated with ADHD may not be typical of these other disorders (Pennington & Ozonoff, 1996).

Research using psychophysiological measures of central and autonomic nervous system electrical activity (galvanic skin responses, heart rate deceleration, etc.) have proven largely in-

consistent in demonstrating group differences between children with ADHD and control children in resting arousal. Where differences from controls are found, they are consistently in the direction of diminished reactivity to stimulation, as in evoked responses, in those with ADHD (Beauchaine, Katkin, Strassberg, & Snarr, 2001; Borger & van der Meere, 2000; Herpertz et al., 2001); these findings may point to impaired right prefrontal mechanisms underlying response inhibition (Pliszka, Liotti, & Woldorff, 2000). Far more consistent have been the results of quantitative electroencephalographic (QEEG) and evoked response potential (ERP) measures, sometimes taken in conjunction with vigilance tests (El-Sayed, Larsson, Persson, & Rydelius, 2002; Monastra et al., 1999; see Loo & Barkley, in press, for a review). The most consistent pattern in the EEG research is increased slow-wave or theta activity, particularly in the frontal lobe, and excess beta activity—all indicative of a pattern of underarousal and underreactivity in ADHD (Monastra et al., 2001). Children with ADHD have also been found to have smaller amplitudes in the late positive and negative components of their ERPs. These late components are believed to be a function of the prefrontal regions of the brain, are related to poorer performances on inhibition and vigilance tests, and are corrected by stimulant medication (Johnstone, Barry, & Anderson, 2001; Pliszka, Liotti, & Woldorff, 2000). The EEG improvements seen with stimulant medication have been recently shown to be partly a function of the DAT1 gene allele, particularly in its 10-repeat form (Loo et al., 2003), which some studies suggest may be overrepresented in some forms of ADHD (Levy & Hay, 2001).

Several studies have examined cerebral blood flow, using single-photon emission computed tomography, in children with ADHD and control children (see Hendren, De Backer, & Pandina, 2000, for a review). They have consistently shown decreased blood flow to the prefrontal regions (particularly in the right frontal area) and pathways connecting these regions to the limbic system via the striatum (specifically, its anterior region, known as the caudate) and with the cerebellum. Degree of blood flow in the right frontal region has been correlated with behavioral severity of the disorder and with reduced EEG activity, while that in more posterior regions and in the cerebellum seems related to degree of motor impairment (Gustafsson, Thernlund, Ryding, Rosen, & Cederblad, 2000).

Studies using positron emission tomography to assess cerebral glucose metabolism have found diminished metabolism in adults, particularly in the frontal region (Schweitzer et al., 2000; Zametkin et al., 1990) but have been far less consistent with teens and children (for reviews, see Ernst, 1996; Tannock, 1998). Using a radioactive tracer that indicates dopamine activity, Ernst and colleagues (1999) were able to show abnormal dopamine activity in the right midbrain region of children with ADHD; severity of symptoms was correlated with the degree of this abnormality. These demonstrations of an association between the metabolic activity of certain brain regions and symptoms of ADHD and associated executive deficits is critical to proving a connection between the findings pertaining to brain activation and the behaviors constituting ADHD.

Studies using magnetic resonance imaging find differences in the structure (mainly size) of selected brain regions in those with ADHD relative to control groups (Tannock, 1998). These studies have indicated significantly smaller anterior right frontal regions, smaller size of the caudate nucleus, possibly reversed asymmetry in the size of the head of the caudate, and smaller globus pallidus regions in children with ADHD than in control subjects (Aylward et al., 1996; Castellanos et al., 2002; Filipek et al., 1997). Besides reduced size, there is some evidence of reduced neurometabolite activity in the right frontal region (Yeo et al., 2003), with degree of this activity being associated with degree of attention problems on a continuous-performance test. The size of the basal ganglia and right frontal lobe has been shown in other studies as well to correlate with the degree of impairment in inhibition and attention in children with ADHD (Casey et al., 1997; Semrud-Clikeman et al., 2000). Numerous studies (Castellanos et al., 1996, 2001, 2002; Durston et al., 2004) also found smaller cerebellar volume in those with ADHD, especially in a central region known as the vermis. This would be consistent with the view that the cerebellum plays a major role in executive functioning and the motor presetting aspects of sensory perception that derive from planning and other executive actions (Diamond, 2000), and that these functions may be deficient in children with ADHD.

Studies using functional MRI find children with ADHD to have different patterns of activation during attention and inhibition tasks from those of control children, particularly in the right prefrontal region, the basal ganglia (striatum and putamen), and the cerebellum (Rubia et al., 1999; Teicher et al., 2000; Vaidya et al., 1998; Yeo et al., 2003). Again, the demonstrated linkage of brain structure and function with psychological measures of ADHD symptoms and executive deficits is exceptionally important in such research, to permit causal inferences to be made about the role of these brain abnormalities in the cognitive and behavioral deficits constituting ADHD. A recent study (Durston et al., 2004) suggests that the reduced size of the brain (about 3–5%), particularly in the right frontal area, found in ADHD may be evident as well in siblings without ADHD; perhaps this is consistent with the increased familial risk for the disorder and a spectrum of the phenotype for ADHD within these families. But the reduced volume of the cerebellum was also found to be specific to the children with ADHD and was not evident in the unaffected siblings, implying that this region may be directly related to the pathophysiology of the disorder.

Possible neurotransmitter dysfunction or imbalances in ADHD have been proposed for quite some time (see Pliszka, McCracken, & Maas, 1996, for a review). Initially, these rested chiefly on the responses of children with ADHD to dopamine and norepinephrine reuptake inhibitors, such as methylphenidate and atomoxetine, respectively. Medications such as these are reviewed in detail later in this chapter. For present purposes, suffice it to say that studies have used blood and urinary metabolites of brain neurotransmitters to infer deficiencies in ADHD, largely related to dopamine regulation (Halperin et al., 1997). What limited evidence there is from this literature seems to point to a selective deficiency in the availability of both dopamine and norepinephrine, but this evidence cannot be considered conclusive at this time.

Pregnancy and Birth Complications

Some studies have found a greater incidence of pregnancy or birth complications for children with ADHD than for control children. For instance, Claycomb, Ryan, Miller, and

Schnakenburg-Ott (2004) found that mother's age at delivery (younger), educational level (lower), time between onset of labor and birth (longer), and presence of delivery complications accounted for 42% of the variance in ADHD. The study, however, did not control for maternal ADHD symptoms, which may have resulted in the younger age at delivery and lower educational level of the mothers. The latter maternal characteristics may simply be markers for maternal ADHD and so might explain their being associated with child ADHD.

Prematurity has been associated with later risk for ADHD (Breslau et al., 1996; Schothorst & van Engeland, 1996). After controlling for other factors that may be associated with low birthweight and ADHD (maternal smoking, alcohol use, ADHD, socioeconomic status, etc.), Mick, Biederman, Faraone, Sayer, and Kleinman (2002) continued to find low birthweight to be three times more common in children with ADHD than in control children, perhaps accounting for nearly 14% of all ADHD diagnoses. Thus low birthweight associated with prematurity may be a particularly salient marker for later ADHD. Furthermore, the extent of white matter abnormalities due to birth injuries, such as parenchymal lesions and/or ventricular enlargement, seems especially contributory to later ADHD among prematurely born babies (Whittaker et al., 1997). Several studies suggest that mothers of children with ADHD are younger when they conceive these children than are mothers of control children, and that such pregnancies may have a greater risk of adversity (Claycomb et al., 2004; Denson, Nanson, & McWatters, 1975; Hartsough & Lambert, 1985).

GENETIC FACTORS

Evidence for a genetic basis to ADHD is now overwhelming and comes from three sources: family studies, twin studies, and (most recently) molecular genetic studies identifying individual candidate genes. Nearly all of this research applies to the combined type of ADHD, and most of it has occurred with children rather than adolescents. Between 10% and 35% of the immediate family members of children with ADHD are also likely to have the disorder, with the risk to siblings of these children being approximately 32% (Levy & Hay, 2001). If a parent has ADHD, the risk to the offspring is 57% (Biederman et al., 1995). These elevated rates of disorders have also been noted in African American samples with ADHD (Samuel et al., 1999), as well as in girls with ADHD compared to boys (Faraone & Doyle, 2001). Some research suggests that ADHD with CD may be a distinct familial subtype of ADHD (Faraone, Biederman, Mennin, Russell, & Tsuang, 1998). Using sibling pairs in which both siblings had ADHD, Smalley and colleagues (2000) have also recently supported this view through findings that CD significantly clusters among the families of only those pairs having CD. Some research has also suggested that females who manifest ADHD may need to have a greater genetic loading (higher family member prevalence) than do males with ADHD (Smalley et al., 2000; Faraone & Doyle, 2001).

Twin studies of ADHD and its behavioral dimensions have proven strikingly consistent. Large twin studies have found a very high degree of heritability for ADHD, ranging from .75 to .97 (for reviews, see Levy & Hay, 2001; Thapar, 1999; see also Coolidge et al., 2000; Kuntsi & Stevenson, 2000). The average heritability of ADHD (degree of variance in the trait due to genetic effects) is at least .80. This is about the same as that for human height (.80–.91), and higher than that found for intelligence (.55–.70) or the major personality traits (.40–.50). These studies consistently find little if any effect for shared (rearing) environment on the traits of ADHD; this refutes any effort to attribute ADHD to poor parenting, family diet, household television exposure, or other popularly held causes of the disorder.

The twin studies have sometimes found a small significant contribution for unique (nonshared) environmental events. Factors in the nonshared environment are those events or conditions that have uniquely affected only one twin or child in a family and not others. Such unique factors not only include those typically thought of as involving the social environment (differing schools, peer groups, etc.), but also all biological factors that are nongenetic in origin (lead poisoning, head injury, etc.). Approximately 9–20% of the variance in hyperactive–impulsive–inattentive behavior or ADHD symptoms can be attributed to such nonshared environmental (nongenetic) factors (Levy & Hay, 2001). If researchers are interested in identifying environmental contributors to ADHD, these twin studies suggest that such researchers should focus on those biological, interactional, and social experiences that are specific and unique to the individual and are not part of the common family environment to which other siblings have been exposed.

Most investigators suspect that multiple genes contribute to risk for the disorder, given the complexity of the traits underlying ADHD and their dimensional nature. The dopamine transporter gene (DAT1) has been implicated (Cook, Stein, & Leventhal, 1997), but has not been consistently associated with the disorder (Swanson et al., 1997). Another gene related to dopamine, the DRD4 (repeater gene), has been the most reliably found in samples of children with ADHD (Faraone et al., 1999). The 7-repeat or longer forms (alleles) of this gene are the ones that have been found to be over-represented in children with ADHD (Lahoste et al., 1996). This gene has previously been associated with the personality trait of high novelty-seeking behavior, affects pharmacological responsiveness, and has an impact on post-synaptic sensitivity (primarily in frontal and prefrontal cortical regions) (Swanson et al., 1997). More recently, the long allele of the DBH gene has also been implicated in Barkley and Fischer's Milwaukee longitudinal study of hyperactive children followed to adulthood (Mueller et al., 2003).

Environmental Toxins

As noted above, variance in the expression of ADHD that may be due to environmental sources means variance attributable to all non-genetic sources more generally. These include pre-, peri-, and postnatal complications; malnutrition; diseases; trauma; toxin exposure; and other neurologically compromising events that may occur during the development of the nervous system before and after birth. Such events are likely to happen to one child in a family but not to others, and so they probably fall under the unique or nonshared variance found in twin studies to have some significant association with the variation of ADHD symptoms in the population. Among these various biologically compromising events, several have been repeatedly linked to risks for inattention and hyperactive behavior. One such factor is exposure to environmental toxins, and one such toxin is lead (Needleman, Schell, Bellinger, Leviton, & Alfred, 1990). But an even stronger case has been subsequently made for

prenatal exposure to alcohol and tobacco (Maughan, Taylor, Taylor, Butler, & Bynner, 2001; Mick et al., 2002; Milberger, Biederman, Faraone, Chen, & Jones, 1996; Streissguth, Bookstein, Sampson, & Barr, 1995). The relationship between maternal smoking during pregnancy and ADHD remains significant even after symptoms of ADHD in the parent are controlled for (Mick et al., 2002; Milberger et al., 1996), and maternal smoking shows the strongest association with risk for ADHD, whereas maternal alcohol consumption has been less reliably documented as a risk factor (Linnet et al., 2003).

CONCEPTUALIZATION OF THE DISORDER

Until recently, ADHD has lacked a reasonably credible scientific theory to explain its basic nature and associated symptoms, and to link it with typical developmental processes. Consequently, the vast majority of research into the treatment of ADHD has remained exploratory or descriptive in nature, rather than being based on any theory of the disorder. Treatments were tried principally because they had shown some efficacy for other disorders (e.g., behavior modification for mental retardation) or were discovered to have beneficial effects primarily by accident (e.g., stimulant medications). Thus treatment decisions have not been guided so much by a scientific theory but by pragmatics; whatever seems to work is retained, and whatever doesn't is discarded, with little guidance from any sound theoretical rationale.

The field of ADHD has reached a point, however, where the neuropsychological, neuroimaging, and genetic studies cited above are coming to set clear limits on theorizing not only about the origins of ADHD, but about its nature as well. Any credible theory on the nature of ADHD must now posit neuropsychological constructs that are related to the typical development of inhibition, self-regulation, and executive functioning, and must explain how these may go awry in ADHD. And such a theory will need to argue that these constructs arise from the functions of the prefrontal–striatal network and its interconnections with other brain regions that appear to subserve the executive functions and self-control, such as the cerebellum. Those cognitive functions will be shown to have a substantial hereditary contribution to individual differences in them, given the results of twin studies on the genetic contribution to variation in ADHD symptoms.

Barkley has been working on just such a theoretical conceptualization of ADHD for well over 10 years (see Barkley, 1997a, 2006). It is briefly discussed below, followed by its implications for the management of ADHD. Research continues on the merits of this model for ADHD, but we include it here because of its far greater implications for treatment than any prior theories founded solely on ADHD arising from deficits in response inhibition (Quay, 1997), delay aversion (Sonuga-Barke, Taylor, & Hepinstall, 1992), or arousal and energetic pools (Sergeant & van der Meere, 1988, 1994).

The model is founded on the premise that ADHD consists mainly of a developmental delay in behavioral inhibition that disrupts self-regulation—an assertion for which there is substantial research support (see Barkley, 1997a; Nigg, 2001; Nigg, Goldsmith, & Sachek, 2004). This theory links behavioral inhibition to the executive functions and shows them to provide for self-regulation. Behavioral inhibition occupies a foundation in relationship to four other executive functions that are dependent upon it for their own effective execution. "Self-regulation" is defined as any self-directed action used to change one's own behavior so as to alter the probability of a delayed (future) consequence. The executive functions are seen as forms of "behavior to the self"—the actions one uses to change oneself so as to change the future.

Four executive functions are theorized to exist and to permit self-regulation—bringing behavior (motor control) progressively more under the control of internally represented information (forms of self-directed action), time, and the probable future, and wresting it from control by the immediate external context and temporal now. Such self-control functions to maximize future consequences for the individual over merely immediate ones. The model applies only to the combined type of ADHD to date.

"Behavioral inhibition" involves, first, the capacity to inhibit prepotent responses, creating a delay in the response to an event (response inhibition). There may be two other inhibitory processes related to it; at least for the moment, Barkley has combined these into a single construct concerning inhibition. These two other processes are the capacity to inter-

rupt ongoing responses given feedback about performance, particularly those response patterns that are proving ineffective; and the protection of this delay in responding, of the self-directed actions occurring within it, and of the goal-directed behaviors they create from interference by competing events and their prepotent responses (interference control). Through the postponement of the prepotent response and the creation of this protected period of delay, the occasion is set for the four executive functions (covert, self-directed actions) to act effectively in modifying the individual's eventual response(s) to the event. The chain of goal-directed, temporally governed, and future-oriented behaviors set in motion by these acts of self-regulation is then protected during performance by interference control. And even if the chain is disrupted, the individual retains the capacity or intention (via working memory) to return to the goal-directed actions until the outcome is successfully achieved or judged to be no longer necessary. The four executive functions are listed below, first by their more common labels in the neuropsychological literature, and then by Barkley's redefinitions of the self-directed actions comprising them (in parentheses).

1. *Nonverbal working memory (covert self-directed sensing).* "Nonverbal working memory" is the ability to maintain mental information online that will be used subsequently to control a motor response. These prolonged mental representations of events, achieved by covertly sensing to the self, serve to recall past events for the sake of preparing a current response; they represent "hindsight" or the "retrospective function" of working memory (Fuster, 1997). The chief forms of sensing that are being self-directed are visual imagery and private audition, or rehearing. Individuals are reactivating and using the images and sounds (and other sensory information) associated with past events to guide present- and future-directed behavior.

Past events are retained in a temporal sequence, and this sequence has been shown to contribute to the subjective estimation of psychological time (Michon, 1985). Analysis of temporal sequences of events for recurring patterns can be used to conjecture hypothetical future events—the individual's best guess as to what may happen next or later in time, based on the detection of recurring patterns in past event sequences. This extension of hindsight forward into time also creates "forethought" or the "prospective function" of working memory, forming a temporally symmetrical counterpart to the retrospective function of hindsight (Fuster, 1997). And from this sense of the future probably emerges the increasing valuation of future consequences over immediate ones that takes place throughout child development into young adult life (Green, Fry, & Meyerson, 1994).

This self-directed sensing (seeing the past so as to see the future) gives rise to hindsight and forethought, thereby permitting the individual to create a preparation or intention to act, called an "anticipatory set" (Fuster, 1997). In so doing, individuals are now capable of the cross-temporal organization of behavior—that is, the linking of events, responses, and their eventual consequences via their representation in working memory, despite what may be considerable gaps among them in real time. Thus self-regulation relative to time arises, at least initially, as a consequence of nonverbal working memory and the internally represented information it provides for the control and guidance of behavior over time.

2. *Verbal working memory (internalized, self-directed speech).* During the early preschool years, speech, once developed, is initially employed for communication with others. Language is now not just a means of influencing the behavior of others, but a means of reflection (self-directed description) as well as a means for controlling one's own behavior (Berk, 1992, 1994; Diaz & Berk, 1992). Self-directed speech progresses from being public, to being subvocal, to finally being private, all over the course of perhaps 6–10 years. With this progressive privatization of speech comes the increasing control it permits over behavior. Self-speech now provides a tremendously increased capacity for self-control, planfulness, and goal-directed behavior, which augments that being provided by the first executive function, self-directed imagery and hearing.

3. *Self-regulation of affect/motivation/ arousal (self-directed emotion).* The occasion is now set for the self-regulation of affect, motivation, and arousal through the use of the first two executive abilities (self-sensing and self-speech). Individuals now possess the capacity to present images (and other sensory information), along with words to themselves that can be used to manipulate emotional states. This is because images and other sensory information from the past come automatically with emotional valences welded to them (i.e., the ways we felt about them) (Damasio, 1995). Yet it is not just affect that is being managed by the use of self-speech and self-sensing (especially imagery). Emotion is, by definition, a motivational state. And so this re-presenting of words and images to the self creates a capacity for self-motivation (Fuster, 1997), because emotion and motivation are inherently linked (Ekman & Davidson, 1994; Lang, 1995). By privately manipulating and modulating emotional and motivational states, a child can induce drive or motivational states that may be required for the initiation and maintenance of goal-directed behavior (Barkley, 1997a).

4. *Planning or reconstitution (self-directed play).* Bronowski (1977) reasoned that the use of images and language to represent the objects, the actions, and their properties that exist in the world around us provides a means by which the world can be taken apart into pieces. These pieces can then be combined to create novel recombinations. Internal speech and imagery permit "analysis" (taking apart), and out of this process comes its complement, "synthesis" (recombination), to create entirely new ideas about the world (Bronowski, 1977) and entirely new responses to that world. The analysis–synthesis process provides a means to create novel behavioral sequences in the service of problem solving and goal-directed action, particularly when obstacles are encountered in pursuit of a goal and new behaviors must be generated to solve the problem (Barkley, 1997a; Fuster, 1997). Barkley has hypothesized that, like the other executive functions, this one is also a form of self-directed behavior that, like the internalization of speech, becomes turned on the self during development and is eventually privatized.

The development of increasingly more powerful executive functions during maturation protects increasingly lengthy, complex, hierarchically organized, and novel chains of goal-directed behavior, from being disrupted by interference. This is achieved by generating internally represented information that serves to take over the control of behavior from the moment and immediate setting and direct behavior toward time and the probable or anticipated future. Such internal control over behavior creates not only a greater purposeful-ness or intentionality to behavior, but also a greater flexibility. The executive functions grant behavior a more determined, persistent, reasoned, intentional, and purposive quality, while also permitting greater shifting of behavior as needed to achieve one's goals—an appearance of volition, choice, and will arising from internally guided behavior (James, 1890/1950).

The impairment in behavioral inhibition occurring in ADHD is hypothesized to disrupt the efficient execution of these executive functions, thereby limiting the capacity for self-regulation they provide. The result is impairment in the cross-temporal organization of behavior and in the guidance and control of behavior by internally represented information. This inevitably leads to a reduction in the maximization of long-term consequences for the individual. In other words, individuals with ADHD have temporal myopia such that they do not readily recognize long-term consequences and therefore overfocus on relatively immediate outcomes. This theory, if correct, provides a much deeper insight into the nature of ADHD and a much broader perspective on its likely impairments, along with a litany of implications for its management (see below). In essence, ADHD is not so much an attention disorder from this perspective as it is a disorder of executive functioning—of internally guided and regulated behavior across time and toward future events. It leaves the individual to be more affected by external events of the moment, and more governed by concerns for immediate than for delayed gratification.

TREATMENT APPROACHES

Research on the treatment of ADHD over the past decade has focused largely on evaluating multimodal treatment packages (MTA Cooperative Group, 1999a, 2004a). The primary innovations have been the development of new delivery systems within psychopharmacology and even of new drugs, rather than the development of new psychosocial treatments. This is not to say that more information on the prevailing psychosocial treatments has not been gained over this decade; this is hardly the case. It is to say that no significant breakthroughs in the psychosocial treatment of the disorder have been forthcoming. Most of the psychosocial treatment research has served to clarify the effi-

cacy (or lack of it) of already extant treatment approaches, or their combinations.

A major problem in the ADHD treatment literature is a lack of documentation of long-term treatment effectiveness. Almost all of the research has focused on short-term effects (i.e., within 3 months), with a few studies providing intervention for up to 14 months (MTA Cooperative Group, 1999a; Shelton et al., 2000) and follow-up evaluations for several years thereafter (Barkley, Shelton, et al., 2002; MTA Cooperative Group, 2004a). Thus, at the time of the preceding edition of this book, long-term effects beyond a few years had been largely unstudied. This situation has since been remedied somewhat by the Multimodal Treatment Study of ADHD, commonly called the MTA (MTA Cooperative Group, 1999a, 2004a), and by the New York–Montreal (NYM) multimodal treatment study (Abikoff, Hechtman, Klein, Gallacher, et al., 2004; Abikoff, Hechtman, Klein, Weiss, et al., 2004; Hechtman, Abikoff, Klein, Greenfield, et al., 2004; Hechtman, Abikoff, Klein, Weiss, et al., 2004). The results of the 24-month follow-ups for both projects were published in the spring of 2004. These long-term studies have provided some important insights about treatment, and especially about the efficacy of combining psychosocial and pharmacological treatment.

Another concern regarding the treatment research on ADHD has been that despite consistent findings of improvement in core symptoms of ADHD, there have been few reports of psychosocial treatment effects on key indicators of functioning, such as academic achievement or social skills. For any treatment of ADHD to be considered truly effective, there needs to be documentation of its long-term effectiveness on key ecological indicators of functioning in major life activities (school grades, sustained peer relations, etc.). Again, this situation has been somewhat remedied by the MTA project and, to a lesser extent, by the NYM study. Although the former study seems to suggest some minor benefits of multimodal (combined medication and psychosocial) treatment for ADHD, the latter study found no such advantage. Because of the MTA's methodological advantages (to be described later in this chapter), we posit that more weight should be given to the MTA results than to those of the NYM study. Nevertheless, the NYM study has provided some important insights into the evaluation of long-term effects of treatments for children with ADHD.

Before we venture into a more detailed discussion of the efficacy of specific treatments for ADHD, it will be helpful to reexamine some traditional assumptions about the treatment of this disorder. They are being called into question by the theoretical model of Barkley (discussed above), as well as by the results of research on etiologies and on the efficacy of particular treatments.

Reexamining Treatment Assumptions

Advances in research on the etiologies of ADHD and in theoretical models about the disorder seem to suggest why few treatment breakthroughs, especially in the psychosocial arena, have occurred. The information yielded from these sources points increasingly to ADHD as being a developmental disorder of probable neurogenetic origins in which some unique environmental factors play a role in the expression of the disorder, though a far smaller role than genetic ones play. Therefore, unless new treatments address the underlying neurological substrates or genetic mechanisms that are contributing so strongly to it, the treatments will have fleeting or minimal impact on remedying this disorder.

We are not suggesting that prevention of ADHD is an impossible goal. For instance, some have suggested that reshaping the environments of young preschoolers, such as by limiting television watching, might help to prevent some cases of ADHD (Christakis, Zimmerman, DiGiuseppe, & McCarty, 2004). However, we doubt that this will prove effective, given that there are serious questions concerning the direction of causality in such correlational findings (Barkley, 2004a). Others have made a more compelling case for the reduction of environmental lead, given the contribution of lead poisoning before age 3 years to the risk for later ADHD (Needleman et al., 1990). Certainly the reduction of maternal use of alcohol and tobacco products during pregnancy would seem to be useful, in view of the linkages noted earlier between these fetal neurotoxins and risk for ADHD in the offspring of pregnancies affected by them. This type of preventive research and related interventions should be encouraged. However, this is a chapter on treatment—and by the time individuals meet diagnostic criteria for ADHD, we believe that

they are on a chronic course and need to be treated accordingly. Therefore, the treatment of ADHD is actually management of a chronic developmental condition. As such, it involves finding means to cope with, compensate for, and accommodate to the developmental deficiencies, so as to reduce the numerous secondary harms that can accrue from the unmanaged disorder. These means also include the provision of symptomatic relief, such as that obtained with various medications.

Given the relatively greater contribution of genotype than of environment to explaining individual differences in the symptoms of the disorder, it is highly likely that treatments for ADHD, while providing improvements in the symptoms, do little to change the relative rank ordering of such individuals in their posttreatment levels of ADHD (for general discussions of this issue in developmental psychology and clinical interventions, see Rutter, 1997; Scarr, 1992; Scarr & McCartney, 1983). It is also likely that such treatments, particularly in the psychosocial realm, will prove to be specific to the treatment setting; that is, minimal generalization will occur unless generalization to other settings is actively planned for and encouraged.

Some psychosocial treatments for ADHD may have carryover effects, mostly in the form of parents' or teachers' providing external structure that ameliorates ADHD-related symptoms. Ideally, these environmental adjustments will alter the developmental trajectory of a child or adolescent with ADHD. However, such interventions are not expected to produce fundamental changes in the underlying deficits of ADHD; they only prevent an accumulation of failures and problems secondary to ADHD. Thus researchers and clinicians should anticipate that long-term studies are more likely to find treatment effects on problems secondary to ADHD than on deficits specific to ADHD.

The results of the MTA project lend some support to the assertions above. For instance, this study has found stronger treatment effects on core symptoms of ADHD during the intensive phases of treatment. Also, the trend in the follow-up seems to be toward showing advantages of combined pharmacological and psychosocial treatment on constructs other than core symptoms of ADHD. However, such findings were not evident in the 24-month follow-up of the NYM study (Abikoff, Hechtman, Klein, Weiss, et al., 2004;

Hechtman, Abikoff, Klein, Weiss, et al., 2004). One possible explanation for the difference is that the psychosocial treatments in the MTA were much more intensive, whereas the efficacy of the psychosocial treatments used in the NYM study was not established by the authors (this is discussed in greater detail later in the chapter). Thus only strong, empirically supported treatments might be expected to have the kind of carryover effects discussed above.

The theoretical model of ADHD described earlier suggests other reasons why treatment effects may be so limited. According to this model, ADHD does not result from a lack of skill, knowledge, or information; therefore, it will not respond well to interventions emphasizing the transfer of knowledge or of skills, as might occur in psychotherapy, social skills training, cognitive therapies, or academic tutoring. Instead, in Barkley's (2006) model, ADHD is viewed as a disorder of performance—not doing what one knows, rather than not knowing what to do. Like patients with injuries to the frontal lobes, those with ADHD find that intellect has been partially cleaved or dissociated from action, or knowledge from performance. Thus individuals with ADHD may know how to act, but may not act that way when placed in social settings where such action would be beneficial to them. The timing and timeliness of behavior are also disrupted more in ADHD than the basic knowledge or skill about that behavior is.

From this vantage point, treatments for ADHD will be most helpful when they assist with the execution of a particular behavior at the *point of performance* in the natural environments where and when such behavior should be performed. A corollary of this is that the further away in space and time a treatment is from this point of performance, the less effective it is likely to be in assisting with the management of ADHD (Goldstein & Ingersoll, 1993). Not only is assistance at the point of performance going to prove critical to treatment efficacy, but so is assistance with the time, timing, and timeliness of behavior in those with ADHD, not just in the training of the behavior itself (Barkley, 2006). Nor will there necessarily be any lasting value or maintenance of treatment effects from such assistance, if it is summarily removed within a short period of time once the individual is performing the desired behavior. The value of such treatments lies not only in providing assistance with eliciting be-havior that is already likely to be in the individual's repertoire at the point of performance where its display is critical, but in maintaining the performance of that behavior over time in that natural setting.

ADHD and other disorders of performance thus pose great challenges for mental health and educational services. At the core of such problems is the vexing issue of how to get people to behave in ways that they know are good for them, but that they seem unlikely, unable, or unwilling to perform. Conveying more knowledge does not prove as helpful as altering the motivational parameters associated with the performance of that behavior at its appropriate point of performance. Coupled with this is the realization that such changes in behavior are maintained only as long as those environmental adjustments or accommodations are maintained as well. To expect otherwise would seem to approach the treatment of ADHD with outdated or misguided assumptions about its essential nature.

The conceptual model of ADHD introduced above brings with it many other implications for the management of ADHD (see Barkley, 2006). Some of these are briefly mentioned here:

1. If the process of regulating behavior by internally represented forms of information (working memory or the internalization of behavior) is delayed in those with ADHD, then they will be best assisted by "externalizing" those forms of information; the provision of physical representations of that information will be needed in the setting at the point of performance. Since covert or private information is weak as a source of stimulus control, making that information overt and public may assist with strengthening control of behavior by that information.

2. Disrupted organization of an individual's behavior both within and across time is one of the ultimate disabilities caused by the disorder. ADHD is to time what nearsightedness is to spatial vision; it creates a temporal myopia in which the individual's behavior is governed even more than usual by events close to or within the temporal now and the immediate context, rather than by internal information that pertains to longer-term, future events. It may thus be possible to assist those with ADHD by making time itself more externally represented; by reducing or eliminating gaps in

time among the components of a behavioral contingency (event, response, outcome); and by working to bridge such temporal gaps related to future events, with the assistance of caregivers and others.

3. Given that the model hypothesizes a deficit in the internally generated and represented forms of motivation that are needed to drive goal-directed behavior, those with ADHD will require the provision of externalized sources of motivation. For instance, the provision of artificial rewards, such as tokens, may be needed throughout the performance of a task or other goal-directed behavior when there are otherwise few or no such immediate consequences associated with that performance. Such artificial reward programs become for children with ADHD like prosthetic devices (braces, mechanical limbs, etc.) for children with physical disabilities—allowing them to perform more effectively in some tasks and settings with which they otherwise would have considerable difficulty. The motivational disability created by ADHD makes such "motivational prostheses" nearly essential for most children with the disorder.

4. Given the above-listed considerations, parents and teachers should reject any approach to intervention for ADHD that does not involve helping them provide a child or adolescent with an active intervention at the point of performance. Many parents and teachers seek what might be called the "garage mechanic approach." According to this model, a child can be dropped off someplace and be "fixed" by the "mechanic" without the parents' or teachers' "getting their hands dirty." Such an approach is untenable, and a hands-on approach to intervention is strongly recommended. This is true for all interventions, including pharmacotherapy.

Trends in Treatment Provision

The provision of treatment services to children with ADHD has increased dramatically over the past 20 years, owing in large part to four national trends: (1) the recognition by special education laws (circa 1991) that ADHD is eligible for identification as a disability and for specialized services in public schools; (2) the growth of formally organized advocacy groups (such as Children and Adults with ADHD; see www.chadd.org) in the late 1980s; (3) the growth of advertising and educational efforts

by pharmaceutical companies promoting new stimulant delivery systems, and more recently new types of medication, for the management of ADHD; and (4) increased continuing education programs for educational and mental health professionals on the disorder. For instance, between 1986 and 1996, stimulant prescriptions for ADHD increased to such an extent that they accounted for three-fourths of all physician visits for children with ADHD; a 10-fold increase in related services such as health counseling, and a 3-fold increase in diagnostic services, were also found (Hoagwood, Kelleher, Feil, & Comer, 2000). Nevertheless, this report also documented a decline in the use of follow-up care, apparently due to insurance obstacles, lengthy waiting lists, and limited access to pediatric specialists. Treatment appears to be increasingly provided by primary care professionals, who are likely to utilize only medication management. Only a third of children with ADHD are being referred to and treated by mental health professionals (Bussing, Zima, & Belin, 1998). Those who are referred to specialists are more likely to have comorbid disorders, greater impairment, and greater family burdens.

We now present the major treatment approaches employed with ADHD that have some scientifically established effectiveness. These include (1) psychopharmacology; (2) parent training in child behavior (contingency) management methods; (3) teacher implementation of these and other child behavior management tactics; and (4) combinations of these approaches into multimodal therapy programs. As part of our discussion of these combined approaches, we give special consideration to the historic MTA project and its results. Given the weaknesses inherent in any single treatment modality, the multimodal approach is preferred here for treating most cases of ADHD, because of the inability of medication to provide adequate help for all children with ADHD—especially those with coexisting disorders, such as learning disabilities, anxiety, depression, or CD.

Psychopharmacology

Research suggests that the three most commonly used drugs for the management of ADHD symptoms are the stimulants, the antidepressants, and the antihypertensives (Zito et al., 2003). Until recently, however, use of each of these types of medications has been founded on virtual chance discoveries of their effectiveness, and not as yet on any theoretical rationale (Bradley, 1937; Winsberg, Bialer, Kupietz, & Tobias, 1972). A rationale may be emerging, though, in view of recent theoretical models (see above) that emphasize poor behavioral inhibition as probably being central to the nature of the disorder. Brain regions subserving inhibition appear to be involved in the etiology of ADHD; these regions are largely dopaminergic, and stimulants (which increase extracellular dopamine) seem to produce their greatest effects within these same brain regions (Volkow et al., 1995, 1997). Atomoxetine increases extracellular norepinephrine but produces an indirect increase in dopamine in the prefrontal cortex, which may also explain its therapeutic benefit.

Until recently, it was not clear precisely how these medications affected brain function, and particularly what their sites and neurochemical modes of action were. It now appears as if the major therapeutic effects of the drugs are achieved through alterations in frontal–striatal activity (Volkow et al., 1997), via their impact on at least three or more neurotransmitters important to the functioning of this region and related to response inhibition—these being dopamine, norepinephrine, and epinephrine (Pliszka et al., 1996). The direct rationale, then, for employing some medications with children with ADHD may be that they directly (if only temporarily) improve the deficiencies in these neural systems related to behavioral inhibition and self-regulation.

Stimulant Medication

Since Bradley (1937) first accidentally discovered their successful use for children with behavior problems, the stimulants have received an enormous amount of research (Greenhill, Halperin, & Abikoff, 1999). Meta-analyses indicate that stimulants provide a clear benefit in managing the disorder in the short term (Schachter, Pham, King, Langford, & Moher, 2001), and some continuing benefit in symptomatic management (but not necessarily academic achievement) in the long term (Schachar et al., 2002). As long as clients comply with treatment, benefits can be found over as long as 5 years (Charach, Ickowicz, & Schachar, 2004). The results of research on

stimulants indicate overwhelmingly that these medications are quite effective for the management of ADHD symptoms in most children older than 5 years (Connor, 2006b; Greenhill & Osman, 1991; Solanto, Arnsten, & Castellanos, 2001). For youngsters between 4 and 5 years of age, the drugs are equally as effective as in older children (Connor, 2002), with some 82% of cases responding positively (Short, Manos, Findling, & Schubel, 2004). The drugs are not recommended for use with children under 3 years of age, however, as little or nothing is known about medication effects in this age group. Guidelines for the use of stimulant medications for children with ADHD have been issued by both the American Academy of Pediatrics (2001) and the American Academy of Child and Adolescent Psychiatry (2002).

Research by Safer, Zito, and colleagues has documented dramatic increases in the overall rate of stimulant medication use among children and adolescents with ADHD (e.g., Zito et al., 2003). During the 1990s, stimulant prescription rates more than tripled. This is part of a general boom in the diagnosis and treatment of ADHD. For example, as noted earlier, surveys comparing physician practices in 1986 and 1999 found a 3-fold increase in diagnoses of ADHD and a 10-fold increase in treatment services for ADHD (Hoagwood et al., 2000). Comparing 1987 with 1997 records in the National Medical Expenditure Survey, Olfson, Gameroff, Marcus, and Jensen (2003) documented a marked expansion of access to treatment among children with ADHD, from 0.9 per 100 children to 3.4 per 100 receiving outpatient treatment. Despite this improvement in access to care, there was a decline in the intensity of treatment, as determined by number of visits and forms of treatment recommended other than medication. The authors interpret these changes as probably arising from increased access to special education services during this period, the growth of managed health care and its emphasis on brief visits and treatments, and increased public acceptance of medication use for the disorder.

The most rapid expansion of stimulant use has been with preschoolers (Zito et al., 2003), with low-income children (Olfson et al., 2003), and with adolescents (Olfson et al., 2003; Safer, Zito, & Fine, 1996), most likely due to these groups' having been markedly undertreated in prior years relative to elementary-age and to middle- and upper-income children. By the end of the 1990s, several studies concluded that 2–6% of American school children (ages 5–15) had been treated with stimulants (Greydanus, Pratt, Sloane, & Rappley, 2003), with the largest databases placing the figure at 1.3–3.8% (Jensen et al., 1999; Safer & Malever, 2000; Zito et al., 2003) by the late 1990s. Thus there is clearly a strong trend toward increased use of stimulants, but the exact rate of stimulant use is hard to describe, for various reasons: the rapid rate of change, widely varied use among various providers and communities, and the lack of any national database that might address the issue.

The most commonly prescribed stimulants are shown in Table 2.2. They include methylphenidate (e.g., Ritalin), dextroamphetamine (e.g., Dexedrine), and a combination of amphetamine salts marketed under the name Adderall. Some other stimulants are on the market, including pemoline and various types of amphetamines, but these are infrequently prescribed. Because methylphenidate and the

amphetamines share similar characteristics, these drugs are discussed collectively in this section. By virtue of its unique chemical properties and some unique risks, pemoline is discussed separately.

Methylphenidate and amphetamines are rapidly acting stimulants. In their immediate-release formulations, the stimulants produce effects on behavior within 30–45 minutes after oral ingestion and peak in their behavioral effects within 2–4 hours (Connor, 2006b). The utility of these immediate-release formulations in managing behavior quickly dissipates within 3–7 hours, although minuscule amounts of the medications may remain in the blood for up to 24 hours (Greenhill & Osman, 1991; Solanto et al., 2001). Because of their short halflife, they are often prescribed in twice- or thrice-daily doses. Claims that Adderall lasts longer than methylphenidate and the other stimulants have not been fully substantiated, and dosing protocols for Adderall often involve twice-daily administration (Greydanus et al., 2003).

TABLE 2.2. Stimulant Preparations for ADHD

Preparation	Active agent	Dose availability	Dosing schedule
Immediate-release for 4- to 6-hour coverage			
Adderall tablets	Neutral sulfate salts of dextroamphetamine saccharate and dextro,levoamphetamine aspartate	5, 7.5, 10, 12.5 15, 20, 30 mg	b.i.d. to t.i.d.
Desoxyn tablets[a]	Methamphetamine HCl	5 mg	b.i.d. to t.i.d.
Dexedrine tablets	Dextroamphetamine sulfate	5 mg	b.i.d. to t.i.d.
Dextrostat tablets	Dextroamphetamine sulfate	5, 10 mg	b.i.d. to t.i.d.
Focalin tablets	Dexmethylphenidate HCl	2.5, 5, 10 mg	b.i.d. to t.i.d.
Ritalin HCl tablets	Methylphenidate HCl	5, 10, 20 mg	b.i.d. to t.i.d.
Intermediate-acting for 8-hour coverage			
Dexedrine spansule	Dextroamphetamine sustained-release	5, 10, 15 mg	b.i.d.
Metadate CD	Methylphenidate HCl extended-release	20 mg	b.i.d.
Metadate ER	Methylphenidate HCl extended-release	10, 20 mg	b.i.d.
Ritalin SR	Methylphenidate HCl sustained-release	20 mg	b.i.d.
Long-acting for 10- to 12-hour coverage			
Adderall XR capsules	Neutral salts of dextroamphetamine and amphetamine with dextroamphetamine saccharate and dextro,levoamphetamine aspartate monohydrate extended-release	5, 10, 15, 20, 25, 30 mg	q.d. A.M.
Concerta tablets	Methylphenidate HCl extended-release	18, 27, 36, 54 mg	q.d. A.M.

Note. b.i.d., twice a day; t.i.d., three times a day; g.d., every day (once a day).
From Connor (2006a). Copyright 2006 by The Guilford Press. Reprinted by permission.
[a]High abuse potential.

An important recent development in the treatment of ADHD is the availability of effective extended-release forms of methylphenidate. These do not represent new drugs, but new delivery systems for sustaining blood levels of a drug over longer periods, so as to reduce dosing to once per day where possible. Intermediate-duration versions of methylphenidate that have therapeutic effects for 6–8 hours include Ritalin SR, Metadate ER, Methylin ER, Ritalin LA, and Metadate CD. Adderall is considered by some to be an intermediate duration stimulant. Once-daily stimulants include Dexedrine spansules (dextroamphetamine), Concerta (oral-osmotic-release [OROS] methylphenidate), and Adderall XR (a mixture of dextro- and levoamphetamines) that may last up to 12 hours.

There is some variability in the effectiveness of these longer-acting preparations. For example, the initial version of sustained-release methylphenidate (Ritalin SR) had erratic effects on some children (Greydanus et al., 2003) and often reduced therapeutic efficacy relative to immediate-release forms of the medication, resulting from a truncation of the peak blood level below that required for an acceptable treatment response. This limitation has been overcome in the recently approved extended-release preparations, such as Concerta, Metadate CD, and Adderall XR. Another unique feature of some of these new delivery packages, such as Concerta, is that they provide a steady increase in the amount of medicine delivered during the day, thus overcoming problems with diminished effect later in the day. Possibly due to the emphasis on sustained effects, some of the once-daily preparations may have limited effectiveness in the first hour or so following administration. In cases of delayed effect, earlier daily administration can be employed (e.g., 6:30 instead of 7:30 A.M.), or a small "booster dose" of standard stimulant of the same type can be given to increase effectiveness (e.g., 5 mg of methyphenidate with Metadate CD in the morning).

Although the stimulants were once used predominantly for school days, there is an increasing clinical trend toward usage throughout the week as well as school vacations, particularly for children with more severe ADHD and conduct problems. This treatment option appears to have a favorable cost–benefit ratio. Benefits have been supported by some well-designed, randomized studies. The putative costs of treatment over weekends and school holidays, mostly concern about possible growth suppression, may not be as serious as was once believed (Greydanus et al., 2003; Spencer et al., 1996). Nevertheless, research on the potential long-term effects of stimulants is in its early stages, and the possibility of a correlation between lifetime dose of stimulants and problems such as growth suppression is a nagging concern.

The behavioral improvements produced by stimulants include sustained attention, improved impulse control, and reduction of task-irrelevant activity, especially in settings demanding restraint of behavior (Barkley, 1977; Connor, 2006b; Rapport & Kelly, 1993; Solanto et al., 2001). Generally noisy and disruptive behavior also diminishes with medication. Children with ADHD may become more compliant with parental and teacher commands, are better able to sustain such compliance, and often increase their cooperative behavior toward others with whom they may have to accomplish a task as a consequence of stimulant treatment (see Danforth et al., 1991, for a review). Research also suggests that children with ADHD are able to perceive the medication as beneficial to the reduction of ADHD symptoms and even describe improvements in their self-esteem (DuPaul, Anastopoulos, Kwasnik, Barkley, & McMurray, 1996; Pelham et al., 2002), though they may report somewhat more side effects than do their parents and teachers.

Improvements in other domains of behavior in children with ADHD have also been demonstrated. Both overt and covert aggressive behavior are often reduced by stimulant treatment of children with ADHD who demonstrate abnormally high levels of pretreatment aggressiveness (Connor, Glatt, Lopez, Jackson, & Melloni, 2002), though the effect on overt aggression may be somewhat less if CD is present. The quality of the children's handwriting may also improve with medication (Lerer, Lerer, & Artner, 1987). Academic productivity, or the number of problems completed, and accuracy of work completion also increase—in some cases, dramatically—as a function of medication (Pelham, Bender, Caddell, Booth, & Moorer, 1985; Rapport, DuPaul, Stoner, & Jones, 1986). But longer-term effects on academic achievement (level of difficulty of material mastered) have not been documented to date in the few long-term studies available (Schachar et al., 2002; Schachter et al., 2001).

It should be strongly emphasized that the effects of stimulant medication are idiosyncratic (see Rapport, DuPaul, et al., 1986). Although reported response rates vary across studies, many reviewers have concluded that 70–82% of children show a clinically beneficial response to any single stimulant. However, with a trial of a second stimulant, the positive response rate may approach 90% (Pliszka, Greenhill, et al., 2000). Unfortunately, there is no way to predict in advance which children will respond to which stimulant. Similarly, among the students who do respond positively to stimulants, there is no basis for predicting which dose will be best. Most children and adolescents show maximal improvement at low to moderate doses of stimulants, but others are most improved at higher doses (Pelham et al., 1998; Smith, Pelham, Evans, et al., 1998). In addition to this between-subject variability in doses, there is considerable variability in the domains that respond to medication. For instance, some children may improve in one domain (e.g., behavior) when treated with stimulants, but may show no change or even deteriorate in other domains (e.g., academic performance). For this reason, we strongly recommend that clinicians assess treatment with stimulant medication on a case-by-case basis, using measures that sample a broad range of domains of functioning.

Even when careful evaluations show a positive response, caution is warranted about the implications of such a response. Much controversy remains over whether immediate improvements in academic performance translate into greater gains in academic achievement over longer-term use of the medications (Barkley & Cunningham, 1978; Schachar & Tannock, 1993; Schachar et al., 2002). Nevertheless, the stimulants appear to remain useful in the management of ADHD symptoms over extended periods of time.

The most frequently occurring side effects of the stimulants are mild insomnia and appetite reduction (particularly at the noon meal), as well as subjective reports of stomachache, headache, and dizziness or jitteriness (Barkley, McMurray, Edelbrock, & Robbins, 1990; Connor, 2006b; Greenhill et al., 1999; Greydanus et al., 2003). These subjective side effects tend to dissipate within a few weeks of beginning medication or can be managed by

reducing the dose. Temporary growth suppression (loss of 1–4 pounds in the first year) may accompany stimulant treatment, but is not generally severe or especially common (Spencer et al., 1996). It can be managed by ensuring that adequate caloric and nutritional intake is maintained—for example, by shifting the distribution of food intake to other times of the day, when the child is more amenable to eating (Taylor, 1986).

Some children become irritable and prone to crying late in the afternoon, when their medication may be wearing off. This may be accompanied by an increase in hyperactivity. This apparent "rebound" phenomenon appears to be rare and might be controlled by adjusting doses and dose schedules (Greydanus et al., 2003).

In approximately 1–2% of children with ADHD treated with stimulants, motor or vocal tics may occur (Connor, 2006b; Greenhill & Osman, 1991). This is well within the base rate prevalence for tics in the general population. In instances where tics already exist, they can be mildly exacerbated by stimulant treatment in some cases, but may even be improved in others (Gadow, Sverd, Sprafkin, Nolan, & Ezor, 1995). It now appears to be relatively safe to use stimulant medications with children who have ADHD and comorbid tic disorders, but to be prepared to reduce the dose or discontinue medication if the children experience a drug-related exacerbation of their tic symptoms.

To avoid potential dose-dependent side effects, we recommend a "low–slow–go" approach to titrating doses. That is, one begins with a low dose, slowly titrates the dose upward, and goes further until the most appropriate dose for that child is reached. We believe that this dose should be the *lowest possible level that produces satisfactory clinical improvement*. This is contrary to some clinical practices of titrating doses to the highest tolerable level. Finding the lowest effective dose may be more difficult, but it has the potential to save money on medication, to reduce the risk of side effects, and perhaps to improve compliance due to increased comfort on medication.

As mentioned previously, it has been difficult to establish any reliable predictors of response to stimulant medication in children with ADHD. Those characteristics having the most consistent relationship to response have been pretreatment levels of poor sustained attention and hyperactivity (Barkley, 1976; Buitelaar, van der Gaag, Swaab-Barneveld, & Kuiper,

1995; Taylor, 1983). The more children differ from typical children on such factors, the better their response to medication. Predictors of adverse responding have not been as well studied. Some research suggests that pretreatment levels of anxiety are associated with poorer responding to stimulants (Buitelaar et al., 1995; DuPaul, Barkley, & McMurray, 1994; Taylor, 1983). However, Pliszka (2003) argues that response to stimulants for treating ADHD is not affected by anxiety, but that children with ADHD plus anxiety may show greater benefit from psychosocial interventions than children with ADHD alone.

There is little doubt now that the stimulant medications are the most studied and most effective treatment for the symptomatic management of ADHD and its secondary consequences (Connor, 2006b; Greydanus et al., 2003). As a result, for many children with moderate to severe levels of ADHD, this may be the first type of treatment employed in their clinical management. And for some, who have no (or no significant) comorbid disorders, it may be the only treatment required. The NYM study, in fact, found that among stimulant-responsive children with ADHD, adding various forms of psychosocial treatments (such as parent training, social skills training, psychotherapy, or academic tutoring) provided no benefits beyond that achieved by medication alone (Abikoff, Hechtman, Klein, Gallacher, et al., 2004; Abikoff, Hechtman, Klein, Weiss, et al., 2004; Hechtman, Abikoff, Klein, Greenfield, et al., 2004; Hechtman, Abikoff, Klein, Weiss, et al., 2004). On the other hand, the results of the MTA project suggest that a more intensive multimodal treatment may produce a broader range of positive results than those achieved by medication alone (e.g., Pelham, 1999).

Despite some conflicting studies and opinions, there seems to be a general consensus that stimulant treatment is not always effective (i.e., the 20–30% nonresponse rate), or always necessary (i.e., in some cases psychosocial treatment is sufficient), or always sufficient (i.e., many children meet criteria for improvement, but not for recovery, on stimulants). The issue of insufficiency is particularly salient with regard to the appropriate management of the comorbid conditions often seen in ADHD, such as learning disabilities, depression, anxiety, or CD. Given that medication typically does not address all of these presenting problems shown by many children with ADHD, other treatments may be required as adjuncts.

The following issues should be considered in the decision to employ medication for the management of ADHD: (1) the age of the child; (2) duration and severity of symptoms; (3) the risk of injury to the child (through either accident or abuse) that the present severity of untreated symptoms poses; (4) the success of prior treatments; (5) the absence of atypical levels of anxiety (perhaps); (6) the absence of stimulant abuse in both the child or adolescent and the caregivers; (7) the likelihood that the caregivers will employ the medication responsibly, in compliance with physician recommendations; and (8) the child or adolescent's living arrangements (in a group setting such as a dormitory, supervision of the medication may be poor, and diversion of the medication to students without ADHD may be more likely). Some of these latter concerns related to stimulant abuse (i.e., points 6–8) may be somewhat ameliorated by the longer-acting preparations of stimulants, such as Concerta, which have lower abuse potential than immediate-release preparations.

Several suggested paradigms for evaluating stimulant drug response in individual cases have been reported (Barkley et al., 1988; Pelham, 1987; Rapport, DuPaul, et al., 1986). We recognize that these are not always practical or available in clinical practice, but recommend them as exemplars toward which practitioners should strive. The trial includes the traditional and mandatory initial medical checkup of the child, to ensure that there are no preexisting conditions that might contraindicate or complicate the medication trial (cardiac problems, unusually high levels of anxiety, prior history of stimulant abuse, etc.). This is followed by the child's receiving a baseline evaluation on the measures (often rating scales) to be collected across the weeks of the trial. Such a baseline evaluation (which is highly recommended) must include ratings of potential side effects of the medication, given that many of these are frequently preexisting problems that, if not assessed at baseline, could be misconstrued as drug side effects (Barkley, McMurray, et al., 1990; Connor, 2002). The child's participation is then scheduled for a 4-week drug–placebo trial, during which the child is tested on three different doses of medication (typically methylphenidate at 5, 10, and 15 mg given at morning and noon or 18, 27, and 36 mg of Concerta given in the morning) and a placebo (lactose powder placed in gelatin capsule; optional). Arrangements are made to have the noon dose of medication given at school on school days, if an immediate-release formulation of the medication is being used. The parents, teachers, child, and clinical assistant conducting the assessments of the child are all kept unaware of the order of medication doses and placebo until the end of the trial.

The major outcome variables are typically ratings completed by parents, teachers, and (for a child over age 8) the child receiving the medication. The frequency of ratings should match the frequency of switches between dose levels in the medication trial. For example, weekly dose switches can be paired with weekly ratings, but daily dose switches need to be paired with daily ratings.

One rating scale assesses the symptoms of ADHD as well as ODD, while another is used to obtain information about side effects the child may have experienced that week (see Barkley & Murphy, 2006). A third rating scale, completed only by the teacher, assesses work productivity and accuracy (the Academic Performance Rating Scale; see DuPaul & Stoner, 2003). Another potentially useful pair of measures that has repeatedly been shown to be sensitive to intervention are the Child Daily Report and Parent Daily Report (Dishion & Kavanagh, 2003; also available at www.cfc.uoregon.edu). Furthermore, the clinical team should solicit nonstandardized information relevant to impairment and other clinically or academically meaningful phenomena. For example, teacher comments can be collected by telephone or via the Internet, as can parent comments during weekly clinic visits during the medication assessment. Forms for soliciting parent and teacher comments, as well as some other useful forms for monitoring medication effects, are available from Pelham and colleagues (www.wings.buffalo.edu/psychology/adhd).

The ratings may be supplemented by objective data (if available and if collection is practical), such as grades and direct observations of behavior in school or in a clinic room. For example, during each weekly clinic visit, the child can be given a set of math problems of appropriate grade level to perform while seated alone in a clinic playroom. Observations can be taken of the child from behind a one-way mirror or with a video camera, and the observations can be coded for behaviors related to ADHD (i.e., off task, fidgets, plays with objects, out of seat, etc.). In addition, the amount of work attempted and the accuracy of that work can be scored. Computerized measures such as continuous-performance tasks may also be used to assess response to medication, but the ecological validity of these measures is questionable (Barkley, 1991), and therefore the value of such measures may be limited. We recognize that for the busy private or clinic-based practitioner, these supplemental measures may not be available or cost-effective. But the use of rating scales to evaluate ADHD and related symptoms, side effects, and even academic productivity is strongly recommended.

Different dosing schedules can be evaluated. For example, in one procotol, each drug condition lasts for 7–10 days before the child progresses to the next drug condition. The order of the drug conditions is random, except that the middle and high doses—say, 10 and 15 mg of immediate-release methylphenidate—are paired, such that the 10-mg condition always precedes the 15-mg condition. This is done to reduce the possibility of provoking unnecessary side effects by beginning the trial at an initially excessive dose. An alternative approach is to switch doses daily in a counterbalanced, random order. Compared to the former, the daily crossover design provides better control for unusual events or spurious improvement over time. However, it incurs a much higher response burden than weekly ratings do and may reduce compliance with the protocol. Furthermore, the daily crossover design may also miss cumulative effects.

At the end of the 4-week trial, the results are tabulated, and a recommendation is made concerning possible continuation of the medication and, if so, which dose seems most effective. Children not found to be responsive to this stimulant may be tried on another, and if a second stimulant does not work, other medications may be considered (see Pliszka, Greenhill, et al., 2000). Furthermore, consistent with the "low–slow–go" approach, children should be routinely tested on a lower dose than selected in the titration trial to see whether the lower dose is sufficient. If there is still room for improvement relative to the higher dose, then the higher dose is well justified.

EFFECTIVENESS, SAFETY, AND PRACTICALITY OF STIMULANT MEDICATIONS

The rise in the use of stimulant medications is supported by numerous studies documenting the efficacy of these medications (Greenhill et al., 1999; Schachter et al., 2001). A meta-analytic review of 62 high-quality studies (Schachter et al., 2001) found a medium-sized effect of stimulants on parent-rated behavior (mean effect size = 0.54) and a large effect on teacher-rated behavior (0.78). Most of these studies were conducted in university or medical school research programs by experts, and therefore speak more to treatment efficacy than to effectiveness as applied in typical community settings. Yet the substantial supportive research across labs, investigators, regions, and even countries, combined with the long-standing successful and ever-increasing use of this treatment in clinical practice, speaks (albeit indirectly) to both effectiveness and practicality. According to the Biglan and colleagues (2003) criteria, stimulant treatment is a grade A intervention, meaning that stimulants have a level of support most appropriate for widespread dissemination.

The stimulants used to treat ADHD are very safe (Rapport & Moffitt, 2002). At therapeutic doses, stimulants produce few negative side effects—and in almost all cases, either youths develop tolerance for the negative effects, or these can be reduced to a tolerable level by lowering the dose or changing to a different stimulant or a nonstimulant (e.g., as atomoxetine). Long-term negative consequences are not evident in the research literature (Greenhill et al., 1999), but the potential for mild growth suppression is an issue of ongoing investigation and debate (MTA Cooperative Group, 2004b). Concerns about predisposing stimulant-treated children to later substance use disorders have been refuted by more than 14 studies, despite a single study implying otherwise (see Barkley, Fischer, Smallish, & Fletcher, 2003; Wilens, Faraone, Biederman, & Gunawardene, 2003). When absorbed rapidly (e.g., inhaled nasally or injected intravenously) or taken at high doses, stimulants may result in euphoric effects and health risks similar to those of cocaine. Such use is uncommon and is less likely with the longer-acting preparations. Mortality or serious morbidity from prescribed stimulants is rare. Indeed, compared to many other commonly prescribed psychiatric medications, stimulants are among the safest drugs given to children. Nevertheless, safety may be diminished when stimulants are taken in combination with other medications (e.g., clonidine), or when potent stimulants (e.g., Adderall XR) or high doses are used with children having preexisting cardiac abnormalities or family histories of sudden cardiac arrest.

Research specific to practical issues with stimulant medication is limited, and the preliminary findings raise some questions about the effectiveness of this treatment in primary care settings. Although taking pills seems to be a simple intervention, there are some significant barriers to daily administration of stimulant medication—including limited access to prescribing physicians, cost, inconvenience, uncertainty about dose or type of medication, side effects, and parent or child resistance to taking medication. Research on compliance is limited, but it suggests that children and adolescents with ADHD tend to take less medication than prescribed, due to missed doses and termination of treatment against medical advice (Jensen et al., 1999). The high cost of some new formulations of stimulants ($60–$100 per month) may contribute to an already tenuous compliance situation, though their once-daily extended-release delivery systems may counteract such a problem. The problems with compliance are clinically important, because stimulants exert their effects only when taken as prescribed. Even the longest-acting stimulants have no measurable effect 24 hours after administration, so missed doses mean that a child is essentially untreated. Thus, although stimulants get high marks for safety and effectiveness, there are some practical barriers to their effective use.

SPECIAL CONSIDERATIONS WITH ADOLESCENTS

Although there has been much less research on stimulant treatment for adolescents than for children (Smith, Waschbush, Willoughby, & Evans, 2000), there is enough research to document that stimulants have similar efficacy from childhood to adolescence (Smith, Pelham, Evans, et al., 1998; Smith, Pelham, Gnagy, & Yudell, 1998). However, due to teens' more frequent involvement with recreational drugs that could be associated with stimulant abuse or could lead to interactions between therapeutic stimulants and recreational drugs, caution should be taken when prescribing stimulants to adolescents. Also, clinicians need to be aware of the potential for diversion of prescribed stimulant medication by a teen with ADHD to other teens for recreational misuse when the teens all reside in a dormitory or other group-living situation.

A major threat to the effectiveness of stimulant medication is the tendency for adolescents to discontinue medication as they get older. Thus more vigorous monitoring and promotion of compliance are necessary in work with adolescents than with children. To avoid premature termination of effective stimulant treatment, parents and physicians should encourage adolescents to participate in treatment decisions and self-monitoring during periodic trials of stimulants. For adolescents who do not recognize the value of taking stimulants (in cases when individualized medication trial unambiguously supports the efficacy of a stimulant), it may be necessary to negotiate behavioral contingency contracts related to the appropriate use of stimulants (see Robin, 1998). In some cases, therefore, multimodal treatment with an emphasis on compliance issues may be necessary for effective stimulant treatment of ADHD in adolescents. Unfortunately, the efficacy of multimodal treatments for adolescents with ADHD has yet to be tested in a major controlled trial.

PEMOLINE

A controversial stimulant treatment for ADHD is pemoline (Cylert). This medication has several advantages over other stimulants. One advantage is convenience, because this drug only has to be taken once a day. Another unique and desirable characteristic of pemoline is that, unlike the other stimulants, it has a low abuse potential. All of the other commonly used stimulant medications are classified by the U.S. Food and Drug Administration (FDA) in the category of prescription drugs that have the highest abuse potential (i.e., Schedule II). This complicates the process of prescribing and purchasing stimulants other than pemoline. Because of its low abuse potential, pemoline has been recommended for use with adolescents with ADHD and a comorbid substance use disorder (Riggs, Leon, Mikulich, & Pottle, 1996). However, a better treatment in such cases may be the use of atomoxetine or bupropion (see below), in view of pemoline's risk for liver impairment (Safer, Zito, & Gardner, 2001) and the requirement of liver function monitoring, which is not an issue with atomoxetine or bupropion.

Given its many positive attributes, it is unfortunate that pemoline has been associated with at least 13 cases of liver failure since 1975. Surveillance data suggest that the rate of liver failure is 4–17 times the rate in the general population (Safer et al., 2001). These findings have required prominent warnings, written informed consent prior to taking the medication, and bimonthly liver functioning tests. Due to the inconvenience, cost, and pain of recommended monitoring procedures, and the risk of life-threatening liver failure, pemoline is now considered a last-choice medication for management of ADHD. A grade of B would be assigned to this treatment if it were not for this newly imposed requirement of liver function monitoring and its attendant inconvenience.

Atomoxetine (Strattera)

Atomoxetine was approved by the FDA in January 2003 for use in children with ADHD 6 years of age and older, and in adolescents and adults with ADHD. This makes it the first such drug so approved for use in the adult stage of the disorder, and the first new drug approved for ADHD in more than 25 years (pemoline having been the last such medication). The drug is a highly selective inhibitor of norepinephrine reuptake, with minimal to no action at other neurotransmitter sites. Its effectiveness has been established in more than 10 large-scale published studies involving various randomized, controlled clinical trials. These samples included 3,264 children and adolescents, and 471 adults, with all types of ADHD (Kratochvil et al., 2001, Michelson et al., 2001, 2002, 2003; Spencer et al., 1998). The clinical trials clearly established both the efficacy and safety of atomoxetine for use in the management of ADHD.

Atomoxetine is not a stimulant, in that it is not a dopamine agonist. It has no abuse potential, as studies show that it is not preferred over placebo by individuals who abuse stimulants and does not result in symptoms of craving, dependence, or addiction. It is therefore not scheduled, whereas the stimulants are classified as Schedule II agents. Consequently, atomoxetine is a more convenient medication: It can be prescribed without the special prescription pads needed in the United States for Schedule II agents, can be prescribed with refills, and can be distributed to patients by physicians as samples. The fact that it is unscheduled and has no abuse potential can make it an attractive alternative to families of children with ADHD concerned about the use of Schedule II medications for their children.

Atomoxetine may assist in the management of ADHD via its inhibition of the norepinephrine transporter, thereby making more norepinephrine available in the extracellular space. This results in a secondary increase of dopamine in the prefrontal cortex. The fact that it does not increase dopamine levels in the nucleus accumbens (the primary dopamine-mediated reward pathway) may explain why it does not have reinforcing or otherwise addictive properties. Because it does not appear to increase dopamine levels in the striatum, which helps control motor movements, it seems to have no exacerbating effect on motor and vocal tics.

Research shows that atomoxetine reduces both inattentive and hyperactive–impulsive symptoms of ADHD in over 70% of cases. The overall effect size (degree of change in group mean scores) of atomoxetine appears to be the same as that for Concerta among children previously untreated with stimulants, but it may have a smaller effect size than that seen with the stimulants in the treatment of individuals with ADHD who have had prior stimulant exposure (D. Michelson, personal communication, September 2004). In controlled studies, atomoxetine has an effect size of about 0.9–1.0 among stimulant-naive cases, but an effect size of 0.6–0.8 (standard deviations) in cases with prior stimulant treatment. The effect size for the stimulants ranges from 0.8 to 1.2 (Michelson et al., 2001).

Peak plasma concentrations for atomoxetine occur in 1–2 hours after oral ingestion and persist for 6–10 hours (half-life of 4 hours). The medication may therefore be given in either once- or twice-daily dosing. When given in twice-daily divided doses, atomoxetine shows much longer daily coverage for ADHD symptoms than do stimulant medications. In contrast to the tricyclic antidepressants (see below), atomoxetine demonstrates no cardiovascular toxicity or abnormalities on electrocardiogram. Atomoxetine appears to improve ODD symptoms as well in children with ADHD who have significant levels of these symptoms (Newcorn, Michelson, Spencer, & Milton, 2002). It also results in significant improvements in parent–child relations, peer relations, school behavior and academic performance, and coexisting internalizing symptoms (such as depression or anxiety).

Atomoxetine can be considered a first-line agent in the treatment of ADHD in children, adolescents, and adults. Whether it is the first or second choice of a starting medication will depend on several patient and social-ecological characteristics that may exist at the time of a clinical trial. For instance, in patients with ADHD and comorbid generalized anxiety, obsessive–compulsive behavior, or tic disorders (e.g., Tourette syndrome), atomoxetine may be a first-choice agent, given that the stimulants may exacerbate such preexisting conditions. In cases where someone with a history of drug abuse resides with the child, or where the child or adolescent has a substance use disorder or history of such, atomoxetine may be the preferred agent because of its lack of abuse potential. When a child or teen with ADHD resides in a dormitory during the school year (at boarding school or college), atomoxetine may be considered before stimulants because of its lack of potential for diversion to dorm-mates for their own recreational use. Obviously, in cases where prior stimulant response has been poor, atomoxetine would be the next medication in line to consider, ahead of the tricyclic antidepressants or antihypertensive agents (which have a greater potential for more serious side effects). And because atomoxetine does not have an adverse impact on sleep onset, it should be considered as an alternative to stimulants in cases where stimulant-induced insomnia is significantly problematic or where sleep problems are preexisting. Also, in cases where parents are concerned about the use of a Schedule II agent in the management of their child's behavior—often as a consequence of adverse publicity in the popular media about Ritalin and other stimulants—atomoxetine may prove useful, given its unscheduled status and hence greater acceptability among such consumers. However, where there exists an urgent need to gain control over disruptive, hyperactive–impulsive, or otherwise externalizing behavior due to imminent adverse consequences (school suspension, potential abuse of the child by caregivers, etc.), or where none of these preexisting conditions are problematic, then stimulants would be the first-choice agents because of their shorter titration period and the apparently greater rapidity of onset of a therapeutic response.

Atomoxetine is prescribed by body weight in young children (Spencer, 2006). In children and adolescents weighing up to 70 kg, atomoxetine is initiated at a total daily dose of 0.5 mg/kg. Dose titration occurs at a minimum of every 3 days to a target total daily dose of approximately 1.2 mg/kg, administered either as a single daily dose in the morning or as evenly divided doses in the morning and late afternoon or early evening. In children, adolescents, and adults who weigh more than 70 kg, atomoxetine is initiated at a total daily dose of 40 mg and increased after a minimum of 3 days to a target total daily dose of approximately 80 mg, given in the morning as two evenly divided daily doses. If no treatment benefit occurs after 2–4 weeks, the dose of atomoxetine may be increased to a maximum of 100 mg/day. The total daily dose of atomoxetine in children and adolescents should not exceed 1.4 mg/kg/day or 100 mg, whichever is less. During atomoxetine initiation and dose titration, contact with the prescribing physician should occur regularly. Pulse and blood pressure should be assessed on full dose. Height and weight should be followed twice yearly.

The side effects of atomoxetine are well documented and generally benign, like those of the stimulants. They include chiefly sedation, gastrointestinal disturbance (nausea), decreased appetite, and upper abdominal pain. Some weight loss may be present over the first 2–4 months of atomoxetine treatment, but tends not to persist beyond the first year. Slight increases in blood pressure and heart rate may occur, as they do with the stimulants, but are typically benign unless hypertension was a preexisting problem—in which case neither stimulants nor atomoxetine should be considered.

To summarize, atomoxetine should be considered at least a grade B+ treatment in terms of efficacy. This drug has only recently been released, so information on effectiveness and safety is growing steadily. What is known at this writing is that it appears to be at least as safe as the stimulants.

Antidepressants

TRICYCLIC ANTIDEPRESSANTS

The next stage in the choice of medications where the stimulants or atomoxetine prove unsuccessful may be a trial of either tricyclic antidepressants or the unique antidepressant bupropion. Because these medications are so different, they are reviewed separately here. Initially, clinicians began turning to the use of the tricyclic antidepressants, such as imipramine, nortriptyline, and desipramine, for the management of ADHD symptoms where stimulants had not been successful. In part, this trend was also due to the occasional negative (and often undeserving) publicity in the popular media about the stimulants, especially Ritalin.

Less is known about the pharmacokinetics and behavioral effects of the antidepressants in children with ADHD than about those of the stimulants or atomoxetine. However, research on these compounds generally supports their efficacy in the management of ADHD (Werry & Aman, 1999; Wilens et al., 1996; see Greydanus et al., 2003, for a review). Nevertheless, with the recent approval of atomoxetine and its greater safety and efficacy, atomoxetine is likely to replace the tricyclic antidepressants in the management of ADHD.

Often given twice daily (morning and evening), the tricyclic antidepressants are longer-acting than the stimulants. As a result, it takes longer to evaluate the therapeutic value of any given dose (Viesselman, Yaylayan, Weller, & Weller, 1999). Some research suggests that low doses of the tricyclics may mimic stimulants in increasing vigilance and sustained attention and decreasing impulsivity. As a result, disruptive and aggressive behavior may also be reduced. Elevation in mood may also occur, particularly in those children in whom significant pretreatment levels of depression and anxiety exist (Pliszka, 1987). Rapoport and Mikkelsen (1978) as well as Ryan (1990) reported that treatment effects may diminish over time, however; it is possible that the tricyclics cannot be used as long-term therapy for ADHD, unlike the stimulants.

The most common side effects of the tricyclics are drowsiness during the first few days of treatment, dry mouth and constipation, and flushing. Less likely but more important are the cardiotoxic effects, such as possible tachycardia or arrhythmia, and (in cases of overdose) coma or death (Viesselman et al., 1999). Some children may develop sluggish reactions in focusing of the optic lens that may mimic nearsightedness. The reaction is not permanent, dissipating when treatment is withdrawn. Skin rash is occasionally reported and usually warrants ceasing drug treatment.

In general, it seems that the tricyclic antidepressants may be useful in the shortterm treatment of children with ADHD when the stimulants cannot be used, when atomoxetine has not proven effective, or where significant mood disturbances accompany the ADHD symptoms (Pliszka, 1987; Ryan, 1990). However, the cardiac functioning of children must be properly evaluated before treatment begins, and then such functioning must be periodically monitored throughout the course of treatment, given the apparent risks of the tricyclic antidepressants for impairing cardiac functioning. (See Wilens et al., 1996, for a review and guidelines for monitoring children on tricyclic antidepressants.)

EFFICACY, SAFETY, AND PRACTICALITY OF TRICYCLIC ANTIDEPRESSANTS

Several controlled studies of tricyclics have found significant therapeutic effects, often as large as those with methylphenidate. However, this research has focused on efficacy, so effectiveness data are lacking. Thus the tricyclics are a grade B– intervention. Unfortunately, there have been some reports of deaths, cardiac arrhythmia problems, and a high rate of very unpleasant side effects at therapeutic doses (Greydanus et al., 2003). Moreover, at high doses tricyclic antidepressants are very toxic, and this class of drugs figures prominently among the drugs causing fatal intentional overdoses. The problems with desipramine were severe enough that this medication was deliberately omitted from the Texas Medication Algorithm (Pliszka, Greenhill, et al., 2000). In terms of practicality, annoying side effects such as drowsiness, dry mouth, and inhibited elimination of bodily wastes are major barriers to compliance with these drugs. Cost and inconvenience of treatment are other problems, with baseline and follow-up electrocardiograms required every 3–6 months. On a positive practical note, elimination is slow enough that therapeutic levels can be maintained even if the occasional dose is missed.

The most significant consideration with adolescents relative to children is the increased likelihood of comorbid depression or substance abuse in adolescents. Several studies have shown that tricyclic antidepressants are not effective in treating depression in adolescents (Greydanus et al., 2003). Therefore, medications other than the tricyclics should be considered for treating depression. On a more positive note, due to the low abuse potential of tricyclics, these drugs at one time were thought to be a viable alternative to stimulants if there are concerns about stimulant abuse. With the advent of atomoxetine, however, tricyclic antidepressants will probably be relegated to the bottom of the list of acceptable treatments and, like pemoline, considered only as a last resort.

BUPROPION (WELLBUTRIN)

Bupropion is FDA-approved for treatment of depression and nicotine addiction in adults, but not for ADHD. It is believed to be effective in improving attention, reducing irritability, and ameliorating depression (Greydanus et al., 2003; Spencer, 2006); however, the research on bupropion's effects in children and adolescents should be treated with caution, due to the small number of studies (two) and small sample sizes in those studies (a total of 36). One study with 15 adolescents found that bupropion was equivalent to methylphenidate in treating ADHD (Barrickman et al., 1995). A single-blind study with 24 adolescents who had ADHD and comorbid depression found statistically significant changes in parent and child ratings, but not teacher ratings (see Spencer, 2006). In this study, clinically significant change (as rated by clinicians who were aware of the treatment conditions) was reported for about 60% of the participants. An open-label study found that bupropion might be effective with adolescents with ADHD and substance use disorders (Riggs et al., 1998). Although these results are promising, and suggest that bupropion might be effective in treating ADHD in adolescents with or without comorbid depression or substance abuse, the current state of the literature supports only a grade of C for the quality of research on bupropion as a treatment for adolescents with ADHD. At best, a grade of D is warranted for treatment of children with ADHD. We should note that these low efficacy grades are due to limited research, as opposed to negative findings.

Although the adverse effects of bupropion are rare, they include nausea, anorexia, restlessness, agitation, drowsiness, headaches, exacerbation of tics, and seizures. Due to these side effects, bupropion is not appropriate for treating individuals with epilepsy or eating disorders. The risk of seizures can presumably be controlled through slow titration, taking doses more than 8 hours apart, and using sustained-release formulations (Greydanus et al., 2003). Bupropion overdose is tolerated far better than overdose of tricyclic antidepressants. Furthermore, there appear to be few drug-to-drug interactions with bupropion. The availability of once-a-day dosing (Wellbutrin XL) simplifies the administration of this drug. Thus, pending further research, bupropion could be the drug of choice for treating adolescents with comorbid depression or substance use disorders. However, because the research is currently limited, bupropion is the third or fourth medication to consider when the primary presenting problem is ADHD.

Antihypertensive Medications

Two drugs originally marketed as alpha-andrenergic agonists for treating hypertension, clonidine (Catapres) and guanfacine (Tenex), have become increasingly popular for treating ADHD (Connor, 2006a). These drugs have primarily been used as alternatives or adjuncts to stimulants such as methylphenidate. Studies have found that clonidine is superior to placebo in reducing ADHD symptoms and conduct problems (see Connor, Fletcher, & Swanson, 1999, for a meta-analysis; see also Hazell & Stuart, 2003; Pliszka, Greenhill, et al., 2000). Empirical support for guanfacine exists (Scahill et al., 2001) but is similarly weak, earning these drugs a grade of C (i.e., efficacy based primarily on studies with serious methodological limitations and on a few randomized, controlled studies).

The most commonly reported side effect of clonidine is drowsiness, which occurs in about 50% of cases (Connor, 2006a; Greydanus et al., 2003). This side effect is sometimes used to therapeutic advantage in children with ADHD who have difficulty falling asleep or exhibit symptom rebound after a day of taking stimulant medication. Safety concerns about the combination of stimulants and clonidine appear to be diminishing over time, following some reports of deaths in the mid-1990s that were associated with, but not proven to be caused by, combining clonidine and methylphenidate. Nevertheless, there are lingering concerns about the potential electrocardiographic effects of clonidine and its potential

to worsen preexisting cardiac arrhythmias (Greydanus et al., 2003).

The need for electrocardiograms at baseline, every dose change, and every 6 months when clonidine is used is a serious threat to the practicality of this medication. Also, due to possible decreased glucose tolerance, monitoring of blood glucose levels at least every 6 months is warranted (Greydanus et al., 2003). Furthermore, the many unpleasant side effects reported with this drug may hamper compliance, including headache, dry mouth, itchy eyes, weight gain, dizziness, and postural hypotension. In some cases, treatment with clonidine may create new problems that mimic psychiatric disorders. For instance, there have been some reports of irritability, dysphoria, and attention impairment in children on clonidine. Although side effects may be reduced and compliance may be improved with the availability of a patch, this delivery system runs the risk of causing a rash at the site of the patch. Finally, rapid withdrawal from clonidine may cause serious problems with symptom rebound and tachycardia. Adverse effects of guanfacine appear to be similar to those of clonidine, with possibly less sedation and more agitation and headaches (Connor, 2006a; Greydanus et al., 2003; Werry & Aman, 1999).

To summarize, compared to all other medications evaluated in this chapter, the risk–benefit ratio of clonidine and guanfacine appears to be poor. Pending further research to the contrary, we do not recommend these drugs for the treatment of ADHD.

Behavioral Interventions

A Rationale

We now turn our attention to the nonpharmacological therapies, which have been largely dominated by behavior modification programs. These methods were initially employed for children with ADHD largely on an atheoretical basis; their success for children with mental retardation and other developmental disabilities (e.g., autism) encouraged their use for children with behavioral disorders. However, with the recent theory of ADHD as a problem in response inhibition and self-regulation, and the secondary consequences this may create in terms of poor self-motivation to persist at assigned tasks (Barkley, 1997d), a persuasive theoretically based rationale for employing behavioral interventions for children with ADHD now exists. ADHD appears to be a developmental delay in the self-regulation of behavior by internal means of representing information (working memory) and motivating goal-directed behavior. If so, then interventions that provide more externally represented information to prompt and guide behavior, and that enhance motivation via an increased density of external consequences, greater immediacy in their timing, and greater salience for a child, should be useful—at least for symptomatic reduction in some settings and tasks. Such procedures for the artificial manipulation of antecedent and consequent events are precisely those provided by the behavior therapies.

A logical extension of this argument holds, however, that such socially arranged means of addressing this neurologically based disorder of self-regulation would not be likely to alter the underlying neurophysiological basis for it. These techniques must be employed across situations over extended time intervals (months to years), much as prosthetic devices (e.g., hearing aids, mechanical limbs) are employed to compensate for physically disabling conditions. Premature removal of the socially arranged stimulus prompts and motivational programs would predictably result in an eventual return to pretreatment levels of the behavioral symptoms, just as removal of a ramp that permits persons in wheelchairs to enter public buildings would cease to allow them such successful entry. Also, use of the behavioral techniques in only one environment would be unlikely to affect rates of ADHD symptoms in other, untreated settings, unless generalization had been intentionally programmed to occur across such settings. The research reviewed below for the various behavioral techniques seems to support this interpretation.

Important to note from Barkley's theoretical stance is that behavioral interventions are not implemented chiefly to increase skills or information, as if children with ADHD were ignorant of them, but are being implemented to enhance the motivation of these children to show what they already know. From this perspective, ADHD is a disorder of performance, not of knowledge of skills. Therefore, behavioral interventions are used to cue the use of those skills at key points of performance in natural settings, and to motivate their display through

the use of artificial consequences that ordinarily do not exist at those points.

Direct Application of Behavior Therapy Methods in the Laboratory

A number of early studies evaluated the effects of reinforcement and punishment, usually response cost, on the behavior and cognitive performance of children with ADHD. These studies usually indicated that the performance of these children on lab tasks measuring vigilance or impulse control could be immediately and significantly improved by the use of contingent consequences (Firestone & Douglas, 1975, 1977; Patterson, 1965). In some cases, the behavior of children with ADHD approximated that of nondisabled control children. For example, Paniagua (1987) evaluated the contribution of stimulus control to the management of children with ADHD. Using a method known as "correspondence training," he attempted to establish greater control over ADHD symptoms by commands and rules previously stated publicly by the children. "Correspondence" in this context referred to the degree of concordance between public statements by children as to what they would do and the actual behavior they subsequently displayed in that setting—in essence, the degree of agreement between "saying" and "doing."

In this paradigm, children with ADHD were requested to state publicly how they would behave in an immediately subsequent situation. Their behavior in that situation was then observed, after which they were reinforced or punished for the degree of correspondence. Paniagua's (1987) results suggested that under such conditions, children with ADHD significantly reduced their levels of inattention and overactivity during task performance, and their levels of aggressive behavior during peer interactions. These preliminary findings with a small sample ($n = 3$) of 7- to 10-year-old children were quite promising, suggesting that self-instruction followed by reinforcement for the degree of rule–behavior correspondence might be yet another way of improving the performance of children with ADHD through stimulus manipulations. However, work by Hayes and colleagues (1985) suggested that such self-statements would need to be publicly made in order to be effective, because they served as a form of public goal setting for which social consequences could be made contingent. Further research would have needed to show that the children's own statements were serving as the controlling stimuli in such paradigms, rather than the presence of the examiner during the task.

However, none of these studies examined the degree to which such changes generalized to the natural environments of the children, and this omission called into question the clinical effectiveness of such an approach. It is highly unlikely that behavioral techniques implemented only in the clinic or laboratory have carried over into the home or school settings of these children without formal programming for such generalization. As a result, there has been no further research interest shown in the direct training of children with ADHD via behavioral means in clinical or laboratory settings. This early work remains of historical significance, however, it presaged and instigated later efforts to train parents and teachers in the application of behavioral methods in home and school settings, thereby partly addressing the problem of generalization of treatment effects that limited these early laboratory demonstrations.

Direct Training of Attention in the Clinic

More recently, a few neuropsychologists have begun to explore the direct training of attentional skills for children with ADHD in clinical settings. These approaches have been founded largely on the success of cognitive rehabilitation and training programs for individuals with head injuries or other neurological impairments (Kerns, Eso, & Thomson, 1999). One specific cognitive rehabilitation protocol for attention training is the "attention process training" (APT) system developed by Sohlberg and Mateer (1989) for adults with brain injuries. The APT involves a series of cards containing drawings of family situations involving different ages, sexes, dress, and social circumstances; the cards are of different colors, so that they can be sorted on a variety of stimulus characteristics as specified by the trainer. The APT also includes auditory tasks of a similar nature that require trainees to attend to specified stimuli on the sound track. The tasks become faster over the training sessions and include distracting stimuli. Children are reinforced for meeting specific success criterion during each session, but no strategies for attending to and succeed-

ing at these tasks are taught to the children. Studies to date have involved very small samples of children with ADHD (ages 6–14), with training occurring two to four times per week for 1- to 2-hour sessions over periods of 5–18 weeks (Kerns et al., 1999; Semrud-Clikeman, Harrington, Clinton, Connor, & Sylvester, 1998). These studies typically find significant improvement on both the attention training tasks (as one might expect) and on untrained comparable tasks used to assess attention given by the same examiners in the clinic lab setting. But none have been able to document significant improvements on measures of academic efficiency given in the same clinic, or on parent or teacher rating scales of ADHD symptoms or related behavior at home or school. Hence it appears that training effects are limited to the training environment and tasks, with no evidence to date of generalization to untreated settings or more ecologically important activities (e.g., academic performance).

Training Parents in Child Behavior Management Methods

A plethora of research exists on parent training in child behavior modification (Kazdin, 1997; see Serketich & Dumas, 1996, for a meta-analysis); this research has been primarily conducted with children having conduct or disruptive behavior problems (see McMahon, Wells, & Kotler, Chapter 3, this volume). More recent studies have shown behavioral parent training (BPT) programs to be effective for such children, whether or not they have co-occurring attentional/hyperactive difficulties (Bor, Sanders, & Markie-Dadds, 2002; Hartman, Stage, & Webster-Stratton, 2003). A growing number of studies have examined the efficacy of this approach with children either specifically diagnosed having as ADHD or judged to be having high levels of hyperactive or ADHD symptoms (Chronis, Chacko, Fabiano, Wymbs, & Pelham, 2004). What research exists (Anastopoulos, Guevremont, Shelton, & DuPaul, 1993; Chronis et al., 2004; Sonuga-Barke, Daley, & Thompson, 2002; Sonuga-Barke, Daley, Thompson, Laver-Bradbury, & Weeks, 2001; Strayhorn & Weidman, 1989, 1991) supports the clinical efficacy of BPT for children with ADHD, but with some apparent caveats.

One such caveat is that most studies were of short duration and did not examine either for generalization of treatment effects to no-treatment settings or for maintenance of treatment effects once training was discontinued (Eyberg, Edwards, Boggs, & Foote, 1998; Kazdin, 1997). One of the few studies to conduct a follow-up reevaluation 1 year after treatment, however, found that the families receiving BPT were no longer different from the families in the control group, although the children's school behavior was rated by teachers as significantly better than that of the control children (Strayhorn & Weidman, 1991). Another caveat is that the studies to date have been largely university- or medical-school-based programs implemented by expert trainers; thus they attest to the efficacy of BPT, but there is little research evidence for its effectiveness in more natural clinical service delivery settings.

As a further caveat, the high genetic contribution to the disorder ensures that a number of parents undergoing training may have ADHD themselves. One study has found that maternal ADHD can significantly limit the improvement shown during BPT by children with ADHD (Sonuga-Barke et al., 2002). Hence the treatment of parental ADHD may be a prerequisite to successful training outcomes for children with ADHD. Other forms of parental psychological maladjustment, such as maternal depression, antisocial personality and drug use, parenting stress, or marital/couple distress, exist with greater frequency among parents of children with ADHD, could likewise limit the success of BPT; however, these factors have been largely unstudied in families of children with ADHD (Chronis et al., 2004).

Studies that supplement basic BPT with additional psychological treatments designed to address such parental problems in children with ODD have shown mixed success at doing so. Apparently most families have benefited from the supplemented intervention, whether or not they had these preexisting parental problems (Chronis et al., 2004). Single-parent status and fathers' participation in treatment have also been shown to limit the effectiveness of BPT for children with ODD and disruptive behavior (see McMahon et al., Chapter 3, this volume), but have not been directly investigated in children specifically having ADHD.

A third caveat is that BPT appears in some studies to result in more dramatic improvements in child oppositional behavior than in ADHD symptoms per se, suggesting that the treatment is most useful when parent–child

conflict exists in families having children with ADHD (Anastopoulos et al., 1993). Such findings, however, may be specific to children of elementary school age or older; studies of preschool children with ADHD have found significant improvements in symptoms of ADHD (Sonuga-Barke et al., 2001, 2002).

The treatment techniques used to date have primarily consisted of training parents in general contingency management tactics, such as contingent application of reinforcement or punishment following appropriate or inappropriate behaviors, respectively. Reinforcement procedures have typically relied on praise, privileges, or tokens. Punishment methods have usually been either loss of positive attention, privileges, or tokens, or formal time out from reinforcement.

Several similar, though not identical, BPT programs have been studied with children having ADHD. These include Cunningham's Community Parent Education (COPE) program (Cunningham, Bremner, & Secord, 1997); the program outlined in the book *The Incredible Years* by Webster-Stratton (1992); Eyberg's parent–child interaction therapy (Eyberg & Boggs, 1998); and Barkley's program as described in his book *Defiant Children* (Barkley, 1997d). The core methods taught in these programs are quite similar—not surprisingly, since all of the developers trained either directly with Constance Hanf at the Oregon Health Sciences University or with one of her former students. Hanf developed one of the original BPT programs for disruptive children based largely on two procedures: enhanced parental attention to compliant child behavior, coupled with immediate time out for noncompliant behavior (see Forehand & McMahon, 1981; McMahon & Forehand, 2003). Though these subsequent programs vary from this original program in their format and in the procedures they have added to supplement the basic two steps, all are founded on a social learning model of disruptive child behavior (disrupted parenting and social coercion). And all have demonstrated efficacy for disruptive children, including those with ADHD (Chronis et al., 2004).

The rationale for Barkley's version as applied to children with ADHD, however, is twofold and is not based solely on social learning theory. First, Barkley (1997a) has hypothesized that children with ADHD may have deficits in self-regulation and executive functioning, and specifically in rule-governed behavior, or the stimulus control of behavior by commands, rules, and self-directed speech. Unlike a similar theory by Willis and Lovaas (1977), Barkley's theory does not stipulate that the problem has arisen from poor child management by parents, but instead proposes that a neurophysiological deficiency underlies the problem with rules. As noted earlier (see "A Rationale," above), children with ADHD have limitations in the internally represented information and motivation that instruct, guide, and support behavior, and therefore require more externally represented information and artificially arranged consequences to compensate for these executive deficits. Consequently, parents of children with ADHD are going to need to use more explicit, systematic, externalized, and compelling forms of presenting rules and instructions and providing consequences for their compliance with them than are likely to be needed with nondisabled children.

As second unique feature of Barkley's approach to parent training is that a considerable number of clinic-referred children with ADHD also exhibit oppositional defiant behavior, and such children are recognized to have poorer adolescent and young adult outcomes (Hinshaw, 1987; Paternite & Loney, 1980; Weiss & Hechtman, 1993). ODD is recognized to originate at least partially in disrupted parenting and coercive family interactions (see McMahon et al., Chapter 3). Hence appropriate training of parents must be provided for the oppositional defiant behaviors associated with ADHD in such cases. The most useful vehicle for accomplishing both purposes seems to be training parents in behavioral techniques applied contingently for compliance or noncompliance (Barkley, 1997d).

The BPT program by Barkley, for instance, consists of 10 steps, with 1- to 2-hour weekly training sessions provided either to individual families or in groups. Each step is described in detail elsewhere (Barkley, 1997a), but is briefly presented below.

1. *Review of information on ADHD.* In the first session, the therapist provides a succinct overview of the nature, developmental course, prognosis, and etiologies of ADHD. Providing the parents with additional reading materials, such as a book for parents (Barkley, 2000), can be a useful addition to this session. Professional videotapes are also available

(Barkley, 1992a, 1992b) that present such an overview; these can be loaned to parents for review at home and sharing with relatives or teachers, as needed. Such a session is essential in BPT to dispel a number of misconceptions parents often have about ADHD in children. Research suggests that just this provision of information can result not only in improved parental knowledge about ADHD, but also in improved parental perceptions of the degree of deviance of their child's behavioral difficulties (Andrews, Swank, Foorman, & Fletcher, 1995).

2. *The causes of oppositional defiant behavior.* Next, parents are provided with an indepth discussion of those factors identified in past research as contributing to the development of defiant behavior in children. Essentially, four major contributors are discussed: (a) child characteristics, such as health, developmental disabilities, and temperament; (b) parent characteristics similar to those described for the child; (c) situational consequences for oppositional and coercive behavior; and (d) stressful family events. Parents are taught that where problems exist in (a), (b), and (d), they increase the probability of children displaying bouts of coercive, defiant behavior. However, the consequences for such defiance, (c) seem to determine whether that behavior will be maintained or even increased in subsequent situations where commands and rules are given. Such behavior appears to function primarily as escape/avoidance learning, in which oppositional behavior results in a child escaping from aversive parent interactions and task demands, negatively reinforcing the child's coercion. As in the first session, this content is covered so as to correct parents' potential misconceptions about defiance (i.e., that it is primarily attention-getting in nature). This session can be augmented by the use of two professional videotapes on the nature of oppositional defiant behavior and its management (Barkley, 1997e, 1997f).

3. *Developing and enhancing parental attention.* Patterson (1965, 1982) has suggested that the value of verbal praise and social reinforcement is greatly reduced for oppositional or hyperactive children, making it weak as a reinforcer for their compliance. In this session, parents are trained in more effective ways of attending to child behavior, so as to enhance the value of their attention to their children. The technique consists of verbal narration and oc-

TOURO COLLEGE LIBRARY

casional positive statements to a child, with attention being strategically deployed only when appropriate behaviors are displayed by the child. Parents are taught to reduce the amount of attention to inappropriate behaviors, including ignoring as much negative behavior as possible, while greatly increasing their attention to ongoing prosocial and compliant child behaviors. This is a critical step, because many parenting programs result in reductions of rates of negative behavior without corresponding increases in rates of positive behavior (Bor et al., 2002). One of the most effective results of BPT is to increase rates of positive behaviors that are incompatible with the negative behaviors the parents wish to terminate.

4. *Attending to child compliance and independent play.* This session extends the techniques developed in session 3 to instances when parents issue direct commands to children. Parents are trained in methods of giving effective commands, such as reducing questionlike commands (e.g., "Why don't you pick up your toys now?"), increasing imperatives, eliminating setting activities that compete with task performance (e.g., television), reducing task complexity, and so on. They are then encouraged to begin using a more effective command style and to pay immediate positive attention when compliance is initiated by the child. As part of this assignment, parents are asked to increase the frequency with which they give brief commands to their child this week and to reinforce each command obeyed. Research suggests that these brief commands are more likely to be obeyed, thereby providing excellent training opportunities for attending to compliance. In this session, parents are also trained to provide more positive attention frequently and systematically when their children are engaged in nondisruptive activities while the parents must be occupied with some other work or activity. Essentially, the method taught here amounts to a shaping procedure, in which parents provide frequent praise and attention for progressively longer periods of a child's nondisruptive activities.

5. *Establishing a home token economy.* As noted above, the theoretical model of ADHD posits that children with the disorder may require more frequent, immediate, and salient consequences for appropriate behavior and compliance in order to maintain it. If this is correct, then instituting a home token economy is critical to addressing these difficulties with

intrinsically generated and represented motivation by bringing more salient, more immediate, and more frequent external consequences to bear on child compliance than is typically the case. In establishing this program, the parents list most of the child's home responsibilities and privileges, and then assign values of points or chips to each. The parents are encouraged to have at least 12–15 reinforcers on the menu so as to maintain the motivating properties of the program. Generally, plastic chips are used with children age 8 or younger, as they seem to value the tangible features of the token. For children age 9 or older, points recorded in a notebook seem sufficient.

During the first week of this program, the parents are not to fine the child or remove points for misconduct. The program is used for rewarding good behavior only. Parents are also asked to be liberal in awarding chips to the child for even minor instances of appropriate conduct. However, chips are given only for obeying first requests. If a command must be repeated, it must still be obeyed, but the opportunity to earn chips has been forfeited. Parents are also encouraged to give bonus chips for good attitude or emotional regulation. For instance, if a command is obeyed quickly, without complaint, and with a positive attitude, parents may give the child additional chips beyond those typically given for that job. Where this is used, parents are to note expressly that the awarding of the additional chips is for a positive attitude. Families are encouraged to establish and maintain such programs for at least 6–8 weeks, to allow for the newly developed interaction patterns spawned by such programs to become habitual patterns in dealing with child compliance.

6. *Implementing time out for noncompliance.* Parents are now trained to use response cost (removal of points or chips) contingent on noncompliance. In addition, they are trained in an effective time-out-from-reinforcement technique for use with two serious forms of defiance that may continue to be problematic, despite the use of the home token economy. These two misbehaviors are selected in consultation with the parents and typically involve a type of command or household rule that the child continues to defy, despite parental use of previous treatment strategies. Time out is limited to these two forms of misconduct, so as to keep it from being used excessively during the next week.

The time-out procedure taught in this program often differs from that commonly used by parents. First, the time out is to be implemented shortly after a child's noncompliance begins. Parents often wait until they are very upset with a child before instituting punishment, often repeating their commands frequently to the child in the interim. In this program, parents issue a command, wait 5 seconds, issue a warning, wait another 5 seconds, and then take the child to time out immediately if compliance has not yet begun to these commands or warnings. Second, children are not given control over the time-out interval, as they often are in many households. For instance, parents often place a child in time out and then say that the child can leave time out when he or she is quiet, when the child is ready to do as the parent asked, or when a timer signals the end of the interval. In each of these cases, determination of when the time-out interval ends is no longer under the parent's control. This program teaches parents simply to tell the child not to leave the time-out chair until a parent gives permission for this. Three conditions must be met by the child before time out ends, and these are in a hierarchy: (1) The child must serve a minimum sentence in time out, usually 1–2 minutes for each year of his or her age; (2) the child must then become quiet for a brief period of time, so as not to have disruption associated with the parents approaching the time-out chair and talking to the child; and (3) the child must then agree to obey the command. Failure of the child to remain in time out until all three conditions are met is dealt with by additional punishment. The consequence is tailored to meet parental wishes but may consist of a fine within the home token system, extension of the time-out interval an additional 5 or 10 minutes, or placement of the child in his or her bedroom. In the latter case, toys or other entertaining activities are previously removed from the bedroom, and the door to the room may be closed and locked to preclude further escape from the punishment.

7. *Extending time out to additional noncompliant behaviors.* In this session, no new material is taught to parents. Instead, any problems with previously implementing time out are reviewed and corrected. Parents may then extend their use of time out to one or two additional noncompliant behaviors with which the child may still have trouble.

8. *Managing noncompliance in public places.* Parents are now taught to extrapolate their home management methods to troublesome public places, such as stores, places of worship, restaurants, and the like. Using a "think aloud, think ahead" paradigm, parents are taught to stop just before entering a public place, review two or three rules with the child that the child may previously have defied, explain to the child what reinforcers are available for obedience in the place, then explain what punishment may occur for disobedience, and finally assign the child an activity to perform during the outing. Parents then enter the public place and immediately begin attending to and reinforcing ongoing child compliance with the previously stated rules. Time out or response cost is used immediately for disobedience.

Time out in a public place may require slight modification from its use at home. For instance, parents may be taught to use the farthest wall from the central aisle of a store as the time-out location. If this is inconvenient, then taking the child to a restroom or having him or her face the side of a display cabinet may be adequate substitutes. If unavailable, then taking the child outside the building to face the front wall or returning to the car can be used for time out. When none of these locations seem appropriate, parents can be trained to use a delayed punishment contingency. In this case, the parent carries a small spiral notebook to the public place and, before entering the building, indicates that rule violations will be recorded in the book and that the child will serve time out for them upon return home from this trip. Barkley (1997b) encourages parents to keep a picture of the child sitting in time out at home with this notebook and to show it to the child before entering the public building. This serves as a reminder to the child of what will be in store if a rule is violated. Whenever time out is used in a public place, it need not be for as long an interval as at home. Barkley suggests that half of the usual time-out interval may be sufficient for public misbehavior, given the richly reinforcing activities in public places from which the child has just been removed.

9. *Improving child school behavior from home: The daily school behavior report card.* This session is a fairly recent addition (Barkley, 1997d) to the original BPT program and is designed to help parents assist their child's teacher with the management of classroom behavior problems. The session focuses on training parents in the use of a home-based

reward program, in which children are evaluated on a daily school behavior report card by their teachers. This card serves as the means by which consequences later in the day will be dispensed at home for classroom conduct. The card can be designed to address class behavior, recess or free-time behavior, or more specific behavioral or academic targets for any given child. The consequence provided at home typically consist of the rewarding or removal of tokens or points within the home token system as a function of the ratings the child has received from teachers on this daily behavioral report card. To emphasize the importance of the school-to-home communication, and to prevent the child from escaping consequences if he or she "loses" the school behavior report card, it is best to set up a contingency such that "no news is worse than bad news." Thus the most austere level in the contingency system should be implemented when the card is incomplete or missing.

10. *Managing future misconduct.* By now, parents should have acquired an effective repertoire of child management techniques. The goal of this session is to get parents to think about how they might be implemented in the future if some other forms of noncompliance developed. The therapist challenges the parents with misbehaviors they have not seen yet, and then asks them to explain how they might use their recently acquired skills to manage these problems. Behavioral rehearsals (i.e., role plays) surrounding anticipated barriers to implementation of existing parenting plans, as well as making modifications or innovations to deal with new and different behaviors, are strongly recommended as a means to prepare for future misconduct.

11. *One-month review/booster session.* In what is typically the final session, the concepts taught in earlier sessions are briefly reviewed; problems that have arisen in the last month are discussed; and plans are made for their correction. Other sessions may be needed to deal with additional issues that persist, but for most families, the 10 sessions described above appear adequate for improving rates of compliant behavior in children with ADHD.

Barkley's program is intended for children ages 2–11 years for whom oppositional or defiant behavior is an issue. Studies examining the efficacy of this particular BPT program for children with ADHD have consistently reported significant improvements in child behavior as a function of the parents' acquisition of these child management skills (Anastopoulos et al., 1993; Johnston, 1992; Pisterman et al., 1989). Indeed, this was the program that was selected and modified for use in the MTA project (discussed below). Results suggest that up to 64% of families experience clinically significant change or recovery ("normalization") of their children's disruptive behavior as a consequence of this program (Anastopoulos et al., 1993; Sonuga-Barke et al., 2002). However, improvements in behavior may be more concentrated in the realm of aggressive and defiant child behavior than in the realm of inattentive and hyperactive symptoms (Johnston, 1992). All of these studies have relied on clinic-referred families, most of whom sought the assistance of mental health professionals for their children.

In contrast to the results of research with such motivated families, Barkley and colleagues (2000) found that if such a clinic-based BPT program was offered to parents whose preschool children were identified at kindergarten enrollment as having significant levels of aggressive–hyperactive–impulsive behavior, most did not attend training or did not attend reliably, and no treatment effect was evident. Moreover, no significant improvements in child behavior were found even among those who did attend at least some of the training sessions. Studies with disruptive children or those at high risk for externalizing behavior suggest that BPT may be more cost-effective, may reach more severely disruptive children and more minority families, and possibly may be more effective for them if they are provided as group training classes offered through neighborhood public schools in the evenings, with paraprofessionals as trainers (Cunningham, Bremer, & Boyle, 1995; van de Wiel, Matthys, Cohen-Kettenis, & van Engeland, 2003). This may prove to be the case for children specifically having ADHD as well.

For teenagers with ADHD and oppositional behavior, there is little research on BPT. We have often recommended a family training program that includes the problem-solving communication training (PSCT) program developed by Robin and Foster (1989), combined with variations of Barkley's BPT program. The efficacy of the Robin and Foster program when used specifically for teenagers with ADHD has been examined (Barkley, Guevremont,

Anastopoulos, & Fletcher, 1992). This program was compared against the BPT program described above (Barkley, 1997d), which was modified somewhat for use with adolescents (e.g., token systems became point systems, time out was changed to grounding to the home, etc.). It was also compared against the family therapy program developed by Minuchin and Fishman (1981). Families in each group received 8–10 sessions of therapy, and multiple outcome measures of family conflict were collected, including videotaped parent–teen interactions. Results indicated that all three treatments produced statistically significant improvements in the various self-report ratings of family conflict, but no significant improvements in the direct observations of parent–teen interactions. When statistics evaluating individual change and recovery were applied to these data, they revealed that only 5–30% of the families in these programs improved reliably during treatment and that only 5–20% had recovered ("normalized") in their level of conflicts, with no significant differences among the groups in these reliable change and recovery percentages. Such results are quite disappointing and suggest that the power of treatment needs to be enhanced in various ways, if it is to be of much value to most families of adolescents with ADHD experiencing significant family conflict.

A subsequent study by Barkley and colleagues enhanced this treatment by increasing the number of sessions to 18, encouraging greater father involvement in therapy, and combining the BPT and PSCT programs, among other changes (Barkley, Edwards, Laneri, Fletcher, & Metevia, 2001a). The study compared PSCT/BMT with PSCT alone for clinically referred teenagers having both ADHD and ODD. Results were essentially the same as those of the initial study. Both treated groups showed improvement over time at the group level of analysis, with there being no differences between them; however, only 30% or fewer families in these groups were demonstrating clinically reliable change at the end of treatment. The combined PSCT/BMT approach was superior to the PSCT-alone approach in just one respect, that being fewer dropouts from treatment.

To summarize the efficacy of training parents in behavior management methods, these methods receive a grade of B to A for use with children of elementary school age, depending on which parenting approach is used. However, these approaches have not been as effective for preschoolers or adolescents with ADHD. Practical barriers, such as parental engagement, have limited studies with preschoolers. Innovations to improve the efficacy of parent-based interventions with teenagers with ADHD are sorely needed. BPT suffers from several practical limitations, such as the need for training providers, numerous demands placed on families, a commitment to use the methods consistently and persistently over a long period of time, and the need to tailor techniques in response to changing developmental and social factors. When used properly, these techniques can be very safe, but overly punitive or haphazard programs can actually make things worse. Paradoxically, some worsening of behavior (e.g., transient increases in tantrums when a parent starts ignoring the behavior) may suggest that parents are on the right track. This example also illustrates the fact that these behavior methods, which seem so simple at their basic conceptual level, can be fraught with subtleties that confuse and frustrate parents. A limitation of these approaches is that many therapists do not have the skills and training to provide the sophisticated guidance that most parents need. Consequently, even though behavioral methods can be used to get whales to jump through burning hoops, past failures with other providers may cause many parents to complain that their children's behavior is completely impervious to change through behavioral methods. This is a significant limitation to the effectiveness of BPT programs, and it must be handled delicately to recruit and retain parents in such programs. Intensive professional education and widespread public education to overcome ignorance and stigma associated with BPT may be necessary for this to become a truly grade A intervention for ADHD and related problems.

Training Teachers in Classroom Behavior Management

Somewhat more research has occurred on the application of behavior management methods in the classroom for children with ADHD than on BPT. Moreover, there is a voluminous literature on the application of classroom management methods to disruptive child behaviors, many of which include the typical symptoms of ADHD. This research clearly indicates the effectiveness of behavioral techniques in the shortterm treatment of academic performance problems in children with ADHD.

A meta-analysis of the research literature on school interventions for ADHD, which included 70 separate experiments of various within- and between-subjects designs as well as single-case designs, was conducted (DuPaul & Eckert, 1997). This review found an overall mean effect size for contingency management procedures of 0.60 for between-subject designs, nearly 1.00 for within-subject designs, and approximately 1.40 for single-case experimental designs. Interventions aimed at improving academic performance through the manipulation of the curriculum, antecedent conditions, or peer tutoring produced approximately equal or greater effect sizes. In contrast, cognitive-behavioral treatment (CBT) approaches when used in the school setting were significantly less effective than these other two forms of interventions. Thus, despite some initial findings of rather limited impact of classroom behavior management on children with ADHD (Abikoff & Gittelman, 1984), later studies (Carlson, Pelham, Milich, & Dixon, 1992; Pelham & Hoza, 1996; Pelham et al., 1998), and the totality of the extant literature reviewed by DuPaul and Eckert (1997, 1998) suggest that behavioral and academic interventions in the classroom can be effective in improving behavioral problems and academic performance in children with ADHD. The greatest and most reliable improvements across studies are evident with contingency management and peer-tutoring approaches, while studies of curriculum modifications, strategy training, and other CBT approaches are less reliable (DuPaul & Eckert, 1997, 1998). Moreover, even the most effective classroom interventions may not make the behavior of children with ADHD fully comparable to that of nondisabled children.

As noted above in regard to laboratory applications of behavior therapy techniques, research suggests some promise in the use of stimulus control procedures for children with ADHD, and many of these can be readily adapted to the classroom. For example, reducing task length, "chunking" tasks into smaller units to fit more readily within a child's attention span, and setting quotas for a child to achieve within shorter time intervals may increase these children's success with academic work (see Ayllon & Rosenbaum, 1977; DuPaul & Stoner, 2003; Pfiffner, Barkley, & DuPaul,

2006). As Zentall (1985) has already documented, the use of increased stimulation within a task (e.g., color, shape, texture, rate of stimulus presentation) may enhance attention to academic tasks in children with ADHD. Teaching styles may also play an important role in how well such children attend to lectures by a teacher. More vibrant, enthusiastic teachers who move about more, engage children frequently while teaching, and allow greater participation of the children in the teaching activity may increase sustained attention to the task at hand. Zentall has also shown that permitting children with ADHD to move or participate motorically while learning a task may improve attention and performance. The use of written, displayed rules and timers for setting task time limits, as already described, may further benefit these children in the classroom.

A number of studies have also shown that the contingent application of reinforcers for reduced activity level or increased sustained attention can rapidly alter the levels of these ADHD symptoms (DuPaul & Eckert, 1997, 1998; DuPaul & Stoner, 2003). Usually these programs incorporate token rewards, as some research suggests that praise may not be sufficient to increase levels of on-task behavior or to maintain increased levels in children with ADHD (Pfiffner et al., 2006). Several studies have shown that group-administered rewards, where all children in class receive a reward contingent on the performance of one child, are as effective as individually administered rewards (O'Leary, Pelham, Rosenbaum, & Price, 1976). One of the problems arising in early research on this topic, however, was the demonstration that simply reinforcing greater on-task behavior and decreased activity levels did not necessarily translate into increased work productivity or accuracy (Marholin & Steinman, 1977). Since the latter are the ultimate goals of behavioral intervention in the classroom, these results were somewhat dismaying. Research now suggests that reinforcing the products of classroom behavior (i.e., number and accuracy of problems completed) not only results directly in increased productivity and accuracy, but also indirectly in declines in offtask and hyperactive behavior (see DuPaul & Stoner, 2003).

A serious limitation to these promising results has been the lack of followup on the maintenance of these treatment gains over time. In addition, none of these studies examined whether generalization of behavioral control occurred in other school settings where no treatment procedures were in effect. Other studies employing a mixture of CBT and contingency management techniques have failed to find such generalization for children with ADHD (Barkley, Copeland, & Sivage, 1980), suggesting that improvements derived from classroom management methods are quite situation-specific and may not generalize or be maintained once treatment has been terminated.

The role of punishment in the management of classroom behavior in children with ADHD has been less well studied. Pfiffner, O'Leary, Rosen, and Sanderson (1985) evaluated the effects of continuous and intermittent verbal reprimands and response cost on offtask classroom behaviors. They found that while each of these treatments significantly reduced disruptive and offtask behavior, the continuous use of response cost (loss of recess time) was most effective. Ayllon and Rosenbaum (1977) also report on the initial success of adding response cost contingencies to an ongoing classroom token economy. However, after less than 1 week, disruptive behavior returned to baseline levels despite the punishment contingency.

In a later paper, Pfiffner and O'Leary (1987) determined that the sole use of positive reinforcement for controlling ADHD behaviors in the classroom was not sufficient to maintain improved behavior in these children unless punishment in the form of response cost was added to the program. The addition of response cost further increased rates of ontask behavior and academic accuracy. These gains in behavior could then be maintained by an all-positive program once the response cost procedure was gradually withdrawn. However, abrupt withdrawal of the punishment contingency resulted in declines in on-task behavior and accuracy, suggesting that the manner in which response cost techniques are implemented and then faded out of classroom management programs is important in the maintenance of initial treatment gains. In general, the efficacy of response cost procedures for children with ADHD has been well documented (DuPaul, Guevremont, & Barkley, 1992; Gordon, Thomason, & Cooper, 1990; Rapport, Murphy, & Bailey, 1982).

What conclusions can be drawn from this literature indicate that contingency management methods can produce immediate, significant, shortterm improvement in the behavior, pro-

ductivity, and accuracy of children with ADHD in the classroom. Secondary or tangible reinforcers are more effective in reducing disruptive behavior and increasing performance than attention or other social reinforcers are. The use of positive reinforcement programs alone does not seem to result in as much improvement, nor does it maintain that improvement over time, as well as does the combination of token reinforcement systems with punishment, such as response cost (i.e., removal of tokens or privileges). Such findings would be expected from the theory of ADHD discussed earlier, which suggest a decreased power to self-regulate motivation and a delay in the development of internalized speech and the rule-governed behavior it affords in children with this disorder. What little evidence there is, however, suggests that treatment gains are unlikely to be maintained in these children once treatment has been withdrawn, and that improvements in behavior probably do not generalize to other settings where no treatment is in effect.

Another promising method deserving of further evaluation is the use of home-based contingencies for in-class behavior and performance. Atkinson and Forehand (1979), in an early review of this literature, found that the method offered some usefulness for managing disruptive classroom behavior, but that much more rigorous research would be required to evaluate its promise. Despite the lack of research demonstrating the unique contributions of home-based contingencies designed to improve classroom behavior, this is probably one of the most commonly recommended interventions for children having behavior problems in school. This commonsense intervention is vulnerable to delays in rewards or punishment, teacher and child resistance or inconsistency in submitting reports, and parental inconsistency in delivering consequences. Thus, the efficacy of school-to-home reports for managing classroom behavior should not be taken for granted. In the absence of well-conducted research in peer-reviewed journals, clinicians are advised to evaluate the efficacy of school-to-home reports on a case-by-case basis. An example of such a program is given below.

As discussed above in connection with Barkley's BPT program (Barkley, 1997d), the method involves having a teacher rate a child's daily school performance one or more times throughout a school day. These ratings are then sent home with the child for review by the parents. The parents then dispense rewards and punishments (usually response cost) at home, contingent upon the content of these daily ratings. O'Leary and colleagues (1976) employed this procedure for 10 weeks with nine hyperkinetic children and documented significant improvements on teacher ratings of classroom conduct and hyperkinesis as compared to a no-treatment control group. Others have similarly found such home–school behavioral report cards to be useful, either alone or in combination with parent and teacher training in behavior management, in the treatment of children with ADHD (Ayllon, Garber, & Pisor, 1975; MTA Cooperative Group, 1999a; O'Leary & Pelham, 1978; Pelham et al., 1988).

Some recent innovative treatment approaches, exploratory in nature, are of note. Hook and DuPaul (1999) evaluated the beneficial effects of parent tutoring on the reading performance of four students with ADHD, using a multiple-baseline-across-participants design. Parental tutoring of the students in reading resulted in improved reading performance both at home and in school, and stable or improved attitudes toward reading, with two of the four students reaching average levels of reading performance at least once during the training. However, overall, these children did not reach average performance levels consistently.

Ota and DuPaul (2002) examined the effects of using game-like math software to supplement mathematics instruction in three students with ADHD, again using a multiple-baseline-across-participants design. Behavioral observations and curriculum-based math probes revealed significant improvements in math performance with the software supplementation. Both of these studies employing small-scale, single-case designs offer some promise of additional supplemental interventions to those discussed above. And both are now in need of replication with larger samples, a more diverse population of students with ADHD, and examination of clinical (educational) effectiveness, not just efficacy.

To summarize the efficacy of classroom-focused contingency management, this should be considered a grade A or B treatment, depending on which techniques are used. Cognitive or CBT techniques and skills training appear to be failed interventions unless the techniques or skills are specifically reinforced

at the point of performance. Behavior modification methods that use a combination of reward and punishment seem to have the best results, but there is still some uncertainty about which methods are best and for whom. It does seem to be clear that the effects of these interventions are transient and that the interventions need to be implemented over a very long term. Approaches that train parents to set up reinforcement contingencies based on teacher-to-parent communication (e.g., daily behavior reports) may be the best hope for sustained intervention across the life span. All of the significant barriers to the effectiveness of behavioral management discussed previously for parents apply to teachers. There is widespread ignorance, neglect, or poor implementation of these methods. Intensive efforts to educate and support parents and teachers in the use of these methods could make a huge difference in the functioning of many children with learning or behavior problems at school. Unfortunately, even school psychologists may not have the time or expertise to assist in setting up proper behavior management programs, so there is a quite a bit of work to be done to make this a grade A intervention that is widely available.

Cognitive-Behavioral Treatment

The provision of CBT, or cognitive therapy, was previously felt to hold some promise for children with ADHD (Douglas, 1980; Kendall & Braswell, 1985; Meichenbaum & Goodman, 1971). Such treatment involves training children to give themselves instructions overtly in how to approach a task, strategies to employ during the task, and self-statements of evaluation and self-reinforcement at the end of the task. A few small-scale studies suggested some benefits to this form of treatment for children with ADHD (Fehlings, Roberts, Humphries, & Dawe, 1991). But CBT has been challenged as being seriously flawed from the conceptual (Vygotskian) point of view on which the treatment was initially founded (Diaz & Berk, 1995). Whether or not the self-statements of children with ADHD during task performance are actually deficient and in need of such correction is also open to question. And its efficacy for impulsive children or those with ADHD has been repeatedly challenged by the rather poor or limited results of empirical research (Abikoff, 1985, 1987; Abikoff & Gittelman, 1985).

Reviews of the CBT literature using meta-analyses have typically found the effect sizes to be only about a third of a standard deviation, and in many studies even less than this (Baer & Nietzel, 1991; DuPaul & Eckert, 1997; Dush, Hirt, & Schroeder, 1989). Although such treatment effects may at times rise to the level of statistical significance, they are nonetheless of only modest clinical importance and usually are to be found mainly on relatively circumscribed lab measures (Brown, Wynne, et al., 1986), rather than more clinically important measures of functioning in natural settings.

A large-scale, well-controlled study of CBT conducted in the Minneapolis public school system found no effect on children with ADHD. The study involved substantial training of parents, teachers, and children, and 2 years of this multicomponent intervention. But the researchers found no significant treatment effects on any of a variety of dependent measures at the 1-year assessment, with the exception of class observations of off-task/disruptive behavior, and no effects after 2 years of treatment (Bloomquist, August, & Ostrander, 1991; Braswell et al., 1997). Even the treatment effect on class observations was not maintained at the 2-year follow-up. Therefore, given the extant research findings of limited effect sizes in most clinical studies and the absence of treatment effects in the largest study, this treatment is given a grade of D, and no further discussion of CBT for ADHD is presented here.

Social Skills Training

Early reviews of social skills training (SST) as applied specifically to children with ADHD were quite discouraging (Hinshaw, 1992; Hinshaw & Erhardt, 1991; Whalen & Henker, 1991). Children with ADHD certainly have serious difficulties in their social interactions with peers (Bagwell et al., 2001; Cunningham & Siegel, 1987; Erhardt & Hinshaw, 1994; Hubbard & Newcomb, 1991; Whalen & Henker, 1992). This seems to be especially true for the subgroup having significant levels of comorbid aggression (Erhardt & Hinshaw, 1994; Hinshaw, 1992), for whom more than 50% of the variance in peer ratings of children they disliked was predicted by the aggressive behavior alone. As Hinshaw (1992) has summarized, the social interaction problems of children with ADHD are quite heterogeneous; such problems are thus not likely to respond to

a treatment package that focuses only on social approach strategies, and that treats all children with ADHD as if they shared common problems in their peer relationship difficulties. Nor is it especially clear at this time what the actual source of these peer difficulties happens to be or the mechanism by which it operates, with the exception of aggressive behavior as noted above. For instance, do children with ADHD actually lack the knowledge of proper social skills, or is it that they know how to act with others but do not do so at the points of performance in social interactions, where such skills would be useful to perform? The theoretical model presented earlier would suggest that the latter is likely to be more of a problem than the former, at least for children having ADHD without significant aggression. Teaching them additional skills is not so much the issue as is assisting them in performing the skills they have *when* it would be useful to do so *at the point of performance*, where such skills are most likely to prove useful to the long-term social acceptance of the individual.

Those children with ADHD and comorbid aggression may well have additional problems with peer perceptions—particularly in the motives they attribute to others for their behavior, as well as in information processing about social interactions (Dodge, 1989; Milich & Dodge, 1984). This combination of perceptual/information-processing deficits with problems in performing appropriate social skills in social interactions with others may make children with ADHD and aggression particularly resistant to SST (Hinshaw, 1992).

Actual research on SST for ADHD has produced rather mixed results. Early studies suggested that at-risk groups of children responded better to such programs (i.e., larger effect sizes were found) than did children with externalizing or disruptive behavioral problems (Beelmann, Pfingsten, & Losel, 1994). Frankel, Myatt, and Cantwell (1995) subsequently examined an SST program for outpatient children with disruptive disorder, half of whom were diagnosed with ADHD. Nearly half of the children in the treated and wait-list control groups were receiving medication. Treatment assignment was not random, but was associated with various clinical factors (date of intake, class starting date, class space available). Mothers' ratings showed improved social skills in the treated children compared to the wait-list control children; teachers' ratings revealed decreased aggression and withdrawal in the treated group, but only among those who did not have ODD. A later study by this same research team provided SST to children already receiving medication. Children with ADHD ($n = 35$) were compared to a wait-list control group ($n = 12$) of children with ADHD who were also receiving medication. Parents were trained in strategies to help with generalization to the home setting. It is not clear how participants were assigned to treatment groups, or to what extent this study included data from participants in the earlier study. Significant benefits on both parent and teacher ratings were found in the treated compared to the wait-list children, with the presence of ODD having no moderating effects, as it had in the earlier report (Frankel, Myatt, Cantwell, & Feinberg, 1997).

A study of young children (ages 4–8 years) having either ODD or CD, some of whom also had ADHD (Webster-Stratton, Reid, & Hammond, 2001), showed positive benefits of an SST/problem-solving training program on conduct problem behavior, both on teacher ratings and on home behavioral observations, but not on parent ratings of conduct problems. Treatment effects remained at a 1-year follow-up. Likewise, Pfiffner and McBurnett (1997) found evidence for the efficacy of an SST program for children with ADHD, but only on parent ratings and not teacher ratings. Children were randomly assigned to receive SST alone, SST supplemented with parent training in generalization strategies, or a wait-list control group. Both SST groups improved in parent rated social behavior relative to control children, with improvements being maintained at a 4-month follow-up. But there was little evidence that these benefits generalized to the school setting. The addition of parent training in generalization strategies did not result in any further benefits over SST alone.

All of these studies indicate some benefits of SST for children with conduct problems, including those with ADHD, particularly when parent ratings serve as the outcome measure. Yet many suffer from significant limitations in their methods. Bear in mind that several of these studies did not employ randomized assignment to treated or untreated groups (the Frankel et al. studies), and that parents were aware of the intervention being received (all studies). Moreover, all of the studies used wait-list control groups for their comparisons. It is

not clear whether such positive results would be found if efforts were made to control for therapist attention, as in attention placebo groups, or if alternative treatment approaches were also employed. Effects on teacher ratings of school social behavior are also not as encouraging as results from parent ratings, but they do imply that some children in some studies may have demonstrated reduced social withdrawal and possibly aggression in school.

More sobering results are revealed in two other studies of children with ADHD. Sheridan, Dee, Morgan, McCormack, and Walker (1996) found no evidence that SST generalized to peer interactions in the school setting. A more recent study using a clinic-referred sample of 120 children having ADHD found no significant benefits for most of the children on a variety of measures of social functioning (Antshel & Remer, 2003). The children with the primarily inattentive type of ADHD may have improved in their assertion skills following treatment, but not on any other measures of social interaction. Contrary to the Webster-Stratton and colleagues (2001) study, children having comorbid ODD did not benefit as much as those children with ADHD but no ODD. Moreover, some evidence of "peer deviancy training" was evident in the study. This refers to the peer reinforcement of aggressive and antisocial behavior among the children in the group, such that children actually increased their levels of aggressive behavior as a result of group participation. Earlier studies did not examine this possibility of a detrimental impact of group SST. Such an adverse impact is certainly worthy of further examination in future research with children having ADHD.

At this time, SST for children with ADHD might receive a grade of C, reflecting the inconsistent nature of the results, the limited number of studies using randomized assignment to treatment groups, the parents' and teachers' awareness of treatment conditions, the absence of attention placebo or alternative treatment groups, the limited evidence of generalization to the school setting, and the fact that studies to date have mainly involved efficacy rather than effectiveness in actual clinical contexts. In addition to the questionable efficacy of SST, it is worth noting that there may be some risk of accelerating antisocial behavior, or deviancy training, in SST training when delinquent youths are placed together in groups (Dishion, McCord, & Poulin, 1999).

Combined Interventions[1]

Psychopharmacological and behavioral treatments are not, by themselves, typically or completely adequate to address all of the difficulties likely to be presented by clinic-referred children or adolescents with ADHD. Optimal treatment is likely to comprise a combination of many of these approaches for maximal effectiveness (Carlson et al., 1992; Pelham et al., 1998; Phelps, Brown, & Power, 2002). However, the extent to which combined treatments are superior to medication alone is a controversial issue, especially given the relatively high cost of many psychosocial interventions. Nevertheless, findings emerging from the MTA project discussed below imply some potential advantages of combined treatment, although some other multisite studies may challenge that conclusion. We first present some of the historical studies on combined treatments, as well as some more recent efforts at intensive multimodal treatment; we then review the MTA project in depth, along with qualifications offered by another multisite combined treatment project, the NYM study.

Early Research

Some early research studies examined the utility of combining psychosocial and pharmacological treatment packages, with interesting results. It appeared that in many of these studies, the combination of contingency management training of parents or teachers with stimulant drug therapies was generally little better than either treatment alone for the management of ADHD symptoms (Firestone, Kelly, Goodman, & Davey, 1981; Gadow, 1985; Pollard, Ward, & Barkley, 1983; Wolraich, Drummond, Salomon, O'Brien, & Sivage, 1978). Several studies also found impressive results for classroom behavior management methods (Carlson et al., 1992; DuPaul & Eckert, 1997; Pelham et al., 1988), but found that the addition of medication provided some improvements beyond those achieved by behavior management alone. Moreover, the combination might result in the need for less intense behavioral interventions or lower doses of medication than might have been the case if either intervention were used alone. Where there was an advantage for behavioral interventions, it appeared to be related to functioning rather than symptom relief, such as reliably increasing rates of aca-demic productivity and accuracy (DuPaul & Stoner, 2003). Despite some failures in these early studies to obtain additive effects for these two treatments, their combination may still be advantageous, given that the stimulants are not usually used in the late afternoons or evenings (when parents may need effective behavior management tactics to deal with the ADHD symptoms). Moreover, a minority of children (10–25%) do not respond positively to these medications (Connor, 2006b), making behavioral interventions one of the few scientifically proven alternatives for these cases.

Several studies examined the combined effects of stimulant medication with CBT interventions. Horn, Chatoor, and Conners (1983) examined the separate and combined effects of dextroamphetamine and self-instructional training for a 9-year-old inpatient with ADHD. The combined program was more effective in increasing ontask behavior during classwork, and decreasing teacher ratings of ADHD symptoms. However, academic productivity was improved only by the use of direct reinforcement for correct responses. In contrast, using group comparison designs, Brown, Borden, Wynne, Schleser, and Clingerman (1986) and Brown, Wynne, and Medenis (1985) found no benefits of combined drug and CBT interventions over either treatment alone for similar domains of functioning in children with ADHD. Similarly, a later study by Horn and colleagues (1991) did not find the combination of treatments to be superior to medication alone.

Some success for combined medication and self-evaluation procedures has been reported (Hinshaw, Henker, & Whalen, 1984a) when social skills, such as cooperation, have been targets of intervention. Yet, when these same investigators attempted to teach anger control strategies to children with ADHD to enhance self-control during peer interactions, no benefits of combined intervention were found beyond those achieved by self-control training alone (Hinshaw, Henker, & Whalen, 1984b). The self-control techniques were the most successful in teaching these children specific coping strategies to employ in provocative interactions with peers, which usually led to angry reactions from the children with ADHD. Medication, in contrast, served only to lower the overall level of anger responses, but did not enhance the application of specific anger control strategies. These studies suggest that each form of treatment may have highly specific and unique effects on some aspects of social behavior but not on others.

Limited research has evaluated the effects of BPT, either alone or combined with child training in self-control strategies (Horn, Ialongo, Popovich, & Peradotto, 1987), on home and school behavioral problems. The results failed to find any significant advantage for the combined treatments. Both self-control training and BPT alone improved home behavior problems, but neither resulted in any generalization of treatment effects to the school, where no treatment had occurred. Since a no-treatment group was not employed in this study, however, it is not possible to conclude that these effects were due to treatment rather than to nonspecific effects (e.g., maturation, therapist attention, regression effects, etc.). A later study by Horn, Ialongo, Greenberg, Packard, and Smith-Winberry (1990) did find such a combination to be superior to either treatment used alone in producing a significantly larger number of children responding to treatment. Once again, however, no generalization of the results to the school setting occurred.

Satterfield, Satterfield, and Cantwell (1980) attempted to evaluate the effects of individualized multimodality intervention provided over extensive time periods (up to several years) on the outcome of boys with ADHD. Interventions included medication, BPT, individual counseling, special education, family therapy, and other programs as needed by the individual. Results suggested that such an individualized program of combined treatments continued over longer time intervals could produce improvements in social adjustment at home and school, rates of antisocial behavior, substance abuse, and academic achievement. These results seemed to be sustained across at least a 3-year follow-up period (Satterfield, Cantwell, & Satterfield, 1979; Satterfield, Satterfield, & Cantwell, 1981; Satterfield, Satterfield, & Schell, 1987). Although this research suggested great promise for the possible efficacy of multimodality treatment extended over years for children with ADHD, the lack of random assignment and more adequate control procedures in this series of studies limited the ability to attribute the improvements directly to the treatments employed. And these limitations certainly precluded establishing which of the treatment components was most effective. Still, studies such as these and others (Carlson et al., 1992; Pelham et al., 1988) raised hopes that intensive multimodality treatment could be effective for ADHD if extended over long intervals of time.

Intensive Multimodal Treatment Programs

Two of the most well-known and well-regarded multimodality intervention programs are the summer treatment program (STP) developed by William Pelham and colleagues and conducted at Western Psychiatric Institute in Pittsburgh (Pelham & Hoza, 1996), and the University of California–Irvine/Orange County Department of Education (UCI/OCDE) intervention developed by James Swanson, Linda Pfiffner, Keith McBurnett, and Dennis Cantwell (see Pfiffner et al., 2006). The latter program incorporates a number of features of the program developed by Pelham, as well as some components of the multimodal program conducted by Stephen Hinshaw, Barbara Henker, and Carol Whalen at the University of California–Los Angeles. Both of these programs rely on four major components of treatment: (1) parent training in child behavior management; (2) classroom implementation of behavior modification techniques; (3) SST (typically centered around sports); and (4) stimulant medication, in some cases. Whereas the Pelham STP is a day camp–style program conducted during the summer months, the UCI/OCDE program is a year-round, school-style program. These two programs, plus a third project conducted under the auspices of the University of Massachusetts Medical School (UMASS) and the Worcester (Massachusetts) Public Schools (WPS), are described below.

THE SUMMER TREATMENT PROGRAM

The STP was largely developed by Pelham and colleagues and is conducted in a day-treatment environment with a summer school/day camp–like format. Daily activities include a few hours of classroom instruction, which also incorporates behavior modification methods (such as token economies, response cost, and time out from reinforcement). In addition, 3–4 hours of sports and recreational activities are arranged each day, during which behavioral management programs are operative. The program also includes parent training, peer relationship training, and a follow-up protocol to enhance the likelihood that treatment gains will be maintained after children leave the program.

During their stay at the camp, some children may be tested on stimulant medication. A double-blind, placebo-controlled procedure is used, in which a child is tested on several different doses of medication while teacher ratings and behavioral observations are collected across the different camp activities.

Pelham and colleagues have used this setting and larger programmatic context to conduct more focused research investigations into the effectiveness of classroom behavior management procedures alone, stimulant medication alone, and their combination in managing ADHD symptoms and improving academic performance and social behavior. Some of the components of the STP have been evaluated previously, such as classroom contingency management, and have been found to produce significant short-term improvements in children with ADHD (see DuPaul & Eckert, 1997, 1998; Pfiffner et al., 2006). And so they clearly seem to do in the STP itself (Carlson et al., 1992; Pelham et al., 1988). The STP, in fact, was a part of the intensive multimodal treatment program for children with ADHD studied in the MTA project (see below). But other components of the program have not been so well evaluated previously for their efficacy with children having ADHD, such as SST. And while results from parent ratings before and after their children's participation indicate that 86% believe their children have improved through their participation in the program, no data have been published as yet on whether the gains made during the treatment program are maintained in the subsequent typical school and home settings after the children terminate their participation in this program.

THE UCI/OCDE PROGRAM

The UCI/OCDE program (see Pfiffner et al., 2006) provides weekday treatment for children with ADHD in kindergarten through fifth grade in a school-like atmosphere, using classes of 12–15 children. The clinical interventions rely chiefly on a token economy program for the management of behavior in the classrooms, and a parent training program conducted through both group and individual treatment sessions. Some training of self-monitoring, evaluation, and reinforcement also occurs as part of the class program. In addition, children receive daily group instruction in social skills as part of the classroom curriculum, and some of

these behaviors may be targeted for modification outside of the group instruction time by using consequences within the classroom token economy. Before returning to their regular public schools, some children may participate in a transitional school program that focuses on more advanced social skills, as well as behavior modification programs to facilitate the transfer of learning to their regular school setting. Some children within this program also may receive stimulant medication as needed for management of their ADHD symptoms.

Although this program has served as an exemplar for many others, published research on its efficacy is not available. Granted, the parent training program and classroom behavior modification methods are highly similar to those used in published studies that have found them to be effective at least in the short term, so long as they are in use (Barkley, 1997d; DuPaul & Eckert, 1997; Pelham & Sams, 1992). But the actual extent to which this particular program achieves its stated goals—and, specifically, the generalization of treatment gains to nontreatment settings, as well as the maintenance of those gains after children return to their public schools—has not been systematically evaluated or published.

THE UMASS/WPS EARLY INTERVENTION PROJECT

Barkley, Shelton, and colleagues completed a multimethod early intervention program for kindergarten children (ages 4–6 years) having significant problems with hyperactivity and aggression (see Barkley et al., 2000; Shelton et al., 2002). This program did not utilize clinic-referred children, whose parents and even teachers may be highly motivated to cooperate with treatment. Instead, children were identified at kindergarten registration as displaying significantly high levels of hyperactive and aggressive behavior (93rd percentile) and being at high risk for both ADHD and ODD. Indeed, more than 70% of them met criteria for these disorders upon subsequent clinical evaluation with structured psychiatric interviews. They were randomly assigned to one of four intervention groups for their entire kindergarten year. One group received a 10-week group parent training program, followed by monthly booster session group meetings. Otherwise, the children participated in the standard (WPS) kindergarten program. The second group was assigned to a special enrichment kindergarten classroom, in which they received accelerated instruction in academic skills, SST, classroom contingency management procedures (token systems and other reinforcements, response cost, time out, etc.), and cognitive therapy (self-instruction training) as part of their full-day kindergarten program. These special classes contained 12–16 hyperactive–aggressive children in each and were held in two neighborhood elementary schools in the WPS system (to which the children were provided busing). Children in this special classroom also received several months of follow-up consultation to their teachers when they returned to their regular public schools for their first grade year. A third group received both the parent training and enrichment classroom treatments, while a fourth group received no special services except for the initial evaluation and periodic reevaluations.

All children were followed for 2 years after their participation in these treatment programs. Results indicated no beneficial effect of the parent training program, in large part because more than 60% of the parents did not attend the training classes regularly, if at all. The enrichment classroom produced a significant improvement in the children's classroom behavior and social skills during the kindergarten year, but did not result in any change in behavior in the home as rated by parents. Nor did it produce greater gains in academic achievement skills than had been experienced by the control groups not receiving this classroom program. Moreover, the results of the classroom appear to have been attenuated during the follow-up period. Such results once again show that intensive classroom behavioral interventions can be effective in the short term for addressing the disruptive behavior of children. Yet these same results are rather sobering in view of the large investment of money, time, and staff training. Parent training programs for children at high risk for school and home behavior problems may not be especially effective in families identified through such community screening programs, largely due to poor parental motivation and investment in the training program. And even where classroom interventions are successful in the short-term "active" treatment phase, their effects may diminish or disappear with time after children leave the treatment environment. This study suggests that the rather positive treatment outcome results for families whose members seek

treatment and, by inference, are motivated to change themselves and their children with ADHD may not be readily extrapolated to families with similarly deviant children whose members have not sought treatment but were identified through community screening programs.

The Historic MTA Project

The National Institute of Mental Health (NIMH) collaborative multisite Multimodal Treatment Study of Children with ADHD (MTA) project is the first major clinical trial by NIMH with a focus on a childhood disorder (MTA Cooperative Group, 1999a, 1999b). Although much research has documented the short-term effectiveness of medication and behavioral interventions to treat ADHD, significant questions remain unanswered about long-term effectiveness of these interventions, alone or in combination, on the multiple functional outcome areas affected by ADHD. Questions also remain about which types of youths with ADHD may benefit most from which types of treatment. The ambitious and groundbreaking MTA was designed to help answer some of these major questions by randomly assigning children to four treatment groups: medication alone (MedMgt), behavior modification alone (Beh), the combination of medication and behavior modification (Comb), and community comparison (CC). In order to obtain a sufficiently large and diverse sample of youths with ADHD to begin to address these questions, a multisite study was initiated by NIMH (along with funding from the U.S. Department of Education) in 1992. Six proposals were funded; after 1 year, a common intervention protocol was created and then implemented at six sites in the United States and one collaborative site in Canada.

MTA DESIGN/METHODOLOGY

In order to be eligible for the study, children had to be between ages 7 and 9.9; to be in grades 1–4; to meet DSM-IV diagnostic criteria for ADHD, combined type, via the Parent version of the Diagnostic Interview Schedule for Children (supplemented by teacher-reported symptoms if a case was near the diagnostic threshold); and to be living with the same caretaker for at least the previous 6 months. Youths with comorbid internalizing or externalizing psychiatric disorders were included, as long as these conditions did not require treatment incompatible with study treatments. The schools the children attended also had to express cooperation with both the treatment and assessment protocols. Other exclusionary criteria included situations that would prevent full participation in the study, such as not having a phone, intellectual and adaptive functioning in the borderline range or below, or major medical illness (for complete information on the screening and selection procedures, see MTA Cooperative Group, 1999a). Important characteristics of the sample selected for the study included variables identified a priori as potential moderators of treatment: gender (20% female); prior medication status (31%); ODD or CD diagnoses (40% and 14%); DSM-III-R anxiety disorder (34% with simple phobia alone were not included); and numbers of youths whose families were receiving welfare, public assistance, or Supplemental Security Income (19%). Important to note is that the 579 children represented only 13% of those initially contacting the project, 25% of those passing an initial rating scale screening, and 62% of those completing the diagnostic interview and evaluation of school cooperation.

Once selected, participants were randomly assigned to one of the four conditions. Treatments were delivered over a 14-month period; comprehensive assessments of functioning in multiple domains were conducted at baseline prior to randomization, as well as at 3, 9, and 14 months (with the 14-month assessment constituting the treatment endpoint assessment) (MTA Cooperative Group, 1999a). The MTA Cooperative Group (2004a, 2004b) recently published results of a 24-month follow-up, and 36- and 48-month follow-ups are currently underway or planned for the future.

Behavioral treatments (in both the Beh and Comb conditions) encompassed parent, child, and school domains. BPT was provided by experienced training consultants and based on models by Barkley (1997d) and Forehand and McMahon (1981; McMahon & Forehand, 2003). This intervention consisted of 27 group and 8 individual sessions. Child behavioral treatment consisted of an intensive summer treatment program (based on the Pelham STP model) as well as school consultation services (similar to the UCI/OCDE model). The STP was an intensive 8-week, 9-hour-per-day program; study training consultants supervised

staff members working with the children and continued to provide parent interventions during the summer. The same training consultants provided school consultation services (10–16 sessions of teacher consultation and establishment of a daily report card), and the staff members working with the children in the STP worked in the schools in the fall as paraprofessional aides (12 weeks at half time under supervision of the training consultants and the children's teachers). Families attended an average of 77.8% of parent training sessions, 36.2 of 40 possible STP days, 10.7 teacher consultation visits, and 47.6 (of 60) possible days with a classroom aide. Delivery of behavioral treatments was faded over the course of treatment, so that by the endpoint assessment at 14 months, therapist contact with parents had ended or was reduced to once per month.

Like the intensive behavioral interventions, the medication treatments (in both the MedMgt and Comb conditions) provided in the MTA occurred in a much more rigorous and intensive way than is typical in clinical practice. All medication treatment provided by the MTA included an initial 28-day double-blind, placebo-controlled titration consisting of placebo plus four different doses of methylphenidate (5, 10, 15, and 20 mg) randomly given over the titration period. Three-times-per-day dosing was used in the titration (and typically during treatment), in which the full dose was given in the morning and at lunch, as well as a half dose in the midafternoon. Parent and teacher daily ratings were collected during the titration; graphs portraying the results were rated by a cross-site panel of experienced clinicians. A "best dose" was chosen, and the blind was broken; that dose became the initial dose for treatment. If the dose chosen was placebo, alternative medications were openly titrated until a satisfactory medication was chosen (or, in the case of a robust placebo response, the child was not medicated). Approximately 89% of youths assigned to MedMgt or Comb successfully completed titration; of these, 68.5% were assigned to initial doses of methylphenidate averaging 30.5 mg/day divided across doses given three times per day. Of the remaining group of youths who completed titration but were not started on methylphenidate, 26 received an unblinded titration of dextroamphetamine because of unsatisfactory methylphenidate response, and 32 were given no medication because of a robust placebo response.

Of note is that of the 289 subjects assigned to MedMgt or Comb, 17 families refused titration, and another 15 subjects did not complete titration (11 due to side effects or problems with titration, and 4 because inadequate titration data were gathered) (MTA Cooperative Group, 1999a).

Youths assigned to the CC condition received no intervention by the MTA staff, but sought treatment as usually provided in the community. Referrals to non-MTA providers were made as necessary for these families; all CC youths and families returned for assessments at the same time as youths in the other three conditions of the study. Initially, it was thought that the CC group would provide a minimal- or no-treatment comparison group. However, as described later in this section, about two-thirds of the children in the CC group received medication for ADHD.

Outcomes in this study were assessed with a large number of measures in multiple domains, including verbal report information (via interview and paper/pencil measures) by parents, teachers, and children; direct observation in the clinic and school; and computerized assessments of attention. Given the large number of measures, settings, and informants used in the study, data reduction methods were conducted to condense measures into outcome domains. The major outcome domains that have received attention in the literature are as follows: ADHD symptoms, oppositional/aggressive symptoms, social skills, internalizing symptoms, parent–child relations, parental discipline, and academic achievement.

MAJOR FINDINGS FROM THE MTA ON ADHD SYMPTOMS

All four MTA groups showed symptom reduction over time. In our opinion, the trends in the data favored the Comb treatment over the other three conditions, but this conclusion may depend on how those data are analyzed. When an idiographic approach that looks at individual outcomes is used, there is a clear advantage of combined treatment. Swanson and colleagues (2001) created a categorical measure of treatment outcome, based on composite ADHD and ODD symptom scores from teachers and parents who completed the Swanson, Nolan, and Pelham Questionnaire–IV (SNAP-IV). Treatment success was identified as an average composite SNAP-IV score of 1 or below at the end of treatment (representing symptoms falling in the "not at all" or "just a little" range of categories at treatment endpoint). Success rates were as follows: 68% for Comb, 56% for MedMgt, 34% for Beh, and 25% for CC. A similar, but less robust, pattern of results was observed at the 24-month follow-up. Specifically, the success rates at follow-up were 48%, 37%, 32%, and 28%, for Comb, MedMgt, Beh, and CC, respectively (MTA Cooperative Group, 2004a).

Another way to look at the MTA data is in terms of statistical significance of the group means, which is the analysis that has received the most attention in the published literature. When using this approach on the 14- and 24-month follow-up data, the MTA Collaborative Group reached the conclusion that treatments involving MedMgt (i.e., MedMgt and Comb) were superior to those that did not include the intensive medication management (i.e., Beh and CC). Based on significance tests of means, the Beh and CC conditions were statistically equivalent. Likewise, the MedMgt and Comb groups were comparable, thus indicating no advantage of Comb relative to intensive MedMgt (MTA Cooperative Group, 1999a, 2004a). A few comments on these findings are warranted, however.

Some effects on ADHD symptoms were apparently mediated by medication (MTA Cooperative Group, 2004b). Therefore, it is important to note that 67% of the children in the CC group were taking medication. Thus the CC group was an active treatment group rather than a no-treatment control, and the group that received only behavior modification (Beh) was being compared to this group that received medications in the community. It is also important to consider the implications of the fact that there were some substantial differences in the doses of medication across the treatment groups. For instance, at the 14-month follow-up, the average daily dose for Comb was 31.2 mg, while the average daily dose for MedMgt was 37.7 mg (MTA Cooperative Group, 1999a). Given that Comb and MedMgt had identical medication titration procedures, the difference in dose at 14 months suggests that the intensive behavioral intervention allowed individuals to take lower doses of medication. Lower doses are a considerable therapeutic advantage, because most stimulant side effects, including the mild growth suppression observed in the MTA, are dose-dependent (i.e., lower doses lessen the risk and severity of side effects; MTA Cooperative Group, 2004b).

When one is examining the group data, it is tempting to conclude that the MedMgt condition was superior to CC, even though most of the CC participants were medicated. Such a conclusion implies that the package of procedures in the MedMgt protocol, which includes monthly supportive contact and decisions supported by high-quality data, is superior to routine community care. Indeed, this has been one of the major messages from the MTA Cooperative Group (e.g., 2004a). However, it is noteworthy that the average dose for those in the CC group who sought treatment in the community was 22.6 mg/day (MTA Cooperative Group, 1999a). The fact that children receiving intensive medication management in the MTA (i.e., MedMgt and Comb) were taking the equivalent of 10–15 mg more methylphenidate each day than the CC group is perplexing. In this situation, it is unclear whether the higher dose or some other aspect of the MedMgt intervention, such as dosing three times per day in some cases, resulted in the better outcomes.

Another consideration in comparing the Beh and Comb conditions with the MedMgt and CC conditions is that intensive behavioral treatments were faded by the study endpoint (Pelham, 1999). Due to this unequal treatment activity, it is plausible that the comparison of Beh and Comb to MedMgt at the 14-month follow-up may have been biased in favor of the MedMgt. This issue has been argued on theoretical grounds (see Pelham, 1999) and is consistent with observation that the therapeutic effect size of intensive MedMgt diminished by 50% from the intensive phase to the follow-up phase (i.e., from the 14- to the 24-month follow-up; MTA Cooperative Group, 2004a).

In our reading of the MTA data, as the fading becomes an increasingly distant past event, the trend in the data seems to be for the Comb group to outperform the other groups. However, according to the MTA Cooperative Group's statistical conclusion criteria, the differences between Comb and MedMgt are not yet statistically significant. Moreover, it appears that all treatments declined in effectiveness at the 2-year follow-up. Therefore, our conclusions regarding the superior efficacy of combined treatment in the MTA are open to alternative interpretation, particularly in light of a more recently reported multisite study discussed below.

MTA OUTCOMES OTHER THAN ADHD SYMPTOMS

When measures of other disorders or domains of impairment than those of ADHD symptoms are considered, most of the trends favor the Comb condition. For instance, the results when the MTA Cooperative Group ordered treatments by the number of times each group placed first, compared with all others, on 19 outcome measures were as follows: Comb, 12; MedMgt, 4; Beh, 2; and CC, 1. The four times that MedMgt was superior were for parent ratings of symptoms of inattention and hyperactivity, and classroom observation of hyperactivity and impulsivity (MTA Cooperative Group, 1999a). Although such data appear to strongly favor combined treatment over unimodal or community interventions, this analysis does not take into account the relative importance of the outcome measures. We submit that the areas tapped, including oppositional/aggressive symptoms, internalizing symptoms, social skills, parent–child relations, and academic achievement, are very important. This finding is critically important, as the non-ADHD domains assessed tap areas that are important in daily functioning and greatly affect quality of life for youths with ADHD and those who interact with them on a daily basis.

It is also noteworthy that at the 14-month follow-up, satisfaction scores by parents for the Comb and Beh conditions were equal to each other and significantly better than parent satisfaction scores for the MedMgt condition (MTA Cooperative Group, 1999a). Given the emphasis placed on consumer satisfaction in terms of third-party payments, this is not a trivial matter. Indeed, the highest attrition rates were for the MedMgt condition.

The relative superiority of combined treatment was highlighted by Conners and colleagues (2001), who conducted a post hoc analysis using a composite outcome measure. This was done in an effort to further examine the relative impact of MedMgt versus Comb, which did not differ statistically, due to the presence of multiple outcome measures in the primary analyses. When the composite measure was used, a statistically significant difference was detected: Comb outperformed MedMgt, with an effect size of 0.28 (low to moderate). In addition, use of the composite resulted in reduced effect sizes for comparisons of MedMgt versus Beh alone (0.26), and a moderate effect size of 0.35 for MedMgt versus

CC. Use of the composite therefore places combined treatment in the lead, albeit by only about a quarter of a standard deviation on the composite measure. Also, composite measures do result in more reliable estimates of effects, but effects could be obscured if treatments had idiosyncratic impacts on different aspects of functioning that were included in the composite.

In the 24-month MTA outcome, the investigators focused on ADHD symptoms plus four other areas of outcome deemed to be important and validly measured (MTA Cooperative Group, 2004a). These areas were oppositional symptoms, social skills, negative/ineffective parenting, and reading achievement. In this analysis, which focused on group means, the MTA intensive medication groups experienced a greater reduction in oppositional/aggressive symptoms. The mean for Comb was lower than that for MedMgt (0.83 vs. 0.96, respectively), and the p was .081. Thus, a directional one-tailed test with an alpha of .05 would have been statistically significant. However, the MTA Cooperative Group chose a two-tailed alpha of .01 for this particular comparison.

For the other three variables examined, best results in terms of ordering of group means were achieved with Comb treatment. However, the omnibus F-ratios for social skills, negative/ineffective parenting, and reading achievement were not statistically significant. Planned contrasts of two of the five outcomes reached borderline statistical significance for Comb versus MedMgt. Specifically, Comb was better than MedMgt for social skills ($p = .05$) and negative/ineffective parenting ($p = .03$). No such differences were found for Beh versus CC. These results suggest that there may be clinically meaningful advantages of combined treatment over unimodal treatments.

MODERATORS AND MEDIATORS OF TREATMENT EFFECTS

Mediators and moderators are often confused, and therefore we begin this discussion with a brief review (see Holmbeck, 1997, for more on the mediator–moderator distinction). Moderators include participant characteristics that could influence outcome, positively or negatively. Mediators are intervening variables operating during treatment that could affect outcome. Knowledge of moderators helps in making decisions about who benefits from what treatment. Knowledge of mediators can

help identify causal pathways from intervention to outcomes. The MTA Cooperative Group (1999b) is careful to note that mediator and moderator defined subgroup analyses are exploratory, as they are affected by sample size/power limitations, as well as suffering from the effects of repeated analyses.

Moderators were selected a priori and included gender, prior medication status, ODD or CD diagnoses, DSM-III-R anxiety disorder, and receipt of public assistance, as noted earlier. Study outcomes did not vary as a function of gender, prior history of medication, or comorbid disruptive disorders. There were some differences for youths with comorbid anxiety disorders and those who received public assistance. In the group with comorbid anxiety, all MTA treatments outperformed treatment in the community (CC). This is an interesting finding, because the MTA treatments did not target anxiety. The reasons for the differential response pattern are not well understood (see Jensen et al., 1999).

For the families on public assistance, parents in the MedMgt condition reported less closeness in parent–child interactions, and teachers reported better social skills for the Comb group. As with the other moderator effect, the reasons for the apparent effect have been explored but remain elusive. For example, no differences were seen between the treatment conditions in terms of positive parenting or family stress measures (see Wells et al., 2000).

A mediator analysis that examined the role of medication in mediating outcomes has been reported (MTA Cooperative Group, 2004b). Another mediator analysis in the MTA focused on treatment acceptance and attendance (MTA Cooperative Group, 1999b). In this second analysis, mediators were defined as acceptance of treatment and attendance at treatment sessions, defined as either "as intended" or "below intended." Operational definitions included accepting the treatment assignment, as well as percentage of treatment sessions attended: for MedMgt, 80% medical visits attended with prescriptions written/delivered during the sessions; and for Beh, 75% attendance at group parent training sessions and STP days, as well as a child and a paraprofessional being present together in the classroom for 75% of the possible days of this aspect of the intervention. (Comb families needed to meet both sets of unimodal criteria in order for their acceptance and attendance to be considered "as intended.") Interestingly, neither individual parent training session attendance nor teacher/therapist consultation visits, both vital portions of the intensive behavioral intervention, were counted. In the "as intended" subgroup, the main intent-to-treat analyses held (MedMgt = Comb, and both were better than CC and Beh). However, in the "below intended" subgroup, Comb was superior in terms of ADHD symptom reduction, with MedMgt = Beh (MTA Cooperative Group, 1999b). Thus there was an effect of compliance with treatment outcome, and the Comb condition was apparently more robust to noncompliance.

The NYM Multimodal Treatment Study

The results of a multimodal treatment study that was completed prior to the MTA and that also involved large samples and several treatment sites, have recently been reported. These results conflict with the findings of the MTA concerning the benefits of combined treatment over medication management alone. The New York–Montreal (NYM) study selected 103 children with ADHD (ages 7–9 years) who were free of CD and learning disorders, and who had shown an initial positive response to methylphenidate (abbreviated in this study as MPH) during a short-term trial. Hence, unlike the MTA, the NYM study focused exclusively on stimulant-responsive children having far less comorbidity. These children were randomly assigned to receive 2 years of treatment in one of three treatment arms: (1) MPH alone, (2) MPH plus intensive multimodal psychosocial treatment, or (3) MPH plus an attention placebo psychosocial treatment. The latter approach to controlling for professional attention was not used in the MTA. The intensive 2-year psychosocial treatment consisted of BPT, parent counseling, SST, psychotherapy, and extra academic assistance. Treatment contact during the first year was twice weekly, with fading of treatment to a considerable degree during the second year.

Assessments involved parent, teacher, and psychiatrist ratings; children's self-ratings; children's ratings of their parents; observations collected in school settings; and academic tests. The domains assessed included symptoms of ADHD and other behavioral problems (ODD), home and school functioning, social functioning, and academic performance. The results were consistent across all domains: No support

was found for combining intensive psychosocial treatments of any sort with MPH in children with ADHD who were initially shown to be responsive to MPH (Abikoff, Hechtman, Klein, Gallacher, et al., 2004; Abikoff, Hechtman, Klein, Weiss, et al., 2004; Hechtman, Abikoff, Klein, Greenfield, et al., 2004; Hechtman, Abikoff, Klein, Weiss, et al., 2004). Nor was it found that MPH could be discontinued successfully in those who were receiving the combination treatment. Thus it appears that the set of psychosocial treatments used in this study produced no incremental benefit in children who were shown to have strong and unambiguous responses to stimulant medication. Although the authors made some statements that there may have been improvement from MPH, the study was not designed to test for benefit from medication, and uncontrolled confounds (such as maturation or regression to the mean) are plausible alternative explanations for what may seem like sustained improvement associated with MPH across the 2 years of treatment.

In contrast to the MTA project, the NYM study did not include treatment within the children's usual school setting, nor did the children attend an intensive STP. Also unlike the MTA project, the NYM study intervened over a 24-month rather than a 14-month period. Lacking in both the MTA and the NYM study was documentation that the specific individual components of the psychosocial treatments were effective. This contrasts with the assessment of medication effects, because each child received very well-controlled individualized trials that determined whether medication worked. Based on the reviews in previous sections of this chapter, several of the interventions in the NYM study are not thought to be effective for children with ADHD (e.g., SST and individual therapy). Furthermore, although the BPT was shown to achieve significant improvements in knowledge of behavioral methods, there was no reported change in parenting behavior (Hechtman, Abikoff, Klein, Greenfield, et al., 2004). Thus there was no evidence that the psychosocial treatments met the requirement of showing activity at the point of performance.

Overall, the results of the NYM study may not represent a fair comparison of treatments, because grade A treatment with methylphenidate was compared with psychosocial treatments of unknown quality. A reasonable comparison of medication and psychosocial treatment should pit equivalent-quality treatments against each other (i.e., grade A medication and grade A psychosocial treatments). Such studies need to document that both treatments were delivered as intended, with appropriate implementation at the point of performance. This is key with medication, because according to the NYM study, poor compliance (as seen with the discontinuation probe) very rapidly results in deterioration. Psychosocial treatments should be evaluated with equal rigor (e.g., through experimental analysis of the effectiveness of behavior contingencies by using reversal designs in the context in individual case studies). To our knowledge, no such study has yet been conducted, but some insights might be gained for further analysis of compliance data in the MTA project and the NYM study. Until studies of the highest-quality interventions and with the most rigorous quality control are conducted and properly analyzed, there will be lingering questions about the relative merits of intensive multimodal treatment relative to excellent medication management for the treatment of ADHD and related problems.

Efficacy, Safety, and Practicality of Combined Treatment

Using the grading system for level of empirical validation described at the beginning of this chapter, we give the combination of stimulant medication and behavioral intervention the grade of B or lower. Let us clarify. Although the literature indicates that each of these treatments separately deserves a grade of A, what is being graded here is the superiority of their combination relative to either alone, based on the evidence. Is the evidence for the combined treatment sufficient to warrant this grade? Combined treatments have been shown to be superior to unimodal treatment on some measures in some subsets of children with ADHD in at least two well-designed studies by independent investigators. However, the fact that the NYM study found no advantages for intensive multimodal treatment may raise some doubts. Due to the relative methodological strengths of the MTA compared to the NYM study, we believe that greater weight should be given to the MTA. Because the MTA is a multisite study, some may consider the cross-site results as evidence of replication. However, replications within MTA were not independent. Pending replication or extension of the MTA findings, the highest grade possible for intensive, multimodal treatment is a grade of B. If the key outcome is symptoms of ADHD or equal weight is given to the NYM study as is to the MTA, the appropriate grade for multimodal treatment is C.

The grade of B to C for intensive multimodal treatment is also intended to convey the message that the practicality of combined treatments is unknown. Indeed, there are several reasons to believe that these treatments would be very difficult to replicate in most applied settings. For instance, the acceptance and attendance data from the MTA found 81% compliance for the medication component, but only 64% compliance for the behavioral component (MTA Collaborative Group, 1999b). This suggests that some important issues related to therapist expectations and family participation in the treatment need to be worked out. Moreover, the studies of combined treatment used some unique treatments that are difficult to find in many regions of the country or to replicate in applied clinical settings, such as Pelham and colleagues' STP. Until barriers to access to and participation in these treatments are overcome, the effectiveness of these treatments is open to doubt.

Generally speaking, combined treatment that uses family-based behavioral interventions and stimulant medication or atomoxetine should be very safe. Some possible safety concerns related to the multimodal treatments of ADHD have been studied. For example, some prominent theories related to conduct problems posit that placing children with behavior problems in groups with other disruptive children could lead to some harmful effects mediated by peer facilitation of antisocial behavior (Dishion et al., 1999). This was recently found to occur in an SST program for children with ADHD, particularly among those who were not manifesting significant conduct problems prior to treatment (Antshel & Remer, 2003). Also, Barkley and colleagues have twice documented an adverse effect (escalation of conflicts) during behavioral family therapy for teens with ADHD/ODD in a subset of participating families (Barkley, Edwards, et al., 2001a; Barkley, Guevremont, et al., 1992). Researchers studying behavioral interventions typically do not examine their data for such subsets of adverse responses, but should be encouraged by these results to do so.

Side effects of the medications warrant attention as well. Approximately 2.9% of children in the MTA reported having severe side effects, which apparently remitted with discontinuation of medication. Also, the MTA Cooperative Group (2004b) estimated that there was a growth suppression effect related to medication of approximately −1.23 cm/year in height and −2.48 kg/year in weight. Thus, although the treatments studied generally seem to be effective, potential risks warrant individual monitoring of potential iatrogenic effects—both for medications and for some psychosocial treatments.

Ineffective or Unproved Therapies

Numerous questionable treatments for children with ADHD have been attempted over the past century (for reviews, see Ingersoll & Goldstein, 1993; Pelham et al., 1998; Ross & Ross, 1976, 1982). Vestibular stimulation (Arnold, Clark, Sachs, Jakim, & Smithies, 1985), biofeedback and relaxation training (Richter, 1984), EEG biofeedback or neurofeedback (Linden, Habib, & Radojevic, 1996; Loo, 2003), and sensory integration exercises (Vargas & Camilli, 1999), among others, have been described as potentially effective in either uncontrolled case reports, small series of case studies, or some treatment versus no-treatment comparisons; however, all of these are lacking in well-controlled experimental replications of their efficacy. A meta-analysis of studies examining the benefits of physical exercise and suggesting that it may be preferentially beneficial for participants with hyperactivity warrants further study of this effect in better-controlled research (Allison, Faith, & Franklin, 1995).

Many dietary treatments—such as removal of additives, colorings, or sugar from the diet, or addition of high doses of vitamins, minerals, or other "health food" supplements—have proven very popular (Chan, Rappaport, & Kemper, 2003), and some reviews of research claim that there is evidence for their effectiveness (Schnoll, Burshteyn, & Cea-Aravena, 2003). But a careful reading of such reviews, as well as the existence of better-controlled research, shows little or no scientific support (Conners, 1980; Ingersoll & Goldstein, 1993; Milich, Wolraich, & Lindgren, 1986; Wolraich, Wilson, & White, 1995). Certainly traditional psychotherapy and play therapy have not proven especially effective for ADHD (see Pelham et al., 1998; Ross & Ross, 1976).

CONCLUSION

The treatment of children and teens with ADHD is an often complex and certainly longer-term enterprise than was previously thought to be necessary. Viewed now as a chronic disorder for most children, ADHD requires treatments that must be combined and sustained in order to have a long-term impact on these children's quality of life and developmental outcomes. Treatments appear to succeed by temporarily reducing or ameliorating symptoms for as long as treatments are in effect, so as to reduce the numerous secondary harms associated with unmanaged ADHD. Though numerous therapies have been proposed for this disorder, those having the greatest empirical support are contingency management methods applied in classrooms and elsewhere (summer camps); training of parents in these same methods (BPT), to be used in the home and elsewhere (e.g., community settings); psychopharmacology, particularly stimulants and atomoxetine; and, to a lesser extent, the combination of behavioral treatments with medication. Evidence for CBT is lacking at this time, while that for SST programs is mixed and is based mainly on studies with significant methodological limitations. Better-controlled and larger studies appear to show few or no treatment effects when the skills or behaviors are not cued and reinforced for occurring at the specific point of performance. Treatments that are popular among laypeople, such as dietary manipulations, do not have compelling evidence for their efficacy; nor do several other professionally popular treatments, such as EEG biofeedback or sensory integration training.

Among children who are already stimulant-responsive, it is not clear to what extent intensive psychosocial treatments provide added benefit. However, medication is neither necessary nor always sufficient for treating ADHD. Some children do not respond positively to pharmacological treatment for ADHD, and therefore their only treatment option is psychosocial intervention. Some children show only partial responses to medication, and need additional evidence-based intervention to achieve clinically significant improvement. Also, there are some issues, such as specific skill deficits, that no reasonable person should consider to be changed by medication alone. Thus, in many cases it is plausible that multimodal treatments for ADHD are necessary and appropriate. In these cases, which is likely to be most cases, interventions will need to be high-quality and sustained over several years (or more), and reintervention is highly likely, as new developmental transitions occur and new domains of potential impairment become available to individuals with ADHD across the life span.

NOTE

1. Portions of this section are adapted from Smith, Barkley, and Shapiro (2006). Copyright 2006 by The Guilford Press. Adapted by permission.

REFERENCES

Abikoff, E. (1987). An evaluation of cognitive behavior therapy for hyperactive children. In B. Lahey & A. Kazdin (Eds.), *Advances in clinical child psychology* (Vol. 10, pp. 171–216). New York: Plenum Press.

Abikoff, H. (1985). Efficacy of cognitive training interventions in hyperactive children: A critical review. *Clinical Psychology Review, 5*, 479–512.

Abikoff, H., & Gittelman, R. (1984). Does behavior therapy normalize the classroom behavior of hyperactive children? *Archives of General Psychiatry, 41*, 449–454.

Abikoff, H., & Gittelman, R. (1985). Hyperactive children treated with stimulants: Is cognitive training a useful adjunct? *Archives of General Psychiatry, 42*, 953–961.

Abikoff, H., Hechtman, L., Klein, R. G., Gallacher, R., Fleiss, K., Etcovitch, J., et al. (2004). Social functioning in children with ADHD treated with long-term methylphenidate and multimodal psychosocial treatment. *Journal of the American Academy of Child and Adolescent Psychiatry, 43*, 820–829.

Abikoff, H., Hechtman, L., Klein, R. G., Weiss, G., Fleiss, K., Etcovitch, J., et al. (2004). Symptomatic improvement in children with ADHD treated with long-term methylphenidate and multimodal psychosocial treatment. *Journal of the American Academy of Child and Adolescent Psychiatry, 43*, 802–811.

Abikoff, H., Jensen, P. S., Arnold, L. L., Hoza, B., Hechtman, L., Pollack, S., et al. (2002). Observed classroom behavior of children with ADHD: Relationship to gender and comorbidity. *Journal of Abnormal Child Psychology, 30*, 349–359.

Accardo, P. J., Blondis, T. A., Whitman, B. Y., & Stein, M. A. (2000). *Attention deficits and hyperactivity in children and adults*. New York: Dekker.

Achenbach, T. M. (2001). *Manual for the Child Behavior Checklist and Revised Child Behavior Profile.*

Burlington: University of Vermont, Research center for Children, Youth, and Families.

Allison, D. B., Faith, M. S., & Franklin, R. D. (1995). Antecedent exercise in the treatment of disruptive behavior: A meta-analytic review. *Clinical Psychology: Science and Practice, 2*, 279–304.

American Academy of Child and Adolescent Psychiatry. (2002). Practice parameter for the use of stimulant medications in the treatment children, adolescents, and adults. *Journal of the American Academy of Child and Adolescent Psychiatry, 41*(2, Suppl.), 26S–49S.

American Academy of Pediatrics. (2001). Clinical practice guideline: Treatment of the school-aged child with attention-deficit/hyperactivity disorder. *Pediatrics, 108*, 1033–1044.

American Psychiatric Association. (1968). *Diagnostic and statistical manual of mental disorders* (2nd ed.). Washington, DC: Author.

American Psychiatric Association. (1980). *Diagnostic and statistical manual of mental disorders* (3rd ed.). Washington, DC: Author.

American Psychiatric Association. (1987). *Diagnostic and statistical manual of mental disorders* (3rd ed., rev.). Washington, DC: Author.

American Psychiatric Association. (2000). *Diagnostic and statistical manual of mental disorders* (4th ed., text rev.). Washington, DC: Author.

Anastopoulos, A. D., Guevremont, D. C., Shelton, T. L., & DuPaul, G. J. (1992). Parenting stress among families of children with attention deficit hyperactivity disorder. *Journal of Abnormal Child Psychology, 20*, 503–520.

Anastopoulos, A. D., Shelton, T. L., DuPaul, G. J., & Guevremont, D. C. (1993). Parent training for attention-deficit hyperactivity disorder: Its impact on parent functioning. *Journal of Abnormal Child Psychology, 21*, 581–596.

Andrews, J. N., Swank, P. R., Foorman, B., & Fletcher, J. M. (1995). Effects of educating parents about ADHD. *The ADHD Report, 3*(4), 12–13.

Angold, A., Costello, E. J., & Erkanli, A. (1999). Comorbidity. *Journal of Child Psychology and Psychiatry, 40*, 57–88.

Antshel, K. M., & Remer, R. (2003). Social skills training in children with attention deficit hyperactivity disorder: A randomized–controlled clinical trial. *Journal of Clinical Child and Adolescent Psychology, 32*, 153–165.

Applegate, B., Lahey, B. B., Hart, E. L., Waldman, I., Biederman, J., Hynd, G. W., et al. (1997). Validity of the age-of-onset criterion for ADHD: A report of the DSM-IV field trials. *Journal of the American Academy of Child and Adolescent Psychiatry, 36*, 1211–1221.

Arnold, L. E., Clark, D. L., Sachs, L. A., Jakim, S.., & Smithies, C. (1985). Vestibular and visual rotational stimulation as treatment for attention deficit and hyperactivity. *American Journal of Occupational Therapy, 39*, 84–91.

Atkinson, B. M., & Forehand, R. (1979). Home-based reinforcement programs designed to modify classroom behavior: A review and methodological evaluation. *Psychological Bulletin, 86,* 1298–1308.

Ayllon, T., Garber, S., & Pisor, K. (1975). The elimination of discipline problems through a combined school–home motivational system. *Behavior Therapy, 6,* 616–626.

Ayllon, T., & Rosenbaum, M. (1977). The behavioral treatment of disruption and hyperactivity in school settings. In B. Lahey & A. Kazdin (Eds.), *Advances in clinical child psychology* (Vol. 1, pp. 83–118). New York: Plenum Press.

Aylward, E. H., Reiss, A. L., Reader, M. J., Singer, H. S., Brown, J. E., & Denckla, M. B. (1996). Basal ganglia volumes in children with attention-deficit hyperactivity disorder. *Journal of Child Neurology, 11,* 112–115.

Baer, R. A., & Nietzel, M. T. (1991). Cognitive and behavioral treatment of impulsivity in children: A meta-analytic review of the outcome literature. *Journal of Clinical Child Psychology, 20,* 400–412.

Bagwell, C. L., Molina, B., Pelham, W. E., & Hoza, B. (2001). Attention-deficit hyperactivity disorder and problems in peer relations: Predictions from childhood to adolescence. *Journal of the American Academy of Child and Adolescent Psychiatry, 40,* 1285–1292.

Ball, J. D., & Koloian, B. (1995). Sleep patterns among ADHD children. *Clinical Psychology Review, 15,* 681–691.

Barkley, R. A. (1976). Predicting the response of hyperkinetic children to stimulant drugs: A review. *Journal of Abnormal Child Psychology, 4,* 327–348.

Barkley, R. A. (1977). A review of stimulant drug research with hyperactive children. *Journal of Child Psychology and Psychiatry, 18,* 137–165.

Barkley, R. A. (1988). Attention. In M. Tramontana & S. Hooper (Eds.), *Assessment issues in child neuropsychology* (pp. 145–176). New York: Plenum Press.

Barkley, R. A. (1991). The ecological validity of laboratory and analogue assessment methods of ADHD symptoms. *Journal of Abnormal Child Psychology, 19*(2), 149–178.

Barkley, R. A. (1992a). *ADHD: What can we do?* [Videotape]. New York: Guilford Press.

Barkley, R. A. (1992b). *ADHD: What do we know?* [Videotape]. New York: Guilford Press.

Barkley, R. A. (1997a). *ADHD and the nature of self-control.* New York: Guilford Press.

Barkley, R. A. (1997b). Attention-deficit/hyperactivity disorder. In E. J. Mash & L. Terdal (Eds.), *Assessment of childhood disorders.* New York: Guilford Press.

Barkley, R. A. (1997c). Behavioral inhibition, sustained attention, and executive functions: Constructing a unifying theory of ADHD. *Psychological Bulletin, 121,* 65–94.

Barkley, R. A. (1997d). *Defiant children: A clinician's manual for assessment and parent training.* New York: Guilford Press.

Barkley, R. A. (1997e). *Managing the defiant child* [Videotape]. New York: Guilford Press.

Barkley, R. A. (1997f). *Understanding the defiant child.* [Videotape]. New York: Guilford Press.

Barkley, R. A. (2000). *Taking charge of ADHD: The complete, authoritative guide for parents* (rev. ed.). New York: Guilford Press.

Barkley, R. A. (2004a). ADHD and television viewing: Correlations as causes. *The ADHD Report, 12*(4), 1–4.

Barkley, R. A. (2004b). Driving impairments in teens and adults with attention-deficit/hyperactivity disorder. *Psychiatric Clinics of North America, 27*(2), 233–260.

Barkley, R. A. (2006). *Attention-deficit hyperactivity disorder: A handbook for diagnosis and treatment* (3rd ed.). New York: Guilford Press.

Barkley, R. A., Anastopoulos, A. D., Guevremont, D. G., & Fletcher, K. F. (1992). Adolescents with attention deficit hyperactivity disorder: Mother–adolescent interactions, family beliefs and conflicts, and maternal psychopathology. *Journal of Abnormal Child Psychology, 20,* 263288.

Barkley, R. A., & Biederman, J. (1997). Towards a broader definition of the age of onset criterion for attention deficit hyperactivity disorder. *Journal of the American Academy of Child and Adolescent Psychiatry, 36,* 1204–1210.

Barkley, R. A., Cook, E. H., Diamond, A., Zametkin, A. J., Thapar, A. J., Teeter, P. A., et al. (2002). International consensus statement on ADHD. *Clinical Child and Family Psychology Review, 5,* 89–111.

Barkley, R. A., Copeland, A. P., & Sivage, C. (1980). A self-control classroom for hyperactive children. *Journal of Autism and Developmental Disorders, 10,* 75–89.

Barkley, R. A., & Cunningham, C. E. (1978). Do stimulant drugs improve the academic performance of hyperkinetic children?: A review of outcome research. *Journal of Clinical Pediatrics, 17,* 85–92.

Barkley, R. A., DuPaul, G. J., & McMurray, M. B. (1990). A comprehensive evaluation of attention deficit disorder with and without hyperactivity. *Journal of Consulting and Clinical Psychology, 58,* 775–789.

Barkley, R. A., Edwards, G., Laneri, M., Fletcher, K., & Metevia, L. (2001a). The efficacy of problem-solving training alone, behavior management training alone, and their combination for parent–adolescent conflict in teenagers with ADHD and ODD. *Journal of Consulting and Clinical Psychology, 69,* 926–941.

Barkley, R. A., Edwards, G., Laneri, M., Fletcher, K., & Metevia, L. (2001b). Executive functioning, temporal discounting, and sense of time in adolescents with attention deficit hyperactivity disorder and oppositional defiant disorder. *Journal of Abnormal Child Psychology, 29,* 541–556.

Barkley, R. A., Fischer, M., Edelbrock, C. S., & Smallish, L. (1990). The adolescent outcome of hyperactive children diagnosed by research criteria, I: An 8 year prospective followup study. *Journal of the American Academy of Child and Adolescent Psychiatry, 29*, 546–557.

Barkley, R. A., Fischer, M., Edelbrock, C. S., & Smallish, L. (1991). The adolescent outcome of hyperactive children diagnosed by research criteria: III. Mother–child interactions, family conflicts, and maternal psychopathology. *Journal of Child Psychology and Psychiatry, 32*, 233–256.

Barkley, R. A., Fischer, M., Newby, R., & Breen, M. (1988). Development of a multi-method clinical protocol for assessing stimulant drug responses in ADHD children. *Journal of Clinical Child Psychology, 17*, 14–24.

Barkley, R. A., Fischer, M., Smallish, L., & Fletcher, K. (2002). The persistence of attention-deficit/hyperactivity disorder into young adulthood as a function of reporting source and definition of disorder. *Journal of Abnormal Psychology, 111*, 279–289.

Barkley, R. A., Fischer, M., Smallish, L., & Fletcher, K. (2003). Does the treatment of ADHD with stimulant medication contribute to illicit drug use and abuse in adulthood?: Results from a 15-year prospective study. *Pediatrics, 111*, 109–121.

Barkley, R. A., Fischer, M., Smallish, L., & Fletcher, K. (2004a). Young adult follow-up of hyperactive children: Antisocial activities and drug use. *Journal of Child Psychology and Psychiatry, 45*, 195–211.

Barkley, R. A., Fischer, M., Smallish, L., & Fletcher, K. (2004b). *Young adult outcome of hyperactive children: Adaptive functioning.* Manuscript submitted for publication.

Barkley, R. A., Guevremont, D. C., Anastopoulos, A. D., & Fletcher, K. E. (1992). A comparison of three family therapy programs for treating family conflicts in adolescents with attention-deficit hyperactivity disorder. *Journal of Consulting and Clinical Psychology, 60*, 450–462.

Barkley, R. A., Karlsson, J., & Pollard, S. (1985). Effects of age on the mother-child interactions of hyperactive children. *Journal of Abnormal Child Psychology, 13*, 631–638.

Barkley, R. A., McMurray, M. B., Edelbrock, C. S., & Robbins, K. (1990). The side effects of Ritalin in ADHD children: A systematic, placebo controlled evaluation. *Pediatrics, 86*, 184–192.

Barkley, R. A., & Murphy, K. R. (2006). *Attention-deficit hyperactivity disorder: A clinical workbook* (3rd ed.). New York: Guilford Press.

Barkley, R. A., Murphy, K. R., & Bush, T. (2001). Time perception and reproduction in young adults with attention deficit hyperactivity disorder. *Neuropsychology, 15*, 351–360.

Barkley, R. A., Shelton, T. L., Crosswait, C., Moorehouse, M., Fletcher, K., Barrett, S., et al. (2000). Early psycho-educational intervention for children with disruptive behavior: Preliminary post-treatment outcome. *Journal of Child Psychology and Psychiatry, 41*, 319–332.

Barkley, R. A., Shelton, T. L., Crosswait, C., Moorehouse, M., Fletcher, K., Barrett, S., et al. (2002). Preschool children with high levels of disruptive behavior: Three-year outcomes as a function of adaptive disability. *Development and Psychopathology, 14*, 45–68.

Barrickman, L. L., Perry, P. J., Allen, A. J., Kuperman, S., Arndt, S. V., Herrmann, K. J., et al. (1995). Buproprion versus methylphenidate in the treatment of attention-deficit hyperactivity disorder. *Journal of the American Academy of Child and Adolescent Psychiatry, 34*(5), 649–657.

Bayliss, D. M., & Roodenrys, S. (2000). Executive processing and attention deficit hyperactivity disorder: An application of the supervisory attentional system. *Developmental Neuropsychology, 17*, 161–180.

Beauchaine, T. P., Katkin, E. S., Strassberg, Z., & Snarr, J. (2001). Disinhibitory psychopathology in male adolescents: Discriminating conduct disorder from attention-deficit/hyperactivity disorder through concurrent assessment of multiple autonomic states. *Journal of Abnormal Psychology, 110*, 610–624.

Beelmann, A., Pfingsten, U., & Losel, F. (1994). Effects of training social competence in children: A meta-analysis of recent evaluation studies. *Journal of Clinical Child Psychology, 23*, 260–271.

Berk, L. E. (1992). Children's private speech: An overview of theory and the status of research. In R. M. Diaz & L. E. Berk (Eds.), *Private speech: From social interaction to self-regulation* (pp. 17–54). Hillsdale, NJ: Erlbaum.

Berk, L. E. (1994, November). Why children talk to themselves. *Scientific American*, pp. 78–83.

Biederman, J., Faraone, S. V., Mick, E., Moore, P., & Lelon, E. (1996). Child Behavior Checklist findings further support comorbidity between ADHD and major depression in a referred sample. *Journal of the American Academy of Child and Adolescent Psychiatry, 35*, 734–742.

Biederman, J., Faraone, S. V., Mick, E., Spencer, T., Wilens, T., Kiely, K., et al. (1995). High risk for attention deficit hyperactivity disorder among children of parents with childhood onset of the disorder: A pilot study. *American Journal of Psychiatry, 152*, 431–435.

Biederman, J., Faraone, S. V., Mick, E., Wozniak, J., Chen, L., Ouellette, C., et al. (1996). Attention-deficit hyperactivity disorder and juvenile mania: An overlooked comorbidity. *Journal of the American Academy of Child and Adolescent Psychiatry, 35*, 997–1008.

Biederman, J., Faraone, S. V., Milberger, S., Guite, J., Mick, E., Chen, L., et al. (1996). A prospective 4-year follow-up study of attention-deficit hyperactivity and related disorders. *Archives of General Psychiatry, 53*, 437–446.

Biederman, J., Milberger, S., Faraone, S. V., Guite, J., & Warburton, R. (1994). Associations between childhood asthma and ADHD: Issues of psychiatric comorbidity and familiality. *Journal of the American*

Academy of Child and Adolescent Psychiatry, 33, 842–848.

Biglan, A., Mrazek, P., Carnine, D., & Flay, B. (2003). The integration of research and practive in the prevention of youth problem behaviors. *American Psychologist, 58,* 433–440.

Bloomquist, M. L., August, G. J., & Ostrander, R. (1991). Effects of a school-based cognitive-behavioral intervention for ADHD children. *Journal of Abnormal Child Psychology, 19,* 591–605.

Bor, W., Sanders, M. R., & Markie-Dadds, C. (2002). The effects of the Triple P-Positive Parenting Program on preschool children with co-occurring disruptive behavior and attentional/hyperactive difficulties. *Journal of Abnormal Child Psychology, 30,* 571–587.

Borger, N., & van der Meere, J. (2000). Visual behaviour of ADHD children during an attention test: An almost forgotten variable. *Journal of Child Psychology and Psychiatry, 41,* 525–532.

Bradley, W. (1937). The behavior of children receiving Benzedrine. *American Journal of Psychiatry, 94,* 577–585.

Braswell, L., August, G. J., Bloomquist, M. L., Realmuto, G. M., Skare, S. S., & Crosby, R. D. (1997). School-based secondary prevention for children with disruptive behavior: Initial outcomes. *Journal of Abnormal Child Psychology, 25,* 197–208.

Breslau, N., Brown, G. G., DelDotto, J. E., Kumar, S., Exhuthachan, S., Andreski, P., et al. (1996). Psychiatric sequelae of low birth weight at 6 years of age. *Journal of Abnormal Child Psychology, 24,* 385–400.

Breton, J., Bergeron, L., Valla, J. P., Berthiaume, C., Gaudet, N., Lambert, J., et al. (1999). Quebec children mental health survey: Prevalence of DSM-III-R mental health disorders. *Journal of Child Psychology and Psychiatry, 40,* 375–384.

Briggs-Gowan, M. J., Horwitz, S. M., Schwab-Stone, M. E., Leventhal, J. M., & Leaf, P. J. (2000). Mental health in pediatric settings: Distribution of disorders and factors related to service use. *Journal of the American Academy of Child and Adolescent Psychiatry, 39,* 841–849.

Bronowski, J. (1977). Human and animal languages. In J. Bronowski, *A sense of the future* (pp. 104–131). Cambridge, MA: MIT Press.

Brown, R. T., Borden, K. A., Wynne, M. E., Schleser, R., & Clingerman, S. T. (1986). Methylphenidate and cognitive therapy with ADD children: A methodological reconsideration. *Journal of Abnormal Child Psychology, 14,* 481–497.

Brown, R. T., Wynne, M. E., Borden, K. A., Clingerman, S. R., Geniesse, R., & Spunt, A. L. (1986). Methylphenidate and cognitive therapy in children with attention deficit disorder: A double-blind trial. *Journal of Developmental and Behavioral Pediatrics, 7,* 163–170.

Brown, R. T., Wynne, M. E., & Medenis, R. (1985). Methylphenidate and cognitive therapy: a comparison of treatment approaches with hyperactive boys. *Journal of Abnormal Child Psychology, 13,* 69–88.

Buitelaar, J. K., van der Gaag, R. J., Swaab-Barneveld, H., & Kuiper, M. (1995). Prediction of clinical response to methylphenidate in children with attention-deficit hyperactivity disorder. *Journal of the American Academy of Child and Adolescent Psychiatry, 34,* 1025–1032.

Bussing, R., Gary, F., Mason, D. M., Leon, C. E., Sinha, K., & Garvan, C. W. (2003). Child temperament, ADHD, and caregiver strain: Exploring relationships in an epidemiological sample. *Journal of the American Academy of Child and Adolescent Psychiatry, 42,* 184–192.

Bussing, R., Zima, B. T., & Belin, T. R. (1998). Variations in ADHD treatment among specual education students. *Journal of the American Academy of Child and Adolescent Psychiatry, 37,* 968–976.

Campbell, S. B. (2002). *Behavior problems in preschool children* (2nd ed.). New York: Guilford Press.

Carlson, C. L., Pelham, W. E., Jr., Milich, R., & Dixon, J. (1992). Single and combined effects of methylphenidate and behavior therapy on the classroom performance of children with attention-deficit hyperactivity disorder. *Journal of Abnormal Child Psychology, 20,* 213–232.

Casey, B. J., Castellanos, F. X., Giedd, J. N., Marsh, W. L., Hamburger, S. D., Schubert, A. B., et al. (1997). Implication of right frontostriatal circuitry in response inhibition and attention-deficit/hyperactivity disorder. *Journal of the American Academy of Child and Adolescent Psychiatry, 36,* 374–383.

Castellanos, F. X., Giedd, J. N., Berquin, P. C., Walter, J. M., Sharp, W., Tran, T., et al. (2001). Quantitative brain magnetic resonance imaging in girls with attention-deficit/hyperactivity disorder. *Archives of General Psychiatry, 58,* 289–295.

Castellanos, F. X., Giedd, J. N., Marsh, W. L., Hamburger, S. D., Vaituzis, A. C., Dickstein, D. P., et al. (1996). Quantitative brain magnetic resonance imaging in attention-deficit hyperactivity disorder. *Archives of General Psychiatry, 53,* 607–616.

Castellanos, F. X., Lee, P. P., Sharp, W., Jeffries, N. O., Greenstein, D. K., Clasen, L. S., et al. (2002). Developmental trajectories of brain volume abnormalities in children and adolescents with attention-deficit/hyperactivity disorder. *Journal of the American Medical Association, 288,* 1740–1748.

Chan, E., Rappaport, L., & Kemper, K. J. (2003). Complementary and alternative therapies in childhood attention and hyperactivity problems. *Journal of Developmental and Behavioral Pediatrics, 24,* 4–8.

Charach, A., Ickowicz, A., & Schachar, R. (2004). Stimulant treatment over five years: Adherence, effectiveness, and adverse effects. *Journal of the American Academy of Child and Adolescent Psychiatry, 43,* 559–567.

Chi, T. C., & Hinshaw, S. P. (2002). Mother–child relationships of children with ADHD: The role of maternal depressive symptoms and depression-related distortions. *Journal of Abnormal Child Psychology, 30,* 387–400.

Christakis, D. A., Zimmerman, F. J., DiGiuseppe, D. L., & McCarty, C. A. (2004). Early television exposure and subsequent attentional problems in children. *Pediatrics, 113,* 708–713.

Chronis, A. M., Chacko, A., Fabiano, G. A., Wymbs, B. T., & Pelham, W. E., Jr. (2004). Enhancements to the behavioral parent training paradigm for families of children with ADHD: Review and future directions. *Clinical Child and Family Psychology Review, 7,* 1–27.

Chronis, A. M., Lahey, B. B., Pelham, W. E., Jr., Kipp, H. I., Baumann, B. L., & Lee, S. S. (2003). Psychopathology and substance abuse in parents of young children with attention-deficit/hyperactivity disorder. *Journal of the American Academy of Child and Adolescent Psychiatry, 42,* 1424–1432.

Claycomb, C. D., Ryan, J. J., Miller, L. J., & Schnakenberg-Ott, S. D. (2004). Relationships among attention deficit hyperactivity disorder, induced labor, and selected physiological and demographic variables. *Journal of Clinical Psychology, 60,* 689–693.

Conners, C. K. (1980). *Food additives and hyperactive children.* New York: Plenum Press.

Conners, C. K. (1998). *Conners Adult ADHD Rating Scale.* North Tonawanda, NY: Multi-Health Systems.

Conners, C. K., Epstein, J. N., March, J. S., Angold, A., Wells, K. C., Klaric, J., et al. (2001). Multimodal treatment of ADHD in the MTA: An alternative outcome analysis. *Journal of the American Academy of Child and Adolescent Psychiatry, 40,* 159–167.

Connor, D. F. (2002). Preschool attention deficit hyperactivity disorder: A review of prevalence, diagnosis, neurobiology, and stimulant treatment. *Journal of Developmental and Behavioral Pediatrics, 23,* S1–S9.

Connor, D. F. (2006a). Other medications. In R. A. Barkley, *Attention-deficit hyperactivity disorder: A handbook for diagnosis and treatment* (3rd ed., pp. 658–677). New York: Guilford Press.

Connor, D. F. (2006b). Stimulants. In R. A. Barkley, *Attention-deficit hyperactivity disorder: A handbook for diagnosis and treatment* (3rd ed., pp. 608–647). New York: Guilford Press.

Connor, D. F., Fletcher, K. E., & Swanson, J. M. (1999). A meta-analysis of clonidine for symptoms of attention-deficit hyperactivity disorder. *Journal of the American Academy of Child and Adolescent Psychiatry, 38,* 1551–1559.

Connor, D. F., Glatt, S. J., Lopez, I. D., Jackson, D., & Melloni, R. H. (2002). Psychopharmacology and aggression. I: A meta-analysis of stimulant effects on overt/covert aggression-related behaviors in ADHD. *Journal of the American Academy of Child and Adolescent Psychiatry, 41,* 253–261.

Cook, E. H., Stein, M. A., & Leventhal, D. L. (1997). Family-based association of attention-deficit/hyperactivity disorder and the dopamine transporter. In K. Blum & E. P. Noble (Ed.), *Handbook of psychiatric genetics* (pp. 297–310). Boca Raton, FL: CRC Press.

Coolidge, F. L., Thede, L. L., & Young, S. E. (2000). Heritability and the comorbidity of attention deficit hyperactivity disorder with behavioral disorders and executive function deficits: A preliminary investigation. *Developmental Neuropsychology, 17,* 273–287.

Cunningham, C. E., & Boyle, M. H. (2002). Preschoolers at risk for attention-deficit hyperactivity disorder and oppositional defiant disorder: Family, parenting, and behavioral correlates. *Journal of Abnormal Child Psychology, 30,* 555–569.

Cunningham, C. E., Bremmer, R., & Boyle, M. (1995). Large group community-based parenting programs for families of preschoolers at risk for disruptive behaviour disorders: Utilization, cost effectiveness, and outcome. *Journal of Child Psychology and Psychiatry, 36,* 1141–1159.

Cunningham, C. E., Bremmer, R., & Secord, M. (1997). COPE: *The Community Parent Education Program. A school-based family systems oriented workshop for parents of children with disruptive behavior disorders.* Hamilton, ON, Canada: COPE Works.

Cunningham, C. E., & Siegel, L. S. (1987). Peer interactions of normal and attention-deficit disordered boys during freeplay, cooperative task, and simulated classroom situations. *Journal of Abnormal Child Psychology, 15,* 247–268.

Damasio, A. R. (1995). Structure and function of the human prefrontal cortex. *Annals of the New York Academy of Sciences, 769,* 241–251.

Danforth, J. S., Barkley, R. A., & Stokes, T. F. (1991). Observations of parent–child interactions with hyperactive children: Research and clinical implications. *Clinical Psychology Review, 11,* 703–727.

Denson, R., Nanson, J. L., & McWatters, M. A. (1975). Hyperkinesis and maternal smoking. *Canadian Psychiatric Association Journal, 20,* 183–187.

Diamond, A. (2000). Close interrelation of motor development and cognitive development and of the cerebellum and prefrontal cortex. *Developmental Psychology, 71,* 44–56.

Diaz, R. M., & Berk, L. E. (Eds.). (1992). *Private speech: From social interaction to self-regulation.* Hillsdale, NJ: Erlbaum.

Diaz, R. M., & Berk, L. E. (1995). A Vygotskian critique of self-instructional training. *Development and Psychopathology, 7,* 369–392.

Dishion, T. J., & Kavanagh, K. (2003). *Intervening in adolescent problem behavior: A family-centered approach.* New York: Guilford Press.

Dishion, T. J., McCord, J., & Poulin, F. (1999). When interventions harm: Peer groups and problem behavior. *American Psychologist, 54,* 755–764.

Dodge, K. A. (1989). Problems in social relationships. In E. J. Mash & R. A. Barkley (Eds.), *Treatment of childhood disorders* (pp. 222–246). New York: Guilford Press.

Douglas, V. I. (1980). Higher mental processes in hyperactive children: Implications for training. In R.

Knights & D. Bakker (Eds.), *Treatment of hyperactive and learning disordered children* (pp. 65–92). Baltimore: University Park Press.

Douglas, V. I. (1983). Attention and cognitive problems. In M. Rutter (Ed.), *Developmental neuropsychiatry* (pp. 280–329). New York: Guilford Press.

Draeger, S., Prior, M., & Sanson, A. (1986). Visual and auditory attention performance in hyperactive children: Competence or compliance. *Journal of Abnormal Child Psychology, 14,* 411–424.

DuPaul, G. J., Anastopoulos, A. D., Kwasnik, D., Barkley, R. A., & McMurray, M. B. (1996). Methylphenidate effects on children with attention deficit hyperactivity disorder: Self-report of symptoms, side-effects, and self-esteem. *Journal of Attention Disorders, 1,* 3–15.

DuPaul, G. J., Barkley, R. A., & McMurray, M. B. (1994). Response of children with ADHD to methylphenidate: Interaction with internalizing symptoms. *Journal of the American Academy of Child and Adolescent Psychiatry, 93,* 894–903.

DuPaul, G. J., & Eckert, T. L. (1997). The effects of school-based interventions for attention deficit hyperactivity disorder: A meta-analysis. *School Psychology Digest, 26,* 5–27.

DuPaul, G. J., & Eckert, T. L. (1998). Academic interventions for students with attention-deficit/hyperactivity disorder: A review of the literature. *Reading and Writing Quarterly: Overcoming Learning Difficulties, 14,* 59–82.

DuPaul, G. J., Guevremont, D. C., & Barkley, R. A. (1992). Behavioral treatment of attention-deficit hyperactivity disorder in the classroom: The use of the Attention Training System. *Behavior Modification, 16,* 204–225.

DuPaul, G. J., McGoey, K. E., Eckert, T., & VanBrakle, J. (2001). Preschool children with attention-deficit/hyperactivity disorder: impairments in behavioral, social, and school functioning. *Journal of the American Academy of Child and Adolescent Psychiatry, 40,* 508–515.

DuPaul, G. J., Power, T. J., Anastopoulos, A. D., & Reid, R. (1998). *The ADHD Rating Scale–IV: Checklists, norms, and clinical interpretation.* New York: Guilford Press.

DuPaul, G. J., & Stoner, G. (2003). *ADHD in the schools: Assessment and intervention strategies* (2nd ed.). New York: Guilford Press.

DuPaul, G. R. (1991). Parent and teacher ratings of ADHD symptoms: Psychometric properties in a community-based sample. *Journal of Clinical Child Psychology, 20,* 232–253.

Durston, S., Hulshoff, H. E., Schnack, H. G., Buitelaar, J. K., Steenhuis, M. P., Minderaa, R. B., et al. (2004). Magnetic resonance imaging of boys with attention-deficit/hyperactivity disorder and their unaffected siblings. *Journal of the American Academy of Child and Adolescent Psychiatry, 43,* 332–240.

Dush, D. M., Hirt, M. L., & Schroeder, H. E. (1989). Self-statement modification in the treatment of child behavior disorders: A meta-analysis. *Psychological Bulletin, 106,* 97–106.

Edwards, G., Barkley, R., Laneri, M., Fletcher, K., & Metevia, L. (2001). Parent–adolescent conflicts and parent and teen psychological adjustment in teenagers with ADHD and ODD: The role of maternal depression. *Journal of Abnormal Child Psychology, 29,* 557–572.

Ekman, P., & Davidson, R. J. (1994). *The nature of emotion: Fundamental questions.* New York: Oxford University Press.

El-Sayed, E., Larsson, J. O., Persson, H. E., & Rydelius, P. (2002). Altered cortical activity in children with attention-deficit/hyperactivity disorder during attentional load task. *Journal of the American Academy of Child and Adolescent Psychiatry, 41,* 811–819.

Erhardt, D., & Hinshaw, S. P. (1994). Initial sociometric impressions of attention-deficit hyperactivity disorder and comparison boys: Predictions from social behaviors and from nonbehavioral variables. *Journal of Consulting and Clinical Psychology, 62,* 833–842.

Ernst, M. (1996). Neuro-imaging in attention-deficit/hyperactivity disorder. In G. R. Lyon & J. M. Rumsey (Eds.), *Neuro-imaging: A window to the neurological foundations of learning and behavior in children.* Baltimore: Brookes.

Ernst, M., Zametkin, A. J., Matochik, J. A., Pascualvaca, D., Jons, P. H., & Cohen, R. M. (1999). High midbrain [^{18}F]DOPA accumulation in children with attention deficit hyperactivity disorder. *American Journal of Psychiatry, 156,* 1209–1215.

Eyberg, S. M., & Boggs, S. R. (1998). Parent–child interaction therapy: A psychosocial intervention for the treatment of young conduct-disordered children. In J. M. Briesmeister & C. E. Schaefer (Eds.), *Handbook of parent training: Parents as co-therapists for children's behavior problems* (2nd ed., pp. 61–97). New York: Wiley.

Eyberg, S. M., Edwards, D., Boggs, S. R., & Foote, R. (1998). Maintaining the treatment effects of parent training: The role of booster sessions and other maintenance strategies. *Clinical Psychology: Science and Practice, 5,* 544–554.

Faraone, S. V., Biederman, J., Mennin, D., Russell, R., & Tsuang, M. T. (1998). Familial subtypes of attention deficit hyperactivity disorder: A 4-year follow-up study of children from antisocial–ADHD families. *Journal of Child Psychology and Psychiatry, 39,* 1045–1053.

Faraone, S. V., Biederman, J., Weiffenbach, B., Keith, T., Chu, M. P., Weaver, A., et al. (1999). Dopamine D4 gene 7–repeat allele and attention deficit hyperactivity disorder. *American Journal of Psychiatry, 156,* 768–770.

Faraone, S. V., & Doyle, A. E. (2001). The nature and heritability of attention-deficit/hyperactivity disorder. *Child and Adolescent Psychiatric Clinics of North America, 10,* 299–316.

Fehlings, D. L., Roberts, W., Humphries, T., & Dawe,

G. (1991). Attention deficit hyperactivity disorder: Does cognitive behavioral therapy improve home behavior? *Journal of Developmental and Behavioral Pediatrics, 12,* 223–228.

Filipek, P. A., Semrud-Clikeman, M., Steingard, R. J., Renshaw, P. F., Kennedy, D. N., & Biederman, J. (1997). Volumetric MRI analysis comparing subjects having attention-deficit hyperactivity disorder with normal controls. *Neurology, 48,* 589–601.

Firestone, P., & Douglas, V. I. (1975). The effects of reward and punishment on reaction times and autonomic activity in hyperactive and normal children. *Journal of Abnormal Child Psychology, 3,* 201–216.

Firestone, P., & Douglas, V. 1. (1977). The effects of verbal and material reward and punishers on the performance of impulsive and reflective children. *Child Study Journal, 7,* 71–78.

Firestone, P., Kelly, M. J., Goodman, J. T., & Davey, J. (1981). Differential effects of parent training and stimulant medication with hyperactives. *Journal of the American Academy of Child Psychiatry, 20,* 135–147.

Fischer, M. (1990). Parenting stress and the child with attention deficit hyperactivity disorder. *Journal of Clinical Child Psychology, 19,* 337–346.

Fischer, M., Barkley, R. A., Smallish, L., & Fletcher, K. (2002). Young adult follow-up of hyperactive children: Self-reported psychiatric disorders, comorbidity, and the role of childhood conduct problems. *Journal of Abnormal Child Psychology, 30,* 463–475.

Fischer, M., Barkley, R. A., Smallish, L., & Fletcher, K. (in press). Hyperactive children as young adults: Driving abilities, safe driving behavior, and adverse driving outcomes. *Accident Analysis and Prevention.*

Fletcher, K., Fischer, M., Barkley, R. A., & Smallish, L. (1996). A sequential analysis of the mother–adolescent interactions of ADHD, ADHD/ODD, and normal teenagers: Neutral and conflict discussions. *Journal of Abnormal Child Psychology, 24,* 271–298.

Forehand, R., & McMahon, R. (1981). *Helping the noncompliant child: A clinician's guide to parent training.* New York: Guilford Press.

Frankel, F., Myatt, R., & Cantwell, D. P. (1995). Training outpatient boys to conform with the social ecology of popular peers: Effects on parent and teacher ratings. *Journal of Clinical Child Psychology, 24,* 300–310.

Frankel, F., Myatt, R., Cantwell, D. P., & Feinberg, D. T. (1997). Parent-assisted transfer of children's social skills training: Effects on children with and without attention deficit hyperactivity disorder. *Journal of the American Academy of Child and Adolescent Psychiatry, 36,* 1056–1064.

Frazier, T. W., Demaree, H. A., & Youngstrom, E. A. (2004). Meta-analysis of intellectual and neuropsychological test performance in attention-deficit/hyperactivity disorder. *Neuropsychology, 18,* 543–555.

Fuster, J. M. (1997). *The prefrontal cortex* (3rd ed.). New York: Raven Press.

Gabel, S., Schmitz, S., & Fulker, D. W. (1996). Comorbidity in hyperactive children: Issues related to selection bias, gender, severity, and internalizing symptoms. *Child Psychiatry and Human Development, 27,* 15–28.

Gadow, K. D. (1985). Relative efficacy of pharmacological, behavioral., and combination treatments for enhancing academic performance. *Clinical Psychology Review, 5,* 513–533.

Gadow, K. D., Sprafkin, J., & Nolan, E. E. (2001). DSM-IV symptoms in community and clinic preschool children. *Journal of the American Academy of Child and Adolescent Psychiatry, 40,* 1383–1392.

Gadow, K. D., Sverd, J., Sprafkin, J., Nolan, E. E., & Ezor, S. N. (1995). Efficacy of methylphenidate for attention-deficit hyperactivity disorder in children with tic disorder. *Archives of General Psychiatry, 52,* 444–455.

Gerdes, A. C., Hoza, B., & Pelham, W. E. (2003). Attention-deficit/hyperactivity disordered boys' relationships with their mothers and fathers: Child, mother, and father perceptions. *Development and Psychopathology, 15,* 363–382.

Gershon, J. (2002). A meta-analytic review of gender differences in ADHD. *Journal of Attention Disorders, 5,* 143–153.

Gioia, G. A., Isquith, P. K., Guy, S. C., & Kenworthy, L. (2000). *Behavior Rating Inventory of Executive Function (BRIEF).* Lutz, FL: Psychological Assessment Resources.

Goldman, L. S., Genel, M., Bezman, R. J., & Slanetz, P. J. (1998). Diagnosis and treatment of attention-deficit/hyperactivity disorder in children and adolescents. *Journal of the American Medical Association, 279*(14), 1100–1107.

Goldstein, S., & Ingersoll, B. (1993). Controversial treatments for ADHD: Essential information for clinicians. *The ADHD Report, 1*(3), 4–5.

Gordon, M., Thomason, D., & Cooper, S. (1990, August). *Non-medical treatment of ADHD/hyperactivity: The Attention Training System.* Paper presented at the 98th annual convention of the American Psychological Association, Boston.

Green, L., Fry, A. F., & Meyerson, J. (1994). Discounting of delayed rewards: A life-span comparison. *Psychological Science, 5,* 33–36.

Greydanus, D. E., Pratt, H. D., Sloane, M. A., & Rappley, M. D. (2003). Attention-deficit/hyperactivity disorder in children and adolescents: Interventions for a complex costly conundrum. *Pediatric Clinics of North America, 50,* 1049–1092.

Greene, R. W., Biederman, J., Faraone, S. V., Ouellette, C. A., Penn, C., & Griffin, S. M. (1996). Toward a psychometric definition of social disability in children with attention-deficit hyperactivity disorder. *Journal of the American Academy of Child and Adolescent Psychiatry, 35,* 571–578.

Greenhill, L. L., Halperin, J. M., & Abikoff, H. (1999). Stimulant medications. *Journal of the American*

Academy of Child and Adolescent Psychiatry, 38, 503–512.

Greenhill, L. L., & Osman, B. B. (Eds). (1991). *Ritalin: Theory and patient management.* New York: Liebert.

Gustafsson, P., Thernlund, G., Ryding, E., Rosen, I., & Cederblad, M. (2000). Associations between cerebral blood-flow measured by single photon emission computer tomography (SPECT), electro-encephalogram (EEG), behaviour symptoms, cognition and neurological soft signs in children with attention-deficit hyperactivity disorder (ADHD). *Acta Paediatrica, 89,* 830–835.

Halperin, J. M., Newcorn, J. H., Koda, V. H., Pick, L., McKay, K. E., & Knott, P. (1997). Noradrenergic mechanisms in ADHD children with and without reading disabilities: A replication and extension. *Journal of the American Academy of Child and Adolescent Psychiatry, 36,* 1688–1697.

Harrison, C., & Sofronoff, K. (2002). ADHD and parental psychological distress: Role of demographics, child behavioral characteristics, and parental cognitions. *Journal of the American Academy of Child and Adolescent Psychiatry, 41,* 703–711.

Hart, E. L., Lahey, B. B., Loeber, R., Applegate, B., & Frick, P. J. (1995). Developmental changes in attention-deficit hyperactivity disorder in boys: A four-year longitudinal study. *Journal of Abnormal Child Psychology, 23,* 729–750.

Hartman, R. R., Stage, S. A., & Webster-Stratton, C. (2003). A growth curve analysis of parent training outcomes: Examining the influence of child risk factors (inattention, impulsivity, and hyperactivity problems), parental and family risk factors. *Journal of Child Psychology and Psychiatry, 44,* 388–398.

Hartsough, C. S., & Lambert, N. M. (1985). Medical factors in hyperactive and normal children: Prenatal, developmental, and health history findings. *American Journal of Orthopsychiatry, 55,* 190–201.

Hartung, C. M., Willcutt, E. G., Lahey, B. B., Pelham, W. E., Loney, J., Stein, M. A., et al. (2002). Sex differences in young children who meet criteria for attention deficit hyperactivity disorder. *Journal of Clinical Child and Adolescent Psychology, 31,* 453–464.

Hayes, S. C. (1989). *Rule-governed behavior.* New York: Plenum Press.

Hayes, S. C., Rosenfarb, I., Wulfert, E., Munt, E. D., Korn, Z., & Zettle, R. D. (1985). Self-reinforcement effects: An artifact of social standard setting? *Journal of Applied Behavior Analysis, 18,* 201–214.

Hazell, P. L., & Stuart, J. E. (2003). A randomized controlled trial of clonidine added to psychostimulant medication for hyperactive and aggressive children. *Journal of the American Academy of Child and Adolescent Psychiatry, 42,* 886–894.

Hechtman, L., Abikoff, H., Klein, R. G., Greenfield, B., Etcovitch, J., Cousins, L., et al. (2004). Children with ADHD treated with long-term methylphenidate and multimodal psychosocial treatment: Impact on parental practices. *Journal of the American Academy of Child and Adolescent Psychiatry, 43,* 830–838.

Hechtman, L., Abikoff, H., Klein, R. G., Weiss, G., Respitz, C., Kouri, J., et al. (2004). Academic achievement and emotional status in children with ADHD treated with long-term methylphenidate and multimodal psychosocial treatment. *Journal of the American Academy of Child and Adolescent Psychiatry, 43,* 812–819.

Hendren, R. L., De Backer, I., & Pandina, G. J. (2000). Review of neuroimaging studies of child and adolescent psychiatric disorders from the past 10 years. *Journal of the American Academy of Child and Adolescent Psychiatry, 39,* 815–828.

Henggeler, S. W., Melton, G. B., Brondino, M. J., Scherer, D. G., & Hanley, J. H. (1997). Multisystemic therapy with violent and chronic juvenile offenders and their families: The role of treatment fidelity in successful dissemination. *Journal of Consulting and Clinical Psychology, 65,* 821–833.

Herpertz, S. C., Wenning, B., Mueller, B., Qunaibi, M., Sass, H., & Herpetz-Dahlmann, B. (2001). Psychological responses in ADHD boys with and without conduct disorder: Implications for adult antisocial behavior. *Journal of the American Academy of Child and Adolescent Psychiatry, 40,* 1222–1230.

Hervey, A. S., Epstein, J. N., & Curry, J. F. (2004). Neuropsychology of adults with attention-deficit/hyperactivity disorder: A meta-analytic review. *Neuropsychology, 18,* 485–503.

Hinshaw, S. P. (1987). On the distinction between attentional deficits/hyperactivity and conduct problems/aggression in child psychopathology. *Psychological Bulletin, 101,* 443–447.

Hinshaw, S. P. (1992). Interventions for social competence and social skill. *Child and Adolescent Psychiatric Clinics of North America, 1*(2), 539–552.

Hinshaw, S. P., & Erhardt, D. (1991). Attention-deficit hyperactivity disorder. In P. C. Kendall (Ed.), *Child and adolescent therapy: Cognitive-behavioral procedures* (pp. 98–128). New York: Guilford Press.

Hinshaw, S. P., Henker, B., & Whalen, C. K. (1984a). Cognitive-behavioral and pharmacologic interventions for hyperactive boys: Comparative and combined effects. *Journal of Consulting and Clinical Psychology, 52,* 739–749.

Hinshaw, S. P., Henker, B., & Whalen, C. K. (1984b). Self-control in hyperactive boys in anger-inducing situations: Effects of cognitive-behavioral training and of methylphenidate. *Journal of Abnormal Child Psychology, 12,* 55–77.

Hoagwood, K., Kelleher, K. J., Feil, M., & Comer, D. M. (2000). Treatment services for children with ADHD: A national perspective. *Journal of the American Academy of Child and Adolescent Psychiatry, 39,* 198–206.

Holmbeck, G. N. (1997). Toward terminological, conceptual, and statistical clarity in the study of mediators and moderators: Examples from the child-clinical and pediatric psychology literatures. *Journal of Consulting and Clinical Psychology, 65,* 599–610.

Hook, C. L., & DuPaul, G. J. (1999). Parent tutoring

for students with attention-deficit/hyperactivity disorder: Effects on reading performance at home and school. *School Psychology Review, 28*, 60–75.

Horn, W. F., Chatoor, I., & Conners, C. K. (1983). Additive effects of Dexedrine and self-control training: A multiple assessment. *Behavior Modification, 7*, 383–402.

Horn, W. F., Ialongo, N., Greenberg, G., Packard, T., & Smith-Winberry, C. (1990). Additive effects of behavioral parent training and self-control therapy with attention deficit hyperactivity disordered children. *Journal of Clinical Child Psychology, 19*, 98–110.

Horn, W. F., Ialongo, N., Pascoe, J. M., Greenberg, G., Packard, T., Lopez, M., et al. (1991). Additive effects of psychostimulants, parent training, and self-control therapy with ADHD children. *Journal of the American Academy of Child and Adolescent Psychiatry, 30*, 233–240.

Horn, W. F., Ialongo, N., Popovich, S., & Peradotto, D. (1987). Behavioral parent training and cognitive-behavioral self-control therapy with ADD-H children: Comparative and combined effects. *Journal of Clinical Child Psychology, 16*, 57–68.

Hoza, B., Gerdes, A. C., Hinshaw, S. P., Arnold, L. E., Pelham, W. E., Jr., Molina, B. S. G., et al. (2004). Self-perceptions of competence in children with ADHD and comparison children. *Journal of Consulting and Clinical Psychology, 72*, 382–391.

Hubbard, J. A., & Newcomb, A. F. (1991). Initial dyadic peer interaction of attention deficit-hyperactivity disorder and normal boys. *Journal of Abnormal Child Psychology, 19*, 179–195.

Ingersoll, B. D., & Goldstein, S. (1993). *Attention deficit disorder and learning disabilities: Realities, myths, and controversial treatments.* New York: Doubleday.

James, H. (1950). *The principles of psychology* (2 vols.). New York: Dover. (Original work published 1890)

Jensen, P. S., Kettle, L., Roper, M. T., Sloan, M. T., Dulcan, M. K., Hoven, C., et al. (1999). Are stimulants overprescribed?: Treatment of ADHD in four U.S. communities. *Journal of the American Academy of Child and Adolescent Psychiatry, 38*(7), 797–804.

Jensen, P. S., Shervette, R. E., III, Xenakis, S. N., & Richters, J. (1993). Anxiety and depressive disorders in attention deficit disorder with hyperactivity: New findings. *American Journal of Psychiatry, 150*, 1203–1209.

Johnston, C. (1992, February). *The influence of behavioral parent training on inattentive–overactive and aggressive–defiant behaviors in ADHD children.* Poster presented at the annual meeting of the International Society for Research in Child and Adolescent Psychopathology, Sarasota, FL.

Johnston, C., & Mash, E. J. (2001). Families of children with attention-deficit/hyperactivity disorder: Review and recommendations for future research. *Clinical Child and Family Psychology Review, 4*, 183–207.

Johnston, C., Murray, C., Hinshaw, S. P., Pelham, W. E., Jr., & Hoza, B. (2002). Responsiveness in interactions of mothers and sons with ADHD: Relations to maternal and child characteristics. *Journal of Abnormal Child Psychology, 30*, 77–88.

Johnstone, S. J., Barry, R. J., & Anderson, J. W. (2001). Topographic distribution and developmental timecourse of auditory event-related potentials in two subtypes of attention-deficit hyperactivity disorder. *International Journal of Psychophysiology, 42*, 73–94.

Kadesjo, B., & Gillberg, C. (2001). The comorbidity of ADHD in the general population of Swedish school-age children. *Journal of Child Psychology and Psychiatry, 42*, 487–492.

Kashdan, T. B., Jacob, R. G., Pelham, W. E., Lang, A. R., Hoza, B., Blumenthal, J. D., et al. (2004). Depression and anxiety in parents of children with ADHD and varying levels of oppositional defiant behaviors: Modeling relationships with family functioning. *Journal of Clinical Child and Adolescent Psychology, 33*, 169–181.

Kazdin, A. E. (1997). Parent management training: Evidence, outcomes, and issues. *Journal of the American Academy of Child and Adolescent Psychiatry, 36*, 1349–1356.

Kendall, P. C., & Braswell, L. (1985). *Cognitive-behavioral therapy for impulsive children.* New York: Guilford Press.

Keown, L. J., & Woodward, L. J. (2002). Early parent–child relations and family functioning of preschool boys with pervasive hyperactivity. *Journal of Abnormal Child Psychology, 30*, 541–553.

Kerns, K. A., Eso, K., & Thomson, J. (1999). Investigation of a direct intervention for improving attention in young children with ADHD. *Developmental Neuropsychology, 16*, 273–295.

Kratochvil, C. J., Heiligenstein, J. H., Dittmann, R., Spencer, T. J., Biederman, J., Wernicke, J., et al. (2002). Atomoxetine and methylphenidate treatment in children with ADHD: A prospective, randomized, open-label trial. *Journal of the American Academy of Child and Adolescent Psychiatry, 41*, 776–784.

Kuntsi, J., & Stevenson, J. (2000). Hyperactivity in children: A focus on genetic research and psychological theories. *Clinical Child and Family Psychology Review, 3*, 1–23.

Lahey, B. B., Applegate, B., McBurnett, K., Biederman, J., Greenhill, L., Hynd, G., et al. (1994). DSM-IV field trials for attention deficit/hyperactivity disorder in children and adolescents. *Journal of the American Academy of Child and Adolescent Psychiatry, 151*, 1673–1685.

Lahoste, G. J., Swanson, J. M., Wigal, S. B., Glabe, C., Wigal, T., King, N., et al. (1996). Dopamine D4 receptor gene polymorphism is associated with attention deficit hyperactivity disorder. *Molecular Psychiatry, 1*, 121–124.

Lang, P. J. (1995). The emotion probe: Studies of motivation and attention. *American Psychologist, 50*, 372–385.

Lerer, R. J., Lerer, P., & Artner, J. (1977). The effects of methylphenidate on the handwriting of children with minimal brain dysfunction. *Journal of Pediatrics, 91,* 127–132.

Levy, F., & Hay, D. (Eds.). (2002). *Attention, genes and attention deficit hyperactivity disorder.* Philadelphia: Psychology Press.

Lewinsohn, P. M., Hops, H., Roberts, R. E., Seeley, J. R., & Andrews, J. A. (1993). Adolescent psychopathology: I. Prevalence and incidence of depression and other DSM-III-R disorders in high school students. *Journal of Abnormal Psychology, 102,* 133–144.

Linden, M., Habib, T., & Radojevic, V. (1996). A controlled study of the effects of EEG biofeedback on cognition and behavior of children with attention deficit disorder and learning disabilities. *Biofeedback and Self-Regulation, 21,* 35–50.

Linnet, K. M., Dalsgaard, S., Obel, C., Wisborg, K., Henriksen, T. B., Rodriguez, A., et al. (2003). Maternal lifestyle factors in pregnancy risk for attention deficit hyperactivity disorder and associated behaviors: Review of the current evidence. *American Journal of Psychiatry, 160,* 1028–1040.

Loeber, R., Green, S. M., Lahey, B. B., Christ, M. A., G., & Frick, P. J. (1992). Developmental sequences in the age of onset of disruptive child behaviors. *Journal of Child and Family Studies, 1,* 21–41.

Loo, S. K. (2003). EEG and neurofeedback findings in ADHD. *The ADHD Report, 11*(3), 1–6.

Loo, S. K., & Barkley, R. A. (2005). Clinical utility of EEG in attention deficit hyperactivity disorder. *Applied Developmental Neuropsychology, 12,* 64–76.

Loo, S. K., Specter, E., Smolen, A., Hopfer, C., Teale, P. D., & Reite, M. L. (2003). Functional effects of the DAT1 polymorphism on EEG measures in ADHD. *Journal of the American Academy of Child and Adolescent Psychiatry, 42,* 986–993.

Lorch, E. P., Sanchez, R. P., van den Broek, P., Baer, S., & Hooks, K. (2000). Comprehension of televised stories in boys with attention deficit/hyperactivity disorder and nonreferred boys. *Journal of Abnormal Psychology, 109*(2), 321–330.

Luk, S. (1985). Direct observations studies of hyperactive behaviors. *Journal of the American Academy of Child Psychiatry, 24,* 338–344.

Mannuzza, S., Gittelman-Klein, R., Bessler, A., Malloy, P., & LaPadula, M. (1993). Adult outcome of hyperactive boys: Educational achievement, occupational rank, and psychiatric status. *Archives of General Psychiatry, 50,* 565–576.

Mannuzza, S., Klein, R. G., Bonagura, N., Malloy, P., Giampino, T. L., & Addalli, K. A. (1991). Hyperactive boys almost grown up: V. Replication of psychiatric status. *Archives of General Psychiatry, 48,* 77–83.

Marholin, D., & Steinman, W. M. (1977). Stimulus control in the classroom as a function of the behavior reinforced. *Journal of Applied Behavior Analysis, 10,* 465–478.

Mariani, M. A., & Barkley, R. A. (1997). Neuropsychological and academic functioning in preschool boys with attention deficit hyperactivity disorder. *Developmental Neuropsychology, 13,* 111–129.

Mash, E. J., & Johnston, C. (1982). A comparison of the mother–child interactions of younger and older hyperactive and normal children. *Child Development, 53,* 1371–1381.

Mash, E. J., & Johnston, C. (1983). Parental perceptions of child behavior problems, parenting self-esteem, and mothers' reported stress in younger and older hyperactive and normal children. *Journal of Consulting and Clinical Psychology, 51,* 68–99.

Matthys, W., Cuperus, J. M., & van Engeland, H. (1999). Deficient social problem-solving in boys with ODD/CD, with ADHD, and with both disorders. *Journal of the American Academy of Child and Adolescent Psychiatry, 38,* 311–321.

Maughan, B., Taylor, C., Taylor, A., Butler, N., & Bynner, J. (2001). Pregnancy smoking and childhood conduct problems: A causal association? *Journal of Child Psychology and Psychiatry, 42,* 1021–1028.

McClellan, J. M., & Werry, J. S. (2003). Evidence-based treatments in child and adolescent psychiatry: An inventory. *Journal of the American Academy of Child and Adolescent Psychiatry, 42*(12), 1388–1400.

McGee, R., Stanton, W. R., & Sears, M. R. (1993). Allergic disorders and attention deficit disorder in children. *Journal of Abnormal Child Psychology, 21,* 79–88.

McKee, T. E., Harvey, E., Danforth, J. S., Ulaszek, W. R., & Friedman, J. L. (2004). The relation between parental coping styles and parent–child interactions before and after treatment for children with ADHD and oppositional disorder. *Journal of Clinical Child and Adolescent Psychology, 33,* 158–168.

McMahon, R. J., & Forehand, R. L. (2003). *Helping the noncompliant child: Family-based treatment for oppositional behavior* (2nd ed.). New York: Guilford Press.

Meichenbaum, D., & Goodman, J. (1971). Training impulsive children to talk to themselves: A means of developing self-control. *Journal of Abnormal Psychology, 77,* 115–126.

Michelson, D., Adler, L., Spencer, T., Reimherr, F. W., West, S. A., Allen, A. J., et al. (2003). Atomoxetine in adults with ADHD: Two randomized, placebo-controlled studies. *Biological Psychiatry, 53,* 112–120.

Michelson, D., Allen, A. J., Busner, J., Casat, C., Dunn, D., Kratochvil, C., et al. (2002). Once-daily atomoxetine treatment for children and adolescents with attention deficit hyperactivity disorder: A randomized, placebo-controlled study. *American Journal of Psychiatry 159,* 1896–1901.

Michelson, D., Faries, D., Wernicke, J., Kelsey, D., Kendrick, K., Sallee, F. R., et al. (2001). Atomoxetine in the treatment of children and adolescents with attention deficit hyperactivity disorder: A randomized, placebo-controlled, dose–response study. *Pediatrics, 108,* e83.

Michon, J. (1985). Introduction. In J. Michon & T.

Jackson (Eds.), *Time, mind, and behavior*. Berlin: Springer-Verlag.

Mick, E., Biederman, J., Faraone, S. V., Sayer, J., & Kleinman, S. (2002). Case–control study of attention-deficit hyperactivity disorder and maternal smoking, alcohol use, and drug use during pregnancy. *Journal of the American Academy of Child and Adolescent Psychiatry, 41,* 378–385.

Mikami, A., & Hinshaw, S. (2003). Buffers of peer rejection among girls with and without ADHD: The role of popularity with adults and goal-directed solitary play. *Journal of Abnormal Child Psychology, 31*(4), 381–397.

Milberger, S., Biederman, J., Faraone, S. V., Chen, L., & Jones, J. (1996). Is maternal smoking during pregnancy a risk factor for attention deficit hyperactivity disorder in children? *American Journal of Psychiatry, 153,* 1138–1142.

Milich, R., & Dodge, K. A. (1984). Social information processing in child psychiatry populations. *Journal of Abnormal Child Psychology, 12,* 471–490.

Milich, R., Wolraich, M., & Lindgren, S. (1986). Sugar and hyperactivity: A critical review of empirical findings. *Clinical Psychology Review, 6,* 493–513.

Minuchin, S., & Fishman, H. C. (1981). *Family therapy techniques.* Cambridge, MA: Harvard University Press.

Mirsky, A. F. (1996). Disorders of attention: A neuropsychological perspective. In R. G. Lyon & N. A. Krasnegor (Eds.), *Attention, memory, and executive function* (pp. 71–96). Baltimore: Brookes.

Monastra, V. J., Lubar, J. F., & Linden, M. (2001). The development of a quantitative electroencephalographic scanning process for attention deficit-hyperactivity disorder: Reliability and validity studies. *Neuropsychology, 15,* 136–144.

Monastra, V. J., Lubar, J. F., Linden, M., VanDeusen, P., Green, G., Wing, W., et al. (1999). Assessing attention deficit hyperactivity disorder via quantitative electroencephalography: An initial validation study. *Neuropsychology, 13,* 424–433.

MTA Cooperative Group. (1999a). A 14-month randomized clinical trial of treatment strategies for attention-deficit/hyperactivity disorder. *Archives of General Psychiatry, 56,* 1073–1086.

MTA Cooperative Group. (1999b). Moderators and mediators of treatment response for children with attention-deficit/hyperactivity disorder. *Archives of General Psychiatry, 56,* 1088–1096.

MTA Cooperative Group. (2004a). National Institute of Mental Health Multimodal Treatment Study of ADHD follow-up: 24-month outcomes of treatment strategies for attention-deficit/hyperactivity disorder. *Pediatrics, 113,* 754–761.

MTA Cooperative Group. (2004b). National Institute of Mental Health Multimodal Treatment Study of ADHD follow-up: Changes in effectiveness and growth after the end of treatment. *Pediatrics, 113,* 762–769.

Mueller, K., Daly, M., Fischer, M., Yiannoutsos, C. T., Bauer, L., Barkley, R., et al. (2003). Association of the dopamine beta hydroxylase gene with attention deficit hyperactivity disorder: Genetic analysis of the Milwaukee longitudinal study. *American Journal of Medical Genetics, 119B,* 77–85.

Murphy, K. R., Barkley, R. A., & Bush, T. (2001). Executive functioning and olfactory identification in young adults with attention deficit hyperactivity disorder. *Neuropsychology, 15,* 211–220.

Needleman, H. L., Schell, A. Bellinger, D. C., Leviton, L., & Alfred, E. D. (1990). The long-term effects of exposure to low doses of lead in childhood: An 11-year follow-up report. *New England Journal of Medicine, 322,* 83–88.

Newcorn, J., Michelson, D., Spencer, T., & Milton, D. (2002, October). *Atomoxetine treatment in child/adolescent ADHD with comorbid ODD.* Poster presented at the annual meeting of the American Academy of Child and Adolescent Psychiatry, San Francisco.

Nigg, J. T. (1999). The ADHD response-inhibition deficit as measured by the stop task: Replication with DSM-IV combined type, extension, and qualification. *Journal of Abnormal Child Psychology, 27,* 393–402.

Nigg, J. T. (2000). On inhibition/disinhibition in developmental psychopathology: Views from cognitive and personality psychology and a working inhibition taxonomy. *Psychological Bulletin, 126,* 220–246.

Nigg, J. T. (2001). Is ADHD an inhibitory disorder? *Psychological Bulletin, 125,* 571–596.

Nigg, J. T., Blaskey, L. G., Huang-Pollock, C. L., & Rappley, M. D. (2002). Neuropsychological executive functions in DSM-IV ADHD subtypes. *Journal of the American Academy of Child and Adolescent Psychiatry, 41,* 59–66.

Nigg, J. T., Goldsmith, H. H., & Sachek, J. (2004). Temperament and attention deficit hyperactivity disorder: The development of a multiple pathway model. *Journal of Clinical Child and Adolescent Psychology, 33,* 42–53.

Nolan, E. E., Gadow, K. D., & Sprafkin, J. (2001). Teacher reports of DSM-IV ADHD, ODD, and CD symptoms in schoolchildren. *Journal of the American Academy of Child and Adolescent Psychiatry, 40,* 241–249.

O'Leary, R. D., Pelham, W. E., Rosenbaum, A., &, Price, G. H. (1976). Behavioral treatment of hyperkinetic children: An experimental evaluation of its usefulness. *Clinical Pediatrics, 15,* 510–515.

O'Leary, S. G., & Pelham, W. E. (1978). Behavior therapy and withdrawal of stimulant medication in hyperactive children. *Pediatrics, 61,* 211–216.

Olfson, M., Gameroff, M. J., Marcus, S. C., & Jensen, P. S. (2003). National trends in the treatment of attention deficit hyperactivity disorder. *American Journal of Psychiatry, 160,* 1071–1077.

Ota, K. R., & DuPaul, G. J. (2002). Task engagement

and mathematics performance in children with attention-deficit hyperactivity disorder: Effects of supplemental computer instruction. *School Psychology Quarterly, 17,* 242–257.

Paniagua, F. A. (1987). Management of hyperactive children through correspondence training procedures: A preliminary study. *Behavioral Residential Treatment, 2,* 1–23.

Paternite, C., & Loney, J. (1980). Childhood hyperkinesis: Relationships between symptomatology and home environment. In C. K. Whalen & B. Henker (Eds.), *Hyperactive children: The social ecology of identification and treatment* (pp. 105–141). New York: Academic Press.

Patterson, G. R. (1965). Responsiveness to social stimuli. In L. Krasner & L. P. Ullman (Eds.), *Research in behavior modification: New developments and implications* (pp. 157–178). New York: Holt, Rinehart & Winston.

Patterson, G. R. (1982). *Coercive family process.* Eugene, OR: Castalia.

Pelham, W. E. (1987). What do we know about the use and effects of CNS stimulants in the treatment of ADD? In J. Loney (Ed.), *The hyperactive child: Answers to about prognosis and treatment* (pp. 99–110). New York: Haworth Press.

Pelham, W. E. (1999). The NIMH Multimodal Treatment Study for Attention-Deficit Hyperactivity Disorder: Just say yes to drugs alone? *Canadian Journal of Psychiatry, 44,* 981–990.

Pelham, W. E., Bender, M. E., Caddell, J., Booth, S., & Moorer, S. R. (1985). Methylphenidate and children with attention deficit disorder. *Archives of General Psychiatry, 42,* 948–952.

Pelham, W. E., & Hoza, B. (1996). Intensive treatment: A summer treatment program for children with ADHD. In E. Hibbs & P. Jensen (Eds.), *Psychosocial treatments for child and adolescent disorders: Empirically based strategies for clinical practice* (pp. 311–340). Washington, DC: American Psychological Association.

Pelham, W. E., Hoza, B., Pillow, D. R., Gnagy, E. M., Kipp, H. L., Greiner, A. R., et al. (2002). Effects of methylphenidate and expectancy on children with ADHD: Behavior, academic performance, and attributions in a summer treatment program and regular classroom settings. *Journal of Consulting and Clinical Psychology, 70(2),* 320–335.

Pelham, W. E., & Sams, S. E. (1992). Behavior modification. *Child and Adolescent Psychiatric Clinics of North America, 1(2),* 255.

Pelham, W. E., Schnedler, R. W., Bender, M. E., Nilsson, D. E., Miller, J., Budrow, M. S., et al. (1988). The combination of behavior therapy and methylphenidate in the treatment of attention deficit disorders: A therapy outcome study. In L. Bloomingdale (Ed.), *Attention deficit disorders* (Vol. 3, pp. 29–48) New York: Pergamon Press.

Pelham, W. E., Jr., Wheeler, T., & Chronis, A. (1998). Empirically supported psychosocial treatments for attention deficit hyperactivity disorder. *Journal of Clinical Child Psychology, 27(2),* 190–205.

Pennington, B. F., & Ozonoff, S. (1996). Executive functions and developmental psychopathology. *Journal of Child Psychology and Psychiatry, 37,* 51–87.

Pfiffner, L. J., Barkley, R. A., & DuPaul, G. J. (2006). Treatment of ADHD in school settings. In R. A. Barkley, *Attention-deficit hyperactivity disorder: A handbook for diagnosis and treatment* (3rd ed., pp. 547–589). New York: Guilford Press.

Pfiffner, L. J., & McBurnett, K. (1997). Social skills training with parent generalization: Treatment effects for children with attention deficit disorder. *Journal of Consulting and Clinical Psychology, 65,* 749–757.

Pfiffner, L. J., & O'Leary, S. G. (1987). The efficacy of all-positive management as a function of the prior use of negative consequences. *Journal of Applied Behavior Analysis, 20,* 265–271.

Pfiffner, L. J., O'Leary, S. G., Rosen, L. A., & Sanderson, W. C. Jr. (1985). A comparison of the effects of continuous and. intermittent response cost and reprimands in the classroom. *Journal of Clinical Child Psychology, 14,* 348–352.

Phelps, L., Brown, R. T., & Power, T. J. (2002). *Pediatric psychopharmacology: Combining medical and psychosocial interventions.* Washington, DC: American Psychological Association

Pisterman, S., McGrath, P., Firestone, P., Goodman, J. T., Webster, I., & Mallory, R. (1989). Outcome of parent-mediated treatment of preschoolers with attention deficit disorder with hyperactivity. *Journal of Consulting and Clinical Psychology, 57,* 628–635.

Pliszka, S. R. (1987). Tricyclic antidepressants in the treatment of children with attention deficit disorder. *Journal of the American Academy of Child and Adolescent Psychiatry, 26,* 127–132.

Pliszka, S. R. (2003). Non-stimulant treatment of attention-deficit hyperactivity disorder. *CNS Spectrums, 8,* 253–258.

Pliszka, S. R., Greenhill, L. L., Crimson, M. L., Sedillo, S., Carlson, C., Conners, S. K., et al. (2000). The Texas Children's Medication Algorithm Project: Report of the Texas Consensus Conference on Medication Treatment of Childhood Attention-Deficit/Hyperactivity Disorder. Part 1. *Journal of the American Academy of Child and Adolescent Psychiatry, 39(7),* 908–919.

Pliszka, S. R., Liotti, M., & Woldorff, M. G. (2000). Inhibitory control in children with attention-deficit/hyperactivity disorder: Event-related potentials identify the processing component and timing of an impaired right-frontal response-inhibition mechanism. *Biological Psychiatry, 48,* 238–246.

Pliszka, S. R., McCracken, J. T., & Maas, J. W. (1996). Catecholamines in attention-deficit hyperactivity disorder: Current perspectives. *Journal of the American Academy of Child and Adolescent Psychiatry, 35,* 264–272.

Pollard, S., Ward, E. M., & Barkley, R. A. (1983). The effects of parent training and Ritalin on the parent–

child interactions of hyperactive boys. *Child and Family Behavior Therapy, 5,* 51–69.

Porrino, L. J., Rapoport, J. L., Behar, D., Sceery, W., Ismond, D. R., & Bunney, W. E. (1983). A naturalistic assessment of the motor activity of hyperactive boys. *Archives of General Psychiatry, 40,* 681–687.

Quay, H. C. (1997). Inhibition and attention deficit hyperactivity disorder. *Journal of Abnormal Child Psychology, 25,* 7–13.

Quinn, P. O., & Rapoport, J. L. (1974). Minor physical anomalies and neurologic status in hyperactive boys. *Pediatrics, 53,* 742–747.

Rapoport, J., & Mikkelsen, E. (1978). Antidepressants. In J. Werry (Ed.), *Pediatric psychopharmacology* (pp. 208–233). New York: Brunner/Mazel.

Rapport, M. D., DuPaul, G. J., Stoner, G., & Jones, J. T. (1986). Comparing classroom and clinic measures of attention deficit disorder: Differential, idiosyncratic, and dose–response effects of methylphenidate. *Journal of Consulting and Clinical Psychology, 54,* 334–341.

Rapport, M. D., & Kelly, K. L. (1993). Psychostimulant effects on learning and cognitive function. In J. L. Matson (Ed.), *Handbook of hyperactivity in children* (pp. 97–135). Boston: Allyn & Bacon.

Rapport, M. D., & Moffitt, C. (2002). Attention deficit/hyperactivity disorder and methylphenidate. A review of height/weight, cardiovascular, and somatic complaint side effects. *Clinical Psychology Review, 22,* 1107–1131.

Rapport, M. D., Murphy, A., & Bailey, J. S. (1982). Ritalin versus response cost in the control of hyperactive children: A within-subject comparison. *Journal of Applied Behavior Analysis, 15,* 205–216.

Rapport, M. D., Tucker, S. B., DuPaul, G. J., Merlo, M., & Stoner, G. (1986). Hyperactivity and frustration: The influence of control over and size of rewards in delaying gratification. *Journal of Abnormal Child Psychology, 14,* 191–204.

Richter, N. C. (1984). The efficacy of relaxation training with children. *Journal of Abnormal Child Psychology, 12,* 319–344.

Riggs, P. D., Leon, S. L., Mikulich, M. S., & Pottle, L. C. (1998). An open trial of buproprion for ADHD in adolescents with substance use disorders and conduct disorder. *Journal of the American Academy of Child and Adolescent Psychiatry, 37*(12), 1271–1278.

Robin, A. L. (1998). *ADHD in adolescents: Diagnosis and treatment.* New York: Guilford Press.

Robin, A. L., & Foster, S. (1989). *Negotiating parent–adolescent conflict.* New York: Guilford Press.

Roizen, N. J., Blondis, T. A., Irwin, M., & Stein, M. (1994). Adaptive functioning in children with attention-deficit hyperactivity disorder. *Archives of Pediatric and Adolescent Medicine, 148,* 1137–1142.

Romano, E., Tremblay, R. E., Vitaro, F., Zoccolillo, M., & Pagani, L. (2001). Prevalene of psychiatric diagnoses and the role of perceived impairment: Findings from an adolescent community sample. *Journal of Child Psychology and Psychiatry, 42,* 451–462.

Ross, D. M., & Ross, S. A. (1976). *Hyperactivity: Research, theory, and action.* New York: Wiley.

Ross, D. M., & Ross, S. A. (1982). *Hyperactivity: Current issues, research, and theory* (2nd ed.). New York: Wiley.

Rubia, K., Overmeyer, S., Taylor, E., Brammer, M., Williams, S. C. R., Simmons, A., et al. (1999). Hypofrontality in attention deficit hyperactivity disorder during higher-order motor control: A study with functional MRI. *American Journal of Psychiatry, 156,* 891–896.

Rutter, M. (1997). Nature–nurture integration: The example of antisocial behavior. *American Psychologist, 52,* 390–398.

Ryan, N. D. (1990). Heterocyclic antidepressants in children and adolescents. *Journal of Child and Adolescent Psychopharmacology, 1,* 21–32.

Safer, D. J., & Malever, M. (2000). Stimulant treatment in Maryland public schools. *Pediatrics, 106,* 533–539.

Safer, D. J., Zito, J. M., & Fine, E. M. (1996). Increased methylphenidate usage for attention deficit disorder in the 1990s. *Pediatrics, 98,* 1084–1088.

Safer, D. J., Zito, J. M., & Gardner, J. F. (2001). Pemoline hepatoxicity and postmarketing surveillance. *Journal of the American Academy of Child and Adolescent Psychiatry, 40,* 622–629.

Samuel, V. J., George, P., Thornell, A., Curtis, S., Taylor, A., Brome, D., et al. (1999). A pilot controlled family study of DSM-III-R and DSM-IV ADHD in African-American children. *Journal of the American Academy of Child and Adolescent Psychiatry, 38,* 34–39.

Satterfield, J. H., Cantwell, D. P., & Satterfield, B. T. (1979). Multimodality treatment: A one-year follow-up of 84 hyperactive boys. *Archives of General Psychiatry, 36,* 965–974.

Satterfield, J. H., Satterfield, B. T., & Cantwell, D. P. (1980). Multimodality treatment: A two-year evaluation of 61 hyperactive boys. *Archives of General Psychiatry, 37,* 915–919.

Satterfield, J. H., Satterfield, B. T., & Cantwell, D. P. (1981). Three-year multimodality treatment study of 100 hyperactive boys. *Journal of Pediatrics, 98,* 650–655.

Satterfield, J. H., Satterfield, B. T., & Schell, A. M. (1987). Therapeutic interventions to prevent delinquency in hyperactive boys. *Journal of the American Academy of Child and Adolescent Psychiatry, 26,* 56–64.

Satterfield, J. H., Swanson, J., Schell, A., & Lee, F. (1994). Prediction of antisocial behavior in attention-deficit hyperactivity disorder boys from aggression/defiance scores. *Journal of the American Academy of Child and Adolescent Psychiatry, 33,* 185–190.

Scahill, L., Chappell, P. B., Kim, Y. S., Schultz, R. T., Katsovich, L., Shepherd, E., et al. (2001). A placebo-controlled study of guanfacine in the treatment of children with tic disorders and attention deficit hyperactivity disorder. *American Journal of Psychiatry, 158,* 1067–1074.

Scarr, S. (1992). Developmental theories for the 1990s: Development and individual differences. *Child Development, 63,* 1–19.

Scarr, S., & McCartney, K. (1983). How people make their own environments: A theory of genotype–environment effects. *Child Development, 54,* 424–435.

Schachar, R., Jadad, A. R., Gauld, M., Boyle, M., Booker, L., Snider, A., et al. (2002). Attention-deficit hyperactivity disorder: Critical appraisal of extended treatment studies. *Canadian Journal of Psychiatry, 47,* 337–348.

Schachar, R. J., & Tannock, R. (1993). Childhood hyperactivity and psychostimulants: A review of extended treatment studies. *Journal of Child and Adolescent Psychopharmacology, 3,* 81–98.

Schachar, R. J., Tannock, R., & Logan, G. (1993). Inhibitory control, impulsiveness, and attention deficit hyperactivity disorder. *Clinical Psychology Review, 13,* 721–740.

Schachter, H., Pham, B., King, J., Langford, S., & Moher, D. (2001). How efficacious and safe is short-acting methylphenidate for the treatment of attention-deficit disorder in children and adolescents?: A meta-analysis. *Canadian Medical Association Journal, 165*(11), 1475–1488.

Schnoll, R., Burshteyn, D., & Cea-Aravena, J. (2003). Nutrition in the treatment of attention-deficit hyperactivity disorder: A neglected but important aspect. *Applied Psychophysiology and Biofeedback, 28,* 63–75.

Schothorst, P. F., & van Engeland, H. (1996). Long-term behavioral sequelae of prematurity. *Journal of the American Academy of Child and Adolescent Psychiatry, 35,* 175–183.

Schweitzer, J. B., Faber, T. L., Grafton, S. T., Tune, L. E., Hoffman, J. M., & Kilts, C. D. (2000). Alterations in the functional anatomy of working memory in adult attention deficit hyperactivity disorder. *American Journal of Psychiatry, 157,* 278–280.

Seidman, L. J., Biederman, J., Faraone, S. V., Milberger, S., Norman, D., Seiverd, K., et al. (1995). Effects of family history and comorbidity on the neuropsychological performance of children with ADHD: Preliminary findings. *Journal of the American Academy of Child and Adolescent Psychiatry, 34,* 1015–1024.

Seidman, L. J., Biederman, J., Faraone, S. V., Wever, W., & Oullete, C. (1997). Toward defining a neuropsychology of attention-deficit/hyperactivity disorder: Performance of children and adolescents from a larger clinic referred sample. *Journal of Consulting and Clinical Psychology, 65,* 150–160.

Seidman, L. J., Doyle, A., Fried, R., Valera, E., Crum, K., & Matthews, L. (2004). Neuropsychological function in adults with attention-deficit/hyperactivity disorder. *Psychiatric Clinics of North America, 27,* 261–282.

Semrud-Clikeman, M., Harrington, K., Clinton, A., Connor, R. T., & Sylvester, L. (1998, February). *Attention functioning in two groups of ADHD children with and without attention training interventions.* Paper presented at the 26th annual conference of the International Neuropsychological Society, Honolulu, HI.

Semrud-Clikeman, M., Steingard, R. J., Filipek, P., Biederman, J., Bekken, K., & Renshaw, P. F. (2000). Using MRI to examine brain–behavior relationships in males with attention deficit disorder with hyperactivity. *Journal of the American Academy of Child and Adolescent Psychiatry, 39,* 477–484.

Sergeant, J. A., & van der Meere, J. (1988). What happens when the hyperactive child commits an error? *Psychiatry Research, 24,* 157–164.

Sergeant, J. A., & van der Meere, J. P. (1994). Toward an empirical child psychopathology. In D. K. Routh (Ed.), *Disruptive behavior disorders in children* (pp. 59–86). New York: Plenum Press.

Serketich, W. J., & Dumas, J. E. (1996). The effectiveness of behavioral parent training to modify antisocial behavior in children: A meta-analysis. *Behavior Therapy, 27,* 171–186.

Shelton, T. L., Barkley, R. A., Crosswait, C., Moorehouse, M., Fletcher, K., Barrett, S., et al. (2000). Multimethod psychoeducational intervention for preschool children with disruptive behavior: Two-year post-treatment follow-up. *Journal of Abnormal Child Psychology, 28,* 253–266.

Sheridan, S. M., Dee, C. C., Morgan, J. C., McCormick, M. E., & Walker, D. (1996). A multi-method introduction for social skills deficits in children with ADHD and their parents. *School Psychology Review, 25,* 401–416.

Short, E. J., Manos, M. J., Findling, R. L., & Schubel, E. A. (2004). A prospective study of stimulant response in preschool children: Insights from ROC analyses. *Journal of the American Academy of Child and Adolescent Psychiatry, 43,* 251–259.

Smalley, S. L., McGough, J. J., Del'Homme, M., Newdelman, J., Gordon, E., Kim, T., et al. (2000). Familial clustering of symptoms and disruptive behaviors in multiplex families with attention-deficit/hyperactivity disorder. *Journal of the American Academy of Child and Adolescent Psychiatry, 39,* 1135–1143.

Smith, A. J., Brown, R. T., Bunke, V., Blount, R. L., & Christophersen, E. (2002). Psychological adjustment and peer competence of siblings of children with attention-deficit/hyperactivity disorder. *Journal of Attention Disorders, 5,* 165–176.

Smith, B. H., Barkley, R. A., & Shapiro, C. J. (2006). Combined child therapies. In R. A. Barkley, *Attention-deficit hyperactivity disorder: A handbook for diagnosis and treatment* (3rd ed., pp. 678–691). New York: Guilford Press.

Smith, B. H., Pelham, W. E., Evans, S., Gnagy, E., Molina, B., Bukstein, O., et al. (1998). Dosage effects of methylphenidate on the social behavior of adolescents diagnosed with attention-deficit hyperactivity disorder. *Experimental and Clinical Psychopharmacology, 6*(2), 187–204.

Smith, B. H., Pelham, W. E., Gnagy, E., & Yudell, R. S. (1998). Equivalent effects of stimulant treatment for attention-deficit hyperactivity disorder during childhood and adolescence. *Journal of the American Academy of Child and Adolescent Psychiatry, 37*(3), 314–321.

Smith, B. H., Waschbusch, D., Willoughby, M., & Evans, S. (2000). The efficacy, safety, and practicality of treatments for adolescents with attention-deficit/hyperactivity disorder. *Clinical Child and Family Therapy Review, 3*(4), 243–267.

Sohlberg, M. M., & Mateer, C. A. (1989). *Attention process training*. Puyallup, WA: Association for Neuropsychological Research and Development.

Solanto, M. V., Arnsten, A. F. T., & Castellanos, F. X. (2001). *Stimulant drugs and ADHD: Basic and clinical neuroscience*. New York: Oxford University Press.

Sonuga-Barke, E. J. S., Daley, D., & Thompson, M. (2002). Does maternal ADHD reduce the effectiveness of parent training for preschool children's ADHD? *Journal of the American Academy of Child and Adolescent Psychiatry, 41*, 696–702.

Sonuga-Barke, E. J. S., Daley, D., Thompson, M., Laver-Bradbury, C., & Weeks, A. (2001). Parent-based therapies for preschool attention-deficit/hyperactivity disorder: A randomized, controlled trial with a community sample. *Journal of the American Academy of Child and Adolescent Psychiatry, 40*, 402–408.

Sonuga-Barke, E. J. S., Taylor, E., & Hepinstall, E. (1992). Hyperactivity and delay aversion: II. The effect of self versus externally imposed stimulus presentation periods on memory. *Journal of Child Psychology and Psychiatry, 33*, 399409.

Spencer, T. J. (Ed.). (2004). Adult attention-deficit/hyperactivity disorder [Special issue]. *Psychiatric Clinics of North America, 27*(2).

Spencer, T. J. (2006). Antidepressants and specific norepinephrine reuptake inhibitor treatments. In R. A. Barkley, *Attention-deficit hyperactivity disorder: A handbook for diagnosis and treatment* (3rd ed., pp. 648–657). New York: Guilford Press.

Spencer, T. J., Biederman, J., Harding, M., O'Donnell, D., Faraone, S. V., & Wilens, T. E. (1996). Growth deficits in ADHD children revisited: Evidence for disorder-associated growth delays? *Journal of the American Academy of Child and Adolescent Psychiatry, 35*, 1460–1469.

Spencer, T. J., Biederman, J., Wilens, T., Prince, J., Hatch, M., Jones, J., et al. (1998). Effectiveness and tolerability of tomoxetine in adults with attention deficit hyperactivity disorder. *American Journal of Psychiatry, 155*, 693–695.

Spitzer, R. L., Davies, M., & Barkley, R. A. (1990). The DSMIIIR field trial for the disruptive behavior disorders. *Journal of the American Academy of Child and Adolescent Psychiatry, 29*, 690697.

Stein, M. A., Szumowski, E., Blondis, T. A., & Roizen, N. J. (1995). Adaptive skills dysfunction in ADD and

ADHD children. *Journal of Child Psychology and Psychiatry, 36*, 663–670.

Strayhorn, J. M., & Weidman, C. S. (1989). Reduction of attention deficit and internalizing symptoms in preschoolers through parent–child interaction training. *Journal of the American Academy of Child and Adolescent Psychiatry, 28*, 888–896.

Strayhorn, J. M., & Weidman, C. S. (1991). Follow-up one year after parent–child interaction training: Effects on behavior of preschool children. *Journal of the American Academy of Child and Adolescent Psychiatry, 30*, 138–143.

Streissguth, A. P., Bookstein, F. L., Sampson, P. D., & Barr, H. M. (1995). Attention: Prenatal alcohol and continuities of vigilance and attentional problems from 4 through 14 years. *Development and Psychopathology, 7*, 419–446.

Stroes, A., Alberts, E., & van der Meere, J. J. (2003). Boys with ADHD in social interaction with a nonfamiliar adult: An observational study. *Journal of the American Academy of Child and Adolescent Psychiatry, 42*, 295–302.

Swanson, J. M., Kraemer, H. C., Hinshaw, S. P., Arnold, L. E., Conners, C. K., Abikoff, H. B., et al. (2001). Clinical relevance of the primary findings of the MTA: Success rates based on severity of ADHD and ODD symptoms at the end of treatment. *Journal of the American Academy of Child and Adolescent Psychiatry, 40*, 168–179.

Swanson, J. M., Sunohara, G. A., Kennedy, J. L., Regino, R., Fineberg, E., Wigal, E., et al. (1997). Association of the dopamine receptor D4 (DRD4) gene with a refined phenotype of attention deficit hyperactivity disorder (ADHD): A family-based approach. *Molecular Psychiatry, 3*, 38–41.

Szatmari, P. (1992). The epidemiology of attention-deficit/hyperactivity disorders. *Child and Adolescent Psychiatric Clinics of North America, 1*(2), 361–372.

Szatmari, P., Offord, D. R., & Boyle, M. H. (1989). Correlates, associated impairments, and patterns of service utilization of children with attention deficit disorders: Findings from the Ontario Child Health Study. *Journal of Child Psychology and Psychiatry, 30*, 205–217.

Tallmadge, J., & Barkley, R. A. (1983). The interactions of hyperactive and normal boys with their mothers and fathers. *Journal of Abnormal Child Psychology, 11*, 565–579.

Tannock, R. (1998). Attention deficit hyperactivity disorder: Advances in cognitive, neurobiological, and genetic research. *Journal of Child Psychology and Psychiatry, 39*, 65–100.

Tannock, R. (2000a). Attention deficit disorders with anxiety disorders. In T. E. Brown (Ed.), *Attention deficit disorders and comorbidities in children, adolescents, and adults*. Washington, DC: American Psychiatric Press.

Tannock, R. (2000b). Attention deficit disorders with learning disabilities. In T. E. Brown (Ed.), *Attention deficit disorders and comorbidities in children, ado-*

lescents, and adults. Washington, DC: American Psychiatric Press.

Taylor, E. A. (1983). Drug response and diagnostic validation. In M. Rutter (Ed.), Developmental neuropsychiatry (pp. 348–368). New York: Guilford Press.

Taylor, E. A. (1986). Childhood hyperactivity. British Journal of Psychiatry, 149, 562–573.

Teicher, M. H., Anderson, C. M., Polcari, A., Glod, C. A., Maas, L. C., & Renshaw, P. F. (2000). Functional deficits in basal ganglia of children with attention-deficit/hyperactivity disorder shown with functional magnetic resonance imaging relaxometry. Nature Medicine, 6, 470–473.

Teicher, M. H., Ito, Y, Glod, C. A., & Barber, N. I. (1996). Objective measurement of hyperactivity and attentional problems in ADHD. Journal of the American Academy of Child and Adolescent Psychiatry, 35, 334–342.

Thapar, A. J. (1999). Genetic basis of attention deficit and hyperactivity. British Journal of Psychiatry, 174, 105–111.

Thompson, L. L., Riggs, P. D., Mikulich, S. K., & Crowley, T. J. (1996). Contribution of ADHD symptoms to substance problems and delinquency in conduct-disordered adolescents. Journal of Abnormal Child Psychology, 24, 325–347.

Vaidya, C. J., Austin, G., Kirkorian, G., Ridlehuber, H. W., Desmond, J. E., Glover, G. H., et al. (1998). Selective effects of methylphenidate in attention deficit hyperactivity disorder: A functional magnetic resonance study. Proceedings of the national Academy of Science USA, 95, 14494–14499.

van de Wiel, N. M. H., Matthys, W., Cohen-Kettenis, P., & van Engeland, H. (2003). Application of the Utrecht Coping Power Program and care as usual for children with disruptive behavior disorders in outpatient clinics: A comparative study of cost and course of treatment. Behavior Therapy, 34, 421–436.

Vargas, S., & Camilli, G. (1999). A meta-analysis of research on sensory-integration treatment. Journal of Occupational Therapy, 53, 189–198.

Viesselman, J. O., Yaylayan, S., Weller, E. B., & Weller, R. A. (1999). Antidysthymic drugs (antidepressants and antimanics). In J. S. Werry & M. G. Aman (Eds.), A practitioner's guide to psychoactive drugs for children and adolescents (2nd ed., pp. 239–268). New York: Plenum Press.

Volkow, N. D., Ding, Y., Fowler, J. S., Wang, G., Logan, J., Gatley, J. S., et al. (1995). Is methylphenidate like cocaine?: Studies on their pharmacokinetics and distribution in the human brain. Archives of General Psychiatry, 52, 456–463.

Volkow, N. D., Wang, G., Fowler, J. S., Logan, J., Angrist, B., Hitzemann, R., et al. (1997). Effects of methylphenidate on regional brain glucose metabolism in humans: Relationship to dopamine D_2 receptors. American Journal of Psychiatry, 154, 50–55.

Webster-Stratton, C. (1992). The incredible years. Toronto: Umbrella Press.

Webster-Stratton, C., Reid, J., & Hammond, M. (2001). Social skills and problem-solving training for children with early-onset conduct problems: Who benefits? Journal of Child Psychology and Psychiatry, 42, 945–952.

Weiss, G., & Hechtman, L. (1993). Hyperactive children grown up (2nd ed.). New York: Guilford Press.

Weisz, J. R. (2004). Psychotherapy for children and adolescents: Evidence-based treatments and case examples. New York: Cambridge University Press.

Wells, C. K., Epstein, J. N., Hinshaw, S. P., Conners, C. K., Klaric, J., Abikoff, H. B., et al. (2000). Parenting and family stress treatment outcomes in attention deficit hyperactivity disorder (ADHD): An empirical analysis in the MTA Study. Journal of Abnormal Child Psychology, 28(6), 543–553.

Werry, J. S., & Aman, M. G. (Eds.). (1999). A practitioner's guide to psychoactive drugs for children and adolescents (2nd ed.). New York: Plenum Press.

Werry, J. S., Elkind, G. S., & Reeves, J. S. (1987). Attention deficit, conduct, oppositional, and anxiety disorders in children: III. Laboratory differences. Journal of Abnormal Child Psychology, 15, 409–428.

Werry, J. S., Reeves, J. C., & Elkind, G. S. (1987). Attention deficit, conduct, oppositional, and anxiety disorders in children: I. A review of research on differentiating characteristics. Journal of the American Academy of Child and Adolescent Psychiatry, 26, 133–143.

Whalen, C. K., & Henker, B. (1991). Therapies for hyperactive children: Comparisons, combinations, and compromises. Journal of Consulting and Clinical Psychology, 59, 126–137.

Whalen, C. K., & Henker, B. (1992). The social profile of attention-deficit hyperactivity disorder: Five fundamental facets. Child and Adolescent Psychiatric Clinics of North America, 1(2), 395–410.

Whalen, C. K., Henker, B., & Dotemoto, S. (1980). Methylphenidate and hyperactivity: Effects on teacher behaviors. Science, 208, 1280–1282.

Whittaker, A. H., Van Rossem, R., Feldman, J. F., Schonfeld, I. S., Pinto-Martin, J. A., Torre, C., et al. (1997). Psychiatric outcomes in low-birth-weight children at age 6 years: Relation to neonatal cranial ultrasound abnormalities. Archives of General Psychiatry, 54, 847–856.

Wilens, T. E., Biederman, J., Baldessarini, R. J., Geller, B., Schleifer, D., Spencer, T. J., et al. (1996). Cardiovascular effects of therapeutic doses of tricyclic antidepressants in children and adolescents. Journal of the American Academy of Child and Adolescent Psychiatry, 35, 1491–1501.

Wilens, T. E., Faraone, S. V., Biederman, J., & Gunawardene, S. (2003). Does stimulant therapy of attention-deficit/hyperactivity disorder beget later substance abuse?: A meta-analytic review of the literature. Pediatrics, 111, 179–185.

Willis, T. J., & Lovaas, I. (1977). A behavioral approach to treating hyperactive children: The parent's role. In

J. B. Millichap (Ed.), *Learning disabilities and related disorders* (pp. 119–140). Chicago: Year Book Medical.

Winsberg, B. G., Bialer, I., Kupietz, S., & Tobias, J. (1972). Effects of imipramine and dextroamphetamine on behavior of neuropsychiatrically impaired children. *American Journal of Psychiatry, 128,* 1425–1431.

Wolraich, M. L., Drummond, T., Saloman, M. K., O'Brien, M. L., & Sivage, C. (1978). Effects of methylphenidate alone and in combination with behavior modification procedures on the behavior and academic performance of hyperactive children. *Journal of Abnormal Child Psychology, 6,* 149–161.

Wolraich, M. L., Hannah, J. N., Baumgaerel, A., & Feurer, I. D. (1998). Examination of DSM-IV criteria for attention-deficit/hyperactivity disorder. *Journal of Developmental and Behavioral Pediatrics, 19,* 162–168.

Wolraich, M. L., Wilson, D. B., & White, J. W. (1995). The effect of sugar on behavior or cognition in children; A meta-analysis. *Journal of the American Medical Association, 274,* 1617–1621.

Yeo, R. A., Hill, D. E., Campbell, R. A., Vigil, J.,

Petropoulos, H., Hart, B., et al. (2003). Proton magnetic resonance spectroscopy investigation of the right frontal lobe in children with attention-deficit/hyperactivity disorder. *Journal of the American Academy of Child and Adolescent Psychiatry, 42,* 303–310.

Zalecki, C. A., & Hinshaw, S. P. (2004). Overt and relational aggression in girls with attention deficit hyperactivity disorder. *Journal of Clinical Child and Adolescent Psychology, 33,* 125–137.

Zametkin, A. J., Nordahl, T. E., Gross, M., King, A. C., Semple, W. E., Rumsey, J., et al. (1990). Cerebral glucose metabolism in adults with hyperactivity of childhood onset. *New England Journal of Medicine, 323,* 1361–1366.

Zentall, S. S. (1985). A context for hyperactivity. *Advances in Learning and Behavioral Disabilities, 4,* 273–343.

Zentall, S. S., Cassady, J. C., & Javorsky, J. (2001). Social comprehension of children with hyperactivity. *Journal of Attention Disorders, 5,* 11–24.

Zito, J., Safer, D., DosReis, S., Gardner, J., Magder, L., Soeken, K., et al. (2003). Psychotropic practice patterns for youth: a 10-year perspective. *Archives of Pediatric and Adolescent Medicine, 157*(1), 14–26.

3

Conduct Problems

Robert J. McMahon, Karen C. Wells, and Julie S. Kotler

Conduct problems in children and adolescents constitute a broad range of "acting-out" behaviors, ranging from annoying but relatively minor oppositional behaviors (such as yelling and temper tantrums) to more serious forms of antisocial behavior (including aggression, physical destructiveness, and stealing). Typically, these behaviors do not occur in isolation but as a complex or syndrome, and there is strong evidence to suggest that oppositional behaviors (e.g., noncompliance in younger children) are developmental precursors to antisocial behaviors in adolescence. However, it is also the case that for some youths, these behaviors first appear during adolescence. When displayed as a cluster, these behaviors have been referred to as "oppositional," "antisocial," "conduct-disordered," and, from a legal perspective, "delinquent" (see Hinshaw & Lee, 2003, and Tremblay, 2003, for discussions of terminology). In this chapter, we use the term "conduct problems" (CP) to refer to this constellation of behaviors. Terminology from the *Diagnostic and Statistical Manual of Mental Disorders* (DSM; American Psychiatric Association [APA], 1994, 2000) is used only in those instances in which a formal DSM diagnosis is being discussed or referred to (e.g., conduct disorder [CD], oppositional defiant disorder [ODD]).

The primary purpose of this chapter is to present and critically evaluate evidence-based interventions currently in use for addressing CP in children and adolescents. After a brief look at the historical context of CP, we present an overview of CP in children and adolescents,

followed by a section on the assessment of CP. The overview provides a description of CP, including diagnostic issues, associated comorbidities and child characteristics, epidemiology, contextual influences (including the family, peer group, and neighborhood), and developmental pathways. In the section on assessment, we describe methods and processes that are currently employed with children and adolescents with CP in different contexts.

BRIEF HISTORICAL CONTEXT

How to define and deal with CP in children and adolescents has a long and checkered history. Costello and Angold (2001) present an intriguing historical account from religious, legal, and medical perspectives of how society has attempted to deal with "bad" children over the centuries. They note that many of the same issues first described by Plato 2,500 years ago pertaining to how best to ascribe responsibility and culpability for such behavior, as well as the relative roles of the family and state, are still sources of debate.

The formal recognition of CP as a diagnostic entity (or entities) is fairly recent. CD first appeared in the second edition of the DSM (DSM-II; APA, 1968), and what was then called "oppositional disorder" appeared 12 years later in DSM-III (APA, 1980). It was relabeled as ODD in DSM-III-R (APA, 1987). The specific symptoms and the number required to make these diagnoses have fluctuated across the various versions of the DSM. For example, only a single symptom was required for a CD diagnosis in DSM-III, whereas 3 of 13 symptoms were required in DSM-III-R, and 3 of 15 symptoms are required in the most recent versions of the DSM (DSM-IV and DSM-IV-TR; APA, 1994, 2000). The subtypes of CD presented in the DSM have also differed in various editions. For example, DSM-III had four subtypes based on crossing aggressive–nonaggressive and socialized–undersocialized dimensions, whereas the basis for subtyping in DSM-IV and DSM-IV-TR has to do with age of onset (i.e., childhood- vs. adolescent-onset).

An issue of current concern is whether rates and severity of CP have been increasing over the past 50 years or so. One perspective on this question involves official statistics concerning juvenile crime. Based on an extensive analysis of crime records in both Europe and North America from 1950 through the mid-1990s, Rutter and colleagues (Rutter, Giller, & Hagell, 1998; Rutter & Smith, 1995) concluded that juvenile crime did increase in these countries from the 1950s through the 1980s, with a plateau occurring in the 1990s. Findings in the 1990s are less clear-cut because of various policy changes regarding the handling of offending juveniles. In addition, there is evidence that the proportion of violent to nonviolent crime has increased, that proportionally more juvenile crime is being committed by females, and that the peak age of offending has moved from middle to late adolescence. In the United States, both the total number and the rates of juvenile arrests for violent crime (including homicides) dropped annually from 1994 to 2000 (Howell, 2003).

Another perspective on whether there have been changes in the occurrence of CP behaviors involves data presented by Achenbach and colleagues with respect to the renorming of the Child Behavior Checklist from 1976 to 1999 (Achenbach, Dumenci, & Rescorla, 2003a). In brief, there were slight but significant increases in the various indicators of CP behavior (the Externalizing broad-band scale, the Rule-Breaking Behavior and Aggressive Behavior narrow-band syndrome scales, and the Oppositional Defiant Problems and Conduct Problems DSM-oriented scales) from 1976 to 1989 and decreases from 1989 to 1999. However, effect sizes (ES) ranged from 1% to 2%. Results were similar when analyses were conducted with national samples in 1989 and 1999 that included referred children. The Aggressive Behavior and Externalizing Scales had more positive scores in 1999 than in 1989; however, the DSM-oriented scale of Oppositional Defiant Problems increased from 1989 to 1999 (ES = 1%). In contrast, the Conduct Problems scale was the only DSM-oriented scale to show a significant reduction from 1989 to 1999, when percentage of scores in the deviant range was the variable of interest (9.2% to 6.8%). Achenbach and colleagues (2003a) concluded that there is no evidence to suggest that the overall functioning of children in the United States is steadily worsening. When their findings and those related to juvenile crime rates are considered together, a similar conclusion appears to apply with respect to CP: CP does seem to have increased from 1950 through the 1980s, but during the 1990s, it seems to have plateaued or in some cases decreased.

DESCRIPTION

There are a number of current approaches to the description and classification of CP. We begin by first describing the diagnostic criteria delineated in DSM-IV-TR (APA, 2000) for various disorders related to CP. We then describe a number of ways in which CP (or certain aspects of CP, such as aggression) have been subtyped. This is followed by a section on the various disorders and conditions that are most commonly associated with CP.

Diagnostic Criteria

In DSM-IV-TR (APA, 2000), CP is classified in the category of disruptive behavior disorders (see Angold & Costello, 2001, for a consideration of nosological issues related to CD and ODD). The two diagnostic categories that are most relevant to CP are ODD and CD. The essential feature of ODD is a "recurrent pattern of negativistic, defiant, disobedient, and hostile behavior toward authority figures" (p. 100). The pattern of behavior must have a duration of at least 6 months, and at least four of the following eight behaviors must be present: losing temper, arguing with grownups, defying or not complying with grownups' rules or requests, deliberately doing things that annoy other people, blaming others for own mistakes, being touchy or easily becoming annoyed by others, exhibiting anger and resentment, and showing spite or vindictiveness. The behaviors must have a higher frequency than is generally seen in other children of similar developmental level and age. Furthermore, the behaviors must lead to meaningful impairment in academic and social functioning.

Although the prototypical presentation of ODD is in a preschool-age child (e.g., McMahon & Forehand, 2003), it is possible for ODD to begin in early adolescence (APA, 2000). Because the behaviors described above can be typical of many young children and adolescents, DSM-IV-TR emphasizes the frequency and impairment criteria noted above.

The essential feature of CD is a "repetitive and persistent pattern of behavior in which the basic rights of others or major age-appropriate societal norms or rules are violated" (APA, 2000, p. 93). At least 3 of the 15 behaviors listed below must have been present in the past 12 months, with at least one of the behaviors present in the past 6 months. The behaviors are categorized into four groups: aggressiveness to people and animals (bullying, fighting, using a weapon, physical cruelty to people, physical cruelty to animals, stealing with confrontation of victim, forced sexual activity); property destruction (firesetting, other destruction of property); deceptiveness or theft (breaking and entering, lying for personal gain, stealing without confronting victim); and serious rule violations (staying out at night [before age 13], running away from home, being truant [before age 13]). It is important to note that ODD includes behaviors (e.g., noncompliance) that are also included in CD. However, ODD does not involve the more serious behaviors that represent violations of either the basic rights of others or age-appropriate societal norms or rules. Thus, if a youth meets the diagnostic criteria for both disorders, only the diagnosis of CD is made.

Two subtypes of CD are described in DSM-IV-TR (APA, 2000); these are differentiated on the basis of the child's age at the appearance of the first symptom of CD. The childhood-onset type is defined by the onset of at least 1 of the 15 behaviors prior to 10 years of age, whereas CD behavior does not appear until age 10 or older in the adolescent-onset type. It is important to note that clinicians working with adolescents with CP will encounter both subtypes. Indeed, distinguishing adolescents with CP on the basis of age of onset is one of the most clinically important tasks for the clinician, given differences in likely causal and maintaining factors and prognosis (see below).

Field trials for assessing the psychometric properties of the DSM-IV diagnoses of ODD and CD demonstrated that the internal consistency and test–retest reliabilities of the DSM-IV versions were higher than those of their DSM-III-R counterparts (Lahey et al., 1994). The validity of the childhood-onset and adolescent-onset types of CD was also supported, in that children with the childhood-onset type were more likely to display more aggressive symptoms, to be boys, to have a family history of antisocial behavior, to experience neurocognitive and temperamental difficulties, and to have additional psychiatric diagnoses, whereas adolescent-onset type CD was more highly related to ethnic minority status and exposure to deviant peers (e.g., Lahey et al., 1998; McCabe, Hough, Wood, & Yeh, 2001; Moffitt & Caspi, 2001; Waldman & Lahey, 1994).

Additional Subtypes of CP

In addition to the distinction between ODD and CD and subtypes based on age of onset, several other subtypes of CP are salient when diagnosis and treatment are considered. Loeber and Schmaling (1985a) proposed a bipolar unidimensional typology of "overt" and "covert" CP behaviors. Overt CP behaviors include those that involve direct confrontation with or disruption of the environment (e.g., aggression, temper tantrums, argumentativeness), whereas covert CP behaviors include those that usually occur without the awareness of adult caretakers (e.g., lying, stealing, firesetting).

In an extension of this investigation, Frick and colleagues (1993) conducted a meta-analysis of 60 factor analyses with more than 28,000 children. They identified a similar "overt–covert" dimension, but also extracted a second bipolar dimension of "destructive–nondestructive." When individual CP behaviors were plotted, four subtypes were obtained: "property violations," "aggression," "status violations," and "oppositional" (see Figure 3.1). Symptoms of CD fell into the first three quadrants, whereas symptoms of ODD fell into the fourth quadrant. Cluster analyses of an independent sample of clinic-referred boys ages 7–12 indicated one group of boys who displayed high elevations on the oppositional quadrant score and moderate elevations on the aggression quadrant score, and another group of boys who showed high elevations on the

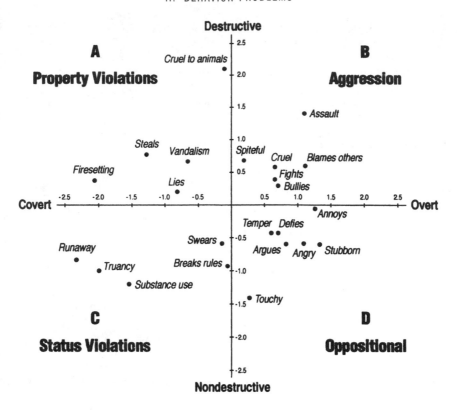

FIGURE 3.1. Meta-analysis of parent and teacher ratings of child conduct problems, using multidimensional scaling. From Frick et al. (1993, p. 327). Copyright 1993 by Elsevier Science Ltd. Reprinted by permission.

property violations, oppositional, and aggression quadrant scores. These clusters approximated those groups of boys who received diagnoses of ODD and CD, respectively.

More recent studies (e.g., Tiet, Wasserman, Loeber, Larken, & Miller, 2001; Tolan, Gorman-Smith, & Loeber, 2000; Willoughby, Kupersmidt, & Bryant, 2001) have provided additional validation for this typology. For example, the earlier phase of the developmental trajectory of childhood-onset type CD consists primarily of overt CP, followed by a rapid increase in covert CP (Patterson & Yoerger, 2002).

Noncompliance (i.e., excessive disobedience to adults) appears to be a keystone behavior in the development of both overt and covert CP. Loeber and Schmaling (1985a) found that noncompliance was positioned near the zero point of their unidimensional overt–covert scale of CP behaviors. Patterson and his colleagues at the Oregon Social Learning Center (OSLC; e.g., Chamberlain & Patterson, 1995; Patter-

son, Reid, & Dishion, 1992) have developed a comprehensive theoretical model for the development and maintenance of CP; in their model, early child noncompliance not only is the precursor of severe manifestations of CP behaviors later in childhood and adolescence, but plays a role in these children's subsequent academic and peer relationship problems as well. Walker and Walker (1991) have stressed the role of compliance and noncompliance in the classroom. There is also empirical support for the premise that noncompliance appears early in the progression of CP, and continues to be manifested in subsequent developmental periods (e.g., Chamberlain & Patterson, 1995; Loeber et al., 1993; McMahon & Forehand, 2003). Low levels of compliance are also associated with referral for services in children with CP (Dumas, 1996). Furthermore, intervention research has shown that when child noncompliance is targeted, there is often concomitant improvement in other CP behaviors as well (Parrish, Cataldo, Kolko, Neef, & Egel, 1986;

Russo, Cataldo, & Cushing, 1981; Wells, Forehand, & Griest, 1980).

There appear to be several different forms of aggressive behavior. One of the most robust distinctions is between "reactive" and "proactive" forms of aggression (e.g., Crick & Dodge, 1996; Dodge & Coie, 1987; Poulin & Boivin, 2000). The former is a response to perceived provocation, whereas the latter occurs as a means of obtaining some self-serving outcome or to influence and coerce others (e.g., bullying). This reactive–proactive subtyping of aggression has been found to have good criterion validity, to differ in terms of antecedent characteristics (e.g., a temperament characterized by angry reactivity/emotional dysregulation and inattention is more closely related to reactive aggression), and to differentially predict maladaptive outcomes (e.g., proactive aggression tends to predict more delinquency and disruptive behavior) (e.g., Hubbard et al., 2002; Vitaro, Brendgen, & Tremblay, 2002; Vitaro, Gendreau, Tremblay, & Oligny, 1998; Waschbusch, Willoughby, & Pelham, 1998). Youths who display reactive aggression are more likely to display social information-processing deficits (e.g., hostile attributional bias, poor social problem-solving skills) (Crick & Dodge, 1996; Dodge, Lochman, Harnish, Bates, & Pettit, 1997). There is also a subgroup of children who are both proactively and reactively aggressive and who have more difficulties than their nonaggressive and proactively aggressive peers, but fewer difficulties than reactively aggressive children in terms of social information-processing deficits (Dodge & Coie, 1987) and on dimensions of reactivity, attention, and depression (Vitaro et al., 2002).

Bullying is a form of proactive aggression, occurring primarily in school settings, that has received increasing attention. It is notable that some authors (e.g., Pikas, 1989) have suggested that some bullying may also be provoked; thus such bullying behavior might also be appropriately categorized as reactive rather than proactive. Several authoritative reviews have appeared on the topic of bullying (e.g., Farrington, 1993; Olweus, 1993a; Smith et al., 1999). The general definition of "bullying" has included physical, verbal, or psychological attack or intimidation that is intended to cause fear, distress, or harm to the victim. Direct bullying, which is more characteristic of boys, involves physical and direct verbal attacks. Indirect bullying, which is more characteristic of

girls, includes efforts to isolate and exclude the victim from the social group and involves behaviors such as slandering, spreading rumors, and manipulating friendships (similar to the construct of "relational aggression" discussed below). In addition, whether direct or indirect, these bullying behaviors are generally carried out repeatedly over time and are characterized by an imbalance of power between the perpetrator and the victim (Olweus, 1999). A cross-national comparison of bullying definitions demonstrated that adolescents (age 14) discriminate between direct and indirect, and between verbal and nonverbal, bullying more effectively than do younger children (age 8), who mostly distinguish aggressive from nonaggressive acts (Smith, Cowie, Olafsson, & Liefooghe, 2002). Furthermore, according to Smith and colleagues (2002), gender differences in youths' conceptualization of bullying are much less appreciable than these developmental differences.

Throughout both childhood and adolescence, the prevalence of bullying is alarmingly high. A number of studies have examined the prevalence of bullying behaviors. With respect to bullying during the elementary school years, Kochenderfer and Ladd (1997) found that approximately 50% of kindergarten children reported experiencing some form of peer victimization. In a study of third graders, 40% of children reported experiencing physical or verbal aggression in a 1-month period, while 14% identified themselves as perpetrators of bullying (Silvernail, Thompsom, Yang, & Kopp, 2000). A cross-national study including data from 35 countries participating in a World Health Organization survey indicated that for adolescents ages 11–16, the prevalence rates of two or three bullying occurrences in the last month ranged from 2% to 37% for bullying and from 2% to 36% for being victimized (Craig & Yossi, 2003). Additional data suggest that, in a given year, 75% of youths report at least one bullying incident (Glover, Gough, Johnson, & Cartwright, 2000). Furthermore, in a recent U.S. study that included a survey of 15,686 students in grades 6 through 10, Nansel and colleagues (2001) found that 29.9% of the sample reported frequent involvement in bullying, with 13% as perpetrators, 10.6% as victims, and 6% as both. Nansel and colleagues also found that the typical developmental trajectory of bullying included an increase and peak during early adolescence, and a decrease during high school. Although bullying is often studied independently of other CP behaviors, some findings suggest that it may also be a part of a more general pattern of violent and aggressive behavior (Andershed, Kerr, & Stattin, 2001; Baldry & Farrington, 2000). Researchers in this area emphasize that adults (teachers and parents) are relatively unaware of the extent of or harm created by the problem, and that teachers intervene to help victims very infrequently. Peers intervene approximately three times more often than teachers to stop bullying (Craig & Pepler, 1995), but even they are more likely to observe or even collaborate than to help the victims. Involvement in bullying as a perpetrator, a victim, or both is associated with a range of negative psychological outcomes (e.g., anger, depression, low self-esteem, unhappiness at school, suicidal ideation) (Bosworth, Espelage, & Simon, 1999; Duncan, 1999; Kaltiala-Heino, Rimpela, Marttunen, Rimpela, & Rantanen, 1999; Nansel et al., 2001), and youths involved in bullying are four times as likely to have criminal convictions by early adulthood (Olweus, 1993b).

In contrast to proactive and reactive forms of aggression, both of which are primarily overt in nature, Crick and colleagues have identified a form of aggression called "relational aggression," which involves manipulation of relationships and may be overt or covert (e.g., Crick & Grotpeter, 1995; Crick & Werner, 1998; Geiger, Zimmer-Gembeck, & Crick, 2004). It includes strategies such as social isolation and exclusion, and behaviors including slandering, rumor spreading, and friendship manipulation. Relational aggression occurs more frequently in girls, although the evidence for this gender difference is less clear during adolescence (Underwood, 2003). Recent evidence suggests that it may be possible to divide relational aggression into proactive and reactive forms as well (Little, Jones, Henrich, & Hawley, 2003).

Some authors have proposed that unique subtypes of CP can even be identified within the childhood-onset pathway. Frick and colleagues suggest that youths described as "early starters" are quite a heterogeneous group and can be distinguished based on their affective and interpersonal style (Frick & Ellis, 1999). Specifically, these authors have identified two groups of youths that differ according to the presence or absence of "callous and unemotional" (CU) traits (e.g., lack of guilt and empathy, callous use of others) (e.g., Caputo, Frick,

& Brodsky, 1999; Christian, Frick, Hill, Tyler, & Frazer, 1997; Frick, Bodin, & Barry, 2000). Within groups of youths diagnosed with CD, Frick and colleagues have identified youths who also have high scores on the dimension of CU traits and have found that these youths (1) engage in more diverse and serious CP; (2) have a more stable constellation of CP; (3) are more likely to have had police contact; (4) engage in patterns of violence that are more severe, premeditated, and instrumental; and (5) have an increased likelihood of parental antisocial personality disorder (APD) (Christian et al., 1997; Frick, Cornell, Barry, Bodin, & Dane, 2003; Kruh, Frick, & Clements, 2005). In contrast, youths with CP who are low on CU traits are less likely to be aggressive, and their aggression is more likely to be reactive in nature (Frick, Cornell, Barry, et al., 2003). Also, youths with CP who are low on CU traits are more likely to have experienced dysfunctional parenting practices (Oxford, Cavell, & Hughes, 2003; Wootton, Frick, Shelton, & Silverthorn, 1997) and to have deficits in verbal intelligence (Loney, Frick, Ellis, & McCoy, 1998).

There is also evidence that the subgroup of youths with CU traits may exhibit some unique temperamental attributes. In general, these youths have higher levels of behavioral dysregulation and lower levels of behavioral inhibition, compared to children with CP who are low on CU traits (Frick, Cornell, Barry, et al., 2003). Specifically, they seem to prefer novel, exciting, and dangerous activities (Frick, Cornell, Barry, et al., 2003; Frick, Lilienfeld, Ellis, Loney, & Silverthorn, 1999) and are less reactive to emotionally distressing stimuli than other youths with CP (Blair, 1999; Frick, Cornell, Barry, et al., 2003). Furthermore, children with CU traits have been shown to be less sensitive to punishment cues (Barry et al., 2000; Fisher & Blair, 1998), to have poor perspective-taking skills, and to expect more positive rewards from aggression (Pardini, Lochman, & Frick, 2003).

Relatively less research has been conducted on covert types of CP, and has focused on youths who steal and who set fires. Lying is significantly underresearched compared to other forms of covert CP. There is a paucity of longitudinal research on youths who steal, although retrospective reports suggest developmental sequences for stealing, such that minor forms of theft (e.g., shoplifting) seem to occur prior to more serious forms of theft (e.g., car theft)

(LeBlanc & Fréchette, 1989; Loeber, 1988). Much of the work on stealing has been conducted by Patterson and his colleagues. Youths who steal exhibit levels of aversive behavior comparable to those of nonreferred youths, although youths who engage in both stealing and social aggression are even more aversive than youths who are socially aggressive but who do not steal (Loeber & Schmaling, 1985b; Patterson, 1982). It also appears that youths who steal are older at time of referral than youths referred for overt types of CP (Moore, Chamberlain, & Mukai, 1979; Reid & Hendricks, 1973) and are at greater risk for committing delinquent offenses as adolescents (Loeber & Schmaling, 1985b; Moore et al., 1979). In one study of incarcerated juveniles, stealing was the most common first offense, accounting for 42% of the cases (Taylor et al., 2001).

Patterson (1982) has reported that the parents of youths who steal are more distant and less involved in interactions with their offspring than parents of nonreferred youths or parents of youths who are aggressive. The mothers and siblings of aggressive youths are more coercive than their counterparts in nonreferred families or families in which the youths steal. Loeber and Schmaling (1985b) have found that families with aggressive youths and those with youths who both fight and steal were more likely to demonstrate poorer monitoring skills and to have rejecting mothers. Fathers of youths who steal also appear to be less involved in the discipline process than fathers of aggressive or nonreferred youths (Loeber, Weissman, & Reid, 1983).

Lying, defined as a "verbal statement intended to deceive" (Stouthamer-Loeber, 1986, p. 268), may be one of the first covert CP behaviors to appear (Edelbrock, 1985) and is highly correlated with stealing (especially in adolescents). For example, the correlations between lying and stealing in 4th-, 7th-, and 10th-grade boys were .39, .59, and .74, respectively (Stouthamer-Loeber & Loeber, 1986). Based on the findings of the meta-analytic study conducted by Loeber and Schmaling (1985a), Stouthamer-Loeber (1986) concluded that although lying loads most heavily on the covert dimension of CP, it is also related (albeit less strongly) to overt CP. Lying did correlate significantly with fighting in a community sample of boys in 4th to 10th grades (r's = .50–.65) (Stouthamer-Loeber & Loeber, 1986), particu-

larly when it occurred in conjunction with stealing. Furthermore, early lying has been shown to be predictive of later recidivism (Loeber & Dishion, 1983).

Childhood firesetting is quite common and potentially very serious in its effects. Prevalence estimates have ranged from 3% to 35% across epidemiological, outpatient, and inpatient samples (Achenbach & Edelbrock, 1981; Heath, Hardesty, Goldfine, & Walker, 1983; Kolko & Kazdin, 1988). Juveniles are arrested for a greater share of arsons than any other type of crime, accounting for 50% of the firesetting arrests according to the Federal Bureau of Investigation's *Uniform Crime Reports* (Snyder, 1999). Approximately two-thirds of those arrested are adolescents (i.e., ages 13 to 18).

In the last 20 years, three general domains of risk factors associated with firesetting have emerged: child characteristics, parenting, and the broader family climate (e.g., Kolko & Kazdin, 1992; McCarty, McMahon, & Conduct Problems Prevention Research Group, 2005). Child factors that have been identified as risk factors for firesetting behavior include being male, having higher impulsivity or traits of attention-deficit/hyperactivity disorder (ADHD), having social skill deficits and poor peer relations, displaying other CP behaviors, demonstrating poorer academic performance, and having been abused.

Firesetting has been consistently associated with other CP behaviors. Although only a relatively small proportion of youths with CP engage in firesetting behavior (e.g., 5% in Jacobson's [1985] outpatient sample in London), most, but not all, such youths demonstrate other CP behaviors (i.e., can be considered to display the "syndrome" of CP). For example, 74% of the youths who set fires in both outpatient (Jacobson, 1985) and inpatient (Kazdin & Kolko, 1986) samples received a diagnosis of CD. In addition, juveniles with other offenses who also set fires seem to have more severe levels of CP behavior, to have a history of previous firesetting, and to be arrested at younger ages (Becker, Stuewig, Herrera, & McCloskey, 2004; Forehand, Wierson, Frame, Kemptom, & Armistead, 1991; Hanson, Mackay-Soroka, Staley, & Poulton, 1994; Stickle & Blechman, 2002).

Parenting factors that have been empirically linked to firesetting behavior include harsh or lax discipline, lack of parental involvement, less parental acceptance of the child, and limited monitoring and supervision. Family factors associated with firesetting behavior include low socioeconomic status (SES), marital discord, parental psychopathology/depression, and stressful life events.

The number and nature of risk factors associated with firesetting may vary according to age of onset and persistence of firesetting. McCarty and colleagues (2005) classified youths from a community-based sample into four groups (which they labeled "nonfiresetters," "desisters," "late-onset firesetters," and "persisters"), based on their reported firesetting behavior during two developmental periods: prior to fourth grade and between fourth and sixth grades. Firesetters differed from nonfiresetters on 13 of 19 risk factors. Within firesetting groups, most of the differences were between persisters and desisters. Persisters were more likely to exhibit impulsivity/hyperactivity, and their parents demonstrated lower levels of appropriate discipline, higher levels of harsh discipline, and higher levels of maternal depression and spousal hostility. Persisters and desisters had significantly more risk factors than nonfiresetters. The cumulative number of risk factors had a linear relationship with an increased likelihood of firesetting. The percentages of youths who engaged in firesetting were 1.5%, 13.2%, 19.6%, and 40.3% for zero, one, two, and three or more risk factors.

In the clinical literature, several typologies of juvenile firesetting exist. For example, Humphreys, Kopet, and Lajoy (1993) described typologies that include "curiosity firesetting" (typically exhibited by younger children), "crisis firesetting" (associated with stress or high negative affect), "delinquent firesetting" (involving deliberate violations of others' rights), and "severely disturbed firesetting" (associated with major affective instability or disturbed thinking). Although these typologies of firesetting have a certain appeal in terms of face validity, there has been relatively little empirical validation.

Comorbidity and Associated Characteristics

Youths with CP are at increased risk for manifesting a variety of other behavior disorders and adjustment problems as well. These include ADHD; various internalizing disorders, such as anxiety and depressive disorders; somatization disorder (e.g., Loeber & Keenan,

1994); substance use disorders; and academic underachievement (Hinshaw, 1992). In their review of the relationship of CP to various comorbid conditions, Loeber and Keenan (1994) stressed the importance of considering the temporal ordering of comorbid conditions, as well as the different patterns and influences of these comorbid disorders for boys versus girls. For example, although girls are less likely to display CP than are boys, when girls do display CP, they may be more likely than boys to develop one or more of these comorbid disorders.

ADHD is the comorbid condition most commonly associated with CP, and is thought to precede the development of CP in the majority of cases. In fact, some investigators consider ADHD (or, more specifically, the impulsivity or hyperactivity components of ADHD) to be the "motor" that drives the development of early-onset CP, especially for boys (e.g., Burns & Walsh, 2002; Coie & Dodge, 1998; Loeber, Farrington, Stouthamer-Loeber, & Van Kammen, 1998; White et al., 1994). Coexisting ADHD also predicts a more negative life outcome than does CP alone (see Waschbusch, 2002). For example, children with both ADHD and CD seem to show a greater variety of delinquent acts in adolescence (Loeber, Brinthaupt, & Green, 1990), a greater number of aggressive acts in adolescence (Moffitt, 1993), and increased APD and more violent offending in adulthood (Fischer, Barkley, Smallish, & Fletcher, 2002; Klinteberg, Andersson, Magnusson, & Stattin, 1993). Some have suggested that comorbid ADHD and CP warrant separate diagnostic status (e.g., Angold & Costello, 2001).

Internalizing disorders, such as the depressive and anxiety disorders, and somatization disorder, also co-occur with CP at rates higher than expected by chance (Zoccolillo, 1992). In most cases, CP precedes the onset of depressive symptoms (Loeber & Keenan, 1994), although in some cases depression may precede CP behavior (e.g., Kovacs, Paulauskas, Gatsonis, & Richards, 1988). However, this relationship between CP and depression may be due to common risk factors as opposed to a causal relationship (Fergusson, Lynskey, & Horwood, 1996). Also, the relationship appears to differ for boys and girls, at least during middle to late adolescence. Wiesner (2003) found a reciprocal relationship between delinquent behaviors and depressive symptoms for girls, whereas for boys there was a unidirectional effect of delinquent behavior on depressive symptoms. Risk for suicidality has been shown to increase as a function of preexisting CP (e.g., Capaldi, 1991, 1992), and this risk appears to be higher for girls than for boys (Loeber & Keenan, 1994). In addition, Loeber and Keenan (1994) indicate that the co-occurrence of anxiety disorders with CP is especially likely for girls. In some studies, children with CP and a comorbid anxiety disorder are less seriously impaired than are children with CP alone (e.g., J. L. Walker et al., 1991); in other studies, the presence of a comorbid anxiety disorder has not been shown to have a differential effect (e.g., Campbell & Ewing, 1990); and in yet others, comorbid anxiety is associated with increased risk (e.g., Serbin, Moskowitz, Schwartzman, & Ledingham, 1991). Recent investigators (e.g., Hinshaw & Lee, 2003; Lahey & Waldman, 2003) have noted the importance of distinguishing between anxiety based on inhibition and fear (which appear to be protective) and anxiety based on social withdrawal due to emotional negativity (which seems to increase risk) as a means of interpreting these apparently contradictory findings. It is notable that although the base rate of somatization disorder alone is much higher in girls than in boys, its comorbid occurrence with CP may actually be higher in boys (Lilienfeld, 1992; Offord, Alder, & Boyle, 1986).

In a review of 20 population-based studies examining the comorbidity of CD/ODD with other disorders, Angold and Costello (2001) noted that the joint odds ratio (OR) of CD/ODD with either ADHD (OR = 10.7) or depression (OR = 6.6) was significantly higher than the OR with anxiety (OR = 3.1). They concluded that the apparent comorbidity of CD/ODD with anxiety may be due to the co-occurrence of anxiety with depression and ADHD, rather than representing an independent comorbid relationship with CD/ODD (Angold, Costello, & Erkanli, 1999).

Both longitudinal and cross-sectional studies have documented that preexisting CP constitutes a significant risk factor for substance use (e.g., Angold et al., 1999; Hawkins, Catalano, & Miller, 1992). This may be particularly true for girls (Loeber & Keenan, 1994). The comorbidity between CP and substance abuse is important, because when youths with CP also abuse substances, they tend to show an early onset of substance use and are more likely to abuse multiple substances (Lynskey & Fergusson, 1995). They may be at increased risk of more serious delinquent behavior as well (Angold et al., 1999). Although most of the research on the association between CP and substance abuse prior to adulthood has been conducted with adolescents, the association between CP and substance use may begin much earlier in development (Van Kammen, Loeber, & Stouthamer-Loeber, 1991).

An association between CP and academic underachievement has long been noted. In a comprehensive review, Hinshaw (1992) concluded that during preadolescence, this relationship is actually a function of comorbid ADHD rather than of CP per se. In adolescence, the relationship is more complex, with preexisting ADHD (and perhaps other neuropsychological deficits), a history of academic difficulty and failure, and long-standing socialization difficulties with family and peers all playing interacting roles. It is also important to note that the relationship between CP and academic achievement is a transactional one that plays out across the developmental period (Hinshaw & Lee, 2003).

An issue of ongoing debate concerns the extent to which CP in adolescence is most appropriately conceptualized as part of a unitary behavior problem syndrome ("problem behavior theory"; Jessor, 1998; Jessor & Jessor, 1977) or as one of several different but related types of behavior problems (e.g., Fergusson, Horwood, & Lynskey, 1994). The range of behavior problems considered in problem behavior theory has typically included CP, various forms of substance use, and risky sexual behavior (Biglan, Brennan, Foster, & Holder, 2004), although others (e.g., Jessor, 1998; Loeber et al., 1998) have more recently broadened the theory to include ADHD and internalizing disorders, school failure, and health behavior. Space considerations preclude a thorough examination of this issue. Although it is quite clear that CP behavior is associated with a variety of other behavior problems and disorders during childhood *and* adolescence, the evidence that this spectrum of behaviors reflects a single underlying dimension is mixed. For example, Fergusson and colleagues (1994) found four latent classes of problem behavior in their sample of 15-year-olds from New Zealand: (1) low problem behaviors of any type (85.4% of the sample); (2) high risk of precocious sexual behavior, alcohol use, and marijuana use (5.2%); (3) high risk of CP, police contact, and marijuana use (6.7%); and (4) elevated risks for all problem behaviors (2.7%). The model applied equally well for boys and girls, but among girls, the predominant pattern was that of precocious sexual activity and alcohol and marijuana use (9.4%, vs. 3.6% for boys). For boys, the CP pattern was predominant (6.1%, vs. 3.6% for girls). The multiproblem class included 3.3% of boys and 2.0% of girls. Fergusson et al. concluded that their findings were not generally supportive of problem behavior theory. Although there was a group of multiproblem youths, they accounted for fewer than 20% of the youths engaging in problem behaviors.

EPIDEMIOLOGY

Prevalence

CP is among the most frequently occurring child behavior disorders. However, determining accurate estimates of prevalence has proven to be quite difficult as a function of the various changes in diagnostic criteria for both ODD and CD over the various DSM revisions; the inclusion (or not) of an impairment criterion; the informant (i.e., youth, parent, teacher, clinician); and the method of combining information from various informants (Essau, 2003). Averaging across 20 population-based studies conducted in the United States, Puerto Rico, Holland, and New Zealand, Angold and Costello (2001) reported that from 5% to 10% of youths ages 8–16 years demonstrated CD or ODD (the diagnoses were combined in their analyses). Prevalence rates generally range from 1% to 9% for CD and from 2% to 10% for ODD in various nonclinic samples (e.g., Essau, 2003; Lahey, Miller, Gordon, & Riley, 1999). Adolescents tend to report more frequent engagement in CD behaviors than do their parents. For example, in a sample of 13- to 18-year-old Dutch adolescents, the 6-month prevalence of CD was 5.6% and 1.2% based on adolescent and parent reports, respectively (Verhulst, van der Ende, Ferdinand, & Kasius, 1997). This difference is probably due at least in part to parents' unawareness of their offspring's engagement in covert forms of CP behavior. The prevalence figures for ODD were the same for adolescent and parent informants (0.7% and 0.6%, respectively).

Age of Onset and Sex Differences

Prevalence rates have been shown to vary as a function of age and sex of the child, as well as the type of CP behavior. For example, younger children are more likely to engage in oppositional, overt behaviors, whereas older children and adolescents are more likely to engage in more covert CP behaviors (e.g., stealing) (Patterson & Yoerger, 2002). Because the specific CP behaviors required for a DSM diagnosis of CD generally occur much more frequently in older children and adolescents, it is much more difficult for younger children to receive a CD diagnosis. In fact, there are few data concerning the diagnostic criteria for ODD and CD as they might be applied to children younger than age 7 (Angold & Costello, 2001; Keenan & Wakschlag, 2002), although the ability to identify an externalizing broad-band syndrome of CP in these younger children is well established (e.g., Campbell, 2002).

In general, boys are more likely to begin engaging in overt CP behaviors earlier and at higher rates than girls throughout the developmental period (Archer & Cote, 2005). In fact, gender is the most consistently documented risk factor for CP (Robins, 1991). Perhaps due to the lower rates of antisocial behavior in girls, much of the research on CP either has focused exclusively on boys or, when girls have been included, has failed to consider possible gender effects. Many questions about the onset and development of CP behavior in girls remain unanswered. However, some evidence does suggest that girls' CP behavior tends to be less chronic, more experimental, and more likely to desist than boys' CP behavior. Most of the sex differences in CD are probably due to the increased prevalence of physical aggression among boys (Angold & Costello, 2001). As noted above, even this sex difference may be attenuated or disappear when more socially oriented forms of aggression (e.g., relational aggression), which occur more frequently among girls, are incorporated into the definition of aggression. During adolescence, gender differences in prevalence decrease dramatically; this seems to be largely accounted for by an increase in the number of girls engaging in covert CP behaviors. However, gender differences in ODD, in which more boys than girls are diagnosed prior to adolescence, also disappear for the most part during adolescence (APA, 2000). There is an increase in oppositional behavior during adolescence for both boys and girls (e.g., McDermott, 1996). For a comprehensive discussion of CP in girls, the reader is referred to recent volumes by Putallaz and Bierman (2004); Moretti, Odgers, and Jackson (2004); Pepler, Madsen, Webster, and Levene (2005); and Underwood (2003).

Continuity and Adult Outcomes

There is a high degree of continuity in CP behaviors from infancy to early childhood (e.g., Keenan, Shaw, Delliquadri, Giovannelli, & Walsh, 1998), from early childhood to later childhood (e.g., Campbell, 1995), from childhood to adolescence (e.g., Lahey, Loeber, Burke, & Rathouz, 2002; Offord et al., 1992), and from adolescence to adulthood (e.g., Farrington, 2003; Rutter, Harrington, Quinton, & Pickles, 1994). There is also evidence for cross-generational consistency (e.g., Huesmann, Eron, Lefkowitz, & Walder, 1984; Loeber et al., 2003). Furthermore, stability appears comparable for boys and girls (e.g., Coie & Dodge, 1998; Stanger, Achenbach, & Verhulst, 1997). In general, youths with CP are at increased risk for a broad spectrum of negative outcomes that extend beyond APD and criminal activity to family instability, and poor educational and health outcomes (see Maughan & Rutter, 2001, for a review). Both boys and girls with CP are at increased risk as adults for engaging in criminal activity (e.g., Keenan, Loeber, & Green, 1999; Kratzer & Hodgins, 1997; Pajer, 1998); girls also seem to be more at risk for a broad array of other adverse outcomes, including various internalizing disorders (e.g., Bardone, Moffitt, Caspi, Dickson, & Silva, 1996; Pajer, 1998). One outcome of adolescent CP in girls is increased risk for early pregnancy, which, in conjunction with other risk factors associated with adolescent pregnancy (and the mothers' own CP), increases the risk for the eventual development of CP in the offspring (e.g., Stack, Serbin, Schwartzman, & Ledingham, 2005; Zoccolillo, Paquette, & Tremblay, 2005).

DEVELOPMENTAL COURSE, OUTCOMES, AND POTENTIAL ETIOLOGICAL FACTORS

The preceding description of CP and various comorbid conditions fails to convey three different but related considerations that must guide assessment and intervention procedures for children and adolescents with CP: the developmental, contextual, and transactional aspects of CP (McMahon & Estes, 1997). With respect to developmental considerations, it is clear that the behavioral manifestations of CP (as well as the base rates of various comorbid disorders) change over time. With respect to context, the development and maintenance of CP are influenced by genetic/constitutional characteristics of the child, family, peers, and broader ecologies. Ethnicity and cultural considerations may also apply to these contexts (e.g., Prinz & Miller, 1991). By "transactional," we mean that these developmental and contextual processes unfold over time and continuously influence one another.

Space considerations preclude an extensive description of the roles these various developmental, contextual, and transactional influences play in the development and maintenance of CP. Instead, we present summary descriptions of two developmental progressions of CP as a means of illustrating many of these influences. The reader is referred to several recent excellent sources for more extensive treatment of these issues (Dodge & Pettit, 2003; Lahey, Moffitt, & Caspi, 2003; Moffitt, 2003; Patterson & Yoerger, 2002; Thornberry & Krohn, 2003).

Early-Starter Pathway

The most thoroughly delineated pathway, and the one that seems to have the most negative long-term prognosis, has been referred to as the "early-starter" (Patterson, Capaldi, & Bank, 1991) or "life-course-persistent" (Moffitt, 1993, 2003) pathway. The childhood-onset type of CD in DSM-IV-TR (APA, 2000) would seem to be a likely diagnostic outcome of this pathway. The early-starter pathway is characterized by the onset of CP in the preschool and early school-age years, and by a high degree of continuity throughout childhood and into adolescence and adulthood. It is thought that these youths progress from relatively less serious to more serious CP behaviors over time; that overt behaviors appear earlier than covert behaviors; and that later CP behaviors expand the youths' behavioral repertoire rather than replace earlier behaviors (Edelbrock, 1985; Loeber & Farrington, 2000; Patterson, Forgatch, Yoerger, & Stoolmiller, 1998; Patterson & Yoerger, 2002). Furthermore, there is an expansion of the settings in which the CP behaviors occur over time—from the home to other settings, such as the school and the broader community. The risk for continuing on this developmental pathway through the elementary school years and into adolescence may be as high as 50% for children who display CP behaviors at ages 3 and 4 (Campbell, 1995). In the Dunedin study, this pathway was much more common in boys than girls (5–10% vs. 1%) (Moffitt, Caspi, Rutter, & Silva, 2001).

As we present in detail below, characteristics of the child (e.g., temperament, social-cognitive skills) and the family (e.g., insecure attachment, coercive patterns of interaction) can lead to the development of high levels of child noncompliance and other CP behaviors in the preschool years. Upon school entry, the child's coercive style of interaction with parents and siblings is likely to extend to interactions with teachers and peers, resulting in frequent disciplinary confrontations with school personnel, rejection by peers, and continued coercive interchanges with parents (some of which now center around school-related problems) (e.g., Patterson et al., 1992). Difficulties in the acquisition of basic academic skills are most likely consequences of preexisting neuropsychological deficits (which now may be manifested as verbal deficits, self-control difficulties, social-cognitive deficits and biases, and/or ADHD), as well as the child's coercive interactional style. The CP behaviors may become more serious, more frequent, and more covert (e.g., stealing) during the elementary school years.

By age 10 or 11, this recurrent constellation of negative events places the child at increased risk for association with deviant peer groups in middle school and high school (with a likely escalation in the CP behaviors) and/or for depression. The role of the peer group in the maintenance and escalation of CP behaviors during middle and late childhood and early adolescence has been documented in several longitudinal investigations, in terms of both peer rejection (e.g., Coie, Lochman, Terry, & Hyman, 1992) and subsequent involvement with antisocial peers (e.g., Dishion, Patterson, Stoolmiller, & Skinner, 1991). Peer rejection in childhood may operate to increase subsequent CP behavior in several ways: through exclusion from opportunities for peer socialization, through modeling of CP behavior by other rejected children, or through demoralization

(Hinshaw & Lee, 2003). Association with a deviant peer group provides multiple and repeated opportunities for the modeling of, practice in, and reinforcement of a wide variety of CP behaviors (e.g., Dishion, Patterson, & Griesler, 1994; Lacourse, Nagin, Tremblay, Vitaro, & Claes, 2003).

Children with CP are also at increased risk for depression by the time they reach adolescence. Capaldi (1991, 1992) found co-occurrence of CP and depressive symptoms in an at-risk community sample of early adolescent boys in sixth grade. Over the next 2 years, the boys with CP and depressive symptoms displayed higher levels of suicidal ideation than boys with only CP or only depressive symptoms. They also displayed poor academic achievement and a high arrest rate (65%) by eighth grade. The boys with CP who were depressed also appeared to initiate substance use at an earlier age than boys with only CP. Adolescent girls' risk for both CP and depressive behavior at age 16 was associated with family and sibling coercive processes in childhood and adolescence (Compton, Snyder, Schrepferman, Bank, & Shortt, 2003). (The coercive processes predicted CP but not depressive behavior for boys.)

Early menarche appears to be a significant risk factor for CP in adolescent girls, particularly if they already have a history of CP (Moffitt, Caspi, Belsky, & Silva, 1992). An increased likelihood of exposure to older males with CP is a potential consequence (Caspi, Lynam, Moffitt, & Silva, 1993).

It is not surprising that youths who have progressed along the early-starter pathway are at significant risk for continuing to engage in more serious CP behaviors throughout adolescence and into adulthood (e.g., Farrington, 2003; Moffitt, Caspi, Harrington, & Milne, 2002; Rutter et al., 1994). As adults, not only are such individuals at high risk for subsequent diagnosis of APD; they are also at increased risk for other psychiatric diagnoses and a variety of negative life outcomes (e.g., lower occupational adjustment and educational attainment, poorer physical health) (e.g., Farrington, 2003; Kratzer & Hodgins, 1997; Moffitt et al., 2002). For example, in the Dunedin Multidisciplinary Health Study, at age 26, males who exhibited this early-starter pattern of CP had two to three times as many convictions than did the late-starting youths; were more likely to exhibit substance use problems and APD symptoms; engaged in more domestic violence; and were more likely to lack minimal education credentials, to have a poor work history in low-status, unskilled jobs, and to have married antisocial women (Moffitt et al., 2002).

Risk Factors

There is a growing body of evidence concerning the many individual, familial, and broader contextual factors that may increase the likelihood of a child's entering and progressing along the early-starter pathway (for reviews, see Dodge & Pettit, 2003; Leve & Chamberlain, 2005; Loeber & Farrington, 2000; Patterson et al., 1998; Shaw, Bell, & Gilliom, 2000). Child factors that may increase risk for entering the early-starter pathway include hyperactivity (e.g., Loeber & Keenan, 1994; Moffitt, 1993) and a difficult temperament (Frick & Morris, 2004; Moffitt, 1993). Moffitt posits that subtle neuropsychological variations in an infant's central nervous system, which could be due to a variety of prenatal, perinatal, and/or postnatal difficulties (e.g., exposure to toxic agents, birth complications, heredity), increase the likelihood that the infant will be "temperamentally difficult"—displaying characteristics such as irritability, hyperactivity, impulsivity, and the like.

The role of child temperament (usually viewed as involving relatively stable innate personality characteristics) has received increased attention from clinicians as a possible contributing factor to CP (e.g., Frick & Morris, 2004). Of particular interest is the temperamentally difficult child who, from very early in life, is intense, irregular, negative, and nonadaptable (Thomas, Chess, & Birch, 1968). Such a child is thought to be predisposed to the development of subsequent behavior problems, due to the increased likelihood of maladaptive interactions with family members. However, temperament has often been found to have a low to moderate relation to subsequent CP in early and middle childhood at best (e.g., Bates, Bayles, Bennett, Ridge, & Brown, 1991), and in some cases to have no relation (Aguilar, Sroufe, Egeland, & Carlson, 2000). Other investigators have shown that the combination of difficult temperament in infancy with other concurrently measured risk factors—such as maternal perception of difficulty, male gender,

prematurity, and low SES (Sanson, Oberklaid, Pedlow, & Prior, 1991), or inappropriate parenting (Bates et al., 1991)—is what best predicts subsequent CP.

The development of the child's social-cognitive skills may also be affected by these neuropsychological deficits (e.g., Coie & Dodge, 1998; Crick & Dodge, 1994).[1] Children with CP have deficits in encoding (e.g., lack of attention to relevant social cues, hypervigilant biases), make more hostile attributional biases and errors in the interpretation of social cues, have deficient quantity and quality of generated solutions to social situations, evaluate aggressive solutions more positively, and are more likely to decide to engage in aggressive behavior. These deficiencies and biases in social-cognitive skills predict the subsequent development of CP in kindergarten, and are associated with parental report of earlier harsh disciplinary practices (Weiss, Dodge, Bates, & Pettit, 1992).

A difficult temperamental style may increase risk for the development of both an insecure attachment to the parent (DeKlyen & Speltz, 2001; Greenberg, 1999) and a coercive style of interaction with family members (Patterson et al., 1992; Snyder & Stoolmiller, 2002). Both of these interaction patterns have been implicated in the development of CP. However, the relationship between security of attachment in infancy and later CP has been inconsistent. Attachment researchers (e.g., Greenberg, 1999) have noted the necessity of adopting a transactional perspective, in that attachment security is probably mediated by other risk or protective factors (e.g., parenting practices, maternal depression, family adversity) over time.

The critical role of parenting practices in the development and maintenance of CP has been well established. Types of parenting practices that have been closely associated with the development of child CP include inconsistent discipline, irritable/explosive discipline, low supervision and involvement, and inflexible/rigid discipline (Chamberlain, Reid, Ray, Capaldi, & Fisher, 1997). Indeed, physical abuse is a clear risk factor for the development of CP (Dodge, Bates, & Pettit, 1990; Jaffee, Caspi, Moffitt, & Taylor, 2004).

The most comprehensive family-based formulation for the early-starter pathway has been the coercion model developed by Patterson and his colleagues (e.g., Patterson, 1982,

2002; Patterson et al., 1992; Snyder, Reid, & Patterson, 2003). The model describes a process of "basic training" in CP behaviors that occurs in the context of an escalating cycle of coercive parent–child interactions in the home, beginning prior to school entry. The proximal causes for entry into the coercive cycle are thought to be ineffective parental management strategies, particularly in regard to child compliance with parental directives during the preschool period. As this process continues over long periods, significant increases in the rate and intensity of these coercive behaviors occur as family members are reinforced by engaging in aggressive behaviors. Furthermore, the child observes his or her parents engaging in coercive responses, and this provides the opportunity for modeling of aggression to occur (Patterson, 1982). Coercive interactions with siblings also play an important role in the development of CP (Garcia, Shaw, Winslow, & Yaggi, 2000; Snyder & Stoolmiller, 2002). Siblings of children with CP often engage in comparable levels of coercive behavior, and coercive parent–child interactions interact with sibling coercion and conflict to predict subsequent child CP. Although the coercion process begins early in the developmental period, it continues into adolescence (Snyder et al., 2003).

Various other risk factors that may have an impact on the family and serve to precipitate or maintain child CP have been identified. These include familial factors such as parental social cognitions, parental personal and marital adjustment, and other familial stressors; they also include certain extrafamilial factors, such as low SES, neighborhood risk, and parental insularity/low social support (e.g., Capaldi, DeGarmo, Patterson, & Forgatch, 2002; Coie & Jacobs, 1993; Ingoldsby & Shaw, 2002; Leve & Chamberlain, 2005; Wakschlag & Keenan, 2001). Less clear are the mechanisms by which these factors exert their effects on CP and on one another, the extent to which child CP may reciprocally influence them, and the role of timing and duration (Kazdin, 1995b). For example, these risk factors may have a direct effect on child CP, or they may exert their effects by disrupting parenting practices (Patterson et al., 1992). In some cases, a "risk" factor may be a *result* of CP, rather than a potential cause. With these caveats in mind, we note some of the relationships of these factors to CP.

Parents of children with CP display more maladaptive social cognitions, and they experience more personal (e.g., depression, antisocial behavior), interparental (marital problems), and extrafamilial (e.g., isolation) distress, than do parents of nonreferred children. It has been suggested that these stressors may interact to impede parental tracking of child behavior and lead to perceptual biases (Wahler & Dumas, 1989). With respect to social cognitions, Johnston (1996) has proposed a model that places parental cognitions (expectancies, perceptions, and attributions concerning child behavior and sense of parenting efficacy) in a mediational role vis-à-vis parenting behavior. Parents of clinic-referred children with CP are more likely to misperceive child behaviors (Holleran, Littman, Freund, & Schmaling, 1982; Middlebrook & Forehand, 1985; Wahler & Sansbury, 1990), to have fewer positive and more negative family-referent cognitions (Sanders & Dadds, 1992), and to perceive CP behaviors as intentional and to attribute them to stable and global causes (Baden & Howe, 1992; MacBrayer, Milich, & Hundley, 2003). Furthermore, these negative perceptions of the children are associated with higher levels of maternal anger and overreactivity in child discipline (Slep & O'Leary, 1998). Sense of parenting efficacy has been shown to relate negatively to child CP in both clinic-referred and nonreferred samples (e.g., Johnston & Mash, 1989; Roberts, Joe, & Rowe-Hallbert, 1992).

Maternal depression is related to a broad spectrum of child behavior disorders, including CP (e.g., Cummings & Davies, 1994b; Goodman & Gottlib, 1999). Some evidence suggests that maternal depression not only may adversely affect the mothers' parenting behavior, but may also negatively bias maternal perceptions of children with CP (e.g., Dumas & Serketich, 1994; Fergusson, Lynskey, & Horwood, 1993; Forehand, Lautenschlager, Faust, & Graziano, 1986). However, others have presented evidence suggesting that depressed mothers do not possess a negative perceptual bias in their reports of their children's CP behaviors, and that they may be accurate reporters (Richters, 1992). There is evidence of a reciprocal relationship between maternal depression and child adjustment problems, including CP (Elgar, McGrath, Waschbusch, Stewart, & Curtis, 2004). Chronicity of maternal depression may be particularly related to child CP (Alpern & Lyons-Ruth, 1993; Fergusson & Lynskey, 1993).

Parental antisocial behavior has received increasing attention as both a direct and an indirect influence on the development and maintenance of CP. Links between parental criminality, aggressive behavior, and a diagnosis of APD, and childhood delinquency, aggression, and CD/ODD diagnoses, have been reported by a number of investigators (see Frick & Loney, 2002, for a review; see Leve & Chamberlain, 2005, for a consideration of this risk factor in girls). This association appears specific to CP, occurs more frequently in parents whose children are diagnosed with CD rather than ODD (but see Frick et al., 1993), and is not associated with increased occurrence of ADHD or other child disorders (Frick et al., 1992). There is some evidence to suggest that parental antisocial behavior may play a more central role than other risk factors in its effect on parenting practices and child CP (e.g., Capaldi et al., 2002; Frick et al., 1992; Leve & Chamberlain, 2005; Patterson et al., 1992). For example, in a sample of boys at high risk for CP, Patterson and colleagues (1992) reported that both paternal and maternal antisocial behavior was negatively correlated with parenting practices; furthermore, parental antisocial behavior mediated the effect of social disadvantage and divorce/remarriage transitions in predicting parental practices. Thus parental antisocial behaviors may have a direct impact on child behavior, may have an indirect impact on child behavior through parenting, and may play a role in the relationship between other family and extrafamilial variables and parenting.

Similarly, parental substance abuse has been associated with youth CP and substance use, at least partly because of its association with disrupted parenting practices (Dishion, Reid, & Patterson, 1988; Wills, Schreibman, Benson, & Vaccaro, 1994). Observations of parent–child interactions in families with parental alcohol problems suggest that these parents are less able to engage their children and are less congenial (Jacob, Krahn, & Leonard, 1991; Whipple, Fitzgerald, & Zucker, 1995). Furthermore, alcohol consumption by parents can influence parental perceptions of children's behavior and has a negative impact on parenting behaviors displayed toward children (e.g., inadequate monitoring, inconsistent and harsh discipline, indulgence, less problem solving) (El-Sheikh & Flanagan, 2001; Lang, Pelham, Atkeson, & Murphy, 1999; Pelham & Lang,

1993; Whipple et al., 1995). In a review of laboratory studies examining the effects of alcohol consumption on parent–child interaction, Pelham and Lang (1993) concluded not only that alcohol consumption had a deleterious effect on parenting practices, but that the children's inappropriate behavior increased parental alcohol consumption (for parents with a positive family history of alcohol problems) and distress (for all parents), thus perpetuating the cycle.

Marital distress and conflict have been shown to be associated with child CP, negative parenting behavior, and parental perceptions of child maladjustment (Amato & Keith, 1991; Cummings & Davies, 1994a). The most commonly offered hypothesis for the relationship has been that such distress or conflict interferes with the parents' ability to engage in appropriate parenting practices, which then leads to child CP (e.g., Emery, 1999); however, other explanations are possible (see Rutter, 1994). These include direct modeling of aggressive and coercive behavior, and the cumulative stressful effects of such conflict, including maternal depression. It has been suggested that both child CP and parental marital distress or conflict may be the result of parental antisocial behavior (Frick, 1994). Child characteristics such as age and gender appear to moderate the relationship between specific aspects of marital adjustment and CP (Dadds & Powell, 1991; Katz & Gottman, 1993). Some investigators (e.g., Abidin & Brunner, 1995; Jouriles et al., 1991; Porter & O'Leary, 1980) have focused more narrowly on specific aspects of marital conflict that relate directly to parenting, such as disagreement over child-rearing practices, conflict in a child's presence, or the strength of the parenting alliance. There is some indication that these more narrowly focused constructs may demonstrate stronger relationships to CP than may broader constructs such as marital distress.

Parents of children with CP also appear to experience higher frequencies of stressful events, both minor ones (e.g., daily hassles) and those of a more significant nature (e.g., unemployment, major transitions) (Capaldi et al., 2002; Leve & Chamberlain, 2005; Webster-Stratton, 1990b). The effects of stress on child CP may be mediated through maladaptive parental social cognitions (e.g., Johnston, 1996; Wahler & Dumas, 1989) and parenting practices such as disrupted parental discipline (e.g.,

Forgatch, Patterson, & Skinner, 1988; Snyder, 1991), although the role of parenting behavior in mediating the association between parenting stress and child adjustment has not yet been rigorously tested (Deater-Deckard, 1998).

CP has been associated with a number of extrafamilial factors (Capaldi et al., 2002; Coie & Jacobs, 1993), such as low SES (Dodge, Pettit, & Bates, 1994), neighborhood risk (Ingoldsby & Shaw, 2002), and parental insularity/low social support (Jennings, Stagg, & Connors, 1991; Wahler, Leske, & Rogers, 1979). However, it is important to note that the relationship of SES with CP appears to be largely mediated by parenting practices (e.g., Capaldi & Patterson, 1994). On the other hand, neighborhood risk has been shown to operate as an independent risk factor (e.g., Gorman-Smith, Tolan, & Henry, 2000). Some parents of children with CP may be quite isolated from friends, neighbors, and the community. Wahler and his colleagues have developed a construct called "insularity," which is defined as a "specific pattern of social contacts within the community that is characterized by a high level of negatively perceived coercive interchanges with relatives and/or helping agency representatives and by a low level of positively perceived supportive interchanges with friends" (Wahler & Dumas, 1984, p. 387). Insularity is positively related both to negative parent behavior directed toward children and to oppositional child behavior directed toward parents (Dumas & Wahler, 1985; Wahler, 1980). It has also been associated with poor maintenance of treatment effects (e.g., Dumas & Wahler, 1983). Thus, when a mother has a large proportion of aversive interactions outside the home, the interactions between the mother and her child in the home are likely to be negative as well.

Not surprisingly, youths who follow the early-starter pathway are at greatly increased risk for negative outcomes as adults. In their follow-up of individuals with CP at age 26, Moffitt and colleagues (2002) found criminal conviction rates to be two to three times greater for the early-starter group than for the late-starter group. This was especially the case for more serious offenses, including violence. Family violence is also more common in the early-starter group (Moffitt et al., 2002; Woodward, Fergusson, & Horwood, 2002). As adults, the early-starter individuals were also more likely to work in low-status, unskilled jobs; to lack minimal education credentials; and to have increased levels of substance use problems.

Late-Starter Pathway

A second major pathway for the development of CP has been proposed, but there has been less consistency in how it has been described. In general, this second pathway begins in adolescence rather than early childhood; it is also thought to result in less serious forms of CP (e.g., property offenses rather than violent offenses) and to have a higher rate of desistance. However, more children are involved in this pathway than in the early-starter pathway (e.g., 24% vs. 7%, respectively, in the Dunedin study; Moffitt, Caspi, Dickson, Silva, & Stanton, 1996), and it is roughly comparable between boys and girls (Moffitt et al., 2001). It has been referred to as the "late-starter" (Patterson et al., 1991) or "adolescence-limited" (Moffitt, 1993) pathway. The adolescent-onset type of CD in DSM-IV-TR (APA, 2000) would seem to be a likely diagnostic outcome of this pathway.

Empirical support for the late-starter pathway has been provided in both epidemiological (e.g., McGee, Feehan, Williams, & Anderson, 1992; Moffitt, 1990; Moffitt et al., 1996; Piquero & Brezina, 2000) and high-risk (e.g., Loeber et al., 1993) samples. In the Dunedin sample, a large increase in nonaggressive (but not aggressive) CP behaviors was noted between ages 11 and 15 for both boys and girls (McGee et al., 1992). Moffitt (1990) found that the late-starter group made up 73% of her delinquent sample of boys at age 13, and had levels of CP behaviors at age 13 comparable to those displayed by the early-starter boys. However, in contrast to the early-starter boys, the late-starter boys had engaged in very low levels of CP in childhood, and there was no evidence of Verbal IQ deficits, reading difficulties, preexisting family adversity, temperamental difficulty (Moffitt et al., 1996), or perinatal or motor skills difficulties. Furthermore, they were less likely to have been convicted of violent criminal offenses than were the early-starter boys (Moffitt et al., 1996). Moffitt and colleagues (2001) found that the risk factors associated with the late-starter pathway were comparable for boys and girls. Capaldi and Patterson (1994) presented data on a high-risk sample indicating that late-starter boys were less likely than early-starter boys to live in families characterized by inappropriate parental discipline practices, unemployment, divorce, parental antisocial behavior, and low SES. Association with a deviant peer group was especially salient for the late-starter boys.

Moffitt (1993, 2003) posits that participation in CP behaviors by late-starter youths is a form of social mimicry of early-starter youths and is one way of asserting independence from the family. Initial empirical support for this proposition was provided by Piquero and Brezina (2000), who found that late-starter youths were more likely to commit "rebellious" than aggressive offenses, and that both maturational timing and aspects of personal autonomy related to peers were associated with this form of CP behavior. The basis for desistance among the late-starter group is thought to be the gradual increase in opportunities to engage in more legitimate adult roles and activities as these adolescents grow older. However, the likelihood of desistance is decreased to the extent that adolescents are caught in "snares" (e.g., incarceration, dropout). Patterson and colleagues (e.g., Patterson & Yoerger, 2002) have hypothesized that the process leading to the late-starter pathway begins in families that have marginally effective family management skills. Inadequate parental supervision in middle and high school increases the likelihood of significant involvement in a deviant peer group. However, because these adolescents have a higher level of social skills and a longer learning history of employing such skills successfully than do early-starter youths, they are far less likely to continue to engage in CP behaviors.

Nonetheless, there is evidence suggesting that adolescents who develop CP through the late-starter pathway may still be at substantial risk for future maladjustment. Moffitt and colleagues (2002) reported that at age 26, the original adolescent-limited boys had elevated convictions for property and drug offenses. They postulated that these individuals were still in a "maturity gap" that prevented them from assuming adult roles. Hämäläinen and Pulkkinen (1996) found that late-starter youths constituted nearly one-third of their group of young adults (age 27) with criminal offenses. At age 32, males in the late-starter group reported that they continued to fight, commit various offenses, and abuse substances, although this was not reflected in official records (Nagin, Farrington, & Moffitt, 1995).

Other Developmental Pathways

Identification of the early-starter and late-starter pathways nearly 15 years ago has stimulated a tremendous amount of research concerning developmental pathways of CP. In addition to validating and clarifying the nature of these two pathways, this research has identified other pathways. For example, Loeber and colleagues (1993, 2003) have identified three pathways: authority conflict (i.e., noncompliance, defiance), overt CP (i.e., fighting, severe violence), and covert CP (i.e., property damage, serious delinquency). Movement across pathways for individual youths is fluid, and some will be on more than one pathway at a given point in development. These pathways have been replicated in European American, African American, and Hispanic samples (Loeber et al., 2003; Tolan et al., 2000).

Hinshaw and Lee (2003) suggest that there are at least three developmental pathways that have childhood onset of CP as a common starting point: (1) "early starters" (who persist in their CP behavior), (2) "desisters," and (3) "low-level chronics," who engage in relatively low but persistent levels of CP throughout the developmental period and into adulthood (e.g., Fergusson, Horwood, & Nagin, 2000). With respect to the desister pathway, as noted above, it is estimated that 50% of children who demonstrate high levels of CP behavior during the preschool period will not follow the early starter progression of increasingly severe CP as they get older (Campbell, 1995). With respect to the low-level chronic pathway, in Moffitt's earlier work (e.g., Moffitt et al., 1996) she identified a third group of youths in the Dunedin sample that was originally labeled as the "recovery" group. This group was characterized by high levels of CP during childhood, but only moderate levels during adolescence. However, at the age 26 follow-up, these individuals were engaging in low but consistent levels of offending (Moffitt et al., 2002). In addition, they displayed high levels of internalizing problems such as depression and anxiety disorders, and were impaired on a variety of life outcome indicators such as education, occupational status, and degree of optimism.

Other hypothesized pathways include a delayed-onset pathway for CP in girls (Silverthorn & Frick, 1999), and as noted above, Frick and colleagues (2000) have suggested that youths with CP who display CU traits represent a specific subtype of the early-starter pathway. Other investigators have identified multiple trajectories for individual forms of CP behavior, such as physical aggression, vandalism, and stealing (e.g., Broidy et al., 2003; Lacourse et al., 2002).

Although ongoing research will most certainly lead to further development and delineation of the pathways described above, current versions illustrate the value of adopting a developmental perspective for constructing an accurate and useful conceptual framework for the assessment and treatment of children and adolescents with CP. We now turn to a discussion of the assessment process itself.

ASSESSMENT

The delineation of different developmental pathways of CP has a number of important implications for the assessment of youths with CP (McMahon & Estes, 1997; McMahon & Frick, 2005). First, the assessment must be developmentally sensitive—not only with respect to a child's age and sex, but also in terms of the child's status and progression on a particular developmental pathway of CP. The heterogeneity of CP requires that the assessment of these behaviors be focused broadly. In adolescence, this also includes the assessment of delinquent behaviors. The possibility of comorbid conditions such as ADHD, internalizing disorders, and substance use should also be investigated. Furthermore, the assessment must be contextually sensitive; that is, it should cover not only CP behavior and other behavior problems, but also other youth characteristics, as well as familial and peer influences. Furthermore, this assessment must examine the broader ecologies of home, school, neighborhood, and community to the extent that each is warranted. Cultural sensitivity in the development, administration, acceptability, and interpretation of assessment instruments also requires increased attention (Forehand & Kotchick, 1996; Prinz & Miller, 1991). Finally, the clinician needs to recognize the transactional nature of these developmental and contextual processes, and conduct the assessment accordingly. In addition to focusing on each of these issues, a proper assessment of a youth with CP must make use of multiple methods completed by multiple informants in the various settings and contexts in which the youth functions (McMahon & Estes, 1997; McMahon & Frick, 2005).

CP Behavior Per Se and in an Interactional Context

In order to obtain an accurate representation of the referred youth's CP behavior, the therapist must rely on multiple assessment methods, including interviews with the parents, youth, and other relevant parties (e.g., teachers); behavior rating scales completed by the same individuals; and direct behavioral observations of the youth in the clinic, home, and/or school settings (McMahon & Estes, 1997; McMahon & Frick, 2005).

Interviews

Interviews conducted with youths with CP and their families, and other important adults (e.g., teachers), can be divided into two general categories: clinical interviews and structured diagnostic interviews. Clinical interviews with a parent and youth provide a method for assessing (1) the type, severity, and impairment associated with CP; (2) typical parent–child interactions that may be contributing to the CP; and (3) relevant antecedent and consequent events. Some of the interview formats, such as those presented by McMahon and Forehand (2003) and Wahler and Cormier (1970), are structured around problematic situations (e.g., bedtime, sibling interactions), whereas others are structured according to different child behaviors (e.g., Patterson, Reid, Jones, & Conger, 1975).

An individual interview with a youth may or may not provide useful content-oriented information, depending on the age and/or developmental level of the youth and the nature of the specific CP behaviors. Children below the age of 9 are not usually reliable reporters of their own behavioral symptoms (Loney & Frick, 2003). However, an informal interview can be extremely useful even with a younger child, in that it can provide the therapist with an opportunity to assess the child's perception of why he or she has been brought to the clinic and can provide a subjective evaluation of the child's cognitive, affective, and behavioral characteristics (e.g., Bierman, 1983). In assessment of overt CP behaviors, Loeber and Schmaling (1985b) have suggested that maternal and teacher reports may be preferable to youth reports, because youths often underestimate or minimize their own aggressive behaviors. However, in regard to covert types of CP, more valid reports are likely to be obtained from the youths.[2]

When the presenting problems include classroom behavior or academic underachievement, an interview with a youth's teacher or teachers is also appropriate. Breen and Altepeter (1990) have provided an outline for a brief interview with a teacher, which can be conducted at the school or by telephone. Situationally formatted interview guides based on Barkley's (1997) School Situations Questionnaire or Wahler and Cormier's (1970) preinterview checklists can be employed in conjunction with specific questions related to the child's problem behaviors. Contextual factors, such as classroom rules of conduct, teacher expectations, and the behavior of other children in the classroom, are important as well. (See McMahon & Forehand, 2003, and Walker, 1995, for additional discussions of teacher interviewing procedures.)

Historically, much of the treatment research conducted in school settings has failed to include a comprehensive assessment of children referred for school problems to ascertain whether they meet objective and/or clinical criteria for the diagnosis of CD or ODD; behavior often was defined loosely as "inappropriate" and worthy of intervention if teachers and/or parents defined it as such. More recently, researchers and practitioners are increasingly using functional behavioral assessment (FBA) methods to assess children's needs in school and to match intervention strategies to behavioral functions in order to enhance treatment effectiveness (Walker, Ramsey, & Gresham, 2004). This innovation has come about as a result of the increasing emphasis on utilization of evidence-based best practices, as well as from amendments made to federal legislation in the Individuals with Disabilities Education Act Amendments of 1997, which now mandate the use of FBA. Use of these methods is also endorsed by the National Association of School Psychologists and by the National Institutes of Health. These methods involve specifying problem behaviors in school in operational terms, as well as identifying events that reliably predict and control behavior through an exam-

ination of antecedents and consequences. Information relevant to FBA is gathered through FBA interviews, as well as through direct observation of classroom behavior by teachers or school psychologists. Use of these methods has been shown to contribute to beneficial outcomes for children and adolescents in school (Walker et al., 2004).

Structured interviews have been used in efforts to improve the reliability and validity of diagnostic (using DSM criteria) interviewing. They can be employed with multiple informants. Two structured diagnostic interviews that are frequently employed in the diagnosis of youths with CP are the Diagnostic Interview Schedule for Children (e.g., Shaffer, Fisher, Lucas, Dulcan, & Schwab-Stone, 2000) and the Diagnostic Interview for Children and Adolescents (e.g., Reich, 2000). For reviews of these and other structured diagnostic interviews, see Loney and Frick (2003) and McClellan and Werry (2000). However, structured interviews have their own limitations, including length of administration, inadequate reliability from child informants below the age of 9, and evidence that the number of symptoms reported declines over the course of the interview (McMahon & Frick, 2005).

An alternative approach to interviewing youth has been developed by McConaughy and Achenbach (2001). The Semistructured Clinical Interview for Children and Adolescents is a broad interview administered to youths (ages 6–18) that employs a protocol of open-ended questions to assess various areas of functioning. Dimensional scores similar to those obtained from various instruments in the Achenbach System of Empirically Based Assessment (ASEBA; Achenbach & Rescorla, 2000, 2001; see below) can also be derived from these items. Kolko and colleagues have developed several semistructured interviews for parents and children that have been used to assess various aspects of firesetting and matchplay in inpatient, outpatient, and community samples of children. Examples include the Firesetting History Screen, the Firesetting Risk Interview, and the Children's Firesetting Interview (Kolko, Nishi-Strattner, Wilcox, & Kopet, 2002; Wilcox & Kolko, 2002). Evidence for the reliability and validity of these interviews is encouraging.

The interview as an assessment tool does not end with the first contact, but continues throughout treatment formulation and implementation. The interview is used to obtain information necessary for the development of interventions, to assess the effectiveness of the intervention and its implementation, and to alter the intervention if necessary (Breen & Altepeter, 1990).

Behavior Rating Scales

Behavior rating scales completed by adults or youths are very useful as screening devices for covering a broad range of CP behaviors and for assessing the presence of other child behavior disorders or adjustment difficulties that can be used to evaluate the level of impairment associated with CP. In addition, they provide the best norm-referenced assessment concerning a youth's CP behavior. Although there are many behavior rating scales, several have been recommended as most appropriate for clinical and research use with youths with CP (McMahon & Estes, 1997; McMahon & Frick, 2005). Several instruments in the ASEBA are applicable for use with children and adolescents (Achenbach & Rescorla, 2000, 2001). There are parallel forms for parents (Child Behavior Checklist [CBCL/1½–5, CBCL/6–18]), teachers (Caregiver Report Form for Ages 1½–5 [C-TRF]; Teacher's Report Form [TRF/6–18]), youths (Youth Self-Report [YSR/11–18]), and observers (Direct Observation Form [DOF/5–14]). These instruments are similar in terms of structure, items, scoring, and interpretation. They are designed to be self-administered, and each can usually be completed in 10–20 minutes. The instruments include sections concerning Competence and Problem items (the CBCL/1½–5 includes Problem items and a Language Development Survey; the DOF includes only Problem items). Competence scales include items related to various activities, social relationships, and success in school. With respect to the Problem items, the various ASEBA instruments typically yield Total, Internalizing, and Externalizing broad-band scales, and a number of narrow-band scales. With respect to CP, the narrow-band scales constituting the Externalizing scale (e.g., Rule-Breaking Behavior and Aggressive Behavior on the CBCL/6–18) are of particular interest. The ASEBA now also includes DSM-oriented scales, such as Oppositional Defiant Problems and Conduct Problems on the CBCL/6–18 (Achenbach, Dumenci, & Rescorla, 2003b). The psychometric properties of the various ASEBA instruments are de-

scribed thoroughly in their respective manuals (Achenbach & Rescorla, 2000, 2001). The CBCL and the TRF are sensitive to treatment changes resulting from parent training and child cognitive-behavioral therapy as interventions for CP (e.g., DeGarmo, Patterson, & Forgatch, 2004; Eisenstadt, Eyberg, McNeil, Newcomb, & Funderburk, 1993; Kazdin, Bass, Siegel, & Thomas, 1989; Kendall, Reber, McLeer, Epps, & Ronan, 1990; Scott, Spender, Doolan, Jacobs, & Aspland, 2001). Other broad-band rating scales include the Behavior Assessment System for Children, Second Edition (Reynolds & Kamphaus, 2004), the Conners Rating Scales—Revised (Conners, 1997), the Revised Behavior Problem Checklist (Quay & Peterson, 1996), and the Child Symptom Inventory-4 (Gadow & Sprafkin, 1995).

Various other behavior rating scales, completed by parents, teachers, or youths, focus on specific aspects of CP. Two examples of parent or teacher report measures are the Eyberg Child Behavior Inventory and Sutter–Eyberg Student Behavior Inventory (ECBI and SESBI; Eyberg & Pincus, 1999). The ECBI is completed by parents and is intended for use with children ages 2–16. The 36 items describe specific CP behaviors (primarily overt) and are scored on both a frequency-of-occurrence scale and a yes–no problem identification scale. Both scales have been shown to discriminate children with CP from other clinic-referred children and from nonreferred children (Burns & Patterson, 1990, 2000b; Burns, Patterson, Nussbaum, & Parker, 1991; Eyberg, 1992; Eyberg & Colvin, 1994; Rich & Eyberg, 2001), and to be sensitive to treatment effects from parent training interventions with young children (e.g., Eisenstadt et al., 1993; McNeil, Eyberg, Eisenstadt, Newcomb, & Funderburk, 1991; Nixon, Sweeney, Erickson, & Touyz, 2003; Webster-Stratton & Hammond, 1997). Recently, evidence for longer-term (10-month) test–retest reliability has also been obtained for the ECBI (Funderburk, Eyberg, Rich, & Behar, 2003).

The SESBI is identical in format to the ECBI. Standardization studies have been done on the SESBI with preschoolers (Burns, Sosna, & Ladish, 1992; Funderburk & Eyberg, 1989; Funderburk et al., 2003), with children in kindergarten through sixth grade (Burns & Owen, 1990; Burns & Patterson, 2000b; Burns, Walsh, & Owen, 1995), and with middle school and high school students (Floyd,

Rayfield, Eyberg, & Riley, 2004). The SESBI has also been shown to be sensitive to the effects of a parent training intervention (McNeil et al., 1991). Eyberg and colleagues have begun to evaluate a revised version of the SESBI (SESBI-R; Eyberg & Pincus, 1999) that includes the addition of items derived from the disruptive behavior categories of the DSM-III-R (APA, 1987) and the deletion of items with low item-to-total correlations. Initial results suggest that the SESBI-R has adequate psychometric properties (Querido & Eyberg, 2003) and may have a more distinct factor structure than its predecessor (Rayfield, Eyberg, & Foote, 1998).

Children whose scores exceed the cutoff points on the ECBI or the SESBI are probably a heterogeneous group who may present with ADHD as well as ODD or CD. Given the increasing attention paid to comorbidity of ADHD and CP, this represents a potentially serious limitation of the ECBI. However, the ECBI and SESBI show promise as useful rating scales in clinical settings, where they can be employed as screening instruments and as treatment outcome measures for disruptive behavior (broadly defined) as rated by parents and teachers.

In order to begin to address limitations resulting from the unidimensional nature of the ECBI, Burns and Patterson (2000a) conducted factor analyses of this measure in 1,263 children and adolescents. They identified a three-factor model with good fit across multiple analysis groups and across gender and age. The three factors included Oppositional Defiant Behavior toward Adults, Inattentive Behavior, and Conduct Problem Behavior. This additional information on the factor structure of the ECBI may increase its utility as a screening instrument. However, for situations in which a broader screening is desired or when information pertinent to differential diagnosis is sought, then use of the CBCL and related ASEBA instruments is recommended.

An example of an adolescent self-report measure that focuses specifically on CP is the Self-Report Delinquency Scale (SRD; Elliott, Huizinga, & Ageton, 1985). The SRD is probably the most widely used self-report measure of CP behavior. It consists of 47 items that are derived from offenses listed in the *Uniform Crime Reports* (e.g., Federal Bureau of Investigation, 2004) and covers property, status, drug, and violent offenses. The SRD is intended for use by 11- to 19-year-olds, who report on the frequency of engagement in each behavior over the past year. It has been employed primarily in epidemiological and community samples to assess prevalence of CP (e.g., Elliott et al., 1985; Loeber, Stouthamer-Loeber, Van Kammen, & Farrington, 1989), but it has also been employed as a measure of intervention outcome in clinic-referred samples (e.g., Henggeler, Melton, Brondino, Scherer, & Hanley, 1997; Kazdin, Mazurick, & Siegel, 1994; Kazdin, Siegel, & Bass, 1992). Pretreatment levels of CP behavior as assessed by the SRD were predictive of teacher ratings of youth behavior problems following a cognitive-behavioral therapy intervention (Kazdin, 1995a).

Behavioral Observation

Direct behavioral observation has long been a critical component of the assessment of youths with CP and their families, both for delineating specific patterns of maladaptive parent–child or teacher–child interaction and for assessing change in those interactions as a function of treatment. More recently, observational data have been compared with data gathered via other methods to assist the clinician in determining whether the focus of treatment should be on the adult–youth interaction or on adult perceptual and/or personal adjustment issues.

Space limitations preclude an extensive review of the many behavioral observation systems currently in use for assessing interactions of children with CP in the clinic, home, and school settings. Two widely used, structured, microanalytic observation procedures available for assessing parental interactions with younger (3- to 8-year-old children) in the clinic and home are the Behavioral Coding System (BCS; Forehand & McMahon, 1981) and the Dyadic Parent–Child Interaction Coding System II (DPICS II; Eyberg, Bessmer, Newcomb, Edwards, & Robinson, 1994). As employed in the clinic setting, the BCS and DPICS II place the parent–child dyad in standard situations that vary in the degree to which parental control is required, ranging from a free-play situation to one in which the parent directs the child's activity. In each system, various parent and child behaviors are scored, many of which emphasize parental antecedents (e.g., commands) and consequences (e.g., praise, time out) for child compliance or noncompliance. Both systems have adequate psychometric properties

(McMahon & Metzler, 1998) and have been extensively employed as intervention outcome measures (e.g., Eisenstadt et al., 1993; McMahon, Forehand, & Griest, 1981; Webster-Stratton & Hammond, 1997).

For older children and adolescents, structured clinical observational paradigms have been developed for the direct assessment of parent–child communication and problem solving (see Foster & Robin, 1997, for a review). For example, Martinez and Forgatch (2001) employed a series of tasks that included a parent–child problem-solving discussion and teaching tasks with elementary-school-age children. These tasks were coded for various parenting practices and child aversive behavior and noncompliance, using both microanalytic and global rating systems.

The use of observation systems in the home setting for practicing clinicians is desirable, but rare for obvious reasons. The coding systems are relatively complex, and lengthy periods are required to train observers and to maintain adequate levels of reliability. The observations themselves are usually lengthy as well. As a consequence, the use of structured clinical observations to assess parent–child interactions is recommended (McMahon & Frick, 2005; Roberts, 2001). In addition, simplified versions of both the DPICS II and the BCS have been developed (Eyberg et al., 1994; McMahon & Estes, 1994). These adaptations are designed to reduce training demands, and may ultimately prove to be more useful to clinicians.

Behavioral observation systems designed specifically for assessing CP types of behavior in the school setting have received relatively less attention. The DOF/5–14 (Achenbach & Rescorla, 2001) may be used as part of a multimodal assessment with the other ASEBA instruments described above. Yielding Internalizing, Externalizing, and Total Problem scores as well as scores for six narrow-band problem scales and a measure of on-task behavior, the DOF is relatively simple to use; it has been shown to discriminate between referred and nonreferred children in the classroom, as well as between children with externalizing behavior problems and children with other behavior problems. The BCS (Forehand & McMahon, 1981) has been modified for use in the classroom to assess teacher–child interaction (e.g., Breiner & Forehand, 1981), both alone and in combination with a measure of academic engaged time (AET). AET is the amount of time

a child is appropriately engaged in on-task behavior during class time and is assessed via a simple stopwatch procedure (Walker, Colvin, & Ramsey, 1995). AET has been shown to correlate positively with academic performance (Walker, 1995) and to discriminate boys at risk for CP from boys not at risk (e.g., Walker, Shinn, O'Neill, & Ramsey, 1987). The Revised Edition of the School Observation Coding System (Jacobs et al., 2000), which has been used with 3- to 6-year-old clinic-referred children with ODD and nonreferred children in preschool and kindergarten classrooms, may be particularly appropriate for classroom observations of young noncompliant children.

An alternative to observations by independent observers in the natural setting is to train significant adults in a youth's environment to observe and record certain types of behavior. An added advantage is the opportunity to assess low-rate behaviors such as stealing or fire setting. The most widely used procedure of this type is the Parent Daily Report (PDR; Chamberlain & Reid, 1987), a parent observation measure that is typically administered during brief telephone interviews. Parents are asked which of various overt and covert behaviors have occurred in the past 24 hours. The PDR has been employed on a pretreatment basis to assess the magnitude of CP behaviors, to monitor the progress of the family during therapy, and to assess treatment outcome (e.g., Bank, Marlowe, Reid, Patterson, & Weinrott, 1991; Chamberlain & Reid, 1991; Webster-Stratton & Hammond, 1997). An added advantage is its brevity, and, because of the 24-hour reporting frame, it may also provide more objective data than those obtained from interviews or behavior rating scales.

Few assessment instruments have focused primarily on covert, as opposed to overt, forms of CP behavior (Miller & Klungness, 1989). Jones (1974) developed a brief daily interview similar to the PDR for collecting parent report data on stealing. The Telephone Interview Report on Stealing and Social Aggression (TIROSSA) has adequate test–retest reliability and is sensitive to the effects of treatment procedures designed to reduce stealing (Reid, Hinojosa Rivera, & Lorber, 1980). Hinshaw and colleagues have developed and evaluated an analogue observational procedure to assess stealing and property destruction in children ages 6–12 years (Hinshaw, Heller, & McHale, 1992; Hinshaw, Simmel, & Heller, 1995;

Hinshaw, Zupan, Simmel, Nigg, & Melnick, 1997). Kolko, Watson, and Faust (1991) employed a very brief (1-minute) observation to assess children's preference for fire-related stimuli. Both of these temptation provocation tasks demonstrated high interobserver agreement and sensitivity to treatment.

Associated Youth Characteristics

A brief developmental and medical history of each youth should be obtained, in order to determine whether any medical factors might be associated with the development or maintenance of the youth's CP behaviors and whether the youth's early temperament may have contributed to the development of a coercive style of parent–child interaction. Several standardized ratings of temperament may have utility in assessing youths with CP (Frick & Morris, 2004). Because youths with CP may also present with a variety of other behavior disorders, behavior rating scales that provide information about a wide range of narrow-band behavior disorders (e.g., the ASEBA family of instruments; Achenbach & Rescorla, 2001) can serve as useful screening devices, but will probably need to be supplemented with a clinical or structured interview and/or a disorder-specific behavior rating scale (McMahon & Frick, 2005). As noted above, ADHD, internalizing disorders, and substance use are of particular interest. With preschool-age children, if CP may be occurring in the context of language impairment, then a developmental assessment is warranted (Wakschlag & Danis, 2004). The Antisocial Process Screening Device (Frick & Hare, 2002), which is a behavior rating scale completed by parents and/or teachers, can be used to identify youths with CP who also exhibit CU traits (e.g., Christian et al., 1997; Frick et al., 2000).

In addition to having comorbid behavior disorders, youths with CP frequently have problems with peer interactions and classroom behavior. Demaray and colleagues (1995) review several behavior rating scales for the assessment of social competence. Other measures, such as peer sociometric ratings, are difficult to employ outside of elementary school settings. Research-based measures to assess youths' social-cognitive processes (e.g., Dodge & Coie, 1987) may have clinical utility for treatment planning, given that the processes are targeted in many cognitively oriented interventions (McMahon & Frick, 2005). Clinically useful measures to assess associations with a deviant peer group are limited currently to youth or parent report, although Dishion and colleagues (e.g., Dishion, Andrews, & Crosby, 1995) have developed a structured observational paradigm for research purposes that may be adaptable to the clinical setting (McMahon & Frick, 2005).

If the presenting problem concerns classroom behavior, then the youth's academic functioning and behavior should also be included in the assessment. Although interviews, observations, and behavior rating scales can provide information concerning the youth's academic behavior, additional evaluation in the form of standardized intelligence test and academic achievement test screeners is necessary to determine whether the youth may have learning difficulties in addition to CP. Walker (1995) also discusses the use of a standardized method for retrieving and using school records (School Archival Records System; H. M. Walker, Block-Pedego, Todis, & Severson, 1991) for youths with CP. Kaufman and Kaufman (2001) provide a comprehensive review of assessment strategies with which to evaluate level of intellectual functioning and learning problems.

Familial and Extrafamilial Factors

McMahon and Estes (1997) have delineated six areas that are relevant to the assessment of youths with CP: parenting practices; parents' (and teachers') social cognitions; parents' perceptions of their own personal and marital adjustment; parental stress; parental functioning in extrafamilial social contexts; and parental satisfaction with treatment. Parenting practices have been assessed through clinical interviews, behavioral observation of parent–child interaction, and parent and youth report on behavior rating scales. Questionnaires that have been specifically designed to assess parenting practices may be quite useful as adjuncts to behavioral observations or as methods for assessing parental behaviors that either occur infrequently or are otherwise difficult to observe (e.g., physical discipline, parental monitoring practices); they may also be used to measure the effects of parent training interventions. Examples include the Parenting Scale (Arnold, O'Leary, Wolff, & Acker, 1993), the Parent Practices Scale (Strayhorn & Weidman, 1988), the Alabama Parenting Questionnaire (Shelton,

Frick, & Wootton, 1996), and the Loeber Youth Questionnaire (Jacob, Moser, Windle, Loeber, & Stouthamer-Loeber, 2000). Although most of these measures of parenting practices have been developed for parents of children ages 2–13, some have also been employed with adolescent samples (e.g., Frick, Christian, & Wootton, 1999; Jacob et al., 2000). Parenting practices questionnaires have been shown to be sensitive to intervention effects (e.g., Feinfeld & Baker, 2004; Sanders, Markie-Dadds, Tully, & Bor, 2000).

Parents' (and teachers') perceptions of the youth and their social cognitions constitute a second important area to be assessed. Perceptions of the youth may be best assessed through the behavior rating scales described above. Several measures that assess aspects of parental self-esteem (e.g., satisfaction, self-efficacy, and locus of control with the parenting role) are the Parenting Sense of Competence Scale (as adapted by Johnston & Mash, 1989), the Cleminshaw–Guidubaldi Parent Satisfaction Scale (Guidubaldi & Cleminshaw, 1985), and the Parental Locus of Control Scale (Campis, Lyman, & Prentice-Dunn, 1986). When examined in the context of behavioral observation data and the clinician's own impressions, these perception measures can be important indicators of whether the informants (parents, teachers) appear to have a perceptual bias in their assessment of the referred youth's behavior; they can also serve as indicators of intervention outcome (e.g., Nixon et al., 2003; Roberts et al., 1992).

The third area involves the assessment of the role that parents' personal and marital adjustment problems may be playing in the youth's presenting behavior problems. Measures of parental depression (e.g., Beck Depression Inventory–II; Beck, Steer, & Brown, 1996), parental antisocial behavior (e.g., Antisocial Behavior Checklist; Zucker & Fitzgerald, 1992), parental substance use (e.g., Drug Abuse Screening Test; Skinner, 1982), marital satisfaction (e.g., Dyadic Adjustment Scale; Spanier, 1976), marital conflict (e.g., Conflict Tactics Scale—Partner; Straus, 1979, 1990), and parenting-related conflict (e.g., Parenting Alliance Inventory; Abidin, 1988) can be employed. Parental screening for both lifetime and current ADHD (e.g., DSM-IV ADHD Rating Scale; Murphy & Gordon, 2006) is recommended when a child presents with comorbid CP and ADHD (McMahon & Frick, 2005).

The fourth area is parenting stress, assessment of which includes both general measures of stress (e.g., Family Events List; Patterson, 1982) and specific measures of parenting-related stress (e.g., Parenting Stress Index; Abidin, 1995). With respect to extrafamilial functioning, the Community Interaction Checklist (Wahler et al., 1979), which is a brief interview designed to assess maternal insularity, has been extensively employed in research with children with CP and their families. The Neighborhood Questionnaire (Greenberg, Lengua, Coie, Pinderhughes, & Conduct Problems Prevention Research Group, 1999) is a brief parent report measure used to assess a parent's perception of the family's neighborhood in terms of safety, violence, drug traffic, satisfaction, and stability. Finally, it is important to evaluate parental satisfaction with treatment, which may be assessed in terms of satisfaction with the outcome of treatment, therapists, treatment procedures, and teaching format (McMahon & Forehand, 1983). The Therapy Attitude Inventory (Brestan, Jacobs, Rayfield, & Eyberg, 1999; Eyberg, 1993) and the Parent's Consumer Satisfaction Questionnaire (McMahon & Forehand, 2003; McMahon, Tiedemann, Forehand, & Griest, 1984) are examples of measures designed to evaluate parental satisfaction with treatment. At present, no single consumer satisfaction measure is appropriate for use with all types of interventions for youths with CP and their families.

An Assessment Model

As described above, the assessment of a youth with CP should be guided by what is currently known about the heterogeneous nature of CP, its comorbid conditions, the relevant risk and protective factors, and the different developmental pathways (McMahon & Estes, 1997; McMahon & Frick, 2005). It is readily apparent that the assessment of a youth with CP must make use of multiple methods (e.g., behavior rating scales, direct observation, interviews) completed by multiple informants (parents, teachers, the youth him- or herself) concerning the youth's behavior in multiple settings (e.g., home, school). However, in cost-effectiveness terms, to conduct such a broad-based assessment with every youth who is referred would be prohibitively expensive, and the incremental utility of each additional assessment measure or content area with respect to improving our treatment-selecting capabilities would be suspect as well (Johnston & Murray, 2003).

"Multiple-gating" approaches to screening constitute one strategy for employing multiple assessment measures that may prove to be cost-effective (e.g., Reid, Baldwin, Patterson, & Dishion, 1988; Walker et al., 2004). In this approach, less costly assessment procedures (e.g., brief interviews, broad-band behavior rating scales) can be employed as screening instruments with all youths who are clinic-referred for the treatment of CP. More expensive methods, such as structured diagnostic interviews and observational methods, can be used to assess only that subgroup of youths for whom the less expensive methods have indicated the desirability of further assessment. An analogous strategy could be followed in the assessment of other youth characteristics and familial and extrafamilial factors. That is, low-cost methods such as interview questions (e.g., concerning a youth's temperament) and/or brief questionnaires (e.g., concerning the presence of substance use) would be employed as screening measures; should additional assessment in these areas be warranted, then a more thorough (and expensive) assessment could be conducted.

The ultimate goal of the assessment process is, of course, to facilitate selection of the most appropriate treatment strategy or strategies. Algorithms for matching clinic-referred families with specific interventions exist (e.g., Blechman, 1981; Embry, 1984), but they have been quite limited in scope, have not been closely tied to underlying assessment strategies, and have yet to be empirically tested. A comprehensive, empirically based treatment selection model for youths with CP is sorely needed. More clinically oriented strategies for integrating and interpreting information from comprehensive assessments, such as those presented by Kamphaus and Frick (2002), are a step in the right direction. Others have suggested that incorporation of an FBA approach into more traditional assessment practices will facilitate integration of information from multiple sources and the selection of appropriate treatments (e.g., Reitman & Hupp, 2003; Scotti, Morris, McNeil, & Hawkins, 1996; Walker et al., 2004).

Another goal of assessment is intervention monitoring and evaluating treatment outcome

(McMahon & Frick, 2005). It is essential for a clinician to ascertain whether interventions have brought about meaningful change in the youth's adjustment, either for better or for worse (i.e., an iatrogenic effect). The very real possibility of iatrogenic effects resulting from interventions to treat CP in adolescents is discussed below. As noted above, various assessment measures have demonstrated sensitivity to intervention effects; however, there is minimal evidence of the successful use of assessment measures to monitor the effects of *ongoing* interventions for youths with CP.

TREATMENT AND PREVENTION

As demonstrated in the preceding material, CP is multifaceted in the diversity of specific behaviors that are manifested, the ages of the youths who engage in those behaviors, and the settings in which the behaviors occur. Not surprisingly, a plethora of interventions have been developed to deal with the various manifestations of CP (e.g., Frick, 1998; Hill & Maughan, 2001; McMahon & Kotler, 2004, 2006; McMahon & Rhule, 2005). In order to impose some structure on our discussion of this array of interventions, we first describe four broad categories of psychosocial interventions that have been developed primarily to treat overt forms of CP behavior: (1) family-based interventions, (2) skills training approaches, (3) community-based programs, and (4) school-based interventions. For each type of program, interventions that are available for and appropriate to preadolescents (3–12 years of age) and adolescents (13 years and older) are described. This is followed by a description of interventions that have been developed for covert CP. In addition, we provide a summary of the relatively limited evidence for pharmacological interventions specific to CP behaviors. We then briefly summarize evidence for the effects of preventive interventions in infancy, childhood, and early adolescence on CP behavior displayed during adolescence. In the next section of the chapter, we discuss a number of issues related to the development, selection, and evaluation of these interventions, such as generalization and social validity, the prediction of outcome, comparative efficacy, and effectiveness and dissemination. We close the chapter with a brief discussion of future directions.

Because available interventions vary widely

in the extent to which they have been empirically validated, we have selected interventions that are generally considered to meet currently accepted criteria for determining whether an intervention is considered efficacious. (See Brestan & Eyberg, 1998, for a discussion of this issue specifically related to CP.) It is important to note that most of the interventions address overt rather than covert CP. Although covert CP behaviors (e.g., lying, stealing, firesetting) are key components of later developmental manifestations of CD, most interventions primarily targeting covert CP do not qualify as empirically supported treatments. However, for the sake of completeness, we provide brief descriptions of interventions for these specific manifestations of CP.

Family-Based Interventions

Family-Based Interventions with Preadolescents

Approaches to treating children with CP in their families have typically been based on a social-learning-based "parent training" model of intervention (e.g., Miller & Prinz, 1990). The underlying assumption of this model is that some sort of parenting skills deficit has been at least partly responsible for the development and/or maintenance of the CP behaviors. The core elements of the parent training approach have been delineated by a number of authors (e.g., Dumas, 1989; Kazdin, 1995b; Miller & Prinz, 1990). They include the following:

1. Intervention is conducted primarily with the parents, with relatively less therapist–child contact.
2. There is a refocusing from a preoccupation with CP behavior to an emphasis on prosocial goals.
3. The content of these programs typically includes instruction in the social learning principles underlying the parenting techniques; training in defining, monitoring, and tracking child behavior; positive reinforcement procedures, including praise and other forms of positive parent attention and token or point systems; extinction and mild punishment procedures such as ignoring, response cost, and time out in lieu of physical punishment; training in giving clear instructions or commands; and problem solving.

4. Extensive use is made of didactic instruction, modeling, role playing, behavioral rehearsal, and structured homework exercises.

Parent training interventions have been successfully utilized in the clinic and home settings, have been implemented with individual families or with groups of families, and have involved some or all of the instructional techniques listed above. O'Dell (1985) has provided an extensive review of the myriad parametric considerations involved in parent training.

Although the short-term efficacy of behavioral parent training in producing changes in both parent and child behaviors has been demonstrated repeatedly (e.g., O'Dell, 1974; Serketich & Dumas, 1996), the generalization of those effects has been less consistently documented. Forehand and Atkeson (1977) discussed four major types of generalization relevant to parent training interventions with children. "Setting generalization" refers to the transfer of treatment effects to settings in which treatment did not take place (e.g., from the clinic to the home), whereas "temporal generalization" pertains to the maintenance of treatment effects following termination. "Sibling generalization" concerns the transfer of the newly acquired parenting skills to untreated siblings in the family, and the siblings' responding in the desired manner. "Behavioral generalization" refers to whether targeted changes in specific CP behaviors are accompanied by improvements in other nontargeted behaviors.

Pertinent to the generalization of effects is the "social validity" of the intervention, which refers to whether therapeutic changes are "clinically or socially important" for the client (Kazdin, 1977a, p. 429). Parent training interventions for the treatment of children with CP have demonstrated their generalizability and social validity to varying degrees—some quite impressively, others not at all. As a consequence of this emphasis on the generalization and social validity of treatment effects, and the increased awareness of the multiple causal and maintaining factors of CP, the parent training model has been broadened to what is referred to as "behavioral family therapy" (Griest & Wells, 1983; Wells, 1985). This model is an attempt to acknowledge and incorporate into treatment the variety of child and parent variables that have been implicated in the development and maintenance of CP, such as parental personal adjustment and perceptions of the child, and child characteristics such as temperament and attributional style. Johnston (1996) has presented a model for conceptualizing various types of parental cognitions and their role in family-based interventions with children with CP. Miller and Prinz (1990) provide a thorough discussion and review of various enhancements to the basic parent training model as a means of enhancing generalization and social validity.

We present several parent training/behavioral family therapy programs as examples of state-of-the-art family-based interventions for preadolescent children with CP. Descriptions of the clinical procedures utilized in these programs are widely available, and each of the programs has been extensively evaluated.

HELPING THE NONCOMPLIANT CHILD

The first parent training program is specifically designed to treat noncompliance in younger children (3–8 years of age). As noted above, noncompliance is regarded as a keystone behavior in the development and maintenance of CP. The program was originally developed by Hanf (1969, 1970; Hanf & Kling, 1973), but has been modified and subsequently evaluated by several independent groups of clinical researchers, including Forehand and his colleagues (Forehand & McMahon, 1981; McMahon & Forehand, 2003), Webster-Stratton (2000), and Eyberg (e.g., Brinkmeyer & Eyberg, 2003). The Helping the Noncompliant Child (HNC) parent training program (Forehand & McMahon, 1981; McMahon & Forehand, 2003) employs a controlled learning environment in which the parent is taught to change maladaptive patterns of interaction with the child. Sessions are typically conducted in a clinic setting with individual families rather than in groups. Ideally, treatment occurs in playrooms equipped with one-way mirrors for observation, sound systems, and "bug-in-the-ear" devices by which a therapist can communicate unobtrusively with a parent, although these are not necessary for successful implementation of the program. A number of discrete parenting skills are taught to the parent by way of didactic instruction, modeling, and role playing. The parent also practices the skills in the clinic with the child while receiving prompting and feedback from the therapist. Finally, the parent employs these newly acquired skills in the home setting.

The HNC program consists of two phases. During the differential-attention phase of treatment (Phase I), the parent learns to break out of the coercive cycle of interaction with the child by increasing the frequency and range of positive attention to the child and ignoring minor inappropriate behaviors. The primary goal is to establish a positive, mutually reinforcing relationship between the parent and child. The parent is first taught to attend to and describe the child's appropriate behavior while eliminating commands, questions, and criticisms. The second segment of Phase I consists of teaching the parent to use verbal and physical attention contingent upon compliance and other appropriate behaviors, and to actively ignore minor inappropriate behaviors. Homework is assigned in the form of daily 10-minute practice sessions with the child, using the skills taught in the clinic. The parent is also required to develop programs for use outside the clinic, designed to increase at least three child behaviors by means of the new skills.

In Phase II (compliance training), the primary parenting skills are taught in the context of the clear instructions sequence. This involves teaching the parent to use appropriate commands and a time-out procedure to decrease noncompliant behavior exhibited by the child. The parent is taught to give direct, concise commands one at a time, and to allow the child sufficient time to comply. If compliance is initiated, the parent is taught to praise or attend to the child. If compliance is not initiated, the parent learns to implement a 3-minute time-out procedure. Following time out, the command that originally elicited noncompliance is repeated. Compliance is followed by contingent attention from the parent. When the parent is able to administer the command–warning–time-out sequence successfully in the clinic, he or she is instructed to begin using the procedure for noncompliance at home. Finally, parents are taught to use permanent "standing rules" as an occasional supplement to this sequence.

Progression to each new skill in the HNC program is determined by the use of behavioral and temporal (number of sessions) criteria. These criteria ensure that a parent has attained an acceptable degree of competence in a particular skill before being taught additional parenting techniques, and allow for the individualization of the treatment program by allocating training time more efficiently. For complete details of the HNC parent training program, see McMahon and Forehand (2003).

The HNC parent training program has been extensively evaluated in terms of its short-term effectiveness, generalization, and social validity (see McMahon & Forehand, 2003). Short-term effectiveness and setting generalization from the clinic to the home have been demonstrated for both parent and child behaviors, as well as parents' perceptions of their children (e.g., Peed, Roberts, & Forehand, 1977). Furthermore, these improvements occur regardless of families' SES (Rogers, Forehand, Griest, Wells, & McMahon, 1981) or age of the children (within the 3- to 8-year-old age range) (McMahon, Forehand, & Tiedemann, 1985). Two studies have failed to find evidence for setting generality to the classroom, but there was also no evidence of a behavioral contrast effect, since there were no systematic increases or decreases in child deviant behavior in the classroom (Breiner & Forehand, 1981; Forehand et al., 1979).

The temporal generalization of the HNC program has been documented in several studies (Baum & Forehand, 1981; Forehand & Long, 1988; Forehand, Rogers, McMahon, Wells, & Griest, 1981; Forehand, Steffe, Furey, & Walley, 1983; Forehand et al., 1979; Long, Forehand, Wierson, & Morgan, 1994), with follow-up assessments ranging from 6 months to 14 years after treatment termination. Forehand and Long (1988) demonstrated that, relative to a nonreferred "normal" sample, a sample of children who had participated in the parent training program 4.5–10.5 years earlier (and who were now between the ages of 11 and 15) were functioning well. Long et al. (1994) reported similar findings at a 14-year follow-up. Sibling generalization has been demonstrated by Humphreys, Forehand, McMahon, and Roberts (1978), who showed that mothers employed the skills they had learned in the parent training program with untreated siblings, who responded by being more compliant to maternal directives. Finally, improvement in child compliance has been shown to be accompanied by decreases in other overt CP behaviors, such as aggression, tantrums, destructiveness, and inappropriate verbal behavior, thereby supporting the behavioral generalization of the program (Wells, Forehand, & Griest, 1980).

With respect to the social validity of the HNC program, child compliance and inappropriate behavior have improved to within the "normal" range by the end of treatment, although mothers' perceptions of the children's adjustment appear to lag slightly behind the children's behavioral improvements (Forehand, Wells, & Griest, 1980). However, by 2 months after the conclusion of treatment, mothers' perceptions are consistent with the children's improved behavior and are comparable to those of mothers of "normal" children. High parental ratings of the acceptability of (Cross Calvert & McMahon, 1987) and satisfaction with (Baum & Forehand, 1981; Forehand et al., 1980; McMahon et al., 1984) the HNC program in general and its components have also been documented.

Several procedures have been evaluated as adjuncts to the basic HNC program. These include maternal (Wells, Griest, & Forehand, 1980) and child (Baum, Reyna McGlone, & Ollendick, 1986) self-control procedures; training the parents in the social learning principles underlying the parent training program (McMahon, Forehand, & Griest, 1981); expanded exemplars of common parent–child situations ("simulation training"; Powers & Roberts, 1995); and a multimodal treatment package ("parent enhancement therapy") designed to enhance general family functioning, which includes components related to parental perceptions of the child's behavior, marital adjustment, parental personal adjustment, and the parents' extrafamilial relationships (Griest et al., 1982). In general, these studies have supported the efficacy of these adjunctive procedures in enhancing the generalization and/or maintenance of treatment effects, over and above those gains obtained in the basic HNC program.

Two studies have compared the effects of the HNC program with those of other treatments for children with CP. Wells and Egan (1988) found that the HNC program was more effective than family systems therapy on observational measures of parent and child behaviors. The two treatment groups did not differ on parental self-report measures of personal (depression, anxiety) or marital adjustment. Baum and colleagues (1986) reported that a group version of the HNC program (with or without the child self-control adjunct noted above) was more effective at posttreatment and at a 6- to 8-month follow-up than a parent discussion group based on the Systematic Training for Effective Parenting (STEP) program (Dinkmeyer & McKay, 1976).

PARENT–CHILD INTERACTION THERAPY

A second parent training program closely modeled after the Hanf approach is Parent–Child Interaction Therapy (PCIT; e.g., Bell & Eyberg, 2002; Brinkmeyer & Eyberg, 2003; Eyberg, 1988). In additional to being grounded in social learning theory, the development of PCIT has been influenced by attachment theory (Foote, Eyberg, & Schuhmann, 1998). Thus, when compared to other Hanf-based models of parenting training, PCIT could be described as being somewhat more explicit in its focus on the enhancement of a nurturing parent–child relationship (although the skills taught in PCIT and the intervention procedures do not differ substantially from other Hanf-based parenting training approaches). PCIT is generally appropriate for families with children in the 2- to 8-year-old range. Treatment typically includes approximately 13 one-hour sessions, although the specific number of sessions is based on the needs of the individual family.

Similar to the HNC parent training program (McMahon & Forehand, 2003), PCIT is divided into two phases. The first phase, child-directed interaction (CDI), is based on Hanf's Child's Game. During this phase, parents are encouraged to follow the child's lead using nondirective "PRIDE" skills, including (1) praising the child, (2) reflecting child statements, (3) imitating the play, (4) describing child behavior, and (5) using enthusiasm in play with the child. As with the HNC program, the therapist coaches the parent in these skills, and criteria for mastery are met through behavioral observations of parent–child interactions. In the second phase of PCIT, parent-directed interaction (PDI), parents take the lead in the play and are coached in giving appropriate commands and directives to the child and enforcing consequences for compliance and noncompliance. Labeled praise is also introduced in this phase (whereas in the HNC program, labeled praise is introduced in the initial phase of the intervention). A primary component of PDI includes training parents in the appropriate use of time out. "House rules" (equivalent to standing rules in the HNC program) are also introduced and implemented during PDI.

In an early test of the intervention, Eyberg and Robinson (1982) conducted PCIT with seven families of children with behavior problems (ages 2–7). Children in this study also had siblings between the ages of 2 and 10 years who did not receive treatment. Changes were observed from pre- to posttest in targeted parent training skills, and there were significant improvements on observer ratings of child behavior, untreated sibling behavior, and parental adjustment.

A second study conducted by McNeil and colleagues (1991) included control groups (although children were not randomly assigned to conditions). Ten children were treated with PCIT, and this intervention group was compared with a normative control group ($n = 10$) and a problem behavior control group ($n = 10$). Compared to the control groups, the PCIT group had reduced levels of behavior problems at home; moreover, there were significant improvements on a number of classroom measures of disruptive behavior (observation and teacher report), compared to the control groups. It is important to note that the PCIT group had higher levels of problem behavior prior to the intervention than either of the control groups; thus the group comparison results in this study must be interpreted cautiously. Eyberg, Funderburk, Hembree-Kigin, McNeil, and Querido (2001) examined the maintenance of treatment effects in the home for 13 families at 1 and 2 years posttreatment. Based on parent report and observational data, treatment effects were maintained for eight families at the 1-year follow-up, while nine families had maintained treatment effects at the 2-year follow-up. Funderburk and colleagues (1998) examined the maintenance of the classroom treatment effects in 12 children at 12 and 18 months posttreatment. At the 12-month follow-up, children had maintained improvements in teacher ratings and classroom observations of disruptive behavior. However, at the 18-month follow-up, children had maintained improvements in compliance, but all other measures of CP and social competence had returned to pretreatment levels.

A randomized controlled trial of PCIT was conducted by Schuhmann, Foote, Eyberg, Boggs, and Algina (1998). In this study, 64 families with 3- to 6-year-old children with ODD were assigned to PCIT or a waiting-list control. At the conclusion of therapy, compared to the control group, the PCIT group showed greater reductions in child behavior problems (problems were within the typical range at the conclusion of treatment), and parents reported experiencing less stress and feeling more in control. Gains were maintained at a 4-month follow-up. Hood and Eyberg (2003) reported maintenance of maternal reports of child behavior and parental locus of control for 23 families from the Schuhmann and colleagues study at 3–6 years posttreatment. Boggs and colleagues (2004) compared these 23 families that completed PCIT in the Schuhmann and colleagues study to 23 families that dropped out (follow-up was approximately 20 months after treatment intake). Overall, families that had completed treatment had maintained gains at follow-up, while the children in families that had dropped out of treatment had returned to pretreatment levels of CP.

Recently, Nixon and colleagues (2003) conducted a study comparing PCIT to an abbreviated PCIT protocol that involved the use of didactic videotapes, telephone consultation, and abbreviated in-person sessions. Fifty-four preschool children and their mothers were assigned to the standard PCIT condition, the abbreviated PCIT condition, or a waiting-list control. A group of normative preschoolers was also included. At the conclusion of treatment, according to parent report, children in both PCIT groups had reduced externalizing behavior, and there were improvements in parental stress levels and discipline practices compared to the waiting-list control group. The standard PCIT was superior to the abbreviated PCIT at the postintervention assessment, based on an observational measure (i.e., percentage of change in maternal criticisms); however, the two groups were comparable at a 6-month follow-up, based on results from both parent report instruments and observational measures. Follow-up assessments at 1 and 2 years were also conducted (Nixon, Sweeney, Erickson, & Touyz, 2004). Parent report and observational measures at these assessments indicated that treatment gains were largely maintained, and little difference was noted between the two treatment conditions.

When analyzed as part of a cost–benefit study conducted by the Washington State Institute of Public Policy (Aos, Lieb, Mayfield, Miller, & Pennucci, 2004), PCIT was shown to save taxpayers approximately $3,427 per participant in the program, compared to the cost of one offense (including the crime itself, associated law enforcement costs, adjudication, and punishment/rehabilitation).

INCREDIBLE YEARS

A third parent training program for young (3- to 8-year-old) children with CP, which includes some components of the Hanf (1969) and HNC (Forehand & McMahon, 1981; McMahon & Forehand, 2003) programs, is the Incredible Years program developed by Webster-Stratton (2000; Webster-Stratton & Reid, 2003). The core parent training component of this program is a videotape modeling/group discussion intervention (BASIC; Webster-Stratton, 2000; Webster-Stratton & Reid, 2003). What is unique about this particular intervention is its use of a standard package of videotape programs of modeled parenting skills, shown by a therapist to groups of parents. The 250 video vignettes (each of which lasts approximately 2 minutes), presented during the 12- to 14-week program, include examples of parents interacting with their children in both appropriate and inappropriate ways. After each vignette, the therapist leads a discussion of the relevant interactions and solicits parental responses to the vignettes. In this particular program, the children do not attend the therapy sessions, although parents are given homework exercises to practice various parenting skills with their children. The videotapes and associated therapist manuals are commercially available.

A number of outcome studies have evaluated the immediate and longer-term effects of the Incredible Years program. The first study of the BASIC program (Webster-Stratton, 1981, 1982a, 1982b) employed a sample of nonreferred mothers; it reported positive changes in mothers' and children's behaviors and in maternal perceptions of the children's adjustment at posttreatment, compared to a waiting-list control group. Mothers also reported high levels of satisfaction with the treatment program. At a 1-year follow-up, most of the parental perceptions and mother and child behaviors were maintained or continued to improve; however, there was a significant decrease in mothers' confidence in their parenting skills and perceived ability to manage their children's behavior problems.

In the second study, Webster-Stratton (1984) randomly assigned mothers of clinic-referred children with CP to the BASIC program, an individual parent training program (with similar content), or a waiting-list control. Positive changes in both treatment conditions compared to the waiting-list control condition were obtained on a variety of treatment outcome measures at posttreatment, and most of these changes were maintained at a 1-year follow-up. There were virtually no differences between the two treatment groups at posttreatment and at the follow-up. Given that therapist time per client was significantly greater for the individual parent training condition than for the BASIC condition, the latter program represents a cost-effective alternative to the traditional parent training format of individual consultation with a single family, at least for families of young children with CP.

A component analysis of the BASIC program was conducted with a sample of mothers and fathers of 114 children with CP (Webster-Stratton, 1989, 1990a; Webster-Stratton, Hollinsworth, & Kolpacoff, 1989; Webster-Stratton, Kolpacoff, & Hollinsworth, 1988). Parents were randomly assigned to the BASIC program, self-administered videotape modeling (with no therapist feedback or group discussion), group discussion alone, or a waiting-list control condition. Each of the three treatment conditions was superior to the waiting-list control condition on most of the various outcome measures (Webster-Stratton et al., 1988), and these improvements were maintained at a 1-year follow-up (Webster-Stratton et al., 1989). However, the BASIC program appeared to be somewhat more effective than the other two treatment conditions, and both mothers and fathers reported somewhat greater satisfaction with the BASIC program than with the other conditions (Webster-Stratton, 1989). At a 3-year follow-up, only the parents in the BASIC condition reported stable improvements in their children's behavior problems (Webster-Stratton, 1990a). These findings again support the short-term effectiveness and temporal generalization of Webster-Stratton's parent training program and suggest the power of the videotape modeling component.

The BASIC program has also been compared to treatment as usual in a community mental health center (Taylor, Schmidt, Pepler, & Hodgins, 1998). In addition to being conducted by an independent group of researchers, this study provided a test of the effectiveness of the BASIC program because it was conducted

in a community clinic setting with on-site staff. Children ($n = 108$) were assigned to the BASIC program, the usual treatment of the clinic, or a waiting list. Both the BASIC group and the treatment-as-usual group showed greater reductions in child CP compared to the waiting-list control group. Furthermore, compared to the treatment-as-usual group, children with parents in the BASIC group had significantly fewer behavioral concerns (as assessed by two parent report measures of child CP). Consumer satisfaction was also higher for the BASIC program than for treatment as usual.

In a cross-cultural test of the BASIC program, Scott and colleagues (2001) tested the effectiveness of the BASIC program, using therapists in community mental health centers in the United Kingdom. Children were assigned to the BASIC program or a waiting-list control. Parents in the BASIC program showed improvements in parenting behavior, whereas parents in the waiting-list control group actually showed decreases in positive parenting. CP was also significantly reduced for children with parents in the BASIC program.

Webster-Stratton (2000; Webster-Stratton & Reid, 2003) has described the development of several adjuncts to the BASIC program. Two adjunct programs (the ADVANCE program and the SCHOOL program) are administered to the parents. There is also a teacher-focused adjunct (the Teacher Training Program) and a child-focused adjunct (Dinosaur School). The ADVANCE program, which consists of 8–10 sessions and 60 videotaped vignettes, focuses on the enhancement of parental interpersonal skills (i.e., self-control strategies, problem solving, communication, ways to give and get support). Parents who received the ADVANCE component following participation in the BASIC parent training program reported greater improvements in communication, problem-solving skills, and consumer satisfaction than did parents who received only the BASIC program (Webster-Stratton, 1994). The SCHOOL program typically requires three or four additional sessions (although this material can also be incorporated into the BASIC program) and includes two additional training videos. It was developed to teach parents strategies to enhance child reading and academic readiness and to develop effective partnerships with teachers. The Teacher Training Program is a 42-hour training unit (conducted as a 6-day workshop, a 1-day-per-month in-service session, or 18–20 weekly sessions) for teachers (as well as school counselors and psychologists), which includes the use of 11 videotapes of vignettes. This program is designed to promote effective classroom management techniques for addressing misbehavior. "Transition plans," which include behavior management strategies and goals, are developed for each child in the Incredible Years program. In the Dinosaur School program, small groups of five to six children with CP are pulled from the classroom for 2 hours per week (if administered in a clinic setting, these sessions can be conducted simultaneously with the parent BASIC program) and receive a skills training and problem-solving intervention designed to promote appropriate classroom behavior, social skills, conflict resolution skills, and positive peer interactions. This program can also be conducted as a classroom-based curriculum. Videotaped vignettes are used in each session and are narrated by human and animal puppets. Role playing of appropriate responses, feedback, and reinforcement are also used throughout the training.

The child-focused adjunct treatment (Dinosaur School), whether alone or in conjunction with BASIC and ADVANCE, resulted in child improvements in problem solving and conflict management skills with peers (Webster-Stratton & Hammond, 1997; Webster-Stratton, Reid, & Hammond, 2001b, 2004). However, the combined parent and child intervention had the most robust improvements in child behavior at a 1-year follow-up. Moreover, studies combining the parent training components with both the child-focused treatment and the Teacher Training Program (e.g., Reid & Webster-Stratton, 2001; Webster-Stratton et al., 2004) have shown that these additional programs further enhance the effects of the parent training components (see Webster-Stratton & Reid, 2003, for a review of these studies). Two-year follow-up data have also been examined for a group of children ($n = 159$) who were assigned to either the BASIC program alone or this program with one or more adjunct treatments. Across the intervention groups, approximately 75% of children were functioning in the normative range, according to parent and teacher report (Reid, Webster-Stratton, & Hammond, 2003).

In addition to being studied in a variety of clinical populations, the Incredible Years parent training program and some of its adjunct programs have been used as a selective pre-ventive intervention with Head Start mothers (Webster-Stratton, 1998; Webster-Stratton, Reid, & Hammond, 2001a). Compared to control groups, intervention groups showed improvement in parenting skills, reductions in child CP behaviors, increases in child social competence, and improvements in teachers' classroom management skills. Additional follow-up analyses demonstrated that program response did not significantly differ by ethnicity (samples included African American, Asian American, European American, and Hispanic mothers; Reid, Webster-Stratton, & Beauchaine, 2001).

Recently, Webster-Stratton and colleagues (Beauchaine, Webster-Stratton, & Reid, 2005) have compiled data from six randomized clinical trials of various modules from the Incredible Years program, in order to examine mediators, moderators, and predictors of treatment outcome at 1-year follow-up. Separate latent growth curve models for child externalizing behavior were based on mother report data and observational data. In the mother report model, children of younger mothers, children of fathers with substance abuse histories, and children with comorbid anxiety/depression symptoms exhibited more positive treatment responses. In the observational model, comorbid anxiety/depression symptoms were again predictive of positive treatment response, as was a history of maternal substance abuse. Moderators of treatment outcome were also identified and included marital adjustment, maternal depression, social class, paternal substance abuse, marital status, comorbid attention problems, and comorbid anxiety/depression symptoms.

TRIPLE P

Developed by Sanders and colleagues (Sanders, Markie-Dadds, & Turner, 2003) in Australia, the Triple P-Positive Parenting Program consists of five levels of intervention, ranging from a universal prevention program to an intensive and individualized treatment targeting children with serious CP. This program combines parent training strategies with a range of family support materials and services. The group of interventions was designed originally for use with parents of children from birth to age 12. Recently, Triple P has been extended to include intervention strategies appropriate for youths ages 12–16.

The Level 1 intervention (Universal Triple P) is a universal prevention program designed to provide all parents with easy access to parenting information using media sources (e.g., newspaper, radio, TV), a set of "tip sheets," and videotapes that demonstrate particular parenting strategies. Level 2 (Selected Triple P) is a brief (one- or two-session) intervention conducted by a primary health care provider. This level of intervention is designed for parents of children with mild CP behaviors or for parents who have a specific behavioral concern. The Selected Triple P intervention includes the provision of problem-specific advice as well as developmental guidance, and also incorporates tip sheets and videotapes demonstrating positive parenting strategies. Level 3 (Primary Care Triple P) is a four-session intervention, again conducted by a primary health care provider. This level is appropriate for parents of children with mild to moderate CP behaviors and includes the provision of parenting advice and opportunities for parents to learn and practice skills designed to address problem behavior. Level 4 (Standard Triple P) is a more intensive intervention, including 8–10 sessions for parents of children with more severe CP. This level includes many components of traditional parent training programs, such as a focus on parent–child interaction and training in a set of parenting skills designed to be applicable to a range of problem behavior. It is notable that there are individual, group, and self-directed treatment options for Level 4. The Level 5 intervention (Enhanced Triple P) is appropriate when there is family dysfunction (e.g., parental depression, marital conflict) in addition to serious youth CP. At this level, a behavioral family intervention is individually tailored to families' needs, and treatment strategies often include home visits focused on parenting practices, training in coping skills, and management of mood problems, marital conflict, and/or family stress. Mental heath practitioners typically administer Level 4 and Level 5 interventions. Currently, in addition to widespread implementation in Australia, the Triple P program is being disseminated and replicated in a number of countries, including Canada, New Zealand, Singapore, the United Kingdom, and the United States.

A number of randomized controlled trials have been used to evaluate the Triple P program. Most of these studies have focused on Level 4 (Standard Triple P) and/or Level 5 (En-

hanced Triple P) interventions. An initial trial compared child management training with Standard Triple P in 20 children ages 2–7 years (Sanders & Christensen, 1985). Based on in-home observational data, both interventions lead to reductions in aversive parenting strategies and child CP behavior. Effects were maintained at a 3-month follow-up, and there were no significant differences in CP behavior between intervention youths and controls without identified behavior problems.

A second study compared Standard Triple P with an initial version of the Enhanced Triple P intervention (i.e., Standard Triple P plus a partner support module) in 24 families with children ages 2–5 (Dadds, Schwartz, & Sanders, 1987). Again, using in-home observations as well as parent report measures (e.g., a questionnaire for marital satisfaction), these authors found that aversive parenting strategies and child CP were reduced and marital satisfaction increased in both groups. However, in families with partner conflict, the addition of the partner support module resulted in less relapse in terms of both child CP and marital satisfaction.

Further investigating multiple forms of the Standard Triple P intervention as well as the enhanced program, a third study of 305 families compared Standard Triple P, a self-directed format for Standard Triple P, Enhanced Triple P, and a waiting-list control (Sanders et al., 2000). Compared to the control group, all intervention groups showed reductions in parent-reported child CP. However, only children in the Standard Triple P program and the Enhanced Triple P program showed improvements on observational measures of child CP. The intervention groups did not differ from the control group in terms of observed aversive mother behavior, although mothers in the intervention groups did self-report using fewer dysfunctional parenting practices. There were no intervention effects on maternal reports of parental and marital adjustment. Interestingly, at a 1-year follow-up, children of parents in the self-directed form of Standard Triple P had made additional behavioral improvements, and the intervention groups no longer differed on measures of child CP. In another randomized controlled trial of families with 3-year-olds (n = 87; Bor, Sanders, & Markie-Dadds, 2002), Standard Triple P, Enhanced Triple P, and a waiting-list control group were again compared. In this study, parents in both of the intervention conditions reported reduced child behavior problems (although significant improvements in observed child behavior could only be demonstrated when the Enhanced Triple P group was compared with the control group). In comparison to the control group, parents in the intervention groups also reported reductions in aversive parenting practices. However, observational measures of parenting practices did not show similar group differences. Obtained intervention gains were maintained at a 1-year follow-up.

A group version of the Standard Triple P intervention has also been examined. In a cross-cultural evaluation of the Triple P program conducted in Hong Kong, Leung, Sanders, Leung, Mak, and Lau (2003) compared Group Triple P to a waiting-list control. Ireland, Sanders, and Markie-Dadds (2003) compared Group Triple P with and without a partner support module. Based on parent report, disruptive child behavior was reduced in all intervention groups, as were dysfunctional parenting strategies and parenting conflict. However, differences between Group Triple P with and without the partner support module were not found.

Recently, an effectiveness trial for Group Triple P has been conducted. Group Triple P was implemented in one high-risk health region, with a comparable region used as a control ($n = 1,615$ families; Zubrick et al., in press). Study results were complicated by the fact that the intervention region had significantly higher preintervention levels of dysfunctional parenting strategies. However, at the postintervention assessment and at 1- and 2-year follow-ups, these dysfunctional parenting strategies decreased significantly in the intervention region and were actually lower than those of parents in the control region. Based on parent report measures, child CP in the intervention region was also significantly reduced compared to the control region; again, these changes were maintained at 1- and 2-year follow-up assessments.

Two recent studies have focused specifically on the self-directed forms of the Standard Triple P intervention (Markie-Dadds & Sanders, 2004a, 2004b). Compared to a waiting-list control, the Self-Directed Triple P intervention resulted in reduced parent reports of child CP behaviors and decreased aversive parenting practices. Improvements in child CP behavior and parenting practices were even more pronounced when limited telephone sessions with

a mental health practitioner were added to the self-directed program. Results were generally maintained at a 6-month follow-up.

Limited research has also been conducted to evaluate the lower-level Triple P interventions. Turner and Sanders (in press) compared Primary Triple P and a waiting-list control in a sample of 30 families (children ages 2–5). Based on parent monitoring and report instruments, children of parents in the intervention group showed significant improvement in targeted CP behaviors, and mothers reported reduced aversive parenting practices, decreased anxiety and stress, and increased satisfaction with their parenting role compared to the control group. Gains were mostly maintained at a 6-month follow-up. Sultana, Matthews, De Bortoli, and Cann (2004) compared Selected Triple P, Primary Care Triple P, and a waiting-list control in a sample of 1- to 5-year-olds ($n = 50$). Compared to waiting-list controls, parents in the Primary Care Triple P intervention reported significantly fewer child CP behaviors and the use of fewer aversive parenting strategies. However, although some positive changes were noted, the Selected Triple P intervention did not result in behavioral changes for parents or children that were significantly different from those of waiting-list controls.

OSLC PARENT TRAINING

As noted above, the work of Gerald Patterson and his associates at OSLC with children with CP and their families has been seminal in the development of the theoretical and empirical knowledge base concerning CP. Patterson's efforts over the past 35 years have also been extremely influential with respect to the development and evaluation of family-based intervention strategies for children with CP. Here, we briefly review Patterson's parent training program for preadolescent children (3–12 years of age) who engage in overt CP. OSLC intervention programs for adolescents and for children who steal are described later in the chapter.

The parent training program for preadolescent aggressive children is delineated in the treatment manual by Patterson and colleagues (1975) and has been summarized by Forgatch (1991). Prior to beginning treatment, parents are given a copy of either *Living with Children* (Patterson, 1976) or *Families* (Patterson, 1975), to provide a conceptual background for the specific skills training in the treatment sessions and to facilitate generalization and maintenance. After completion of the reading assignment, the next step is to teach the parents to pinpoint the problem behaviors of concern and then to track the child's behavior. Once the parents are pinpointing and tracking child behavior appropriately, they are assisted in establishing a positive reinforcement system, using points, backup reinforcers such as privileges or treats, and social reinforcement (i.e., praise). Over time, the tangible reinforcers are faded. After the point system is well established, the parents are taught to use a 5-minute time-out procedure for noncompliance or aggressive behavior. Response cost (e.g., loss of privileges) and work chores are also sometimes used with older children. As treatment progresses, parents become increasingly responsible for designing and implementing behavior management programs for various child behaviors. Parents are also taught to monitor or supervise their children, even when they are away from home. Problem-solving and negotiation strategies are taught to the parents at this point in treatment. Patterson and Chamberlain (1988) estimate that approximately 30% of treatment time is devoted to dealing with problems such as marital difficulties, parental personal adjustment problems, and family crises.

This parent training program has been extensively evaluated at OSLC and in community settings. Patterson, Cobb, and Ray (1973) treated 13 consecutive referrals of boys with CP and their families. Behavioral observation data indicated that 9 of the 13 families demonstrated improvements equal to or greater than 30% reduction from baseline levels of observed deviant behavior. In subsequent replication studies, similar effects were obtained (Patterson, 1974; Patterson & Reid, 1973). Improvements in maternal perceptions of children's adjustment have also been reported, and there is evidence for generalization across settings, time (up to 2 years posttreatment), behavior, and siblings (e.g., Arnold, Levine, & Patterson, 1975; Horne & Van Dyke, 1983; Patterson, 1974; Patterson & Fleischman, 1979; Patterson & Forgatch, 1995). The program has been shown to have comparable effects for families with older children (6.5–12.5 years old) and younger children (2.5–6.5 years old), although families with older children were more likely to drop out of treatment (Dishion & Patterson, 1992).

Findings comparable to those reported by Patterson (1974) have been obtained in a mixed sample of children who stole or who were socially aggressive (Fleischman, 1981), and for a subset of children who were socially aggressive (Weinrott, Bauske, & Patterson, 1979). These families were treated by clinicians who, although affiliated with Patterson, had not participated in the 1974 investigation and were not supervised by the OSLC staff during the course of the studies. Not only were positive treatment effects maintained at a 1-year follow-up, but standardization of treatment procedures and use of a group format in the replication studies reduced treatment time per family from 31 hours to 13–16 hours. Fleischman and Szykula (1981) conducted another replication study in a community setting with 50 families, and reported comparable improvements at posttreatment and at a 1-year follow-up.

The OSLC group has also conducted a number of comparison studies. Early investigations comparing the parent training program with attention placebo (Walter & Gilmore, 1973) and waiting-list control (Wiltz & Patterson, 1974) conditions reported significant reductions in targeted deviant child behaviors, whereas there were no significant changes for the comparison groups. A later study (Patterson, Chamberlain, & Reid, 1982) randomly assigned 19 families to parent training or waiting-list control conditions. The control condition actually became a comparison treatment condition by default, since eight of nine families obtained treatment from various clinicians in the community. This other treatment ranged from "eclectic" to behavioral in orientation. Observational data in the home indicated significant reductions in child deviant behavior for the parent training program only. However, both groups demonstrated significant improvements on the PDR with respect to frequency of parent-reported problem behaviors.

Findings from a comparative study at OSLC were reported by Patterson and Chamberlain (1988) and by Reid (1987). Seventy families of children with CP (ages 6–12 years) were randomly assigned to parent training ($n = 50$) or to a community agency employing eclectic family therapy ($n = 20$). Preliminary findings based on the first 34 families in the study indicated significant reductions in child CP behavior for families in the parent training condition, but no significant reduction for children in the family therapy condition (Reid, 1987). Only mothers in the parent training condition also demonstrated significant reductions in self-reported levels of depression.

More recently, Forgatch and DeGarmo (1999) examined the efficacy of a group-based format of the OSLC parent training program (Forgatch, 1994) in a sample (n = 238) of divorcing mothers and their sons (mean age = 7.8 years). Two-thirds of the sample was assigned to the intervention group, and the remaining third of the sample constituted the control group. Fourteen group sessions were conducted, and professionals made midweek telephone calls to encourage use of the procedures and to troubleshoot problems with the weekly assigned homework. Observational findings indicated that the intervention resulted in reductions in coercive parenting, maintenance of positive parenting, and increases in effective parenting, compared to the control group. These improved parenting practices were significantly related to improvements in teacher-reported school adjustment and child- and parent-reported maladjustment. Models based on child report and, to a lesser degree, on teacher report indicated that improvements in parenting practices mediated positive changes in child adjustment. Direct effects of the intervention on child outcomes were not observed.

Additional work with this sample focused on the efficacy on the intervention in terms of discipline and child noncompliance. Martinez and Forgatch (2001) found that, compared to the control group, mothers in the intervention group demonstrated reductions in coercive discipline, and boys' noncompliance was reduced. This reduction in noncompliance was mediated by the impact of the intervention on coercive discipline and positive parenting (although, of the two mediating variables, positive parenting was more strongly associated with reductions in boys' noncompliance). To further clarify the nature of these observed intervention effects, DeGarmo and colleagues (2004) conducted analyses to test hypothesized mechanisms of change. Parenting changed within the first 12 months of the baseline assessment, followed by changes in boys' behaviors and reductions in maternal depression within 30 months. As expected from previous analysis, increases in effective parenting mediated improvements in boys' externalizing behavior. However, these changes in externalizing behavior were also mediated by improvements in boys' depression (which was in turn partially mediated by increases in effective parenting). Reductions in maternal depression were mediated by improvements in boys' externalizing behavior.

A cross-cultural replication of the OSLC parent training model is currently underway in Norway (Ogden, 2000; Ogden, Forgatch, Askeland, Patterson, & Bullock, 2005). With a final goal of nationwide program implementation, pilot programs have been initiated in the elementary school system and the child welfare system. Within this context, randomized effectiveness trials (including multimethod assessment) are in progress.

Family-Based Interventions with Adolescents

We describe five family-based intervention models that have been employed with adolescents with CP: the OSLC parent training model as adapted for adolescents (Bank et al., 1991); Functional Family Therapy (FFT; Alexander & Sexton, 2002); Brief Strategic Family Therapy (BSFT; Szapocznik & Williams, 2000); Problem-Solving Communication Training (PSCT; Robin & Foster, 1989); and Multi-Systemic Therapy (MST; Henggeler, Schoenwald, Borduin, Rowland, & Cunningham, 1998).

OSLC PARENT TRAINING

Patterson and his colleagues have modified their parent training intervention for use with adolescents with CP (Bank et al., 1991; Forgatch & Patterson, 1989; Patterson & Forgatch, 1987). Modifications for delinquent adolescents include (1) targeting any behaviors that put an adolescent at risk for further delinquency; (2) emphasizing parental monitoring/ supervision; (3) revising punishment procedures to include work details, point loss, restriction of free time, and restitution of stolen/ damaged property; (4) encouraging parents to report legal offenses to juvenile authorities, and then to act as advocates for the adolescent in court; and (5) promoting greater involvement of the adolescent in treatment sessions (Bank et al., 1991). A study of the efficacy of this modification (Bank et al., 1991) revealed that although adolescents in the parent training condition did have fewer offenses during the treatment year than those in the control condition (i.e., community treatment as usual), offense rates for the two conditions were comparable by the first year after treatment, and remained so throughout the 3-year follow-up. Despite these somewhat positive findings, Bank et al. were pessimistic as to the feasibility of this approach on a larger scale, given the extreme distress of the families and the high likelihood of therapist burnout. Instead, they argued for intervention with these families at an earlier stage, before the problems have increased to such severity and duration.

FUNCTIONAL FAMILY THERAPY

A family-based intervention for adolescents engaging in CP behaviors has been developed and evaluated by Alexander and his colleagues. FFT (Alexander & Parsons, 1982; Barton & Alexander, 1981) represents a unique integration and extension of family systems and behavioral perspectives. The model has also incorporated cognitive and affective perspectives (Alexander, Jameson, Newell, & Gunderson, 1996).

FFT consists of three main phases (e.g., Alexander & Sexton, 2002; Sexton & Alexander, 2002). The engagement/motivation phase is concerned with family members' expectations prior to therapy and in the initial sessions. Factors enhancing the perception that positive change is possible are maximized, while factors that might lessen this perception are minimized. During this phase, the clinician identifies the behavioral, cognitive, and emotional expectations of each family member and the family processes in need of change (e.g., interpersonal functions such as closeness and distance). In addition, the clinician takes steps to modify the inappropriate attributions and expectations of family members. Various cognitive therapy techniques, especially relabeling of "negative" behavior as more positive or benign, are employed. This reattribution process among family members is seen as necessary, but not sufficient, for successful treatment. Actual behavior change must follow. In the behavior change phase, various behavioral techniques are employed, including communication skills training, behavioral contracting, and contingency management. In the generalization phase, the therapist's job is to facilitate maintenance of therapeutic gains while also fostering the family's independence from the therapy context through gradual disengagement. It is also during this phase that relevant extra-

familial factors (e.g., school, the legal system) are dealt with as necessary.

Much of the empirical research on the efficacy of FFT was conducted in the 1970s, prior to the inclusion of the cognitive and affective components described above. A series of three studies was conducted, using a single sample of 86 delinquent juveniles with status offenses and their families (Alexander & Parsons, 1973; Klein, Alexander, & Parsons, 1977; Parsons & Alexander, 1973). At the conclusion of treatment, families in the FFT condition performed better than families in the comparison conditions on a number of communication variables assessed in a 20-minute family discussion. An examination of juvenile court records 6–18 months after treatment indicated that adolescents in the FFT condition had a significantly lower recidivism rate (26%) than adolescents in comparison conditions (50% for no-treatment controls, 47% for client-centered family groups, and 73% for eclectic psychodynamic family therapy) (Alexander & Parsons, 1973). Within the FFT condition, a poorer outcome on the behavioral family interaction measures was associated with an increased likelihood of recidivism, thus lending direct support to the relationship between the two measures.

These early investigations focused on the families of delinquent adolescents with relatively minor status offenses. The current version of FFT, in conjunction with supportive adjuncts such as remedial education and job training, has been shown to be effective with multiply offending, previously incarcerated adolescents (Barton, Alexander, Waldron, Turner, & Warburton, 1985). In this investigation, adolescents who participated in FFT were less likely to be charged with committing an offense in the 15-month follow-up period than were adolescents placed in group homes (60% vs. 93%, respectively). FFT participants who did commit additional offenses committed significantly fewer offenses than adolescents in the group home condition.

Gordon, Arbuthnot, and their colleagues (Gordon, Arbuthnot, Gustafson, & McGreen, 1988; Gordon, Graves, & Arbuthnot, 1995) successfully employed a slightly modified version of FFT (longer treatment, treatment in the home as opposed to a clinic, and longer training and supervision of therapists) with a sample of 27 disadvantaged rural families of delinquent adolescents, many of whom had multiple offenses. Recidivism rates for the FFT and comparison (probation-only) groups at a 2.5-year follow-up were 11% and 67%, respectively. In a subsequent follow-up when the subjects were 20 to 22 years old, Gordon and colleagues (1995) reported a recidivism rate of 9% (vs. 41% for the FFT and comparison groups, respectively).

A cross-cultural replication of FFT with delinquent juveniles was completed recently in Sweden by Hansson, Cederblad, and Alexander (2002). In this study, 49 youths received FFT while 40 comparison subjects received treatment as usual (e.g., counseling, case management, referral to other treatment resources). At a 1-year follow-up, only 33% of the FFT group had relapsed, compared to 65% of the comparison group. This pattern was maintained at the 2-year follow-up (a 41% relapse rate in the FFT group, compared to an 83% relapse rate in the group that received treatment as usual).

When examined as part of the Aos and colleagues (2004) cost–benefit study, FFT was shown to save taxpayers between approximately $14,351 (in Washington State) and $26,216 (excluding Washington State) per participant in the program, compared to the cost of one offense.

BRIEF STRATEGIC FAMILY THERAPY

BSFT began as a response to increasing drug use in the Hispanic adolescent population in the 1970s (Robbins, Szapocznik, et al., 2003; Szapocznik & Williams, 2000). The initial goal was to develop a culturally appropriate intervention for behavior problems in Cuban American youths. Eventually, a time-limited treatment approach that included both structural and strategic interventions was developed and refined. According to Szapocznik and Williams (2000), "The goal of BSFT is to target repetitive interactions within or between systems in the family social ecology that are unsuccessful at achieving the goals of the family or its individual members" (p. 119).

BSFT interventions are strategic in that they are practical and problem-focused (Szapocznik & Williams, 2000). When a practical intervention is selected, the goal is to move the family toward desired objectives, and these interventions often involve positive or negative reframing. Problem-focused interventions involve targeting only family interaction patterns

that are directly relevant to the behavior problem of concern.

The content of BSFT involves a number of key steps (Robbins, Szapocznik, et al., 2003). The first step is the establishment of a therapeutic alliance with each family member and the family as a whole. Steps 2–5 involve diagnosing the strengths and weaknesses of a family and developing a treatment plan. Step 6 is called "restructuring" and involves using change strategies to "transform" family relations. In addition to reframing, other interventions employed at this step might include directing, redirecting, or blocking communication; shifting family alliances; giving parents more control; building conflict resolution skills; developing behavior management skills; and fostering effective parenting skills.

In the early years of its implementation, three adaptations to BSFT were developed in order to better serve high-risk families. First, BSFT was adapted for use with an individual client in a family therapy framework. Szapocznik and colleagues (Szapocznik, Kurtines, Foote, Perez-Vidal, & Hervis, 1983, 1986) compared this adapted form of BSFT, termed "one-person family therapy," to traditional BSFT in 72 families with an adolescent between the ages of 12 and 17 who was currently abusing drugs. The treatments were equally effective in reducing substance use and behavior problems and improving family functioning.

One of the most troubling problems in treating families with adolescents with CP and/or substance abuse problems is that many of these families never become engaged in therapy (Robbins, Szapocznik, et al., 2003). To address this problem, a second adaptation of BSFT was designed. Specifically, a set of specialized engagement procedures for addressing treatment resistance was developed to add to the core BSFT intervention. These strategies include allying with the adolescent and asking the mother for permission to talk to the most "resistant" family member (Robbins, Szapocznik, et al., 2003). In order to test the value of these specialized engagement procedures, Szapocznik and colleagues (1988) assigned 108 families with adolescents with CP and/or substance use problems to either a BSFT-engagement-as-usual condition (the control group) or a BSFT-enhanced-engagement condition. Whereas only 42% of the families in the control condition were successfully engaged into treatment, 93%

of the families in the enhanced condition were engaged into treatment. Of these engaged cases, only 59% of the control families completed treatment, compared to 83% of the families in the enhanced-engagement group. Additional studies conducted by Szapocznik and colleagues have replicated and extended these findings (Coatsworth, Santisteban, McBride, & Szapocznik, 2001; Santisteban et al., 1996).

In order to better adapt BSFT to serve the immigration and acculturation needs of recent-immigrant Hispanic families, a psychoeducational intervention was developed based on BSFT principles. This intervention, called "bicultural effectiveness training," was compared to traditional BSFT in a sample of 41 Cuban American families of adolescents with behavior problems (Szapocznik et al., 1986). Both interventions led to improvements in adolescent problem behavior and family functioning.

Several clinical trials have also compared BSFT to alternative treatments. Szapocznik and colleagues (1989) compared BSFT to individual psychodynamic child-centered psychotherapy and a recreational control condition. The sample included 69 preadolescent boys (ages 6–11 years) with moderate behavioral and/or emotional problems. Family retention was significantly better in the two treatment conditions than in the recreation condition. Furthermore, both treatment conditions were equivalent in terms of the reduction in emotional and behavior problems. However, BSFT was more effective than child-centered psychotherapy at improving family functioning at the 1-year follow-up.

The efficacy of BSFT was also examined in a clinical trial in which 126 adolescents (ages 12–18, 77% male) with CP and/or substance use problems were assigned to BSFT or a control group condition (Santisteban et al., 2003). In the control condition, adolescents were in a group and were encouraged to discuss and solve problems among themselves with the guidance of a facilitator. Of the 126 families entered in the study, 79 families completed treatment. Youths receiving BSFT demonstrated significantly greater reductions in CP, socialized aggression, and delinquency (as assessed by parent report) than the control group did. BSFT was also more effective at reducing marijuana use than the control group (although there was no treatment effect with respect to alcohol use), and families in the BSFT group also demonstrated significantly more improvement in observer ratings and self-reports of family functioning.

PROBLEM-SOLVING COMMUNICATION TRAINING

PSCT (Robin & Foster, 1989) is an intervention for adolescents with mild to moderate CP that directly addresses family members' discussions of conflict situations (Foster & Robin, 1998). This intervention is rooted in a behavioral–family systems model of parent–adolescent conflict, which posits that family conflict is driven by a combination of adolescent developmental factors, family skill deficits and structural difficulties, and problematic interaction patterns (Robin & Foster, 1989). Specifically, family members receive direct training in problem solving, communications skills, and cognitive restructuring in the context of sessions that focus on specific family problems (Foster & Robin, 1998; Robin & Foster, 1989). Less complex and anger-provoking issues are addressed before the family members proceed to more difficult issues.

Problem-solving skills are taught didactically, modeled, and rehearsed by family members. Basic problem-solving skills addressed include problem definition, generation of alternative solutions, decision making, and implementation of a solution. The therapist provides feedback on these skills and helps to guide feedback between family members. Generally, communication training is tailored to address communication deficits specific to the family. Communication problems are addressed when they occur in sessions, and instruction and modeling of more appropriate communication strategies is provided. The cognitive restructuring component of PSCT involves teaching techniques that can be used to change problematic perceptions, beliefs, and attributions. Reframing and relabeling techniques, and experiments designed to disconfirm unreasonable beliefs, are common therapy techniques for this intervention component. The complete treatment is generally conducted in 8–12 sessions. Homework is completed between sessions and involves communication and problem-solving practice (including implementing solutions generated during therapy).

The first studies evaluating PSCT used samples of families recruited through public notices advertising treatment for "families in conflict" (Foster, Prinz, & O'Leary, 1983; Robin, Kent,

O'Leary, Foster, & Prinz, 1977). Robin and colleagues (1977) trained 12 mother–adolescent dyads (the adolescents were 11–14 years old) with PSCT utilizing both hypothetical and real problems, and compared this group to 12 control dyads. Compared to the control group, improvements in observed communication were noted in the intervention group. However, reports of home conflict did not decrease. Foster and colleagues (1983) replicated and extended this first study by including fathers in the treatment and focusing solely on actual problems rather than hypothetical problems (n = 28 families divided into a control group, a PSCT group, and a group receiving "enhanced" PSCT [PSCT plus homework discussions and discussions of home use of communication skills]). In contrast to the previous study, results from the Foster et al. (1983) study showed no change in observed skills in the PSCT group or the enhanced-PSCT group compared to the control group. However, intervention groups did demonstrate significant improvements on questionnaire measures assessing family relationships. Gains were maintained at a 6- to 8-week follow-up. Although the enhanced-PSCT condition was designed to improve home generalization, there was no evidence that generalization in this group was superior than that of the PSCT-only intervention group.

Robin (1981) compared PSCT, an alternative family therapy (AFT) treatment, and a control condition in a sample of families with adolescents experiencing parent–adolescent conflict (n = 31 families, divided into the three groups). The AFT condition consisted of typical treatment that might be obtained from therapists with psychodynamic, family systems, or eclectic orientations. Compared to the control group, both treatment groups improved on observational measures of problem-solving communication skills and on self-report conflict measures. PSCT resulted in significantly larger improvements on observational measures of problem-solving behavior than did either AFT or the control condition. Gains on questionnaire measures were maintained at a 10-week follow-up.

More recently, Barkley, Edwards, Laneri, Fletcher, and Metevia (2001) compared 18 sessions of PSCT alone to a combined treatment composed of 9 sessions of behavior management training followed by 9 sessions of PSCT, in a sample of 97 families with adolescents

(ages 12–18 years) meeting criteria for both ADHD and ODD. In the discussion of results that follows, both therapies produced equivalent results except where noted. At the midpoint of treatment and at posttreatment, there were improvements on participant ratings of parent–adolescent conflicts (compared to pretreatment measures). Improvements in observational measures of communication and problem solving were evident at posttreatment but not at the midpoint of treatment, and these improvements were only significant for mothers. At a 2-month follow-up, improvements in observational measures were significant for fathers and adolescents but not for mothers. Only 23% of families showed significant improvements on a measure of "reliable change." However, a contrasting measure of "normalization" (i.e., the percentage of families that were brought into the "normal" range on outcome measures as a consequence of treatment) suggested that from 31% to 71% of families improved. It is notable that significantly more families dropped out of the PSCT-alone condition than the combined treatment condition.

MULTISYSTEMIC THERAPY

Although the family unit has clearly been a successful focus of interventions for youths with CP, adolescents with CP and their families commonly present with a range of problems that are demonstrated in multiple settings. This is especially the case with adolescents who display the early-starting manifestations of CP. Thus there is increasing recognition of the value of family interventions that have been shown to successfully address adolescents' CP behavior in multiple settings. MST (Henggeler & Lee, 2003; Henggeler et al., 1998) is a family-based intervention that has been extensively tested with adolescents with CP and multiproblem juveniles with serious offenses. The MST approach to treating adolescents with CP emphasizes both the interactional nature of adolescent psychopathology and the role of the multiple systems in which an adolescent is embedded, such as the family, school, and peer group (Henggeler & Borduin, 1990; Henggeler et al., 1998). The family is viewed as a core focus of the intervention. Assessment and treatment are concerned with the adolescent as an individual, his or her role in the various systems, and the interrelationships among those systems. Therapists intervene at one or more levels as required, and employ various therapy approaches (e.g., family therapy, school consultation, peer intervention strategies, marital therapy, and/or individual therapy). Treatment techniques are similarly wide-ranging, and may include traditional family therapy procedures (e.g., paradoxical intent) as well as behavioral and cognitive-behavioral techniques (e.g., reinforcement, contingency contracting, self-instructions) (Schoenwald, Henggeler, Pickrel, & Cunningham, 1996). Clinicians are guided by a set of nine treatment principles (e.g., "Focus on systemic strengths," "Promote responsible behavior and decrease irresponsible behavior among family members," "Interventions should be developmentally appropriate") (Henggeler et al., 1998; Schoenwald, Brown, & Henggeler, 2000).

MST has been evaluated in multiple studies across problems, therapists, and settings (Henggeler et al., 1998; Henggeler & Lee, 2003; Schoenwald et al., 2000). Most of the evaluations of MST have been conducted with samples of offending juveniles (often with chronic and/or violent offenses), although the efficacy of MST has also been investigated for adolescents with sexual offenses, offending juveniles who meet criteria for substance abuse or dependence, youths presenting with psychiatric emergencies, and youths who have been physically abused. MST has been shown to be generally efficacious in treating these youth populations (including minority populations; see Borduin et al., 1995; Henggeler, Melton, & Smith, 1992; Henggeler, Pickrel, & Brondino, 1999, for results indicating that MST outcomes are not moderated by race). However, results regarding the effectiveness of MST in broader community applications (i.e., using community therapists rather than graduate student therapists supervised by program developers) are less robust.

In an initial examination of MST's efficacy, Henggeler and colleagues (1986) conducted an evaluation of MST with inner-city delinquent adolescents, most of whom had repeat offenses, and their families ($n = 57$). At the conclusion of treatment, parents in the MST condition reported fewer CP behaviors, whereas parents of adolescents in an alternative mental health services condition ($n = 23$) and in the normative control condition ($n = 44$) reported no change. Families in the MST condition had also improved at posttreatment on several observational measures of family interaction,

whereas the families in the alternative treatment condition either did not change or deteriorated on those measures from pretreatment to posttreatment.

Henggeler and colleagues (1992) assessed the efficacy of MST in a sample of 84 juveniles with violent, chronic offenses (mean age = 15.2 years). The juveniles were randomly assigned to receive either MST or "usual services" through the Department of Youth Services. One year following referral, youths whose families had participated in MST reported fewer CP behaviors and were less likely to have been arrested or incarcerated than youths in the comparison group. Families who received MST also reported greater cohesion and less peer aggression than families in the comparison group. In a follow-up study conducted 2.4 years after referral (Henggeler, Melton, Smith, Schoenwald, & Hanley, 1993), survival analyses indicated that MST continued to be the superior treatment: 39% of the MST group had not been rearrested, compared to 20% of the comparison group.

In a second randomized trial with 200 seriously delinquent adolescents (mean age = 15) (Borduin et al., 1995), youths were assigned to MST or a treatment-as-usual condition that consisted of community individual therapy. At the end of treatment, the MST group demonstrated decreased CP, decreased parent psychopathology, and improved parent–youth interaction, whereas the treatment-as-usual group either showed no improvement or grew worse on these measures. In a 4-year follow-up, adolescents in the MST group had much lower rates of rearrest (26%, compared to 71% in the treatment-as-usual group), and those adolescents who were rearrested were arrested less often and for less serious and violent offenses than adolescents in the treatment-as-usual group. A recently published long-term follow-up study (Schaeffer & Borduin, 2005) examined arrest and incarceration data from 176 of the participants in the original study approximately 13.7 years after the intervention (mean follow-up age = 28.8 years). Intervention participants had significantly lower recidivism rates (50%, compared to 81% in the treatment-as-usual group), 54% fewer arrests, and 57% fewer days in adult detention facilities.

In an application of MST to a sample of offending juveniles with substance abuse or dependence, youths were randomly assigned to

MST or community services as usual, consisting of outpatient substance use treatment (Henggeler et al., 1999). Compared to the youths receiving community services as usual, the youths receiving MST had higher treatment completion (Henggeler, Pickrel, Brondino, & Crouch, 1996) and increased mainstream school attendance (Brown, Henggeler, Schoenwald, Brondino, & Pickrel, 1999). Treatment with MST also resulted in cost savings compared to treatment with community services as usual (Schoenwald, Ward, Henggeler, Pickrel, & Patel, 1996). Although significant treatment effects for substance abuse were reported at posttreatment, they were not maintained at a 6-month follow-up (Henggeler et al., 1999). A 4-year follow-up revealed significant reductions in aggressive criminal behavior (Henggeler, Clingempeel, Brondino, & Pickrel, 2002). Findings in terms of long-term reductions in illicit drug use were mixed. Although biological indices of drug use (i.e., urine and head hair samples) indicated the superiority of MST, self-report measures did not distinguish MST from community services as usual.

A cross-cultural evaluation of MST has also recently been completed in Norway (Ogden & Halliday-Boykins, 2004). Male and female adolescents (n = 100; mean age = 15.0 years) with serious antisocial behavior were randomly assigned to MST or treatment as usual (i.e., child welfare services). At posttreatment, MST was more effective than treatment as usual at reducing internalizing and externalizing behaviors and out-of-home placements. Compared to treatment as usual, MST also led to higher youth social competence, and MST families were more satisfied with treatment.

However, not all outcome research on MST has supported its effectiveness. Leschied and Cunningham (2002; Cunningham, 2002) conducted a carefully designed multisite effectiveness trial of MST, using teams of community therapists at four sites in Ontario, Canada. Across the sites, 409 youths (largely on probation and with court referrals; mean age = 14.6 years) and their families participated in the study, with half of the youths receiving community treatment as usual and half receiving MST. According to the currently available follow-up data (collected at 6 months and 1, 2, and 3 years), the MST group and the treatment as usual group were not statistically distinguishable on any outcome measure of offending (e.g., convictions, prosecutions, time before a first conviction, time to first custody admission, overall incarceration rate, length of sentence). Important caveats for these results include the fact that not all subjects had serious or chronic offenses (unlike most of the other MST studies). Furthermore, broader outcome measures (e.g., school completion, need for residential treatment) were not explored, and treatment fidelity was not specifically examined (Cunningham, 2002). Finally, collection and analysis of longer-term outcome data are still underway.

A meta-analysis of MST conducted by Curtis, Ronan, and Borduin (2004) may shed some light on discrepant findings related to the efficacy and effectiveness of MST. Examining seven MST treatment studies (but not including the ongoing Canadian study conducted by Leschied & Cunningham [2002; Cunningham, 2002]), Curtis and colleagues found that overall, youths and their families treated with MST were functioning better and offending less than 70% of their counterparts who received alternative treatments. These treatment effects were sustained for up to 4 years. MST demonstrated larger effects on measures of family relations than on peer measures or individual measures. However, Henggeler (2004) notes that the most significant finding from this meta-analysis demonstrated that treatment effect size was moderated by differences in study conditions (i.e., efficacy trials with MST developers as clinical supervisors and graduate student therapists had ES = 0.81 on average, while community effectiveness trials had much lower effect sizes [ES = 0.26]). Henggeler also indicates that the results underlined the importance of (1) conducting research on optimizing treatment transportability, and (2) considering factors that may influence effectiveness in real-world settings during efficacy trials (e.g., site characteristics, funding, organizational structure).

The Aos and colleagues (2004) cost–benefit analysis suggested that MST saved taxpayers approximately $9,316 per participant in the program. A cost-efficiency analysis for the study conducted by Leschied and Cunningham (2002) is also planned, but results are not available at this time (Cunningham, 2002).

Skills Training Approaches

Several systematic programs of research have evaluated skills training programs for children and adolescents with CP (see reviews and meta-analyses by Bennett & Gibbons, 2000; Lösel & Beelmann, 2003; Nangle, Erdley, Carpenter, & Newman, 2002; Taylor, Eddy, & Biglan, 1999). Although the particular foci of these programs may vary, they share an emphasis on remediating or changing skill deficiencies and dysfunctions displayed by youths with CP. The historical evolution of this research has followed a path from early emphasis on the behavioral aspects of social skills to a later emphasis on the cognitive aspects of social/interpersonal behavior; the most recent emphasis has been on comprehensive, multicomponent skills training programs. As the interventions have become more complex, so too have the theoretical models underpinning these interventions. The following is a brief overview of some of the current major skills training models of intervention for youths with CP.

Social Skills Training Programs

One of the first skills-based models of intervention for youths with CP was social skills training. As noted above, youths with CP often evidence problematic peer relations (including involvement with deviant peer groups) and display social skills deficits. Theoretical models underpinning social skills training have emphasized that youths who display such skill deficits will engage in CP behavior in order to secure rewards from the social environment. Therefore, direct training in social skills was hypothesized to be a potentially viable treatment method for these youths. Social skills training typically involves modeling, role playing, coaching and practice, feedback, and positive reinforcement.

One of the first evaluations of a social skills training approach was the well-designed investigation reported by Spence and Marzillier (1981), in which 76 male delinquents (ages 10–16) were randomly assigned to a social skills training group, an attention placebo group, or a no-treatment group. The social skills training program included 12 one-hour sessions with youths in groups of four. Training procedures included instructions, discussion, live and videotaped modeling, role plays, videotaped feedback, social reinforcement, and homework tasks. Skills taught were individually tailored to each adolescent, based on a needs assessment. Results of both multiple-baseline-across-behaviors and group comparison designs indicated specific improvements in many indi-

vidual social skills on the analogue assessment tests for the social skills training group, but not for the attention placebo or no-treatment control groups. Furthermore, these improvements were maintained at a 3-month follow-up assessment. However, there was no evidence of generalized differential changes in the following: staff ratings of social skills; self-report of social problems; observer ratings of friendliness, social anxiety, social skills, and employability; social workers' ratings of improvements in family work, school, and social relationships; self-report of delinquent offenses; or police convictions.

Subsequent studies of youths with CP have also found positive effects for social skills training. Michelson and colleagues (1983), studying a clinical population of 61 boys (ages 8–12 years) with CP, compared social skills training, interpersonal problem solving, and a nondirective control condition. Using a comprehensive assessment strategy, the study indicated that the social skills and interpersonal problem-solving treatments resulted in significant changes on parent, teacher, and self-report ratings, and on peer sociometric ratings at posttreatment. At the 1-year follow-up, the social skills treatment group maintained gains and continued to show modest improvement, whereas the other two groups manifested significant declines. Bierman and her colleagues (Bierman, 1989; Bierman, Miller, & Staub, 1987) engaged aggressive/rejected boys in grades 1–3 and competent peers in enjoyable activities, and provided individual and group reinforcement, coaching, and shaping of social skills. Following a 10-session program, these investigators reported reduced CP behavior and improved peer acceptance at a 1-year follow-up.

Cognitive-Behavioral Skills Training

Several of the programs of skills-based intervention research have been based on cognitive models of psychopathology in youths, which began to gain prominence after the earlier models that focused more exclusively on behavior (e.g., social skills). One cognitive model evolved quite directly from social skills training approaches. It was hypothesized that social skills deficits were at least partially driven by immaturity in moral reasoning and judgment (Chandler & Moran, 1990; Gregg, Gibbs, & Basinger, 1994; Nelson, Smith, &

Dodd, 1990). Therefore, direct training in moral reasoning was suggested as a potentially viable treatment method. Two studies found that higher levels of moral reasoning could be facilitated by relatively brief (8- to 20-session) discussion groups composed of behavior-disordered (Arbuthnot & Gordon, 1986) or incarcerated delinquent (Gibbs, Arnold, Ahlborn, & Cheesman, 1984) adolescents. However, only the Arbuthnot and Gordon study included measures of behavioral functioning to assess whether changes in moral reasoning were associated with behavior change. Following participation in a "moral dilemma discussion group" that met for 45 minutes per week over 16–20 weeks in the school, adolescents with CP had fewer referrals to the principal for disciplinary reasons, were less tardy, had higher grades in the humanities and social sciences, and had fewer police or court contacts than adolescents in a no-treatment control condition. At a 1-year follow-up, these between-group differences were still evident, although both groups had virtually eliminated any police or court contacts. It should also be noted that there were no differences between the groups on teacher ratings of the adolescents' behavior, either at posttreatment or at the 1-year follow-up.

Other studies using this approach have shown that while intervention may stimulate more mature moral judgment, the reduction of CP behavior does not necessarily follow (Gibbs et al., 1984; Power, Higgins, & Kohlberg, 1989). Interestingly, the Arbuthnot and Gordon (1986) study, which did find positive changes on indices of CP behavior, also included techniques to develop social skills. Insofar as the Arbuthnot and Gordon intervention included such techniques, it may be that the singular results in terms of changes in indices of CP may be mainly attributable to the social skills training rather than the moral reasoning component.

Somewhat more comprehensive cognitive models for skills deficits have been articulated most forcefully by Kendall (1985, 1991; Kendall & MacDonald, 1993) and by Dodge and his associates in the latter's social information-processing model of social competence in children (Crick & Dodge, 1994; Dodge, 2003). A fundamental assumption of these models is that when youths with CP encounter an anger- or frustration-arousing event (often an interpersonal interaction), their emotional, phys-iological, and behavioral reactions are determined by their cognitive perceptions and appraisals of that event, rather than by the event itself. Intervening at the level of these cognitive processes then becomes the most important focus of treatment (e.g., Guerra & Slaby, 1990; Hudley & Graham, 1993). Evidence supporting these more complex cognitive models indicates that youths with CP appear to display both deficiencies (a lack or insufficient amount of cognitive activity in situations in which this would be useful) and distortions (active but maladaptive cognitive content and processes) in their cognitive functioning (Crick & Dodge, 1994; Kendall, 1991; Kendall & MacDonald, 1993).

Guerra and Slaby (1990) developed and evaluated a 12-session program based on Dodge's (1986) social information-processing model and targeted male and female adolescents incarcerated for aggressive offenses. In this program, adolescents learned social problem-solving skills, addressed and modified beliefs supporting a broad and extensive use of aggression as a legitimate activity, and learned cognitive self-control skills to control impulsive responding. Relative to an attention placebo control group, the aggressive adolescents who received treatment showed greater social problem-solving skills, greater reductions in some beliefs associated with aggression, and greater reductions on staff ratings of aggressive, impulsive, and inflexible behavior. In addition, posttreatment aggression was related to change in cognitive factors. However, no differences were noted between groups on recidivism rates 24 months after release from the institution, although there seemed to be a trend toward lower recidivism for those who received the active treatment.

Kendall and colleagues (1990) evaluated a 20-session cognitive-behavioral treatment program also anchored in the cognitive model of youth psychopathology described above and based on the Kendall and Braswell (1985, 1993) treatment manual. The program was implemented with 6- to 13-year-old youths who had been psychiatrically hospitalized and formally diagnosed with CD. Cognitive-behavioral treatment was compared to supportive and insight-oriented therapy, commonly used in psychiatric hospitals, in a cross-over design. Results indicated the superiority of cognitive-behavioral treatment on measured teacher ratings of self-control and prosocial behavior, and self-report of perceived social competence. However, not all measures evidenced gains. Nevertheless, the difference between the percentage of children who moved from the deviant range to within the nondeviant range of behavior was significantly higher for the cognitive-behavioral program, supporting the greater clinical significance of this treatment. In a similar study with psychiatrically hospitalized inpatient children, Kolko, Loar, and Sturnick (1990) found improvements in dimensions of children's assertiveness, staff sociometric ratings, role-play performances, and *in vivo* behavioral observations of individual social skills for children who received social-cognitive skills training, relative to children receiving an activity group.

PROBLEM-SOLVING SKILLS TRAINING

Another line of programmatic skills-based research heavily influenced by the cognitive-behavioral model is that of Kazdin and his colleagues. These authors have developed a cognitive-behavioral skills training program (problem-solving skills training, or PSST), which they combine with a behavioral parent training approach (parent management training, or PMT) (see Kazdin, 2003, for a review) to treat preadolescent children (i.e., ages 7–13) with CD. PSST emphasizes teaching skills related to the latter stages of the information-processing model (skills for problem identification, solution generation and evaluation, solution selection, and enactment) and utilizes skills training and *in vivo* practice techniques. PSST is administered individually over 20 sessions, each of which lasts approximately 45–50 minutes. PMT is a traditional behavioral parent training approach, focusing on the parent as the agent of change and clearly defining child target behaviors; it uses role plays of parent behavior, homework, monitoring, and reinforcement techniques. PMT is administered individually over approximately 15 sessions, with each session lasting 1.5–2 hours. When these two protocols are combined, procedures are individualized to address a particular family's structure and needs (e.g., single- or dual-parent status, number of children in the home, parents' work schedule).

In a first evaluation of PSST alone (Kazdin, Esveldt-Dawson, French, & Unis, 1987b), 56 children (ages 7–13) who were inpatients on a psychiatric unit were randomly assigned to PSST, a nondirective relationship therapy condition, or an attention placebo control condition. Parent and teacher ratings on both behavior problem and social adjustment scales were collected at pre- and posttreatment and at a 1-year follow-up. PSST demonstrated a clear superiority over the relationship therapy and attention placebo control conditions on both parent and teacher ratings at posttreatment and the 1-year follow-up. Children in the PSST condition were also more likely to move to within or near the normative range on these measures, although it is important to note that most of the children in this group were still outside this range on measures of behavior problems in the home and school. Kazdin and colleagues (1989) reported no difference in 1-year follow-up effects obtained from PSST with or without *in vivo* practice in a mixed sample of inpatient and outpatient children. Children who received client-centered relationship therapy did not improve. Thus PSST seems to produce improvements in children with serious, aggressive CP, as well as in children with mild to moderate CP treated on an outpatient basis.

A second study compared the effects of combined PSST and PMT to those of nondirective relationship therapy (Kazdin, Esveldt-Dawson, French, & Unis, 1987a) in an inpatient sample of children ages 7–12. At posttreatment and 1-year follow-up, children in the combined condition showed significantly less aggression and externalizing behavior at home and school, as well as demonstrating improved prosocial behavior and improvements in overall adjustment.

Kazdin and colleagues (1992) evaluated the unique and combined effects of PSST and PMT. At 1-year follow-up, the combined treatment was more effective than either one alone. Children in the combined group fell within the normative range of CP behavior according to parent report; all treatment groups were rated in the normative range by teacher report. In a further analysis of the data from this study, Kazdin and Wassell (2000b) found that in addition to improvements in child functioning, several aspects of family life improved (quality of family relationships, functioning of the family as a system, and perceived social support). Parent functioning also improved (i.e., decreases in depression, overall symptoms, and stress).

More recently, Kazdin and Whitley (2003) have developed an adjunctive therapy for PSST that is designed to address parent stress during treatment. This adjunct, parent problem solving (PPS), consists of five sessions in which a therapist helps a parent to develop and implement problem-solving skills to better cope with the parent's identified sources of stress. A combined PSST and PMT condition was compared to a condition with these two treatments plus the PPS adjunct in 127 children (ages 6–14) and their families referred for treatment because of child aggressive and antisocial behavior. Although both groups improved with treatment, the inclusion of the PPS adjunct was related to a reduction in barriers to treatment participation and to higher levels of therapeutic change.

INTERVENTIONS FOR ANGER MANAGEMENT

A number of skills training interventions have been specifically designed to address issues with anger control. Sukhodolsky, Kassinove, and Gorman (2004) conducted a meta-analysis to examine intervention results for anger-related problems. This analysis involved 50 studies (21 published and 19 unpublished) that used cognitive-behavioral therapy to treat anger in children and adolescents. Youth age ranged from 7 to 17.2 years (mean age = 12.5). In all, there were 51 treatment versus control comparisons, and approximately 25 of these involved adolescents. Overall, the mean ES for the cognitive-behavioral interventions was in the medium range (ES = 0.67). Age of subjects in the studies and the magnitude of ES were not correlated. However, the authors conducted a qualitative examination of ES means for the first age quartile and the fourth age quartile, and found a 0.2 increase in ES for the older age group. Skills training, problem-solving, and multimodal interventions were more effective than affective education. Skills training and multimodal interventions were particularly effective in reducing aggressive behavior and improving social skills. Problem-solving interventions were more effective in reducing youths' self-reports of anger. Specific treatment techniques involving modeling, feedback, and homework were related to larger ES.

An example of a well-validated anger control program is that developed by Lochman and his colleagues. Based originally on Novaco's (1978) model of anger arousal and subsequently heavily influenced by Dodge's (1986; Crick & Dodge, 1994) social information-processing model, this treatment program has evolved from a 12-session school-based program called Anger Coping (Lochman, Lampron, Gemmer, & Harris, 1987) to a 33-session program called Coping Power (the latter is also supplemented by a parent training intervention) (Lochman & Wells, 1996). Elementary-school-age children with CP meet once a week in pull-out groups of six during the school day and participate in sessions that have specific goals, objectives, and exercises. Although it is designed for use in school, the program can be implemented in a clinic setting as well.

The exercises in the Anger Coping and Coping Power interventions are designed to provide children with practice in cognitive and behavioral skills associated with each stage of the social information-processing model. Children practice reviewing examples of social encounters and discussing social cues and possible motives of people in the situations. As weeks go by, they receive *in vivo* practice in problem-solving elements: identifying problems, generating many possible solutions to problems, and using prosocial judgment criteria to evaluate solutions. They role-play enactments of behavioral responses to social situations and receive reinforcement and feedback. Children also receive training in strategies for increasing awareness of feelings and physiological states.

After skills for managing anger arousal in problem situations are practiced, exercises designed to induce affective arousal in the groups are introduced. Children are supported in the use of anger control strategies and anger-reducing self-talk. In the Coping Power intervention (Lochman & Wells, 1996), sessions have been expanded in number and complexity to focus on an expanded range of skills and social contexts that children must negotiate (e.g., family interactions, sibling interactions, organization skills for homework completion).

Lochman and colleagues have conducted a series of studies aimed at evaluating the effects of the Anger Coping program for boys with CP (Lochman, 1985; Lochman, Burch, Curry, & Lampron, 1984; Lochman & Curry, 1986; Lochman, Nelson, & Sims, 1981). In their first uncontrolled study (Lochman et al., 1981), 12 children who participated in the cognitive-behavioral intervention showed significant decreases from pre- to posttreatment on teacher ratings of aggressiveness in the classroom and increases in on-task behavior. The children tended to have fewer acting-out behaviors on a teacher-completed behavior rating scale. A subsequent controlled evaluation (Lochman et al., 1984) confirmed that the cognitive-behavioral program was more effective than either goal setting alone or no treatment in reducing disruptive, aggressive, and off-task behavior in the classroom. Also, the addition of a goal-setting strategy (in which children set daily behavioral goals that were monitored and reinforced by their teachers) to the cognitive-behavioral intervention resulted in greater reductions in aggressive behavior than did the cognitive-behavioral intervention alone. In a subsequent study looking at the parameters of treatment, Lochman (1985) found that longer-duration treatment (18 sessions) produced more significant changes in classroom behavior than did a 12-session intervention.

Maintenance effects of the Anger Coping intervention have also been examined. Lochman and Lampron (1988) examined a subsample of boys in the original Lochman and colleagues (1984) study. Maintenance effects were examined on independently observed classroom behavior at a 7-month follow-up. Boys with CP who had received the Anger Coping intervention had significantly higher levels of on-task behavior and lower levels of passive off-task behavior than untreated controls. However, significant posttreatment reductions in disruptive off-task behavior were not maintained at the 7-month follow-up.

Subsequently, Lochman (1992) examined the 3-year follow-up effects of the Anger Coping intervention. Follow-up effects were most evident on substance use outcomes. Treated boys with CP had significantly lower levels of drug and alcohol use than untreated boys with CP; furthermore, the treated boys' level of substance use was within the level displayed by typical boys. Three-year maintenance effects were not observed for independently observed classroom behavior except for boys who had received booster sessions in the second year, who did show lower levels of off-task behavior. These booster session effects have served as part of the rationale for extending the Anger Coping program to its current iteration (Coping Power), which covers 33 sessions over 2 school years.

Lochman and Wells (1996) have examined the effects of the Coping Power program, which, in addition to being a longer and more extensive program than Anger Coping, also includes a par-

ent intervention component involving 16 group parent training sessions over the same 2-year period. Parent sessions are coordinated with child sessions so that, in addition to addressing parenting skills, parents also learn material that will help them support the skills learned by children in their group sessions. In a study of the Coping Power program, Lochman and Wells (2004) randomly assigned at-risk aggressive boys to receive the child component alone, both the child and parent components, or a control (no-intervention) condition. Coping Power produced lower rates of covert delinquent behavior and of parent-rated substance use 1 year after the intervention than did the control condition. These effects were most apparent for the combined child and parent condition.

Lochman and Wells (2002, 2003) have examined the interaction of the Coping Power intervention (both child and parent components) with a universal teacher and parent intervention offered to all teachers and parents of children in intervention classrooms. When compared to a no-treatment control, all three interventions (Coping Power alone, universal intervention alone, and the combination of Coping Power and the universal intervention) resulted in lower rates of substance use, as well as positive effects on children's social competence and self-regulation and on parents' parenting skills at postintervention (Lochman & Wells, 2002). A subsequent 1-year follow-up study (Lochman & Wells, 2002) demonstrated that the earlier-reported postintervention improvement led to preventive effects on substance use for the older children in the sample (13.4 years or older) and for moderate-risk children.

Skills Training Based on a Coping–Competence Model

Another line of theoretically driven programmatic intervention research has been reported by Blechman, Prinz, and Dumas (Blechman, 1996; Blechman, Dumas, & Prinz, 1994; Prinz, Blechman, & Dumas, 1994). The coping–competence model organizes the empirically identified correlates of a high-risk developmental trajectory into first-order and second-order constructs, and specifies interdependent pathways of influence among surface characteristics of individuals, risk–protection variables, competence, and life outcomes (Blechman, Prinz, & Dumas, 1995).

The program is a school-based intervention designed to support prosocial coping (rather than to remediate skills deficits) with emotional, social, and achievement challenges faced by high-risk *and* competent youths. The program includes competent, low-risk youths in groups with highly aggressive youths in order to provide role models in prosocial coping. Without any public labeling, youths identified as competent and aggressive are invited to participate in self-management "clubs." The primary goal of self-management club meetings is to encourage prosocial coping through "information exchange," in which children are encouraged to share information about controllable and uncontrollable challenges in their lives. Information exchange centers around describing situations, sharing thoughts and feelings, and cooperating in discussing possible coping mechanisms (Blechman et al., 1994). Ideally, families are engaged in a process that begins with home visits and proceeds to parent training with parents of both high-risk and competent youths.

Prinz and colleagues (1994) evaluated the Peer Coping Skills (PCS) training program based on the model (with the exception that no family intervention was provided in this study) described above with 100 first- to third-grade children with and without CP. The children were compared to 96 similarly identified children who received minimal classroom intervention. In each PCS intervention group, half of the children engaged in CP and half did not. After 22 sessions of intervention (posttreatment) and at a 6-month follow-up, children in the PCS group (both those with and without CP) significantly improved in prosocial coping via information exchange, and their social skills improved compared to control subjects who showed no improvement. For children with CP, PCS training produced a significant reduction in teacher-rated aggression in comparison to controls, although the mean level of aggression at posttreatment was still in the clinical range. Peer ratings of social acceptance did not show significant change. No iatrogenic effects were noted on the children without CP by virtue of their being in groups with children with CP. In fact, as noted earlier, the children with CP also showed significant improvements in prosocial coping, compared to their counterparts who did not participate in the PCS intervention (Prinz et al., 1994).

More recently, Rohde, Jorgensen, Seeley, and Mace (2004) have also developed an intervention for youths with CP focused on the enhancement of coping skills. The Coping Course is a group intervention designed to foster coping and problem-solving skills in incarcerated youths; it is a modified version of the Adolescent Coping with Depression Course (Clarke, Lewinsohn, & Hops, 1990), which was not effective in reducing CP in youths with comorbid depression and CD (Rohde, Clarke, Mace, Jorgensen, & Seeley, 2004). The Coping Course intervention focuses on developing coping skills to control a range of negative emotions (e.g., sadness, anger) and includes didactic instruction, handouts, structured learning tasks, and homework assignments. In a pilot evaluation of this program, 76 incarcerated male adolescents were assigned to either the Coping Course or usual care (e.g., group drug/alcohol treatment, group treatment for sex offenses). Compared to youths receiving usual care, the youths in the Coping Course program had reduced self-reported externalizing problems and suicide proneness, as well as increased self-esteem.

Multicomponent Skills Training

Because single-component programs may produce limited results, some investigators have combined different skills training interventions into multicomponent treatment approaches. Goldstein and his colleagues have developed one such approach—Aggression Replacement Training (ART; Goldstein, Glick, & Gibbs, 1998; Goldstein, Glick, Reiner, Zimmerman, & Coultry, 1986), which originally combined interventions designed to enhance social skills (structured learning training; Goldstein & Pentz, 1984), anger control (anger control training; Feindler, Marriott, & Iwata, 1984), and moral reasoning (moral education) in a 10-week curriculum. This was subsequently expanded to a 50-skill curriculum (Goldstein & Glick, 1994).

Preliminary evaluations in two juvenile correctional facilities suggested differential improvements on analogue measures of social skills (and sometimes on the moral development measure) for adolescent males who participated in ART as opposed to those in either a brief-instruction or a no-treatment control group (Glick & Goldstein, 1987). Subsequent evaluations in community settings employing

ART with adolescents with CP showed evidence of significantly improved skills across a variety of domains targeted in treatment (Goldstein, Glick, Irwin, McCartney, & Rubama, 1989). Evidence for generalization to the community after release was limited to global ratings completed by probation officers in initial studies. In subsequent reports, 3-month rearrest data showed significantly fewer arrests for youths receiving ART (Goldstein & Glick, 1994). At a 1-year follow-up, social workers rated youths who had received ART more highly on various indices of adjustment.

Independent investigators have also conducted evaluations of ART (as reported by Goldstein et al., 1998). Coleman, Pfeiffer, and Oakland (1991) evaluated the effectiveness of a 10-week ART program for behaviorally disordered adolescents in a residential treatment center. Improvements in skills knowledge were evident, but there were not significant changes in overt skill behaviors. However, Jones (1990) compared ART to moral education and a no-treatment control in a sample of aggressive male high school students in Brisbane, Australia, and found that students in the ART program showed significant decreases in aggressive behavior and significant improvements in coping behaviors and social skills.

Taken together, this body of research suggests that ART does have the potential for facilitating improvement across a broad array of skills deficits, and may also be useful for reducing recidivism rates in offending adolescents with CP. When analyzed as part of the Aos and colleagues (2004) cost–benefit study, ART was shown to be cost-effective as well. It saved taxpayers between approximately $8,805 (in Washington State) and $14,846 (excluding Washington State) per participant in the program.

Another multicomponent skills training approach that integrates methods from ART with an approach based on the concept of "positive peer culture" has been described by Gibbs, Potter, Barriga, and Liau (1996). This treatment model, called EQUIP, combines social skills training, moral reasoning, and problem solving in group meetings that emphasize positive peer culture. Behavioral methods such as self-monitoring in daily homework assignments are also included. The effectiveness of EQUIP has been evaluated in a controlled outcome study with 15- to 18-year-old incarcerated males (Leeman, Gibbs, & Fuller, 1993). The experimental condition was compared to both no-treatment and attention placebo (a brief motivational induction) control conditions. Outcome measures assessed institution and postrelease conduct, as well as mediating processes of social skills and moral judgment. Improvements in institutional conduct were significant for the EQUIP group relative to the control groups in terms of self-reported misconduct, staff-filed incident reports, and unexcused absences from schools. Twelve months after subjects' release from the institution, the recidivism rate for EQUIP participants remained low and stable (15%), whereas the likelihood of recidivism for untreated subjects (41%) climbed. Social skills also improved significantly for EQUIP participants and were significantly correlated with self-reported improvements in institutional conduct. Both the ART and the EQUIP studies of intervention efficacy suggest that multicomponent skills training programs are more effective than single-component programs and may result in more significant long-term effects as well.

Finally, Webster-Stratton (Webster-Stratton, 2000; Webster-Stratton & Reid, 2003) has also developed a multicomponent skills training intervention for early conduct problems (Dinosaur School). Please refer to the earlier section on family-based interventions with preadolescents for descriptions of this program.

Additional Considerations

Although skills training approaches are quite commonly used to treat CP in youths, reviews of the literature in this area indicate that there is generally weak empirical support for the use of skills training as an isolated intervention for the treatment of serious CP (Taylor et al., 1999). Specifically, Taylor and colleagues (1999) reviewed several of the interventions discussed above and concluded that although they appeared to result in short-term improvements for minor CP, there was little empirical evidence for longer-term improvements in more serious CP (e.g., violence, property damage, parole violations). In addition, Bennett and Gibbons (2000) conducted a meta-analysis of 30 skills training studies for children and adolescents, and generally found that skills training interventions resulted in a fairly small treatment effect (mean weighted ES = 0.23). However, it is notable that Bennett and Gibbons also identified a trend in the studies they evaluated suggesting that skills training may be more effective with older children and adolescents than with younger children. Finally, results from a cost-efficacy study provide some evidence that skills training may be useful even in adolescents with more serious CP as compared to other possible community treatments. Blechman, Maurice, Buecker, and Helberg (2000) found that a skills training program with offending juveniles was more cost-effective than a mentoring approach or a standard juvenile-diversion program. Specifically, the skills training program reduced the recidivism rate of juveniles in the study to 37% (vs. 51% and 46% for the other two programs, respectively), resulting in a cost savings of approximately $33,600 per 100 youths.

Clinicians who employ skills training interventions (or any group intervention component) with adolescents with CP must be aware of, and take steps to minimize, the possibility of iatrogenic effects for group-based approaches to treatment. (See a recent special issue of the *Journal of Abnormal Child Psychology* [2005, Vol. 33, Number 3] for an excellent discussion of this topic.) Dishion and colleagues (e.g., Dishion, McCord, & Poulin, 1999) have focused on this concern, citing evidence suggesting that the placement of high-risk adolescents in at least some peer group interventions may result in increases in both CP behavior and negative life outcomes, compared to control youths. For example, Poulin, Dishion, and Burraston (2001) demonstrated that increases in both teacher-reported delinquency and self-report of smoking were associated with participation in prevention-oriented groups of high-risk youths 3 years earlier. The putative mechanism of influence is so-called "deviancy training," in which youths receive group attention for engaging in various problem behaviors (Dishion, Spracklen, Andrews, & Patterson, 1996; Gifford-Smith, Dodge, Dishion, & McCord, 2005). These findings have led to the development and promotion of interventions that minimize the influence of groups of high-risk adolescent peers and involve the youngsters in conventional peer activities (e.g., sports teams, school clubs) with low-risk peers. New evidence suggests that iatrogenic effects may also occur with groups of younger children (Boxer, Guerra, Huesmann, & Morales, 2005; Hanish, Martin, Fabes, Leonard, & Herzog, 2005; Lavallee, Bierman, Nix, & Conduct Problems Prevention Research Group, 2005) and may be more prevalent in prevention programs than in treatment programs (Dishion & Dodge, 2005). Taken together, these findings send a clear message to clinicians working with children and adolescents at risk for CP. In some cases, alternatives to group treatment may need to be considered, and when group formats are deemed the best approach, specific steps should be taken to minimize the risk of unintended negative effects (see Dodge, Dishion, & Lansford, 2005, for suggested approaches).

Community-Based Programs

The systematic development and evaluation of community-based residential programs for aggressive and delinquent adolescents began over 35 years ago, arising from several national directives (e.g., Presidential Commission on Law Enforcement and the Administration of Justice, 1967) that highlighted the inhumane, expensive, and ineffective nature of traditional institutional programs. Since that time, numerous programs have been developed to address the challenges presented by offending juveniles who also often display other emotional or behavioral conditions.

Achievement Place/Teaching Family Model

The Achievement Place program (currently known as the Teaching Family Model, or TFM) was originally developed in 1967 and has become the prototypical community-based residential program for aggressive and delinquent adolescents. Each TFM group home is run by a young married couple, referred to as "teaching parents," who undergo a rigorous 1-year training program. While living in the group home, the adolescents, most of whom are adjudicated as delinquent, attend local schools and are involved in community activities. The primary treatment components of TFM include a multilevel point system, self-government procedures, social skills training, academic tutoring, and a home-based reinforcement system for monitoring school behavior. The average stay for a participant in the program is about 1 year (Kirigin, 1996).

In terms of effectiveness, the TFM approach appears to be more effective than comparison programs while the adolescents are active participants. Specifically, the developers of TFM compared TFM to other community-based programs (nearly all of which were group homes) and found that during treatment, a lower percentage of TFM participants engaged in offenses, and fewer offenses were recorded (Kirigin, Braukmann, Atwater, & Wolf, 1982). Independent evaluators (Weinrott, Jones, & Howard, 1982) found that participants in TFM showed slightly more academic improvement than participants in community-based comparison programs. However, once the adolescents complete treatment and leave the group home setting, these differences have generally been found to disappear (Kirigin, 1996). It is notable that results from a recent evaluation of TFM at Girls and Boys Town (Larzelere et al., 2001) suggest that some improvements in youth functioning are maintained at a 10-month follow-up. However, as this study did not include a control group, it is difficult to compare these results to those of youths in other types of treatment settings. In a meta-analytic study of intervention efficacy with offending juveniles (Lipsey, 1999; see "Issues in Intervention Effectiveness," below, for additional coverage of meta-analytic research), TFM produced consistently positive effects on recidivism (approximately 6-month follow-up) in populations of institutionalized youth, and was generally found to be more effective than a variety of behavioral programs and community residential placements. With respect to cost-effectiveness, TFM is cheaper than alternative group homes. However, both approaches are very expensive; only 45% of the adolescents complete treatment; and by 2–3 years later, there are few meaningful differences between treatment completers and dropouts (Weinrott et al., 1982).

A cross-cultural replication of TFM was conducted in the Netherlands (Slot, Jagers, & Dangel, 1993). Comparisons of pre- and posttreatment scores indicated that the 58 adolescents (ages 14–19 years) in the program showed improvements in social competence and decreases in delinquent behavior. An analysis of program costs indicated that the TFM program was about one-quarter as costly as placements in a Dutch correctional institute.

Multidimensional Treatment Foster Care

Treatment foster care models are seeing a proliferation in use and evaluation. In a meta-analytic review, Reddy and Pfeiffer (1997) analyzed 40 published studies encompassing 12,282 subjects that employed some kind of treatment foster care model for a variety of child and adolescent populations. There were large positive effects on increasing placement permanency of difficult-to-place and difficult-to-maintain youths and on improving the youths' social skills, and medium positive effects on reducing behavior problems, improving psychological adjustment, and reducing restrictiveness of postdischarge placement.

The therapeutic foster care model that has the greatest evidence of empirical support for youths with CP is Multidimensional Treatment Foster Care (MTFC), developed by Chamberlain and her colleagues at OSLC (e.g., Chamberlain, 1994, 2003; Chamberlain & Moore, 1998; Chamberlain & Reid, 1994, 1998; Eddy & Chamberlain, 2000). This model is based on previous intervention work at OSLC and was also influenced by the work of Hawkins and colleagues (Hawkins, 1989; Hawkins, Meadowcroft, Trout, & Luster, 1985), who were the first to use treatment foster care in community-based settings. The key components of MTFC include (1) recruitment and up to 20 hours of preservice training (which is both didactic and experiential) for foster parents in a social-learning-based parent training model; (2) ongoing case management, consisting of individualized consultation to foster parents, weekly group foster parent meetings, and 24-hour on-call services for crisis management and support to foster parents; (3) daily structure and telephone contact support; (4) school consultation, consisting of teaching foster parents school advocacy skills and setting up a home–school daily report card for each adolescent; (5) family therapy with biological parents (or relatives) to coordinate gradual transfer of care from the MTFC parents to the home, if possible; and (6) individual therapy for skills training in problem solving, anger management, educational issues, and other individual issues. A hallmark of the program is the provision of some adjunctive services that are individualized to meet the needs of youths and their families, similar to MST.

The MTFC program has been evaluated in a number of experimental trials that have supported its effectiveness (Chamberlain & Mihalic, 1998). In an early pilot study of the program, Chamberlain and Reid (1991) randomly assigned 19 adolescents with CP who had been discharged from the state hospital to either postdischarge MTFC or control treatment consisting of traditional community placements (e.g., group homes, training school). There were significantly greater reductions in PDR ratings of behavior problems at 3 months for MTFC youths compared to control subjects, and a trend for differences at 7 months. There was also a significantly shorter time from referral to placement for MTFC subjects, with associated cost savings. However, social competency and problem-solving skills did not improve for either group.

Another study was conducted with a sample of regular foster parents and the children placed in their care (Chamberlain, Moreland, & Reid, 1992). This study compared one group of foster parents who received the MTFC model of training and support plus a small increase in their monthly stipend to a control group of foster parents who received only the increased stipend. The enhanced MTFC group had increased foster parent retention rates, increased ability to manage child CP, decreased reports of child CP, and decreased number of disrupted placements over the 2-year study period.

In more recent work, Chamberlain and Reid (1998) randomly assigned 79 boys (ages 12–17), referred for out-of-home care due to chronic delinquency, to either MTFC or one of 11 group care placements that involved individual, group, and family therapy (Chamberlain & Reid, 1998; Fisher & Chamberlain, 2000). During the 1-year follow-up, significant differences were found in length of time in placement, runaway rates, arrest rates, days incarcerated, and self-reported delinquency, all in favor of MTFC. Two-year follow-up showed that, according to self-report, significantly more boys in the MTFC condition were working at legal jobs, had positive relationships with their parents, refrained from unprotected sex, and had less drug use. Four-year follow-up data showed that boys in MTFC continued to have significantly fewer arrests (Chamberlain, Fisher, & Moore, 2002). Family management skills and peer associations mediated the effect of MFTC on antisocial behavior and delinquency, accounting for approximately one-third of the variance in boys' subsequent antisocial behavior (Eddy & Chamberlain, 2000).

Chamberlain and colleagues (Chamberlain & Smith, 2003; Leve & Chamberlain, 2005) have also just completed a 5-year randomized trial of MTFC with 12- to 17-year-old females who had an average of 11 offenses prior to referral. Girls were randomly assigned to MTFC or treatment-as-usual settings (e.g., group home, hospital, inpatient drug and alcohol treatment). Preliminary 12-month follow-up data for 61 girls showed a greater decrease in arrests, and fewer days in the hospital for mental-health-related problems for girls treated with MTFC compared to girls receiving treatment as usual. Notably, however, girls in MTFC still reported participating in high-risk sexual activities and using alcohol and drugs at high rates. Chamberlain and colleagues (Chamberlain & Smith, 2003; Leve & Chamberlain, 2005) are currently conducting a study in which they have added components to MTFC to address these concerns.

With respect to the financial benefits of MTFC, the Aos and colleagues (2004) cost–benefit analysis estimated that the MTFC model saved taxpayers approximately $24,290 per participant in the program. In sum, these studies indicate that MTFC is an efficacious and cost-effective intervention for seriously delinquent and aggressive youths requiring out-of-home placement. Although the program is staff- and time-intensive, it still results in greater cost savings than traditional group home and residential placements.

Case Management Services

Case management is best described as a set of functions intended to mobilize, coordinate, and maintain the services and resources necessary to meet an individual's needs over time (Bloomquist & Schnell, 2002; Stroul, 1995). With regard to children with CP, case management services provide parents, foster parents, or caregivers the assistance they may require in accessing whatever support services that may be needed for the child. Case management can provide a critical function, since accessing the service system with its myriad venues, providers, payment requirements, and systemic barriers can prove daunting for many caregivers. As identified by Burns and her colleagues (1995), case management services optimally involve (1) assessment, to determine the strengths and needs of the child; (2) planning, to develop a service plan; (3) linking, a critical case management function of connecting the child and family with the services identified in steps 1 and 2; (4) advocacy, to help the family overcome the barriers to obtaining the needed services; and (5) support, to provide supportive services through the process.

Case management services are difficult to evaluate, because it is difficult to separate the effects of the various services provided from the effects of the case management process. Partly as a result of this, evidence for the effectiveness of case management services with children with CP is mixed. Results from the Fort Bragg project did not find positive effects associated with case management services (Bickman, Lambert, Andrade, & Penaloza, 2000). However, a project reported by Burns, Farmer, Angold, Costello, and Behar (1996) investigating case management services for 8- to 17-year-old youths, the majority of whom had CP, showed that such services resulted in fewer days in the hospital and greater parental satisfaction than services provided through primary mental health care. Such research defining and evaluating the most appropriate strategies for case management should continue to be done, because this is an approach that is currently used in many community mental health settings, and because the approach has face validity in assisting families to overcome barriers to effective utilization of services needed by youths with CP.

Day Treatment Programs

Another type of community-based intervention that falls at a more intermediate level of care is the day treatment program. Although these programs represent a wide array of services, we present the following description of a multi-component approach to day treatment with preadolescent children with CP presented by Kolko (1995). The program is oriented toward maintaining each child in the community; meeting for several hours per week; providing exposure to peer and staff role models and multimodal services (e.g., cognitive-behavioral skills training, contingency management, parent training, school consultation); addressing multiple clinical targets (e.g., children, parents, and teachers); and conducting routine weekly monitoring and follow-up. The program is conducted after school, on Saturday mornings, and during the summer. Children participating in the day treatment program improved with respect to in-program assessments of aggression and property destruction; however, noncompliance was not affected. There was some evidence for setting generalization to the home and to the school, based on parent and teacher reports. The children and parents both re-

ported high levels of consumer satisfaction with the program.

Grizenko, Papineau, and Sayegh (1993) reported that preadolescent children with CP who participated in their day treatment program reported greater gains on parental ratings of child measures of behavior (including CP) and child self-perception of adjustment, compared to a waiting-list control group. Peer, family, and academic functioning was not differentially affected by the intervention at the posttreatment assessment. By a 6-month follow-up, children who had participated in the day treatment program had improved significantly on all of the measures except academics.

School-Based Treatment

There is substantial empirical evidence that school systems vastly underserve the needs of school-age children with CP (Walker, Nishioka, Zeller, Severson, & Feil, 2000). Historically, these children were excluded from the definition of "emotional disturbance" by federal mandate, and therefore could not receive special education services. In addition, schools have a financial incentive not to certify these children as needing services, since they are then obligated to pay for the special education programs that might be needed.

In spite of historical weaknesses in identification of CP problems in schools, there is adequate reason to believe that the literature can provide useful guidelines for the treatment of children with CP in school settings. Although these children are often globally described as "disruptive," as "socially maladjusted," and as displaying "high rates of inappropriate behavior," an examination of the behaviors identified through FBA procedures that are the targets of treatment in these studies reveals such overt CP behaviors as noncompliance to teacher requests or classroom rules, disturbing others, aggression, tantrums, and excessive verbal outbursts. The few investigations that have dealt with covert CP behaviors in the school are described later in the chapter.

Even if CP behaviors are not occurring initially in the school setting, research on behavioral covariation and setting generality in behavioral treatment programs indicates that when such behaviors are treated in the clinic or home environment, similar behaviors in school may remain unchanged (e.g., Breiner & Forehand, 1981; Forehand et al., 1979); a behavioral contrast effect may occur, in which deviant school behaviors increase as home disruption decreases (e.g., Johnson, Bolstad, & Lobitz, 1976; Walker, Hops, & Johnson, 1975); or setting generalization may occur (e.g., Fellbaum, Daly, Forest, & Holland, 1985; McNeil et al., 1991). Because some children do not show generalization of positive treatment effects to the school setting when CP behavior is treated in the clinic or at home, it is necessary to monitor the school behavior of these children throughout and following treatment to ascertain whether interventions specific to the school setting are needed. It is also necessary to have an armamentarium of treatment strategies available for school intervention once the need for treatment is identified.

In this section of the chapter, we highlight some of the major types of psychosocial interventions that have been applied to overt CP behaviors in the school. A comprehensive review of the myriad intervention procedures that have been employed for these and related problems (such as academic achievement per se and peer relationship difficulties) is beyond the scope of this chapter. The reader is referred to Goldstein (1995), Pfiffner and Barkley (2006), and Walker and colleagues (2004).

Classroom Management Strategies

In their classic book on classroom behavior management strategies, O'Leary and O'Leary (1977) discuss the importance of teacher behavior in modifying disruptive classroom behavior of children. Many of the earliest studies in classroom behavior therapy focused on contingency arrangements in the interactions of teachers and students. For example, a number of studies have shown that teacher praise for appropriate behavior, especially when coupled with ignoring of inappropriate behaviors, can effectively reduce classroom disruption (Becker, Madsen, Arnold, & Thomas, 1967; Brown & Elliot, 1965). In these strategies, teachers are taught to notice instances of appropriate behavior that are the prosocial opposites of the child's target CP behaviors, and to praise and otherwise reward the child when prosocial behaviors occur. Although teachers often protest that "I routinely praise my students," naturalistic observation studies show that rates of positive teacher attention to prosocial behavior are surprisingly low, and may be insufficient for increasing and maintaining

the prosocial behavior of children with mild levels of CP who enter the classroom with problems in this domain (Martens & Hiralall, 1997; Strain, Lambert, Kerr, Stagg, & Lenkner, 1983; White, 1975). Walker and colleagues (2004) recommend that the ratio of teacher praise statements to criticisms be at least 4:1, and higher if possible. A technical manual on teacher praise that provides detailed guidelines on how to use this technique was developed for the Utah BEST Project (Reavis et al., 1996).

It is also important to note that studies with children engaging in more severe negative/aggressive behaviors have shown that praise alone can have a neutral or even negative effect (Walker et al., 2004), because of a long history of negative interactions with adults. Pairing of praise with other incentives such as points exchangeable with privileges will eventually increase the reinforcing value of praise alone (Walker et al., 2004).

Other elements of effective classroom management include the establishment of clear rules and directions; use of programmed instructional materials that pace the student's academic progress at his or her own rate; provision of positive and corrective feedback; use of classroom token economies; and, for disruptive behaviors that cannot be ignored, the use of reprimands, time out, and response cost procedures contingent upon the occurrence of CP behavior. Although some studies demonstrate that each of these procedures alone can exert control over CP behaviors (e.g., Proctor & Morgan, 1991), clinically significant changes are most likely to occur when treatment strategies are combined (Greenwood, Hops, Delquadri, & Guild, 1974; O'Leary, Becker, Evans, & Saudargas, 1969). In fact, results of a body of research indicate that combining positive and negative approaches to contingency management produces more powerful effects than either positive-alone or negative-alone approaches (e.g., Pfiffner & O'Leary, 1987; Pfiffner, Rosen, & O'Leary, 1985; Shores, Gunter, & Jack, 1993; Walker & Hops, 1993; Walker et al., 2004).

Although instituting changes in teacher social behavior can be an effective approach for modifying some children's CP behavior, there are a number of disadvantages to such an approach. First, some teachers resent the implication that somehow their behavior is responsible for some children's misconduct, and they are resistant to consultation regarding how to change their own social behavior. In addition, some investigators have shown that teachers who have higher baseline levels of teaching self-efficacy are less accepting of behavioral consultation (Dunson, Hughes, & Jackson, 1994) and perceive less positive outcomes from consultation (Hughes, Grossman, & Barker, 1990). Other investigators have discussed the fact that changes in teacher social behavior alone may be effective with mildly disruptive children, but for children displaying more severely deviant classroom behavior, more powerful procedures are necessary (O'Leary et al., 1969; Walker, Hops, & Fiegenbaum, 1976). As noted earlier, several studies have demonstrated that changing teacher social behavior alone is not sufficient to change extremely disruptive child behavior, and that combined strategies are necessary for these students.

For these reasons, researchers have also investigated the use of token reinforcement systems in the classroom. Token reinforcement programs typically involve three basic ingredients: (1) a set of instructions to the class about the behaviors that will be reinforced; (2) a means of making a potentially reinforcing stimulus (usually called a "token") contingent upon behavior; and (3) a set of rules governing the exchange of tokens for backup reinforcers (O'Leary & Drabman, 1971). Typical examples of classroom target behaviors have been paying attention, remaining seated, raising hands before speaking, facing the front of the room, not running, not talking out, and accurately completing class assignments. Many of these behaviors are incompatible with the aggressive and oppositional behaviors of children with CP.

A variety of systems can be developed for the delivery of tokens to children; specific details should always be worked out with each individual classroom teacher, so that the system fits as smoothly as possible into ongoing classroom routine. For example, in special education classrooms with a small teacher-to-pupil ratio, the teacher(s) may be able to monitor and rate children's behavior every 10–15 minutes. In large classrooms, teachers may do well to rate behavior and dispense tokens at the end of each class.

Token reinforcement programs have been evaluated singly and in combination with other classroom management strategies by a number of investigators showing substantial behavioral improvement with use of token systems (for

reviews, see Abramowitz & O'Leary, 1991; Kazdin, 1977b). There may be differences in the effectiveness of token programs when individual versus group contingencies are used. Pigott and Heggie (1986) reviewed 20 studies that directly compared these two strategies. In individual contingencies, individual children are reinforced solely on the basis of their own performance. In group contingencies, three or more children are reinforced on the basis of the overall performance of the group or a significant proportion thereof. Group contingencies were superior to individual ones when academic performance was the target behavior, whereas there was no consistent differential effect when social responses were the target behaviors. Group contingencies have been associated with an increase in verbal threats among classmates, however, and this potential effect should be strongly considered in deciding between the use of group or individual contingencies.

An example of a program employing interdependent group contingencies bears special mention. The Good Behavior Game (Barrish, Saunders, & Wolf, 1969; Deitz, 1985; Medland & Stachnik, 1972) is an approach that capitalizes on team competitiveness and group social conformity. The classroom is divided into two or more teams. Each team receives marks against itself when violations of posted rules by individual team members occur. Reinforcement is provided to both teams if a maximum threshold of total marks is not exceeded by both teams. Otherwise, the team with the fewest marks wins and receives reinforcement. A variant of this procedure, the Good Behavior Game Plus Merit (Darveaux, 1984), also allows students to earn merit points for their team for accurate academic assignment completion.

The effectiveness (Barrish et al., 1969) and acceptability to teachers (Tingstrom, 1994) of the Good Behavior Game have been demonstrated. Interestingly, teachers evaluated the Good Behavior Game Plus Merit as less acceptable than the basic version. Tingstrom speculates that because the former is more complex and requires more time to implement, teachers are less accepting of the procedure, even though it targets positive behaviors in addition to negative behaviors. The Good Behavior Game also has been implemented in a large-scale, preventive intervention program (see "Prevention," below).

As noted above, Webster-Stratton (Webster-Stratton, 2000; Webster-Stratton & Reid, 2003) has developed a school-based intervention program and a teacher training program for addressing early conduct problems as adjuncts to her parent training program. Please refer to the earlier section on family-based interventions with preadolescents for descriptions of these interventions.

A number of investigators have examined the extent to which the effects of multicomponent treatment programs involving teacher training and token economies generalize across time and settings. In some of the earliest studies to examine these questions, little evidence for generalization was found (Kuypers, Becker, & O'Leary, 1968; O'Leary et al., 1969; Walker & Hops, 1976). On the other hand, there is some evidence that positive treatment effects will be maintained across time, although the duration of follow-up has ranged only from 3 to 12 weeks (Greenwood et al., 1974; Greenwood, Hops, & Walker, 1977; Walker & Hops, 1976). Treatment-acquired gains do not appear to generalize well from one academic year to the next when no attempts at facilitating generalization are implemented (Walker et al., 1975).

For all these reasons, Walker, Hops, and their colleagues have conducted a number of studies evaluating strategies to enhance generalization and maintenance of treatment effects acquired in multicomponent classroom programs. Walker and Buckley (1972) treated children for 2 months in a token economy classroom and then randomly assigned them to one of three maintenance strategies or a control group before returning them to their regular classrooms: a "peer reprogramming" strategy, in which classroom peers were trained to support positive behavior; an "equating stimulus conditions" strategy, in which experimental class procedures were transferred to the regular classroom; and a "teacher training" strategy. The peer reprogramming and equating stimulus conditions were significantly more effective than teacher training or no generalization programming in facilitating transfer of positive treatment effects to the regular classroom. In another study, Walker and colleagues (1975) showed that providing teachers with feedback and credit hours resulted in greater generalization than no maintenance strategies.

One of the most comprehensive systems for school-based behavior management is the four-component system developed by the Center at Oregon for Research in the Behavioral Education of the Handicapped (CORBEH) during the 1970s for children in mainstream kindergarten through fourth-grade classrooms (Hops & Walker, 1988; Walker, Hops, & Greenwood, 1984). Two of the four components are specifically designed to deal with CP behaviors such as acting-out disruptive behavior and social aggression. The other two components address low academic survival skills and social withdrawal. Each component uses a teacher consultant (e.g., counselor, school psychologist) as the primary delivery agent, with control ultimately transferred to the classroom teacher and/or playground supervisor.

The Contingencies for Learning Academic and Social Skills (CLASS) program is designed to decrease disruptive behaviors in various school settings (i.e., classroom cafeteria, hallways, playground). It is designed as a behavior management template to be overlaid on the curricular content and instructional routines of educational settings (Walker et al., 2004). CLASS has two phases: a consultant phase in days 1–6, and a teacher phase in days 6–30. Behavioral techniques include a token economy with a response cost component, contingency contracting, teacher praise, school and home rewards, and 1-day suspensions for certain serious acting-out behaviors (Hops & Walker, 1988; Walker & Hops, 1979). During the first week, the consultant implements the procedures; then the program is shifted to the classroom teacher, who assumes primary control of the daily procedures with the support and assistance of the consultant. Over the next 5 weeks, the program is extended over the entire day, and there is a gradual fading from tangible rewards to social reinforcement in the natural environment. Because a child's progress through the program is performance-based, the actual length of the program varies from 6 to 10 weeks (Walker & Hops, 1979).

The Reprogramming Environmental Contingencies for Effective Social Skills (RECESS) program, also developed by Walker and his colleagues, is a comprehensive intervention for aggressive behavior that focuses on the remediation of social aggression with peers on the playground and in the classroom (Walker, Hops, & Greenwood, 1993; Walker et al., 2004). It is designed for children in kindergarten through grade 3. RECESS consists of four program components: (1) systematic training in cooperative, positive, social behavior via prepared scripts, discussion, and role playing for the child with CP and the entire class; (2) a response cost system in which points are lost for aggressive social behavior and rule infractions; (3) praise by the RECESS consultant, teacher, and playground supervisor for positive, cooperative, interactive behavior; and (4) concurrent group and individual reward contingencies, with group activity rewards available at school and individual rewards available at home (Walker et al., 2004). The program is administered in four phases: recess only, extension to the classroom, fading, and then maintenance. It requires 40–45 hours of program consultant time over a 2- to 3-month intervention period. The program has been successfully applied to hundreds of aggressive students (Walker et al., 1984, 1993, 2004). The program has a powerful impact and is probably the most successful program of its kind. It is generally reserved for the most aggressive students, due to the time and effort to implement it. However, for school systems willing to make the investment and to implement the maintenance phase over the long term, this program can be expected to produce very significant reductions in aggressive behavior (Walker et al., 2004).

All of the CORBEH packages were developed and evaluated through a systematic three-phase process of component evaluation and package development in an experimental classroom, adaptation and standardization of package components, and field testing under typical conditions of use (Walker et al., 1984). The CLASS program has been implemented and evaluated with 119 children in this process in both urban and rural settings (Walker et al., 1984). Field trial evaluations indicate not only that the CLASS program was effective in increasing the level of appropriate behaviors among children in the classroom, compared to acting-out children who did not participate in the program, but that these effects were maintained at a 1-year follow-up (Hops et al., 1978). Furthermore, examination of student files 1.5–3 years after the program indicated that students who had participated in the CLASS program were less likely to have been placed in special education settings. The CLASS program has also been successfully implemented in Costa Rica, although the magnitude of treatment effects was somewhat reduced (Walker, Fonseca Retana, & Gersten,

1988). Most recently, the CLASS program has been included in a multicomponent prevention program for high-risk children in kindergarten (Walker et al., 2004).

The RECESS program has also been extensively validated in experimental and field settings (Walker, Hops, & Greenwood, 1981; Walker et al., 2004). As noted above, the program is quite effective in reducing the rates of negative/aggressive social responses of the target children, compared to those of untreated controls. Maintenance is achieved as long as the maintenance phase is implemented over the long term (Walker et al., 2004).

At an even broader level of systems conceptualization and intervention, Sugai, Horner, and colleagues (Sugai & Horner, 1999; Sugai, Horner, & Gresham, 2002) have developed a schoolwide intervention model, called Positive Behavior Support (PBS), to enable special and general educators to meet classroom and schoolwide disciplinary needs. PBS is a system that seeks to transform the overall culture and effectiveness of a school. As such it requires support from a majority of school staff in order to be effective (and thus the commitment of the school and/or district administration). The PBS approach consists of four linked systems. There is an overarching schoolwide discipline system with clearly defined expectations for staff and students, and procedures for increasing positive behavior and preventing negative behavior. At the classroom level, teachers must organize their classrooms in ways that support academic instruction. In nonclassroom settings (e.g., playground, cafeteria, hallways), proactive supervision is essential. Finally, individualized student support systems provide a more intensive and individualized approach that is based on FBA. The nine-step PBS program teaches mastery of key social competencies across three core skill areas stated as schoolwide expectations: (1) Be safe, (2) be respectful, and (3) be responsible. Target behaviors are designated in each core skill domain, and all staff members are trained to monitor rewards and reinforce instances of these behaviors in multiple settings across the school environment. There is heavy emphasis on teacher and peer modeling of both successful and unsuccessful examples of the specific behavioral expectations that exemplify the skill areas in each school setting (e.g., the bus area, recess, classroom, lunchroom). Successful installation and implementation of the PBS program requires 2 years (Horner, Sugai, Lewis-Palmer, & Todd, 2001; Sugai & Horner, 1999; Sugai et al., 2002).

The PBS approach has been enthusiastically received by school leaders in recent years and has been adopted in over 400 U.S. schools (Walker et al., 2004). Longitudinal data collected across years at schools where the system has been implemented show reductions in disciplinary referrals to the principal's office, which is a sensitive measure of schoolwide intervention effects (Sugai, Sprague, Horner, & Walker, 2000). In addition, as the culture and atmosphere of middle schools improve, such schools become more orderly, manageable environments (Walker et al., 2004). Although such interventions require considerable commitment at a systems level, behavioral consultants may find districts and schools increasingly willing to make such a commitment, as the prevalence of CP displayed in schools has risen and schools find themselves confronted with management of increasing numbers of youths with CP.

In summary, it is clear that teacher training and consultant-assisted implementation of behavior therapy programs in the classroom and across multiple school settings can significantly improve socially aggressive and disruptive behavior in the school environment, and in some cases can improve these children's academic achievement as well. In addition, maintenance and generalization strategies can be built into treatment to enhance the probability that treatment-acquired gains will transfer to other class periods and even into the next academic year. Obviously, these programs can be quite expensive in terms of the amount of consultant time necessary to train teachers and schools to install and implement programs appropriately. In addition, the studies by Walker and his colleagues (2004) show that maintenance procedures must be in place in the long term in order to maintain gains achieved in intensive treatment phases.

Home-Based Reinforcement Programs

In schools or districts that are not able or willing to make the commitment to a classroom-level or schoolwide intervention program, other procedures, though less comprehensive and effective, may be needed. One procedure that has proven useful in regular classrooms is the use of home-based reinforcement programs (see Kelley, 1990). With home-based reinforcement programs, a concerted effort is made to relieve the teacher of many of the aspects of managing a behavioral system, and to place some of the responsibility for implementation of the program on the parents and even on the child him- or herself. The steps involved in initiating a home-based reinforcement system involve (1) deciding which behaviors (academic, social, behavioral) to target; (2) selecting a monitoring interval agreeable to the teacher; (3) preparing monitoring sheets or index cards; and (4) setting up backup consequences at home. Coordination between the teacher and the parent is necessary to accomplish these steps.

Studies have varied in the extent to which the clinician or experimenter has consulted with the parents regarding the home backup reinforcers. Ayllon, Garber, and Pisor (1975) had a single 2-hour meeting with parents, and in some cases only telephone contact. Parents were informed about the home-based reward system for their children, and they were told to use their own judgment in selecting rewards and sanctions that had worked for them in the past. At the other end of the spectrum, Schumaker, Hovell, and Sherman (1977) sent a clinician to students' homes to draw up lists of privileges and to negotiate systems for exchanging points earned at school for privileges at home. Weekly home visits occurred throughout the study, and twice-weekly telephone contact was made with each family. Although the procedure followed by Schumaker et al. may not be clinically feasible, the one followed by Ayllon et al. may not be sufficient or appropriate for some families. For example, in families in which rewards are scarce and punishment is impulsive, irrational, or abusive, clinicians need to take greater responsibility for working out the details of the backup system of consequences with the parents in therapy sessions.

A number of studies have evaluated the efficacy of home-based reinforcement programs for school behavior problems (for reviews, see Abramowitz & O'Leary, 1991; Atkeson & Forehand, 1979; Kelley, 1990). Target populations have ranged from kindergarteners (Budd, Liebowitz, Riner, Mindell, & Goldfarb, 1981; Lahey et al., 1977) to middle school students (Schumaker et al., 1977) to predelinquent youths in group home placement (Bailey, Wolf, & Phillips, 1970). Backup reinforcers have ranged from praise delivered by teachers and/

or parents to concrete, detailed home-based reinforcement systems. Thus positive effects of the daily report card systems have been demonstrated across a variety of subject and treatment parameters.

Other studies have generally confirmed the positive effects of home-based reinforcement systems that involve a child's own parents. Ayllon and colleagues (1975) implemented a home-based reinforcement system with disruptive third graders in public school after a teacher-administered token system failed to effect sustained improvements in classroom behavior. The system involved one global daily report and minimal parent consultation regarding home consequences. Nevertheless, the system was highly effective in reducing classroom disruption.

Schumaker and colleagues (1977) also demonstrated the efficacy of a home-based reinforcement program involving daily report, praise, and home privileges in a multiple-baseline-across-subjects design, using "problem" junior high school students. In addition, these investigators showed that although praise alone may result in transient improvements in school behavior, the greatest, most sustained improvements are achieved when contingent privileges are provided at home. Similarly, Budd and colleagues (1981) found that praise in the absence of home-based privileges was not sufficient to reduce the disruptive behavior of kindergarten children with serious behavior disorders. By contrast, Lahey and colleagues (1977) showed that praise alone delivered by parents contingent upon receipt of daily report cards was sufficient to improve the behavior of mildly disruptive kindergarten students. The discrepancy in the results of these three studies is probably related to the different ages of the subject populations (parental praise is more likely to function as a powerful reinforcer for younger than for older students) and to behavior problem severity (more severe behavior problems may require more concrete backup reinforcers). Rosen, Gabardi, Miller, and Miller (1990) showed that the combination of reinforcement plus response cost may be more effective than reinforcement alone in home-based reinforcement programs, mimicking the effects obtained with classroom-based contingencies.

The social validity of home-based reinforcement systems has been examined with respect to acceptability. Teachers rated home-based reinforcement as more acceptable than token economies, time out, and ignoring, and less acceptable than praise or response cost (Witt, Martens, & Elliott, 1984). Students (fifth to ninth graders) preferred home-based praise over home-based reprimands, teacher praise, and teacher reprimands (Turco & Elliott, 1986).

In this section, we have reviewed individual strategies as well as more comprehensive systemwide interventions for addressing CP behaviors in the school. The review has focused on interventions that have the greatest evidence for beneficial outcomes. However, the reader is cautioned that single techniques and interventions are seldom sufficient to deal with CP behavior in school (Greenberg, Domitrovich, & Bumbarger, 2001; Reid, Patterson, & Snyder, 2002). Interventions with the best chance of powerful effects are comprehensive programs that target positive skills as well as problem behavior, that are implemented over time, that have built-in and long-term strategies for maintenance, and that occur in schools that have made a schoolwide commitment to reform (Miller, Brehm, & Whitehouse, 1998; Walker et al., 2004). In addition to specific interventions to decrease CP behavior, schools must also focus on positive replacement behaviors and skills that are adaptive and functional, such as study skills, social skills, and health awareness, as these areas represent risks that affect nearly all children and youths with CP (Walker et al., 2004).

Techniques for Increasing Compliance and Decreasing Noncompliance

As noted above, noncompliance is considered to be a keystone behavior in the development of CP. Walker and Walker (1991) report that child compliance and noncompliance are rated by teachers as among the most and least acceptable classroom behaviors, respectively. They provide a number of guidelines and procedures for increasing compliance and decreasing noncompliance in the classroom. These include structuring the classroom in terms of classroom rules that communicate teacher expectations concerning academic performance and behavior; posting a daily schedule of classroom activities; making classwide and/or individual activity rewards available for following classroom rules; and planning the physical arrangement of the classroom to accommodate different activities. In addition, concrete suggestions for improving teacher relationships with students and managing difficult teacher–student interactions that involve noncompliance are provided.

Interventions for Bullying

Bullying interventions have, for the most part, been implemented in the school setting. Large-scale efforts to introduce and evaluate school-wide antibullying programs have occurred in Scandinavia (Olweus, 1993a), England (Smith & Sharp, 1994a), Canada (Pepler, Craig, Ziegler, & Charach, 1993, 1994), and Belgium (Stevens, De Bourdeaudhuij, & Van Oost, 2000). These programs are both systems- and person-oriented (Olweus, 1992); that is, they are directed at both the school as a system and at the level of individual perpetrators, victims, and their parents. Although component analyses have not been conducted, Olweus believes that both major components are necessary, and that the typical clinical approach of intervening at the individual level will not be sufficient to achieve a meaningful outcome.

Key elements of the whole-school approach are the school taking responsibility for bullying and giving it a high priority; increasing awareness of bullying by teachers, peers, and parents; publicizing explicit school policies and classroom rules that devalue and communicate low tolerance and negative consequences for bullying; discussing bullying in the curriculum; encouraging peer disapproval of bullying; and encouraging bystanders to help victims and report bullying to teachers (Farrington, 1993; Olweus, 1992). Examples of interventions at the individual level include serious talks with perpetrators; letters home to parents and parent meetings; implementation of negative consequences for bullying (e.g., privilege removal); social skills training for victims; encouraging victims to report bullying incidents to adults; and assigning older children to "shadow" victims to observe the bullying and report it to teachers (Farrington, 1993; Pepler et al., 1993).

Pepler (2005) has recently presented a reconceptualization of whole-school interventions for bullying. Pepler describes bullying as a "relationship problem" and suggests that two concepts—"scaffolding" and "social architecture"—are important in developing effective bullying interventions that include individuals, parents and teachers, peers, the classroom, and the whole school. Scaffolding provides a child with the support needed to function slightly above his or her current skill level. Scaffolding for children who bully might include empathy development, increasing emotional and behavioral regulation, and encouraging positive leadership. Scaffolding for victims might include providing protection, increasing social skills, and developing domains of competence. Social architecture involves creating a "dynamic health promoting social context for children and youth." Social architecture for bullies involves decreasing positive support for bullying by intervening with the peer group. Social architecture for victims includes developing positive peer support at home and school. On the classroom level, social architecture uses classroom management strategies to promote positive peer groupings and discourage negative ones. Social architecture at the school level includes developing a whole-school antibullying policy in the context of a supportive and harmonious school environment.

The first large-scale evaluation of the whole-school approach to bullying was conducted by Olweus (1990, 1991, 1996) in Norway. Olweus's intervention, called the Core Program against Bullying and Antisocial Behavior, was a nationwide campaign to intervene in grades 4–7 with an antibullying, whole-school approach to intervention, following the suicides of several victims of bullying. This program aimed to "restructure the social environment" by targeting the school, classroom, and individuals, in order to provide fewer opportunities and rewards for aggression and bullying. The intervention emphasized positive teacher and parent involvement; enhanced communication, awareness, and supervision; firm limits to unacceptable behavior; and consistent, nonphysical sanctions for rule breaking. At the school level, components included dissemination of an anonymous student questionnaire that assessed the extent of bullying in each school, formal discussion of the problem, formation of a committee to plan and deliver the program, and a system of supervision of students between classes and during recess. At the classroom level, teachers provided clear, "no-tolerance" rules for bullying and held regular classroom meetings for students and parents. Finally, individual interventions were provided for perpetrators, victims, and parents to ensure that the bullying stopped and that victims were supported and protected.

Evaluation of the effects of the intervention was based on data from approximately 2,500 students in Bergen schools, using a quasi-experimental design. Outcome data were derived from a student self-report questionnaire. Results after 8 and 20 months of intervention showed marked reductions in the level of bully–victim problems for both boys and girls. Similar effects were found on an aggregated peer rating variable. There was also a reduction in covert CP behaviors, such as vandalism, theft, and truancy. This was an interesting, unintended effect that may have arisen from the general increase in adult monitoring and supervision. Finally, there was an increase in student satisfaction with school life. Marked reductions in aggressive behavior have been demonstrated in a subsequent intervention trial, with effects maintained 2 years later (see Olweus, 2001, for an overview).

A similar program, based closely on the model implemented in Norway, was introduced in 23 schools in the United Kingdom by Smith and his colleagues (Smith & Sharp, 1994a, 1994b). In addition to the basic Olweus program elements, this variation also included so-called "bully courts" and the "Heartstone Odyssey" (a story that introduces experiences of racial harassment). The U.K. program has produced results similar to those presented by Olweus (Smith & Sharp, 1994a), although in contrast with the results from Olweus and colleagues, there were larger program outcomes in primary schools than in secondary schools. In addition, Easley and Smith (1998) followed up four of the original primary schools and found that the program had been effective in reducing bullying by boys, but not by girls.

Pepler, Craig, and their colleagues (Pepler et al., 1993, 1994) conducted an evaluation of the Toronto Anti-Bullying Intervention, a whole-school approach modeled after the Olweus program and developed and implemented with the cooperation of the Toronto Board of Education. As the Olweus program did, the Toronto program involved intervention components at the school, parent, classroom/peer, and individual levels, similar to those described above. Results of this study confirmed that bullying is a stable and pervasive problem in schools. Over an 18-month whole-school intervention program implemented in four Toronto schools, there were some improvements in students' reports of bullying as assessed at individual, peer, and school levels, as well as increases

in teachers' interventions to stop bullying. However, there were no differences in students' discussions of bully–victim problems with their parents, and, unfortunately, victim reports of racial bullying actually increased.

Although the programs described have tested school bullying interventions with substantial numbers of youths, Stevens and colleagues (2000) also included a nonintervention control group in their study of a whole-school bullying program in primary and secondary schools. They found significant improvements in the experimental group, but only in the primary school setting. Stevens et al. suggested that the lack of results in the secondary school setting may have been due in part to adolescents' tendency to conform less with antibullying rules (a key component of these programs). They also commented that administering and maintaining these interventions in secondary schools was much more complicated, because of the less structured secondary school setting. Taken together, this group of studies suggests that whole-school bullying interventions have promise, but that they currently appear to be more efficacious with preadolescent populations than with adolescents.

Given these findings, some recent work has specifically targeted the primary school setting. Orpinas, Home, and Staniszewski (2003) conducted an antibullying program in one large public elementary school in the southwestern United States. This intervention focused on bringing together school personnel, parents, and university consultants to develop a collaborative program that (1) modified the school environment, (2) educated students in conflict resolution and effective communication, and (3) provided 20 hours of training for teachers on schoolwide bullying prevention strategies and on conflict resolution and behavior management. To assess intervention effects, students ($n = 541$) completed an anonymous survey before and after the implementation of the program. Among children in kindergarten to second grade, there was a 40% reduction in self-reported aggression and a 19% reduction in self-reported victimization. For children in third to fifth grades, there was no significant difference in self-reported aggression, but there was a 23% reduction in self-reported victimization.

Whereas Orpinas and colleagues (2003) worked with school personnel to tailor a bullying intervention for a specific primary school population, DeRosier (2004) took a somewhat different approach, evaluating whether a less customized, more broadly focused intervention could also reduce bullying. In this study, a general group social skills intervention was implemented with third-grade children (n = 187) in 11 elementary schools who were selected from a pool of children experiencing peer dislike, social anxiety, and bullying (both perpetrators and victims). Compared to the control group (n = 194), the intervention increased overall peer liking and decreased aggression and bullying in a subgroup of children with higher levels of aggression. At a 1-year follow-up (DeRosier & Marcus, 2005), posttreatment effects were maintained for all areas of adjustment (including aggression) except for self-reported bullying. Compared to the control group, the treatment group demonstrated additional improvements in levels of social acceptability, self-esteem, depression, and anxiety. These effects were more robust for girls than for boys.

As described previously, many of the findings reported in this section suggest that bullying interventions are more effective with younger populations. However, it should be noted that Baldry (2001), using a somewhat more individualistic approach, obtained contrasting results. She developed a bullying program that was directed toward students and their peer groups and was designed to enhance awareness of violence and its negative effects. Using videos and a three-part booklet combined with role playing, group discussions, and focus groups, participants were taught about the negative effects of bullying; intervention components focused on enhancing empathy, building perspective-taking skills, and encouraging peers to support victims rather than ignoring or downplaying bullying. Baldry and Farrington (2004) evaluated this intervention with 237 students (control n = 106, intervention n = 131) ages 11–15. Victimization (e.g., direct victimization, having belongings stolen, being called nasty names) decreased for older students, but not for younger students.

Interventions for Covert CP

Whereas psychosocial interventions for overt CP behaviors have been evaluated extensively in home, school, and community settings, there are relatively fewer data concerning interventions of any type for covert types of CP be-

havior, especially with respect to adolescents. However, the attention being given to some of these covert behaviors (especially firesetting) and their treatment is increasing, due to the rising recognition that when both overt and covert behaviors are present, a youth's CP is more serious and may have a poorer long-term outcome. In addition, covert CP often represents serious violations of the rights of others, provoking concern from the community. In this section of the chapter, we describe interventions that have been designed to treat stealing, lying, and firesetting.

Stealing

There is a consensus that the identification/labeling of stealing is the key to developing a successful intervention for this behavior (Barth, 1987; Miller & Klungness, 1989; Patterson et al., 1975). Because of its low base rate and covert nature, immediate firsthand detection of all stealing events by parents, teachers, or others is not a feasible goal. Therefore, stealing is operationally defined as "the child's taking, or being in possession of, anything that does not clearly belong to him [or her]" (Barth, 1987, p. 151). Table 3.1 contains an elaboration of this definition, as well as instructions for caregivers on how to respond to stealing behavior. Although adoption of this definition of stealing may result in instances in which a youth is incorrectly labeled as having stolen, the alternative of not being able to treat the stealing behavior effectively is regarded as the greater of the two evils.

The most systematic work on the treatment of covert CP has been conducted by Patterson, Reid, and their colleagues at OSLC with respect to family-based interventions for treating stealing. The OSLC group developed a specialized approach to parent training for youths who display stealing and other covert CP behaviors (Patterson et al., 1975; Reid et al., 1980). This approach takes into account the definitional and detection problems inherent in treating covert CP behaviors, and also attempts to have a direct impact on the parenting variables strongly associated with delinquency (i.e., parental involvement, monitoring, and parental discipline practices). The failure of parents of youths who steal to monitor their youths' whereabouts or to be involved with the youths to any great extent compounds the difficulty of designing effective family-based interventions.

TABLE 3.1. Instructions to Caregivers for Defining and Providing Consequences for Stealing

1. The most important part of working to decrease stealing is *defining stealing as stealing. Stealing is defined as the child's taking, or being in possession of, anything that does not clearly belong to him [or her]*. Parents, teachers, or other adults are the only judges. They may label an act as stealing by observing, it, by having it reported to them, or by noticing that something is missing. There is no arguing about guilt or innocence. It is the child's job to be sure that he [or she] is not accused. The value of the object is irrelevant. Trading and borrowing are not permissible. Any "purchases" that the child brings home must be accompanied by a receipt. Otherwise they are to be returned and consequences instituted.

2. Once the behavior of stealing has been labeled, then the consequences are to be applied. Avoid discussions, shaming, or counseling.

3. *Every* stealing event must be so labeled and consequences given.

4. Avoid using excessive detective tactics (such as searches); just keep your eyes open, and investigate the origins of new property.

5. Consequences for stealing should be work restrictions and loss of privileges for the day of the stealing, and basic privileges only on the following weekend. There should be no other consequences such as humiliations or beatings. Special privileges can be earned again on the following day.

6. *Remember*: Stealing goes hand in hand with wandering and with your not knowing the whereabouts of your child. Check-in times are recommended if stealing is a problem.

7. Do not tempt your child. Keep items like those that your child has stolen in the past away from him or her. For example, avoid leaving your wallet or cigarette packs in view or unwatched.

8. Stealing may occur no matter how many possessions your child has, so giving him or her everything is not a successful approach to ending stealing. Your child should, however, have some way of earning his or her own money so that he or she may have a choice of things to buy.

Note. From Barth (1987). Copyright 1987 by Plenum Publishing Corporation. Reprinted by permission from the author and Springer Science and Business Media.

In the OSLC approach to the treatment of stealing, the standard parent training program for treating overt CP behaviors is implemented first, because these behaviors covary with the lower-rate covert CP behaviors in many youths. In addition, the standard OSLC program addresses two important parenting practices: poor discipline practices and low parental involvement with the child. Next, parents are taught to identify stealing (using an operational definition similar to the one presented above) and to monitor its occurrence on a daily basis. Much discussion and role playing of these procedures occur in therapy sessions.

Once the operational definition of stealing is accepted by the parents, parents are taught to administer a mild consequence immediately contingent upon each and every suspected stealing event. The consequence (e.g., 1–2 hours of hard work around the home) is kept at a mild level, because the youth will be inaccurately accused from time to time. The implementation of this approach involves much support, telephone contact, and discussion. Check-in systems are instituted for families in which infrequent monitoring occurs. In addition, it would seem important to incorporate therapeutic strategies for involving fathers in the therapy process, given the relationship between uninvolved fathers and stealing (Frick, 1994; Loeber et al., 1983).

In a study that remains the most systematic evaluation of treatment focused specifically on stealing behavior, Reid and colleagues (1980) evaluated the effectiveness of this modified approach to parent training for 5- to 14-year-old youths with CP who were referred for stealing. In this study, 28 families of children with CP who stole received treatment. The mean amount of therapist contact was 32 hours. Outcome measures consisted of parent reports of stealing on the TIROSSA, parent reports of other referral problems on the PDR, and a deviant behavior summary score in home observations conducted by trained independent observers. There were significant decreases in parent-reported stealing events and other referral problems from pre- to posttreatment and at a 6-month follow-up. Observed deviant behavior scores decreased nonsignificantly. However, as might be expected, aversive social behaviors in the families were not high to begin with in this sample of youths who stole. A waiting-list control group, in which parent report data on stealing were collected at baseline, at the end of the parent training program for dealing with overt CP, and following the treatment package for stealing, indicated that significant reductions in parent-reported stealing did not occur until after the treatment for stealing was implemented. However, large differences in baseline levels of stealing limit the utility of this comparison.

In another study with chronic delinquents from the OSLC group, described earlier in this chapter, Bank and colleagues (1991) found some empirical support for the efficacy of this family-based approach with the subset of adolescents who engaged in both overt and covert CP behaviors. Parent-reported stealing (as noted on the PDR) was reduced to zero at treatment termination. In addition, the preventive intervention implemented by Tremblay and colleagues (see below), which employed an adaptation of the OSLC model of parent training and children's social skills training, successfully reduced stealing through age 17 (e.g., Lacourse et al., 2002).

Stealing has also been approached from a more traditional family therapy model. Seymour and Epston (1989) treated 45 consecutive cases (20% of whom were adolescents ages 13–15) of childhood stealing with an approach that "regraded" the child from "stealer" to "honest person." Therapists focused questions in such a way as to "externalize the symptom," a framework promulgated by White (1986), and assisted the child and the parents to engage together in working against the stealing. Thereafter, techniques were very similar to those employed by Reid and colleagues (1980). Emphasis was placed on suspicion of stealing; on responding to stealing with work chore consequences; and on "honesty tests," in which items of interest were left around the house, and the child was reinforced by parents for not stealing. Although no control group was employed, Seymour and Epston reported significant pre- to posttreatment changes in stealing. Fifty-four percent of the cases reported no stealing at a 2-month follow-up, and an additional 40% reported only one to three instances. At a 1-year follow-up, levels of stealing remained low. Sixty-two percent of parents reported no instances of stealing, and 19% of parents reported that stealing was "substantially reduced." A similar family-based intervention is described by Pawsey (1996). An initial period of parental monitoring of stealing was followed by the sequential presentation of up to four additional interventions: contracting, restitution, punishment, and honesty tests. The intervention was successful for 12 of 14 youths (ages 7–15 years) referred to an outpatient child psychiatry clinic; effects were maintained for 10 of the 12 youths at a 3-month follow-up. Effects were comparable for preadolescents and adolescents. More recently,

Venning, Blampied, and France (2003) presented a case study describing the effects of the Triple P-Positive Parenting Program (Sanders, Turner, & Markie-Dadds, 2002) on stealing with two preadolescent boys. Using similar procedures to those described above, they reported rapid cessation of stealing that was maintained at a 10-week follow-up.

Although the results of family-based intervention studies are suggestive, the effects of treatment on stealing were assessed primarily from parent report measures. Given the problems these parents have with respect to effective monitoring of their children's behavior, future investigators should attempt to include some treatment component directed specifically to parental monitoring (see Dishion & McMahon, 1998). Not only is this a worthwhile target of intervention in its own right, but effective monitoring of these youths' behavior and whereabouts would seem to be a prerequisite for accurate recording on measures such as the TIROSSA and PDR. Another critical issue that must be addressed pertains to the generalizability of family-based interventions for stealing in other settings, such as the school or the community at large. Although there are effective treatment procedures for dealing with stealing in the elementary school setting (see below), identifying and stopping stealing in public places such as stores is very difficult.

Henderson (1981, 1983) has developed an individualized combined treatment (ICT) approach for children and adolescents who report that they want to stop stealing. This approach has three broad components: (1) self-control of the internal environment, (2) adult or responsible-other control of the external environment, and (3) personalization of the program by the therapist. The first component teaches relaxation skills in an effort to countercondition internal arousal stimuli, which Henderson maintains are often associated with stealing. In therapy sessions, the youth is asked to imagine him- or herself in theft situations, and then to relax and imagine walking away. In this way, relaxation and imagery are also conceptualized as self-control techniques, which are later extended to the external environment. Heart rate biofeedback is used to facilitate relaxation. Parents are asked to provide stealing opportunities or "traps" for the youth in the home, so that the youth has an opportunity to practice self-control strategies. Bonuses in a reward system are provided for not stealing. The "traps" are gradually made less obvious and easier to take without being caught.

To provide external controls for not stealing, some system for monitoring "not stealing" must be implemented. Henderson (1981) advocates the use of a "not-stealing diary." Two types of entries are made in the diary: (1) any length of time that a youth has been observed by a responsible adult not to have stolen; and (2) times of departure and arrival noted by responsible adults at both ends of a journey (e.g., from home to school). If the times logged in conform to appropriate travel time, then an assumption is made that no stealing has occurred. Daily time "not stealing" is computed, and this time is rewarded with backup privileges and activities. These reinforcers are selected so that they are related in some way to the youth's motive for stealing (see Barth, 1987). For example, if the youth seems to steal for "kicks," then an appropriate backup reinforcer might be a roller-coaster ride at an amusement park.

Henderson (1981, 1983) presented descriptive data on 10 youths (ages 8–15 years) who received the ICT program. Compared to 17 other youths who were treated for stealing at the same clinic using a variety of other treatment procedures, only 20% of the youths who received the ICT program were reported to have stolen in the 2-year period following treatment, whereas 60–75% of the other youth were reported to have stolen. Although the descriptive data on this approach to treatment are certainly encouraging, systematic evaluation of the program with appropriate controls needs to be undertaken.

A few studies have focused on the reduction of stealing in elementary school classrooms. To our knowledge, similar work has not been conducted with adolescent samples in school settings. Because of its relatively controlled and geographically confined nature, the classroom may be amenable to more systematic monitoring of stealing behavior and to the implementation of differential reinforcement procedures for not stealing than is the case when treatment is implemented in the home (cf. Reid, 1984). Classroom interventions have included some form of response cost for stealing and positive reinforcement for periods of nonstealing (Brooks & Snow, 1972; Rosen & Rosen, 1983; Switzer, Deal, & Bailey, 1977). In all cases, the frequency of stealing was significantly reduced when either group or individual contingencies were applied. Group contingencies that are applied to an entire classroom may be considered as adjuncts to individualized sets of contingencies when an intervention for stealing by an individual youth is being designed. Behavioral generalization of the effects of other school-based interventions to stealing has been demonstrated in at least one instance. As noted above, reductions in stealing at school (as well as other covert behaviors, such as vandalism and truancy) were found as a result of implementing the antibullying program designed by Olweus (1990, 1991, 1996).

In their review of the treatment of nonconfrontative stealing in elementary-school-age children, Miller and Klungness (1986) raise some important issues that must be considered in the detection, monitoring, and treatment of stealing in the classroom. The use of unannounced theft probes (Switzer et al., 1977) or systematic searches (Rosen & Rosen, 1983) raises important legal and ethical issues. The use of group contingencies has the potential for several undesirable side effects, such as increased negative peer pressure and/or rejection (Pigott & Heggie, 1986), and the possibility that children may eventually choose not to report stealing because they do not want to lose access to the reward. In the Switzer and colleagues (1977) investigation, peer sociometric ratings prior to and after the implementation of the group contingency, and unobtrusive audiotaping of the children's conversations when the teacher left the classroom after each stealing incident, did not indicate the presence of any of these negative effects. However, more systematic and practical methods of monitoring such potential negative side effects are essential.

Miller and Klungness (1989) make several recommendations about interventions to reduce the occurrence of stealing. First, they recommend that therapists emphasize the accurate labeling and consistent detection of stealing. Second, therapists should emphasize the promotion of effective child management skills with parents. Third, with motivated youths, Miller and Klungness recommend the use of self-control procedures by the youths in addition to external controls employed by parents. Fourth, the intervention should designate alternative behaviors to reinforce in order to counteract the withdrawal of reinforcement that has been attendant to stealing. Fifth, it is important to implement systemic-level changes in the school setting, such as increased supervision of youths at recess and in school hallways. Although the recommendations of Miller and Klungness have not been evaluated, they are consistent with the treatment package designed and evaluated by Reid and colleagues (1980).

Lying

Stouthamer-Loeber (1986) has suggested that younger children, whose lies are more transparent and easily detectable, should be easier to treat than older children who lie. She advocates an educational approach in which a parent instructs a child in the difference between what is true and not true, and provides training in empathy and/or perspective taking. For older children and adolescents, she suggests an approach similar to that described above by Reid and colleagues (1980) for stealing: If a parent suspects that a child is lying, the child must prove that he or she is being truthful to avoid a negative consequence. Stouthamer-Loeber also stresses the necessity of focusing on increasing parental monitoring of the child in interventions designed to decrease lying. To our knowledge, there has only been a single report of a formalized intervention to deal with lying. Venning and colleagues (2003) presented data in which the Triple P parenting intervention (Sanders et al., 2002) was used successfully to decrease lying (and stealing) in a 10-year-old male. Intervention procedures paralleled those employed to decrease stealing; they included good-behavior charts, immediate parental response when lying was suspected, and various consequences (such as time out, restitution, and loss of privileges). At a 10-week follow-up, parental concerns about lying had been eliminated over the 3-week data collection period.

Firesetting

Although firesetting is often (but not always) associated with a diagnosis of CD and indicates a more advanced, extreme, or complex form of CP (Forehand et al., 1991; Hanson et al., 1994; Stickle & Blechman, 2002), it has been recognized as requiring a specific treatment focus in addition to standard psychosocial treatments for CP.

There are a number of case studies and a few experimental studies involving both behavioral and nonbehavioral treatments (see Kolko,

2002b, and Stadolnik, 2000, for reviews). Treatments have included contingency management procedures, negative practice in firesetting as a satiation and extinction procedure, prosocial skills training in the expression of anger and other emotional arousal, and family therapy. A brief cognitive-behavioral skills training curriculum implemented with psychiatrically hospitalized children (ages 4–8) was associated with significantly greater reductions in contact with fire-related toys and matches in an analogue task and an increase in firesetting knowledge, compared to a firesetting discussion group control (Kolko et al., 1991). At a 6-month follow-up, parents reported less involvement with fire for children in the cognitive-behavioral condition.

In addition to the psychological treatments just reviewed, another approach to intervention has been developed outside the realm of mental health and is implemented by trained firefighters in the community. Two such programs are those sponsored by the U.S. Federal Emergency Management Agency (FEMA) and by the National Firehawk Foundation. These programs emphasize detection and assessment of firesetters, and rely heavily on fire safety education and mentoring (Kolko, 1988). In addition, several states (e.g., Oregon, Massachusetts) have developed statewide interagency intervention programs (Okulitch & Pinsonneault, 2002), and increasing attention is being paid to residential (Pelletier-Parker, Slate, Moriarty, & Pinsonneault, 1999; Richardson, 2002) and juvenile justice diversion and intervention (Elliott, 2002) programs for adolescents who set fires.

Unfortunately, systematic, controlled evaluations of these programs are scarce. An evaluation of educational materials (a brief brochure) alone or in conjunction with an adaptation of the FEMA program or referral to a mental health specialist showed statistically and clinically significant reductions in frequency and seriousness of firesetting in a sample of 5- to 16-year-olds at a 1-year follow-up assessment, regardless of intervention condition (Adler, Nunn, Northam, Lebnan, & Ross, 1994). Thus the multicomponent FEMA intervention was no more effective than the provision of educational materials.

Because fire safety education alone provides for significant reductions in firesetting, Kolko (2001) conducted an experiment to test the comparative effects of fire safety education as implemented in community settings (such as the FEMA program) and psychosocial treatment as implemented in mental health settings. In this study, psychosocial treatment consisted of cognitive-behavioral procedures designed to modify the characteristics and correlates of firesetting. Specifically, children learned graphing techniques to relate firesetting motives to specific events or affective states, problem-solving skills, and assertion skills. Parents received parent training with special emphasis on child monitoring and consequences. (See Kolko, 2002a, for an extended description of these procedures.) Boys ages 5–13 who had set fires were randomly assigned to the two treatments, each of which consisted of eight sessions. In addition, a third condition, consisting of nonrandomly assigned participants received two fire safety education home visits from a firefighter. All three interventions were associated with significant decreases in a number of indices of firesetting behavior at both posttreatment and at the 1-year follow-up. The cognitive-behavioral and fire safety education interventions demonstrated greater effects than the firefighter visit intervention on several additional indices of firesetting behavior. This study suggests that brief interventions conducted by a trained firefighter are effective in reducing firesetting behavior in preadolescent males, but that more intensive cognitive-behavioral and fire safety education interventions are even more effective.

Psychopharmacological Treatment

Use of psychopharmacological treatment for children and adolescents with primary CP has been steadily increasing over the last two decades. The rationale for the usage of psychopharmacological treatments is the presumption that neurophysiological factors are at least partial contributors to the etiology of CP, or that neurophysiology has a primary role in the mediation of maladaptive behaviors. Aggression, in particular, is thought to be at least partially the behavioral manifestation of abnormalities in the neurochemical functioning of the central nervous system structures associated with behavioral inhibition or behavioral excitation that involve the regulation of impulses or emotions (Mpofu, 2002). Thus there appears to be some empirical support for the involvement of the neurotransmitter serotonin (Halperin et al., 1994; Kruesi et al., 1990) and mixed sup-

port for the involvement of norepinephrine (Magnusson, 1988; Rogeness et al., 1989) in aggressive disorders in youths. Higher levels of the neurohormone testosterone have been observed in violent delinquent adolescents than in a comparable group of nonviolent/nondelinquent controls (Olweus, 1986; Olweus, Mattson, Schalling, & Low, 1980), and low cortisol levels have also been implicated in child aggression (Kruesi, Schmidt, Donnelly, Hibbs, & Hamburger, 1989; Virkunen, 1985). Studies of autonomic arousal point to underarousal as an important correlate of CP in children and adolescents (Kruesi et al., 1992; McBurnett, Swanson, Pfiffner, & Harris, 1991; Raine & Jones, 1987; Raine, Venables, & Williams, 1990).

We briefly review several pharmacological treatments for adolescents with CP for which some empirical support is available. We also recommend three useful reviews, which detail the available literature in this area (Bukstein, 2003; Connor, 2002; Waslick, Werry, & Greenhill, 1999). Before we consider specific classes of drugs often used to treat aspects of CP, an important caveat should be noted: In general, studies on this topic have included only small numbers of children from a wide age range (i.e., preschoolers or young school-age children through adolescents). Furthermore, in the majority of studies, preadolescents (i.e., 11- and 12-year-olds) are the oldest children included. Thus, in reviewing specific studies we have noted age and sample size where appropriate, so that this information can be considered in weighing the applicability of the current research to children and adolescents with CP.

Psychostimulants

Psychostimulants achieve their therapeutic effect on aggression by augmenting norepinephrine and dopamine transmitters that would be associated with a decrease in impulsivity (Julien, 1996). These medications (e.g., methylphenidate, dextroamphetamine, pemoline) have been shown to reduce aggressive behavior as well as some covert CP behaviors in children and adolescents with ADHD. For example, Hinshaw, Henker, Whalen, Erhardt, and Dunnington (1989) examined 25 children with ADHD (ages 6–12 years) and found significant improvements in aggression and related behaviors. Extending these findings into adolescence, Kaplan, Busner, Kupietz, Wasserman, and

Segal (1990) examined six 13- to 16-year-olds and also found improvements in aggression. Hinshaw and colleagues (1992) assessed the effects of methylphenidate on covert CP in boys with ADHD in a laboratory paradigm designed to provide an occasion for stealing, cheating, and property destruction. In a drug–placebo crossover design, drug treatment resulted in significant decreases in stealing and property destruction, observed surreptitiously in the laboratory. However, cheating *increased* when the children were taking methylphenidate. Although ADHD is the only behavioral disorder for which psychostimulants have been clearly shown to be efficacious, this class of drugs may also be useful in the treatment of CP, with or without comorbid ADHD (Barkley, McMurray, Edelbrock, & Robbins, 1989; Connor, Glatt, Lopez, Jackson, & Melloni, 2002; Hinshaw, Buhrmester, & Heller, 1989; Hinshaw, Henker, et al., 1989). Furthermore, because comorbidity of ADHD and CP is probably the rule rather than the exception in clinical samples (Abikoff & Klein, 1992), findings suggesting that psychostimulants may be helpful in cases in which CP and ADHD are co-occurring (e.g., Abikoff, Klein, Kass, & Ganeles, 1987; Connor, Barkley, & Davis, 2000; MTA Cooperative Group, 1999) have significance when treatment options for youths with CP are being considered. Klein, Abikoff, and colleagues have conducted two of the only studies focusing on the use of psychostimulants in youths with CD. Klein, Abikoff, Klass, Shah, and Seese (1994) compared methylphenidate, lithium, and placebo, and found that methylphenidate produced improvement over placebo in measures of CP in 80 children and adolescents diagnosed with CD. Moreover, Klein and colleagues (1997) found that treatment with methylphenidate resulted in reduced aggression and improved symptoms of antisocial behavior in a sample of 84 youths (ages 6–15) diagnosed with CD, regardless of their level of ADHD symptoms. That is, 69% of the youths in the study met criteria for ADHD, but when ADHD was controlled for in the analyses, all findings remained significant, and there was no significant interaction between ADHD and treatment outcome, indicating that initial ADHD ratings did not significantly affect the youths' response to methylphenidate. Likewise, in a double-blind, placebo-controlled trial of methylphenidate in 18 urban children with ADHD, results showed improvements in ADHD symptoms, as

expected, but also less physical aggression, fewer instances of time out for disruptive behavior, and fewer negative peer interactions with methylphenidate (Bukstein & Kolko, 1998). Taken together, these studies provide increasing support for the conclusion that stimulant medications produce reductions in CP in children and adolescents selected on the basis of primary diagnoses of ADHD or CD.

Lithium

Lithium carbonate is an alkali metal that enhances serotonergic activity in the brain. It has been used in children and adolescents for control of severe aggression with an affective component. However, limited and mixed findings regarding its efficacy (see the qualitative review by Connor, 2002, for a complete survey of studies involving the use of lithium in reducing aggression in children and adolescents), as well as concerns about serious toxicity and side effects, have led psychopharmacologists to recommend that lithium be used to treat CP only in a very specific circumstance—with explosively aggressive youths who have failed to improve with other treatments (e.g., Waslick et al., 1999). Recommendations for its use come primarily from two separate, large-scale, double-blind, placebo-controlled studies in preadolescents who were diagnosed with CD characterized by aggressive and explosive behaviors, and who were hospitalized following outpatient treatment failure (Campbell et al., 1984: 21 children ages 5–12; Campbell et al., 1995: 20 children ages 5–12). In both studies, lithium was superior to placebo in reducing aggressive behavior and produced fewer side effects than haloperidol (a commonly prescribed neuroleptic). More recently, Campbell and colleagues (Malone, Delaney, Luebbert, Cater, & Campbell, 2000) have extended these findings into adolescence, again showing lithium to be superior to placebo in reducing aggression and related behaviors in a sample of 20 youths ages 10–17.

In contrast to the positive results reported in studies conducted by Campbell and colleagues, Rifkin and colleagues (1997) conducted a double-blind, placebo-controlled comparison study on the effectiveness of lithium in treating CP in 33 inpatient adolescents and failed to find evidence for effectiveness compared to placebo. Likewise, Klein and colleagues (1994) completed a study in which 80 outpatient children and adolescents with diagnoses of CD were randomly assigned to lithium, methylphenidate, or placebo. Lithium did not produce improvement compared to placebo. However, it is notable that in this study children were outpatients, and "only a few" displayed "explosively dangerous outbursts" (Klein, 1991, p. 120), as opposed to the inpatient population in the Campbell and colleagues (1984, 1995) studies, for whom "explosiveness" was one of the selection criteria. Thus issues of CP subtype as a moderator of treatment outcome for youths treated with lithium may be important, and this question has not been examined experimentally. The usefulness of lithium carbonate in treating CP is in need of further investigation.

Clonidine

Clonidine is an alpha-adrenergic agonist originally used in adults as an antihypertensive agent. It has been used in adult psychiatry to lower activation in various disorders of arousal, such as posttraumatic stress disorder, mania, and anxiety. Although the U.S. Food and Drug Administration (FDA) has not approved any uses of clonidine in the treatment of children and adolescents, and almost no controlled treatment trials have been conducted with children, we mention it here because there is evidence that it is increasingly being prescribed by clinicians for children with CP (Stoewe, Kruesi, & Lelio, 1995).

An open, uncontrolled study of clonidine in 17 children (ages 5–15) with severe, treatment-resistant CP, who manifested cruel behavior and property destruction, showed a significant decrease in aggression in 15 of the 17 children (Kemph, DeVane, Levin, Jarecke, & Miller, 1993). Gamma-aminobutyric acid (GABA) plasma levels increased during clonidine treatment and correlated with the reduction in aggression. Hunt, Minderaa, and Cohen (1986) used clonidine for 10 boys with ADHD. Although the treatment targets were primary ADHD symptoms, teachers reported that children were "less aggressive and explosive." Likewise, in a meta-analysis of studies using clonidine with ADHD conducted between 1980 and 1999, Connor, Fletcher, and Swanson (1999) reported ES of 0.16 to 0.58 on symptoms of ADHD alone and comorbid CD. Connor (1993) also reviewed the literature on the use of beta blockers specifically for treat-

ment of aggression in youths, and reported that 83% of youths in these studies showed improvement, although none of the studies used double-blind control procedures.

These studies, along with the predicted effect of clonidine on adrenergic centers related to the arousal system, may be responsible for the increased usage by clinicians of clonidine for children and adolescents with CP, especially those prone to irritability and explosive outbursts. However, these studies are merely suggestive. Evidence for efficacy from controlled research is lacking, and the increase in prescribing practices is therefore not well justified empirically. Further research on the efficacy of clonidine with CP is greatly needed.

Other Psychopharmacological Agents

ANTIPSYCHOTICS (NEUROLEPTICS)

Neuroleptics are thought to have some potential for treating CP in youths because of their antagonistic actions on dopamine, norepinephrine, acetylcholine, and serotonin receptors (Mpofu, 2002), although the effect may be nonspecific and secondary to sedation. These medications (e.g., chlorpromazine, risperidone, haloperidol) have been used historically to treat CP in children and adolescents, especially those who are hospitalized chronically or who display mental retardation. Several controlled trials have demonstrated the efficacy of antipsychotics in reducing aggression, fighting, explosiveness, and hostility, mostly with inpatient youth populations (e.g., Campbell et al., 1984; Findling, Aman, & Derivan, 2000; Greenhill, Solomon, Pleak, & Ambrosini, 1985). In the Campbell and colleagues (1984) study, haloperidol was as effective as lithium and better than placebo in reducing fighting, bullying, and explosiveness in children with CP. However, it should be noted that of these controlled trials, only that by Findling and colleagues (2000) included adolescents (20 youths ages 5–15 were examined). Thus the applicability of these findings to adolescent populations remains unclear. Double-blind, placebo-controlled studies of risperidone in aggressive children and adolescents with below-average intelligence have shown significant reductions in aggressive behavior (Aman, Findling, Derivan, & Merriman, 1999; Buitelaar, van der Gaag, Cohen-Kettenis, & Melman, 2001). Also, uncontrolled trials (Buitelaar, 2000) and case reports (Schreier,

1998) have reported reduced aggression in youths with average intelligence.

The most common adverse effect of the antipsychotics is weight gain. Sedation is also quite common. Concern about serious adverse side effects (e.g., tardive and withdrawal dyskinesias, neuroleptic malignant syndrome) has limited the use of neuroleptics in both treatment and research in this area. Thus, while there is some limited evidence for the use of neuroleptics to reduce aggressive behavior, the neuroleptics tend to be used with the most complex cases and/or after other medications and psychosocial treatment have failed. Recent reviews by Schur and colleagues (2003) and Pappadopulos and colleagues (2003) provide evidence-based and consensus-based treatment recommendations for the use of antipsychotics for aggressive youths.

ANTICONVULSANTS

The use of anticonvulsants for control of CP emanates from the observation of the sudden onset and episodic nature of rage outbursts in some aggressive individuals, and the speculation that these are secondary to abnormal electrical activity in the limbic system, especially the temporal lobe. These drugs reduce the excitability of neurons, especially when they are overactive.

Carbamazepine has been the most studied anticonvulsant in children with CP, with several open (noncontrolled) trials suggesting positive effects of carbamazepine on symptoms of aggression, hyperactivity, and delinquency, and in severity ratings of assaultiveness (Kafantaris et al., 1992; Mattes, 1990; Vincent, Unis, & Hardy, 1990). However, a double-blind placebo-controlled trial of carbamazepine with children who had well-established diagnoses of CD and symptoms of severe aggressiveness and explosiveness found that carbamazepine was not superior to placebo, even at optimal daily doses (Cueva et al., 1996). In addition, the drug was associated with adverse side effects. The sample was rather small ($n = 22$), probably restricting power to detect a difference in this study. In addition, placebo responders were identified initially and eliminated from the subsequent study, providing a very stringent test of the drug. Meyers and Carrera (1989) reported a worsening of aggression following carbamazepine treatment. Likewise, collateral effects (e.g., decrease in white blood cell count, ataxia, and liver and cognitive toxicities) may contra-

indicate the use of carbamazepine in youths. Cognitive toxicity is especially an issue with school-age youths who already may have learning problems. Taken together, the very mixed results regarding effectiveness plus the concern about side effects suggest that further research is needed to support the use of anticonvulsants in children with CP.

ANTIDEPRESSANTS

Clinical use of antidepressants for treatment of CP in children has been stimulated by the higher than chance comorbidity rates for depression and CP (estimates range from 23% to 37%); by an early clinical report of 13 comorbid boys who experienced improvement in depression and in CP symptoms with imipramine treatment (Puig-Antich, 1982); by evidence for altered serotonergic function in children with CP and in aggression (Reis, 1975); and because of evidence for effectiveness of antidepressants in children with ADHD (Biederman, Baldessarini, Wright, Keenan, & Faraone, 1993).

Case reports indicate that selective serotonin reuptake inhibitor antidepressants may be effective in reducing aggression in young males with various aggressive disorders (Ghaziuddin & Alessi, 1992; Poyurovsky, Halperin, Enoch, Schneidman, & Weisman, 1995). Nevertheless, there are no controlled trials of antidepressants in treatment of children with primary diagnoses related to CP. One open trial of trazodone with three children presenting with serious problems of aggression showed significant decreases in aggression (Ghaziuddin & Alessi, 1992). In another open trial of trazodone with hospitalized children displaying a variety of disruptive behavior disorders, CP improved significantly (Zubieta & Alessi, 1992). However, as we have concluded for other drug classes, further controlled research with children with primary CP is needed before strong conclusions of efficacy can be drawn. In addition, because of the potential for cardiac arrhythmias, as well as rare but disturbing reports of deaths in children treated with antidepressants (Riddle et al., 1991), adverse effects must be strongly considered in the benefit–risk ratio assessment.

Aggression Subtypes and Pharmacological Treatment

Throughout this section, we have repeated the observations of several childhood psychopharmacologists that aggression with an explosive, affective component and/or rage seems to be more responsive to pharmacotherapy than does instrumental, controlled aggression without an affective component. Campbell, Gonzalez, and Silva (1992) go so far as to say that "pharmacotherapy is appropriate *only* for aggressive and destructive behaviors accompanied by explosiveness" (p. 70; emphasis added). Although this recommendation seems extreme, especially in light of studies demonstrating stimulant medication effects in mild to moderate overt CP (i.e., aggression) and on covert CP behaviors, there is a growing opinion among childhood psychopharmacologists that aggression subtypes exist and that these have implications for use of a drug treatment strategy.

Vitiello and Stoff (1997) argue that children with the affective subtype of CP should be more responsive to pharmacological and psychosocial interventions aimed at decreasing arousal, hostility, and impulsivity. In contrast, the predatory subtype, which is more goal-oriented, is less likely to respond to drug treatment and more likely to respond to manipulation of environmental reinforcers via traditional contingency management strategies. These ideas are very intriguing, and we echo the call by other researchers for studies examining the interaction of aggression subtypes with outcome of pharmacological as well as psychosocial treatments.

Any consideration of use of drugs with youths must include careful review of their putative effects against their side effects. Physicians considering pharmacological treatments are referred to other authoritative reviews of drug side effects (Kruesi & Lelio, 1996; Werry & Aman, 1993). Likewise, all clinicians prescribing drugs to children must familiarize themselves with FDA regulations and *Physicians' Desk Reference* guidelines. In addition, Bloomquist and Schnell (2002) and Bukstein (2003) both provide excellent summaries of practical issues worthy of consideration and related "best practices" in the administration and management of psychopharmacological treatments in childhood and adolescence.

Prevention

Although the focus of this chapter is on the *treatment* of children and adolescents with CP, we feel that it is important to briefly describe interventions that are either intended, or have been shown, to *prevent* subsequent CP. The

prevention of CP has received increasing interest and attention over the past 15 years. This has been partly due to advances made in the delineation of developmental pathways of CP (especially the early-starter pathway) and the risk and protective factors associated with progression on this pathway. Increased interest in prevention has also evolved from the successes and limitations of the treatment-focused interventions described in earlier sections of this chapter.

To a certain extent, the distinction between treatment and prevention of CP is often difficult to make, because preventive interventions have usually (although not always) targeted younger children who are already engaging in some type of CP behavior (Coie & Dodge, 1998). One distinction is that treatment involves referral for assistance, whereas participation in prevention is usually done by screening. This is a somewhat tenuous distinction. For example, a number of family-based interventions that were developed as treatments for CP have been identified as model family programs for delinquency prevention (Alvarado, Kendall, Beesley, & Lee-Cavaness, 2000). Such programs include the parent training programs for younger children (ages 3–8 years) developed by Forehand and McMahon (1981; McMahon & Forehand, 2003) and Webster-Stratton (2000; Webster-Stratton & Reid, 2003), and treatments for adolescents such as FFT (Alexander & Sexton, 2002), BSFT (Szapocznik & Williams, 2000), MST (Henggeler et al., 1998), and MTFC (Chamberlain, 1994). As noted earlier, the Incredible Years parent training program and some of its adjunctive interventions have been used as a selective preventive intervention with Head Start mothers (Webster-Stratton, 1998; Webster-Stratton et al., 2001a). The Triple P-Positive Parenting Program (Sanders et al., 2003) also has components (e.g., Universal Triple P) that may serve as preventive interventions.

Two broad classes of interventions are applicable to the prevention of CP: (1) early intervention programs with infants and preschool-age children that are not focused on CP per se, and (2) interventions that specifically target the prevention of CP and have focused on youths ranging from preschool age to early adolescence. Space considerations preclude a detailed description of the many programs that have been developed or that are in progress for the prevention of CP. Reviews of such efforts may be found in LeMarquand, Tremblay, and

Vitaro (2001); McMahon and Rhule (2005); Webster-Stratton and Taylor (2001); and Yoshikawa (1994).

Broad-Based Early Interventions

There is growing evidence that early intervention programs (i.e., those that are implemented during the infancy and/or preschool periods) can have long-term effects on the reduction of CP in adolescence and into adulthood (for reviews, see Yoshikawa, 1994; Zigler, Taussig, & Black, 1992). These long-term effects have been noted in later childhood and adolescence, and in at least one case into adulthood (Schweinhart, Barnes, & Weikart, 1993). This is of particular interest, because prevention of CP has not typically been an explicit goal of these interventions. Yoshikawa (1994) has noted four common elements of these interventions: (1) inclusion of both family support and child education components; (2) implementation during the child's first 5 years; (3) at least 2 years' duration (range = 2–5 years); and (4) short- to medium-term effects on risk factors shown to be associated with CP.

One of the best-known of these early intervention programs is the Infancy and Early Childhood Visitation Program developed by Olds, Kitzman, Cole, and Robinson (1997), which offered extensive home visits from nurses to low-income, first-time mothers and their babies. In order to reduce risk factors for infant prematurity, low birthweight, and neurodevelopmental impairment, visits during pregnancy addressed women's health behaviors (e.g., smoking, drug and alcohol use, and nutrition). Visitation continued until the children were 2 years old and focused on improving caregiving and reducing child maltreatment, preventing future unplanned pregnancies, and promoting the mothers' completion of school and participation in the work force.

Several controlled studies have demonstrated the program's effectiveness in meeting these objectives. However, the program had its primary impact on the most at-risk families (low-income, unmarried women) and offered relatively little benefit for the broader population. In comparison to mothers in the control groups, mothers who received visitation had heavier and fewer preterm babies and showed a greater reduction in smoking. Fifteen years later, visited mothers had fewer subsequent births, fewer reports of child maltreatment and child injuries, a greater increase in labor force participation and decrease in welfare dependence, and fewer arrests. Of particular interest was the finding that although the visitation program did not specifically target child CP, it successfully reduced the children's early antisocial behavior, juvenile delinquency, and other problem behaviors (including arrests, running away, number of sexual partners, smoking and alcohol use, and substance-related behavioral problems) (e.g., Olds et al., 1998).

Preventive Interventions Focused on CP

At least two generations of preventive interventions have been designed specifically to prevent CP. "First-generation" interventions implemented in the 1980s have now reported on long-term outcomes, while "second-generation" interventions implemented in the 1990s have reported short- to medium-term outcomes to date. The Montreal, Seattle, and Baltimore prevention trials were conducted in the 1980s and are representative examples of the first generation of preventive interventions.

MONTREAL LONGITUDINAL–EXPERIMENTAL STUDY

The Montreal Longitudinal–Experimental Study (see Tremblay, Vitaro, Nagin, Pagani, & Seguin, 2003, for a summary) evaluated the effects of a two-component intervention in preventing CP in boys identified as aggressive and disruptive during kindergarten in a randomized trial. The program offered parent training based on the OSLC model developed by Patterson and colleagues (1975), and classroom-based child social skills training focusing on prosocial skills and self-control. Services were provided for 2 years, beginning when boys were in second grade.

By early adolescence (to age 15), boys who received the intervention were less disruptive, showed better elementary school adjustment, and reported fewer delinquent behaviors of their own (including stealing, gang membership, and substance use) and friends' arrests than did boys in the control condition (Tremblay et al., 1992; Tremblay, Masse, Pagani, & Vitaro, 1996; Tremblay, Pagani-Kurtz, Masse, Vitaro, & Pihl, 1995). The combined effects of decreases in postintervention disruptiveness (based on teacher reports) and association with deviant peers over the next 3 years mediated intervention effects on obtaining a diagnosis of CD at age 13 (Vitaro, Brendgen, Pagani, Tremblay, & McDuff,

1999). In a growth curve analysis, Vitaro, Brengden, and Tremblay (2001) demonstrated that the level of self-reported delinquency at age 13 was lower for the intervention boys than for the control boys, and this difference was maintained over the next 3 years. Decreases in disruptiveness and increased parental monitoring at age 11 and association with deviant peers at age 12 mediated the intervention effects at age 13. However, the intervention did not significantly affect delinquency (as measured by juvenile court records) or early sexual intercourse. Although the earlier positive effects in elementary school on school adjustment were not maintained, intervention boys were much less likely than control boys to have dropped out of school by age 17 (10.5% vs. 21.6%) (Vitaro, Brendgen, & Tremblay, 1999). The intervention also altered trajectories of physical aggression, vandalism, and stealing from ages 11 to 17 (Lacourse et al., 2002).

SEATTLE SOCIAL DEVELOPMENT PROJECT

The Seattle Social Development Project (Hawkins et al., 1992; Hawkins, Catalano, & Arthur, 2002) was a universal intervention implemented in regular classrooms in the Seattle public school system. The intervention offered a combination of teacher training, parent training, and social-cognitive skills training for children in grades 1–6. Teachers were instructed in the use of proactive classroom management, interactive teaching, and cooperative learning, and in the implementation of a social-cognitive skills training program based on an interpersonal cognitive problem-solving curriculum (Shure & Spivack, 1980). Tailored to the children's developmental level, the parent component provided skills training in effective monitoring, reinforcement, and consequences; having clear expectations; and the encouragement of greater parental involvement and support of the children's academic success.

At the end of grade 6, girls in the intervention program reported significantly more classroom participation, reported more bonding and commitment to school, and showed a trend toward less initiation of alcohol and marijuana use. Boys showed better social and academic skills, reported more commitment and bonding to school and less initiation of delinquency, and were rated as having fewer antisocial friends (O'Donnell, Hawkins, Catalano, Abbott, & Day, 1995). Six years after the program ended, intervention students reported less school misbehavior, violent delinquent behavior, alcohol use, and sexual activity, as well as greater academic achievement and commitment to school (Hawkins, Catalano, Kosterman, Abbott, & Hill, 1999). Moreover, the intervention demonstrated a dose-dependent effect, in that the students who received the comprehensive 6-year intervention showed better outcomes than those who received the intervention in grades 5 and 6 only.

An additional follow-up assessment was conducted with intervention participants at 21 years of age, 9 years after the intervention ended (Hawkins, Kosterman, Catalano, Hill, & Abbott, 2005). Outcomes were compared among the three intervention conditions (i.e., the full 6-year intervention in grades 1–6, the later 2-year intervention in grades 5–6, and the no-treatment control). Outcome measures included self-report and court records. Broad-based positive effects of the full 6-year intervention were found on measures of school and/or work functioning and emotional/mental health. Only a few significant effects were noted in terms of crime and substance use (e.g., lower variety of crime, less likely to have a court record). The 2-year intervention produced much less robust results, although a few positive effects were noted in the areas of school and/or work functioning and emotional/mental health.

THE BALTIMORE STUDIES

A set of universal preventive intervention trials (formally called the Johns Hopkins University Prevention Intervention Research Center Trials, but referred to here as the Baltimore Studies) was initiated by Kellam and his colleagues with first and second graders, using the Good Behavior Game (Barrish et al., 1969; Deitz, 1985; Medland & Stachnik, 1972) described above (Kellam & Rebok, 1992). (A second intervention, Mastery Learning, was not designed to target CP behavior directly; instead, it focused on curriculum enrichment through the addition of materials designed to increase critical thinking, composition, listening and comprehension skills.) At the end of first grade, boys who participated in the Good Behavior Game were rated as having lower levels of aggression on both teacher ratings and peer sociometrics; girls were rated lower on aggression on the teacher ratings, but not on the sociometrics (Dolan et al., 1993). By the end of sixth grade, effects of the Good Behavior Game on teacher-rated aggression were limited only to boys who had exhibited initially high levels of aggression; there were no effects of the intervention for girls or for boys with lower levels of aggression (Kellam, Rebok, Ialongo, & Mayer 1994).

Kellam and colleagues have more recently conducted a second generation of the Baltimore Studies with two consecutive cohorts of first-grade children in nine elementary schools (Ialongo et al., 1999; Ialongo, Poduska, Werthamer, & Kellam, 2001). In these trials, the Good Behavior Game intervention was combined with the achievement-focused Mastery Learning curriculum (and renamed the "classroom-centered" intervention). In addition, a second universal intervention was conducted (the "family–school partnership" intervention); this focused on improving parent-teacher communication, parental teaching strategies, and parental child behavior management strategies. Within each of the nine participating schools, children were randomly assigned to one of the two intervention classrooms or a control classroom.

In an initial follow-up study (Ialongo et al., 1999), the classroom-centered intervention resulted in significantly fewer teacher-rated total problem behaviors in first and second grades (for both boys and girls), compared to control classrooms. The family–school partnership intervention also had a significant impact on teacher-rated total problem behaviors, but only in the second-grade follow-up. In a sixth-grade follow-up (Ialongo et al., 2001), children in both interventions had significantly lower levels of teacher-rated CP than control children did. Intervention children were also less likely to meet criteria for CD and were less likely to have been suspended in the previous year. Overall, results indicated that the classroom-centered intervention produced larger and more consistent effects than did the family–school partnership intervention. Additional studies conducted by Kellam and colleagues (Furr-Holden, Ialongo, Anthony, Petras, & Kellam, 2004; Storr, Ialongo, Kellam, & Anthony, 2002) have found reduced tobacco use in the classroom-centered intervention group and, to a lesser extent, in the family–school partnership intervention group. The risk of initiating illegal drug use was also reduced in the classroom-centered intervention group (Furr-Holden et al., 2004).

In a cross-cultural examination of the Good Behavior Game, van Lier, Muthén, van der Sar, and Crijnen (2004) implemented this intervention in second-grade classrooms in 13 schools in the Netherlands. In each school there was at least one intervention classroom and one comparison classroom (total number of classrooms = 16 intervention, 15 control). Children's behavior problems were assessed via teacher report. Preintervention measures were collected during the spring and early summer of first grade. Postintervention measures were collected at the end of the second-grade intervention, at a 6-month follow-up, at a 1-year follow-up, and at a 2-year follow-up. Three problem behavior trajectories were created, based on children having low, intermediate, or high levels of problem behaviors at baseline. The intervention had a positive effect on all measured categories of problem behaviors (e.g., attention-deficit/hyperactivity problems, oppositional defiant problems, and CP) in children with intermediate levels of problem behaviors at baseline. For children with high levels of problem behaviors at baseline, a positive impact of the intervention was only evident for CP.

Cost-efficacy data from the Aos and colleagues (2004) cost–benefit analysis suggested that the Good Behavior Game intervention saved taxpayers approximately $196 per participant in the program.

FAST TRACK PROJECT

A second generation of prevention trials specifically focused on CP is currently underway. These trials tend to provide more comprehensive intervention components and to implement the intervention for a longer period of time than the earlier prevention trials did. One example is the Fast Track project (Conduct Problems Prevention Research Group, 1992, 2000). This multisite collaborative study is following a high-risk sample of almost 900 children who have been identified by both teachers and parents as displaying high rates of CP behavior during kindergarten, as well as 387 children constituting a representative sample from the same schools as the high-risk children. The neighborhoods in which these children live are in urban, suburban, and rural communities. There is adequate representation of girls (approximately 30%) and minorities (approximately 50%, most of whom are African American), so that it will be possible to examine both the developmental course and the effects of intervention with various subgroups of children.

Half of the children in the high-risk sample participated in an intensive and long-term intervention that was designed to address the developmental issues involved in the early-starter pathway of CP. The Fast Track project is unique in the size, scope, and duration of the intervention. The intervention began in grade 1 and continued through grade 10. However, there were two periods of more intensive intervention: school entry (grades 1–2) and the transition into middle school (grades 5–6). The intervention at school entry targeted proximal changes in six domains: (1) disruptive behaviors in the home; (2) disruptive and off-task behaviors in the school; (3) social-cognitive skills facilitating affect regulation, as well as social problem-solving skills; (4) peer relations; (5) academic skills; and (6) the family–school relationship. Integrated intervention components included parent training, home visiting, social skills training, academic tutoring, and a teacher-based classroom intervention. (See Bierman, Greenberg, & Conduct Problems Prevention Research Group, 1996, and McMahon, Slough, & Conduct Problems Prevention Research Group, 1996, for detailed descriptions of the first phase of the intervention.) The intervention at the entry into middle school (and through grade 10) included interventions with increasing emphasis on parent/adult monitoring and positive involvement, peer affiliation and peer influence, academic achievement and orientation to school, and social cognition and identity development.

Evaluations of the effects of the intervention through elementary school have been encouraging, with hypothesized changes in the domains described above being obtained, and with other analyses suggesting that changes in child CP behavior and related outcomes are accounted for by changes in the hypothesized parent and child mediating variables (Conduct Problems Prevention Research Group, 1999a, 1999b, 2002a, 2002b, 2004). To date, the intervention appears to have been equally effective through elementary school across child genders, ethnicities, and site locations.

ADOLESCENT TRANSITIONS PROGRAM

Another example of a second-generation prevention trial is the Adolescent Transitions Program (ATP; Dishion & Kavanagh, 2002). ATP is a family-based intervention (integrated into a school setting) that is designed specifically to reduce problem behavior in adolescents. It originated from more than a decade of efforts to combine family treatment experience with research on problem behavior. This "tiered" intervention includes three levels of service for families: a universal intervention, a selected intervention, and an indicated intervention (Dishion & Kavanagh, 2002, 2003). The universal intervention, which is provided to all parents in a school setting, consists of a Family Resource Center. The Family Resource Center is intended to (1) provide an infrastructure for school–parent collaboration; (2) disseminate information and norms about protective parenting practices and family management practices that promote school success; (3) educate school and community professionals about accurate assessment of problem behavior and empirically supported treatments; and (4) reach parents with information about available services. Specific Family Resource Center services include school orientation meetings for parents with a self-checkup, books, and videotapes; media on effective parenting and parenting norms; classroom-based parent–child exercises that support and enhance family management practices; child-specific communication with parents about attendance, behavior, and work completion; and screening and assessment.

For families identified as having at-risk youths, a selected intervention (i.e., the Family Check-Up) is available. This three-session intervention is based on motivational interviewing techniques (Miller & Rollnick, 1991) and offers families (1) an initial interview, (2) a comprehensive assessment, and (3) a feedback session utilizing motivational techniques to encourage maintenance of current positive parenting skills and change of problematic parenting practices.

For families of youths with ongoing problem behavior, an indicated level of intervention is available. A menu of family interventions allows for the provision of direct professional support to parents in dealing with youth adjustment and CP. The available interventions include a brief family intervention, a school monitoring system, parent groups, behavioral family therapy, and case management services. These core intervention components are offered to families as part of the Family Management Curriculum (FMC), which provides a framework for working with families in groups or individually. This curriculum can include a family management group, a home–school card, sessions on special topics, monthly monitoring, individual family management therapy, and referrals to more intensive services.

In an early component analysis of ATP involving 120 families with high-risk adolescents (Dishion & Andrews, 1995), two cognitive-behavioral curricula were examined. The first curriculum was a group intervention for adolescents aimed at improving self-regulation. The second curriculum evaluated was the FMC for parents (described above as the main component in the ATP's indicated level of intervention). Early outcome analyses showed that, contrary to expectations, rates of problem behaviors in the adolescents receiving the group intervention *escalated*, compared to those of the control group (i.e., the adolescent group intervention resulted in iatrogenic effects, as discussed earlier). Thus this adolescent group intervention was dropped from the ATP intervention model. However, the FMC intervention was associated with reductions in parent–child coercion as measured from videotaped parent–child interactions, as well as reductions in teacher-reported antisocial behavior. Reductions in substance use for the FMC group were also noted at immediate follow-up, but faded by the 1-year follow-up and were not evident in later follow-ups. Irvine, Biglan, Metzler, Smolkowski, and Ary (1999) replicated these FMC intervention effects in a sample of high-risk rural families. At the conclusion of the intervention, they found that families in the FMC group showed improved child-rearing practices and reduced adolescent problem behavior.

Project Alliance, a prevention trial initiated in 1996, is currently underway to test the full ATP model (Dishion & Kavanagh, 2003). Two cohorts of sixth-grade youths (*n* = 999 families) in three middle schools were randomly assigned to intervention or control conditions. Initial findings with the first cohort (*n* = 672) indicated that ATP produced a reliable reduction in substance use for both typically developing and high-risk students (Dishion, Kavanagh, Schneiger, Nelson, & Kaufman, 2002). Effects did not differ significantly by ethnicity or gender. Outcomes related to CP have not yet been reported.

In a recent study, the impact of the Family Check-Up (the selected intervention in the ATP model) on parental monitoring was examined in a subset of the Project Alliance sample (*n* = 71 families) (Dishion, Nelson, & Kavanagh, 2003). Families receiving the Family Check-Up intervention increased their monitoring from seventh to eighth grades, whereas control families decreased their monitoring during this period. Furthermore, this increase in monitoring mediated an association between membership in the Family Check-Up intervention group and reduced substance use.

ATP has also been identified as a cost-effective intervention. The Aos and colleagues (2004) cost–benefit analysis showed that ATP saved taxpayers approximately $1,938 per participant in the program.

ISSUES IN INTERVENTION EFFECTIVENESS

In this section of the chapter, we address some of the major issues pertaining to interventions with children with CP. These issues include generalization and social validity; predictors of outcome; comparisons of the relative efficacy of interventions with control conditions (e.g., no treatment, attention placebo) and with other forms of intervention; and the extent to which interventions are being evaluated in effectiveness trials and disseminated.

Generalization and Social Validity

In an earlier section of the chapter, we have employed Forehand and Atkeson's (1977) classification of various types of generalization (setting, temporal, sibling, and behavioral) as an introduction to our evaluation of various family-based interventions for children with CP. With respect to such interventions with preadolescent children and their families (e.g., Brinkmeyer & Eyberg, 2003; McMahon & Forehand, 2003; Patterson et al., 1975; Sanders et al., 2003; Webster-Stratton & Reid, 2003), there have been a number of investigations assessing the various types of generalization; these have, for the most part, supported the effectiveness of behavioral parent training programs.

Each of the five programs described earlier in the chapter has documented setting generalization from the clinic to the home for parent and child behavior and for parents' perception of children's adjustment (e.g., Fleischman, 1981; Peed et al., 1977; Sanders et al., 2000; Schuhmann et al., 1998; Taplin & Reid, 1977;

Webster-Stratton, 1984). Temporal generalization of treatment effects has also been demonstrated over follow-up periods of 1–6 years (e.g., Baum & Forehand, 1981; Bor et al., 2002; Hood & Eyberg, 2003; Patterson & Fleischman, 1979; Patterson & Forgatch, 1995; Reid et al., 2003; Webster-Stratton, 1990a). Maintenance of effects for the HNC (Forehand & McMahon, 1981; McMahon & Forehand, 2003) parent training program has been demonstrated for up to 4.5 years after treatment (Baum & Forehand, 1981), and less rigorous studies done from 4.5 to 14 years after treatment suggest that the children were functioning well compared to their peer group in terms of parent-, teacher-, and self-reported adjustment (Forehand & Long, 1988; Long et al., 1994). Other parent training programs for young children with CP have also demonstrated long-term temporal generalization effects of 3 years or more (e.g., Daly, Holland, Forrest, & Fellbaum, 1985; Strain, Steele, Ellis, & Timm, 1982).

Several investigators have now assessed setting generalization from the clinic or home setting to the school. In their meta-analytic study, Serketich and Dumas (1996) reported an ES of 0.73 for parent training when the outcome was based on teacher report. Whereas several investigators have reported evidence of generalization in the form of teacher ratings of child CP behavior (e.g., Fellbaum et al., 1985; Forgatch & DeGarmo, 1999; Sayger, Horne, & Glaser, 1993; Webster-Stratton et al., 1988), McNeil and colleagues (1991) demonstrated generalization to the classroom via both observational data and teacher ratings of CP behavior (but not of teacher-rated social competence or observed on-task behavior). McNeil and colleagues also demonstrated that change in home behavior was positively correlated with changes in school behavior (based on parent and teacher ratings, respectively). These generalization effects were largely maintained at a 12-month follow-up, although by 18 months, effects were limited to child compliance only (Funderburk et al., 1998). Evidence of behavioral contrast effects (e.g., Johnson et al., 1976; Wahler, 1975) has occasionally been found. Other investigators have failed to find evidence of generalization to the school, or have found that such generalization was not maintained (e.g., Breiner & Forehand, 1981; Forehand et al., 1979; Patterson & Forgatch, 1995; Taylor et al., 1998; Webster-Stratton et al., 1989).

Based on this research, we suggest that when a child presents with problems in both the home and school settings, improvement in school functioning should not necessarily be expected to occur as a function of family-based intervention in the home; rather, intervening directly in the school may be required. Furthermore, the therapist should monitor the child's behavior in the school regardless of whether this was an initial referral problem, because of the possibility of a behavioral contrast effect.

Several parent training programs (HNC, PCIT, OSLC) have demonstrated sibling generalization at the end of treatment (Arnold et al., 1975; Brestan, Eyberg, Boggs, & Algina, 1997; Eyberg & Robinson, 1982; Horne & Van Dyke, 1983; Humphreys et al., 1978), and this generalization has been maintained at 6-month (Arnold et al., 1975) and 1-year (Horne & Van Dyke, 1983) follow-ups for the OSLC program. However, it should be noted that many of the siblings in the Arnold et al. investigation had been directly involved in the actual treatment program.

Behavioral generalization from the treatment of child noncompliance to other deviant behaviors (e.g., aggression, temper tantrums) has been demonstrated for both the HNC (Wells, Forehand, & Griest, 1980) and Incredible Years (Webster-Stratton, 1984) parent training programs for younger children with CP, as well as by other parent trainers (e.g., Russo et al., 1981). Significant reductions in a composite measure of observed coercive child behaviors and in PDR scores over the course of treatment suggest that the OSLC parent training program for preadolescent children with CP also manifests behavioral generality (e.g., Fleischman, 1981; Fleischman & Szykula, 1981; Patterson, 1974), although it should be noted that Patterson and Reid (1973) did not find generalization of treatment effects from targeted to nontargeted observed deviant behaviors.

The social validity of family-based interventions for children with CP has been assessed by a number of methods, including measures of consumer satisfaction completed by the parents (see McMahon & Forehand, 1983), treatment acceptability (e.g., Cross Calvert & McMahon, 1987), and by determining the clinical significance of posttreatment improvements (Sheldrick, Kendall, & Heimberg, 2001). The parent training programs for preadolescents have provided strong evidence of consumer satisfaction at posttreatment and/or follow-up periods of a year or more (e.g., Baum & Forehand, 1981; Brestan et al., 1999; Ireland et al., 2003; Leung et al., 2003; McMahon et al., 1984; Patterson et al., 1982; Taylor et al., 1998; Webster-Stratton, 1989). They have also provided normative comparisons indicating that by the end of treatment, child and/or parent behavior more closely resembles that in nonreferred families (e.g., Forehand et al., 1980; Patterson, 1974; Sanders & Christensen, 1985; Sheldrick et al., 2001). In their meta-analytic review of parent training, Serketich and Dumas (1996) reported that 17 of 19 intervention groups dropped below the clinical range after treatment on at least one measure, and 14 groups did so on all measures.

It is apparent that evidence for the generalization and social validity of family-based interventions with preadolescent children with CP is extensive and, for the most part, positive. A number of studies (many of them conducted by Forehand, Sanders and Dadds, Webster-Stratton, and their colleagues) have examined the role of adjunctive treatments in facilitating generalization and/or social validity, over and above that obtained by standard parent training programs. Adjunctive treatments have included components designed to facilitate maternal self-control/self-management (Sanders, 1982; Sanders & Glynn, 1981; Sanders et al., 2004; Wells, Griest, & Forehand, 1980); child self-control (Baum et al., 1986); maternal depression (Sanders & McFarland, 2000); parental knowledge of social learning principles (McMahon, Forehand, & Griest, 1981); generalization to specific settings in the home and community (Powers & Roberts, 1995; Sanders & Christensen, 1985; Sanders & Dadds, 1982); marital support, communication, and problem solving (Dadds, Sanders, Behrens, & James, 1987; Dadds, Sanders, & James, 1987; Dadds, Schwartz, & Sanders, 1987; Webster-Stratton, 1994); discrimination training for mothers ("synthesis teaching"; Wahler, Cartor, Fleischman, & Lambert, 1993); parental social support (Dadds & McHugh, 1992); and parental stress (Kazdin & Whitley, 2003). One of the more comprehensive adjuncts to date is "parent enhancement therapy" (Griest et al., 1982), which includes components related to parental perceptions of the child's behavior, marital adjustment, parental personal adjustment, and the parents' extrafamilial relationships. Similarly, Prinz and Miller (1994) have developed

an "enhanced" version of parent training that incorporates supportive discussions with the parent about other issues of concern. The utility of these adjunctive treatments when employed in conjunction with the basic parent training programs lends support to the current movement toward a broader behavioral family therapy model of intervention (Griest & Wells, 1983). However, it is important to note that not all of these adjunctive procedures have resulted in enhanced generalization or social validity (e.g., Dadds & McHugh, 1992).

With respect to family-based treatments for adolescents, there have been encouraging developments concerning the generalization and social validity of this approach. However, investigators have either not assessed adolescent and parent behavior in the home (e.g., Alexander & Parsons, 1973; Henggeler et al., 1986) or have not found changes in that setting (Bank et al., 1991). Bank et al. did find significant decreases in targeted delinquent and predelinquent behaviors as reported by parents on the PDR.

Setting and temporal generalization have usually been assessed with some measure of recidivism, the use of which is subject to a number of methodological problems (cf. Gordon & Arbuthnot, 1987). Although the results of the Bank and colleagues (1991) investigation were not supportive of temporal generalization (offense rates for the two conditions were comparable at each of the 3 follow-up years), other family-based interventions have demonstrated temporal generalization effects ranging from 6 months to more than 13 years. Alexander and Parsons (1973) reported reduced recidivism rates at a 6- to 18-month follow-up for adolescents who had participated in FFT, compared to other forms of family therapy. Reduced recidivism over a 5-year posttreatment interval has been documented for juveniles with serious offenses who participated in Gordon's adaptation of FFT (Gordon et al., 1988, 1995). Evidence for the temporal generalization of MST for periods of up to 4 years posttreatment has also been provided (Borduin et al., 1995; Henggeler et al., 1992, 1993), and more recently, Schaeffer and Borduin (2005) have presented evidence of temporal generalization 13.7 years posttreatment. Szapocznik and colleagues (1989) provided evidence for enhanced family functioning at a 1-year follow-up of the effects of BSFT.

FFT also appears to reduce the likelihood of

subsequent court involvement by siblings of the identified client, thus providing some evidence of sibling generalization for this intervention (Gordon & Arbuthnot, 1987; Klein et al., 1977). Henggeler and colleagues (1991) reported that MST also resulted in lower rates of self-reported "soft" drug use and lower rates of substance-related arrests, providing support for behavioral generalization. The social validity of these interventions has not been formally assessed.

With respect to other forms of intervention for children and adolescents with CP, somewhat less attention has been paid to generalization and social validity. Conclusions regarding the generalization of treatment effects for skills training approaches have been somewhat limited by many investigators' reliance on analogue measures and settings to assess treatment effectiveness. Several reviews of the skills training literature (Bennett & Gibbons, 2000; Lösel & Beelmann, 2003; Taylor et al., 1999) have concluded that, overall, there is limited evidence of setting or temporal generalization (exceptions are noted below). In the studies that assessed treatment outcome in naturalistic settings, generalization often either was not assessed or failed to occur (e.g., Guerra & Slaby, 1990; Spence & Marzillier, 1981). Generalization of at least some treatment effects to other settings up to a 1-year follow-up period has been demonstrated for some social skills (e.g., Michelson et al., 1983) and moral reasoning skills (e.g., Arbuthnot & Gordon, 1986) interventions. Evidence of setting generalization to the classroom (e.g., Lochman et al., 1984; Lochman & Wells, 2004), to psychiatric inpatient units (e.g., Feindler, Ecton, Kingsley, & Dubey, 1986), and to community functioning (Goldstein & Glick, 1994) for some of the anger control training interventions has been demonstrated. Maintenance of these effects has been assessed for up to 3 years (Lochman, 1992). Lochman reported that effects were found in the classroom at 3 years posttreatment, but only if the boys had received booster sessions during the second year following intervention. Lower levels of self-reported substance use were found, providing some support for behavioral generalization as well. Lochman and Wells (2002, 2003) have demonstrated continued prevention effects on delinquency and on substance use 1 year after the end of intervention for older children and for moderate-risk children using the Coping Power

program and a universal classroom intervention.

A strong demonstration of generalization for the skills training approaches has been presented by Kazdin (2003). Not only were children who participated in the PSST program while inpatients in a psychiatric unit rated more highly on both parent and teacher report measures (observational measures were not employed) after treatment than children in either relationship therapy or an attention placebo control condition, but this superiority was maintained at a 1-year follow-up (Kazdin et al., 1987b, 1989). Similar findings were obtained when PSST was combined with PMT and compared to an attention placebo control condition (Kazdin et al., 1987a, 1992; Kazdin & Wassell, 2000b). Thus these data provide evidence not only for temporal generalization, but for setting generalization to the home and to school, since intervention occurred primarily with inpatient samples of children.

There is also evidence for the social validity of some skills training approaches. Some social skills researchers (e.g., Willner, Braukmann, Kirigin, & Wolf, 1978) have utilized social validation techniques in a sophisticated manner in their development of teaching procedures for the skills training interventions, and others (e.g., Prinz et al., 1994) have employed assessments of consumer satisfaction from the perspectives of children, parents, and teachers. Kazdin and his colleagues (1987a, 1987b, 1989, 1992) found that children in the PSST condition (alone or in combination with PMT) were more likely to move within or near the normative range on some of the parent and teacher report measures than were children in the other conditions. These data provide evidence for the social validity of PSST; however, using a more rigorous assessment of clinical significance, Sheldrick and colleagues (2001) reported that PSST did not bring posttreatment functioning to within typical limits.

Evaluations of community-based interventions provide evidence for some aspects of generalization and social validity. For example, there is now some evidence to support limited temporal generalization (i.e., 6–10 months) for TFM/Achievement Place (Larzelere et al., 2001; Lipsey, 1999), in contrast to earlier findings that failed to show setting generalization to the home environment or temporal generalization when measures of recidivism were employed (e.g., Kirigin et al., 1982; Kirigin &

Wolf, 1994; Weinrott et al., 1982). These investigations do indicate that TFM possesses a high degree of social validity in how it is perceived by program participants and members of the community. Weinrott et al. demonstrated that although the TFM group homes may not have been more effective than alternative group homes, they were less costly. The data concerning the temporal generalization of MTFC are more encouraging. Long-term follow-up data ranging from 1 to 4 years posttreatment have demonstrated decreased recidivism and increased adaptive functioning (e.g., employment, family relations) for participants in MTFC, compared to residents of traditional group homes (e.g., Chamberlain, 1990; Chamberlain & Reid, 1998; Chamberlain et al., 2002). Some evidence for setting generalization to home and school and temporal generalization has been presented for day treatment programs for children with CP (e.g., Grizenko et al., 1993; Kolko, 1995). Case management services resulted in greater parental consumer satisfaction than did primary mental health care services (Burns et al., 1996).

To our knowledge, the setting generalization to the home of school-based interventions for children with CP has not been assessed. This is potentially of considerable import, given the previously noted findings of occasional generalization or behavioral contrast effects in the school as a function of family-based treatments. Even more restricted forms of setting generalization (e.g., generalization of effects from one class period to another) have usually not been assessed. The available evidence suggests that various school-based interventions often exert their effects only in those classes in which the procedures are implemented (e.g., O'Leary et al., 1969; Walker & Hops, 1976), although use of experimenter-selected material reinforcers (as opposed to child-selected activity reinforcers) did facilitate setting generalization for a token system (Stumpf & Holman, 1985).

Temporal generalization has been largely ignored. Short follow-up intervals (3 to 12 weeks) have been employed in investigations examining token economy and teacher contingency management interventions (e.g., Greenwood et al., 1974, 1977; Walker & Hops, 1976). The CORBEH studies have shown that multicomponent treatment packages do not generalize well from one academic year to the next unless generalization training is attempted

(Walker et al., 1975). The CLASS program has demonstrated maintenance of treatment effects over a 1-year period, but weekly "booster" sessions may need to be held with the teachers during this period (Hops et al., 1978). The temporal generalization of the RECESS program has not been assessed, but Walker et al. (1981) note some anecdotal reports of decay of treatment effects when the program is eventually turned over to the school's playground supervisors. Thus a maintenance phase (Phase 4) is specifically built into the RECESS program, and schools are asked to make a commitment to implementing the maintenance phase over the long run (Walker et al., 2004). When such a commitment is made, greater generalization across time is more likely to occur. Likewise, interventions such as PBS that focus on changing the entire school culture over time and training all school personnel in the essential elements of the program appear to produce the greatest changes over time (Sugai & Horner, 1999; Sugai et al., 2002).

The issue of behavioral generalization of these school-based interventions for overt CP is a critical one. It is essential that investigators who elect to target overt CP behaviors in the classroom not only examine the effects of their interventions on these behaviors, but also determine whether the intervention ultimately leads to adaptive changes in children's academic achievement, social adjustment, and so on (cf. Klein, 1979; Winett & Winkler, 1972). This issue has been largely ignored. (There is at least one study in which changes in academic behavior, as a function of academic tutoring, have led to decreases in CP behavior at school [Coie & Krehbiel, 1984].)

Similarly, the social validity of these school-based interventions has not received systematic attention. The CLASS program appears to reduce demand for special educational services for its participants over at least a 3-year follow-up (Hops et al., 1978), and program consultants perceive their training and the program very positively (e.g., Walker et al., 1988). Teachers perceive the basic Good Behavior Game to be more acceptable than a more complex version (Tingstrom, 1994). The acceptability of home-based reinforcement systems to teachers and students has also been documented (Turco & Elliott, 1986; Witt et al., 1984).

With respect to the various school-based intervention programs for dealing with bullying, there is some evidence for setting, temporal, and behavioral generalization, as well as social validity. In Olweus's (1990, 1991, 1996, 2001) intervention, reductions in bullying were noted not only at school, but on the way to and from school as well. Reductions in bullying were maintained up to 2 years after the program was implemented. (However, it should be noted that the intervention was in effect throughout this period, so, technically speaking, it is not a true maintenance effect.) Reductions were also noted in other forms of CP behavior, including fighting, stealing, truancy, and vandalism. Finally, increases in student satisfaction with the school were noted, providing evidence for the social validity of the intervention.

Other bullying interventions have resulted in behavioral and temporal generalization (e.g., DeRosier, 2004; DeRosier & Marcus, 2005; Orpinas et al., 2003). However, Pepler and colleagues (1993, 1994) noted an increase in racial bullying, even as other forms of bullying decreased. It is not clear whether this was a behavioral contrast effect, or simply an increase that would have occurred regardless of the intervention.

A discussion of the generalization of treatment effects in dealing with covert CP is limited almost entirely to investigations that have dealt with stealing. A study by the OSLC group provides some limited evidence for setting, temporal, and behavioral generalization. Reid and colleagues (1980) noted parent-reported decreases in stealing and other referral problems at posttreatment and at a 6-month follow-up. However, decreases on an observational measure of child aversive behavior were not observed. Furthermore, Moore and colleagues (1979) have presented data suggesting that children referred to OSLC for stealing (only some of whom completed treatment) were at great risk for being labeled as delinquent 2–9 years later. Seymour and Epston (1989) reported decreased frequency of stealing at 2- and 12-month follow-ups, based on parent report. To our knowledge, no one has attempted to assess generalization or behavioral contrast effects of family-based treatments for stealing to other settings, such as the school or community.

In school-based interventions for stealing, Rosen and Rosen (1983) reported maintenance of effects at 1 month for their single subject, and anecdotal reports of decreased stealing of nontargeted items (Switzer et al., 1977) and of disruptive acting-out behaviors (Rosen &

Rosen, 1983) provide minimal support for behavioral generalization. In the latter study, informal teacher and parent reports also suggested a decrease in stealing in other areas of the school and at home. With respect to social validity, methylphenidate reduced levels of stealing (and property damage) to levels comparable to those displayed by a comparison sample of typical boys; however, cheating actually increased as a function of the medication (Hinshaw et al., 1992).

There is minimal evidence concerning the generalization of interventions for firesetting. At a 6-month follow-up, parents reported less overall involvement with fire for children who had participated in a cognitive-behavioral intervention focused on fire safety and prevention skills training than for children who participated in a discussion control condition (Kolko et al., 1991). Adler and colleagues (1994) reported comparable intervention effects at a 1-year follow-up for an educational brochure, whether alone or in conjunction with either a FEMA program or referral to a mental health specialist.

The assessment of the generalization of effects of psychopharmacological treatments has been extremely limited, and most such assessment has been done with methylphenidate. Because the primary clinical use of stimulant medications such as methylphenidate has been to improve attention and decrease impulsivity in children diagnosed with ADHD, the effectiveness of this medication in decreasing both overt (e.g., aggression; Connor et al., 2002) and covert (e.g., stealing; Hinshaw et al., 1992) types of CP might be considered evidence of behavioral generalization. Reductions in aggression have been noted in multiple settings as well, including the lab, classroom, and playground (e.g., Hinshaw, Buhrmester, et al., 1989; Hinshaw, Henker, et al., 1989).

Some preventive interventions have presented impressive evidence for long-term temporal generalization. For example, the Infancy and Early Childhood Visitation Program (Olds et al., 1997) has documented preventive effects on CP behavior in adolescence (e.g., Olds et al., 1998). The effects of the Perry Preschool Project on CP have been demonstrated at age 27 (Schweinhart et al., 1993). Among the preventive interventions that have focused specifically on CP, the Montreal prevention trial (Tremblay et al., 1995, 1996) has demonstrated preventive effects at age 17 (Lacourse et al., 2002), and the Seattle Social Development Project has demonstrated some evidence of temporal generalization at age 21 (Hawkins et al., 2005). The Baltimore Studies have demonstrated temporal generalization of effects up to 5 years postintervention (Ialongo et al., 2001; Kellam et al., 1994).

Predictors of Outcome

We have described a broad spectrum of interventions for the treatment and prevention of CP in children and adolescents. These interventions have varied tremendously in their demonstrated efficacy and effectiveness, both in terms of immediate outcome and in terms of the generalization of these effects. In this section of the chapter, we discuss various predictors of outcome—not only with respect to positive treatment effects, but also with respect to decreasing dropouts (i.e., increasing parent and child engagement). Since the preceding edition of this chapter (McMahon & Wells, 1998), there has been increased attention to attempting to identify mechanisms of outcome (i.e., mediation) as well as moderators of such outcome (e.g., the extent to which intervention effects vary as a function of child age or symptom severity) (Kazdin & Nock, 2003; Weersing & Weisz, 2002). As in other areas, most of the extant research has focused on interventions designed to treat overt CP. Most of that research has been carried out with family-based interventions for preadolescents (i.e., parent training) and with cognitive-behavioral skills training. We have divided our review into child and family characteristics and characteristics of the intervention (e.g., client engagement–resistance, therapist characteristics and behavior). Because of space limitations, our discussion of outcome predictors should be considered illustrative rather than exhaustive.

Child Characteristics

A myriad of characteristics of a child with CP could conceivably affect outcome in a differential manner. These include the nature of the CP behavior (e.g., subtype, severity, duration); comorbid disorders (e.g., ADHD); the child's age, gender, and race; and variables such as temperament, problem-solving abilities, attributional biases, and so on. With the few exceptions described here, there has been a dearth of research in this area. Particularly serious

omissions are the lack of data concerning aspects related to the nature of the CP behavior and to the presence of comorbid disorders, especially ADHD. In terms of CP subtypes, there is some evidence to suggest that children with CP who exhibit "explosive" aggression with an affective component and/or rage may be more responsive to lithium (Campbell et al., 1984, 1995).

More severe or frequent levels of CP at pretreatment have been associated with dropout and negative outcome at posttreatment and at follow-up for parent training interventions (e.g., Dumas, 1984b; Holden, Lavigne, & Cameron, 1990; Patterson & Forgatch, 1995; Ruma, Burke, & Thompson, 1996; Webster-Stratton, 1996b). Similar findings have been noted by Kazdin (1990, 1995a; Kazdin, Mazurick, & Bass, 1993; Kazdin et al., 1994) for skills training, parent training, or their combination, and for interventions to decrease firesetting (Adler et al., 1994; Kolko et al., 1991). Other investigators have not found initial severity of child CP behavior to be associated with treatment outcome or dropout (e.g., Fleischman, 1981; Henggeler et al., 1992). In contrast, Lochman, Lampron, Burch, and Curry (1985) found that greater reductions in disruptive/aggressive off-task behavior in the classroom following their anger control intervention were predicted by higher initial rates of this behavior. Lochman and Wells (2002, 2003) showed greater intervention effects for moderate-risk children following their Coping Power intervention. Similarly, in their school-based preventive intervention, Kellam and colleagues (1994) reported that higher levels of severity of CP behavior in grade 1 were associated with intervention effects (for boys only) at grade 6.

Webster-Stratton and colleagues have examined the extent to which comorbid ADHD and comorbid anxiety/depression may predict treatment outcome in some of the Incredible Years interventions. Comorbid ADHD did not adversely affect treatment outcome either for the BASIC parent training intervention (Hartman, Stage, & Webster-Stratton, 2003) or for the child skills training intervention (i.e., Dinosaur School; Webster-Stratton et al., 2001a), although Beauchaine and colleagues (2005) demonstrated that children with comorbid ADHD responded best when they received an intervention that included a school-based component. Similarly, ADHD symptoms did not predict outcome at 3–6 years posttreatment for PCIT (Hood & Eyberg, 2003). Comorbid anxiety/depression symptoms predicted more positive response to the Incredible Years interventions and also moderated outcome (Beauchaine et al., 2005). Children with comorbid anxiety/depression symptoms responded comparably to all of the various Incredible Years interventions (parent training, child skills, and teacher training), whereas children with low levels of comorbid anxiety/depression symptoms responded most positively to interventions that included parent training.

Several investigators have found that relatively younger children are more likely to succeed in treatment (Strain et al., 1982; Strain, Young, & Horowitz, 1981), and that their families are less likely to drop out of parent training interventions (Dishion & Patterson, 1992; Fleischman, 1981; Scott & Stradling, 1987) than are older children and their families. McMahon and colleagues (1985) reported no differential treatment effects for the HNC parent training program, either at posttreatment or at a 2-month follow-up, as a function of the children's age (which ranged from 3 to 8 years). Beauchaine and colleagues (2005) also reported that age (also ranging from 3 to 8 years) did not predict or moderate 1-year outcomes. However, a meta-analytic study of parent training (Serketich & Dumas, 1996) found larger effect sizes for parent training conducted with elementary-school-age children than with preschool-age children. Similarly, child cognitive-behavioral interventions appear to be more effective for older children and adolescents than for younger, elementary-school-age children (Bennett & Gibbons, 2000). An examination of potential moderators that might account for this conclusion found that children with greater academic dysfunction and higher levels of general (i.e., unspecified) comorbidity at pretreatment had poorer posttreatment outcomes from PSST (Kazdin & Crowley, 1997). Within an elementary-school-age sample, Kolko (1995) found that younger children were more responsive to a day treatment intervention than were older children. In a meta-analytic study, Lipsey (1995) found that older juveniles with more severe histories showed somewhat larger reductions in delinquency as a result of treatment than younger juveniles with less severe histories did. However, Lipsey noted that these findings may have been due to the fact that the youths with more serious offenses had more room for improvement. Kazdin (1995a) reported that age was not related to outcome in his intervention (PSST, PMT, or the combination). Age was also not a significant predictor of response to intervention for firesetting in two different studies (Adler et al., 1994; Kolko et al., 1991).

The questions of whether interventions for CP are equally effective for boys and girls, and whether gender-specific interventions for girls are indicated, have for the most part been ignored. Most investigators have typically either employed samples composed entirely of boys or failed to analyze their outcome data separately by gender of the children. Several investigators have reported no differential effects on outcome as a function of child gender for parent training (e.g., Strain et al., 1981, 1982; Webster-Stratton, 1996); family-based interventions with adolescents (e.g., Henggeler et al., 1992); or skills training, alone or in combination with parent training (e.g., Gibbs et al., 1984; Kazdin, 1995a; Kazdin et al., 1993). The most comprehensive assessment of the effects of child gender on outcome has been presented by Webster-Stratton and colleagues (1996b; Beauchaine et al., 2005). They reported that both boys and girls responded in a similarly favorable fashion to the Incredible Years intervention components, and that these effects were maintained at 1- and 2-year follow-ups. Gordon and colleagues (1988, 1995) reported reduced recidivism rates for both male and female adolescent delinquents following completion of a modified version of FFT; recidivism was virtually eliminated for the girls. Chamberlain and Reid (1994) found that whereas reports of boys' behavior on the PDR improved during their participation in the MTFC intervention, girls' behavior during the intervention actually got worse. However, completion rates of the program and follow-up arrest data were similar. A history of sexual abuse, regardless of gender, was associated with poorer outcome. A gender-specific adaptation of MTFC for girls in the juvenile justice system has shown promising results (Chamberlain & Smith, 2003; Leve & Chamberlain, 2005). Similar findings have been reported with response to a day treatment program (Kolko, 1995). Two of the school-based prevention programs have reported differential effects of intervention, favoring boys over girls (e.g., Hawkins, Von Cleve, & Catalano, 1991; Kellam et al., 1994). In both cases these effects were further qualified, in that effects were found only for boys who had high initial levels of CP behavior (Kellam et al., 1994) or who were white (Hawkins et al., 1991). On the other hand, the Fast Track preventive intervention has not found evidence of moderation of effects throughout the elementary school phase of this 10-year intervention (e.g., Conduct Problems Prevention Research Group, 1999a, 2002a, 2004). DeRosier and Marcus (2005) reported stronger maintenance of effects for girls than for boys from their bullying intervention. Preliminary or interim reports from several gender-specific interventions for girls have recently presented promising results: the Earlscourt Girls Connection for preadolescents (Levene, Walsh, Augimeri, & Pepler, 2004; Pepler, Walsh, & Levene, 2004); the Friend to Friend Program for relationally and physically aggressive elementary-school-age girls (Leff, Angelucci, Grabowski, & Weil, 2004); and the adaptation of MTFC for adolescent girls noted above (Leve & Chamberlain, 2005).

A similar lack of knowledge exists concerning the relative effectiveness of interventions for CP with children of different ethnicities (e.g., Forehand & Kotchick, 1996; Kumpfer, Alvarado, Smith, & Bellamy, 2002; Prinz & Miller, 1991). In many cases, samples consisted of children from different ethnic backgrounds; however, the issue of whether ethnicity served as a predictor or moderator of intervention outcome or of dropout was not examined. In several cases, ethnicity has not been found to be a predictor or moderator of treatment outcome (e.g., Brondino et al., 1997; Conduct Problems Prevention Research Group, 2002b; Reid et al., 2001; Strain et al., 1981, 1982). However, minority status was associated with dropout from another parent training program (Holden et al., 1990) and from Kazdin's (2003) intervention (PSST, PMT, or the combination) (Kazdin et al., 1993). Some investigators have reported positive intervention findings with African American samples for skills training interventions (e.g., Kendall et al., 1990; Lochman et al., 1981). On the other hand, Hawkins and colleagues (1991) reported that effects of their school-based prevention program at the end of second grade were limited to European American boys; the intervention was not shown to be effective with African American children or with European American girls. A meta-analysis of 305 intervention studies with delinquent juveniles (Wilson, Lipsey, & Soydan, 2003) found that interventions for ju-venile delinquency generally had positive effects for minority youths, and that these effects were comparable to those found for non-minority youths. BSFT (Santisteban et al., 2003; Szapocznik et al., 1989) is one of the few ethnically specific interventions (i.e., for Hispanic youths and their families) that has empirical support for the treatment of CP.

Other individual-difference variables have been examined even less frequently. With respect to cognitive interventions, Dodge (1985) has stressed the importance of accurately identifying and assessing an individual child's particular processing deficits. Attributional biases that arise from faulty formal information analysis should respond best to self-instructional interventions, whereas more affectively driven attributions indicate alternative interventions, such as extinguishing the negative affective response. Lochman and colleagues (1985) found that lower initial levels of interpersonal problem-solving abilities and higher parental ratings of a child's somatization predicted a positive response on parental ratings of the child's aggression following participation in anger control training. Children with lower perceived levels of hostility and a more internalized attributional style at pretreatment had a more positive outcome from a cognitive-behavioral social problem-solving intervention (Kendall, Ronan, & Epps, 1991).

A number of individual characteristics have been examined as part of meta-analytic research on treatments for juveniles with serious offenses. Lipsey (1999) found that recidivism was not affected by the gender, ethnicity, or age of the juveniles in the samples. In a subset of studies in which the juveniles were institutionalized, recidivism rates were not affected by the extent of prior offenses or the extent of aggressive history (although variation in prior offenses and aggressive history was somewhat limited, because all of the studies focused on severe delinquency).

Family Characteristics

Characteristics that have been investigated include parent behavior, perceptions of the child's adjustment, and personal and marital adjustment; extrafamilial characteristics such as insularity; and structural variables such as family composition (single-parent vs. two-parent households) and SES.

Parenting behavior has been consistently shown both to predict (e.g., Chamberlain & Moore, 1998; Patterson & Forgatch, 1995; Reid, Webster-Stratton, & Hammond, 2003; Webster-Stratton, 1996) and to mediate (e.g., Beauchaine et al., 2005; Conduct Problems Prevention Research Group, 2002b; DeGarmo et al., 2004) intervention outcome. With adolescent samples, this mediation effect has often been shown to work in concert with decreased association with deviant peers (e.g., Eddy & Chamberlain, 2000; Huey, Henggeler, Brondino, & Pickrel, 2000; Vitaro et al., 2001). Parental perceptions of children's adjustment prior to treatment have not been associated with treatment outcome (Dumas, 1984a; Dumas & Albin, 1986) or with dropout (McMahon, Forehand, Griest, & Wells, 1981); however, maternal shifts to fewer blaming attributions and indiscriminate reactions, and more specific and less global summary descriptions of the children, have been shown to be associated with maintenance of treatment effects (Wahler & Afton, 1980; Wahler et al., 1993).

The role of parental personal and marital adjustment in predicting treatment outcome is somewhat unclear. Parenting locus of control did not influence dropout from the HNC parent training program, although parents who completed the program displayed a more internalized parenting locus of control at posttreatment (Roberts et al., 1992). Maternal adult attachment status moderated the relationship between pretreatment and follow-up (1 to 3.5 years) levels of child CP (Routh, Hill, Steele, Elliott, & Dewy, 1995), in that this relationship held only when mothers were insecurely attached. Maternal depression (as measured by the Beck Depression Inventory) has been shown to predict dropout (McMahon, Forehand, Griest, & Wells, 1981) and failure to participate in an 8-month follow-up assessment (Griest, Forehand, & Wells, 1981) for the HNC parent training program. Both maternal and paternal depression and negative life events have been significant predictors of outcome at either posttreatment or at follow-up for parent training (e.g., Webster-Stratton, 1985b, 1996; Webster-Stratton & Hammond, 1990) and skills training (alone or with parent training) (Kazdin, 1990, 1995a; Kazdin et al., 1993) interventions. Maternal depression also moderated 1-year intervention effects for the Incredible Years interventions, in that children of depressed mothers responded best to interventions that included either parent training or child skills training components (Beauchaine et al., 2005). Kazdin and colleagues (1993) reported that a maternal history of childhood antisocial behavior was also associated with dropout from Kazdin's intervention (PSST, PMT, or the combination). Dumas and Albin (1986) found maternal report of psychopathological symptoms to account for 17% of the variance in predicting treatment outcome in their sample of 82 families; however, Henggeler and colleagues (1992) did not find parental symptomatology to be associated with the outcome of MST. In contrast, both maternal and paternal history of substance abuse was a predictor of more positive treatment outcome for the Incredible Years interventions (Beauchaine et al., 2005). In a nonreferred risk sample, Baydar, Reid, and Webster-Stratton (2003) failed to find a relationship between a composite measure of parental personal adjustment (i.e., depression, anger, history of childhood abuse, substance abuse) and engagement in, or outcome of, the BASIC parent training intervention.

For the most part, level of marital satisfaction has not been found to differentially affect treatment outcome and generalization at posttreatment or brief follow-up assessments (Brody & Forehand, 1985; Dadds, Schwartz, et al., 1987; Forehand, Griest, Wells, & McMahon, 1982). For example, Forehand et al. (1982) reported comparable improvements in parents' and children's behavior and in parental perceptions of the children's behavior at posttreatment and at a 2-month follow-up, regardless of level of marital satisfaction prior to treatment. However, Dadds, Schwartz, and Sanders (1987) failed to find maintenance of the effects of parent training at a 6-month follow-up for maritally distressed families; this suggests that over longer periods of time, marital distress may ultimately impede temporal generalization. In addition, paternal marital satisfaction was found to be a predictor of posttreatment (but not 1-year follow-up) success for both observed paternal and child behavior (Webster-Stratton & Hammond, 1990). More recently, Beauchaine and colleagues (2005) reported that low marital adjustment was associated with more positive outcomes at 1-year follow-up for families that received the parent training component (i.e., BASIC) of the Incredible Years intervention.

Although there is evidence that fathers' behavior and/or perceptions regarding their children with CP change as a function of participation in parent training interventions (e.g., Eyberg & Robinson, 1982; Taplin & Reid, 1977; Webster-Stratton, 1985a, 1994; Webster-Stratton et al., 1988), whether or not such participation enhances outcome and generalization is unclear. The relatively few studies to address this issue have generally not indicated the necessity of including the father in parent training; however, those studies suffer from a number of methodological weaknesses (e.g., small sample size, nonrandom assignment to groups, lack of follow-up data, reliance on self-report data) (Bagner & Eyberg, 2003; Budd & O'Brien, 1982; Coplin & Houts, 1991). Webster-Stratton and Hammond (1990) found that predictors of successful outcome at posttreatment and at a 1-year follow-up were similar for mothers and fathers when parental ratings of child behavior served as the measure of outcome.

Similarly, single-parent status has failed to emerge as a consistent predictor of treatment outcome when examined as an entity. Although a number of investigators have reported single-parent status to be associated with increased risk of dropping out of parent training or with a lack of treatment success (e.g., Dumas & Albin, 1986; Strain et al., 1981, 1982; Webster-Stratton, 1985a, 1985b; Webster-Stratton & Hammond, 1990), other investigators have failed to obtain similar results (e.g., Dumas & Wahler, 1983; Fleischman, 1981; Holden et al., 1990). In one investigation, single mothers were less likely to drop out than were married mothers (Scott & Stradling, 1987). Serketich and Dumas (1996) did not find either single-parent status or SES to be associated with effect size in their meta-analytic study of parent training outcome. Similar findings have been reported with respect to Kazdin's (2003) intervention (PSST, PMT, or the combination) (Kazdin, 1995a) and interventions for firesetting (Kolko et al., 1991), although Kazdin and colleagues (1993) did find that single-parent status was associated with dropout.

Lower SES has been associated with subsequent dropout in at least one parent training program (McMahon, Forehand, Griest, & Wells, 1981), although for mothers who complete that program, SES does not affect treatment outcome (Rogers et al., 1981). Similar findings have been reported with respect to dropout from Kazdin's (2003) intervention (PSST, PMT, or the combination) (Kazdin, 1990; Kazdin et al., 1993), and for outcomes for other parent training interventions (e.g., Holden et al., 1990; Thompson, Grow, Ruma, Daly, & Burke, 1993) and for MST (Henggeler et al., 1992). As noted above, maternal insularity has been associated with failure to maintain improvements in parent and child behavior (Wahler, 1980; Wahler & Afton, 1980). Dumas and Wahler (1983) examined the relative predictive power of maternal insularity and an index of socioeconomic disadvantage at a 1-year follow-up. Each contributed unique variance to predicting outcome, and together they accounted for 49% of the variance in both studies. Noninsular but disadvantaged families (or vice versa) had approximately a 50% chance of having a favorable outcome, whereas those mothers who were both insular and disadvantaged were virtually assured of failure at the 1-year follow-up. Other investigators have reported similar findings with similar indices of socioeconomic disadvantage (Dumas, 1986; Routh et al., 1995; Webster-Stratton, 1985b), and with cumulative counts of total risk factors (e.g., Kazdin et al., 1993; Prinz & Miller, 1994).

Characteristics of Intervention

The attention being paid to the role of engagement in interventions for youths with CP has increased significantly in the past 15 years. Of prime importance has been the development of conceptual frameworks for examining the engagement process in general (e.g., Cunningham & Henggeler, 1999; Kazdin, Holland, & Crowley, 1997; Prinz & Miller, 1996; Webster-Stratton & Herbert, 1993, 1994) and therapist behavior in particular (e.g., Patterson & Chamberlain, 1994). Prinz and Miller (1996) present four domains that they posit affect parental engagement in family-based interventions for CP: (1) parents' personal expectations, attributions, and beliefs (e.g., expectations about the nature of the intervention, attributions about the source of the child's problem and/or about their own self-efficacy) (see also Johnston, 1996); (2) situational demands and constraints (e.g., financial and social stressors, marital and personal adjustment, daily hassles, and competing demands of other activities); (3) intervention characteristics (e.g., group vs. individual parent training, home vs.

clinic delivery, type of intervention, homework); and (4) relationships with the therapist. Prinz and Miller (1994; Miller & Prinz, 2003) demonstrated that externally motivated attributions for treatment (e.g., an expectation that treatment would focus on child change rather than on family issues) and participation variables (e.g., quality of in-session participation, homework completion) were stronger predictors of dropout from family-based intervention than were various child and family characteristics. Kazdin and colleagues (1997) present a similar "barriers-to-treatment" model. Their model focuses on (1) stressors and obstacles that compete with intervention; (2) intervention demands and issues; (3) perceived relevance of the intervention; and (4) relationship with the therapist. In a series of studies, Kazdin and colleagues have demonstrated that these aspects of engagement added explanatory variance to predicting dropout from PSST, PMT, or a combination of the two (Kazdin et al., 1997; Nock & Kazdin, 2001) and to degree of improvement during treatment (Kazdin & Wassell, 1998, 1999, 2000a), over and above that provided by the child, parent, and family factors described above. Furthermore, there was a clear dose–response relationship between the number of barriers experienced by the family and the likelihood of subsequent dropout. Henggeler and colleagues (e.g., Cunningham & Henggeler, 1999) have identified barriers to engagement in MST related to caregivers, therapists, and therapist–caregiver interactions, and provide a number of practical suggestions for overcoming these barriers. As noted above, as a means of enhancing engagement of youths with CP and their families in treatment, Szapocznik and colleagues have developed a "strategic structural systems engagement" approach, which has been shown to successfully increase levels of engagement (i.e., attending initial sessions) and treatment completion (e.g., Szapocznik et al., 1988).

The work of Webster-Stratton and her colleagues (e.g., Webster-Stratton & Herbert, 1994; Webster-Stratton & Spitzer, 1996) has been especially innovative, as it has involved the use of qualitative research methods to describe the process of intervention from the perspective of the parents. Participants in the BASIC version of her parent training program (Webster-Stratton & Reid, 2003) went through five phases during the course of intervention (Spitzer, Webster-Stratton, & Hollinsworth,

1991): acknowledging the problem, alternating despair and hope, "tempering the dream" (settling for less than total recovery), tailoring the program to their own family situations, and coping effectively. Parents' experiences during a 3-year period following the intervention have also been analyzed (Webster-Stratton & Herbert, 1994; Webster-Stratton & Spitzer, 1996).

The importance of a therapist's establishing a collaborative relationship with a parent during parent training has been emphasized, and therapist activities in such a relationship have been delineated (Sanders & Dadds, 1993; Webster-Stratton & Herbert, 1993, 1994). For example, Webster-Stratton and Herbert have delineated a number of roles for the therapist in the context of the BASIC parent training program: building a supportive relationship, empowering parents, active teaching, interpreting, "leading" (e.g., dealing with resistance), and "prophesying" (e.g., anticipating problems and setbacks, resistance to change, and positive change/success). These roles are probably applicable to other family-based interventions for children with CP as well.

Other investigators have examined the role of therapist characteristics in predicting the outcome of interventions with children or adolescents with CP. A number of process studies have been conducted to clarify the mechanisms of therapeutic change associated with FFT (see Sexton & Alexander, 2003, for a detailed review). Alexander, Barton, Schiavo, and Parsons (1976) reported that relationship characteristics (e.g., affect–behavior integration, warmth, humor) accounted for 45% of the variance in predicting treatment outcome (completion of treatment and reduced recidivism). A structuring dimension (directiveness and self-confidence) accounted for an additional 15% of the variance. Examples of additional research from this group include the association of therapist gender with verbal styles of parents, adolescents, and therapists in the first sessions of FFT (Mas, Alexander, & Barton, 1985; Newberry, Alexander, & Turner, 1991); the differential effectiveness of reframing statements on positive within-session attitudes for adolescents versus mothers (Robbins, Alexander, Newell, & Turner, 1996); an examination of the complex impact of family–therapist alliances on dropout rates (Robbins, Turner, Alexander, & Perez, 2003) and an evaluation of several therapy techniques designed to reduce defensive communications between family members (Robbins, Alexander, & Turner, 2000).

Researchers involved with TFM (Achievement Place) have also provided data indicating the importance of a therapist's (in this case, a teaching parent's) behavior to intervention outcome (see Braukmann, Ramp, Tigner, & Wolf, 1984, for a review). Use of teaching behaviors (e.g., description, demonstration, use of rationales, providing opportunities for practicing behaviors, providing positive consequences) and relationship-building behaviors (e.g., joking, showing concern, enthusiasm) are positively correlated with higher levels of youth satisfaction and, for teaching behaviors, also negatively correlated with self-reports of delinquency (Willner et al., 1977).

Patterson and Chamberlain (1994) have presented a conceptualization of parental resistance in the context of the OSLC parent training intervention that includes both within-session (refusal, stated inability to perform) and out-of-session (failure to do homework) resistance. Initial resistance is thought to be a function of a parent's history of parent–child interaction, preexisting parental psychopathology, and social disadvantage, as well as therapist behavior (Patterson & Chamberlain, 1988). Patterson and Chamberlain demonstrated that these contextual variables were associated with parental resistance throughout parent training. According to their "struggle hypothesis," parental resistance is expected to increase initially, but then eventually to decrease as the parent begins to meet with success.

High levels of resistance in the first two therapy sessions are associated with subsequent dropout (Chamberlain, Patterson, Reid, Kavanagh, & Forgatch, 1984). Directive therapist behaviors of "teach" and "confront" increased the likelihood of parental noncooperative behavior within the session, whereas "supportive" and "facilitative" therapist behaviors had the opposite effect (Patterson & Forgatch, 1985). This poses an intriguing paradox for therapists: The directive therapist behaviors that seem to be intrinsic to parent training would also appear to be those that predict parent noncompliance during treatment. Patterson and Forgatch conclude that two sets of therapist skills are required: "standard" parent training skills, and relationship characteristics (to use Alexander et al.'s [1976] term) to deal with parental noncompli-

ance. Growth curve analyses of parental resistance over the course of parent training have shown a pattern of increasing resistance that peaks at about the midpoint, followed by a gradual decrease in resistance (Stoolmiller, Duncan, Bank, & Patterson, 1993). In addition, Stoolmiller et al. reported that chronic maternal resistance (i.e., failure to work through resistance issues) was associated with child arrest over a 2-year follow-up period. In general, these findings are supportive of the struggle hypothesis proposed by Patterson and Chamberlain (1994).

Consistent with these findings, Harwood and Eyberg (2004) found that higher rates of therapist facilitative statements and lower levels of closed-ended questions and supportive statements in early sessions of PCIT were associated with treatment completion.

There has been a significant increase in research over the past 10 years concerning therapist training and supervision, as well as fidelity of implementation, with respect to various interventions for CP. For example, OSLC researchers have developed and evaluated the Fidelity of Implementation Rating System (Knutson, Forgatch, & Rains, 2003) as a means of documenting therapist delivery of their parent training intervention. This observational measure examines five dimensions of adherence to the program: knowledge, structure, teaching skill, clinical skill, and overall quality. High ratings on this measure, based on videotaped samples of intervention sessions, predicted higher rates of change in effective parenting from baseline to a 12-month follow-up (Forgatch, Patterson, & DeGarmo, 2005). Henggeler, Schoenwald, and Pickrel (1995) have addressed aspects of MST that make it particularly effective in community settings (e.g., high levels of training and supervision for community therapists, a very structured and focused treatment model, efforts to maximize the fit between the therapy components and client needs). Henggeler and colleagues (1997) have also demonstrated that high adherence to treatment protocols is a key factor in the success of MST dissemination efforts.

Comparison Studies

We divide our discussion of comparison studies into those comparing interventions with (1) no-treatment, waiting-list, attention placebo, or "normal" control conditions; and (2) other forms of intervention. Some of the meta-analytic studies examining different modes of intervention for CP provide another useful method for comparing treatment approaches; thus consideration of the relevant research in this area is also included in this section.

Control Conditions

Each of the five parent training programs described earlier in the chapter (e.g., Brinkmeyer & Eyberg, 2003; McMahon & Forehand, 2003; Patterson et al., 1975; Sanders et al., 2003; Webster-Stratton & Reid, 2003) has been positively evaluated in comparison with no-treatment and waiting-list control conditions (e.g., Forgatch & DeGarmo, 1999; Peed et al., 1977; Sanders et al., 2000; Schuhmann et al., 1998; Webster-Stratton et al., 2001b; Wiltz & Patterson, 1974) or an attention placebo condition (Walter & Gilmore, 1973). Furthermore, comparisons with groups of nonreferred "normal" children and their parents have indicated greater similarity in parent and child behaviors and/or parental perceptions of children after treatment (e.g., Forehand et al., 1980; Patterson, 1974). Other investigators have also reported the superiority of parent training over waiting-list control conditions (e.g., Bor et al., 2002; Nixon et al., 2003; Scott et al., 2001).

Family-based interventions with adolescents have also demonstrated superiority over no-treatment control conditions. For example, FFT (Alexander & Parsons, 1982) has been shown to lead to greater changes in family communication immediately after treatment and lower recidivism at 6–18 months post-treatment (Alexander & Parsons, 1973; Parsons & Alexander, 1973), as well as to a greater decrease in sibling involvement with the juvenile courts over a 2.5- to 3.5-year follow-up period (Klein et al., 1977). Similarly, BSFT (Szapocznik & Williams, 2000) led to greater reductions in CP, socialized aggression, parent-reported delinquency, and marijuana use (Santisteban et al., 2003). Parents' perceptions of their adolescents' adjustment improved significantly as a function of MST (Henggeler et al., 1986), whereas there was no change in a normative comparison group.

Investigators evaluating skills training approaches to treating children with CP have, for the most part, done an exemplary job of including no-treatment and/or attention placebo comparison conditions in those evaluations.

Both behavioral (e.g., Spence & Marzillier, 1981) and cognitive-behavioral (e.g., Kazdin et al., 1987b; Lochman & Wells, 2002, 2003, 2004; Prinz et al., 1994) interventions have consistently demonstrated superiority over the comparison conditions on a variety of measures. Similarly, multicomponent skills training interventions have also demonstrated their superiority over no-treatment and/or attention placebo comparison conditions (e.g., Glick & Goldstein, 1987; Jones, 1990; Kazdin et al., 1987a; Leeman et al., 1993). Unfortunately, as noted above, generalization of these effects to naturalistic settings and over time has not always occurred.

Grizenko and colleagues (1993) compared children in a multicomponent day treatment program to children in a waiting-list control condition. Children in the intervention condition displayed greater improvements in parents' ratings of child behavior problems and in the children's self-report of personal adjustment.

Several evaluations of school-based interventions with children with CP have employed control groups. For example, children receiving the comprehensive CLASS and RECESS programs developed by the CORBEH group have shown greater improvement than no-treatment control children in the same schools as the treated children (e.g., Hops et al., 1978; Walker et al., 1981, 1988). In evaluating the national implementation of his bullying intervention program in Norway, Olweus (1996) utilized an age cohort quasi-experimental design that permitted time-lagged comparisons between intervention children and children of the same age who had not yet received the intervention. Other bullying interventions have included nonintervention control schools (e.g., DeRosier, 2004; Stevens et al., 2000), and an individualized bullying intervention also included a normative control group (Baldry & Farrington, 2004).

Few studies evaluating the effects of psychosocial interventions for covert CP have included control conditions. Reid and colleagues' (1980) investigation concerning stealing did include a nonrandomly assigned subgroup of families that served as a waiting-list control group. Results from this study suggested that parental reports of decreased stealing were a function of the treatment program and not simply due to the passage of time. Using a drug–placebo crossover design, Hinshaw and colleagues (1992) found that boys with ADHD who were treated with methylphenidate engaged in less stealing and property destruction than when they were receiving a drug placebo; furthermore, these levels were comparable to those exhibited by a normative control sample.

Several other studies have investigated the relative effectiveness of methylphenidate and a drug placebo in affecting overt CP (e.g., Bukstein & Kolko, 1998; Hinshaw, Buhrmester, et al., 1989; Hinshaw, Henker, et al., 1989; Klein et al., 1994). Double-blind placebo trials have also been conducted with lithium (e.g., Campbell et al., 1984, 1995; Klein et al., 1994; Malone et al., 2000; Rifkin et al., 1997), clonidine (e.g., Hunt et al., 1986), antipsychotics (e.g., Buitelaar et al., 2001; Findling et al., 2000), and carbamazepine (e.g., Cueva et al., 1996).

With respect to prevention studies, the large-scale early intervention program conducted by Olds and colleagues (1998; the Infancy and Early Childhood Visitation Program) included a no-treatment control group. As described previously, this intervention resulted in improved outcomes for both mothers (e.g., fewer reports of maltreatment, decreased welfare dependence) and their children (e.g., less early antisocial behavior, juvenile delinquency, and substance use).

Other Interventions as Comparisons

As evidence for the efficacy of various interventions with children with CP has accumulated, increased attention has been focused on comparing these interventions to other forms of treatment. Family-based interventions with preadolescents have been compared with family systems therapies (e.g., Patterson & Chamberlain, 1988; Wells & Egan, 1988), the STEP program (Baum et al., 1986), client-centered therapy (Bernal, Klinnert, & Schultz, 1980), and available community mental health services (e.g., Patterson et al., 1982; Taylor et al., 1998). With the exception of the Bernal et al. investigation, which indicated superiority of behavioral parent training over client-centered therapy on parent report measures at posttreatment but not at 6- and 12-month follow-ups, the other comparative investigations have supported the relative efficacy of behavioral parent training.

Family-based interventions with adolescents have also been compared with a variety of alternative treatments. The OSLC program

(Bank et al., 1991), FFT (Hansson et al., 2002), and MST (e.g., Henggeler et al., 1992, 1997, 1999; Ogden & Halliday-Boykins, 2004) have been favorably compared with "treatment-as-usual" conditions, which provide the standard array of mental health or probation services available to delinquent adolescents in those communities. For example, in the Bank and colleagues (1991) investigation, these services included family therapy of an unspecified nature and, for many of the youths, group sessions concerning drug use. Other studies of family-based interventions for adolescents have included specific alternative treatments. For example, in a series of investigations examining the efficacy of FFT (Alexander & Parsons, 1973; Klein et al., 1977; Parsons & Alexander, 1973), both client-centered and psychodynamic counseling conditions were included. These alternative treatments proved to be no more effective (and sometimes less effective) than the no-treatment control condition for this sample of adolescents with status offenses and their families. Similarly, an efficacy study of BSFT used a psychodynamic child-centered psychotherapy treatment as a comparison (Szapocznik et al., 1989), and a PSCT study used an alternative family therapy condition (Robin, 1981).

Various types of skills training interventions have been compared with each other or with other forms of intervention. For example, Kazdin and colleagues (1987b, 1989) reported the superiority of PSST with inpatient and outpatient children over a nondirective relationship therapy condition, both at treatment termination and at a 1-year follow-up. Similar cognitive-behavioral skills interventions have been shown to be more effective than supportive/insight-oriented therapy (Kendall et al., 1990) and an inpatient activity group (Kolko et al., 1990). Michelson and colleagues (1983) reported that behavioral social skills training was superior to cognitive-behavioral skills training in maintenance of effects. Results from Rohde, Jorgensen, and colleagues (2004) suggested that their Coping Course intervention was superior to treatment as usual for incarcerated youths. Combinations of treatments have also been shown to be more effective than individual treatment components. Kazdin and colleagues (1992) reported that the combination of PMT and PSST was superior to either intervention alone. Similarly, Lochman and Wells (2002, 2003) demonstrated that although the Coping Power child and parent interventions were each superior to the control condition, the combination of these two treatments produced the best result.

Community-based residential programs such as TFM (Achievement Place; Kirigin, 1996) have not, to our knowledge, been compared with no-treatment or attention placebo control conditions. Most evaluations have indicated that the superiority of TFM over other types of group homes is limited for the most part to the period when the youths are active participants in the program (e.g., Kirigin & Wolf, 1994; Kirigin et al., 1982; Weinrott et al., 1982; Wolf, Braukmann, & Kirigin Ramp, 1987).

Therapeutic foster care, as exemplified by MTFC (Chamberlain, 2003), has been compared to a variety of existing community services, such as group homes and/or training schools (e.g., Chamberlain & Reid, 1998; Chamberlain & Smith, 2003). MTFC has also been compared to a condition in which foster parents were untrained (Chamberlain et al., 1992), as well as to individual, group, and family therapy (Chamberlain & Reid, 1998; Fisher & Chamberlain, 2000). As noted above, MTFC has been demonstrated to be more effective in outcome than these alternative services and to contribute to significantly better outcomes at long-term follow-up (2 to 4 years).

Several studies have compared various forms of treatment in the school. For example, studies have shown that combined interventions including both positive and negative contingencies are more effective than either alone (see Rosen et al., 1990; Walker et al., 2004). Other studies have assessed the relative effectiveness of individual versus group contingencies in token programs (see Pigott & Heggie, 1986).

With respect to interventions for covert CP behaviors, several investigators have compared multiple interventions. Henderson (1983) presented descriptive data suggesting that children who received his behavioral ICT program engaged in stealing less frequently over a 2-year period than children who had received a variety of other interventions, either singly or in combination (e.g., counseling, placement in a residential setting or special education class). Kolko and colleagues (1991) reported that a cognitive-behavioral group treatment focusing on fire safety skills training was superior to a discussion group. In a study of the relative effectiveness of fire safety skills training administered in community versus mental health settings, Kolko (2001) reported that both of these interventions were equally effective in reducing firesetting behavior in preadolescent males.

Adler and colleagues (1994) found no advantage of adding an adaptation of the community-based FEMA intervention program to the provision of basic educational materials, whether referral to a mental health specialist was involved or not.

There have been a few studies in which the relative effectiveness of two medications for dealing with CP behavior has been compared. Klein and colleagues (1994) reported methylphenidate to be more effective than lithium, which was comparable to the placebo in an outpatient sample of children diagnosed with CD. However, in an inpatient sample of children with CD, lithium and haloperidol were both more effective than a placebo (Campbell et al., 1984). More children responded positively to lithium than to haloperidol, and there were many fewer side effects.

Preventive interventions focused on CP usually have not been systematically compared with other preventive interventions. However, because these interventions typically include a school-based component (e.g., Conduct Problems Prevention Research Group, 2000; Dishion & Kavanagh, 2002; Hawkins et al., 2002; Ialongo et al., 2001; Tremblay et al., 2003), the array of prevention programs already present in public schools can be considered "treatment-as-usual" comparison conditions. Overall, the various prevention programs presented in this chapter have been shown to be more effective than these de facto treatment-as-usual conditions (e.g., Conduct Problems Prevention Research Group, 1999a; Dishion et al., 2002; Hawkins et al., 2005; Ialongo et al., 2001; Vitaro et al., 2001).

Meta-Analytic Research

As noted at the beginning of this section, meta-analytic research that compares the efficacy of similar interventions (e.g., a variety of skills training interventions) or that aggregates and examines data from a broad array of interventions (e.g., treatments for offending juveniles) can provide a useful alternative approach for comparing treatment outcomes.

For example, as described above, Sukholdosky and colleagues (2004) conducted a meta-analysis of skills training programs for anger-related problems. Although the overall mean ES for these interventions was in the medium range (ES = 0.67), further analysis suggested that some programs were more efficacious than others. Specifically, skills training, problem-solving, and multimodal interventions were more effective than affective education. Furthermore, whereas skills training and multimodal interventions were particularly effective in reducing aggressive behavior and improving social skills, problem-solving interventions were more effective in reducing youths' self-reports of anger.

Lipsey has conducted some of the most extensive and in-depth meta-analytic research on interventions for CP. Several studies have been conducted examining the efficacy (and, where available, effectiveness) of a range of interventions for delinquency in juveniles between the ages of 12 and 21 (Lipsey, 1992, 1995; Lipsey & Wilson, 1998). In a report on 400 of these intervention studies for juvenile delinquency (Lipsey, 1995), recidivism rates in treated groups (at about 6 months posttreatment) were 45% (compared to 50% in control groups). This decrease represents a 10% relative reduction compared to control groups. Compared to control conditions, treatment also led to (1) a 28% relative improvement in psychological outcomes (e.g., attitudes, self-esteem, clinical scales); (2) a 12% relative improvement in interpersonal adjustment (e.g., peer or family relationships, interpersonal skills); (3) a 12% relative improvement in school participation (e.g., attendance, dropout); (4) a 14% relative improvement in academic performance (e.g., grades, achievement tests); and (5) a 10% relative improvement in vocational accomplishment (e.g., job status, wages).

Significant differences in treatment efficacy were attributable to the type of treatment. Interventions that were skill-oriented (i.e., some cognitively oriented skills training approaches, as well as vocational training), multimodal (i.e., broad groups of services that usually combined a number of interventions), and behavioral (i.e., some more behaviorally oriented skills training approaches, as well as some family and community interventions) resulted in a 20–30% improvement compared to control conditions. Several forms of individual counseling were at the other end of the spectrum, resulting in no significant improvement compared to controls.

Examining the subset of intervention studies with at least a partial focus on juveniles with serious offenses ($n = 200$ studies), Lipsey (1999) found that treated youths in this group had a 44% recidivism rate, compared to a 50% recidivism rate for untreated youths. This re-sult, though modest, is actually quite encouraging because it is almost identical to the recidivism rates for the broader group of juveniles discussed above, suggesting that seriously delinquent youths are as "treatable" as other delinquent youths.

In addition, the meta-analytic findings from this study indicated large ES heterogeneity in the 200 studies. Thus Lipsey (1999) conducted further analyses to better understand the factors influencing intervention efficacy. Studies with institutionalized juveniles ($n = 83$) were separated from studies with the noninstitutionalized juveniles ($n = 117$). For both the noninstitutionalized and institutionalized groups, interpersonal skills training (many of the social and cognitive-behavioral skills training intervention strategies discussed previously were included in this category) resulted in consistently positive effects. For the noninstitutionalized juveniles, "individual counseling" approaches (e.g., MST) and behavioral programs (e.g., FFT) also produced consistently positive effects. In contrast, for the institutionalized juveniles, behavioral programs produced less consistent positive effects (community residential programs and programs providing a variety of community services also produced only moderately consistent positive effects), whereas TFM produced consistently positive effects.

Effectiveness/Dissemination

Since the preceding edition of this chapter (McMahon & Wells, 1998), cross-cultural dissemination studies as well as large-scale effectiveness trials have become increasingly common. These research efforts provide essential information on the feasibility of utilizing CP interventions with diverse populations and transporting these interventions to real-world settings. In this section, we provide a selective overview of cross-cultural dissemination and effectiveness data for the interventions described in this chapter.

Currently, several family-based intervention programs for preadolescents have been evaluated in international settings, and several effectiveness trials have also been conducted. For example, cross-cultural replications of the BASIC program of the Incredible Years (Webster-Stratton & Reid, 2003) have been conducted in the United Kingdom (Scott et al., 2001) and Canada (e.g., Patterson et al., 2002; Taylor et al., 1998). Triple P (Sanders et al., 2003) has also been implemented and evaluated in a number of international locations (e.g., Hong Kong—Leung et al., 2003; China—Crisante & Ng, 2003). A cross-cultural implementation of OSLC parent training (Patterson et al., 1975) is also currently underway in Norway (Ogden, 2000; Ogden et al., 2005). Several of these international implementations have also served as effectiveness trials. For example, international implementations of the BASIC program (e.g., Patterson et al., 2002; Scott et al., 2001; Taylor et al., 1998) were conducted in local community mental health centers. The implementation of OSLC parent training in Norway (Ogden, 2000; Ogden et al., 2005) is currently being piloted in the elementary school system and the child welfare system, with the ultimate goal of nationwide implementation. Several other parent training effectiveness trials have been conducted in the countries where the interventions were developed. For example, Group Triple P has been implemented in a high-risk health region in Australia, with another high-risk region used as a control condition (Zubrick et al., in press). In addition, several trials of OSLC parent training have been conducted by community clinicians, unsupervised by OSLC staff (Fleischman, 1981; Fleischman & Szykula, 1981; Weinrott et al., 1979).

Cross-cultural studies and effectiveness trials have also been conducted for adolescent family-based interventions. FFT has been implemented in Sweden (Hansson et al., 2002), and MST has also been implemented internationally (e.g., Norway—Ogden & Halliday-Boykins, 2004; Canada—Cunningham, 2002). In addition to cross-cultural implementation, the effectiveness of MST has been evaluated in the United States and in international settings (e.g., Cunningham, 2002; Ogden & Halliday-Boykins, 2004). As described in the section on MST, a meta-analysis of MST treatment studies conducted by Curtis and colleagues (2004) showed that ES was larger for efficacy studies (in which MST developers provided supervision to graduate student therapists) than for effectiveness trials (ES = 0.81 and 0.26, respectively).

Regarding other forms of intervention with children and adolescents with CP, dissemination and effectiveness research has been less common. However, a few examples are available. TFM has been replicated in the Netherlands (Slot et al., 1993), and Walker and colleagues (1988) implemented the CLASS program in Costa Rica. Although many of the bullying interventions have been developed internationally (e.g., Norway—Olweus, 1993a), the Olweus bullying intervention has served as a model for programs in a number of other international locations (e.g., the United Kingdom—Smith & Sharp, 1994a; Canada—Pepler et al., 1994).

FUTURE DIRECTIONS

In this chapter, we have provided an overview of the characteristics of children with CP and their families, outlined suggested assessment strategies, and described and critically evaluated a variety of interventions. In this section of the chapter, we provide a brief discussion of current research needs and future directions.

Needs Related to Conceptualizing and Understanding CP in Youths

The heterogeneity of CP is perhaps the greatest stumbling block to advancement of knowledge in this area (Bloomquist & Schnell, 2002; Hinshaw & Lee, 2003; McMahon & Frick, 2005). It relates to issues of diagnosis, subtyping, and developmental pathways. It even relates to the question of whether current approaches to describing and classifying CP behavior adequately cover CP behaviors that occur more frequently, or perhaps even primarily, in girls. In adolescence, issues about the definition of delinquency and its partial overlap with the construct of CP also become salient.

Heterogeneity is also an issue in at least two other domains with respect to CP: comorbidity and risk–protective factors. Youths with CP often present with additional difficulties, including ADHD, internalizing disorders, and substance use. In addition, youths with CP (especially adolescents) are functioning in multiple social settings and groups, some or all of which may be playing a role in the development or maintenance of the CP behavior.

An overarching difficulty is that research concerning diagnosis, subtypes, comorbidity, and risk–protective factors has too often occurred in a vacuum. We have stressed the need to employ a developmental pathways perspective as an organizational schema for integrating knowledge about these various aspects of CP in children and adolescents (McMahon & Frick, 2005; McMahon & Kotler, 2006). Although great progress has been made in the past 15 years in the identification and subsequent delineation of some key developmental pathways (most notably the early- and late-starter pathways), it is clear that there is much more to be learned about these pathways, and that identification of additional pathways is needed to provide a more complete picture of CP's phenomenology.

Specific areas that warrant further investigation include the need for additional information concerning covert forms of CP—especially with respect to lying and cheating, which have been significantly underresearched compared to stealing and firesetting. As noted above, ways in which girls develop and manifest CP have also been quite underresearched. We are optimistic that the many research groups that have made this topic a focus of their work will greatly increase our knowledge about this very important issue in the years to come. Similarly, testing the applicability of various developmental pathways to various cultural groups is essential (Dodge & Pettit, 2003).

Needs Related to Assessment and Intervention

General issues and needs with respect to the evidence-based assessment of CP in youths have been delineated recently by McMahon and Frick (2005). They stress the importance of a developmentally sensitive assessment—not only with respect to age and sex, but also with respect to progression along a particular developmental pathway. They also stress the importance of assessing broadly as a means of addressing the heterogeneity of CP, comorbid conditions, and contextual factors discussed above. A clinician needs to recognize the transactional nature of these developmental and contextual processes, and to conduct the assessment accordingly. Finally, use of multiple methods completed by multiple informants in relevant settings is crucial to the success of the assessment process.

Numerous psychosocial interventions have been shown to be efficacious with children and adolescents with CP, and a smaller number have demonstrated effectiveness as well. At present, there is some limited support for the use of psychopharmacological treatment specifically for CP. Also encouraging is the increased attention being paid to examination of

the mediation and moderation of intervention effects.

Psychosocial treatments for CP that work (or that seem to have the best chance of working) share a number of attributes. First, they are based on empirically supported developmental approaches to CP, including coercion theory and social-ecological perspectives of risk and protection. Second, they consider developmental pathways of CP, target both risk and protective factors, and address multiple socialization and support systems (e.g., Bloomquist & Schnell, 2002; Conduct Problems Prevention Research Group, 1992, 2000). In general, multicomponent interventions seem to be particularly indicated for older children and adolescents, primarily because of the multiple social contexts in which they function. These multicomponent interventions should always include family-based interventions as a core component, and it is important for the various intervention components to be well integrated with each other (Conduct Problems Prevention Research Group, 1992, 2000; Rutter et al., 1998). Alternatively, family-based interventions may be sufficient for younger children.

Finally, it is clear that *prevention* of CP can play an important role. Data from both early interventions (i.e., infancy and preschool) and interventions implemented during preadolescence (and even early adolescence) indicate that they can have important effects on decreasing the frequency and severity of CP during adolescence. Furthermore, as the boundaries between prevention and treatment become increasingly blurred, a related issue is the need for an increased focus on developing coherent continua of service and transitioning from prevention efforts to treatment efforts when appropriate (see Prinz & Dumas, 2004).

We feel that several areas concerning interventions for youths with CP are in need of greater attention. Although most of the interventions presented in this chapter have shown documented improvements under controlled and ideal conditions (i.e., efficacy), it is essential to know whether these effects can be maintained when the interventions are moved to real-world settings (i.e., effectiveness). Some of the treatments presented in this chapter (e.g., Incredible Years, OSLC parent training, Triple P, MST, FFT, MTFC) have studies to support effectiveness, and process research has been conducted to examine factors that may influence the success of treatment once it is implemented outside the relatively controlled environment of efficacy trials. However, in most cases, adequate effectiveness trials have yet to be conducted.

Another set of issues deserving increased attention are those relating to the question of whether interventions specifically targeted to subgroups of youths or to subtypes of CP are warranted. With respect to targeting interventions to subgroups of youths, one area of concern has to do with the serious lack of attention paid to issues of comorbidity in the development and evaluation of interventions for children with CP. For example, although it is widely known that there is an extremely high rate of comorbidity between CP and ADHD, most interventions have been developed to deal with one disorder or the other. Webster-Stratton and colleagues (Beauchaine et al., 2005; Hartman et al., 2003; Webster-Stratton et al., 2001b) are among the few investigators to assess whether comorbid ADHD affects intervention outcome. Similar concerns could be raised with respect to various other comorbid disorders, such as depression and anxiety.

A second question is whether gender-specific interventions for girls with CP are indicated (e.g., Craig, 2005; Underwood & Coie, 2004). It is clear that there is a dearth of interventions specifically targeted to relational and other "social" forms of CP. Because at least during some developmental periods girls are more likely to engage in these forms of CP rather than in physical aggression, then they are more likely to be adversely affected by the absence of these types of interventions.

At this point, some general suggestions for interventions with girls with CP can be made. They include (1) increased awareness of parents and teachers of the seriousness of relational aggression; (2) adaptation and expansion of existing interventions for bullying and other forms of CP to directly target relational aggression; and (3) increased focus on gender-specific interventions targeted to girls as they approach adolescence (Geiger et al., 2004; Underwood, 2003; Underwood & Coie, 2004). With respect to the third suggestion, such interventions might target relational aggression (and, more generally, the development of positive same-sex friendships); the tendency of adolescent females with CP to associate with adolescent males with CP; romantic relationships; and sexual risk taking (Craig, 2005; Leve & Cham-

berlain, 2005; Underwood & Coie, 2004). Thus interventions might focus on relationship enhancement strategies and the prevention of relationship violence (e.g., anger management skills, conflict resolution strategies). The common thread underlying all of these suggestions is the emphasis placed on relationship-based issues and interventions. Underwood (2003) provides a thoughtful discussion about a number of content areas for gender-specific interventions with girls.

A related issue is whether current interventions for youths with CP are efficacious or effective for ethnic minority youths. It is well established that most interventions for adolescents with CP have been based primarily on research with European American, middle-class families (Forehand & Kotchick, 1996; Kumpfer et al., 2002; Prinz & Miller, 1991). Important questions that need to be addressed include the extent to which these interventions work with other cultural groups, whether there is a need to adapt these interventions, or whether culturally specific interventions need to be developed. Unfortunately, few data currently address these questions, and the field is divided on this issue (Kumpfer et al., 2002). Many of the interventions described in this chapter have included other ethnic groups in their program evaluations, and some have noted the generalization of effects across groups (i.e., a lack of moderation), including the Incredible Years, MST, Fast Track, and ATP. The Wilson and colleagues (2003) meta-analysis found that interventions for juvenile delinquency generally had positive effects for minority youths, and that these effects were comparable to those found for nonminority youths. However, this is not to say that culturally adapted versions of these interventions would not be even more effective. Finally, some ethnically specific interventions have been developed and shown to be efficacious (e.g., BSFT for Hispanic youths and their families; Szapocznik & Williams, 2000).

With respect to subtypes of CP, treatments for stealing, reactive–proactive aggression, and CU traits require additional attention. There is some empirical support for interventions that specifically target stealing, but they have not tended to be of the same methodological quality or sophistication that characterizes many of the general outcome studies for CP. Smithmyer, Hubbard, and Simons (2000) have proposed using the cognitive deficits that are differentially associated with reactive and proactive aggression to select intervention strategies. Based on their findings with a sample of incarcerated delinquent adolescent males, they suggested that contingency management systems may be more effective for proactive aggression, whereas interventions designed to decrease attributes of hostile intent (e.g., Hudley & Graham, 1993) may be more effective for reactive aggression. To our knowledge, no specific treatments have been developed for CP in the population of youths identified as having CU traits (Stickle & Frick, 2002). However, building on treatment recommendations for adults with psychopathic traits proposed by Wong and Hare (2005), Stickle and Frick suggest a number of treatment strategies that might be more effective for youths with CU traits. These strategies include (1) early intervention to promote the development of empathy; (2) motivational intervention strategies that will engage youths with a reward-oriented response style; and (3) interventions that focus on relationship development and supervision, rather than on discipline and structure.

Finally, it is important to raise the issue of possible iatrogenic effects as a function of intervention. We present two examples in which this may occur. First, as discussed previously, Dishion and colleagues (e.g., Dishion et al., 1999) have focused attention on evidence demonstrating that the inclusion of high-risk adolescents in at least some peer group interventions may result in increases in both CP behavior and negative life outcomes, compared to control youths. The hypothesized mechanism is so-called "deviancy training," in which youths receive peers' attention for engaging in various problem behaviors (Dishion et al., 1996; Gifford-Smith et al., 2005). Evidence also suggests that iatrogenic effects may occur with groups of younger children (e.g., Boxer et al., 2005; Lavallee et al., 2005) and may be more common in prevention programs than in treatment programs (Dishion & Dodge, 2005). These findings suggest that potential risks and benefits should be carefully considered when intervention and prevention programs including group treatments for CP are being designed and evaluated (Dodge et al., in press).

A second example of potential iatrogenic effects pertains to the use of psychopharmacological treatments for CP. Negative physical side effects are a potential risk with any medication. They should be considered in selecting the medication, and should be monitored throughout the intervention. For example, Campbell and colleagues (1984) reported that both lithium and haloperidol were comparable in the extent to which they decreased explosive aggressive behaviors in a sample of inpatient children. However, lithium had significantly fewer adverse side effects than haloperidol, indicating that it would be a better choice. The possibility of psychosocial iatrogenic effects from these medications should also be considered (Gadow, 1991). These might include externalization of child attributions of control, learning to use medication as a way of coping with stress, or possibly increasing the likelihood of later substance use. Hinshaw and colleagues (1992) reported that although methylphenidate reduced stealing and property destruction in a sample of boys with ADHD, cheating was increased.

CONCLUSIONS

Substantial progress has been made in the development and evaluation of efficacious interventions for youths with CP. Various evidence-based approaches are currently available in home, school, clinical, and community settings. However, a number of factors, including the cost and the availability of these treatments and preventive interventions, preclude many youths from receiving the help they need. In addition, even the evidence-based interventions presented in this chapter may not result in the elimination of CP behaviors. Thus the continued development, evaluation, and dissemination of effective interventions that are sensitive to our growing knowledge about the various developmental pathways of CP, and that are designed to address the wide array of CP behaviors, should be primary goals for researchers and clinicians.

In closing, we wish to present the following guidelines for clinicians working with youths with CP. First, know the problem! By this, we mean that clinicians should stay current with respect to knowledge about developmental phenomenology, assessment, and intervention for youths with CP. Second, it is essential to screen youths with CP and assess them broadly, including the CP behaviors, comorbid conditions, risk and protective factors, and (most importantly) developmental pathways. Third, whereas family-based interventions may be sufficient for younger children with CP, multicomponent interventions are probably going to be needed for older children and adolescents. Although the family-based intervention is core, it is likely that intervention will need to be introduced in other settings as well.

We remain encouraged by the significant advances in knowledge that are being made concerning the development of CP, as well as assessment strategies and interventions for children with CP. However, we also remain sobered and challenged by the limitations of what is still unknown about how best to prevent and treat CP. Our continued hope is that the issues raised in this chapter will serve as an impetus for clinicians and researchers alike to address these limitations.

NOTES

1. We should note that some recent research has brought the neuropsychological risk hypothesis into question; it has been found that neuropsychological deficits may not develop until late childhood or adolescence, some time after entry onto the early-starter pathway (Aguilar et al., 2000).
2. However, given the strong positive correlations between stealing and lying noted above, children who steal may not be veridical in their self-reports.

REFERENCES

Abidin, R. R. (1988). *Parenting Alliance Inventory*. Unpublished scale, University of Virginia.

Abidin, R. R. (1995). *Parenting Stress Index—professional manual* (3rd ed.). Odessa, FL: Psychological Assessment Resources.

Abidin, R. R., & Brunner, J. F. (1995). Development of a parenting alliance inventory. *Journal of Clinical Child Psychology, 24,* 31–40.

Abikoff, H., & Klein, R. G. (1992). Attention-deficit hyperactivity and conduct disorder: Comorbidity and implications for treatment. *Journal of Consulting and Clinical Psychology, 60,* 881–892.

Abikoff, H., Klein, R., Klass, E., & Ganeles, D. (1987, October). Methylphenidate in the treatment of conduct disordered children. In H. Abikoff (Chair), *Diagnosis and treatment issues in children with disruptive behavior disorders*. Symposium conducted at the annual meeting of the American Academy of Child and Adolescent Psychiatry, Washington, DC.

Abramowitz, A. J., & O'Leary, S. G. (1991). Behavioral interventions for the classroom: Implications for students with ADHD. *School Psychology Review, 20,* 220–234.

Achenbach, T. M., Dumenci, L., & Rescorla, L. A. (2003a). Are American children's problems still getting worse?: A 23-year comparison. *Journal of Abnormal Child Psychology, 31,* 1–11.

Achenbach, T. M., Dumenci, L., & Rescorla, L. A. (2003b). DSM-oriented and empirically based approaches to constructing scales from the same item pools. *Journal of Clinical Child and Adolescent Psychology, 32,* 328–340.

Achenbach, T. M., & Edelbrock, C. S. (1981). Behavioral problems and competencies reported by parents of normal and disturbed children aged four through sixteen. *Monographs of the Society for Research in Child Development, 46*(Serial No. 188).

Achenbach, T. M., & Rescorla, L. A. (2000). *Manual for the ASEBA preschool forms and profiles*. Burlington: University of Vermont, Department of Psychiatry.

Achenbach, T. M., & Rescorla, L. A. (2001). *Manual for the ASEBA school-age forms and profiles*. Burlington: University of Vermont, Research Center for Children, Youth, & Families.

Adler, R., Nunn, R., Northam, E., Lebnan, V., & Ross, R. (1994). Secondary prevention of childhood firesetting. *Journal of the American Academy of Child and Adolescent Psychiatry, 33,* 1194–1202.

Aguilar, B., Sroufe, A., Egeland, B., & Carlson, E. (2000). Distinguishing the early-onset/persistent and adolescence-onset antisocial behavior types: From birth to 16 years. *Development and Psychopathology, 12,* 109–132.

Alexander, J. F., Barton, C., Schiavo, R. S., & Parsons, B. V. (1976). Systems–behavioral intervention with families of delinquents: Therapist characteristics, family behavior, and outcome. *Journal of Consulting and Clinical Psychology, 44,* 656–664.

Alexander, J. F., Jameson, P. B., Newell, R. M., & Gunderson, D. (1996). Changing cognitive schemas: A necessary antecedent to changing behaviors in dysfunctional families? In K. S. Dobson & K. D. Craig (Eds.), *Advances in cognitive-behavioral therapy* (pp. 174–191). Thousand Oaks, CA: Sage.

Alexander, J. F., & Parsons, B. V. (1973). Short-term behavioral intervention with delinquent families: Impact on family process and recidivism. *Journal of Abnormal Psychology, 81,* 219–225.

Alexander, J. F., & Parsons, B. V. (1982). *Functional Family Therapy*. Monterey, CA: Brooks/Cole.

Alexander, J. F., & Sexton, T. L. (2002). Functional Family Therapy (FFT): A model for treating high-risk, acting-out youth. In F. W. Kaslow (Ed.), *Comprehensive handbook of psychotherapy: Vol. 4. Integrative/eclectic* (pp. 111–132). New York: Wiley.

Alpern, L., & Lyons-Ruth, K. (1993). Preschool children at social risk: Chronicity and timing of maternal depressive symptoms and child behavior problems at school and at home. *Development and Psychopathology, 5,* 371–387.

Alvarado, R., Kendall, K., Beesley, S., & Lee-Cavaness, C. (2000). *Strengthening America's families: Model family programs for substance abuse and delin-*

quency prevention. Salt Lake City: University of Utah.

Aman, M. G., Findling, R. L., Derivan, A., & Merriman, U. (1999). Risperidone versus placebo for severe conduct disorder in children with mental retardation [Abstract]. *Scientific Proceedings of the Annual Meeting of the American Academy of Child and Adolescent Psychiatry and the Canadian Academy of Child Psychiatry*, p. 205.

Amato, P. R., & Keith, B. (1991). Parental divorce and the well-being of children: A meta analysis. *Psychological Bulletin, 110,* 26–46.

American Psychiatric Association (APA). (1968). *Diagnostic and statistical manual of mental disorders* (2nd ed.). Washington, DC: Author

American Psychiatric Association (APA). (1980). *Diagnostic and statistical manual of mental disorders* (3rd ed.). Washington, DC: Author.

American Psychiatric Association (APA). (1987). *Diagnostic and statistical manual of mental disorders* (3rd ed., rev.). Washington, DC: Author.

American Psychiatric Association (APA). (1994). *Diagnostic and statistical manual of mental disorders* (4th ed.). Washington, DC: Author.

American Psychiatric Association (APA). (2000). *Diagnostic and statistical manual of mental disorders* (4th ed., text rev.). Washington, DC: Author.

Andershed, H., Kerr, M., & Stattin, H. (2001). Bullying in school and violence on the streets: Are the same people involved? *Journal of Scandinavian Studies of Criminology and Crime Prevention, 2,* 31–49.

Angold, A., & Costello, E. J. (2001). The epidemiology of disorders of conduct: Nosological issues and comorbidity. In J. Hill & B. Maughan (Eds.), *Conduct disorders in childhood and adolescence* (pp. 126–168). Cambridge, UK: Cambridge University Press.

Angold, A., Costello, E. J., & Erkanli, A. (1999). Comorbidity. *Journal of Child Psychology and Psychiatry, 40,* 57–87.

Aos, S., Lieb, R., Mayfield, J., Miller, M., & Pennucci, A. (2004). *Benefits and costs of prevention and early intervention programs for youth.* Retrieved from www.wsipp.wa.gov/rptfiles/04–07–3901.pdf

Arbuthnot, J., & Gordon, D. A. (1986). Behavioral and cognitive effects of a moral reasoning development intervention for high-risk behavior-disordered adolescents. *Journal of Consulting and Clinical Psychology, 54,* 208–216.

Archer, J., & Cote, S. (2005). Sex differences in aggressive behavior: A developmental and evolutionary perspective. In R. E. Tremblay, W. W. Hartup, & J. Archer (Eds.), *Developmental origins of aggression* (pp. 425–443). New York: Guilford Press.

Arnold, D. S., O'Leary, S. G., Wolff, L. S., & Acker, M. M. (1993). The Parenting Scale: A measure of dysfunctional parenting in discipline situations. *Psychological Assessment, 5,* 137–144.

Arnold, J. E., Levine, A. G., & Patterson, G. R. (1975). Changes in sibling behavior following family inter-

vention. *Journal of Consulting and Clinical Psychology, 43,* 683–688.

Atkeson, B. M., & Forehand, R. (1979). Home-based reinforcement programs designed to modify classroom behavior: A review and methodological evaluation. *Psychological Bulletin, 86,* 1298–1308.

Ayllon, T., Garber, S., & Pisor, K. (1975). The elimination of discipline problems through a combined school–home motivational system. *Behavior Therapy, 6,* 61–626.

Baden, A. D., & Howe, G. W. (1992). Mothers' attributions and expectancies regarding their conduct-disordered children. *Journal of Abnormal Child Psychology, 20,* 467–485.

Bagner, D. M., & Eyberg, S. M. (2003). Parent involvement in parent training: When does it matter? *Journal of Clinical Child and Adolescent Psychology, 32,* 599–605.

Bailey, J. S., Wolf, M. M., & Phillips, E. L. (1970). Home-based reinforcement and the modification of predelinquents' classroom behavior. *Journal of Applied Behavior Analysis, 3,* 223–233.

Baldry, A. C. (2001). Italy. In R. Summers & A. Hoffman (Eds.), *Teen violence: A global view* (pp. 144–196). Westport, CT: Greenwood Press.

Baldry, A. C., & Farrington, D. P. (2000). Bullies and delinquents: Personal characteristics and parental styles. *Journal of Community & Applied Social Psychology, 10,* 17–31.

Baldry, A. C., & Farrington, D. P. (2004). Evaluation of an intervention program for the reduction of bullying and victimization in schools. *Aggressive Behavior, 30,* 1–15.

Bank, L., Marlowe, J. H., Reid, J. B., Patterson, G. R., & Weinrott, M. R. (1991). A comparative evaluation of parent training interventions for families of chronic delinquents. *Journal of Abnormal Child Psychology, 19,* 15–33.

Bardone, A. M., Moffitt, T. E., Caspi, A., Dickson, N., & Silva, P. A. (1996). Adult mental health and social outcomes of adolescent girls with depression and conduct disorder. *Development and Psychopathology, 8,* 811–829.

Barkley, R. A. (1997). *Defiant children: A clinician's manual for assessment and parent training* (2nd ed.). New York: Guilford Press.

Barkley, R. A., Edwards, G., Laneri, M., Fletcher, K., & Metevia, L. (2001). The efficacy of Problem-Solving Communication training alone, behavior management Training alone, and their combination for parent–adolescent conflict in teenagers with ADHD and ODD. *Journal of Consulting and Clinical Psychology, 69,* 926–941.

Barkley, R. A., McMurray, M. B., Edelbrock, C. S., & Robbins, K. (1989). The response of aggressive and nonaggressive ADHD children to two doses of methylphenidate. *Journal of the American Academy of Child and Adolescent Psychiatry, 28,* 873–881.

Barrish, H. H., Saunders, M., & Wolf, M. M. (1969). Good Behavior Game: Effects of individual contingencies for group consequences on disruptive behavior in a classroom. *Journal of Applied Behavior Analysis, 2,* 119–124.

Barry, C. T., Frick, P. J., Grooms, T., McCoy, M. G., Ellis, M. L., & Loney, B. R. (2000). The importance of callous–unemotional traits for extending the concept of psychopathy to children. *Journal of Abnormal Psychology, 109,* 335–340.

Barth, R. P. (1987). Assessment and treatment of stealing. In B. B. Lahey & A. E. Kazdin (Eds.), *Advances in clinical child psychology* (Vol. 10, pp. 137–170). New York: Plenum Press.

Barton, C., & Alexander, J. F. (1981). Functional Family Therapy. In A. S. Gurman & D. P. Kniskern (Eds.), *Handbook of family therapy* (pp. 403–443). New York: Brunner/Mazel.

Barton, C., Alexander, J. F., Waldron, H., Turner, C. W., & Warburton, J. (1985). Generalizing treatment effects of Functional Family Therapy: Three replications. *American Journal of Family Therapy, 13,* 16–26.

Bates, J. E., Bayles, K., Bennett, D. S., Ridge, B., & Brown, M. M. (1991). Origins of externalizing behavior problems at eight years of age. In D. J. Pepler & K. H. Rubin (Eds.), *The development and treatment of childhood aggression* (pp. 93–120). Hillsdale, NJ: Erlbaum.

Baum, C. G., & Forehand, R. (1981). Long-term follow-up assessment of parent training by use of multiple-outcome measures. *Behavior Therapy, 12,* 643–652.

Baum, C. G., Reyna McGlone, C. L., & Ollendick, T. H. (1986, November). *The efficacy of behavioral parent training: Behavioral parent training plus clinical self-control training, and a modified STEP program with children referred for noncompliance.* Paper presented at the annual meeting of the Association for Advancement of Behavior Therapy, Chicago.

Baydar, N., Reid, M. J., & Webster-Stratton, C. (2003). The role of mental health factors and program engagement in the effectiveness of a preventive parenting program for Head Start mothers. *Child Development, 74,* 1433–1453.

Beauchaine, T. P., Webster-Stratton, C., & Reid, M. J. (2005). Mediators, moderators, and predictors of 1-year outcomes among children treated for early-onset conduct problems: A latent growth curve analysis. *Journal of Consulting and Clinical Psychology, 73,* 371–388.

Beck, A. T., Steer, R. A., & Brown, G. K. (1996). *Beck Depression Inventory manual* (2nd ed.). San Antonio, TX: Psychological Corporation.

Becker, K. D., Stuewig, J., Herrera, V. M., & McCloskey, L. A. (2004). A study of firesetting and animal cruelty in children: Family influences and adult outcomes. *Journal of the American Academy of Child and Adolescent Psychiatry, 43,* 905–912.

Becker, W. C., Madsen, C. H., Arnold, C. R., & Thomas, D. R. (1967). The contingent use of teacher attention and praising in reducing classroom problems. *Journal of Special Education, 1,* 287–307.

Bell, S., & Eyberg, S. M. (2002). Parent–Child Interaction Therapy. In L. VanderCreek, S. Knapp, & T. L. Jackson (Eds.), *Innovations in clinical practice: A source book* (Vol. 20, pp. 57–74). Sarasota, FL: Professional Resource Press.

Bennett, D. S., & Gibbons, T. A. (2000). Efficacy of child cognitive-behavioral interventions for antisocial behavior: A meta-analysis. *Child & Family Behavior Therapy, 22,* 1–15.

Bernal, M. E., Klinnert, M. D., & Schultz, L. A. (1980). Outcome evaluation of behavioral parent training and client-centered parent counseling for children with conduct problems. *Journal of Applied Behavior Analysis, 13,* 677–691.

Bickman, L., Lambert, W. E., Andrade, A. R., & Penaloza, R. V. (2000). The Fort Bragg continuum of care for children and adolescents: Mental health outcomes over five years. *Journal of Consulting and Clinical Psychology, 68,* 710–716.

Biederman, J., Baldessarini, R. J., Wright, V., Keenan, K., & Faraone, S. (1993). A double-blind, placebo-controlled study of desipramine in the treatment of ADD: III. Lack of impact of comorbidity and family history factors on clinical response. *Journal of the American Academy of Child and Adolescent Psychiatry, 32,* 199–204.

Bierman, K. L. (1983). Cognitive development and clinical interviews with children. In B. B. Lahey & A. E. Kazdin (Eds.), *Advances in clinical child psychology* (Vol. 6, pp. 217–250). New York: Plenum Press.

Bierman, K. L. (1989). Improving the peer relationships of rejected children. In B. B. Lahey & A. E. Kazdin (Eds.), *Advances in clinical child psychology* (Vol. 12, pp. 53–84). New York: Plenum Press.

Bierman, K. L., Greenberg, M. T., & Conduct Problems Prevention Research Group. (1996). Social skills training in the Fast Track program. In R. D. Peters & R. J. McMahon (Eds.), *Preventing childhood disorders, substance abuse, and delinquency* (pp. 65–89). Thousand Oaks, CA: Sage.

Bierman, K. L., Miller, C. M., & Staub, S. (1987). Improving the social behavior and peer acceptance of rejected boys: Effects of social skill training. *Journal of Consulting and Clinical Psychology, 55,* 194–200.

Biglan, A., Brennan, P. A., Foster, S. L., & Holder, H. D. (2004). *Helping adolescents at risk: Prevention of multiple problem behaviors.* New York: Guilford Press.

Blair, R. J. R. (1999). Responsiveness to distress cues in the child with psychopathic tendencies. *Personality and Individual Differences, 27,* 135–145.

Blechman, E. A. (1981). Toward comprehensive behavioral family intervention: An algorithm for matching families and interventions. *Behavior Modification, 5,* 221–236.

Blechman, E. A. (1996). Coping, competence, and aggression prevention: Part 2. Universal school-based prevention. *Applied and Preventive Psychology, 5,* 19–35.

Blechman, E. A., Dumas, J. E., & Prinz, R. J. (1994). Prosocial coping by youth exposed to violence. *Journal of Child and Adolescent Group Therapy, 4,* 205–227.

Blechman, E. A., Maurice, A., Buecker, B., & Helberg, C. (2000). Can mentoring or skill training reduce recidivism?: Observational study with propensity analysis. *Prevention Science, 1,* 139–155.

Blechman, E. A., Prinz, R. J., & Dumas, J. E. (1995). Coping, competence, and aggression prevention: Part 1. Developmental model. *Applied and Preventive Psychology, 4,* 211–232.

Bloomquist, M. L., & Schnell, S. V. (2002). *Helping children with aggression and conduct problems: Best practices for intervention.* New York: Guilford Press.

Boggs, S. R., Eyberg, S. M., Edwards, D., Rayfield, A., Jacobs, J., Bagner, D., et al. (2004). Outcomes of Parent–Child Interaction Therapy: A comparison of dropouts and treatment completers one to three years after treatment. *Child & Family Behavior Therapy, 26,* 1–22.

Bor, W., Sanders, M. R., & Markie-Dadds, C. (2002). The effects of the Triple P-Positive Parenting Program on preschool children with co-occurring disruptive behavior and attentional/hyperactive difficulties. *Journal of Abnormal Child Psychology, 30,* 571–587.

Borduin, C. M., Mann, B., J., Cone, L. T., Henggeler, S. W., Fucci, B. R., Blaske, D. M., et al. (1995). Multisystemic treatment of serious juvenile offenders: Long-term prevention of criminality and violence. *Journal of Consulting and Clinical Psychology, 63,* 569–578.

Bosworth, K., Espelage, D. L, & Simon, T. (1999). Factors associated with bullying behavior in middle school students. *Journal of Early Adolescence, 19,* 341–362.

Boxer, P., Guerra, N. G., Huesmann, L. R., & Morales, J. (2005). Proximal peer-level effects of a small-group selected prevention on aggression in elementary school children: An investigation of the peer contagion hypothesis. *Journal of Abnormal Child Psychology, 33,* 325–338.

Braukmann, C. J., Ramp, K. K., Tigner, D. M., & Wolf, M. M. (1984). The Teaching-Family approach to training group-home parents: Training procedures, validation research, and outcome findings. In R. F. Dangel & R. A. Polster (Eds.), *Parent training: Foundations of research and practice* (pp. 144–161). New York: Guilford Press.

Breen, M. J., & Altepeter, T. S. (1990). *Disruptive behavior disorders in children: Treatment-focused assessment.* New York: Guilford Press.

Breiner, J. L., & Forehand, R. (1981). An assessment of the effects of parent training on clinic-referred children's school behavior. *Behavioral Assessment, 3,* 31–42.

Brestan, E. V., & Eyberg, S. M. (1998). Effective psychosocial treatments of conduct-disordered children and adolescents: 29 years, 82 studies, and 5,272 kids. *Journal of Clinical Child Psychology, 27,* 180–189.

Brestan, E. V., Eyberg, S. M., Boggs, S. R., & Algina, J. (1997). Parent–Child Interaction Therapy: Parents' perceptions of untreated siblings. *Child & Family Behavior Therapy, 19,* 13–28.

Brestan, E. V., Jacobs, J. R., Rayfield, A. D., & Eyberg, S. M. (1999). A consumer satisfaction measure for parent–child treatments and its relation to measures of child behavior change. *Behavior Therapy, 30,* 17–30.

Brinkmeyer, M., & Eyberg, S. M. (2003). Parent–Child Interaction Therapy for oppositional children. In A. E. Kazdin & J. R. Weisz (Eds.), *Evidence-based psychotherapies for children and adolescents* (pp. 204–223). New York: Guilford Press.

Brody, G. H., & Forehand, R. (1985). The efficacy of parent training with maritally distressed and nondistressed mothers: A multimethod assessment. *Behaviour Research and Therapy, 23,* 291–296.

Broidy, L. M., Nagin, D. S., Tremblay, R. E., Bates, J. E., Brame, B., Dodge, K. A., et al. (2003). Developmental trajectories of childhood disruptive behaviors and adolescent delinquency: A six-site, cross-national study. *Developmental Psychology, 39,* 222–245.

Brondino, M. J., Henggeler, S. W., Rowland, M. D., Pickrel, S. G., Cunningham, P. B., & Schoenwald, S. K. (1997). Multisystemic Therapy and the ethnic minority client: Culturally responsive and clinically effective. In D. K. Wilson, J. R. Rodriguez, & W. C. Taylor (Eds.), *Health-promoting and health compromising behaviors among minority adolescents* (pp. 229–250). Washington, DC: American Psychological Association.

Brooks, R. B., & Snow, D. L. (1972). Two case illustrations of the use of behavior modification techniques in the school setting. *Behavior Therapy, 3,* 100–103.

Brown, P., & Elliot, R. (1965). Control of aggression in a nursery school class. *Journal of Experimental Child Psychology, 2,* 103–107.

Brown, T. L., Henggeler, S. W., Schoenwald, S. K., Brondino, M. J., & Pickrel, S. G. (1999). Multisystemic treatment of substance abusing and dependent juvenile delinquents: Effects on school attendance at posttreatment and 6–month follow-up. *Children's Services Social Policy Research and Practice, 2,* 81–93.

Budd, K. S., Liebowitz, J. M., Riner, L. S., Mindell, C., & Goldfarb, A. L. (1981). Home-based treatment of severe disruptive behaviors: A reinforcement package for preschool and kindergarten children. *Behavior Modification, 5,* 273–298.

Budd, K. S., & O'Brien, T. P. (1982). Father involvement in behavioral parent training: An area in need of research. *The Behavior Therapist, 5,* 85–89.

Buitelaar, J. K. (2000). Open-label treatment with risperidone of 26 psychiatrically-hospitalized children and adolescents with mixed diagnoses and aggressive behavior. *Journal of Child and Adolescent Psychopharmacology, 10,* 19–26.

Buitelaar, J. K., van der Gaag, R. J., Cohen-Kettenis, P., & Melman, C. T. M. (2001). A randomized controlled trial of risperidone in the treatment of aggression in hospitalized adolescents with subaverage cognitive abilities. *Journal of Clinical Psychiatry, 62,* 239–248.

Bukstein, O. G. (2003). Psychopharmacology of disruptive behavior disorders. In C. A. Essau (Ed.), *Conduct and oppositional defiant disorders: Epidemiology, risk factors, and treatment* (pp. 319–355). Mahwah, NJ: Erlbaum.

Bukstein, O. G., & Kolko, D. J. (1998). Effects of methylphenidate on aggressive urban children with attention deficit hyperactivity disorder. *Journal of Clinical Child Psychology, 27,* 340–351.

Burns, B. J., Farmer, E. M. Z., Angold, A., Costello, E. J., & Behar, L. (1996). A randomized trial of case management for youths with serious emotional disturbance. *Journal of Clinical Child Psychology, 25,* 476–486.

Burns, G. L., & Owen, S. M. (1990). Disruptive behaviors in the classroom: Initial standardization data on a new teacher rating scale. *Journal of Abnormal Child Psychology, 18,* 515–525.

Burns, G. L., & Patterson, D. R. (1990). Conduct problem behaviors in a stratified random sample of children and adolescents: New standardization data on the Eyberg Child Behavior Inventory. *Psychological Assessment, 2,* 391–397.

Burns, G. L., & Patterson, D. R. (2000a). Factor structure of the Eyberg Child Behavior Inventory: A parent rating scale of oppositional defiant behavior toward adults, inattentive behavior, and conduct problem behavior. *Journal of Clinical Child Psychology, 29,* 569–577.

Burns, G. L., & Patterson, D. R. (2000b). Normative data on the Eyberg Child Behavior Inventory and Sutter–Eyberg Student Behavior Inventory: Parent and teacher rating scales of disruptive behavior problems in children and adolescents. *Child & Family Behavior Therapy, 23,* 15–28.

Burns, G. L., Patterson, D. R., Nussbaum, B. R., & Parker, C. M. (1991). Disruptive behaviors in an outpatient pediatric population: Additional standardization data on the Eyberg Child Behavior Inventory. *Psychological Assessment, 3,* 202–207.

Burns, G. L., Sosna, T. D., & Ladish, C. (1992). Distinction between well-standardized norms and the psychometric properties of a measure: Measurement of disruptive behaviors with the Sutter–Eyberg Student Behavior Inventory. *Child & Family Behavior Therapy, 14,* 43–54.

Burns, G. L., & Walsh, J. A. (2002). The influence of ADHD-hyperactivity/impulsivity symptoms on the development of oppositional defiant disorder symptoms in a 2-year longitudinal study. *Journal of Abnormal Child Psychology, 30,* 245–256.

Burns, G. L., Walsh, J. A., & Owen, S. M. (1995). Twelve-month stability of disruptive classroom behavior as measured by the Sutter–Eyberg Student Behavior Inventory. *Journal of Clinical Child Psychology, 24,* 453–462.

Campbell, M., Adams, P. B., Small, A. M., Kafantaris, V., Silva, R. R., Shell, J., et al. (1995). Lithium in hospitalized aggressive children with conduct disorder: A double-blind and placebo-controlled study. *Journal of the American Academy of Child and Adolescent Psychiatry, 34,* 445–453.

Campbell, M., Gonzalez, N. M., & Silva, R. R. (1992). The pharmacologic treatment of conduct disorders and rage outbursts. *Psychiatric Clinics of North America, 15,* 69–85.

Campbell, M., Small, A. M., Green, W. H., Jennings, S. J., Perry, R., Bennett, W. G., et al. (1984). Behavioral efficacy of haloperidol and lithium carbonate: A comparison in hospitalized aggressive children with conduct disorder. *Archives of General Psychiatry, 41,* 650–656.

Campbell, S. B. (1995). Behavior problems in preschool children: A review of recent research. *Journal of Child Psychology and Psychiatry, 36,* 113–149.

Campbell, S. B. (2002). *Behavior problems in preschool children: Clinical and developmental issues* (2nd ed.). New York: Guilford Press.

Campbell, S. B., & Ewing, L. J. (1990). Follow up of hard to manage preschoolers: Adjustment at age 9 and predictors of continuing symptoms. *Journal of Child Psychology and Psychiatry, 31,* 871–889.

Campis, L. K., Lyman, R. D., & Prentice-Dunn, S. (1986). The Parental Locus of Control Scale: Development and validation. *Journal of Clinical Child Psychology, 15,* 260–267.

Capaldi, D. M. (1991). Co-occurrence of conduct problems and depressive symptoms in early adolescent boys: I. Familial factors and general adjustment at age 6. *Development and Psychopathology, 3,* 277–300.

Capaldi, D. M. (1992). Co-occurrence of conduct problems and depressive symptoms in early adolescent boys: II. A 2-year follow-up at grade 8. *Development and Psychopathology, 4,* 125–144.

Capaldi, D. M., DeGarmo, D., Patterson, G. R., & Forgatch, M. (2002). Contextual risk across the early life span and association with antisocial behavior. In J. B. Reid, G. R. Patterson, & J. Snyder (Eds.), *Antisocial behavior in children and adolescents: A developmental analysis and model for intervention* (pp. 123–146). Washington, DC: American Psychological Association.

Capaldi, D. M., & Patterson, G. R. (1994). Interrelated influences of contextual factors on antisocial behavior in childhood and adolescence for males. In D. C. Fowles, P. Sutker, & S. H. Goodman (Eds.), *Progress in experimental personality and psychopathology research* (pp. 165–198). New York: Springer.

Caputo, A. A., Frick, P. J., & Brodsky, S. L. (1999). Family violence and juvenile sex offending: Potential mediating roles of psychopathic traits and negative attitudes toward women. *Criminal Justice and Behavior, 26,* 338–356.

Caspi, A., Lynam, D., Moffitt, T. E., & Silva, P. (1993). Unraveling girls' delinquency: Biological, dispositional, and contextual contributions to adolescent misbehavior. *Developmental Psychology, 29,* 19–30.

Chamberlain, P. (1990). Comparative evaluation of specialized foster care for seriously delinquent youths: A first step. *Community Alternatives: International Journal of Family Care, 13,* 21–36.

Chamberlain, P. (1994). *Family connections.* Eugene, OR: Castalia.

Chamberlain, P. (2003). *Treating chronic juvenile offenders: Advances made through the Oregon Multidimensional Treatment Foster Care model.* Washington, DC: American Psychological Association.

Chamberlain, P., Fisher, P. A., & Moore, K. (2002). Multidimensional Treatment Foster Care: Application of the OSLC intervention model to high-risk youth and their families. In J. B. Reid, G. R. Patterson, & J. Snyder (Eds.), *Antisocial behavior in children and adolescents: A developmental analysis and model for intervention* (pp. 203–218). Washington, DC: American Psychological Association.

Chamberlain, P., & Mihalic, S. F. (1998). *Multidimensional Treatment Foster Care.* Boulder: Center for the Study and Prevention of Violence, University of Colorado.

Chamberlain, P., & Moore, K. J. (1998). Models of community treatment for serious juvenile offenders. In J. Crane (Ed.), *Social programs that really work* (pp. 258–276). New York: Russell Sage Foundation.

Chamberlain, P., Moreland, S., & Reid, K. (1992). Enhanced services and stipends for foster parents: Effects on retention rates and outcomes of children. *Child Welfare, 71,* 387–401.

Chamberlain, P., & Patterson, G. R. (1995). Discipline and child compliance in parenting. In M. H. Bornstein (Ed.), *Handbook of parenting: Vol. 4. Applied and practical parenting* (pp. 205–225). Hillsdale, NJ: Erlbaum.

Chamberlain, P., Patterson, G., Reid, J., Kavanagh, K., & Forgatch, M. (1984). Observation of client resistance. *Behavior Therapy, 15,* 144–155.

Chamberlain, P., & Reid, J. B. (1987). Parent observation and report of child symptoms. *Behavioral Assessment, 9,* 97–109.

Chamberlain, P., & Reid, J. B. (1991). Using a specialized foster care community treatment model for children and adolescents leaving the state mental health hospital. *Journal of Community Psychology, 19,* 266–276.

Chamberlain, P., & Reid, J. B. (1994). Differences in risk factors and adjustment for male and female delinquents in treatment foster care. *Journal of Child and Family Studies, 3,* 23–39.

Chamberlain, P., & Reid, J. B. (1998). Comparison of two community alternatives to incarceration for chronic juvenile offenders. *Journal of Consulting and Clinical Psychology, 66,* 624–633.

Chamberlain, P., Reid, J. B., Ray, J., Capaldi, D. M., & Fisher, P. (1997). Parent inadequate discipline (PID). In T. A. Widiger, A. J. Frances, H. A. Pincus, R. Ross, M. B. First, & W. Davis (Eds.), *DSM-IV sourcebook* (Vol. 3, pp. 569–629). Washington, DC: American Psychiatric Association.

Chamberlain, P., & Smith, D. K. (2003). Antisocial behavior in children and adolescents: The Oregon Multidimensional Treatment Foster Care model. In A. E. Kazdin & J. R. Weisz (Eds.), *Evidence-based psychotherapies for children and adolescents* (pp. 282–300). New York: Guilford Press.

Chandler, M., & Moran, T. (1990). Psychopathy and moral development: A comparative study of delinquent and nondelinquent youth. *Development and Psychopathology, 2,* 227–246.

Christian, R. E., Frick, P. J., Hill, N. L., Tyler, L., & Frazer, D. R. (1997). Psychopathy and conduct problems in children: II. Implications for subtyping children with conduct problems. *Journal of the American Academy of Child and Adolescent Psychiatry, 36,* 233–241.

Clarke, G., Lewinsohn, P., & Hops, H. (1990). *Adolescent Coping with Depression Course: Leader's manual for adolescent groups.* Eugene, OR: Castalia.

Coatsworth, J. D., Santisteban, D. A., McBride, C. K., & Szapocznik, J. (2001). Brief Strategic Family Therapy versus community control: Engagement, retention, and an exploration of the moderating role of adolescent symptom severity. *Family Process, 40,* 313–332.

Coie, J. D., & Dodge, K. A. (1998). Aggression and antisocial behavior. In W. Damon (Series Ed.) & N. Eisenberg (Vol. Ed.), *Handbook of child psychology: Vol. 3. Social, emotional, and personality development* (5th ed., pp. 779–862). New York: Wiley.

Coie, J. D., & Jacobs, M. R. (1993). The role of social context in the prevention of conduct disorder. *Development and Psychopathology, 5,* 263–275.

Coie, J. D., & Krehbiel, G. (1984). Effects of academic tutoring on the social status of low-achieving, socially-rejected children. *Child Development, 55,* 1465–1478.

Coie, J. D., Lochman, J. E., Terry, R., & Hyman, C. (1992). Predicting early adolescent disorder from childhood aggression and peer rejection. *Journal of Consulting and Clinical Psychology, 60,* 783–792.

Coleman, M., Pfeiffer, S., & Oakland, T. (1991). *Aggression Replacement Training with behavior disordered adolescents.* Unpublished manuscript, University of Texas.

Compton, K., Snyder, J., Schrepferman, L., Bank, L., & Shortt, J. (2003). The contribution of parents and siblings to antisocial and depressive behavior in adolescents: A double jeopardy coercion model. *Development and Psychopathology, 15,* 163–182.

Conduct Problems Prevention Research Group. (1992). A developmental and clinical model for the prevention of conduct disorder: The FAST Track program. *Development and Psychopathology, 4,* 509–527.

Conduct Problems Prevention Research Group. (1999a). Initial impact of the Fast Track prevention trial of conduct problems: I. The high-risk sample. *Journal of Consulting and Clinical Psychology, 67,* 631–647.

Conduct Problems Prevention Research Group. (1999b). Initial impact of the Fast Track prevention trial of conduct problems: II. Classroom effects. *Journal of Consulting and Clinical Psychology, 67,* 648–657.

Conduct Problems Prevention Research Group. (2000). Merging universal and indicated prevention programs: The Fast Track model. *Addictive Behaviors, 25,* 913–927.

Conduct Problems Prevention Research Group. (2002a). Evaluation of the first three years of the Fast Track prevention trial with children at high risk for adolescent conduct problems. *Journal of Abnormal Child Psychology, 30,* 19–35.

Conduct Problems Prevention Research Group. (2002b). Using the Fast Track randomized prevention trial to test the early-starter model of the development of serious conduct problems. *Development and Psychopathology, 14,* 925–943.

Conduct Problems Prevention Research Group. (2004). The effects of the Fast Track program on serious problem outcomes at the end of elementary school. *Journal of Clinical Child and Adolescent Psychology, 33,* 650–661.

Conners, C. K. (1997). *Conners Rating Scales—Revised manual.* Tonawanda, NY: Multi-Health Systems.

Connor, D. F. (1993). Beta blockers for aggression: A review of the pediatric experience. *Journal of Child and Adolescent Psychopharmacology, 3,* 99–114.

Connor, D. F. (2002). *Aggression and antisocial behavior in children and adolescents: Research and treatment.* New York: Guilford Press.

Connor, D. F., Barkley, R. A., & Davis, H. T. (2000). A pilot study of methylphenidate, clonidine, or the combination in ADHD comorbid with aggressive oppositional defiant or conduct disorder. *Clinical Pediatrics, 39,* 15–25.

Connor, D. F., Fletcher, K. E., & Swanson, J. (1999). A meta-analysis of clonidine for symptoms of attention-deficit hyperactivity disorder. *Journal of the American Academy of Child and Adolescent Psychiatry, 38,* 1551–1559.

Connor, D. F., Glatt, S. J., Lopez, I. D., Jackson, D., & Melloni, R. H. (2002). Psychopharmacology and aggression: I. A meta-analysis of stimulant effects on overt/covert aggression-related behaviors in ADHD. *Journal of the American Academy of Child and Adolescent Psychiatry, 31,* 253–261.

Coplin, J. W., & Houts, A. C. (1991). Father involvement in parent training for oppositional child behavior: Progress or stagnation? *Child & Family Behavior Therapy, 13,* 29–51.

Costello, E. J., & Angold, A. (2001). Bad behaviour: An historical perspective on disorders of conduct. In J. Hill & B. Maughan (Eds.), *Conduct disorders in childhood and adolescence* (pp. 1–31). Cambridge, UK: Cambridge University Press.

Craig, W. M. (2005). The treatment of aggressive girls: Same but different? In D. J. Pepler, K. C. Madsen, C. Webster, & K. S. Levene (Eds.), *The development and treatment of girlhood aggression* (pp. 217–221). Mahwah, NJ: Erlbaum.

Craig, W. M., & Pepler, D. J. (1995). Peer processes in bullying and victimization: An observational study. *Exceptionality Education Canada, 5,* 81–95.

Craig, W. M., & Yossi, H. (2003). Bullying and fighting: Results from the World Health Organization Health and Behavior Survey of school aged children. *International Report for World Health Organization, 29,* 936–941.

Crick, N. R., & Dodge, K. A. (1994). A review and reformulation of social information-processing mechanisms in children's social adjustment. *Psychological Bulletin, 115,* 74–101.

Crick, N. R., & Dodge, K. A. (1996). Social information-processing mechanisms in reactive and proactive aggression. *Child Development, 67,* 993–1002.

Crick, N. R., & Grotpeter, J. K. (1995). Relational aggression, gender, and social-psychological adjustment. *Child Development, 66,* 710–722.

Crick, N. R., & Werner, N. E. (1998). Response decision processes in relational and overt aggression. *Child Development, 69,* 1630–1639.

Crisante, L., & Ng, S. (2003). Implementation and process issues in using Group Triple P with Chinese parents: Preliminary findings. *Australian eJournal for the Advancement of Mental Health, 2*(3).

Cross Calvert, S., & McMahon, R. J. (1987). The treatment acceptability of a behavioral parent training program and its components. *Behavior Therapy, 18,* 165–179.

Cueva, J. E., Overall, J. E., Small, A. M., Armenteros, J. L., Perry, R., & Campbell, M. (1996). Carbamazepine in aggressive children with conduct disorder: A double-blind and placebo-controlled study. *Journal of the American Academy of Child and Adolescent Psychiatry, 35,* 480–490.

Cummings, E. M., & Davies, P. T. (1994a). *Children and marital conflict: The impact of family dispute and resolution.* New York: Guilford Press.

Cummings, E. M., & Davies, P. T. (1994b). Maternal depression and child development. *Journal of Child Psychology and Psychiatry, 35,* 73–112.

Cunningham, A. (2002). *Lessons learned from a randomized study of Multisystemic Therapy in Canada.* Retrieved from www.lfcc.on.ca/One_Step_Forward.pdf

Cunningham, P. E., & Henggeler, S. W. (1999). Engaging multiproblem families in treatment: Lessons learned throughout the development of Multi-Systemic Therapy. *Family Process, 38,* 265–286.

Curtis, N. M., Ronan, K. R., & Borduin, C. M. (2004).

Multisystemic treatment: A meta-analysis of outcome studies. *Journal of Family Psychology, 18*, 411–419.

Dadds, M. R., & McHugh, T. A. (1992). Social support and treatment outcome in behavioral family therapy for child conduct problems. *Journal of Consulting and Clinical Psychology, 60*, 252–259.

Dadds, M. R., & Powell, M. B. (1991). The relationship of interparental conflict and global marital adjustment to aggression, anxiety, and immaturity in aggressive and nonclinic children. *Journal of Abnormal Child Psychology, 19*, 553–567.

Dadds, M. R., Sanders, M. R., Behrens, B. C., & James, J. E. (1987). Marital discord and child behavior problems: A description of family interactions during treatment. *Journal of Clinical Child Psychology, 16*, 192–203.

Dadds, M. R., Sanders, M. R., & James, J. E. (1987). The generalization of treatment effects in parent training with multidistressed parents. *Behavioural Psychotherapy, 15*, 289–313.

Dadds, M. R., Schwartz, S., & Sanders, M. R. (1987). Marital discord and treatment outcome in behavioral treatment of child conduct disorders. *Journal of Consulting and Clinical Psychology, 55*, 396–403.

Daly, R. M., Holland, C. J., Forrest, P. A., & Fellbaum, G. A. (1985). Temporal generalization of treatment effects over a three-year period for a parent training program: Directive parent counseling (DPC). *Canadian Journal of Behavioural Science, 17*, 379–388.

Darveaux, D. X. (1984). The Good Behavior Game Plus Merit: Controlling disruptive behavior and improving student motivation. *School Psychology Review, 13*, 510–514.

Deater-Deckard, K. (1998). Parenting stress and child adjustment: Some old hypotheses and new questions. *Clinical Psychology: Science and Practice, 5*, 314–332.

DeGarmo, D. S., Patterson, G. R., & Forgatch, M. S. (2004). How do outcomes in a specified parent training intervention maintain or wane over time? *Prevention Science, 5*, 73–89.

Deitz, S. M. (1985). Good Behavior Game. In A. S. Bellack & M. Hersen (Eds.), *Dictionary of behavior therapy techniques* (pp. 131–132). New York: Pergamon Press.

DeKlyen, M., & Speltz, M. L. (2001). Attachment and conduct disorder. In J. Hill & B. Maughan (Eds.), *Conduct disorders in childhood and adolescence* (pp. 320–345). Cambridge, UK: Cambridge University Press.

Demaray, M. K., Ruffalo, S. L., Carlson, J., Busse, R. T., Olson, A. E., McManus, S. M., et al. (1995). Social skills assessment: A comparative evaluation of six published rating scales. *School Psychology Review, 24*, 648–671.

DeRosier, M. E. (2004). Building relationships and combating bullying: Effectiveness of a school-based social skills group intervention. *Journal of Clinical Child and Adolescent Psychology, 33*, 196–201.

DeRosier, M. E., & Marcus, S. R. (2005). Building

friendships and combating bullying: Effectiveness of S. S. GRIN at one-year follow-up. *Journal of Clinical Child and Adolescent Psychology, 34*, 140–150.

Dinkmeyer, D., & McKay, G. D. (1976). *Systematic Training for Effective Parenting*. Circle Pines, MN: American Guidance Service.

Dishion, T. J., & Andrews, D. W. (1995). Preventing escalation in problem behaviors with high-risk young adolescents: Immediate and 1-year outcomes. *Journal of Consulting and Clinical Psychology, 63*, 538–548.

Dishion, T. J., Andrews, D. W., & Crosby, L. (1995). Antisocial boys and their friends in early adolescence: Relationship characteristics, quality, and interactional process. *Child Development, 66*, 139–151.

Dishion, T. J., & Dodge, K. A. (2005). Peer contagion in interventions for children and adolescents: Moving toward an understanding of the ecology and dynamics of change. *Journal of Abnormal Child Psychology, 33*, 395–400.

Dishion, T. J., & Kavanagh, K. (2002). The Adolescent Transitions Program: A family-centered prevention strategy for schools. In J. B. Reid, G. R. Patterson, & J. Snyder (Eds.), *Antisocial behavior in children and adolescents: A developmental analysis and model for intervention* (pp. 257–272). Washington, DC: American Psychological Association.

Dishion, T. J., & Kavanagh, K. (2003). *Intervening in adolescent problem behavior: A family-centered approach*. New York: Guilford Press.

Dishion, T. J., Kavanagh, K., Schneiger, A., Nelson, S., & Kaufman, N. (2002). Preventing early adolescent substance use: A family-centered strategy for the public middle-school ecology. *Prevention Science, 3*, 191–201.

Dishion, T. J., McCord, J., & Poulin, F. (1999). When interventions harm: Peer groups and problem behavior. *American Psychologist, 54*, 755–764.

Dishion, T. J., & McMahon, R. J. (1998). Parental monitoring and the prevention of child and adolescent problem behavior: A conceptual and empirical formulation. *Clinical Child and Family Psychology Review, 1*, 61–75.

Dishion, T. J., Nelson, S. E., & Kavanagh, K. (2003). The Family Check-Up with high-risk young adolescents: Preventing early-onset substance use by parental monitoring. *Behavior Therapy, 34*, 553–571.

Dishion, T. J., & Patterson, G. R. (1992). Age effects in parent training outcome. *Behavior Therapy, 23*, 719–729.

Dishion, T. J., Patterson, G. R., & Griesler, P. C. (1994). Peer adaptation in the development of antisocial behavior: A confluence model. In L. R. Huesmann (Ed.), *Current perspectives on aggressive behavior* (pp. 61–95). New York: Plenum Press.

Dishion, T. J., Patterson, G. R., Stoolmiller, M., & Skinner, M. L. (1991). Family, school, and behavioral antecedents to early adolescent involvement with antisocial peers. *Developmental Psychology, 27*, 172–180.

Dishion, T. J., Reid, J. B., & Patterson, G. R. (1988).

Empirical guidelines for a family intervention for adolescent drug use. *Journal of Chemical Dependency Treatment, 1,* 189–224.

Dishion, T. J., Spracklen, K. M., Andrews, D. W., & Patterson, G. R. (1996). Deviancy training in male adolescents' friendships. *Behavior Therapy, 27,* 373–390.

Dodge, K. A. (1985). Attributional bias in aggressive children. In P. C. Kendall (Ed.), *Advances in cognitive behavioral research and therapy* (Vol. 4, pp. 73–110). New York: Academic Press.

Dodge, K. A. (1986). A social information processing model of social competence in children. In M. Perlmutter (Ed.), *Minnesota Symposium on Child Psychology* (Vol. 18, pp. 77–125). Hillsdale, NJ: Erlbaum.

Dodge, K. A. (2003). Do social information-processing patterns mediate aggressive behavior? In B. B. Lahey, T. E. Moffitt, & A. Caspi (Eds.), *Causes of conduct disorder and delinquency* (pp. 254–274). New York: Guilford Press.

Dodge, K. A., Bates, J. E., & Pettit, G. S. (1990). Mechanisms in the cycle of violence. *Science, 250,* 1678–1683.

Dodge, K. A., & Coie, J. D. (1987). Social-information processing factors in reactive and proactive aggression in children's peer groups. *Journal of Personality and Social Psychology, 53,* 1146–1158.

Dodge, K. A., Dishion, T. J., & Lansford, J. (in press). Findings and recommendations: A blueprint to minimize deviant peer contagion in programs designed to benefit youth. In K. A. Dodge, T. J. Dishion, & J. Lansford (Eds.), *Deviant by design: Interventions that aggregate youth.* New York: Guilford Press.

Dodge, K. A., Lochman, J. E., Harnish, J. D., Bates, J. E., & Pettit, G. S. (1997). Reactive and proactive aggression in school children and psychiatrically impaired chronically assaultive youth. *Journal of Abnormal Psychology, 106,* 37–51.

Dodge, K. A., & Pettit, G. S. (2003). A biopsychosocial model of the development of chronic conduct problems in adolescence. *Developmental Psychology, 39,* 349–371.

Dodge, K. A., Pettit, G. S., & Bates, J. E. (1994). Socialization mediators of the relation between socioeconomic status and child conduct problems. *Child Development, 65,* 649–665.

Dolan, L. J., Kellam, S. G., Brown, C. H., Werthamer-Larsson, L., Rebok, G. W., Mayer, L. S., et al. (1993). The short-term impact of two classroom-based preventive interventions on aggressive and shy behaviors and poor achievement. *Journal of Applied Developmental Psychology 14,* 317–345.

Dumas, J. E. (1984a). Child, adult-interactional, and socioeconomic setting events as predictors of parent training outcome. *Education and Treatment of Children, 7,* 351–364.

Dumas, J. E. (1984b). Interactional correlates of treatment outcome in behavioral parent training. *Journal of Consulting and Clinical Psychology, 52,* 946–954.

Dumas, J. E. (1986). Parental perception and treatment outcome in families of aggressive children: A causal model. *Behavior Therapy, 17,* 420–432.

Dumas, J. E. (1989). Treating antisocial behavior in children: Child and family approaches. *Clinical Psychology Review, 9,* 197–222.

Dumas, J. E. (1996). Why was this child referred?: Interactional correlates of referral status in families of children with disruptive behavior problems. *Journal of Clinical Child Psychology, 25,* 106–115.

Dumas, J. E., & Albin, J. B. (1986). Parent training outcome: Does active parental involvement matter? *Behaviour Research and Therapy, 24,* 227–230.

Dumas, J. E., & Serketich, W. J. (1994). Maternal depressive symptomatology and child maladjustment: A comparison of three process models. *Behavior Therapy, 25,* 161–181.

Dumas, J. E., & Wahler, R. G. (1983). Predictors of treatment outcome in parent training: Mother insularity and socioeconomic disadvantage. *Behavioral Assessment, 5,* 301–313.

Dumas, J. E., & Wahler, R. G. (1985). Indiscriminate mothering as a contextual factor in aggressive–oppositional child behavior: "Damned if you do and damned if you don't." *Journal of Abnormal Child Psychology, 13,* 1–17.

Duncan, R. D. (1999). Maltreatment by parents and peers: The relationship between child abuse, bully victimization, and psychological distress. *Child Maltreatment, 4,* 45–55.

Dunson, R. M., Hughes, J. N., & Jackson, T. W. (1994). Effect of behavioral consultation on student and teacher behavior. *Journal of School Psychology, 32,* 247–266.

Easley, M., & Smith, P. K. (1998). The long term effectiveness of anti-bullying work in primary schools. *Educational Research, 40,* 203–218.

Eddy, J. M., & Chamberlain, P. (2000). Family management and deviant peer association as mediators of the impact of treatment condition on youth antisocial behavior. *Journal of Consulting and Clinical Psychology, 68,* 857–863.

Edelbrock, C. (1985). *Conduct problems in childhood and adolescence: Developmental patterns and progressions.* Unpublished manuscript.

Eisenstadt, T. H., Eyberg, S., McNeil, C. B., Newcomb, K., & Funderburk, B. (1993). Parent–Child Interaction Therapy with behavior problem children: Relative effectiveness of two stages and overall treatment outcome. *Journal of Clinical Child Psychology, 22,* 42–51.

Elgar, F. J., McGrath, P. J., Waschbusch, D. A., Stewart, S. H., & Curtis, L. J. (2004). Mutual influences on maternal depression and child adjustment problems. *Clinical Psychology Review, 24,* 441–459.

Elliott, D. S., Huizinga, D., & Ageton, S. S. (1985). *Explaining delinquency and drug use.* Beverly Hills, CA: Sage.

Elliott, E. J. (2002). Juvenile justice diversion and intervention. In D. J. Kolko (Ed.), *Handbook on firesetting in children and youth* (pp. 383–394). San Diego, CA: Academic Press.

El-Sheikh, M., & Flanagan, E. (2001). Parental problem drinking and children's adjustment: Family conflict and parental depression as mediators and moderators of risk. *Journal of Abnormal Child Psychology, 29,* 417–432.

Embry, L. H. (1984). What to do?: Matching client characteristics and intervention techniques through a prescriptive taxonomic key. In R. F. Dangel & R. A. Polster (Eds.), *Parent training: Foundations of research and practice* (pp. 443–473). New York: Guilford Press.

Emery, R. E. (1999). *Marriage, divorce, and children's adjustment* (2nd ed.). Thousand Oaks, CA: Sage.

Essau, C. A. (2003). Epidemiology and comorbidity. In C. A. Essau (Ed.), *Conduct and oppositional defiant disorders: Epidemiology, risk factors, and treatment* (pp. 33–59). Mahwah, NJ: Erlbaum.

Eyberg, S. M. (1988). Parent–Child Interaction Therapy: Integration of traditional and behavioral concerns. *Child & Family Behavior Therapy, 10,* 33–46.

Eyberg, S. M. (1992). Parent and teacher behavior inventories for the assessment of conduct problem behaviors in children. In L. VandeCreek, S. Knapp, & T. L. Jackson (Eds.), *Innovations in clinical practice: A source book* (Vol. 11, pp. 261–270). Sarasota, FL: Professional Resource Press.

Eyberg, S. M. (1993). Consumer satisfaction measures for assessing parent training programs. In L. VandeCreek, S. Knapp, & T. L. Jackson (Eds.), *Innovations in clinical practice: A source book* (Vol. 12, pp. 377–382). Sarasota, FL: Professional Resource Press.

Eyberg, S. M., Bessmer, J., Newcomb, K., Edwards, D., & Robinson, E. (1994). *Dyadic Parent–Child Interaction Coding System II: A manual.* Unpublished manuscript, University of Florida.

Eyberg, S. M., & Colvin, A. (1994, August). *Restandardization of the Eyberg Child Behavior Inventory.* Paper presented at the annual meeting of the American Psychological Association, Los Angeles.

Eyberg, S. M., Funderburk, B. W., Hembree-Kigin, T. L., McNeil, C. B., & Querido, J. G. (2001). Parent–Child Interaction Therapy with behavior problem children: One and two year maintenance of treatment effects in the family. *Child & Family Behavior Therapy, 23,* 1–19.

Eyberg, S. M., & Pincus, D. (1999). *The Eyberg Child Behavior Inventory and Sutter–Eyberg Student Behavior Inventory: Professional manual.* Lutz, FL: Psychological Assessment Resources.

Eyberg, S. M., & Robinson, E. A. (1982). Parent–child interaction training: Effects on family functioning. *Journal of Clinical Child Psychology, 11,* 130–137.

Farrington, D. P. (1993). Understanding and preventing bullying. In M. Tonry (Ed.), *Crime and justice: A review of research* (Vol. 17, pp. 381–458). Chicago: University of Chicago Press.

Farrington, D. P. (2003). Key results from the first forty years of the Cambridge Study in Delinquent Development. In T. P. Thornberry & M. D. Krohn (Eds.), *Taking stock of delinquency: An overview of findings from contemporary longitudinal studies* (pp. 137–183). New York: Kluwer Academic/Plenum.

Federal Bureau of Investigation. (2004). *Uniform crime reports, 2003.* Washington, DC: Author.

Feindler, E. L., Ecton, R. B., Kingsley, D., & Dubey, D. R. (1986). Group anger-control training for institutionalized psychiatric male adolescents. *Behavior Therapy, 17,* 109–123.

Feindler, E. L., Marriott, S. A., & Iwata, M. (1984). Group anger control training for junior high school delinquents. *Cognitive Therapy and Research, 8,* 299–311.

Feinfeld, K. A., & Baker, B. L. (2004). Empirical support for a treatment program for families of young children with externalizing problems. *Journal of Clinical Child and Adolescent Psychology, 33,* 182–195.

Fellbaum, G. A., Daly, R. M., Forrest, P., & Holland, C. J. (1985). Community implications of a home-based change program for children. *Journal of Community Psychology, 13,* 67–74.

Fergusson, D. M., Horwood, L. J., & Lynskey, M. T. (1994). The comorbidities of adolescent problem behaviors: A latent class model. *Journal of Abnormal Child Psychology, 22,* 339–354.

Fergusson, D. M., Horwood, L. J., & Nagin, D. S. (2000). Offending trajectories in a New Zealand birth cohort. *Criminology, 38,* 401–427.

Fergusson, D. M., & Lynskey, M. T. (1993). The effects of maternal depression on child conduct disorder and attention deficit behaviours. *Social Psychiatry and Psychiatric Epidemiology, 28,* 116–123.

Fergusson, D. M., Lynskey, M. T., & Horwood, L. J. (1993). The effect of maternal depression on maternal ratings of child behavior. *Journal of Abnormal Child Psychology, 21,* 245–269.

Fergusson, D. M., Lynskey, M. T., & Horwood, L. J. (1996). Origins of comorbidity between conduct and affective disorders. *Journal of the American Academy of Child and Adolescent Psychiatry, 35,* 451–460.

Findling, R. L., Aman, M., & Derivan, A. (2000). Long-term safety and efficacy of risperidone in children with significant conduct problems and borderline IQ or mental retardation [Abstract]. *Scientific Proceedings of the 39th Annual Meeting of the American College of Neuropsychopharmacology,* p. 224.

Fischer, M., Barkley, R. A., Smallish, L., & Fletcher, K. (2002). Young adult follow-up of hyperactive children: Self-reported psychiatric disorders, comorbidity, and the role of childhood conduct problems and teen CD. *Journal of Abnormal Child Psychology, 30,* 463–475.

Fisher, L., & Blair, R. J. R. (1998). Cognitive impairment and its relationship to psychopathic tendencies in children with emotional and behavioral difficulties. *Journal of Abnormal Child Psychology, 26,* 511–519.

Fisher, P. A., & Chamberlain, P. (2000). Multidimensional Treatment Foster Care: A program for intensive parenting, family support, and skill building. *Journal of Emotional and Behavioral Disorders, 8,* 155–164.

Fleischman, M. J. (1981). A replication of Patterson's "Intervention for boys with conduct problems." *Journal of Consulting and Clinical Psychology, 49,* 342–351.

Fleischman, M. J., & Szykula, S. A. (1981). A community setting replication of a social learning treatment for aggressive children. *Behavior Therapy, 12,* 115–122.

Floyd, E. M., Rayfield, A., Eyberg, S. M., & Riley, J. L. (2004). Psychometric properties of the Sutter–Eyberg Student Behavior Inventory with rural middle school and high school children. *Assessment, 11,* 64–72.

Foote, R., Eyberg, S. M., & Schuhmann, E. (1998). Parent–child interaction approaches to the treatment of child conduct problems. In T. Ollendick & R. Prinz (Eds.), *Advances in child clinical psychology* (Vol. 20, pp. 125–151). New York: Plenum Press.

Forehand, R., & Atkeson, B. M. (1977). Generality of treatment effects with parents as therapists: A review of assessment and implementation procedures. *Behavior Therapy, 8,* 575–593.

Forehand, R., Griest, D. L., Wells, K. C., & McMahon, R. J. (1982). Side effects of parent counseling on marital satisfaction. *Journal of Counseling Psychology, 29,* 104–107.

Forehand, R., & Kotchick, B. A. (1996). Cultural diversity: A wake-up call for parent training. *Behavior Therapy, 27,* 187–206.

Forehand, R., Lautenschlager, G. J., Faust, J., & Graziano, W. G. (1986). Parent perceptions and parent–child interactions in clinic-referred children: A preliminary investigation of the effects of maternal depressive moods. *Behaviour Research and Therapy, 24,* 73–75.

Forehand, R., & Long, N. (1988). Outpatient treatment of the acting out child: Procedures, long term follow-up data, and clinical problems. *Advances in Behaviour Research and Therapy, 10,* 129–177.

Forehand, R., & McMahon, R. J. (1981). *Helping the noncompliant child: A clinician's guide to parent training.* New York: Guilford Press.

Forehand, R., Rogers, T., McMahon, R. J., Wells, K. C., & Griest, D. L. (1981). Teaching parents to modify child behavior problems: An examination of some follow-up data. *Journal of Pediatric Psychology, 6,* 313–322.

Forehand, R., Steffe, M. A., Furey, W. A., & Walley, P. B. (1983). Mothers' evaluation of a parent training program completed three and one-half years earlier. *Journal of Behavior Therapy and Experimental Psychiatry, 14,* 339–342.

Forehand, R., Sturgis, E. T., McMahon, R. J., Aguar, D., Green, K., Wells, K., et al. (1979). Parent behavioral training to modify child noncompliance: Treatment generalization across time and from home to school. *Behavior Modification, 3,* 3–25.

Forehand, R., Wells, K. C., & Griest, D. L. (1980). An examination of the social validity of a parent training program. *Behavior Therapy, 11,* 488–502.

Forehand, R., Wierson, M., Frame, C. L., Kemptom, T., & Armistead, L. (1991). Juvenile firesetting: A unique syndrome or an advanced level of antisocial behavior? *Behaviour Research and Therapy, 29,* 125–128.

Forgatch, M. S. (1991). The clinical science vortex: Developing a theory for antisocial behavior. In D. Pepler & K. H. Rubin (Eds.), *The development and treatment of childhood aggression* (pp. 291–315). Hillsdale, NJ: Erlbaum.

Forgatch, M. S. (1994). *Parenting through change: A training manual.* Eugene: Oregon Social Learning Center.

Forgatch, M. S., & DeGarmo, D. S. (1999). Parenting through change: An effective parenting training program for single mothers. *Journal of Consulting and Clinical Psychology, 67,* 711–724.

Forgatch, M. S., & Patterson, G. R. (1989). *Parents and adolescents living together: Part 2. Family problem solving.* Eugene, OR: Castalia.

Forgatch, M. S., Patterson, G. R., & DeGarmo, D. S. (2005). Evaluating fidelity: Predictive validity for a measure of competent adherence to the Oregon model of parent management training. *Behavior Therapy, 36,* 3–13.

Forgatch, M. S., Patterson, G. R., & Skinner, M. L. (1988). A mediational model for the effect of divorce on antisocial behavior in boys. In E. M. Hetherington & J. D. Arasteh (Eds.), *Impact of divorce, single parenting, and stepparenting on children* (pp. 135–154). Hillsdale, NJ: Erlbaum.

Foster, S. L., Prinz, R. J., & O'Leary, K. D. (1983). Impact of Problem-Solving Communication Training and generalization procedures on family conflict. *Child & Family Behavior Therapy, 5,* 1–23.

Foster, S. L., & Robin, A. L. (1997). Family conflict and communication in adolescence. In E. J. Mash & L. G. Terdal (Eds.), *Assessment of childhood disorders* (3rd ed., pp. 627–682). New York: Guilford Press.

Foster, S. L., & Robin, A. L. (1998). Parent–adolescent conflict and relationship discord. In E. J. Mash & R. A. Barkley (Eds.), *Treatment of childhood disorders* (2nd ed., pp. 601–686). New York: Guilford Press

Frick, P. J. (1994). Family dysfunction and the disruptive behavior disorders: A review of recent empirical findings. In T. H. Ollendick & R. J. Prinz (Eds.), *Advances in clinical child psychology* (Vol. 16, pp. 203–226). New York: Plenum Press.

Frick, P. J. (1998). *Conduct disorders and severe antisocial behavior.* New York: Plenum Press.

Frick, P. J., Bodin, S. D., & Barry, C. T. (2000). Psychopathic traits and conduct problems in community and clinic-referred samples of children: Further development of the Psychopathy Screening Device. *Psychological Assessment, 12,* 382–393.

Frick, P. J., Christian, R. E., & Wootton, J. M. (1999). Age trends in the association between parenting practices and conduct problems. *Behavior Modification, 23*, 106–128.

Frick, P. J., Cornell, A. H., Barry, C. T., Bodin, S. D., & Dane, H. A. (2003). Callous–unemotional traits and conduct problems in the prediction of conduct problem severity, aggression, and self-report of delinquency. *Journal of Abnormal Child Psychology, 31*, 457–470.

Frick, P. J., & Ellis, M. (1999). Callous–unemotional traits and subtypes of conduct disorder. *Clinical Child and Family Psychology Review, 2*, 149–168.

Frick, P. J., & Hare, R. D. (2002). *Antisocial Process Screening Device*. Toronto: Multi-Health Systems.

Frick, P. J., Lahey, B. B., Loeber, R., Stouthamer-Loeber, M., Christ, M. A. G., & Hanson, K. (1992). Familial risk factors to conduct disorder and oppositional defiant disorder: Parental psychopathology and maternal parenting. *Journal of Consulting and Clinical Psychology, 60*, 49–55.

Frick, P. J., Lahey, B. B., Loeber, R., Tannenbaum, L. E., Van Horn, Y., Christ, M. A. G., et al. (1993). Oppositional defiant disorder and conduct disorder: A meta-analytic review of factor analyses and cross-validation in a clinic sample. *Clinical Psychology Review, 13*, 319–340.

Frick, P. J., Lilienfeld, S. O., Ellis, M. L, Loney, B. R., & Silverthorn, P. (1999). The association between anxiety and psychopathy dimensions in children. *Journal of Abnormal Child Psychology, 27*, 381–390.

Frick, P. J., & Loney, B. R. (2002). Understanding the association between parent and child antisocial behavior. In R. J. McMahon & R. D. Peters (Eds.), *The effects of parental dysfunction on children* (pp. 105–126). New York: Kluwer Academic/Plenum.

Frick, P. J., & Morris, A. S. (2004). Temperament and developmental pathways to conduct problems. *Journal of Clinical Child and Adolescent Psychology, 33*, 54–68.

Funderburk, B. W., & Eyberg, S. M. (1989). Psychometric characteristics of the Sutter–Eyberg Student Behavior Inventory: A school behavior rating scale for use with preschool children. *Behavioral Assessment, 11*, 297–313.

Funderburk, B. W., Eyberg, S. M., Newcomb, K., McNeil, C., Hembree-Kigin, T., & Capage, L. (1998). Parent–Child Interaction Therapy with behavior problem children: Maintenance of treatment effects in the school setting. *Child & Family Behavior Therapy, 20*, 17–38.

Funderburk, B. W., Eyberg, S. M., Rich, B. A., & Behar, L. (2003). Further psychometric evaluation of the Eyberg and Behar Rating Scales for Parents and Teachers of Preschoolers. *Early Education and Development, 14*, 67–79.

Furr-Holder, C. D. M., Ialongo, N. S., Anthony, J. C., Petras, H., & Sheppard, K. (2004). Developmentally inspired drug prevention: Middle school outcomes in a school-based randomized prevention trial. *Drug and Alcohol Dependence, 73*, 149–158.

Gadow, K. D. (1991). Clinical issues in child and adolescent psychopharmacology. *Journal of Consulting and Clinical Psychology, 59*, 842–852.

Gadow, K. D., & Sprafkin, J. (1995). *Manual for the Child Symptom Inventory (CSI-4)*. Stony Brook, NY: Checkmate Plus.

Garcia, M. M., Shaw, D. S., Winslow, E. B., & Yaggi, K. E. (2000). Destructive sibling conflict and the development of conduct problems in young boys. *Developmental Psychology, 36*, 44–53.

Geiger, T. C., Zimmer-Gembeck, M. J., & Crick, N. R. (2004). The science of relational aggression: Can we guide intervention? In M. M. Moretti, C. L. Odgers, & M. A. Jackson (Eds.), *Girls and aggression: Contributing factors and intervention principles* (pp. 27–40). New York: Kluwer Academic/Plenum.

Ghaziuddin, N., & Alessi, N. E. (1992). An open clinical trial of trazodone in aggressive children. *Journal of Child and Adolescent Psychopharmacology, 2*, 291–297.

Gibbs, J. C., Arnold, K. D., Ahlborn, H. H., & Cheesman, F. L. (1984). Facilitation of sociomoral reasoning in delinquents. *Journal of Consulting and Clinical Psychology, 52*, 37–45.

Gibbs, J. C., Potter, G. B., Barriga, A. Q., & Liau, A. K. (1996). Developing the helping skills and prosocial motivation of aggressive adolescents in peer group programs. *Aggression and Violent Behavior, 1*, 283–305.

Gifford-Smith, M., Dodge, K. A., Dishion, T. J., & McCord, J. (2005). Peer influence in children and adolescents: Crossing the bridge from developmental to intervention studies. *Journal of Abnormal Child Psychology, 33*, 255–265.

Glick, B., & Goldstein, A. P. (1987). Aggression Replacement Training. *Journal of Counseling and Development, 65*, 356–362.

Glover, D., Gough, G., Johnson, M., & Cartwright, N. (2000). Bullying in 25 secondary schools: Incidence, impact, and intervention. *Educational Research, 42*, 141–156.

Goldstein, A. P., & Glick, B. (1994). Aggression Replacement Training: Curriculum and evaluation. *Simulation and Gaming, 25*, 9–26.

Goldstein, A. P., Glick, B., & Gibbs, J. C. (1998). *Aggression Replacement Training: A comprehensive intervention for aggressive youth*. Champaign, IL: Research Press.

Goldstein, A. P., Glick, B., Irwin, M. J., McCartney, C., & Rubama, I. (1989). *Reducing delinquency: Intervention in the community*. New York: Pergamon Press.

Goldstein, A. P., Glick, B., Reiner, S., Zimmerman, D., & Coultry, T. (1986). *Aggression Replacement Training*. Champaign, IL: Research Press.

Goldstein, A. P., & Pentz, M. A. (1984). Psychological skill training and the aggressive adolescent. *School Psychology Review, 13*, 311–323.

Goldstein, S. (1995). *Understanding and managing children's classroom behavior*. New York: Wiley.

Goodman, S., & Gotlib, I. (1999). Risk for psychopathology in the children of depressed mothers: A developmental model for understanding mechanisms of transmission. *Psychological Review, 106,* 485–490.

Gordon, D. A., & Arbuthnot, J. (1987). Individual, group, and family interventions. In H. C. Quay (Ed.), *Handbook of juvenile delinquency* (pp. 290–324). New York: Wiley.

Gordon, D. A., Arbuthnot, J., Gustafson, K. E., & McGreen, P. (1988). Home-based behavioral-systems family therapy with disadvantaged juvenile delinquents. *American Journal of Family Therapy, 16,* 243–255.

Gordon, D. A., Graves, K., & Arbuthnot, J. (1995). The effect of Functional Family Therapy for delinquents on adult criminal behavior. *Criminal Justice and Behavior, 22,* 60–73.

Gorman-Smith, D., Tolan, P. H., & Henry, D. B. (2000). A developmental–ecological model of the relations of family functioning to patterns of delinquency. *Journal of Quantitative Criminology, 16,* 169–198.

Greenberg, M. T. (1999). Attachment and psychopathology in childhood. In J. Cassidy & P. Shaver (Eds.), *Handbook of attachment: Theory, research, and clinical applications* (pp. 469–496). New York: Guilford Press.

Greenberg, M. T., Domitrovich, C., & Bumbarger, B. (2001). *Preventing mental disorders in school-age children: A review of the effectiveness of prevention programs.* (Available from the Prevention Research Center for the Promotion of Human Development, College of Health and Human Development, Pennsylvania State University, State College, PA, 16802)

Greenberg, M. T., Lengua, L. J., Coie, J., Pinderhughes, E., & Conduct Problems Prevention Research Group. (1999). Predicting developmental outcomes at school entry using a multiple-risk model: Four American communities. *Developmental Psychology, 35,* 403–417.

Greenhill, L. L., Solomon, M., Pleak, R., & Ambrosini, P. (1985). Molindone hydrochloride treatment of hospitalized children with conduct disorder. *Journal of Clinical Psychiatry, 46,* 20–25.

Greenwood, C. R., Hops, H., Delquadri, J., & Guild, J. (1974). Group contingencies for group consequences in classroom management: A further analysis. *Journal of Applied Behavior Analysis, 7,* 413–425.

Greenwood, C. R., Hops, H., & Walker, H. M. (1977). The durability of student behavior change: A comparative analysis at follow-up. *Behavior Therapy, 8,* 631–638.

Gregg, V., Gibbs, J. C., & Basinger, K. S. (1994). Patterns of delay in male and female delinquents' moral judgment. *Merrill–Palmer Quarterly, 40,* 538–553.

Griest, D. L., Forehand, R., Rogers, T., Breiner, J. L., Furey, W., & Williams, C. A. (1982). Effects of parent enhancement therapy on the treatment outcome and generalization of a parent training program. *Behaviour Research and Therapy, 20,* 429–436.

Griest, D. L., Forehand, R., & Wells, K. C. (1981). Follow-up assessment of parent behavioral training: An analysis of who will participate. *Child Study Journal, 11,* 221–229.

Griest, D. L., & Wells, K. C. (1983). Behavioral family therapy with conduct disorders in children. *Behavior Therapy, 14,* 37–53.

Grizenko, N., Papineau, D., & Sayegh, L. (1993). Effectiveness of a multimodal day treatment program for children with disruptive behavior problems. *Journal of the American Academy of Child and Adolescent Psychiatry, 32,* 127–134.

Guerra, N. G., & Slaby, R. G. (1990). Cognitive mediators of aggression in adolescent offenders: 2. Intervention. *Developmental Psychology, 26,* 269–277.

Guidubaldi, J., & Cleminshaw, H. K. (1985). The development of the Cleminshaw–Guidubaldi Parent Satisfaction Scale. *Journal of Clinical Child Psychology, 14,* 293–298.

Halperin, J. M., Sharma, V., Siever, L. J., Schwartz, S. T., Matier, K., Wornell, G., et al. (1994). Serotonergic function in aggressive and nonaggressive boys with attention deficit hyperactivity disorder. *American Journal of Psychiatry, 151,* 243–261.

Hämäläinen, M., & Pulkkinen, L. (1996). Problem behavior as a precursor of male criminality. *Development and Psychopathology, 8,* 443–455.

Hanf, C. (1969). *A two-stage program for modifying maternal controlling during mother–child (M-C) interaction.* Paper presented at the meeting of the Western Psychological Association, Vancouver, BC.

Hanf, C. (1970). *Shaping mothers to shape their children's behavior.* Unpublished manuscript, University of Oregon Medical School.

Hanf, C., & Kling, J. (1973). *Facilitating parent–child interactions: A two-stage training model.* Unpublished manuscript, University of Oregon Medical School.

Hanish, L. D., Martin, C. L., Fabes, R. A., Leonard, S., & Herzog, M. (2005). Exposure to externalizing peers in early childhood: Homophily and peer contagion processes. *Journal of Abnormal Child Psychology, 33,* 267–281.

Hanson, M., Mackay-Soroka, S., Staley, S., & Poulton, L. (1994). Delinquent firesetters: A comparative study of delinquency and firesetting histories. *Canadian Journal of Psychiatry, 39,* 230–232.

Hansson, K., Cederblad, M., & Alexander, J. F. (2002). *A method for treating juvenile delinquents: A cross-cultural comparison.* Manuscript submitted for publication.

Hartman, R. R., Stage, S. A., & Webster-Stratton, C. (2003). A growth curve analysis of parent training outcomes: Examining the influence of child risk factors (inattention, impulsivity, and hyperactivity problems), parental and family risk factors. *Journal of Child Psychology and Psychiatry, 44,* 388–398.

Harwood, M., & Eyberg, S. M. (2004). Therapist verbal behavior early in treatment: Relation to successful completion of Parent–Child Interaction Therapy. *Journal of Clinical Child and Adolescent Psychology, 33,* 601–612.

Hawkins, J. D., Catalano, R. F., & Arthur, M. W. (2002). Promoting science-based prevention in communities. *Addictive Behaviors, 27,* 951–976.

Hawkins, J. D., Catalano, R. F., Kosterman, R., Abbott, R., & Hill, K. G. (1999). Preventing health-risk behaviors by strengthening protection during childhood. *Archives of Pediatrics and Adolescent Medicine, 153,* 226–234.

Hawkins, J. D., Catalano, R. F., & Miller, J. Y. (1992). Risk and protective factors for alcohol and other drug problems in adolescence and early adulthood: Implications for substance abuse prevention. *Psychological Bulletin, 112,* 64–105.

Hawkins, J. D., Kosterman, R., Catalano, R. F., Hill, K. G., & Abbott, R. (2005). Promoting positive adult functioning through social development intervention in childhood. *Archives of Pediatric and Adolescent Medicine, 159,* 25–31.

Hawkins, J. D., Von Cleve, E., & Catalano, R. F. (1991). Reducing early childhood aggression: Results of a primary prevention program. *Journal of the American Academy of Child and Adolescent Psychiatry, 30,* 208–217.

Hawkins, R. P. (1989). The nature and potential of therapeutic foster family care programs. In R. P. Hawkins & J. Breiling (Eds.), *Therapeutic foster care: Critical issues* (pp. 17–36). Washington, DC: Child Welfare League of America.

Hawkins, R. P., Meadowcroft, P., Trout, B. A., & Luster, W. C. (1985). Foster family-based treatment. *Journal of Clinical Child Psychology, 14,* 220–228.

Heath, G. A., Hardesty, V. A., Goldfine, P. E., & Walker, A. M. (1983). Childhood firesetting: An empirical study. *Journal of the American Academy of Child Psychiatry, 22,* 370–374.

Henderson, J. Q. (1981). A behavioral approach to stealing: A proposal for treatment based on ten cases. *Journal of Behavior Therapy and Experimental Psychiatry, 12,* 231–236.

Henderson, J. Q. (1983). Follow-up of stealing behavior in 27 youths after a variety of treatment programs. *Journal of Behavior Therapy and Experimental Psychiatry, 14,* 331–337.

Henggeler, S. W. (2004). Decreasing effect sizes for effectiveness studies—implications for the transport of evidence-based treatments: Comments on Curtis, Ronan, and Borduin (2004). *Journal of Family Psychology, 18,* 420–423.

Henggeler, S. W., & Borduin, C. M. (1990). *Family therapy and beyond: A multisystemic approach to treating the behavior problems of children and adolescents.* Pacific Grove, CA: Brooks/Cole.

Henggeler, S. W., Borduin, C. M., Melton, G. B., Mann, B. J., Smith, L., Hall, J. A., et al. (1991). Effects of Multisystemic Therapy on drug use and abuse in serious juvenile offenders: A progress report from two outcome studies. *Family Dynamics of Addiction Quarterly, 1,* 40–51.

Henggeler, S. W., Clingempeel, G. W., Brondino, M. J., & Pickrel, S. G. (2002). Four-year follow-up of Multisystemic Therapy with substance-abusing and substance-dependent juvenile offenders. *Journal of the American Academy of Child and Adolescent Psychiatry, 41,* 868–874.

Henggeler, S. W., & Lee, T. (2003). Multisystemic treatment of serious clinical problems. In A. E. Kazdin & J. R. Weisz (Eds.), *Evidence-based psychotherapies for children and adolescents* (pp. 301–322). New York: Guilford Press.

Henggeler, S. W., Melton, G. B., Brondino, M. J., Scherer, D. G., & Hanley, J. H. (1997). Multisystemic Therapy with violent and chronic juvenile offenders and their families: The role of treatment fidelity in successful dissemination. *Journal of Consulting and Clinical Psychology, 65,* 821–833.

Henggeler, S. W., Melton, G. B., & Smith, L. A. (1992). Family preservation using Multisystemic Therapy: An effective alternative to incarcerating serious juvenile offenders. *Journal of Consulting and Clinical Psychology, 60,* 953–961.

Henggeler, S. W., Melton, G. B., Smith, L. A., Schoenwald, S. K., & Hanley, J. H. (1993). Family preservation using multisystemic treatment: Long-term follow-up to a clinical trial with serious juvenile offenders. *Journal of Child and Family Studies, 4,* 283–293.

Henggeler, S. W., Pickrel, S. G., & Brondino, M. J. (1999). Multisystemic treatment of substance abusing and dependent delinquents: Outcomes, treatment fidelity, and transportability. *Mental Health Services Research, 1,* 171–184.

Henggeler, S. W., Pickrel, S. G., Brondino, M. J., & Crouch, J. L. (1996). Eliminating (almost) treatment dropout of substance abusing or dependent delinquents through home-based Multisystemic Therapy. *American Journal of Psychiatry, 153,* 427–428.

Henggeler, S. W., Rodick, J. D., Borduin, C. M., Hanson, C. L., Watson, S. M., & Urey, J. R. (1986). Multisystemic treatment of juvenile offenders: Effects on adolescent behavior and family interaction. *Developmental Psychology, 22,* 132–141.

Henggeler, S. W., Schoenwald, S. K., Borduin, C. M., Rowland, M. D., & Cunningham, P. B. (1998). *Multisystemic treatment of antisocial behavior in children and adolescents.* New York: Guilford Press.

Henggeler, S. W., Schoenwald, S. K., & Pickrel, S. G. (1995). Multisystemic Therapy: Bridging the gap between university- and community-based treatment. *Journal of Consulting and Clinical Psychology, 63,* 709–717.

Hill, J., & Maughan, B. (Eds.). (2001). *Conduct disorders in childhood and adolescence.* Cambridge, UK: Cambridge University Press.

Hinshaw, S. P. (1992). Externalizing behavior problems and academic underachievement in childhood and adolescence: Causal relationships and underlying mechanisms. *Psychological Bulletin, 111,* 127–155.

Hinshaw, S. P., Buhrmester, D., & Heller, T. (1989). Anger control in response to verbal provocation: Effects of stimulant medication for boys with ADHD. *Journal of Abnormal Child Psychology, 17,* 393–407.

Hinshaw, S. P., Heller, T., & McHale, J. P. (1992). Covert antisocial behavior in boys with attention-deficit hyperactivity disorder: External validation and effects of methylphenidate. *Journal of Consulting and Clinical Psychology, 60,* 274–281.

Hinshaw, S. P., Henker, B., Whalen, C. K., Erhardt, D., & Dunnington, R. E. (1989). Aggressive, prosocial, and nonsocial behavior in hyperactive boys: Dose effects of methylphenidate in naturalistic settings. *Journal of Consulting and Clinical Psychology, 57,* 636–643.

Hinshaw, S. P., & Lee, S. S. (2003). Conduct and oppositional defiant disorders. In E. J. Mash & R. A. Barkley (Eds.), *Child psychopathology* (2nd ed., pp. 144–198). New York: Guilford Press.

Hinshaw, S. P., Simmel, C., & Heller, T. L. (1995). Multimethod assessment of covert antisocial behavior in children: Laboratory observation, adult ratings, and child self-report. *Psychological Assessment, 7,* 209–219.

Hinshaw, S. P., Zupan, B. A., Simmel, C., Nigg, J. T., & Melnick, S. (1997). Peer status in boys with and without attention-deficit hyperactivity disorder: Predictions from overt and covert antisocial behavior, social isolation, and authoritative parenting beliefs. *Child Development, 68,* 880–896.

Holden, G. W., Lavigne, V. V., & Cameron, A. M. (1990). Probing the continuum of effectiveness in parent training: Characteristics of parents and preschoolers. *Journal of Clinical Child Psychology, 19,* 2–8.

Holleran, P. A., Littman, D. C., Freund, R. D., & Schmaling, K. B. (1982). A signal detection approach to social perception: Identification of negative and positive behaviors by parents of normal and problem children. *Journal of Abnormal Child Psychology, 10,* 547–557.

Hood, K., & Eyberg, S. M. (2003). Outcomes of Parent–Child Interaction Therapy: Mothers' reports on maintenance three to six years after treatment. *Journal of Clinical Child and Adolescent Psychology, 32,* 419–429.

Hops, H., & Walker, H. M. (1988). *CLASS: Contingencies for learning academic and social skills.* Seattle, WA: Educational Achievement Systems.

Hops, H., Walker, H. M., Fleischman, D. H., Nagoshi, J. T., Omura, R. T., Skindrud, K., et al. (1978). CLASS: A standardized in-class program for acting-out children. II. Field test evaluations. *Journal of Educational Psychology, 70,* 636–644.

Horne, A. M., & Van Dyke, B. (1983). Treatment and maintenance of social learning family therapy. *Behavior Therapy, 14,* 606–613.

Horner, R., Sugai, G., Lewis-Palmer, T., & Todd, A. (2001). Teaching school-wide behavioral expectations. *Report on Emotional and Behavioral Disorders in Youth, 1,* 77–79, 93–96.

Howell, J. C. (2003). *Preventing and reducing juvenile delinquency: A comprehensive framework.* Thousand Oaks, CA: Sage.

Hubbard, J. A., Smithmyer, C. M., Ramsden, S. R., Parker, E. H., Flanagan, K. D., Dearing, K. F., et al. (2002). Observational, physiological, and self-report measures of children's anger: Relations to reactive versus proactive aggression. *Child Development, 73,* 1101–1118.

Hudley, C., & Graham, S. (1993). An attributional intervention to reduce peer-directed aggression among African-American boys. *Child Development, 64,* 124–138.

Huesmann, L. R., Eron, L. D., Lefkowitz, M. M., & Walder, L. O. (1984). Stability of aggression over time and generations. *Developmental Psychology, 20,* 1120–1134.

Huey, S. J., Henggeler, S. W., Brondino, M. J., & Pickrel, S. G. (2000). Mechanisms of change in Multisystemic Therapy: Reducing delinquent behavior through therapist adherence and improved family and peer functioning. *Journal of Consulting and Clinical Psychology, 68,* 451–467.

Hughes, J. N., Grossman, P., & Barker, D. (1990). Teachers' expectancies, participation in consultation, and perceptions of consultant helpfulness. *School Psychology Quarterly, 15,* 167–179.

Humphreys, J., Kopet, T., & Lajoy, R. (1993). Clinical considerations in the treatment of juvenile firesetters. *Clinical Child Psychology Newsletter, 9,* 2–3.

Humphreys, L., Forehand, R., McMahon, R., & Roberts, M. (1978). Parent behavioral training to modify child noncompliance: Effects on untreated siblings. *Journal of Behavior Therapy and Experimental Psychiatry, 9,* 235–238.

Hunt, R. D., Minderaa, R. B., & Cohen, D. J. (1986). The therapeutic effect of clonidine in attention deficit disorder with hyperactivity: A comparison with placebo and methylphenidate. *Psychopharmacology Bulletin, 22,* 229–236.

Ialongo, N. S., Poduska, J., Werthamer, L., & Kellam, S. G. (2001). The distal impact of two first-grade preventive interventions on conduct problems and disorder in early adolescence. *Journal of Emotional and Behavioral Disorders, 9,* 146–160.

Ialongo, N. S., Werthamer, L., Kellam, S. G., Brown, C. H., Wang, S., & Lin, Y. (1999). Proximal impact of two first-grade preventive interventions on the early risk behaviors for later substance abuse, depression, and antisocial behavior. *American Journal of Community Psychology, 27,* 599–641.

Individuals with Disabilities Education Act Amendments of 1997, P.L. 105-17, 20 U.S.C. 1400 et seq.

Ingoldsby, E. M., & Shaw, D. S. (2002). The role of neighborhood contextual factors on early-starting antisocial behavior. *Clinical Child and Family Psychology Review, 6,* 21–65.

Ireland, J. L., Sanders, M. R., & Markie-Dadds, C. (2003). The impact of parent training on marital functioning: A comparison of two group versions of the Triple P-Positive Parenting Program for parents of children with early-onset conduct problems. *Behavioural and Cognitive Psychotherapy, 31,* 127–142.

Irvine, A. B., Biglan, A., Metzler, C. W., Smolkowski, K., & Ary, D. V. (1999). The effectiveness of a parenting skills program for parents of middle school students in small communities. *Journal of Consulting and Clinical Psychology, 67,* 811–825.

Jacob, T., Krahn, G. L., & Leonard, K. (1991). Parent–child interactions in families with alcoholic fathers. *Journal of Consulting and Clinical Psychology, 59,* 176–181.

Jacob, T., Moser, R. P., Windle, M., Loeber, R., & Stouthamer-Loeber, M. (2000). New measure of parenting practices involving preadolescent- and adolescent-aged children. *Behavior Modification, 24,* 611–634.

Jacobs, J. R., Boggs, S. R., Eyberg, S. M., Edwards, D., Durning, P., Querido, J. G., et al. (2000). Psychometric properties and reference point data for the Revised Edition of the School Observation Coding System. *Behavior Therapy, 31,* 695–712.

Jacobson, R. R. (1985). Child firesetters: A clinical investigation. *Journal of Child Psychology and Psychiatry, 26,* 759–768.

Jaffee, S. R., Caspi, A., Moffitt, T. E., & Taylor, A. (2004). Physical maltreatment victim to antisocial child: Evidence of an environmentally mediated process. *Journal of Abnormal Psychology, 113,* 44–55.

Jennings, K. D., Stagg, V., & Connors, R. E. (1991). Social networks and mothers' interactions with their preschool children. *Child Development, 62,* 966–978.

Jessor, R. (1998). New perspectives on adolescent risk behavior. In R. Jessor (Ed.), *New perspectives on adolescent risk behavior* (pp. 1–10). New York: Cambridge University Press.

Jessor, R., & Jessor, S. L. (1977). *Problem behavior and psychosocial development.* New York: Academic Press.

Johnson, S. M., Bolstad, O. D., & Lobitz, G. K. (1976). Generalization and contrast phenomena in behavior modification with children. In L. A. Hamerlynck, L. C. Handy, & E. J. Mash (Eds.), *Behavior modification and families* (pp. 160–188). New York: Brunner/Mazel.

Johnston, C. (1996). Addressing parent cognitions in interventions with families of disruptive children. In K. S. Dobson & K. D. Craig (Eds.), *Advances in cognitive-behavioral therapy* (pp. 193–209). Thousand Oaks, CA: Sage.

Johnston, C., & Mash, E. J. (1989). A measure of parenting satisfaction and efficacy. *Journal of Clinical Child Psychology, 18,* 167–175.

Johnston, C., & Murray, C. (2003). Incremental validity in the psychological assessment of children and adolescents. *Psychological Assessment, 15,* 496–507.

Jones, R. R. (1974). *"Observation" by telephone: An economical behavior sampling technique* (Oregon Research Institute Technical Report No. 1411). Eugene: Oregon Research Institute.

Jones, Y. (1990). *Aggression Replacement Training in a high school setting.* Unpublished manuscript, Center for Learning and Adjustment Difficulties, Brisbane, Australia.

Jouriles, E. N., Murphy, C. M., Farris, A. M., Smith, D. A., Richters, J. E., & Waters, E. (1991). Marital adjustment, parental disagreements about child rearing, and behavior problems in boys: Increasing the specificity of the marital assessment. *Child Development, 62,* 1424–1433.

Julien, R. M. (1996). *A primer of drug action: A concise non-technical guide to the actions, uses and side effects of psychoactive drugs.* New York: Freeman.

Kafantaris, V., Campbell, M., Padron-Gayol, M. V., Small, A. M., Locascio, J. J., & Rosenberg, C. R. (1992). Carbamazepine in hospitalized aggressive conduct disorder children: An open pilot study. *Psychopharmacology Bulletin, 28,* 193–199.

Kaltiala-Heino, R., Rimpela, M., Marttunen, M., Rimpela, A., & Rantanen, P. (1999). Bullying, depression, and suicidal ideation in Finnish adolescents: School survey. *British Medical Journal, 319,* 348–351.

Kamphaus, R. W., & Frick, P. J. (2002). *Clinical assessment of child and adolescent personality and behavior* (2nd ed.). Boston: Allyn & Bacon.

Kaplan, S. L., Busner, J., Kupietz, S., Wassermann, E., & Segal, B. (1990). Effects of methylphenidate on adolescents with aggressive conduct disorder and ADHD: A preliminary report. *Journal of the American Academy of Child and Adolescent Psychiatry, 29,* 719–723.

Katz, L. F., & Gottman, J. M. (1993). Patterns of marital conflict predict children's internalizing and externalizing behavior. *Developmental Psychology, 29,* 940–950.

Kaufman, A. S., & Kaufman, N. L. (Eds.). (2001). *Specific learning disabilities and difficulties in children and adolescents: Psychological assessment and evaluation.* New York: Cambridge University Press.

Kazdin, A. E. (1977a). Assessing the clinical or applied importance of behavior change through social validation. *Behavior Modification, 1,* 427–452.

Kazdin, A. E. (1977b). *The token economy: A review and evaluation.* New York: Plenum Press.

Kazdin, A. E. (1990). Premature termination from treatment among children referred for antisocial behavior. *Journal of Child Psychology and Psychiatry, 31,* 415–425.

Kazdin, A. E. (1995a). Child, parent and family dysfunction as predictors of outcome in cognitive-behavioral treatment of antisocial children. *Behaviour Research and Therapy, 33,* 271–281.

Kazdin, A. E. (1995b). *Conduct disorders in childhood and adolescence* (2nd ed.). Thousand Oaks, CA: Sage.

Kazdin, A. E. (2003). Problem-solving skills training and parent management training for conduct disorder. In A. E. Kazdin & J. R. Weisz (Eds.), *Evidence-based psychotherapies for children and adolescents* (pp. 241–262). New York: Guilford Press.

Kazdin, A. E., Bass, D., Siegel, T. C., & Thomas, C. (1989). Cognitive behavioral therapy and relationship therapy in the treatment of children referred for antisocial behavior. *Journal of Consulting and Clinical Psychology, 57,* 522–536.

Kazdin, A. E., & Crowley, M. J. (1997). Moderators of treatment outcome in cognitively based treatment of antisocial children. *Cognitive Therapy and Research, 21,* 185–207.

Kazdin, A. E., Esveldt-Dawson, K., French, N. H., & Unis, A. S. (1987a). Effects of parent management training and problem-solving skills training combined in the treatment of antisocial child behavior. *Journal of the American Academy of Child and Adolescent Psychiatry, 26,* 416–424.

Kazdin, A. E., Esveldt-Dawson, K., French, N. H., & Unis, A. S. (1987b). Problem-solving skills training and relationship therapy in the treatment of antisocial child behavior. *Journal of Consulting and Clinical Psychology, 55,* 76–85.

Kazdin, A. E., Holland, L., & Crowley, M. (1997). Family experience of barriers to treatment and premature termination from child therapy. *Journal of Consulting and Clinical Psychology, 65,* 453–463.

Kazdin, A. E., & Kolko, D. J. (1986). Parent psychopathology and family functioning among childhood firesetters. *Journal of Abnormal Child Psychology, 14,* 315–329.

Kazdin, A. E., Mazurick, J. L., & Bass, D. (1993). Risk for attrition in treatment of antisocial children and families. *Journal of Clinical Child Psychology, 22,* 2–16.

Kazdin, A. E., Mazurick, J. L., & Siegel, T. C. (1994). Treatment outcome among children with externalizing disorder who terminate prematurely versus those who complete psychotherapy. *Journal of the American Academy of Child and Adolescent Psychiatry, 33,* 549–557.

Kazdin, A. E., & Nock, M. K. (2003). Delineating mechanisms of change in child and adolescent therapy: Methodological issues and research recommendations. *Journal of Child Psychology and Psychiatry, 44,* 1116–1129.

Kazdin, A. E., Siegel, T. C., & Bass, D. (1992). Cognitive problem-solving skills training and parent management training in the treatment of antisocial behavior in children. *Journal of Consulting and Clinical Psychology, 60,* 733–747.

Kazdin, A. E., & Wassell, G. (1998). Treatment completion and therapeutic change among children referred for outpatient therapy. *Professional Psychology: Research and Practice, 29,* 332–340.

Kazdin, A. E., & Wassell, G. (1999). Barriers to treatment participation and therapeutic change among children referred for conduct disorder. *Journal of Clinical Child Psychology, 28,* 160–172.

Kazdin, A. E., & Wassell, G. (2000a). Predictors of barriers to treatment and therapeutic change in outpatient therapy for antisocial children and their families. *Mental Health Services Review, 2,* 27–40.

Kazdin, A. E., & Wassell, G. (2000b). Therapeutic changes in children, parents, and families resulting from treatment of children with conduct problems.

Journal of the American Academy of Child and Adolescent Psychiatry, 39, 414–420.

Kazdin, A. E., & Whitley, M. K. (2003). Treatment of parental stress to enhance therapeutic change among children referred for aggressive and antisocial behavior. *Journal of Consulting and Clinical Psychology, 71,* 504–515.

Keenan, K., Loeber, R., & Green, S. (1999). Conduct disorder in girls: A review of the literature. *Clinical Child and Family Psychology Review, 2,* 3–19.

Keenan, K., Shaw, D., Delliquadri, E., Giovannelli, J., & Walsh, B. (1998). Evidence for the continuity of early problem behaviors: Application of a developmental model. *Journal of Abnormal Child Psychology, 26,* 441–454.

Keenan, K., & Wakschlag, L. S. (2002). More than the terrible twos: The nature and severity of behavior problems in clinic-referred preschool children. *Journal of Abnormal Child Psychology, 28,* 33–46.

Kellam, S. G., & Rebok, G. W. (1992). Building developmental and etiological theory through epidemiologically based preventive intervention trials. In J. McCord & R. E. Tremblay (Eds.), *Preventing antisocial behavior: Interventions from birth through adolescence* (pp. 162–191). New York: Guilford Press.

Kellam, S. G., Rebok, G. W., Ialongo, N., & Mayer, L. S. (1994). The course and malleability of aggressive behavior from early first grade into middle school: Results of a developmental epidemiologically-based preventive trial. *Journal of Child Psychology and Psychiatry, 35,* 259–281.

Kelley, M. L. (1990). *School–home notes: Promoting children's classroom success.* New York: Guilford Press.

Kemph, J. P., DeVane, C. L., Levin, G. M., Jarecke, R., & Miller, R. L. (1993). Treatment of aggressive children with clonidine: Results of an open pilot study. *Journal of the American Academy of Child and Adolescent Psychiatry, 32,* 577–581.

Kendall, P. C. (1985). Toward a cognitive-behavioral model of child psychopathology and a critique of related interventions. *Journal of Abnormal Psychology, 13,* 357–372.

Kendall, P. C. (1991). Guiding theory for therapy with children and adolescents. In P. C. Kendall (Ed.), *Child and adolescent therapy: Cognitive-behavioral procedures* (pp. 3–22). New York: Guilford Press.

Kendall, P. C., & Braswell, L. (1985). *Cognitive-behavioral therapy for impulsive children.* New York: Guilford Press.

Kendall, P. C., & Braswell, L. (1993). *Cognitive-behavioral therapy for impulsive children* (2nd ed.). New York: Guilford Press.

Kendall, P. C., & MacDonald, J. P. (1993). Cognition in the psychopathology of youth and implications for treatment. In K. S. Dobson & P. C. Kendall (Eds.), *Psychopathology and cognition* (pp. 387–426). San Diego, CA: Academic Press.

Kendall, P. C., Reber, M., McLeer, S., Epps, J., & Ronan, K. R. (1990). Cognitive-behavioral treatment of conduct-disordered children. *Cognitive Therapy and Research, 14,* 279–297.

Kendall, P. C., Ronan, K. R., & Epps, J. (1991). Aggression in children/adolescents: Cognitive-behavioral treatment perspectives. In D. Pepler & K. H. Rubin (Eds.), *The development and treatment of childhood aggression* (pp. 341–360). Hillside, NJ: Erlbaum.

Kirigin, K. A. (1996). Teaching-Family Model of group home treatment of children with severe behavior problems. In M. C. Roberts (Ed.), *Model programs in child and family mental health* (pp. 231–247). Mahwah, NJ: Erlbaum.

Kirigin, K. A., Braukmann, C. J., Atwater, J. D., & Wolf, M. M. (1982). An evaluation of Teaching-Family (Achievement Place) group homes for juvenile offenders. *Journal of Applied Behavior Analysis, 15,* 1–16.

Kirigin, K. A., & Wolf, M. M. (1994, April). *A follow-up evaluation of Teaching-Family Model participants: Implications for treatment technology.* Paper presented at the meeting of the Southwestern Psychological Association, Tulsa, OK.

Klein, N. C., Alexander, J. F., & Parsons, B. V. (1977). Impact of family systems intervention on recidivism and sibling delinquency: A model of primary prevention and program evaluation. *Journal of Consulting and Clinical Psychology, 45,* 469–474.

Klein, R. D. (1979). Modifying academic performance in the grade school classroom. In M. Hersen, R. M. Eisler, & P. M. Miller (Eds.), *Progress in behavior modification* (Vol. 8, pp. 293–321). New York: Academic Press.

Klein, R. G. (1991). Preliminary results: Lithium effects in conduct disorders [Abstract]. *CME Syllabus and Proceedings Summary, 144th Annual Meeting of the American Psychiatric Association,* pp. 119–120.

Klein, R. G., Abikoff, H., Klass, E., Ganales, D., Seese, L., & Pollack, S. (1997). Clinical efficacy of methylphenidate in conduct disorder with and without attention deficit hyperactivity disorder. *Archives of General Psychiatry, 54,* 1073–1080.

Klein, R. G., Abikoff, H., Klass, E., Shah, M., & Seese, L. (1994). *Controlled trial of methylphenidate, lithium, and placebo in children and adolescents with conduct disorders.* Paper presented at the meeting of the Society for Research in Child and Adolescent Psychopathology, London.

Klinteberg, B. A., Andersson, T., Magnusson, D., & Stattin, H. (1993). Hyperactive behavior in childhood as related to subsequent alcohol problems and violent offending: A longitudinal study of male subjects. *Personality and Individual Differences, 15,* 381–388.

Knutson, N. M., Forgatch, M., & Rains, L. A. (2003). *Fidelity of Implementation Rating System (FIMP): The training manual for PMTO.* Eugene: Oregon Social Learning Center.

Kochenderfer, B. J., & Ladd, G. W. (1997). Victimized children's response to peers' aggression: Behaviors associated with reduced versus continued victimization. *Development and Psychopathology, 9,* 59–73.

Kolko, D. J. (1988). Community interventions for childhood firesetters: A comparison of two national programs. *Hospital and Community Psychiatry, 39,* 973–979.

Kolko, D. J. (1995). Multimodal partial-day treatment of child antisocial behavior: Service description and multi-level program evaluation. *Continuum: Developments in Ambulatory Mental Health Care, 2,* 3–24.

Kolko, D. J. (2001). Efficacy of cognitive-behavioral treatment and fire safety education for children who set fires: Initial and follow-up outcomes. *Journal of Child Psychology and Psychiatry, 42,* 359–369.

Kolko, D. J. (2002a). Child, parent, and family treatment: Cognitive-behavioral interventions. In D. J. Kolko (Ed.), *Handbook on firesetting in children and youth* (pp. 305–336). San Diego, CA: Academic Press.

Kolko, D. J. (2002b). Research studies on the problem. In D. J. Kolko (Ed.), *Handbook on firesetting in children and youth* (pp. 33–56). San Diego, CA: Academic Press.

Kolko, D. J., & Kazdin, A. E. (1988). Prevalence of firesetting and related behaviors among child psychiatric inpatients. *Journal of Consulting and Clinical Psychology, 56,* 628–630.

Kolko, D. J., & Kazdin, A. E. (1992). The emergence and recurrence of child firesetting: A one-year prospective study. *Journal of Abnormal Child Psychology, 20,* 17–37.

Kolko, D. J., Loar, L. L., & Sturnick, D. (1990). Inpatient social-cognitive skills training groups with conduct disordered and attention deficit disordered children. *Journal of Child Psychology and Psychiatry, 31,* 737–748.

Kolko, D. J., Nishi-Strattner, L., Wilcox, D. K., & Kopet, T. (2002). Clinical assessment of juvenile firesetters and their families: Tools and tips. In D. J. Kolko (Ed.), *Handbook on firesetting in children and youth* (pp. 177–212). San Diego, CA: Academic Press.

Kolko, D. J., Watson, S., & Faust, J. (1991). Fire safety/prevention skills training to reduce involvement with fire in young psychiatric inpatients: Preliminary findings. *Behavior Therapy, 22,* 269–284.

Kovacs, M., Paulauskas, S., Gatsonis, C., & Richards, C. (1988). Depressive disorders in childhood. *Journal of Affective Disorders, 15,* 205–217.

Kratzer, L., & Hodgins, S. (1997). Adult outcomes of child conduct problems: A cohort study. *Journal of Abnormal Child Psychology, 25,* 65–81.

Kruesi, M. J. P., Hibbs, E. D., Zahn, T. P., Keysor, C. S., Hamburger, S. D., Bartko, J. J., et al. (1992). A 2-year prospective follow-up study of children and adolescents with disruptive behavior disorders. *Archives of General Psychiatry, 49,* 429–435.

Kruesi, M. J. P., & Lelio, D. F. (1996). Disorders of conduct and behavior. In J. M. Wiener (Ed.), *Diagnosis* and psychopharmacology of childhood and adolescent disorders (2nd ed., pp. 401–447). New York: Wiley.

Kruesi, M. J. P., Rapoport, J. L., Hamburger, S., Hibbs, E., Potter, W. Z., Lenane, M., et al. (1990). Cerebrospinal fluid monoamine metabolites, aggression, and impulsivity in disruptive behavior disorders of children and adolescents. *Archives of General Psychiatry, 47,* 419–426.

Kruesi, M. J. P., Schmidt, M. E., Donnelly, M., Hibbs, E. D., & Hamburger, S. D. (1989). Urinary free cortisol output and disruptive behavior in children. *Journal of the American Academy of Child and Adolescent Psychiatry, 28,* 441–443.

Kruh, I. P., Frick, P. J., & Clements, C. B. (2005). Historical and personality correlates to the violence patterns of juveniles tried as adults. *Criminal Justice and Behavior, 32,* 69–96.

Kumpfer, K. K., Alvarado, R., Smith, P., & Bellamy, N. (2002). Cultural sensitivity and adaptation in family-based prevention interventions. *Prevention Science, 3,* 241–246.

Kuypers, D. S., Becker, W. C., & O'Leary, K. D. (1968). How to make a token system fail. *Exceptional Children, 11,* 101–108.

Lacourse, E., Cote, S., Nagin, D. S., Vitaro, F., Brendgen, M., & Tremblay, R. E. (2002). A longitudinal–experimental approach to testing theories of antisocial behavior development. *Development and Psychopathology, 14,* 909–924.

Lacourse, E., Nagin, D., Tremblay, R. E., Vitaro, F., & Claes, M. (2003). Developmental trajectories of boys' delinquent group membership and facilitation of violent behaviors during adolescence. *Development and Psychopathology, 15,* 183–197.

Lahey, B. B., Applegate, B., Barkley, R. A., Garfinkel, B., McBurnett, K., Kerdyck, L., et al. (1994). DSM-IV field trials for oppositional defiant disorder and conduct disorder in children and adolescents. *American Journal of Psychiatry, 151,* 1163–1171.

Lahey, B. B., Gendrich, J. G., Gendrich, S. I., Schnelle, J. F., Gant, D. S., & McNees, M. P. (1977). An evaluation of daily report cards with minimal teacher and parent contacts as an efficient method of classroom intervention. *Behavior Modification, 1,* 381–394.

Lahey, B. B., Loeber, R., Burke, J., & Rathouz, P. J. (2002). Adolescent outcomes of childhood conduct disorder among clinic-referred boys: Predictors of improvement. *Journal of Abnormal Child Psychology, 30,* 333–348.

Lahey, B. B., Loeber, R., Quay, H. C., Applegate, B., Shaffer, D., Waldman, I., et al. (1998). Validity of the DSM-IV subtypes of conduct disorder based on age of onset. *Journal of the American Academy of Child and Adolescent Psychiatry, 37,* 435–442.

Lahey, B. B., Miller, T. L., Gordon, R. A., & Riley, A. W. (1999). Developmental epidemiology of the disruptive behavior disorders. In H. C. Quay & A. E. Hogan (Eds.), *Handbook of disruptive behavior disorders* (pp. 23–48). New York: Kluwer Academic/Plenum.

Lahey, B. B., Moffitt, T. E., & Caspi, A. (Eds.). (2003). *Causes of conduct disorder and juvenile delinquency.* New York: Guilford Press.

Lahey, B. B., & Waldman, I. D. (2003). A developmental propensity model of the origins of conduct problems during childhood and adolescence. In B. B. Lahey, T. E. Moffitt, & A. Caspi (Eds.), *Causes of conduct disorder and juvenile delinquency* (pp. 76–117). New York: Guilford Press.

Lang, A. R., Pelham, W. E., Atkeson, B. M., & Murphy, D. A. (1999). Effects of alcohol intoxication on parenting behavior and interactions with child confederates exhibiting normal or deviant behavior. *Journal of Abnormal Child Psychology, 27,* 177–189.

Larzelere, R. E., Dinges, K., Schmidt, M. D., Spellman, D. F., Criste, T. R., & Connell, P. (2001). Outcomes of residential treatment: A study of the adolescent clients of Girls and Boys Town. *Child and Youth Care Forum, 30,* 175–185.

Lavallee, K. L., Bierman, K. L., Nix, R. L., & Conduct Problems Prevention Research Group. (2005). The impact of first-grade "friendship group" experiences on child social outcomes in the Fast Track program. *Journal of Abnormal Child Psychology, 33,* 307–324.

LeBlanc, M., & Fréchette, M. (1989). *Male criminal activity from childhood through youth: Multilevel and developmental perspectives.* New York: Springer-Verlag.

Leeman, L. W., Gibbs, J. C., & Fuller, D. (1993). Evaluation of a multicomponent group treatment program for juvenile delinquents. *Aggressive Behavior, 19,* 281–292.

Leff, S. S., Angelucci, J., Grabowski, L., & Weil, J. (2004, July). Using school and community partners to design, implement, and evaluate a group intervention for relationally aggressive girls. In S. S. Leff (Chair), *Using partnerships to design, implement, and evaluate aggression prevention programs.* Symposium conducted at the annual meeting of the American Psychological Association, Honolulu.

LeMarquand, D., Tremblay, R. E., & Vitaro, F. (2001). The prevention of conduct disorder: A review of successful and unsuccessful experiments. In J. Hill & B. Maughan (Eds.), *Conduct disorders in childhood and adolescence* (pp. 449–477). New York: Cambridge University Press.

Leschied, A. W., & Cunningham, A. (2002). *Seeking effective interventions for young offenders: Interim results for a four-year randomized study of Multisystemic Therapy in Ontario, Canada.* London, ON, Canada: Centre for Children and Families in the Justice System.

Leung, C., Sanders, M. R., Leung, S., Mak, R., & Lau, J. (2003). An outcome evaluation of the implementation of the Triple P-Positive Parenting Program in Hong Kong. *Family Process, 42,* 531–544.

Leve, L. D., & Chamberlain, P. (2005). Girls in the juvenile justice system: Risk factors and clinical implications. In D. Pepler, K. Madsen, C. Webster, & K. Levene (Eds.), *Development and treatment of girlhood aggression* (pp. 191–215). Mahwah, NJ: Erlbaum.

Levene, K. S., Walsh, M. M., Augimeri, L. K., & Pepler, D. J. (2004). Linking identification and treatment of early risk factors for female delinquency. In M. M. Moretti, C. L. Odgers, & M. A. Jackson (Eds.), *Girls and aggression: Contributing factors and intervention principles* (pp. 147–163). New York: Kluwer Academic/Plenum.

Lilienfeld, S. O. (1992). The association between antisocial personality and somatization disorders: A review and integration of theoretical models. *Clinical Psychology Review, 12,* 641–662.

Lipsey, M. W. (1992). Juvenile delinquency treatment: A meta-analytic inquiry into the variability of effects. In T. D. Cook, H. Cooper, D. S. Cordray, H. Hartmann, L. V. Hedges, R. J. Light, et al. (Eds.), *Meta-analysis for explanation: A casebook* (pp. 83–127). New York: Russell Sage Foundation.

Lipsey, M. W. (1995). What do we learn from 400 research studies on the effectiveness of treatment with juvenile delinquents? In J. McGuire (Ed.), *What works? Reducing reoffending* (pp. 63–78). New York: Wiley.

Lipsey, M. W. (1999). Can intervention rehabilitate serious delinquents? *Annals of the American Academy of Political and Social Science, 564,* 142–166.

Lipsey, M. W., & Wilson, D. B. (1998). Effective intervention for serious juvenile offenders: A synthesis of research. In R. Loeber & D. P. Farrington (Eds.), *Serious and violent juvenile offenders: Risk factors and successful interventions* (pp. 313–345). Thousand Oaks, CA: Sage.

Little, T. D., Jones, S. M., Henrich, C. C., & Hawley, P. H. (2003). Disentangling the "whys" from the "whats" of aggressive behavior. *International Journal of Behavioural Development, 27,* 122–133.

Lochman, J. E. (1985). Effects of different treatment lengths in cognitive behavioral interventions with aggressive boys. *Child Psychiatry and Human Development, 16,* 45–56.

Lochman, J. E. (1992). Cognitive-behavioral interventions with aggressive boys: Three year follow-up and preventive effects. *Journal of Consulting and Clinical Psychology, 60,* 426–432.

Lochman, J. E., Burch, P. R., Curry, J. F., & Lampron, L. B. (1984). Treatment and generalization effects of cognitive-behavioral and goal-setting interventions with aggressive boys. *Journal of Consulting and Clinical Psychology, 52,* 915–916.

Lochman, J. E., & Curry, J. F. (1986). Effects of social problem-solving training and self-instruction training with aggressive boys. *Journal of Clinical Child Psychology, 15,* 159–164.

Lochman, J. E., & Lampron, L. B. (1988). Cognitive behavioral interventions for aggressive boys: Seven months follow-up effects. *Journal of Child and Adolescent Psychotherapy, 5,* 15–23.

Lochman, J. E., Lampron, L. B., Burch, P. R., & Curry, J. F. (1985). Client characteristics associated with behavior change for treated and untreated aggressive boys. *Journal of Abnormal Child Psychology, 13,* 527–538.

Lochman, J. E., Lampron, L. B., Gemmer, T. C., & Harris, S. R. (1987). Anger coping intervention with aggressive children: A guide to implementation in school settings. In P. A. Keller & S. R. Heyman (Eds.), *Innovations in clinical practice: A source book* (Vol. 6, pp. 339–356). Sarasota, FL: Professional Resource Exchange.

Lochman, J. E., Nelson, W. M., & Sims, J. P. (1981). A cognitive behavioral program for use with aggressive children. *Journal of Clinical Child Psychology, 10,* 146–148.

Lochman, J. E., & Wells, K. C. (1996). A social-cognitive intervention with aggressive children: Prevention effects and contextual implementation issues. In R. D. Peters & R. J. McMahon (Eds.), *Preventing childhood disorders, substance abuse, and delinquency* (pp. 111–143). Thousand Oaks, CA: Sage.

Lochman, J. E., & Wells, K. C. (2002). The Coping Power program at the middle school transition: Universal and indicated prevention effects. *Psychology of Addictive Behaviors, 16,* 40–54.

Lochman, J. E., & Wells, K. C. (2003). Effectiveness of the Coping Power program and of classroom intervention with aggressive children: Outcomes at a 1-year follow-up. *Behavior Therapy, 34,* 493–515.

Lochman, J. E., & Wells, K. C. (2004). The Coping Power program for preadolescent aggressive boys and their parents: Outcome effects at the 1-year follow-up. *Journal of Consulting and Clinical Psychology, 72,* 571–578.

Loeber, R. (1988). Natural histories of conduct problems, delinquency, and associated substance use: Evidence for developmental progressions. In B. B. Lahey & A. E. Kazdin (Eds.), *Advances in clinical child psychology* (Vol. 11, pp. 73–124). New York: Plenum Press.

Loeber, R., Brinthaupt, V. P., & Green, S. M. (1990). Attention deficits, impulsivity, and hyperactivity with or without conduct problems: Relationships to delinquency and unique contextual factors. In R. J. McMahon & R. D. Peters (Eds.), *Behavior disorders of adolescence: Research, intervention, and policy in clinical and school setting* (pp. 39–61). New York: Plenum Press.

Loeber, R., & Dishion, T. S. (1983). Early predictors of male delinquency: A review. *Psychological Bulletin, 94,* 68–99.

Loeber, R., & Farrington, D. P. (2000). Young children who commit crime: Epidemiology, developmental origins, risk factors, early interventions, and policy implications. *Development and Psychopathology, 12,* 737–762.

Loeber, R., Farrington, D. P., Stouthamer-Loeber, M., Moffitt, T. E., Caspi, C., White, H. R., et al. (2003). The development of male offending: Key findings from fourteen years of the Pittsburgh Youth Study. In

T. P. Thornberry & M. D. Krohn (Eds.), *Taking stock of delinquency: An overview of findings from contemporary longitudinal studies* (pp. 93–136). New York: Kluwer Academic/Plenum.

Loeber, R., Farrington, D. P., Stouthamer-Loeber, M., & Van Kammen, W. B. (1998). Multiple risk factors for multi-problem boys: Co-occurrence of delinquency, substance use, attention deficit, conduct problems, physical aggression, covert behavior, depressed mood, and shy/withdrawn behavior. In R. Jessor (Ed.), *New perspectives on adolescent risk behavior* (pp. 90–149). New York: Cambridge University Press.

Loeber, R., & Keenan, K. (1994). Interaction between conduct disorder and its comorbid conditions: Effects of age and gender. *Clinical Psychology Review, 14,* 497–523.

Loeber, R., & Schmaling, K. B. (1985a). Empirical evidence for overt and covert patterns of antisocial conduct problems: A meta-analysis. *Journal of Abnormal Child Psychology, 13,* 337–352.

Loeber, R., & Schmaling, K. B. (1985b). The utility of differentiating between mixed and pure forms of antisocial child behavior. *Journal of Abnormal Child Psychology, 13,* 315–336.

Loeber, R., Stouthamer-Loeber, M., Van Kammen, W. B., & Farrington, D. P. (1989). Development of a new measure of self-reported antisocial behavior for young children: Prevalence and reliability. In M. W. Klein (Ed.), *Cross national research and self-reported crime and delinquency* (pp. 203–225). Dordrecht, The Netherlands: Kluwer-Nijhoff.

Loeber, R., Weissman, W., & Reid, J. B. (1983). Family interactions of assaultive adolescents, stealers, and nondelinquents. *Journal of Abnormal Child Psychology, 11,* 1–14.

Loeber, R., Wung, P., Keenan, K., Giroux, B., Stouthamer-Loeber, M., Van Kammen, W. B., et al. (1993). Developmental pathways in disruptive child behavior. *Development and Psychopathology, 5,* 101–131.

Loney, B. R., & Frick, P. J. (2003). Structured diagnostic interviewing. In C. R. Reynolds & R. W. Kamphaus (Eds.), *Handbook of psychological and educational assessment of children: Personality, behavior, and context* (2nd ed., pp. 235–247). New York: Guilford Press.

Loney, B. R., Frick, P. J., Ellis, M., & McCoy, M. G. (1998). Intelligence, psychopathy, and antisocial behavior. *Journal of Psychopathology and Behavioral Assessment, 20,* 231–247.

Long, P., Forehand, R., Wierson, M., & Morgan, A. (1994). Does parent training with young noncompliant children have long-term effects? *Behaviour Research and Therapy, 32,* 101–107.

Lösel, F., & Beelmann, A. (2003). Effects of child skills training in preventing antisocial behavior: A systematic review of randomized evaluations. *Annals of the American Academy of Political and Social Science, 587,* 84–109.

Lynskey, M. T., & Fergusson, D. M. (1995). Childhood conduct problems, attention deficit behaviors, and adolescent alcohol, tobacco, and illicit drug use. *Journal of Abnormal Child Psychology, 23,* 281–302.

MacBrayer, E. K., Milich, R., & Hundley, M. (2003). Attributional biases in aggressive children and their mothers. *Journal of Abnormal Psychology, 112,* 698–708.

Magnusson, D. (1988). Aggressiveness, hyperactivity, and autonomic activity/reactivity in the development of social maladjustment. In D. Magnusson (Ed.), *Individual development from an interactional perspective: A longitudinal study* (pp. 153–172). Hillsdale, NJ: Erlbaum.

Malone, R. P., Delaney, M. A., Luebbert, J. F., Cater, J., & Campbell, M. (2000). A double-blind placebo-controlled study of lithium in hospitalized aggressive children and adolescents with conduct disorder. *Archives of General Psychiatry, 57,* 649–654.

Markie-Dadds, C., & Sanders, M. R. (2004a). *A controlled evaluation of an enhanced self-directed behavioural family intervention for parents of children with conduct problems in rural and remote areas.* Manuscript submitted for publication.

Markie-Dadds, C., & Sanders, M. R. (2004b). *Self-directed Triple P (Positive Parenting Program) for mothers with children at-risk of developing conduct problems.* Manuscript submitted for publication.

Martens, B. K., & Hiralall, A. S. (1997). Scripted sequences of teacher interaction. *Behavior Modification, 21,* 308–323.

Martinez, C. R., & Forgatch, M. S. (2001). Preventing problems with boys' noncompliance: Effects of a parent training intervention for divorcing mothers. *Journal of Consulting and Clinical Psychology, 69,* 416–428.

Mas, C. H., Alexander, J. F., & Barton, C. (1985). Modes of expression in family therapy: A process study of roles and gender. *Journal of Marital and Family Therapy, 11,* 411–415.

Mattes, J. A. (1990). Comparative effectiveness of carbamazepine and propranolol for rage outbursts. *Journal of Neuropsychiatry and Clinical Neurosciences, 2,* 159–164.

Maughan, B., & Rutter, M. (2001). Antisocial children grown up. In J. Hill & B. Maughan (Eds.), *Conduct disorders in childhood and adolescence* (pp. 507–552). Cambridge, UK: Cambridge University Press.

McBurnett, K., Swanson, J. M., Pfiffner, L. J., & Harris, S. J., (1991, June). *The relationship of prefrontal test performance and autonomic arousal to symptoms of inattention/overactivity and aggression/defiance.* Paper presented at the annual meeting of the Society for Research on Psychopathology, Amsterdam.

McCabe, K. M., Hough, R., Wood, P. A., & Yeh, M. (2001). Childhood and adolescent onset conduct disorder: A test of the developmental taxonomy. *Journal of Abnormal Child Psychology, 29,* 305–316.

McCarty, C. A., McMahon, R. J., & Conduct Problems Prevention Research Group. (2005). Domains of risk in the developmental continuity of firesetting. *Behavior Therapy, 36,* 185–195.

McClellan, J. M., & Werry, J. S. (2000). Introduction to special section: Research psychiatric diagnostic interviews for children and adolescents. *Journal of the American Academy of Child and Adolescent Psychiatry, 39,* 19–27.

McConaughy, S. H., & Achenbach, T. M. (2001). *Manual for the Semistructured Clinical Interview for Children and Adolescents* (2nd ed.). Burlington: University of Vermont, Research Center for Children, Youth, & Families.

McDermott, P. A. (1996). A nationwide study of development and gender prevalence for psychopathology in childhood and adolescence. *Journal of Abnormal Child Psychology, 24,* 53–66.

McGee, R., Feehan, M., Williams, S., & Anderson, J. (1992). DSM-III disorders from age 11 to age 15 years. *Journal of the American Academy of Child and Adolescent Psychiatry, 31,* 50–59.

McMahon, R. J., & Estes, A. (1994). *Fast Track parent–child interaction task: Observational data collection manuals.* Unpublished manuscript, University of Washington.

McMahon, R. J., & Estes, A. M. (1997). Conduct problems. In E. J. Mash & L. G. Terdal (Eds.), *Assessment of childhood disorders* (3rd ed., pp. 130–193). New York: Guilford Press.

McMahon, R. J., & Frick, P. J. (2005). Evidence-based assessment of conduct problems in children and adolescents. *Journal of Clinical Child and Adolescent Psychology, 34,* 477–505.

McMahon, R. J., & Forehand, R. (1983). Consumer satisfaction in behavioral treatment of children: Types issues, and recommendations. *Behavior Therapy, 14,* 209–225.

McMahon, R. J., & Forehand, R. L. (2003). *Helping the noncompliant child: Family-based treatment for oppositional behavior* (2nd ed.). New York: Guilford Press.

McMahon, R. J., Forehand, R., & Griest, D. L. (1981). Effects of knowledge of social learning principles on enhancing treatment outcome and generalization in a parent training program. *Journal of Consulting and Clinical Psychology, 49,* 526–532.

McMahon, R. J., Forehand, R., Griest, D. L., & Wells, K. C. (1981). Who drops out of treatment during parent behavioral training? *Behavioral Counseling Quarterly, 1,* 79–85.

McMahon, R. J., Forehand, R., & Tiedemann, G. L. (1985, November). *Relative effectiveness of a parent training program with children of different ages.* Poster presented at the annual meeting of the Association for Advancement of Behavior Therapy, Houston.

McMahon, R. J., & Kotler, J. S. (2004). Treatment of conduct problems in children and adolescents. In P. M. Barrett & T. H. Ollendick (Eds.), *Handbook of interventions that work with children and adoles-*

cents: Prevention and treatment (pp. 396–426). New York: Wiley.

McMahon, R. J., & Kotler, J. S. (2006). Conduct problems. In D. A. Wolfe & E. J. Mash (Eds.), *Behavioral and emotional disorders in adolescents: Nature, assessment, and treatment* (pp. 153–225). New York: Guilford Press.

McMahon, R. J., & Metzler, C. W. (1998). Selecting parenting measures for assessing family-based preventive interventions. In R. S. Ashery, E. B. Robertson, & K. L. Kumpfer (Eds.), *Drug abuse prevention through family interventions.* (NIDA Research Monograph No. 177, pp. 294–323). Rockville, MD: National Institute on Drug Abuse.

McMahon, R. J., & Rhule, D. M. (2005). The prevention of conduct problems. In P. Graham (Ed.), *Cognitive behaviour therapy for children and families* (2nd ed., pp. 481–503). Cambridge, UK: Cambridge University Press.

McMahon, R. J., Slough, N. M., & Conduct Problems Prevention Research Group. (1996). Family-based intervention in the Fast Track Program. In R. D. Peters & R. J. McMahon (Eds.), *Preventing childhood disorders, substance abuse, and delinquency* (pp. 90–110). Thousand Oaks, CA: Sage.

McMahon, R. J., Tiedemann, G. L., Forehand, R., & Griest, D. L. (1984). Parental satisfaction with parent training to modify child noncompliance. *Behavior Therapy, 15,* 295–303.

McMahon, R. J., & Wells, K. C. (1998). Conduct problems. In E. J. Mash & R. A. Barkley (Eds.), *Treatment of childhood disorders* (2nd ed., pp. 111–207). New York: Guilford Press.

McNeil, C. B., Eyberg, S., Eisenstadt, T. H., Newcomb, K., & Funderburk, B. (1991). Parent–Child Interaction Therapy with behavior problem children: Generalization of treatment effects to the school setting. *Journal of Clinical Child Psychology, 20,* 140–151.

Medland, M. B., & Stachnik, T. J. (1972). Good Behavior Game: A replication and systematic analysis. *Journal of Applied Behavior Analysis, 5,* 45–51.

Meyers, W. C., & Carrera, F. (1989). Carbamazepine induced mania with hypersexuality in a 9-year-old boy. *American Journal of Psychiatry, 146,* 400.

Michelson, L., Mannnarino, A. P., Marchione, K. E., Stern, M., Figueroa, J., & Beck, S. (1983). A comparative outcome study of behavioral social-skills training, interpersonal-problem-solving and non-directive control treatments with child psychiatric outpatients. *Behaviour Research and Therapy, 21,* 545–556.

Middlebrook, J. L., & Forehand, R. (1985). Maternal perceptions of deviance in child behavior as a function of stress and clinic versus non-clinic status of the child: An analogue study. *Behavior Therapy, 16,* 494–502.

Miller, G., Brehm, K., & Whitehouse, S. (1998). Reconceptualizing school-based prevention for antisocial behavior within a resiliency framework. *School Psychology Review, 27,* 364–379.

Miller, G. E., & Klungness, L. (1986). Treatment of

nonconfrontative stealing in school-age children. *School Psychology Review, 15,* 24–35.

Miller, G. E., & Klungness, L. (1989). Childhood theft: A comprehensive review of assessment and treatment. *School Psychology Review, 18,* 82–97.

Miller, G. E., & Prinz, R. J. (1990). Enhancement of social learning family interventions for childhood conduct disorder. *Psychological Bulletin, 108,* 291–307.

Miller, G. E., & Prinz, R. J. (2003). Engagement of families in treatment for childhood conduct problems. *Behavior Therapy, 34,* 517–534.

Miller, W. R., & Rollnick, S. (1991). *Motivational interviewing: Preparing people to change addictive behavior.* New York: Guilford Press.

Moffitt, T. E. (1990). Juvenile delinquency and attention deficit disorder: Boys' developmental trajectories from age 3 to age 15. *Child Development, 61,* 893–910.

Moffitt, T. E. (1993). "Adolescence-limited" and "life-course-persistent" antisocial behavior: A developmental taxonomy. *Psychological Review, 100,* 674–701.

Moffitt, T. E. (2003). Life-course persistent and adolescence-limited antisocial behavior: A 10-year research review and research agenda. In B. B. Lahey, T. E. Moffitt, & A. Caspi (Eds.), *Causes of conduct disorder and juvenile delinquency* (pp. 49–75). New York: Guilford Press.

Moffitt, T. E., & Caspi, A. (2001). Childhood predictors differentiate life-course persistent and adolescence-limited antisocial pathways in males and females. *Development and Psychopathology, 13,* 355–376.

Moffitt, T. E., Caspi, A., Belsky, J., & Silva, P. A. (1992). Childhood experience and the onset of menarche: A test of a sociobiological model. *Child Development, 63,* 47–58.

Moffitt, T. E., Caspi, A., Dickson, N., Silva, P., & Stanton, W. (1996). Childhood-onset versus adolescent-onset antisocial conduct problems in males: Natural history from ages 3 to 18 years. *Development and Psychopathology, 8,* 399–424.

Moffitt, T. E., Caspi, A., Harrington, H., & Milne, B. (2002). Males on the life-course persistent and adolescence-limited antisocial pathways: Follow-up at age 26. *Development and Psychopathology, 14,* 179–206.

Moffitt, T. E., Caspi, A., Rutter, M., & Silva, P. A. (2001). *Sex differences in antisocial behaviour.* Cambridge, UK: Cambridge University Press.

Moore, D., Chamberlain, P., & Mukai, L. (1979). Children at risk for delinquency: A follow-up comparison of aggressive children and children who steal. *Journal of Abnormal Child Psychology, 7,* 345–355.

Moretti, M. M., Odgers, C. L., & Jackson, M. A. (Eds.). (2004). *Girls and aggression: Contributing factors and intervention principles.* New York: Kluwer Academic/Plenum.

Mpofu, E. (2002). Psychopharmacology in the treatment of conduct disorder in children and adolescents: Rationale, prospects, and ethics. *South African Journal of Psychology, 32,* 9–21.

MTA Cooperative Group. (1999). Moderators and mediators of treatment response for children with attention-deficit/hyperactivity disorder. *Archives of General Psychiatry, 56,* 1088–1096.

Murphy, K. R., & Gordon, M. (2006). Assessment of adults with ADHD. In R. A. Barkley, *Attention-deficit hyperactivity disorder: A handbook for diagnosis and treatment* (3rd ed., pp. 425–450). New York: Guilford Press.

Nagin, D. S., Farrington, D. M., & Moffitt, T. E. (1995). Life-course trajectories of different types of offenders. *Criminology, 33,* 111–139.

Nangle, D. W., Erdley, C. A., Carpenter, E. M., & Newman, J. E. (2002). Social skills training as a treatment for aggressive children and adolescents: A developmental-clinical integration. *Aggression and Violent Behavior, 7,* 169–199.

Nansel, T. R., Overpeck, M., Pilla, R. S., Ruan, W. J., Simmons-Morton, B., & Scheidt, P. C. (2001). Bullying behaviors among US youth: Prevalence and association with psychological adjustment. *Journal of the American Medical Association, 285,* 2094–2100.

Nelson, J. R., Smith, D. J., & Dodd, J. (1990). The moral reasoning of juvenile delinquents: A meta analysis. *Journal of Abnormal Child Psychology, 18,* 231–239.

Newberry, A. M., Alexander, J. F., & Turner, C. W. (1991). Gender as a process variable in family therapy. *Journal of Family Psychology, 5,* 158–175.

Nixon, R. D. V., Sweeney, L., Erickson, D. B., & Touyz, S. W. (2003). Parent–Child Interaction Therapy: A comparison of standard and abbreviated treatments for oppositional defiant preschoolers. *Journal of Consulting and Clinical Psychology, 71,* 251–260.

Nixon, R. D. V., Sweeney, L., Erickson, D. B., & Touyz, S. W. (2004). Parent–Child Interaction Therapy: One- and two-year follow-up of standard and abbreviated treatments for oppositional preschoolers. *Journal of Abnormal Child Psychology, 32,* 263–271.

Nock, M. K., & Kazdin, A. E. (2001). Parent expectancies for child therapy: Assessment and relation to participation in treatment. *Journal of Child and Family Studies, 10,* 155–180.

Novaco, R. W. (1978). Anger and coping with stress: Cognitive-behavioral interventions. In J. P. Foreyt & D. P. Rathjen (Eds.), *Cognitive behavioral therapy: Research and application* (pp. 135–173). New York: Plenum Press.

O'Dell, S. L. (1974). Training parents in behavior modification: A review. *Psychological Bulletin, 81,* 418–433.

O'Dell, S. L. (1985). Progress in parent training. In M. Hersen, R. M. Eisler, & P. M. Miller (Eds.), *Progress in behavior modification* (Vol. 9, pp. 57–108). New York: Academic Press.

O'Donnell, J., Hawkins, J. D., Catalano, R. F., Abbott, R. D., & Day, L. E. (1995). Preventing school failure, drug use, and delinquency among low-income children: Long-term intervention in elementary schools. *American Journal of Orthopsychiatry, 65,* 87–100.

Offord, D. R., Alder, R. J., & Boyle, M. H. (1986). Prevalence and sociodemographic correlates of conduct disorder. *American Journal of Social Psychiatry, 6,* 272–278.

Offord, D. R., Boyle, M. H., Racine, Y. A., Fleming, J. E., Cadman, D. T., Blum, H. M., et al. (1992). Outcome, prognosis, and risk in a longitudinal follow-up study. *Journal of the American Academy of Child and Adolescent Psychiatry, 31,* 916–923.

Ogden, T. (2000). *The evaluation of parent management training in Norway (research plan).* Oslo: University of Oslo, The Behavioral Project.

Ogden, T., Forgatch, M. S., Askeland, E., Patterson, G. R., & Bullock, B. M. (2005). Implementation of parent management training at the national level: The case of Norway. *Journal of Social Work Practice, 19,* 317–329.

Ogden, T., & Halliday-Boykins, C. A. (2004). Multisystemic treatment of antisocial adolescents in Norway: Replication of clinical outcomes outside of the U.S. *Child and Adolescent Mental Health, 9,* 77–83.

Okulitch, J. S., & Pinsonneault, I. (2002). The interdisciplinary approach to juvenile firesetting: A dialogue. In D. Kolko (Ed.), *Handbook on firesetting in children and youth* (pp. 57–74). San Diego, CA: Academic Press.

Olds, D., Henderson, C. R., Cole, R., Eckenrode, J., Kitzman, H., Luckey, D., et al. (1998). Long-term effects of nurse home visitation on children's criminal and antisocial behavior: 15-year follow-up of a randomized trial. *Journal of the American Medical Association, 280,* 1238–1244.

Olds, D., Kitzman, H., Cole, R., & Robinson, J. (1997). Theoretical foundations of a program of home visitation for pregnant women and parents of young children. *Journal of Community Psychology, 25,* 9–25.

O'Leary, K. D., Becker, W. C., Evans, M. B., & Saudargas, R. A. (1969). A token reinforcement program in a public school: A replication and systematic analysis. *Journal of Applied Behavior Analysis, 2,* 3–13.

O'Leary, K. D., & Drabman, R. (1971). Token reinforcement programs in the classroom: A review. *Psychological Bulletin, 75,* 379–398.

O'Leary, K. D., & O'Leary, S. G. (1977). *Classroom management: The successful use of behavior modification* (2nd ed.). New York: Pergamon Press.

Olweus, D. (1986). Aggression and hormones: Behavior relationship with testosterone and adrenaline. In D. Olweus, J. Block, & Radke-Yarrow (Eds.), *The development of antisocial and prosocial behavior: Research, theories, and issues* (pp. 51–72). New York: Academic Press.

Olweus, D. (1990). Bullying among children. In K. Hurrelmann & F. Lösel (Eds.), *Health hazards in adolescence: Prevention and intervention in childhood*

and adolescence (Vol. 8, pp. 259–297). Berlin: de Gruyter.

Olweus, D. (1991). Bully/victim problems among schoolchildren: Basic facts and effects of a school based intervention program. In D. J. Pepler & K. H. Rubin (Eds.), *The development and treatment of childhood aggression* (pp. 411–488). Hillsdale, NJ: Erlbaum.

Olweus, D. (1992). Bullying among schoolchildren: Intervention and prevention. In R. D. Peters, R. J. McMahon, & V. L. Quinsey (Eds.), *Aggression and violence throughout the lifespan* (pp. 100–125). Newbury Park, CA: Sage.

Olweus, D. (1993a). *Bullying at school: What we know and what we can do.* Malden, MA: Blackwell.

Olweus, D. (1993b). Victimization by peers: Antecedents and long-term outcomes. In K. H. Rubin & J. B. Asendorf (Eds.), *Social withdrawal, inhibition, and shyness in childhood* (pp. 315–341). Hillsdale, NJ: Erlbaum.

Olweus, D. (1996). Bullying at school: Knowledge base and an effective intervention program. *Annals of the New York Academy of Sciences, 794,* 265–276.

Olweus, D. (1999). Sweden. In P. K. Smith, Y. Morita, J. Junger-Tas, D. Olweus, R. Catalano, & P. Slee (Eds.), *The nature of school bullying: A cross-national perspective* (pp. 7–27). New York: Routledge.

Olweus, D. (2001). Peer harassment: A critical analysis and some important issues. In J. Juvonen & S. Graham (Eds.), *Peer harassment in school: The plight of the vulnerable and victimized* (pp. 1–20). New York: Guilford Press.

Olweus, D., Mattson, A., Schalling, D., & Low, H. (1980). Testosterone, aggression, physical and personality dimensions in normal adolescent males. *Psychosomatic Medicine, 42,* 253–269.

Orpinas, P., Home, A. M., & Staniszewski, D. (2003). School bullying: Changing the problem by changing the school. *School Psychology Review, 32,* 431–444.

Oxford, M., Cavell, T. A., & Hughes, J. N. (2003). Callous–unemotional traits moderate the relation between ineffective parenting and child externalizing problems: A partial replication and extension. *Journal of Clinical Child and Adolescent Psychology, 32,* 577–585.

Pajer, K. A. (1998). What happens to "bad" girls?: A review of the adult outcomes of antisocial adolescent girls. *America Journal of Psychiatry, 155,* 862–870.

Pappadopulos, E., Macintyre, J. C., Crismon, M. L., Findling, R. L., Malone, R. P., Derivan, A., et al. (2003). Treatment recommendations for the use of antipsychotics for aggressive youth (TRAAY): Part II. *Journal of the American Academy of Child and Adolescent Psychiatry, 42,* 145–161.

Pardini, D. A., Lochman, J. E., & Frick, P. J. (2003). Callous/unemotional traits and social cognitive processes in adjudicated youth. *Journal of the American Academy of Child and Adolescent Psychiatry, 42,* 364–371.

Parrish, J. M., Cataldo, M. F., Kolko, D. J., Neef, N. A., & Egel, A. L. (1986). Experimental analysis of response covariation. *Journal of Applied Behavior Analysis, 19,* 241–254.

Parsons, B. V., & Alexander, J. F. (1973). Short-term family intervention: A therapy outcome study. *Journal of Consulting and Clinical Psychology, 41,* 195–201.

Patterson, G. R. (1974). Interventions for boys with conduct problems: Multiple settings, treatments, and criteria. *Journal of Consulting and Clinical Psychology, 42,* 471–481.

Patterson, G. R. (1975). *Families: Applications of social learning to family life* (rev. ed.). Champaign, IL: Research Press.

Patterson, G. R. (1976). *Living with children: New methods for parents and teachers* (rev. ed.). Champaign, IL: Research Press.

Patterson, G. R. (1982). *Coercive family process.* Eugene, OR: Castalia.

Patterson, G. R. (2002). The early development of coercive family process. In J. B. Reid, G. R. Patterson, & J. Snyder (Eds.), *Antisocial behavior in children and adolescents: A developmental analysis and model for intervention* (pp. 25–44). Washington, DC: American Psychological Association.

Patterson, G. R., Capaldi, D., & Bank, L. (1991). An early starter model for predicting delinquency. In D. J. Pepler & K. H. Rubin (Eds.), *The development and treatment of childhood aggression* (pp. 139–168). Hillsdale, NJ: Erlbaum.

Patterson, G. R., & Chamberlain, P. (1988). Treatment process: A problem at three levels. In L. C. Wynne (Ed.), *The state of the art in family therapy research: Controversies and recommendations* (pp. 189–223). New York: Family Process Press.

Patterson, G. R., & Chamberlain, P. (1994). A functional analysis of resistance during parent training therapy. *Clinical Psychology: Science and Practice, 1,* 53–70.

Patterson, G. R., Chamberlain, P., & Reid, J. B. (1982). A comparative evaluation of a parent training program. *Behavior Therapy, 13,* 638–650.

Patterson, G. R., Cobb, J. A., & Ray, R. S. (1973). A social engineering technology for retraining the families of aggressive boys. In H. E. Adams & I. P. Unikel (Eds.), *Issues and trends in behavior therapy* (pp. 139–210). Springfield, IL: Thomas.

Patterson, G. R., & Fleischman, M. J. (1979). Maintenance of treatment effects: Some considerations concerning family systems and follow-up data. *Behavior Therapy, 10,* 168–185.

Patterson, G. R., & Forgatch, M. S. (1985). Therapist behavior as a determinant for client noncompliance: A paradox for the behavior modifier. *Journal of Consulting and Clinical Psychology, 53,* 846–851.

Patterson, G. R., & Forgatch, M. S. (1987). *Parents and adolescents living together: Part 1. The basics.* Eugene, OR: Castalia.

Patterson, G. R., & Forgatch, M. S. (1995). Predicting future clinical adjustment from treatment outcome and process variables. *Psychological Assessment, 7,* 275–285.

Patterson, G. R., Forgatch, M. S., Yoerger, K. L., & Stoolmiller, M. (1998). Variables that initiate and maintain an early-onset trajectory for juvenile offending. *Development and Psychopathology, 10,* 531–547.

Patterson, G. R., & Reid, J. B. (1973). Intervention for families of aggressive boys: A replication study. *Behaviour Research and Therapy, 11,* 383–394.

Patterson, G. R., Reid, J. B., & Dishion, T. J. (1992). *Antisocial boys.* Eugene, OR: Castalia.

Patterson, G. R., Reid, J. B., Jones, R. R., & Conger, R. R. (1975). *A social learning approach to family intervention: Families with aggressive children* (Vol. 1). Eugene, OR: Castalia.

Patterson, G. R, & Yoerger, K. (2002). A developmental model for early and late-onset delinquency. In J. B. Reid, G. R. Patterson, & J. Snyder (Eds.), *Antisocial behavior in children and adolescents: A developmental analysis and model for intervention* (pp. 147–172). Washington, DC: American Psychological Association.

Patterson, J., Barlow, J., Mockford, C., Klimes, I., Pyper, C., & Stewart-Brown, S. (2002). Improving mental health through parenting programmes: Block randomized control trial. *Archives of Disease in Childhood, 87,* 472–477.

Pawsey, R. (1996). A family behavioural treatment of persistent juvenile theft. *Australian Psychologist, 31,* 28–33.

Peed, S., Roberts, M., & Forehand, R. (1977). Evaluation of the effectiveness of a standardized parent training program in altering the interaction of mothers and their noncompliant children. *Behavior Modification, 1,* 323–350.

Pelham, W. E., & Lang, A. R. (1993). Parental alcohol consumption and deviant child behavior: Laboratory studies of reciprocal effects. *Clinical Psychology Review, 13,* 763–784.

Pelletier-Parker, A. Slate, F., Moriarty, D., & Pinsonneault, I. (1999). *The best practice treatment guidelines for adolescent firesetters in residential treatment.* Boston: Option/Commonworks.

Pepler, D. J. (2005, March). *Scaffolding and social architecture: A framework for bullying interventions.* Workshop presented at the Banff International Conference on Behavioural Science: Child and Adolescent Mental Health: Evidence-Based Interventions, Banff, AB, Canada.

Pepler, D. J., Craig, W. M., Ziegler, S., & Charach, A. (1993). A school-based anti-bullying intervention: Preliminary evaluation. In D. Tattum (Ed.), *Understanding and managing bullying* (pp. 76–91). London: Heinemann.

Pepler, D. J., Craig, W. M., Ziegler, S., & Charach, A. (1994). An evaluation of an anti-bullying intervention in Toronto schools. *Canadian Journal of Community Mental Health, 13,* 95–110.

Pepler, D. J., Madsen, K. C., Webster, C., & Levene, K. S. (Eds.). (2005). *The development and treatment of girlhood aggression.* Mahwah, NJ: Erlbaum.

Pepler, D. J., Walsh, M. M., & Levene, K. S. (2004). Interventions for aggressive girls: Tailoring and measuring the fit. In M. M. Moretti, C. L. Odgers, & M. A. Jackson (Eds.), *Girls and aggression: Contributing factors and intervention principles* (pp. 131–145). New York: Kluwer Academic/Plenum.

Pfiffner, L. J., Barkley, R. A., & DuPaul, G. J. (2006). Treatment of ADHD in school settings. In R. A. Barkley, *Attention-deficit hyperactivity disorder: A handbook for diagnosis, assessment, and treatment* (3rd ed., pp. 547–589). New York: Guilford Press.

Pfiffner, L. J., & O'Leary, S. G. (1987). The efficacy of all-positive management as a function of the prior use of negative consequences. *Journal of Applied Behavior Analysis, 20,* 265–271.

Pfiffner, L. J., Rosen, L. A., & O'Leary, S. G. (1985). The efficacy of an all-positive approach to classroom management. *Journal of Applied Behavior Analysis, 18,* 257–261.

Pigott, H. E., & Heggie, D. L. (1986). Interpreting the conflicting results of individual versus group contingencies in classrooms: The targeted behavior as a mediating variable. *Child & Family Behavior Therapy, 7,* 1–14.

Pikas, A. (1989). A pure conception of mobbing gives the best results for treatment. *School Psychology International, 10,* 95–104.

Piquero, A., & Brezina, T. (2000). Testing Moffitt's account of adolescence-limited delinquency. *Criminology, 39,* 353–370.

Porter, B., & O'Leary, K. D. (1980). Marital discord and childhood behavior problems. *Journal of Abnormal Child Psychology, 8,* 287–295.

Poulin, F., & Boivin, M. (2000). Reactive and proactive aggression: Evidence of a two-factor model. *Psychological Assessment, 12,* 115–122.

Poulin, F., Dishion, T. J., & Burraston, B. (2001). 3-year iatrogenic effects associated with aggregating high-risk adolescents in cognitive-behavioral preventive interventions. *Applied Developmental Science, 5,* 214–224.

Power, C., Higgins, A., & Kohlberg, L. (1989). *Lawrence Kohlberg's approach to moral education.* New York: Columbia University Press.

Powers, S. W., & Roberts, M. W. (1995). Simulation training with parents of oppositional children: Preliminary findings. *Journal of Clinical Child Psychology, 24,* 89–97.

Poyurovsky, M. Halperin, E., Enoch, D., Schneidman, M., & Weisman, A. (1995). Fluvoxamine treatment of compulsivity, impulsivity, and aggression. *American Journal of Psychiatry, 152,* 1688–1689.

Presidential Commission on Law Enforcement and the Administration of Justice. (1967). *Task force report: Juvenile delinquency and youth crime.* Washington, DC: U.S. Government Printing Office.

Prinz, R. J., Blechman, E. A., & Dumas, J. E. (1994). An evaluation of peer coping-skills training for childhood aggression. *Journal of Clinical Child Psychology, 23,* 193–203.

Prinz, R. J., & Dumas, J. E. (2004). Prevention of oppositional defiant disorder and conduct disorder in children and adolescents. In P. M. Barrett & T. H. Ollendick (Eds.), *Handbook of interventions that work with children and adolescents: Prevention and treatment* (pp. 475–488). Chichester, UK: Wiley.

Prinz, R. J., & Miller, G. E. (1991). Issues in understanding and treating childhood conduct problems in disadvantaged populations. *Journal of Clinical Child Psychology, 20,* 379–385.

Prinz, R. J., & Miller, G. E. (1994). Family-based treatment for childhood antisocial behavior: Experimental influences on dropout and engagement. *Journal of Consulting and Clinical Psychology, 62,* 645–650.

Prinz, R. J., & Miller, G. E. (1996). Parental engagement in interventions for children at risk for conduct disorder. In R. D. Peters & R. J. McMahon (Eds.), *Preventing childhood disorders, substance abuse, and delinquency* (pp. 161–183). Thousand Oaks, CA: Sage.

Proctor, M. A., & Morgan, D. (1991). Effectiveness of a response cost raffle procedure on the disruptive classroom behavior of adolescents with behavior problems. *School Psychology Review, 20,* 97–109.

Puig-Antich, J. (1982). Major depression and conduct disorder in prepuberty. *Journal of the American Academy of Child and Adolescent Psychiatry, 21,* 118–128.

Putallaz, M., & Bierman, K. L. (Eds.). (2004). *Aggression, antisocial behavior, and violence among girls: A developmental perspective.* New York: Guilford Press.

Quay, H. C., & Peterson, D. (1996). *Revised Behavior Problem Checklist—PAR Edition: Professional manual.* Odessa, FL: Psychological Assessment Resources.

Querido, J. G., & Eyberg, S. M. (2003). Psychometric properties of the Sutter–Eyberg Student Behavior Inventory—Revised with preschool children. *Behavior Therapy, 34,* 1–15.

Raine, A., & Jones, F. (1987). Attention, autonomic arousal and personality in behaviorally disordered children. *Journal of Abnormal Child Psychology, 15,* 583–599.

Raine, A., Venables, P. H., & Williams, M. (1990). Relationship between central and autonomic measures of arousal at age 15 and criminality at age 24 years. *Archives of General Psychiatry, 47,* 1003–1007.

Rayfield, A., Eyberg, S. M., & Foote, R. (1998). Revision of the Sutter–Eyberg Student Behavior Inventory: Teacher ratings of conduct problem behavior. *Educational and Psychological Measurement, 58,* 88–99.

Reavis, H. K., Taylor, M., Jenson, W., Morgan, D., Andrews, D., & Fister, S. (1996). *Best practices: Behavioral and educational strategies for teachers.* Longmont, CO: Sopris West.

Reddy, L. A., & Pfeiffer, S. I. (1997). Effectiveness of

treatment foster care with children and adolescents: A review of outcome studies. *Journal of the American Academy of Child and Adolescent Psychiatry, 36,* 581–588.

Reich, W. (2000). Diagnostic Interview for Children and Adolescents (DICA). *Journal of the American Academy of Child and Adolescent Psychiatry, 39,* 59–66.

Reid, J. B. (1984, November). Stealing and other clandestine activities among antisocial children. In D. J. Kolko (Chair), *Child antisocial behavior research: Current status and implications.* Symposium conducted at the annual meeting of the Association for Advancement of Behavior Therapy, Philadelphia.

Reid, J. B. (1987, March). *Therapeutic interventions in the families of aggressive children and adolescents.* Paper presented at the annual meeting of the Organizzato dalle Cattedre di Psicologia Clinica e delle Teorie di Personalita dell'Universita di Roma, Rome.

Reid, J. B., Baldwin, D. V., Patterson, G. R., & Dishion, T. J. (1988). Observations in the assessment of childhood disorders. In M. Rutter, A. H. Tuma, & I. S. Lann (Eds.), *Assessment and diagnosis in child psychopathology* (pp. 156–195). New York: Guilford Press.

Reid, J. B., & Hendricks, A. F. C. J. (1973). A preliminary analysis of the effectiveness of direct home intervention for treatment of pre-delinquent boys who steal. In L. A. Hamerlynck, L. C. Handy, & E. J. Mash (Eds.), *Behavior change: Methodology, concepts, and practice* (pp. 209–220). Champaign, IL: Research Press.

Reid, J. B., Hinojosa Rivera, G., & Lorber, R. (1980). *A social learning approach to the outpatient treatment of children who steal.* Unpublished manuscript, Oregon Social Learning Center, Eugene.

Reid, J. B., Patterson, G. R., & Snyder, J. J. (Eds.). (2002). *Antisocial behavior in children and adolescents: A developmental analysis and model for intervention.* Washington, DC: American Psychological Association.

Reid, M. J., & Webster-Stratton, C. (2001). The Incredible Years parent, teacher, and child intervention: Targeting multiple areas of risk for a young child with pervasive conduct problems using a flexible, manualized, treatment program. *Cognitive and Behavior Practice, 8,* 377–386.

Reid, M. J., Webster-Stratton, C., & Beauchaine, T. P. (2001). Parent training in Head Start: A comparison of program response among African American, Asian American, Caucasian, and Hispanic mothers. *Prevention Science, 2,* 209–227.

Reid, M. J., Webster-Stratton, C., & Hammond, M. (2003). Follow-up of children who received the Incredible Years intervention for oppositional defiant disorder: Maintenance and prediction of 2-year outcome. *Behavior Therapy, 34,* 471–491.

Reis, D. (1975). *Central neurotransmitters in aggressive behaviors: Neural basis of violence and aggression.* St. Louis, MO: Green.

Reitman, D., & Hupp, S. D. A. (2003). Behavior problems in the school setting: Synthesizing structural and functional assessment. In M. L. Kelley, D. Reitman, & G. H. Noell (Eds.), *Practitioner's guide to empirically based measures of school behavior* (pp. 23–36). New York: Kluwer Academic/Plenum.

Reynolds, C. R., & Kamphaus, K. W. (2004). *BASC-2: Behavior Assessment System for Children, Second Edition.* Circle Pines, MN: American Guidance Service.

Rich, B. A., & Eyberg, S. M. (2001). Accuracy of assessment: The discriminative and predictive power of the Eyberg Child Behavior Inventory. *Ambulatory Child Health, 7,* 249–257.

Richardson, J. P. (2002). Secure residential treatment for adolescent firesetters. In D. Kolko (Ed.), *Handbook on firesetting in children and youth* (pp. 353–381). San Diego, CA: Academic Press.

Richters, J. E. (1992). Depressed mothers as informants about their children: A critical review of the evidence for distortion. *Psychological Bulletin, 112,* 485–499.

Riddle, M. A., Nelson, J. C., Kleinman, C. S., Rasmusson, A., Leckman, J. F., King, R. A., et al. (1991). A case study: Sudden death in children receiving Norpramin: A review of three reported cases and commentary. *Journal of the American Academy of Child and Adolescent Psychiatry, 30,* 104–108.

Rifkin, A., Karajgi, B., Dicker, R., Perl, E., Boppana, V., Hasan, N., et al. (1997). Lithium treatment of conduct disorders in adolescents. *American Journal of Psychiatry, 154,* 554–555.

Robbins, M. S., Alexander, J. F., Newell, R. M., & Turner, C. W. (1996). The immediate effect of reframing on client attitude in family therapy. *Journal of Family Psychology, 10,* 28–34.

Robbins, M. S., Alexander, J. F., & Turner, C. W. (2000). Disrupting defensive family interactions in family therapy with delinquent adolescents. *Journal of Family Psychology, 14,* 688–701.

Robbins, M. S., Szapocznik, J., Santisteban, D. A., Hervis, O. E., Mitrani, V. B., & Schwartz, S. J. (2003). Brief Strategic Family Therapy for Hispanic youth. In A. E. Kazdin & J. R. Weisz (Eds.), *Evidence-based psychotherapies for children and adolescents* (pp. 407–424). New York: Guilford Press.

Robbins, M. S., Turner, C. W., Alexander, J. F., & Perez, G. A. (2003). Alliance and dropout in family therapy for adolescents with behavior problems: Individual and systemic effects. *Journal of Family Psychology, 17,* 534–544.

Roberts, M. W. (2001). Clinic observations of structured parent–child interaction designed to evaluate externalizing problems. *Psychological Assessment, 13,* 46–58.

Roberts, M. W., Joe, V. C., & Rowe-Hallbert, A. (1992). Oppositional child behavior and parental locus of control. *Journal of Clinical Child Psychology, 21,* 170–177.

Robin, A. L. (1981). A controlled evaluation of Problem-Solving Communication Training with parent–adolescent conflict. *Behavior Therapy, 12,* 593–609.

Robin, A. L., & Foster, S. (1989). *Negotiating parent–adolescent conflict.* New York: Guilford Press.

Robin, A. L., Kent, R., O'Leary, K. D., Foster, S. L., & Prinz, R. J. (1977). An approach to teaching parents and adolescents problem-solving communication skills: A preliminary report. *Behavior Therapy, 8,* 639–643.

Robins, L. N. (1991). Conduct disorder. *Journal of Child Psychology and Psychiatry, 32,* 193–209.

Rogeness, G. A., Maas, J. W., Javors, M. A. Macedo, C. A., Fischer, C., & Harris, W. R. (1989). Attention deficit disorder symptoms and urine. *Psychiatry Research, 27,* 241–251.

Rogers, T. R., Forehand, R., Griest, D. L., Wells, K. C., & McMahon, R. J. (1981). Socioeconomic status: Effects on parent and child behaviors and treatment outcome of parent training. *Journal of Clinical Child Psychology, 10,* 98–101.

Rohde, P., Clarke, G. N., Mace, D. E., Jorgensen, J. S., & Seeley, J. R. (2004). An efficacy/effectiveness study of cognitive-behavioral treatment for adolescents with comorbid major depression and conduct disorder. *Journal of the American Academy of Child and Adolescent Psychiatry, 43,* 660–668.

Rohde, P., Jorgensen, J. S., Seeley, J. R., & Mace, D. E. (2004). Pilot evaluation of the Coping Course: A cognitive-behavioral intervention to enhance coping skills in incarcerated youth. *Journal of the American Academy of Child and Adolescent Psychiatry, 43,* 669–676.

Rosen, H. S., & Rosen, L. A. (1983). Eliminating stealing: Use of stimulus control with an elementary student. *Behavior Modification, 7,* 56–63.

Rosen, L. A., Gabardi, L., Miller, C. D., & Miller, L. (1990). Home-based treatment of disruptive junior high school students: An analysis of the differential effects of positive and negative consequences. *Behavioral Disorders, 15,* 227–232.

Routh, C. P., Hill, J. W., Steele, H., Elliott, C. E., & Dewey, M. E. (1995). Maternal attachment status, psychosocial stressors and problem behaviour: Follow-up after parent training courses for conduct disorder. *Journal of Child Psychology and Psychiatry, 36,* 1179–1198.

Ruma, P. R., Burke, R. V., & Thompson, R. W. (1996). Group parent training: Is it effective for children of all ages? *Behavior Therapy, 27,* 159–169.

Russo, D. C., Cataldo, M. F., & Cushing, P. J. (1981). Compliance training and behavioral covariation in the treatment of multiple behavior problems. *Journal of Applied Behavior Analysis, 14,* 209–222.

Rutter, M. (1994). Family discord and conduct disorder: Cause, consequence, or correlate? *Journal of Family Psychology, 8,* 170–186.

Rutter, M., Giller, H., & Hagell, A. (1998). *Antisocial behavior by young people.* Cambridge, UK: Cambridge University Press.

Rutter, M., & Smith, D. J. (1995). *Psychosocial disor-ders in young people: Time, trends, and their causes.* Chichester, UK: Wiley.

Rutter, R., Harrington, R., Quinton, D., & Pickles, A. (1994). Adult outcome of conduct disorder in childhood: Implications for concepts and definitions of patterns of psychopathology. In R. D. Ketterlinus & M. E. Lamb (Eds.), *Adolescent problem behaviors: Issues and research* (pp. 57–80). Hillsdale, NJ: Erlbaum.

Sanders, M. R. (1982). The generalization of parent responding to community settings: The effects of instructions, plus feedback, and self-management training. *Behavioural Psychotherapy, 10,* 273–287.

Sanders, M. R., & Christensen, A. P. (1985). A comparison of the effects of child management and planned activities training in five parenting environments. *Journal of Abnormal Child Psychology, 13,* 101–117.

Sanders, M. R., & Dadds, M. R. (1982). The effects of planned activities and child management procedures in parent training: An analysis of setting generality. *Behavior Therapy, 13,* 452–461.

Sanders, M. R., & Dadds, M. R. (1992). Children's and parents' cognitions about family interaction: An evaluation of video-mediated recall and thought listing procedures in the assessment of conduct-disordered children. *Journal of Clinical Child Psychology, 21,* 371–379.

Sanders, M. R., & Dadds, M. R. (1993). *Behavioral family intervention.* Boston: Allyn & Bacon.

Sanders, M. R., & Glynn, T. (1981). Training parents in behavioral self management: An analysis of generalization and maintenance. *Journal of Applied Behavior Analysis, 14,* 223–237.

Sanders, M. R., Markie-Dadds, C., Tully, L., & Bor, B. (2000). The Triple P-Positive Parenting Program: A comparison of enhanced, standard, and self-directed behavioral family intervention for parents of children with early onset conduct problems. *Journal of Consulting and Clinical Psychology, 68,* 624–640.

Sanders, M. R., Markie-Dadds, C., & Turner, K. M. T. (2003). Theoretical, scientific and clinical foundations of the Triple P-Positive Parenting Program: A population approach to the promotion of parenting competence. *Parenting Research and Practice Monograph, 1,* 1–24.

Sanders, M. R., & McFarland, M. (2000). Treatment of depressed mothers with disruptive children: A controlled evaluation of cognitive behavioral family intervention. *Behavior Therapy, 31,* 89–112.

Sanders, M. R., Pidgeon, A. M., Gravestock, F., Connors, M. D., Brown, S., & Young, R. W. (2004). Does parental attributional retraining and anger management enhance the effects of the Triple P-Positive Parenting Program with parents at risk of child maltreatment? *Behavior Therapy, 35,* 513–535.

Sanders, M. R., Turner, K. M. T., & Markie-Dadds, C. (2002). The development and dissemination of the Triple P-Positive Parenting Program: A multilevel, evidence-based system of parenting and family support. *Prevention Science, 3,* 173–189.

Sanson, A., Oberklaid, F., Pedlow, R., & Prior, M. (1991). Risk indicators: Assessment of infancy predictors of pre-school behavioural maladjustment. *Journal of Child Psychology and Psychiatry, 32,* 609–626.

Santisteban, D. A., Coatsworth, J. D., Perez-Vidal, A., Kurtines, W. M., Schwartz, S. J., LaPerriere, A., et al. (2003). Efficacy of Brief Strategic Family Therapy in modifying Hispanic adolescent behavior problems and substance use. *Journal of Family Psychology, 17,* 121–133.

Santisteban, D. A., Szapocznik, J., Perez-Vidal, A., Kurtines, W. M., Murray, E. J., & LaPerriere, A. (1996). Efficacy of intervention for engaging youth and families into treatment and some variables that may contribute to differential effectiveness. *Journal of Family Psychology, 10,* 35–44.

Sayger, T. V., Horne, A. M., & Glaser, B. A. (1993). Marital satisfaction and social learning family therapy for child conduct problems: Generalization of treatment effects. *Journal of Marital and Family Therapy, 19,* 393–402.

Schaeffer, C. M., & Borduin, C. M. (2005). Long-term follow-up to a randomized clinical trial of Multisystemic Therapy with serious and violent juvenile offenders. *Journal of Consulting and Clinical Psychology, 73,* 445–453.

Schoenwald, S. K., Brown, T. L., & Henggeler, S. W. (2000). Inside Multisystemic Therapy: Therapist, supervisory, and program practices. *Journal of Emotional and Behavioral Disorders, 8,* 113–127.

Schoenwald, S. K., Henggeler, S. W., Pickrel, S. G., & Cunningham, P. B. (1996). Treating seriously troubled youths and families in their contexts: Multi-Systemic Therapy. In M. C. Roberts (Ed.), *Model programs in child and family mental health* (pp. 317–332). Mahwah, NJ: Erlbaum.

Schoenwald, S. K., Ward, D. M., Henggeler, S. W., Pickrel, S. G., & Patel, H. (1996). MST treatment of substance abusing or dependent adolescent offenders: Costs of reducing incarceration, inpatient, and residential placement. *Journal of Child and Family Studies, 5,* 431–444.

Schreier, H. A. (1998). Risperidone for young children with mood disorders and aggressive behavior. *Journal of Child and Adolescent Psychopharmacology, 8,* 49–59.

Schuhmann, E. M., Foote, R., Eyberg, S. M., Boggs, S., & Algina, J. (1998). Parent–Child Interaction Therapy: Interim report of a randomized trial with a short-term maintenance. *Journal of Clinical Child Psychology, 27,* 34–45.

Schumaker, J. B., Hovell, M. F., & Sherman, J. A. (1977). An analysis of daily report cards and parent-managed privileges in the improvement of adolescents' classroom performance. *Journal of Applied Behavior Analysis, 10,* 449–464.

Schur, S. B., Sikich, L., Findling, R. L., Malone, R. P.,

Crismon, M. L., Derivan, A., et al. (2003). Treatment recommendations for the use of antipsychotics for aggressive youth (TRAAY): Part I. A review. *Journal of the American Academy of Child and Adolescent Psychiatry, 42,* 132–144.

Schweinhart, L. J., Barnes, H. V., & Weikart, D. P. (Eds.). (1993). *Significant benefits: The High/Scope Perry Preschool Study through age 27.* Ypsilanti, MI: High/Scope Press.

Scott, M. J., & Stradling, S. G. (1987). Evaluation of a group programme for parents of problem children. *Behavioural Psychotherapy, 15,* 224–239.

Scott, S., Spender, Q., Doolan, M., Jacobs, B., & Aspland, H. (2001). Multicentre controlled trial of parenting groups for child antisocial behaviour in clinical practice. *British Medical Journal, 323,* 1–7.

Scotti, J. R., Morris, T. L., McNeil, C. B., & Hawkins, R. P. (1996). DSM-IV and disorders of childhood and adolescence: Can structural criteria be functional? *Journal of Consulting and Clinical Psychology, 64,* 1177–1191.

Serbin, L. A., Moskowitz, K. S., Schwartzman, A. E., & Ledingham, J. E. (1991). Aggressive, withdrawn, and aggressive/withdrawn children in adolescence: Into the next generation. In D. J. Pepler & K. H. Rubin (Eds.), *The development and treatment of childhood aggression* (pp. 55–70). Hillsdale, NJ: Erlbaum.

Serketich, W. J., & Dumas, J. E. (1996). The effectiveness of behavioral parent training to modify antisocial behavior in children: A meta-analysis. *Behavior Therapy, 27,* 171–186.

Sexton, T. L., & Alexander, J. F. (2002). Functional Family Therapy for at-risk adolescents and their families. In K. W. Kaslow (Series Ed.) & T. Patterson (Vol. Ed.), *Comprehensive handbook of psychotherapy: Vol. 2. Cognitive–behavioral approaches* (pp. 117–140). New York: Wiley.

Sexton, T. L., & Alexander, J. F. (2003). Functional Family Therapy: A mature clinical model for working with at-risk adolescents and their families. In T. L. Sexton, G. R. Weeks, & M. S. Robbins (Eds.), *Handbook of family therapy: The science and practice of working with families and couples* (pp. 323–348). New York: Brunner-Routledge.

Seymour, F. W., & Epston, D. (1989). An approach to childhood stealing with evaluation of 45 cases. *Australian and New Zealand Journal of Family Therapy, 10,* 137–143.

Shaffer, D., Fisher, P., Lucas, C. P., Dulcan, M. K., & Schwab-Stone, M. E. (2000). NIMH Diagnostic Interview Schedule for Children–Version IV (NIMH DISC-IV): Description, differences from previous versions, and reliability of some common diagnoses. *Journal of the American Academy of Child and Adolescent Psychiatry, 39,* 28–38.

Shaw, D. S., Bell, R. Q., & Gilliom, M. (2000). A truly early starter model of antisocial behavior revisited. *Clinical Child and Family Psychology Review, 3,* 155–172.

Sheldrick, R. C., Kendall, P. C., & Heimberg, R. G.

(2001). The clinical significance of treatments: A comparison of three treatments for conduct disordered children. *Clinical Psychology: Science and Practice, 8,* 418–430.

Shelton, K. K., Frick, P. J., & Wootton, J. M. (1996). Assessment of parenting practices in families of elementary school-age children. *Journal of Clinical Child Psychology, 25,* 317–329.

Shores, R., Gunter, P., & Jack, S. (1993). Classroom management strategies: Are they setting events for coercion? *Behavioral Disorders, 18,* 92–102.

Shure, M. B., & Spivack, G. (1980). Interpersonal problem solving as a mediator of behavioral adjustment in preschool and kindergarten children. *Journal of Applied Developmental Psychology, 1,* 29–44.

Silvernail, D. L., Thompsom, A. M., Yang, Z., & Kopp, H. J. P. (2000). *A survey of bullying behavior among Maine third graders.* Gorham: Maine Center for Educational Policy, Applied Research and Evaluation, University of Southern Maine.

Silverthorn, P., & Frick, P. J. (1999). Developmental pathways to antisocial behavior: The delayed onset pathway in girls. *Development and Psychopathology, 11,* 101–126.

Simonoff, E., Pickles, A., Meyer, J., Silberg, J., & Maes, H. (1998). Genetic and environmental influences on subtypes of conduct disorder behavior in boys. *Journal of Abnormal Child Psychology, 26,* 495–510.

Skinner, H. A. (1982). The Drug Abuse Screening Test. *Addictive Behaviors, 7,* 363–371.

Slep, A. M., & O'Leary, S. G. (1998). The effects of maternal attributions on parenting: An experimental analysis. *Journal of Family Psychology, 12,* 234–243.

Slot, N. W., Jagers, H. D., & Dangel, R. F. (1992). Cross-cultural replication and evaluation of the Teaching Family Model of community-based residential treatment. *Behavioral Residential Treatment, 7,* 341–354.

Smith, P. K., Cowie, H., Olafsson, R. F., & Liefooghe, A. P. D. (2002). Definitions of bullying: A comparison of terms used, and age and gender differences, in a fourteen-country international comparison. *Child Development, 73,* 1119–1133.

Smith, P. K., Morita, Y., Junger-Tas, J., Olweus, D., Catalano, R., & Slee, P. (1999). *The nature of school bullying: A cross-national perspective.* New York: Routledge.

Smith, P. K., & Sharp, S. (Eds.). (1994a). *School bullying: Insights and perspectives.* London: Routledge.

Smith, P. K., & Sharp, S. (Eds.). (1994b). *Tackling bullying in your school: A practical handbook for teachers.* London: Routledge.

Smithmyer, C. M., Hubbard, J. A., & Simons, R. F. (2000). Proactive and reactive aggression in delinquent adolescents: Relations to aggression outcome expectancies. *Journal of Clinical Child Psychology, 29,* 86–93.

Snyder, H. N. (1999). *Juvenile arson, 1997* (Fact Sheet No. 91). Washington, DC: U.S. Department of Justice, Office of Justice Programs, Office of Juvenile Justice and Delinquency Prevention.

Snyder, J. (1991). Discipline as a mediator of the impact of maternal stress and mood on child conduct problems. *Development and Psychopathology, 3,* 263–276.

Snyder, J., Reid, J., & Patterson, G. (2003). A social learning model of child and adolescent antisocial behavior. In B. B. Lahey, T. E. Moffitt, & A. Caspi (Eds.), *Causes of conduct disorder and juvenile delinquency* (pp. 27–48). New York: Guilford Press.

Snyder, J., & Stoolmiller, M. (2002). Reinforcement and coercion mechanisms in the development of antisocial behavior: The family. In J. B. Reid, G. R. Patterson, & J. Snyder (Eds.), *Antisocial behavior in children and adolescents: A developmental analysis and model for intervention* (pp. 65–100). Washington, DC: American Psychological Association.

Spanier, G. B. (1976). Measuring dyadic adjustment: New scales for assessing the quality of marriage and similar dyads. *Journal of Marriage and the Family, 38,* 15–28.

Spence, S. H., & Marzillier, J. S. (1981). Social skills training with adolescent male offenders: II. Short-term, long-term, and generalized effects. *Behaviour Research and Therapy, 19,* 349–368.

Spitzer, A., Webster-Stratton, C., & Hollinsworth, T. (1991). Coping with conduct-problem children: Parents gaining knowledge and control. *Journal of Clinical Child Psychology, 20,* 413–427.

Stack, D. M., Serbin, L. A., Schwartzman, A. E., & Ledingham, J. (2005). Girls' aggression across the life course: Long-term outcomes and intergenerational risk. In D. J. Pepler, K. C. Madsen, C. Webster, & K. S. Levene (Eds.), *The development and treatment of girlhood aggression* (pp. 253–283). Mahwah, NJ: Erlbaum.

Stadolnik, R. F. (2000). *Drawn to the flame: Assessment and treatment of juvenile firesetting behavior.* Sarasota, FL: Professional Resource Press.

Stanger, C., Achenbach, T. M., & Verhulst, F. C. (1997). Accelerated longitudinal comparisons of aggressive versus delinquent syndromes. *Development and Psychopathology, 9,* 43–58.

Stevens, V., De Bourdeaudhuij, I., & Van Oost, P. (2000). Bullying in Flemish schools: An evaluation of anti-bullying intervention in primary and secondary schools. *British Journal of Educational Psychology, 70,* 195–210.

Stickle, T. R., & Blechman, E. A. (2002). Aggression and fire: Antisocial behavior in firesetting and nonfiresetting juvenile offenders. *Journal of Psychopathology and Behavioral Assessment, 24,* 177–193.

Stickle, T. R., & Frick, P. J. (2002). Developmental pathways to severe antisocial behavior: Interventions for youth with callous-unemotional traits. *Expert Review of Neurotherapeutics, 2,* 511–522.

Stoewe, J. K., Kruesi, M. J. P., & Lelio, D. F. (1995). Psychopharmacology of aggressive states and features of conduct disorder. *Child and Adolescent Psychiatric Clinics of North America, 4,* 359–379.

Stoolmiller, M., Duncan, T., Bank, L., & Patterson, G. R. (1993). Some problems and solutions in the study of change: Significant patterns in client resistance. *Journal of Consulting and Clinical Psychology, 61,* 920–928.

Storr, C. L., Ialongo, N. S., Kellam, S. G., & Anthony, J. C. (2002). A randomized controlled trial of two primary school intervention strategies to prevent early onset tobacco smoking. *Drug and Alcohol Dependence, 66,* 51–60.

Stouthamer-Loeber, M. (1986). Lying as a problem behavior in children: A review. *Clinical Psychology Review, 6,* 267–289.

Stouthamer-Loeber, M., & Loeber, R. (1986). Boys who lie. *Journal of Abnormal Child Psychology, 14,* 551–564.

Strain, P. S., Lambert, D. L., Kerr, M. M., Stagg, V., & Lenkner, D. A. (1983). Naturalistic assessment of children's compliance to teachers' requests and consequences for compliance. *Journal of Applied Behavior Analysis, 16,* 243–249.

Strain, P. S., Steele, P., Ellis, T., & Timm, M. A. (1982). Long-term effects of oppositional child treatment with mothers as therapists and therapist trainers. *Journal of Applied Behavior Analysis, 15,* 163–169.

Strain, P. S., Young, C. C., & Horowitz, J. (1981). Generalized behavior change during oppositional child training: An examination of child and family demographic variables. *Behavior Modification, 5,* 15–26.

Straus, M. A. (1979). Measuring intrafamily conflict and violence: The Conflict Tactics (CT) Scales. *Journal of Marriage and the Family, 41,* 75–88.

Straus, M. A. (1990). The Conflict Tactics Scales and its critics: An evaluation and new data on validity and reliability. In M. A. Straus & R. J. Gelles (Eds.), *Physical violence in American families: Risk factors and adaptations to violence in 8,145 families* (pp. 49–73). New Brunswick, NJ: Transaction.

Strayhorn, J. M., & Weidman, C. S. (1988). A parent practices scale and its relation to parent and child mental health. *Journal of the American Academy of Child and Adolescent Psychiatry, 27,* 613–618.

Stroul, B. A. (1995). Case management in a system of care. In B. J. Friesen & J. Poertner (Eds.), *From case management to service coordination for children with emotional, behavioural, or mental disorders: Building on family strengths* (pp. 3–25). Baltimore: Brookes.

Stumpf, J., & Holman, J. (1985). Promoting generalization of appropriate classroom behaviour: A comparison of two strategies. *Behavioural Psychotherapy, 13,* 29–42.

Sugai, G., & Horner, R. (1999). Discipline and behavioral support: Preferred process and practices. *Effective School Practices, 17,* 10–22.

Sugai, G., Horner, R., & Gresham, F. (2002). Behaviorally effective school environments. In M. Shinn, H. Walker, & G. Stoner (Eds.), *Interventions for academic and behavior problems: II. Preventive and re-medial approaches* (pp. 315–350). Bethesda, MD: National Association of School Psychologists.

Sugai, G., Sprague, J., Horner, R., & Walker, H. (2000). Preventing school violence: The use of office discipline referrals to assess and monitor school-wide disciplinary interventions. In H. Walker & M. Epstein (Eds.), *Making schools safer and violence free: Critical issues, solutions, and recommended practices* (pp. 50–57). Austin, TX: PRO-ED.

Sukhodolsky, D. G., Kassinove, H., & Gorman, B. S. (2004). Cognitive-behavioral therapy for anger in children and adolescents: A meta-analysis. *Aggression and Violent Behavior, 9,* 247–269.

Sultana, C. R., Matthews, J., De Bortoli, D., & Cann, W. (2004). *An evaluation of two levels of the Positive Parenting Program (Triple P) delivered by primary care practitioners.* Manuscript in preparation.

Switzer, E. B., Deal, T. E., & Bailey, J. S. (1977). The reduction of stealing in second graders using a group contingency. *Journal of Applied Behavior Analysis, 10,* 267–272.

Szapocznik, J., Kurtines, W. M., Foote, F., Perez-Vidal, A., & Hervis, O. E. (1983). Conjoint versus one person family therapy: Some evidence for the effectiveness of conducting family therapy through one person. *Journal of Consulting and Clinical Psychology, 51,* 889–899.

Szapocznik, J., Kurtines, W. M., Foote, F., Perez-Vidal, A., & Hervis, O. E. (1986). Conjoint versus one person family therapy: Further evidence for the effectiveness of conducting family therapy through one person. *Journal of Consulting and Clinical Psychology, 54,* 395–397.

Szapocznik, J., Perez-Vidal, A., Brickman, A., Foote, F. H., Santisteban, D. A., Hervis, O. E., et al. (1988). Engaging adolescent drug abusers and their families in treatment: A strategic structural systems approach. *Journal of Consulting and Clinical Psychology, 56,* 552–557.

Szapocznik, J., Rio, A., Murray, E., Cohen, R., Scopetta, M., Rivas-Vazquez, A., et al. (1989). Structural family versus psychodynamic child therapy for problematic Hispanic boys. *Journal of Consulting and Clinical Psychology, 57,* 571–578.

Szapocznik, J., Santisteban, D., Rio, A., Perez-Vidal, A., Kurtines, W. M., & Hervis, O. E. (1986). Bicultural effectiveness training: A treatment intervention for enhancing intercultural adjustment. *Hispanic Journal of Behavior Sciences, 6,* 317–344.

Szapocznik, J., & Williams, R. A. (2000). Brief Strategic Family Therapy: Twenty-five years of interplay among theory, research and practice in adolescent behavior problems and drug abuse. *Clinical Child and Family Psychology Review, 3,* 117–134.

Taplin, P. S., & Reid, J. B. (1977). Changes in parent consequences as a function of family intervention. *Journal of Consulting and Clinical Psychology, 45,* 973–981.

Taylor, E. R., Kelly, J., Valescu, S., Reynolds, G. S., Sherman, J., & German, V. (2001). Is stealing a gateway crime? *Community Mental Health Journal, 37,* 347–358.

Taylor, T. K., Eddy, J. M., & Biglan, A. (1999). Interpersonal skills training to reduce aggressive and delinquent behavior: Limited evidence and the need for an evidence-based system of care. *Clinical Child and Family Psychology Review, 2,* 169–182.

Taylor, T. K., Schmidt, F., Pepler, D., & Hodgins, H. (1998). A comparison of eclectic treatment with Webster-Stratton's Parent and Children's Series in a children's mental health center: A randomized controlled trial. *Behavior Therapy, 29,* 221–240.

Thomas, A., Chess, S., & Birch, H. G. (1968). *Temperament and behavior disorders in children.* New York: New York University Press.

Thompson, R. W., Grow, C. R., Ruma, P. R., Daly, D. L., & Burke, R. V. (1993). Evaluation of a practical parenting program with middle- and low-income families. *Family Relations, 42,* 21–25.

Thornberry, T. P., & Krohn, M. D. (Eds.). (2003). *Taking stock of delinquency: An overview of findings from contemporary longitudinal studies.* New York: Kluwer Academic/Plenum.

Tiet, Q. Q., Wasserman, G. A., Loeber, R., Larken, S. M., & Miller, L. S. (2001). Developmental and sex differences in types of conduct problems. *Journal of Child and Family Studies, 10,* 181–197.

Tingstrom, D. H. (1994). The Good Behavior Game: An investigation of teacher acceptance. *Psychology in the Schools, 31,* 57–65.

Tolan, P. H., Gorman-Smith, D., & Loeber, R. (2000). Developmental timing of onsets of disruptive behaviors and later delinquency of inner-city youth. *Journal of Child and Family Studies, 9,* 203–220.

Tremblay, R. E. (2003). Why socialization fails: The case of chronic physical aggression. In B. B. Lahey, T. E. Moffitt, & A. Caspi (Eds.), *Causes of conduct disorder and delinquency* (pp. 182–224). New York: Guilford Press.

Tremblay, R. E., Masse, L. C., Pagani, L., & Vitaro, F. (1996). From childhood physical aggression to adolescent maladjustment. In R. D. Peters & R. J. McMahon (Eds.), *Preventing childhood disorders, substance abuse, and delinquency* (pp. 268–299). Thousand Oaks, CA: Sage.

Tremblay, R. E., Pagani-Kurtz, L., Masse, L. C., Vitaro, F., & Pihl, R. O. (1995). A bimodal preventive intervention for disruptive kindergarten boys: Its impact through mid-adolescence. *Journal of Consulting and Clinical Psychology, 63,* 560–568.

Tremblay, R. E., Vitaro, F., Bertrand, L., LeBlanc, M., Beauchesne, H., Boileau, H., et al. (1992). Parent and child training to prevent early onset of delinquency: The Montreal Longitudinal–Experimental Study. In J. McCord & R. E. Tremblay (Eds.), *Preventing antisocial behavior: Interventions from birth through adolescence* (pp. 117–138). New York: Guilford Press.

Tremblay, R. E., Vitaro, F., Nagin, D., Pagani, L., & Seguin, J. R. (2003). The Montreal Longitudinal and

Experimental Study: Rediscovering the power of descriptions. In T. P. Thornberry & M. D. Krohn (Eds.), *Taking stock of delinquency: An overview of findings from contemporary longitudinal studies* (pp. 205–254). New York: Kluwer/Academic/Plenum.

Turco, T. L., & Elliott, S. N. (1986). Students' acceptability ratings of interventions for classroom misbehaviors: A developmental study of well-behaving and misbehaving youth. *Journal of Psychoeducational Assessment, 4,* 281–289.

Turner, K. M. T., & Sanders, M. R. (in press). Help when it's needed first: A controlled evaluation of brief, preventive behavioral family intervention in a primary care setting. *Behavior Therapy.*

Underwood, M. K. (2003). *Social aggression among girls.* New York: Guilford Press.

Underwood, M. K., & Coie, J. C. (2004). Future directions and priorities for prevention and intervention. In M. Putallaz & K. L. Bierman (Eds.), *Aggression, antisocial behavior, and violence among girls: A developmental perspective* (pp. 289–301). New York: Guilford Press.

Van Kammen, W. B., Loeber, R., & Stouthamer-Loeber, M. (1991). Substance use and its relationship to conduct problems and delinquency in young boys. *Journal of Youth and Adolescence, 20,* 399–413.

van Lier, P. A. C., Muthén, B. O., van der Sar, R. M., & Crijnen, A. A. M. (2004). Prevention of disruptive behavior in elementary schoolchildren: Impact of a universal classroom-based intervention. *Journal of Consulting and Clinical Psychology, 72,* 467–478.

Venning, H. B., Blampied, N. M., & France, K. G. (2003). Effectiveness of a standard parenting-skills program in reducing stealing and lying in two boys. *Child & Family Behavior Therapy, 25,* 31–44.

Verhulst, F. C., van der Ende, J., Ferdinand, R. F., & Kasius, M. C. (1997). The prevalence of DSM-III-R diagnoses in a national sample of Dutch adolescents. *Archives of General Psychiatry, 54,* 329–336.

Vincent, J., Unis, A., & Hardy, J. (1990). Pharmacotherapy of aggression. *Journal of the American Academy of Child and Adolescent Psychiatry, 29,* 839–840.

Virkunen, M. (1985). Urinary free cortisol excretion in habitually violent offenders. *Acta Psychiatrica Scandinavica, 72,* 40–42.

Vitaro, F., Brendgen, M., Pagani, L., Tremblay, R. E., & McDuff, P. (1999). Disruptive behavior, peer association, and conduct disorder: Testing the developmental links through early intervention. *Development and Psychopathology, 11,* 287–304.

Vitaro, F., Brengden, M., & Tremblay, R. E. (1999). Prevention of school dropout through the reduction of disruptive behaviors and school failure in elementary school. *Journal of School Psychology, 37,* 205–226.

Vitaro, F., Brengden, M., & Tremblay, R. E. (2001). Preventive intervention: Assessing its effects on the trajectories of delinquency and testing for mediational processes. *Applied Developmental Science, 5,* 201–213.

Vitaro, F., Brendgen, M., & Tremblay, R. E. (2002). Reactively and proactively aggressive children: Antecedent and subsequent characteristics. *Journal of Child Psychology and Psychiatry, 43,* 495–505.

Vitaro, F., Gendreau, P. L., Tremblay, R. E., & Oligny, P. (1998). Reactive and proactive aggression differentially predict later conduct problems. *Journal of Child Psychology and Psychiatry, 39,* 377–385.

Vitiello, B., & Stoff, D. M. (1997). Subtypes of aggression and their relevance to child psychiatry. *Journal of the American Academy of Child and Adolescent Psychiatry, 36,* 307–315.

Wahler, R. G. (1975). Some structural aspects of deviant child behavior. *Journal of Applied Behavior Analysis, 8,* 27–42.

Wahler, R. G. (1980). The insular mother: Her problems in parent–child treatment. *Journal of Applied Behavior Analysis, 13,* 207–219.

Wahler, R. G., & Afton, A. D. (1980). Attentional processes in insular and noninsular mothers. *Child Behavior Therapy, 2*(2), 25–41.

Wahler, R. G., Cartor, P. G., Fleischman, J., & Lambert, W. (1993). The impact of synthesis teaching and parent training with mothers of conduct-disordered children. *Journal of Abnormal Child Psychology, 21,* 425–440.

Wahler, R. G., & Cormier, W. H. (1970). The ecological interview: A first step in out-patient child behavior therapy. *Journal of Behavior Therapy and Experimental Psychiatry, 1,* 279–289.

Wahler, R. G., & Dumas, J. E. (1984). Changing the observational coding styles of insular and noninsular mothers: A step toward maintenance of parent training effects. In R. F. Dangel & R. A. Polster (Eds.), *Parent training: Foundations of research and practice* (pp. 379–416). New York: Guilford Press.

Wahler, R. G., & Dumas, J. E. (1989). Attentional problems in dysfunctional mother–child interactions: An interbehavioral model. *Psychological Bulletin, 105,* 116–130.

Wahler, R. G., Leske, G., & Rogers, E. S. (1979). The insular family: A deviance support system for oppositional children. In L. A. Hamerlynck (Ed.), *Behavioral systems for the developmentally disabled: Vol. 1. School and family environments* (pp. 102–127). New York: Brunner/Mazel.

Wahler, R. G., & Sansbury, L. E. (1990). The monitoring skills of troubled mothers: Their problems in defining child deviance. *Journal of Abnormal Child Psychology, 18,* 577–589.

Wakschlag, L. S., & Danis, B. (2004). Assessment of disruptive behaviors in young children: A clinical–developmental framework. In R. Del Carmen & A. Carter (Eds.), *Handbook of infant and toddler mental health assessment* (pp. 421–440). New York: Oxford University Press.

Wakschlag, L. S., & Keenan, K. (2001). Clinical significance and correlates of disruptive behavior in environmentally at-risk preschoolers. *Journal of Clinical Child Psychology, 30,* 262–275.

Waldman, I. D., & Lahey, B. B. (1994). Design of the DSM-IV disruptive behavior disorder field trials. *Child and Adolescent Psychiatric Clinics of North America, 3,* 195–208.

Walker, H. M. (1995). *The acting-out child: Coping with classroom disruption* (2nd ed.). Longmont, CO: Sopris West.

Walker, H. M., Block-Pedego, A., Todis, B., & Severson, H. (1991). *School Archival Records Search (SARS): User's guide and technical manual.* Longmont, CO: Sopris West.

Walker, H. M., & Buckley, N. K. (1972). Programming generalization and maintenance of treatment effects across time and across settings. *Journal of Applied Behavior Analysis, 5,* 209–224.

Walker, H. M., Colvin, G., & Ramsey, E. (1995). *Antisocial behavior in school: Strategies and best practices.* Pacific Grove, CA: Brooks/Cole.

Walker, H. M., Fonseca Retana, G., & Gersten, R. (1988). Replication of the CLASS program in Costa Rica: Implementation procedures and program outcomes. *Behavior Modification, 12,* 133–154.

Walker, H. M., & Hops, H. (1976). Use of normative peer data as a standard for evaluating classroom treatment effects. *Journal of Applied Behavior Analysis, 9,* 159–168.

Walker, H. M., & Hops, H. (1979). The CLASS program for acting out children: R&D procedures, program outcomes, and implementation issues. *School Psychology Digest, 8,* 370–381.

Walker, H. M., & Hops, H. (1993). *The RECESS program for aggressive children.* Seattle, WA: Educational Achievement Systems.

Walker, H. M., Hops, H., & Fiegenbaum, E. (1976). Deviant classroom behavior as a function of combinations of social and token reinforcement and cost contingency. *Behavior Therapy, 7,* 76–88.

Walker, H. M., Hops, H., & Greenwood, C. R. (1981). RECESS: Research and development of a behavior management package for remediating social aggression in the school setting. In P. S. Strain (Ed.), *The utilization of classroom peers as behavior change agents* (pp. 261–303). New York: Plenum Press.

Walker, H. M., Hops, H., & Greenwood, C. R. (1984). The CORBEH research and development model: Programmatic issues and strategies. In S. C. Paine, G. T. Bellamy, & B. Wilcox (Eds.), *Human services that work: From innovation to clinical practice* (pp. 57–77). Baltimore: Brookes.

Walker, H. M., Hops, H., & Greenwood, C. R. (1993). *RECESS: A program for reducing negative-aggressive behavior.* Seattle, WA: Educational Achievement Systems.

Walker, H. M., Hops, H., & Johnson, S. M. (1975). Generalization and maintenance of classroom treatment effects. *Behavior Therapy, 6,* 188–200.

Walker, H. M., Kavanagh, K., Stiller, B., Golly, A., Severson, H. H., & Feil, E. G. (1998). First Step to Success: An early intervention approach for preventing school antisocial behavior. *Journal of Emotional and Behavioral Disorders, 6,* 66–80.

Walker, H. M., Nishioka, V., Zeller, R., Severson, H., & Feil, E. (2000). Causal factors and potential solutions for the persistent under-identification of students having emotional or behavioral disorders in the context of schooling. *Assessment for Effective Intervention, 26,* 29–40.

Walker, H. M., Ramsey, E., & Gresham, F. M. (2004). *Antisocial behavior in school: Evidence-based practice.* Belmont, CA: Wadsworth/Thomas.

Walker, H. M., Shinn, M. R., O'Neill, R. E., & Ramsey, E. (1987). A longitudinal assessment of the development of antisocial behavior in boys: Rationale, methodology, and first-year results. *Remedial and Special Education, 8,* 7–16, 27.

Walker, H. M., & Walker, J. E. (1991). *Coping with noncompliance in the classroom: A positive approach for teachers.* Austin, TX: Pro-Ed.

Walker, J. L., Lahey, B. B., Russo, M. F., Frick, P. J., Christ, M. A., McBurnett, K., et al. (1991). Anxiety, inhibition, and conduct disorder in children: I. Relations to social impairment. *Journal of the American Academy of Child and Adolescent Psychiatry, 30,* 187–191.

Walter, H. I., & Gilmore, S. K. (1973). Placebo versus social learning effects in parent training procedures designed to alter the behavior of aggressive boys. *Behavior Therapy, 4,* 361–377.

Waschbusch, D. A. (2002). A meta-analytic examination of comorbid hyperactive–impulsive-attention problems and conduct problems. *Psychological Bulletin, 128,* 118–150.

Waschbusch, D. A., Willoughby, M. T., & Pelham, W. E. (1998). Criterion validity and the utility of reactive and proactive aggression: Comparisons to attention deficit hyperactivity disorder, oppositional defiant disorder, conduct disorder, and other measures of functioning. *Journal of Clinical Child Psychology, 27,* 396–405.

Waslick, B., Werry, J. S., & Greenhill, L. L. (1999). Pharmacology and toxicology of oppositional defiant disorder and conduct disorder. In H. C. Quay & A. E. Hogan (Eds.), *Handbook of disruptive behavior disorders* (pp. 455–474). New York: Kluwer Academic/Plenum.

Webster-Stratton, C. (1981). Modification of mothers' behaviors and attitudes through a videotape modeling group discussion program. *Behavior Therapy, 12,* 634–642.

Webster-Stratton, C. (1982a). The long-term effects of a videotape modeling parent-training program: Comparison of immediate and 1-year follow-up results. *Behavior Therapy, 13,* 702–714.

Webster-Stratton, C. (1982b). Teaching mothers through videotape modeling to change their chil-

dren's behavior. *Journal of Pediatric Psychology, 7,* 279–294.

Webster-Stratton, C. (1984). Randomized trial of two parent-training programs for families with conduct-disordered children. *Journal of Consulting and Clinical Psychology, 52,* 666–678.

Webster-Stratton, C. (1985a). The effects of father involvement in parent training for conduct problem children. *Journal of Child Psychology and Psychiatry, 26,* 801–810.

Webster-Stratton, C. (1985b). Predictors of treatment outcome in parent training for conduct-disordered children. *Behavior Therapy, 16,* 223–243.

Webster-Stratton, C. (1989). Systematic comparison of consumer satisfaction of three cost-effective parent training programs for conduct problem children. *Behavior Therapy, 20,* 103–115.

Webster-Stratton, C. (1990a). Long-term follow-up of families with young conduct problem children: From preschool to grade school. *Journal of Clinical Child Psychology, 19,* 144–149.

Webster-Stratton, C. (1990b). Stress: A potential disruptor of parent perceptions and family interactions. *Journal of Clinical Child Psychology, 19,* 302–312.

Webster-Stratton, C. (1994). Advancing videotape parent training: A comparison study. *Journal of Consulting and Clinical Psychology, 62,* 583–593.

Webster-Stratton, C. (1996). Early-onset conduct problems: Does gender make a difference? *Journal of Consulting and Clinical Psychology, 64,* 540–551.

Webster-Stratton, C. (1998). Preventing conduct problems in Head Start children: Strengthening parent competencies. *Journal of Consulting and Clinical Psychology, 66,* 715–730.

Webster-Stratton, C. (2000). *The Incredible Years Training Series bulletin.* Washington, DC: U.S. Department of Justice, Office of Justice Programs, Office of Juvenile Justice and Delinquency Prevention.

Webster-Stratton, C., & Hammond, M. (1990). Predictors of treatment outcome in parent training for families with conduct problem children. *Behavior Therapy, 21,* 319–337.

Webster-Stratton, C., & Hammond, M. (1997). Treating children with early-onset conduct problems: A comparison of child and parent training programs. *Journal of Consulting and Clinical Psychology, 65,* 93–109.

Webster-Stratton, C., & Herbert, M. (1993). "What really happens in parent training?" *Behavior Modification, 17,* 407–456.

Webster-Stratton, C., & Herbert, M. (1994). *Troubled families—problem children.* Chichester, UK: Wiley.

Webster-Stratton, C., Hollinsworth, T., & Kolpacoff, M. (1989). The long-term effectiveness and clinical significance of three cost-effective training programs for families with conduct-problem children. *Journal of Consulting and Clinical Psychology, 57,* 550–553.

Webster-Stratton, C., Kolpacoff, M., & Hollinsworth, T. (1988). Self-administered videotape therapy for families with conduct problem children: Comparison to two other cost effective treatments and a control group. *Journal of Consulting and Clinical Psychology, 56,* 558–566.

Webster-Stratton, C., & Reid, M. J. (2003). The Incredible Years parents, teachers and children training series: A multifaceted treatment approach for young children with conduct problems. In A. E. Kazdin & J. R. Weisz (Eds.), *Evidence-based psychotherapies for children and adolescents* (pp. 224–241). New York: Guilford Press.

Webster-Stratton, C., Reid, M. J., & Hammond, M. (2001a). Preventing conduct problems, promoting social competence: A parent and teacher training partnership in Head Start. *Journal of Clinical Child Psychology, 30,* 238–302.

Webster-Stratton, C., Reid, M. J., & Hammond, M. (2001b). Social skills and problem solving training for children with early-onset conduct problems: Who benefits? *Journal of Child Psychology and Psychiatry, 42,* 943–952.

Webster-Stratton, C., Reid, M. J., & Hammond, M. (2004). Treating children with early-onset conduct problems: Intervention outcomes for parent, child, and teacher training. *Journal of Clinical Child and Adolescent Psychology, 33,* 105–124.

Webster-Stratton, C., & Spitzer, A. (1996). Parenting a young child with conduct problems: New insights using qualitative methods. In T. H. Ollendick & R. J. Prinz (Eds.), *Advances in clinical child psychology* (Vol. 18, pp. 1–62). New York: Plenum Press.

Webster-Stratton, C., & Taylor, T. (2001). Nipping early risk factors in the bud: Preventing substance abuse, delinquency, and violence in adolescence through interventions targeted at young children (0–8 years). *Prevention Science, 2,* 165–192.

Weersing, V. R., & Weisz, J. R. (2002). Mechanisms of action in youth psychotherapy. *Journal of Child Psychology and Psychiatry, 43,* 3–29.

Weinrott, M. R., Bauske, B. W., & Patterson, G. R. (1979). Systematic replication of a social learning approach to parent training. In P. O. Sjoden (Ed.), *Trends in behavior therapy* (pp. 331–351). New York: Academic Press.

Weinrott, M. R., Jones, R. R., & Howard, J. R. (1982). Cost-effectiveness of teaching family programs for delinquents: Results of a national evaluation. *Evaluation Review, 6,* 173–201.

Weiss, B., Dodge, K. A., Bates, J. E., & Pettit, G. S. (1992). Some consequences of early harsh discipline: Child aggression and a maladaptive social information processing style. *Child Development, 63,* 1321–1335.

Wells, K. C. (1985). Behavioral family therapy. In A. S. Bellack & M. Hersen (Eds.), *Dictionary of behavior therapy techniques* (pp. 25–30). New York: Pergamon Press.

Wells, K. C., & Egan, J. (1988). Social learning and systems family therapy for childhood oppositional disorder: Comparative treatment outcome. *Comprehensive Psychiatry, 29,* 138–146.

Wells, K. C., Forehand, R., & Griest, D. L. (1980). Generality of treatment effects from treated to untreated behaviors resulting from a parent training program. *Journal of Clinical Child Psychology, 9,* 217–219.

Wells, K. C., Griest, D. L., & Forehand, R. (1980). The use of a self-control package to enhance temporal generality of a parent training program. *Behaviour Research and Therapy, 18,* 347–358.

Werry, J. S., & Aman, M. G. (1993). *Practitioner's guide to psychoactive drugs for children and adolescents.* New York: Plenum Press.

Whipple, E. F., Fitzgerald, H. E., & Zucker, R. A. (1995). Parent–child interactions in alcoholic and nonalcoholic families. *American Journal of Orthopsychiatry, 65,* 153–159.

White, J. L., Moffitt, T. E., Caspi, A., Bartusch, D. J., Needles, D., & Stouthamer-Loeber, M. (1994). Measuring impulsivity and examining its relationship to delinquency. *Journal of Abnormal Psychology, 103,* 1922–1205.

White, M. (1986). Negative explanation, restraint and double description: A template for family therapy. *Family Process, 25,* 169–184.

White, M. A. (1975). Natural rates of teacher approval and disapproval in the classroom. *Journal of Applied Behavior Analysis, 8,* 367–372.

Wiesner, M. (2003). A longitudinal latent variable analysis of reciprocal relations between depressive symptoms and delinquency during adolescence. *Journal of Abnormal Psychology, 112,* 633–645.

Wilcox, D. K., & Kolko, D. J. (2002). Assessing recent firesetting behavior and taking a firesetting history. In D. J. Kolko (Ed.), *Handbook on firesetting in children and youth* (pp. 161–175). San Diego, CA: Academic Press.

Willner, A. G., Braukmann, C. J., Kirigin, K. A., & Wolf, M. M. (1978). Achievement Place: A community model for youths in trouble. In D. Marholin (Ed.), *Child behavior therapy* (pp. 239–273). New York: Gardner Press.

Willner, A. G., Braukmann, C. J., Kirigin, K. A., Fixsen, D. L., Phillips, E. L., & Wolf, M. M. (1977). The training and validation of youth-preferred social behaviors with child care personnel. *Journal of Applied Behavior Analysis, 10,* 219–230.

Willoughby, M., Kupersmidt, J., & Bryant, D. (2001). Overt and covert dimensions of antisocial behavior in early childhood. *Journal of Abnormal Child Psychology, 29,* 177–187.

Wills, T. A., Schreibman, D., Benson, G., & Vaccaro, D. (1994). Impact of parental substance use on adolescents: A test of a mediational model. *Journal of Pediatric Psychology, 19,* 537–555.

Wilson, S. J., Lipsey, M. W., & Soydan, H. (2003). Are mainstream programs for juvenile delinquency less effective with minority youth than majority youth?: A meta-analysis of outcomes research. *Research on Social Work Practice, 13,* 3–26.

Wiltz, N. A., & Patterson, G. R. (1974). An evaluation of parent training procedures designed to alter inappropriate aggressive behavior of boys. *Behavior Therapy, 5,* 215–221.

Winett, R. A., & Winkler, R. C. (1972). Current behavior modification in the classroom: Be still, be quiet, be docile. *Journal of Applied Behavior Analysis, 5,* 499–504.

Witt, J. C., Martens, B. K., & Elliott, S. N. (1984). Factors affecting teachers' judgments of the acceptability of behavioral interventions: Time involvement, behavior problem severity, and type of intervention. *Behavior Therapy, 15,* 204–209.

Wolf, M. M., Braukmann, C. J., & Kirigin Ramp, K. A. (1987). Serious delinquent behavior as part of a significantly handicapping condition: Cures and supportive environments. *Journal of Applied Behavior Analysis, 20,* 347–359.

Wong, S., & Hare, R. D. (2005). *Guidelines for a psychopathy treatment program.* Toronto: Multi-Health Systems.

Woodward, L. J., Fergusson, D. M., & Horwood, L. J. (2002). Romantic relationships of young people with early and late onset antisocial behavior problems. *Journal of Abnormal Child Psychology, 30,* 231–243.

Wootton, J. M., Frick, P. J., Shelton, K. K., & Silverthorn, P. (1997). Ineffective parenting and childhood conduct problems: The moderating role of callous–unemotional traits. *Journal of Consulting and Clinical Psychology, 65,* 301–308.

Yoshikawa, H. (1994). Prevention as a cumulative protection: Effects of early family support and education on chronic delinquency and its risks. *Psychological Bulletin, 115,* 28–54.

Zigler, E., Taussig, C., & Black, K. (1992). Early childhood intervention: A promising preventative for juvenile delinquency. *American Psychologist, 47,* 997–1006.

Zoccolillo, M. (1992). Co-occurrence of conduct disorder and its adult outcomes with depressive and anxiety disorders: A review. *Journal of the American Academy of Child and Adolescent Psychiatry, 31,* 547–556.

Zoccolillo, M., Paquette, D., & Tremblay, R. (2005). Maternal conduct disorder and the risk for the next generation. In D. J. Pepler, K. C. Madsen, C. Webster, & K. S. Levene (Eds.), *The development and treatment of girlhood aggression* (pp. 217–221). Mahwah, NJ: Erlbaum.

Zubieta, J., & Alessi, N. (1992). Acute and chronic administration of trazodone in the treatment of disruptive behavior disorders in children. *Journal of Clinical Psychopharmacology, 12,* 346–351.

Zubrick, S. R., Northey, K., Silburn, S. R., Lawrence, D., Williams, A. A., Blair, E., et al. (in press). Prevention of child behavioral problems through universal implementation of a group behavioral family intervention. *Prevention Science.*

Zucker, R. A., & Fitzgerald, H. E. (1992). *The Antisocial Behavior Checklist.* (Available from Michigan State University Family Study, Department of Psychology, East Lansing, MI 48824-1117)

III

EMOTIONAL AND SOCIAL DISORDERS

4

Fears and Anxieties

Bruce F. Chorpita and Michael A. Southam-Gerow

Problems related to fears and anxiety in youths are relatively common, with lifetime prevalence rates of clinical disorders ranging from 6% to 15% in epidemiological studies (e.g., Anderson, 1994; Bernstein & Borchardt, 1991; Fergusson, Horwood, & Lynskey, 1993; Silverman & Ginsburg, 1998; U.S. Department of Health and Human Services, 1999). Youths with anxiety problems experience significant and often lasting psychosocial impairments, such as poor school performance, social problems, and familial conflict (e.g., Bell-Dolan & Wessler, 1994; Kendall et al., 1992; Langley, Bergman, McCracken, & Piacentini, 2004; Silverman & Ginsburg, 1998). The co-occurrence of these problems with disruptive behavior problems, depression, or additional anxiety disorders is also quite high, with rates of co-occurrence ranging up to 65% in epidemiological samples (Bird, Gould, & Staghezza, 1993; Fergusson et al., 1993; Zoccolillo, 1992) and up to 84% in clinic samples (e.g., Albano, Chorpita, & Barlow, 2003; Keller et al., 1992; Kendall et al., 1997; Southam-Gerow, Weisz, & Kendall, 2003). Thus the problems found in these youths are typically rather substantial (e.g., Costello, Angold, & Keeler, 1999; Pine, Cohen, Gurley, Brook, & Ma, 1998).

ABOUT FEARS AND ANXIETIES

Overview of Theories

Scientific efforts to understand how and why anxiety becomes problematic can be traced to the beginning of modern psychology. In fact, one focus of Freud's early work was on anxiety in children (e.g., Freud, 1909/1955). Although psychoanalytic and psychodynamic theories of anxiety continue to be elaborated (e.g., Gillett, 2001), the current evidence-based therapies for childhood anxiety are largely based in the behavioral and cognitive theoretical traditions. A comprehensive review of these early theories of anxiety is beyond the scope of this chapter, and the interested reader is referred to recent books on the topic (e.g., Barlow, 2002; Craske, 1999). In this section, we briefly describe the major theories that have influenced the psychological science of anxiety disorders in children and adolescents.

The earliest efforts by behaviorists involved classical conditioning explanations (e.g., Eysenck, 1979; Marks, 1969; Pavlov, 1927; Watson & Morgan, 1917; Watson & Rayner, 1920; Wolpe & Rowan, 1988) and focused on fear induction. One of the most influential early efforts involved the case study of a 3-year-old boy, in which Jones (1924a) demonstrated the successful behavioral treatment of his fear of rabbits. Jones (1924b) thus argued that fear responding can be both learned and unlearned through behavioral means.

Although early research supported this mechanism of fear acquisition, the shortcomings of conditioning theory were outlined by Rachman (1977) and included the recurrent finding that fears could not be reliably established for all stimuli, despite the "proper" circumstances for fear induction. In response to the failings of early respondent conditioning theory, Rachman (1977, 1990, 1991) proposed at least three pathways for fear acquisition: (1) conditioning, (2) vicarious exposures/modeling, and (3) verbal instruction. Psychological scientists continue to pursue all three pathways.

In a related line of theory, several researchers have developed a model based on an evolutionary perspective to explain acquisition of certain fears, called "preparedness" (e.g., Öhman & Mineka, 2001; Seligman, 1970, 1971). Proponents of this perspective posit that certain stimuli possess evolutionary significance by virtue of the long-standing danger they presented to a species. As a result, fear of these stimuli is easily acquired and is resistant to change once established. Fear of stimuli without evolutionary significance can also be established, but not as rapidly. Despite decades of research on preparedness, the theory remains controversial (e.g., McNally, 1987; Öhman & Mineka, 2001), perhaps in part because the theory itself is not directly testable (i.e., it is not possible to determine whether the fears are based in the evolutionary past of the species; e.g., Lovibond, Siddle, & Bond, 1993; McNally, 1987; McNally & Foa, 1986). Öhman and Mineka (2001) have recently updated the theory, suggesting that preparedness is a result of evolutionarily shaped fear modules that are composed of cognitive, behavioral, and neural components. According to work by Öhman and Mineka (e.g., Mineka & Ohman, 2002; Öhman & Mineka, 2001), a fear module demonstrates several characteristics, including (1) input selectivity (i.e., a small, specific set of stimuli can activate the module); (2) automaticity (i.e., the module is activated without higher cognitive involvement); (3) encapsulation from higher cognitive functions (i.e., the acquisition of fear is largely independent of "rational" evaluation of the fear value of the stimuli); and (4) specific neural circuitry (i.e., specific centers of the brain are "designed" for the activation of the fear module). New research will continue to clarify the relevance of the theory.

Another prominent behavioral theory has been two-factor theory (e.g., Mowrer, 1939, 1947, 1960), in which fear is acquired via classical conditioning and maintained by instrumental conditioning. In other words, a stimulus is paired with an unpleasant response (classical conditioning), leading to a fear response. Future exposure to the feared stimulus is avoided, thus leading to a decrease in the fear response. As a result, the avoidance behavior is reinforced, and the fear is strengthened. The theory has considerable intuitive appeal and has had an important influence on treatment development. However, the theory has had a controversial history; indeed, many writers have declared the theory "dead" (e.g., Barrios & O'Dell, 1998; Delprato & McGlynn, 1984). In defending the obituary, researchers point to several lines of research that have questioned the necessity of the link between fear and avoidance. For example, evidence reviewed by Delprato and McGlynn (1984) from human and animal research indicates that avoidance is not extinguished when the feared stimulus no longer provokes fear. Furthermore, avoidance can be acquired without an antecedent. In the theory, avoidance is the conditioned response to some conditioned stimulus. However, laboratory studies have demonstrated that avoidance behavior is exhibited in the absence of a conditioned stimulus (e.g., D'Amato, 1970; Delprato & McGlynn, 1984). Despite these problems, some still champion two-factor theory and have amassed some supportive evidence that attempts to respond to the criticisms of the theory (e.g., Levis & Brewer, 2001). Despite this effort, two-factor theory no longer dominates the theoretical landscape of anxiety as it did a generation ago.

A third model, approach–withdrawal theory, was advanced as an effort to address some of the identified shortcomings of two-factor theory (e.g., Delprato & McGlynn, 1984). The basic contribution of approach–withdrawal theory is the contention that avoidance behavior is maintained by positive and not negative reinforcement. When confronted by a feared stimulus, an organism avoids or withdraws from the stimulus. Avoidance (including the location and associated stimuli) leads to an increase in relaxation; as a result, approach behavior to the avoidance location is positively reinforced. The approach–withdrawal theory explains why avoidance is maintained despite a decrease in or even the absence of anxiety. Furthermore, the theory also offers a conceptual rationale for the use of contingency management approaches for treatment of anxiety in children (e.g., Barrios & O'Dell, 1998; Silverman & Kurtines, 1996). As an example, children who avoid going to school may be positively reinforced in the home environment by attention from their parents and by permission to watch TV or play video games. These positive reinforcers strengthen and maintain the avoidance behavior. Thus treatment strategies aim at reworking the contingencies so that avoidance behavior is punished (or at least not reinforced), and certain approach behaviors (going to school, in the example above) are reinforced.

Social learning theory has also been influential in the area of anxiety disorders, especially concerning treatment. Bandura's (1977, 1986) formulations suggested that fears can be acquired not only through direct conditioning, but also through observation. Thus the basis of some fears and anxieties may involve modeled or vicariously learned, but not directly experienced, contingencies. This supposition has been borne out by empirical evidence with animals (most famously, rhesus monkeys) and with humans (e.g., Bandura, 1969; Zinbarg & Mineka, 2001). Several theories have been forwarded to explain the process by which modeling leads to behavior change in the observer; a review of these theories is beyond the scope of this chapter, and readers are referred to classic analyses of this by Bandura (1969, 1977). This line of thought has produced one of the most widely tested treatment procedures for anxiety—modeling, which we discuss in detail below. The theory has also been used in developing psychoeducational information for families of anxious children. Along these lines, some of the family-involved cognitive-behavioral therapy (CBT) approaches we discuss later emphasize the importance of children's learning about anxiety (and how to cope with it) by observing familial interactions and hearing parental stories.

Recent advances in cognitive theory and research have introduced a variety of concepts with a profound influence on treatments for youths with fears and anxieties. Many different cognitive processes have been studied as related to anxious and fearful behavior, including attributions, expectations, misperceptions, attentional biases, and problem-solving abilities (e.g., Cole, Martin, Peeke, Seroczynski, & Fier, 1999; Dalgleish et al., 2003; Lochman & Wells, 2002; Suarez & Bell-Dolan, 2001; Vasey, 1993). Again, a thorough review of this ample literature is beyond the scope of this chapter; however, we provide a brief overview of some of the major lines of theory in this area.

One of the earliest and most influential of these theories is Bandura's self-efficacy theory. Bandura (e.g., 1978, 1982) postulates that fear

and anxiety are directly linked to expectations of one's efficacy to confront a feared object or situation. This cognitive construct of "self-efficacy" arises from a variety of experiences with the feared stimulus, including direct experiences, vicarious experiences, and verbal persuasion. Although many current cognitive perspectives draw on aspects of this theory as a base, self-efficacy has been challenged by behavior theorists as merely being one factor of a more general "outcome expectancy." Such counterarguments thus posit that the self-efficacy concept has no unique explanatory power over existing behavioral constructs (see Biglan, 1987; Eastman & Marzillier, 1984; Lee, 1989).

Building on the work of Beck and others (e.g., Beck & Emery with Greenberg, 1985), Kendall (e.g., Kendall & MacDonald, 1993; Kendall, Stark, & Adam, 1990) has emphasized the relevance of cognitive "distortions," defined as negatively skewed misinterpretations of social and interoceptive information (Chorpita, Albano, & Barlow, 1996; Vasey, Daleiden, Williams, & Brown, 1995). Negative attributional style has also been associated with anxiety disorders in youths (Bell-Dolan, 1995; Bell-Dolan & Wessler, 1994). However, the association may not be specific to anxiety disorders, because attributional style has been related to other forms of child psychopathology as well (e.g., depression; Gladstone & Kaslow, 1995). "Anxiety sensitivity" (McNally & Reiss, 1985) refers to the extent to which individuals believe that their own anxiety or anxiety-related sensations have harmful consequences, and this is another factor that has been studied as a risk factor for anxiety disorders; however, a review of the literature by Silverman and Weems (1999) leaves the specificity of the findings in question. For example, Rabian, Peterson, Richters, and Jensen (1993) found that although anxiety sensitivity was useful in discriminating youths with anxiety disorders from nondisordered youths, it did not discriminate youths with behavior disorders from those with anxiety disorders (cf. Chorpita & Lilienfeld, 1999). Yet another line of literature has examined the role of attentional bias in anxious youths (e.g., Vasey et al., 1995), showing that youths with clinically elevated anxiety have a tendency to attend to threatening stimuli (Vasey & McLeod, 2001). Another influential information-processing theory is Lang's (1977, 1979) bioinformational conceptualization of anxiety, and particularly the important later work by Foa and Kozak (1986) in applying the model to exposure treatment. In the bioinformational model, there are three components of the memory networks related to fear: (1) information about the feared stimulus; (2) the fear-related responses (behavioral, physiological, and verbal); and (3) the organism's interpretations of the stimulus and response. When conceptualized in this way, the fear-related response components comprise an escape/avoidance program; that is, when the fear memory network is activated, the organism is likely to engage in escape/avoidance behaviors. Foa and Kozak suggested that "pathological [fear] structures involve excessive response elements (e.g., avoidance, physiological activity, etc.) and resistance to modification" (p. 21). Treatment, then, involves evocation of the memory network and the provision of information contrary to information already in the memory network, so that the memory network is "updated" or modified (Foa & Kozak, 1986). Hence exposure therapy would be the critical component in applications of this model, and the exposures would need to be at a sufficient intensity to induce the fear memory. Furthermore, the implied treatment approach would involve reinterpretation or "reprocessing" of information concerning the feared stimuli.

Other work has implicated cognitive-related deficiencies in youths with anxiety, including such problems as deficits in self-control, emotion understanding, and problem solving. Preliminary support of the notion that anxious youths have emotion-processing deficits has been offered by Southam-Gerow and Kendall (2000), who found that youths with anxiety disorders have deficits in their understanding of emotion regulation (i.e., how to hide and change feelings) compared with non-clinic-referred youths. There is also considerable empirical support for the notion that youths with anxiety disorders also exhibit problem-solving deficits. For example, two studies have found that anxious youths tend to generate avoidant solutions to hypothetical situations (Barrett, Dadds, & Rapee, 1996; Chorpita, Albano, & Barlow, 1996). Strengthening these conclusions is some evidence that the bias in problem solving is specific to youths with anxiety disorders, relative to aggressive and nonreferred youths (Barrett et al., 1996). These areas of cognitive deficits all have implications for treatment

that many of the treatments we discuss have incorporated—specifically, in the form of skills training modules for multicomponent CBT approaches.

Clinical Dimensions of Fear and Anxiety

Although the chapter title "Fears and Anxieties" might imply that only two constructs are of primary importance, in fact clinical fears and anxieties appear to be organized along a number of different dimensions. The *Diagnostic and Statistical Manual of Mental Disorders*, fourth edition, text revision (DSM-IV-TR; American Psychiatric Association, 2000) outlines nine principal anxiety disorders: panic disorder, agoraphobia, generalized anxiety disorder (GAD), social phobia, specific phobia, obsessive–compulsive disorder (OCD), posttraumatic stress disorder (PTSD), separation anxiety disorder (SAD), and acute stress disorder. (Although the manual places SAD in the section titled "Disorders Usually First Diagnosed in Infancy, Childhood, or Adolescence" rather than in the "Anxiety Disorders" section, it clearly warrants inclusion with the others here.) Characteristics of the most common of these clinical syndromes in youths are outlined in Table 4.1.

Although the DSM-IV-TR represents an important collection of clinical and empirical knowledge, the validity of clinical syndromes is perhaps best corroborated through statistical analysis (Anastasi & Urbina, 1997). Historically, however, statistical and diagnostic approaches to child psychopathology have not always converged (e.g., Achenbach & Rescorla, 2001), with most statistical models yielding a few general factors related to anxiety and/or depression (e.g., "somatic complaints," "overanxiousness," "concentration problems"), without uniform convergence with DSM syndromes (e.g., Achenbach & Rescorla, 2001; March, Parker, Sullivan, Stallings, & Conners, 1997; Reynolds & Richmond, 1978).

Nevertheless, some recent empirical approaches to assessment have yielded support for the general diagnostic syndromes outlined in the DSM-IV and DSM-IV-TR. Foremost among these is the work of Spence (1998), who designed a self-report measure with items to be consistent with the anxiety disorders as defined by the DSM. Using confirmatory factor analysis, Spence (1997) found support for a six-factor model of anxiety, encompassing the fac-

TABLE 4.1. Selected Anxiety Disorders from the DSM-IV-TR

Separation anxiety disorder (SAD)[a]

SAD is characterized by age-inappropriate anxiety about being separated from a caregiver. It often involves a fear of something threatening happening to oneself or to the caretaker during separation. SAD is more common among younger children (i.e., 12 and under; Albano et al., 2003).

Generalized anxiety disorder (GAD)

GAD is characterized by excessive and uncontrollable worry and associated feelings of tension or restlessness. GAD is common across all ages of children and can involve concerns about family, friends, grades, or things in general. It is important to ensure that the anxiety and worry exhibited by the child are in fact excessive and out of proportion to the situation. For example, a young boy with an abusive father who worries constantly about his mother's and his own safety is demonstrating an appropriate level of anxiety.

Social phobia

Social phobia is characterized by excessive and disabling fear of social or evaluative situations. Although social phobia usually involves a moderate number of social fears, at the extremes it can be discrete, involving only a single feared situation (e.g., giving a speech), or generalized, involving almost all aspects of social functioning. Social phobia is more common among adolescents.

Specific phobia

Specific phobia is characterized by excessive and disabling fear of an object or situation. Phobias can be organized into a number of basic areas: animal (e.g., dogs), natural/environmental (e.g., swimming), situational (e.g., crowds), blood/injury/injection (e.g., getting a shot), and other (e.g., fear of choking on food). Specific phobia is more common among younger children.

Obsessive–compulsive disorder (OCD)

OCD is characterized by repetitive, unwanted thoughts or images, often accompanied by rituals performed to reduce or neutralize the anxious thoughts. OCD is common among children of all ages and can involve a great diversity of fears and obsessions.

Panic disorder

Panic disorder is characterized by sudden feelings of intense fear that can seem to come out of the blue. It is sometimes accompanied by agoraphobia, or the avoidance of places that might trigger feelings of anxiety. Panic disorder is less common in younger children. Panic disorder involves a cycle in which a sensation of anxiety (e.g., fast heartbeat) leads the child to feel as if an attack might begin; this is followed by an escalation of anxiety, which intensifies the sensations, further escalating the anxiety, and so forth until the anxiety spirals out of control.

Posttraumatic stress disorder (PTSD)

PTSD is characterized by frightening thoughts, emotional disturbance, and persistent increased arousal resulting from exposure to a traumatic event or events.

[a]The DSM-IV-TR actually places SAD in its section on "Disorders Usually First Diagnosed in Infancy, Childhood, or Adolescence" rather than in its "Anxiety Disorders" section, but it is included here because of its obvious importance as an anxiety disorder in youngsters.

tors of panic–agoraphobia, social phobia, separation anxiety, obsessive–compulsive problems, generalized anxiety, and fear of physical injury. Evidence for the existence of these factors garnered support for the assumption implicit in DSM-IV that specific subtypes of anxiety disorders can be identified and measured in children (Birmaher et al., 1997; Spence, 1997; Spence, Barrett, & Turner, 2003). These results were replicated in later research using a revised item pool, even more closely indexing constructs as outlined in the DSM-IV (e.g., GAD) and the DSM factors have been confirmed in four additional studies in both clinical and nonclinical samples (Chorpita, Moffitt, & Gray, 2005; Chorpita, Yim, Moffitt, Umemoto, & Francis, 2000; deRoss, Chorpita, & Gullone, 2002). Thus, although the core constructs of fear and anxiety are very important from a theoretical perspective, it is clear that these constructs tend to manifest themselves clinically in terms of various specific dimensions or syndromes. The relations of these clinical dimensions to the broader constructs of fear and anxiety are not entirely straightforward, but contemporary models have emerged that have attempted to articulate these relations in some detail, and these are briefly reviewed below.

Integrative Theories

Gray's Model

Contemporary theories that have attempted to integrate the diversity of findings regarding clinical syndromes, anxious emotion, cognition, affect, and behavior (e.g., Barlow, 2002; Barlow, Chorpita, & Turovsky, 1996; Vasey & Dadds, 2001) often build on the important laboratory work of Gray (1982, 1987; Gray & McNaughton, 1996). At the heart of Gray's model (e.g., Gray, 1982) is a functional brain system that he termed the "behavioral inhibition system" (BIS), involving the septal area, the hippocampus, and the Papez circuit, as well as the neocortical inputs to the septo-hippocampal system, dopaminergic ascending input to the prefrontal cortex, cholinergic ascending input to the septo-hippocampal system, noradrenergic input to the hypothalamus, and the descending noradrenergic fibers of the locus coeruleus (Gray, 1982). According to Gray (1982), the BIS is activated by three classes of inputs: (1) signals for punishment; (2) signals for nonreward (i.e., signals that an expected reward is not going to be delivered); and (3) novelty. The primary, short-term outputs of the BIS involve (1) narrowing of attention; (2) inhibition of gross motor behavior; (3) increased stimulus analysis (e.g., vigilance or scanning); (4) increased central nervous system arousal (e.g., alertness); and (5) priming of hypothalamic motor systems for possible rapid action that may be required (i.e., possible activation of the fight–flight system [FFS]). According to Gray, anxiety is defined as activity of the BIS.

Inputs to the BIS are controlled by what Brooks (1986) and Gray and McNaughton (1996) called the "comparator subsystem." The comparator analyzes information from a number of sources and, based on these analyses, regulates BIS activity. Principally, the information involves (1) the current observed state of the world; (2) the next planned step in the organism's motor program; (3) stored reg-

ularities about the world (stimulus–stimulus associations as determined by Pavlovian conditioning); and (4) stored regularities about the behavior–outcome relations (stimulus–behavior–stimulus associations as determined by instrumental conditioning; see Figure 4.1). According to Gray and McNaughton, the comparator "has the task of predicting the next sensory event to which the animal will be exposed and checking whether it actually does occur; of operating the outputs of the BIS either if there is a mismatch between the actual and predicted events or if the predicted event is aversive; and of testing out alternative strategies . . . which may overcome the difficulty with which the animal is faced" (p. 75).

Gray's model serves as a useful basis for integrating behavioral, biological, cognitive, and emotional literatures, given that the model clearly specifies a role for behavioral inputs and outputs, their biological underpinnings, the influence of stored information (cf. cognition), and the associated experiences of emotion. For example, BIS activity is very much a function of the stored regularities associated

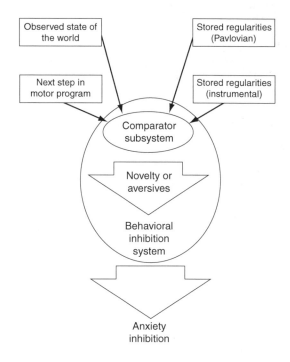

FIGURE 4.1. Activity of the comparator subsystem, which controls inputs to the behavioral inhibition system (BIS) and therefore influences anxiety inhibition.

with conditioning history (i.e., experience), which may be largely established during early development. In more cognitive language, one could use the term "schemas" to describe these information banks of inferred laws about the operations and events in the world (e.g., Beck, Rush, Shaw, & Emery, 1979; Beck et al., 1985). Regardless of their name, these schemas, stored regularities, or records of experience are accessed by the comparator 5–10 times per second, in a constant cycle quantized by the rhythmic theta activity of the hippocampus. The interchange of observed stimuli, stored information, and behavioral outputs is thus tightly organized in the operation of the BIS.

This model bridges some of the existing broad theories related to the development of anxiety (Barlow, 2001; Chorpita, 2001). For example, Kagan's classic work proposed that "behavioral inhibition" (named independently from Gray's model) is a temperamental variable related to a physiological and psychological state of uncertainty, evoked by exposure to unfamiliar objects, people, or stressful situations (Kagan, 1997). Kagan, Snidman, Arcus, and Reznick (1994) showed in two longitudinal cohorts that infants with particular physiological markers for inhibition (e.g., high heart rate, low heart rate variability) were more likely to demonstrate inhibited behavior over the course of development.

A potentially unifying feature of this model involves the role of perceived control in the development and maintenance of anxiety. Chorpita and Barlow (1998) have articulated how the perception of low control at any given time can increase the flow of information along pathways to the comparator subsystem that increase BIS activity. Through increasing or decreasing the probability of accessing relevant information and learning history, perceptions of control over events can stimulate the BIS, thus producing anxiety. Examples of this phenomenon are highly common (Geer, Davison, & Gatchel, 1970; Sanderson, Rapee, & Barlow, 1989). Thus the connection is clear between Gray's BIS activity and Kagan's characterization of inhibition as involving a state of uncertainty. Chorpita and Barlow (1998) have gone on to argue that a history of experience with control has important developmental implications for future experience of anxiety, such that experience with low control can predispose heightened BIS activity later in life. The implications of this notion for intervention are noteworthy, particularly in regard to the role of parenting in encouraging or discouraging experiences with control.

In terms of emotional phenomenology, it is important to note that BIS activity is distinct from some traditional notions of anxiety, in that it does not inherently involve peripheral physiological arousal (e.g., rapid heartbeat, dry mouth). Rather, its phenomenology is mainly characterized by increased caution, vigilance, and processing of threat-relevant information. For this reason, the BIS has sometimes been referred to as the "stop, look, and listen" system (Gray, 1987). In contrast, the FFS is the brain system postulated to underlie the rapid activation of bodily systems designed for engagement with threat or danger. Termed "panic" by Gray, and "fear" by Barlow (1988), this emotion involves such symptoms as rapid heartbeat, dry mouth, dizziness, sweating, and shakiness, among others. Thus, as we return to addressing the title of this chapter, "fear" and "anxiety" are considered two primary, separate, but related types of emotions in the context of this theory. How these two dimensions are related to the clinical syndromes described above is an area to which we now turn.

Integrating the Network of Constructs

The constructs that underlie the operations of fear and anxiety, and their relations to the clinical syndromes introduced above, have become increasingly well understood over the last 15 years. For example, the outputs of the FFS and BIS (i.e., "fear" and "anxiety") are consistent with a number of constructs related to vulnerability for anxiety disorders and depressive disorders from other literatures (Barlow et al., 1996; Brown, Chorpita, & Barlow, 1998; Clark & Watson, 1991; Gray & McNaughton, 1996). Of considerable importance among these literatures, Clark and Watson's (1991) tripartite model of emotion specifies a general factor, negative affect (NA), representing a shared influence on anxiety and depression. It further describes two specific factors: physiological hyperarousal (PH), common to anxiety, and (low) positive affect (PA), common to depression (Clark & Watson, 1991). Initially proposed to account for the high comorbidity of depressive and anxiety disorders and symptoms (Clark, 1989), the tripartite model has become increasingly well specified and has found accumulating empirical support within adult and child samples (e.g., Brown et al., 1998; Chorpita, Albano, & Barlow, 1998; Chorpita & Daleiden, 2002; Joiner, Catanzaro, & Laurent, 1996; Lonigan, Hooe, David, & Kistner, 1999).

The tripartite model has a number of important implications with respect to the understanding of pathological fear and anxiety. Clark, Watson, and Mineka (1994) have described NA as a "stable, highly heritable general trait dimension with a multiplicity of aspects ranging from mood to behavior" (p. 104). Thus NA may be of considerable value in predicting the future emergence of anxious pathology. Furthermore, the model allows for an improved understanding of comorbidity among disorders of emotion, because it offers a theoretical basis for the high co-occurrence of anxiety and depression in children as well as adults. In addition, increased understanding of the core dimensions of affect and arousal related to anxiety disorders offers the possibility for an improved understanding of the nosology for classifying these syndromes. For example, knowledge about whether GAD in children is characterized primarily by negative emotionality or by autonomic arousal has important implications for articulating the key features of that disorder within a diagnostic framework. Finally, recent tests of the model in the context of dimensions of anxiety and depressive disorders have revealed the benefit of moving beyond a single-order assessment strategy to a hierarchical one (Chorpita, 2001). That is, it appears important to assess not only the symptoms of particular

disorders or syndromes, but also the core affective and arousal dimensions related to those syndromes. In this way, the degree to which the symptoms are related to general features of temperament or physiology—which has implications for course, chronicity, and emerging comorbidity—can be determined. This is consistent with the notion of "heterotypic continuity," whereby the symptomatic expression of an underlying, temporally stable pathology differs over the course of development (e.g., Caspi, Elder, & Bem, 1988).

In Clark and Watson's (1991) tripartite model, the construct of negative affectivity bears a notable similarity to Gray's BIS outputs. However, a difficult matter of terminology exists here: Gray (1982, 1987) called these BIS outputs "anxiety," whereas Clark and Watson considered "anxiety" to involve both NA and PH (activity of the autonomic nervous system). As noted above, BIS output (i.e., anxiety) does not explicitly involve autonomic arousal.

A collection of recent research has subsequently outlined the relation between the constructs of NA and PH (cf. BIS and FFS activity), and has resolved the issues of terminology to some degree as well (Brown et al., 1998; Chorpita, 2001; Chorpita, Albano, & Barlow, 1998; Chorpita, Plummer, & Moffitt, 2000; Joiner et al., 1996; Lonigan et al., 1998). Figure 4.2 shows the basic relations identified in children between the dimensions outlined in the DSM-IV-TR and the broader constructs of NA and PH. This general model has been confirmed in four studies in children and adolescents in both clinical and nonclinical samples,

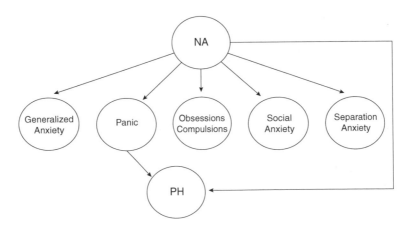

FIGURE 4.2. The relations identified in youths between the primary dimensions of anxiety described in the DSM-IV-TR and the constructs of negative affect (NA) and physiological hyperarousal (PH).

and suggests that NA serves as a risk factor for all of the anxiety syndromes, whereas PH is related only to particular dimensions (Brown et al., 1998). Similar results from an adult clinical sample warranted the reformulation of the tripartite model (Mineka, Watson, & Clark, 1998) to state that PH is not uniformly associated with anxiety; rather, it is associated with particular anxiety syndromes and not with others (Brown et al., 1998).

This integration of the literature on PH and NA, or more generally fear and anxiety, with the diagnostic syndromes also serves to explain the historical divergence of the child assessment literature with the diagnostic classification system. It seems likely that most of the traditional psychometric measures of anxiety in children were designed to assess trait dimensions, and hence converged with the broader constructs of fear, anxiety, and negative emotionality. More recent strategies that were designed to key to diagnostic symptoms yielded confirmation of their respective syndromes. Taken together, these results paint a picture of two conceptual levels on which to consider clinical manifestations of fear and anxiety in youth. Given the current state of the literature, it appears that an understanding of both the general factors (i.e., NA and PH) and the specific syndromes (i.e., clinical disorders) are important in terms of informing the treatment of anxious psychopathology.

When to Treat Fears and Anxieties

Although the various syndromes of clinical fears and anxieties have been outlined above, their symptomatology and structure offer little guidance regarding when to provide a clinical intervention. For example, separation fears, obsessional thinking, worrying, and nearly all types of anxiety are typical parts of the human experience in general (e.g., Borkovec, Shadick, & Hopkins, 1991; Rachman, 1977), and of child development in particular (Bell-Dolan, Last, & Strauss, 1990; Ollendick, 1983). Some of the earliest research on childhood fear and anxiety involved surveys of the number and degree of fears in children; these observations support the notion that fear is a common part of child development, with early studies reporting from four to five fears in 2- to 6-year-olds (Jersild & Holmes, 1935), and five to eight fears in 4- to 16-year-olds (Pintner & Lev, 1940). More recent investigations have found

similar estimates, with children and adolescents collectively reporting between 7 and 17 intense fears (Ollendick, 1983; Ollendick & King, 1994; Ollendick, King, & Frary, 1989; Ollendick, Matson, & Helsel, 1985). Using a slightly different approach, Bell-Dolan and colleagues (1990) found that symptoms of anxiety disorders were endorsed on a diagnostic clinical interview by between 10% and 31% of children ages 5–18. Similarly, studies investigating the prevalence of panic attacks in adolescents have found rates above 60% (e.g., King, Gullone, Tonge, & Ollendick, 1993). These studies together thus suggest that fears and even symptoms of anxiety disorders are highly common among children and adolescents.

The decision regarding whether to intervene must therefore be based on other factors than the mere presence of fear or anxiety. Essentially, it involves three types of considerations; in a practical sense, all three of these considerations are considered necessary and none sufficient to warrant intervention. First, the fear or anxiety should be evaluated to determine whether it is realistic in nature (Barlow, 1988; Marks, 1969)—in other words, whether a youth's response is out of proportion to the actual threat itself. For example, a youth whose parents frequently engage in violence toward one another would be expected to worry about such issues as family and safety, and thus such fears would not typically be addressed through an intervention for the youth's anxiety (although other interventions, such as those targeting the family or parents, would probably be warranted). Barlow (1988, 2002) has referred to anxiety disorders as involving the experience of a natural or appropriate emotion at an unnatural or inappropriate time; he uses the term "false alarm" to refer to episodes of fear or anxiety in the absence of a genuine threat. It is the presence of these "false alarms" that constitutes initial grounds for concern regarding the need for intervention. As discussed earlier, the considerable body of research focused on cognitive correlates of child psychopathology has differentiated several irrational cognitive processes, including cognitive distortions and misattributions (cf. Beck et al., 1979), attentional biases toward threatening stimuli, and problem-solving deficiencies (e.g., over-reliance on avoidance as a solution). Kendall (1992), among others, has proposed that dysfunctional thinking patterns may lead to avoidance of potentially remedial learning experiences in the future, imparting risk for intensification of anxiety across development.

A second consideration is a youth's developmental context. Specifically, is the degree or type of fear outside the range of those fears that are age-appropriate and may resolve on their own with minimal complications? Indeed, research on fears shows that they are common in youths, and that their overall number (although not necessarily their intensity) declines with age (Barrios & O'Dell, 1998; Ollendick et al., 1989). Furthermore, Barrios and O'Dell (1998) point out that children of different ages use different levels of reasoning with regard to evaluating threat. Fears at some ages may be considered out of proportion to the threat from the perspective of an adult. Nevertheless, such a misperception may be one that is normative for a particular age group, and thus likely to resolve on its own over development. The third consideration regarding whether to intervene with fear and anxiety in youths involves the degree of impairment associated with these emotions. For example, a child living in a rural environment who is afraid of elevators—even to the degree of irrationality and out of proportion with developmental norms—may not experience sufficient anxiety to warrant an intervention, because he or she may not encounter elevators with sufficient frequency to provoke distress or interference. As mentioned above, research has shown that anxiety disorders at a clinical level often have a negative impact on multiple areas of a child's performance (e.g., Langley et al., 2004; Pine et al., 1998), that most children with anxiety disorders have at least one other clinical diagnosis (Albano et al., 2003), and that nearly half of these children are considered seriously impaired in terms of their life functioning (Costello et al., 1999). Thus the assessment of distress or interference is critical in making the determination of whether to treat a particular youth.

Recently, some measures of the distress or interference caused by anxiety have emerged (e.g., Hodges & Wong, 1996; Langley et al., 2004). However, most contemporary strategies aimed at assessing life functioning appear to be keyed more toward disruptive behavior and deliberately do not assess for emotional impairment (see Costello et al., 1999), which may be an underappreciated aspect of anxiety in youths relative to some other forms of child psychopathology (Francis, Gray, & Chorpita,

2000). When anxiety was viewed more broadly in terms of interference with the pursuit of goals and realizing one's personal and social potential, Ollendick and King (1994) found that childhood fears interfered at least moderately in daily activities for over 85% of the youths they surveyed. Although definitive measurement strategies have not been determined, the need to examine the degree of emotional and functional impairment associated with children's fear and anxiety is a critical prerequisite to intervention.

TREATMENT STRATEGIES

Following the determination that a youth's fear or anxiety warrants formal intervention, a number of choices exist regarding the types of approaches and strategies. Historically, these strategies organize themselves into a few basic classes, which are reviewed below in some detail. The following section is primarily descriptive in nature, and the quality of these approaches as demonstrated in empirical tests is reviewed later in the chapter.

Exposure and Its Variants

The strategy of "exposure" typically involves a youth's real or imagined confrontation with a feared stimulus. The different variants of exposure involve modifications of the intensity, duration, or order of stimuli, and can involve the addition of other clinical strategies as well, such as relaxation or rewards. Two major variations of exposure involve whether the stimulus is confronted directly or whether it is imagined. Direct confrontation is usually termed "*in vivo* exposure," and requires the youth to rehearse or be in the presence of the actual feared object or situation, such as petting a dog or giving a speech in front of others (e.g., Obler & Terwillinger, 1970). For a variety of reasons, it is sometimes preferable to have the youth imagine the feared object or stimulus—a procedure commonly referred to as "imaginal exposure" or "*in vitro* exposure." This usually involves a therapist describing a scene involving the stimulus, while the youth listens and imagines the details of the scene as fully as possible. Such strategies can be particularly helpful for exposure to stimuli or events that are not easily performed *in vivo*. For example, a child who has a fear of an upcoming surgery may be exposed *in vivo* to the hospital setting or other related stimuli, but confrontation with the event itself (i.e., surgery) is more easily performed through imaginal exposure.

The majority of contemporary protocols for childhood fears and anxiety involve a gradual exposure to increasingly intense stimuli that are rank-ordered on a hierarchy of fears (e.g., Kendall, Kane, Howard, & Siqueland, 1990; Silverman & Kurtines, 1996). For example, a child who is afraid of separation from caregivers may first practice being left alone with the therapist, while the caregiver sits in another room. As the initial practice becomes less anxiety-provoking, the exercises progress to more challenging separation experiences—for example, going to a new place without the caregiver (e.g., the therapist accompanies the child on a walk to a store). Finally, exposure may incorporate such event as sleepovers at other homes or being left in the care of a babysitter. This type of progression is often referred to as "*graduated* exposure," because of its gradually increasing intensity.

In some instances, exposure is performed in such a way that the stimulus is presented all at once. This approach may require the youth to perform only a single exposure exercise; however, the exercise can be very intense and sometimes rather prolonged if fear levels do not decrease quickly. For example, a youth afraid of heights may be taken to a high and very fear-provoking place for an extended period of time until the anxiety subsides.

Another variation of exposure, termed "implosion," involves the imaginal rehearsal of a feared stimulus or event, with added meaning being introduced by the therapist. For example, a script targeting a youth's obsession about leaving the lights on at home (e.g., as in OCD) might describe the youth's anxious internal monologue (e.g., "You know you should not be worrying about the lights, but you cannot stop yourself. You begin to think there is something wrong with you . . . ") or culminate with unrealistic consequences (e.g., "When you return home, there are fire trucks in the street, and your house has been burned down . . . "). Thus implosion typically intensifies the imaginal exposure greatly through the introduction of hypothetical meanings for and/or outcomes to the event, rather than just describing the event itself (Knox, Albano, & Barlow, 1996).

Some of the classic early behavioral work on treatment of anxiety involved a procedure known as "systematic desensitization" (Wolpe, 1958). This procedure is based on the notion of "reciprocal inhibition," which essentially posits that an individual cannot experience incompatible behavioral and affective states simultaneously. Thus a youth is trained in deep muscle relaxation, which is subsequently paired with exposure trials. The rationale is that relaxation induces a state incompatible with anxiety, thereby reducing the conditioned association between the stimulus and the anxious response. Systematic desensitization in its classic form involves the progression from less intensive to more intensive stimuli or events, and is traditionally delivered with imaginal exposure (Wolpe, 1958). When *in vivo* exposure is paired with the incompatible response training, the technique is sometimes referred to as "*in vivo* desensitization" (e.g., Kuroda, 1969). Other variations of systematic desensitization can involve incompatible activities other than relaxation, such as playing games or being in contact with a caregiver (e.g., Bentler, 1962), or the use of positive images (e.g., a supportive superhero or brave cartoon character; Lazarus & Abramovitz, 1962). This latter variation is sometimes referred to as "emotive imagery" (Cornwall, Spence, & Schotte, 1996).

Modeling and Its Variants

Another major class of treatments for anxiety—called "modeling"—involves the youth's observation of another person interacting successfully with the feared stimulus. For example, a therapist may pet a dog to demonstrate to a child that the dog is safe and need not be feared. There are many variations of this basic technique, depending primarily on (1) the nature of the model and (2) the type of behaviors expected of the youth. For example, with "live modeling," the model performs the behaviors directly for the youth (e.g., Bandura, Grusec, & Mendlove, 1967; Murphy & Bootzin, 1973), whereas in "symbolic modeling," the model is shown interacting with the stimulus on a video or in a photograph (e.g., Lewis, 1974). In "covert modeling," the youth is asked to imagine the model interacting with the feared stimulus; in "participant modeling," the youth first observes the model interacting with the stimulus, and is then asked to perform the same behaviors as the model (i.e., participates in *in vivo* exposure; e.g., Ritter, 1968).

Models can also vary in number and in their

degree of similarity to the fearful youth. For example, some studies have used multiple models to demonstrate the interaction with the feared object (Bandura & Menlove, 1968; Lewis, 1974), whereas most have used a single model. Some studies have used peers as models (e.g., Bandura et al., 1967), whereas others have used adults (Murphy & Bootzin, 1973). Models can also differ in their level of fear, with "mastery" models showing minimal fear in the presence of the stimulus (Ritter, 1968), and "coping" models showing fear but overcoming that fear successfully (e.g., Bandura et al., 1967).

Cognitive Techniques and Variants

Variants of cognitive techniques actually predate some of the formal work on cognitive therapy that emerged in the late 1970s, and such procedures were often referred to as "self-management" or "self-talk" strategies. For example, in a study on the treatment of fear of darkness, Kanfer, Karoly, and Newman (1975) tested various strategies to address children's fear of the dark. Participants were assigned to one of three conditions: coping self-talk, stimulus self-talk, or neutral self-talk. In the coping self-talk condition, children were instructed to repeat a phrase to themselves emphasizing their bravery and ability to cope with the dark ("I am brave"). In the stimulus self-talk condition, children repeated positive statements about the dark, without reference to coping (e.g., "The dark is a fun place"). Finally, in the neutral self-talk condition, children repeated a nursery rhyme unrelated to the dark. Results pointed to advantages of both the coping self-talk and stimulus self-talk strategies, suggesting the important role of coping and cognition in the treatment of childhood fears.

More recent protocols have elaborated the procedures intended to alter threat appraisals or anxious cognitions in youths—a process sometimes called "cognitive restructuring." A common first step involves helping a child identify his or her negative self-talk; the child may be asked to think of thoughts running through his or her head as "thought bubbles," similar to those seen in comic strips (Kendall, Kane, et al., 1990). Once the content of the self-talk has been identified, the therapist can help the child consider replacing the maladaptive cognitions with more adaptive ones. "Attribution retraining" is similar, in that a child is trained to distinguish internal from external, global from local, and stable from unstable attributions in his or her own thoughts. Once a child identifies his or her attributions for a given event, the child and therapist can entertain alternative attributions for the given circumstance and test their effect on the child's fear and behavior (Southam-Gerow & Kendall, 2000).

Other Approaches

As interventions have elaborated to encompass more than phobic avoidance—that is, to target such features of anxiety as worrying, fear of separation, and social anxiety—increasing numbers of strategies have been incorporated to address the target syndrome. In fact, the average number of techniques in treatments protocols (e.g., exposure, relaxation, rewards) studied in the 1980s and earlier was roughly two, and in treatments studies from the 1990s onward that number is roughly nine. For example, such well-tested protocols as those developed by Silverman (Silverman & Kurtines, 1996), Kendall (Kendall, Kane, et al., 1990), Deblinger (Deblinger & Heflin, 1996) and others typically involve several strategies in addition to those discussed above. These include rapport building, psychoeducation, emotion skills training, relaxation training, contingency management, self-reinforcement training, and problem-solving training. We discuss each of these briefly here.

Although relationship or nonspecific factors are not discussed in detail in most evidence-based treatments, many recent treatments recognize the importance of rapport building with children and families (e.g., Kendall, 2002). For example, Kendall's CBT program, "Coping Cat," dedicates the first session to building rapport, and the first four sessions—focused on teaching emotion education skills, including relaxation training—are designed to move slowly for the expressed purposes of easing the child into therapy and of building the therapeutic relationship. As Kendall (2002) has noted, "Rapport between the anxious child and the therapist is critical to the success of the therapy, and ample time should be devoted to the establishment of a trusting relationship between the child and therapist" (p. 9). Other treatment approaches similarly emphasize the importance of the treatment relationship (e.g., March & Mulle, 1998; Silverman & Kurtines, 1996).

Psychoeducation is also a component of most treatments for childhood anxiety. It typically focuses on (1) identifying for the child (and his or her family) the various symptoms of anxiety; (2) "normalizing" anxiety, including discussion of the important role of anxiety (i.e., everyone experiences anxiety, and it often serves essential functions, such as protection from danger); and (3) outlining the typical treatment plan in CBT approaches (i.e., skills training and exposure). In addition, many treatment programs include disorder-specific educational content. For instance, March and Mulle's (1998) treatment program for OCD provides the child and family with a neurobehavioral framework from which to understand OCD. As another example, the treatments for PTSD related to sexual abuse usually include education on body safety and sexual health, with the latter adjusted for the age of the child (e.g., Deblinger & Heflin, 1996).

Emotion skills training involves a set of treatment strategies focused on teaching children to identify their characteristic responses to fear-evoking stimuli. These interventions may also involve teaching methods to cope with anxious arousal, including relaxation training (see below). Basic emotion skills training involves teaching the child to recognize, label, and self-monitor various cues (e.g., physiological, behavioral) indicating that the child is feeling anxious. In the Coping Cat program, for example, children generate a list of emotions and their characteristic ways of expressing those emotions. Differentiating anxiety-related from other-emotion-related (e.g., excitement-related) responses is also emphasized in the program. Similarly, Deblinger's CBT program involves teaching children to recognize and interpret the emotion-related cues of others so as to reduce misinterpretations. These sorts of strategies are aimed at fostering a child's awareness of his or her own (and others') feelings, as well as helping the child to recognize the situations likely to evoke those emotions. Furthermore, the interventions are designed to teach children that this awareness is often a first step in coping adaptively with the situation evoking the upset.

As noted above, relaxation training is often paired with emotion skills training as one way to cope with emotional arousal. Several types of relaxation exercises are common in treatment programs, including breathing retraining, progressive muscle relaxation, cue-controlled relaxation, and imagery techniques. Breathing retraining, widely applied in treatment for panic disorder (though with some controversy—see Schmidt et al., 2000), is also used in several CBT programs for other childhood anxiety disorders. In brief, the training involves teaching a child a diaphragmatic breathing technique and then practicing this in sessions as well as in homework assignments. The goal is for the child to experience the relaxing effect of slow, deep breathing. Furthermore, as the exercises can be applied rapidly and privately in public, these exercises are often suggested as a coping strategy in an emergent stressful situation.

Progressive relaxation exercises involve the successive tension and relaxation of major muscle groups (e.g., King, Hamilton, & Ollendick, 1988). The notion is that these exercises help clients perceive bodily tension, with the hope that they will use that tension as a cue to relax. Cue-controlled relaxation involves associating the relaxed state with a personalized cue word, such as "relax" or "calm." In practice, the child repeatedly subvocalizes the cue word while in the relaxed state. Relaxation exercises are frequently accompanied by the incorporation of comforting imagery, such as a beach or forest scene. Using vivid and sensory-rich descriptions, the therapist guides the child through images designed to create a highly relaxed state.

Another common treatment strategy is contingency management, an approach with more widespread application in parent training programs for children with conduct problems (e.g., Barkley, 1997; McMahon & Forehand, 2003). Several intervention developers (e.g., Barrett et al., 1996; Chorpita, Taylor, et al., 2004; King et al., 1998; Silverman & Kurtines, 1996; Silverman, Kurtines, Ginsburg, Weems, Rabian, et al., 1999) have adapted this approach for application to childhood anxiety by teaching parents to examine how the consequences of approach and avoidance in their anxious children's lives have influenced the maintenance of the anxiety-related difficulties. Then parents are taught how to alter the delivery of positive or negative consequences to encourage approach and discourage avoidance behavior. Such interventions are typically paired with exposure and other more traditional techniques as well (although see Heyne et al., 2002, who successfully treated anxious school refusal without formal use of exposure).

Variants have involved providing simple rewards when a child confronts the stimulus (e.g., Leitenberg & Callahan, 1973; Obler & Terwilliger, 1970), or taking away points or privileges when the stimulus is avoided or when previous gains in approach behaviors are not maintained.

Another component of treatment involves training children to self-monitor their "performance" in fear- or anxiety-provoking situations, and to evaluate themselves with an eye toward increasing approach behavior. Children are trained in the behavioral process of "shaping" themselves by rewarding successive approximations toward the desired behavior(s), such as increased approach behavior or improved coping effort (e.g., "did not avoid situation"). In the beginning, concrete "success" (e.g., making a new friend) is downplayed, and effort is rewarded (Kendall et al., 1997; Shortt, Barrett, & Fox, 2001). Children are also trained to reward themselves for their successes, with some rewards being tangible (e.g., a special dinner) and others more subjective and internal (e.g., patting oneself on the back). Parents are often involved in this component, as their intentional and unintentional behaviors sometimes emphasize reward only for the achievement of a goal rather than the process of working toward it.

Finally, some of the treatments for childhood anxiety include problem-solving training (Cohen & Mannarino, 1996; Kendall, 2002). Most problem-solving training involves the presentation of a multistep process: (1) description of the problem and the major goals for the solution; (2) generation of alternative solutions; (3) evaluation of these alternatives in terms of how well they will assist in the achievement of the goal; (4) selection and enactment of the best strategy or strategies identified; and, finally, (5) evaluation of the degree of success of the outcome, with emphasis on problem-solving effort rather than simply on "winning." Such an approach is believed to be useful for children with anxiety disorders for a few reasons. First, it is thought to help these children to realize that their problems are neither unmanageable nor catastrophic. In addition, a problem-solving approach may encourage children to focus on and evaluate several possible solutions to a problem. Finally, research on the correlates of anxiety disorders suggests that anxious children have problem-solving biases that merit remediation.

IDENTIFYING PROMISING INTERVENTIONS

The literature on the treatment of childhood fear and anxiety has matured considerably over the last 15–20 years. In their excellent and comprehensive review, Barrios and O'Dell (1998) referenced over 175 studies involving the interventions for fear or anxiety. Given the growing volume of research in this area, it now seems fitting to employ definitional criteria to select those studies from the literature that are likely to yield the best inferences about promising interventions. That is, without a filter or template by which to extract generalities, it is becoming increasingly difficult to draw inferences from a literature that will soon encompass more than 200 treatment studies. For this chapter, the research on treatments for fear or anxiety is evaluated according to two key dimensions. First, interventions in these studies are evaluated with respect to their "efficacy" (American Psychological Association [APA] Task Force on Psychological Intervention Guidelines, 1995; Chambless & Hollon, 1998), which refers to the degree to which a treatment has an observably reliable effect, due to proper experimental controls and study conditions. Second, the interventions are evaluated with respect to their "effectiveness." This term generally refers to the degree to which conditions in the outcome studies approximate real-world conditions, and are thus likely to suggest generalization of the results to true treatment settings. Because the majority of the clinical trials to date—including those for children with anxiety disorders—have been conducted in university research settings under highly controlled conditions (Weisz & Hawley, 1998), one favored approach to make such inferences about effectiveness is to summarize a variety of study parameters from the entire research base, regardless of the original settings or conditions of the studies (e.g., Chorpita et al., 2002). We have therefore chosen to examine the effectiveness of treatments for childhood fears and anxieties through both a review of their approximation of real-world conditions, and a review of specific study parameters that are relevant to real-world applications. Although one could include in this distinction those studies that included anxiety disorders as compared with those that included fears and anxiety syndromes more generally, we feel that such a distinction is less a reflection of the difference between "real-world" and laboratory applications of treatment than it is a reflection of the evolving nosology and measurement strategies. For example, youths with anxiety disorders can be recruited into treatment studies, and it is unclear that participants in some of the early research did not have anxiety disorders. We feel it is more important to consider client, provider, and context variables in determining the degree to which a study approximates real-world conditions (e.g., Chorpita, 2003; Schoenwald & Hoagwood, 2001b).

Efficacy

The Task Force on Promotion and Dissemination of Psychological Procedures of the APA's Division of Clinical Psychology (1995) has defined two different levels at which an intervention may be deemed efficacious. At the highest level, a "well-established" intervention refers to an intervention that has demonstrated efficacy either (1) in a minimum of two good between-group design experiments, where the intervention is superior to pill or psychological placebo or to another intervention; or (2) in a large series of controlled single-case experiments ($n \geq 9$) that have compared the intervention to another intervention. In either case, interventions must be conducted with a manual, and effects must have been demonstrated by at least two different investigators. At the second level, the status of "probably efficacious" refers to an intervention that has been found to be either (1) superior to a wait-list control group in two experiments; (2) equivalent to an already established intervention or superior to pill placebo, psychological placebo, or another intervention in a single experiment; or (3) superior to pill placebo, psychological placebo, or another intervention in a small series of single-case design experiments ($n \geq 3$).

Here we employ minor adaptations to the definitions of the Task Force on Promotion and Dissemination of Psychological Procedures (1995), as outlined in the work performed by the Hawaii Evidence Based Services Committee (e.g., Chorpita et al., 2002). First, interventions are not defined in this chapter at the level of specific manuals or individual protocols. Rather, interventions sharing a majority of components with similar clinical strategies and theoretical underpinnings are grouped together. For example, different interventions for anxiety that involve self-monitoring, identifying problem thoughts, developing coping

thoughts, and accompanying behavioral exposure exercises are collectively labeled "CBT" and evaluated as a single approach. Second, these levels of empirical support are referred to for simplicity as "Level 1," "Level 2," and "Level 3" (see Table 4.2).

Effectiveness

As noted above, we also review the effectiveness of interventions by summarizing selected aspects of the outcome studies. That is, to allow for inferences about the feasibility, generalizability, and cost–benefit of interventions in real-world settings, specific aspects of these studies are presented, regardless of whether studies were performed in true clinical settings. Effectiveness parameters are selected from those used in the review by Chorpita and colleagues (2002) and are defined in a manner consistent with that of the Task Force on Psychological Intervention Guidelines (1995). The lists of variables coded for each study and the corresponding definitions appear in Table 4.3.

Approach to the Review

The supportive findings from the literature are summarized in four appendices at the end of this chapter. Our approach to reviewing studies allowed for the inclusion of only those conditions or arms within studies that produced an intervention meeting criteria for Level 1, 2, or 3, according to the definitions above. Thus many studies with multiple treatment conditions may have only one condition represented; that is, if the other conditions did not produce an efficacious protocol, they are not indexed as treatments in the appendices, but are listed only as control conditions. We found that 86 study conditions involving an active treatment, drawn from 53 commonly cited studies, failed to produce evidence of an efficacious treatment. The most common reasons for exclusion were (1) equivalence of all study groups at posttreatment (e.g., Last, Hansen, & Franco, 1998; Melamed, Meyer, McGee, & Soule, 1976; Silverman, Kurtines, Ginsburg, Weems, Rabian, et al., 1999), and (2) lack of random assignment to a control group (e.g., Kuroda, 1969; Mendlowitz et al., 1999; Muller & Madson, 1970). Finally, several promising interventions are not noted, simply because they failed to meet criteria for Level 3 by having

TABLE 4.2. Definition of Efficacy Levels

Level 1

I. At least two good between-group-design experiments, demonstrating efficacy in one or both of the following ways:
   a. Superior to pill placebo, psychological placebo, or another treatment.
   b. Equivalent to an already established treatment in experiments with adequate statistical power (about 30 per group; cf. Kazdin & Bass, 1989).

Or

II. A large series of single-case-design experiments ($n \geq 9$) demonstrating efficacy. These experiments must have:
   a. Used good experimental designs.
   b. Compared the intervention to another treatment as in I.a.

And

Further criteria for both I and II:
III. Experiments must be conducted with treatment manuals.
IV. Characteristics of the client samples must be clearly specified.
 V. Effects must have been demonstrated by at least two different investigators or teams of investigators.

Level 2

I. Two experiments showing the treatment is (statistically significantly) superior to a wait-list control group. *Manuals, specification of sample, and independent investigators are not required.*

Or

II. One between-group-design experiment with clear specification of groups and use of manuals, demonstrating efficacy in one or both of these ways:
   a. Superior to pill placebo, psychological placebo, or another treatment.
   b. Equivalent to an already established treatment in experiments with adequate statistical power (about 30 per group; cf. Kazdin & Bass, 1989).

Or

III. A small series of single-case-design experiments ($n \geq 3$) with clear specification of groups; use of manuals; good experimental designs; and comparison of the intervention to pill, psychological placebo, or another treatment.

Level 3

I. One between-group-design experiment with clear specification of groups and treatment approach, demonstrating efficacy in one or both of these ways:
   a. Superior to pill placebo, psychological placebo, or another treatment.
   b. Equivalent to an already established treatment in experiments with adequate statistical power (about 30 per group; cf. Kazdin & Bass, 1989).

Or

II. A small series of single-case-design experiments ($n \geq 3$) with clear specification of groups and treatment approach; good experimental designs; at least two different investigators or teams; and comparison of the intervention to pill, psychological placebo, or another treatment.

Note. These levels are adapted from the Task Force on Promotion and Dissemination of Psychological Procedures (1995). The table itself is adapted from Chorpita et al. (2002). Copyright 2002 by Oxford University Press. Adapted by permission.

TABLE 4.3. Codes for Evaluating Effectiveness

Compliance

Equal to the percentage of children who did not drop out (posttreatment n/pretreatment n) within that treatment condition. For example, if 6 of 30 children drop out during treatment, compliance = 80%.

Gender

The presence of boys or girls within each condition; if information was not reported for a specific treatment condition, this number was estimated from information for the entire study.

Age

Years or months since birth; when range was not reported, it was estimated by using the mean age plus or minus 1.5 SD (approximately 87% of a typical distribution); thus, for mean age = 9.0 and SD = 1.6, the estimated range would be 6–11; if information was not reported for a specific treatment condition, this number was estimated from information for the entire study.

Ethnicity

Ethnic group within condition; if information was not reported for a specific treatment condition, this number was estimated from information for the entire study, under the assumption of the independence of ethnicity and treatment condition; ethnic groups are listed in decreasing order of frequency.

Therapist

The training/profession, if known, for the main provider(s) involved within each treatment condition: PhD, doctoral-level; MA, master's-level, including doctoral-level graduate students; BA, undergraduate degree; undergraduate, enrolled in university but had not completed degree.

Frequency

Frequency of contact with child/family, reported either in sessions per unit time (e.g., "weekly") or in total hours per unit time (e.g., "5 hours/day").

Duration

The length of time from pretreatment to posttreatment assessment.

Contacts

The total number of therapeutic contacts (does not include assessments).

Dose

The length of time in minutes of each therapeutic contact.

Setting

The primary type of location(s) in which treatment was delivered; when setting was not reported, it was sometimes inferred from aspects of the treatment (e.g., "teacher as therapist" implied a school setting).

Format

Whether the treatment was group therapy or individual therapy, and whether it included parents or family members.

Note. From Chorpita et al. (2002). Copyright 2002 by Oxford University Press. Adapted by permission.

only a single demonstration of their efficacy relative to a wait-list or no-treatment condition (e.g., Little & Jackson, 1974). The remaining interventions are summarized in the appendices, and are reviewed in some detail below.

RESEARCH ON INTERVENTIONS FOR FEARS AND ANXIETIES

Exposure and Its Variants

Numerous positive findings have emerged with respect to the treatment of fears and anxieties in children and adolescents, as illustrated in Table 4.4. The majority of the research on exposure and the parameters that influence its efficacy emanates from the 1960s and 1970s, when many of these questions were first being addressed in the treatment context, and much of this information is now well documented. The observation that this research is somewhat dated is not meant to imply, however, that exposure is an "outdated" treatment for anxiety. On the contrary, exposure holds some of the strongest empirical support for its efficacy, and is a treatment of first resort or a component thereof for all childhood fear and anxiety syndromes.

In a large number of controlled studies (see Appendix 4.1), exposure in its various forms has demonstrated superior treatment effects relative to active treatments or no-treatment control conditions (e.g., Chorpita, Vitali, & Barlow, 1997; Mann & Rosenthal, 1969; Menzies & Clarke, 1993; Öst, Alm, Brandberg, & Breitholtz, 2001; Ultee, Griffioen, & Schellekens, 1982). Exposure has been delivered successfully by using either the real stimulus (*in vivo*) or an imaginal form (*in vitro*). In several trials, exposure or variants have shown superiority to modeling (e.g., Bandura, Blanchard, & Ritter, 1969; Lewis, 1974), another efficacious procedure; this comparison represents a highly challenging test of the merits of exposure. Evidence suggests that exposure is more potent when performed *in vivo* (e.g., Ultee et al., 1982) and when paired with relaxation (e.g., Kondas, 1967), but such factors as group or individual delivery (Mann & Rosenthal, 1969), presence or absence of a parent (Öst et al., 2001), presence or absence of modeling (Menzies & Clarke, 1993), and the presence or absence of training study skills (Wilson & Rotter, 1986) have failed to demonstrate a difference in their effects.

Exposure and its variants have been successful with both boys and girls, ranging in age from 3 to 17 years, both individually and in groups. The treatment targets include mainly a variety of fears and phobias. Exposure has shown a very low rate of dropout, suggesting that it can be implemented without great challenges with the appropriate population. Exposure has been used successfully in research with Caucasian and African American youths, and its successful application has ranged in frequency from daily to weekly, with total treatment durations ranging from 1 day to 20 weeks. Exposure has been performed by individuals with minimal professional training, with some studies using undergraduates to perform the exposure exercises with participants (e.g., Menzies & Clarke, 1993).

Modeling and Its Variants

Much in the way that the exposure literature addressed many of the core questions regarding its efficacy 25–35 years ago, so too did the literature on modeling. In fact, we identified only a single study of the efficacy of modeling published within the last 25 years (Faust, Olson, & Rodriguez, 1991). Nevertheless, as in the case of exposure, the fact that the literature on modeling is older does not reflect negatively on its efficacy. Rather, modeling procedures have support for their use in isolation (as will be described below), and they are commonly part of more current multimodal treatment approaches (described further below in the section on CBT procedures).

In dozens of controlled demonstrations (see Appendix 4.2), modeling has demonstrated superior treatment effects relative to active treatments or no-treatment control conditions (Bandura et al., 1969; Blanchard, 1970; Murphy & Bootzin, 1973; Ritter, 1968). The models used have included parents, other adults, characters in slides and films/videos, and peers. The collective evidence points to the following patterns relative to the efficacy of modeling: (1) Live modeling is superior to symbolic modeling (e.g., Bandura et al., 1969); (2) modeling is more efficacious when paired with exposure (e.g., Klingman, Melamed, Cuthbert, & Hermecz, 1984); (3) child models are more effective than adult models (e.g., Kornhaber & Schroeder, 1975); and (4) modeling with real stimuli is more effective than modeling with

TABLE 4.4. Efficacy Levels and Aggregate Effectiveness Parameters of Interventions for Fears and Anxieties

Intervention	Compliance	Gender	Age	Ethnicity	Therapist	Frequency	Duration	Format	Setting
Level 1									
Cognitive techniques and variants	92%	Both	2–17	European American, African American, Hispanic, Asian American, Native American, Pacific Islander	Undergraduate, MA, PhD	Daily to weekly	1 day to 20 weeks	Group, individual, group with parent, individual with parent	Clinic, school, community, dental office
Exposure and variants	97%	Both	3–17	European American, African American	Undergraduate, BA, MA, PhD	Daily to weekly	1 day to 20 weeks	Group, individual	Clinic, community, school
Modeling and variants	100%	Both	2–18	European American, African American	MA, PhD	Twice per day to weekly	1 day to 18 weeks	Group, individual, child with parent	Clinic, community, school, laboratory, dental office, hospital
Level 2									
Tutoring plus self-instruction	100%	Both	12–13	N/R	MA	Twice weekly	3 weeks	Group	School
Level 3									
Education (with and without self-instruction training)	100%	Both	7–10	N/R	BA, MA	Once	1 day	School	Group
Elaborative rehearsal	100%	Both	9	N/R	Undergraduates	Daily	3 days	School	Group
Group play therapy	100%	Boys	8–9	European American	N/R	Weekly	14 weeks	Child group, parent group	N/R
Parent and teacher training	90%	Both	7–14	N/R (Australian national)	MA	Twice weekly	4 weeks	Clinic, school	Individual, and parent and school consults
Study habits training	100%	Both	11–13	African American, European American	PhD	Twice weekly	3 weeks	N/R	Group

Note. N/R, not reported.

replicas of the stimuli (e.g., Weissbrod & Bryan, 1973).

Other factors appear not to add to the effects of modeling in the reduction of fear and anxiety. For example, the following patterns have also been noted: (1) Coping/fearful models appear to be no more effective than mastery/fearless models (e.g., Kornhaber & Schroeder, 1975; Klorman, Hilpert, Michael, LaGana, & Sveen, 1980); (2) single versus multiple models do not account for a difference in effects (e.g., Bandura & Menlove, 1968; Mann & Rosenthal, 1969); (3) adding reinforcement to modeling does not appear to add effects (e.g., O'Connor, 1972); and (4) the age or gender of other child models does not appear to alter the effects (e.g., Weissbrod & Bryan, 1973).

Overall, modeling has been demonstrated to be successful with both boys and girls, ranging in age from 2 to 18 years. The treatment targets include mainly phobic disorders and childhood fears. Based on the studies observed, it is associated with a low or possibly zero rate of dropout, although the majority of studies in support of modeling procedures have been conducted in analogue laboratory clinics (rather than in community clinics), which carry high demand characteristics and would be expected to have higher retention rates than would be expected in more applied contexts. Modeling has been used successfully in research with Caucasian and African American youths, and its successful application has ranged in frequency from twice per day to weekly, with durations ranging from 1 day to 18 weeks. It appears to be effective in both group and individual formats.

Cognitive Techniques and Variants

Consistent with a multicomponent conceptualization of anxiety, there is growing interest in the notion that a combination of treatment strategies might be most efficacious in treating children with anxiety disorders (Kendall et al., 1992; Ollendick & King, 1998). Given the empirical support demonstrated for modeling and exposure described above, it is not surprising that multicomponent treatment packages including such procedures have also proven efficacious. As Appendix 4.3 indicates, we found dozens of studies finding CBT to be superior to a control condition at improving outcomes for treated youths across several target problems, including such anxiety disorders as GAD, SAD, social phobia, OCD, and PTSD. Individual

(child) and group approaches were the two most common formats. Also common were child and parent sessions; often these were conducted in parallel fashion, though some studies involved conjoint sessions as well, which involve working simultaneously with a parent and child. Although ages in the studies ranged from 2 to 17, the typical study included youths ages 7–14; only 11 studies included children below age 7, and only two included children below age 5. Evidence is also sparse for adolescents, with only six studies including youths ages 15 and above. In contrast to modeling and exposure protocols, CBT as a whole has demonstrated success in research with a diversity of ethnic groups, including Caucasian, African American, Hispanic, Asian American, Native American, and Pacific Island youths. More than two-thirds of the treatments tested involved weekly sessions, and the number of client contacts ranged from 1 to 30, though most studies included between 10 and 16 sessions. One notable gap in the literature is the relative lack of non-CBT comparison treatments. Thus there is little evidence that CBT is better than other active treatments—an issue we return to later.

We listed studies as involving CBT if the treatment involved cognitive (e.g., cognitive restructuring, self-statement training) *and* behavioral (e.g., exposure, modeling) interventions. Some early studies did not use the moniker "CBT," and yet, given their composition, are included in that section of our review (e.g., Kanfer et al., 1975; Rosenfarb & Hayes, 1984; Sheslow, Bondy, & Nelson, 1982). Furthermore, although we refer to these treatments collectively as "CBT," there is variability in the strategies employed. Because of this variability, in the following three subsections we examine the "typical" treatment approach for three different categories of anxiety disorders and their therapeutic approaches: (1) generalized and social anxiety disorders (i.e., GAD/overanxious disorder [OAD], SAD, and social phobia/avoidant disorder), (2) OCD, and (3) PTSD.

CBT for Generalized and Social Anxiety Disorders

One of the most widely recognized CBT packages is the Coping Cat program, developed by Kendall and colleagues (Kendall, Kane, et al., 1990). Coping Cat is a primarily youth-focused, 16- to 20-session treatment that includes a skills training component and an exposure component. First, youth are taught a four-step coping plan called the FEAR steps (an acronym for the experience of anxious distress and for steps to take to alleviate it: Feeling frightened, Expecting bad things to happen, Actions and attitudes to take, and Results and rewards). The specific steps include (1) recognition of anxious feelings and somatic reactions; (2) the role of cognition and self-talk in exacerbating anxious situations; (3) the use of problem-solving and coping skills to manage anxiety; and (4) the employment of self-evaluation and self-reinforcement strategies to facilitate the maintenance of coping. After the FEAR steps are mastered, the remaining 8–12 sessions are dedicated to the implementation of the coping plan in increasingly anxiety-provoking situations that are tailored to each child's concerns. Throughout, behavioral strategies such as coping modeling, *in vivo* exposure, role plays, relaxation training, and contingent reinforcement are used (see also Kendall, Kane, et al., 1990).

The empirical support for the program and its variants is strong: multiple baseline studies (Howard & Kendall, 1996; Kane & Kendall, 1989), two large-scale randomized controlled trials (RCTs) (Kendall, 1994; Kendall et al., 1997), and two long-term follow-ups (Kendall, Safford, Flannery-Schroeder, & Webb, 2004; Kendall & Southam-Gerow, 1996). Furthermore, the treatment has recently been adapted in an individual format for an adolescent population (the C.A.T. Project; Kendall, Choudhury, Hudson, & Webb, 2002), though its efficacy for that population awaits empirical confirmation. Other independent investigators have tested variants to Coping Cat that involved (1) fewer sessions, (2) increased parental involvement, and/or (3) a group format (e.g., Barrett, 1998; Barrett et al., 1996; Cobham, Dadds, & Spence, 1998; Flannery-Schroeder & Kendall, 2001; Howard & Kendall, 1996; Mendlowitz et al., 1999; Silverman, Kurtines, Ginsburg, Weems, Lumpkin, et al., 1999). We examine one of the parent-involved and one of the group treatments, as examples of variants of the individual CBT approach.

The Barrett and colleagues (1996) study provides an example of a parent-involved variant. The "Coping Koala" program involved fewer sessions (12 instead of 16–20) and involved teaching a parent three sets of skills: (1) contingency management training, including how to reward courageous behavior and extinguish

fearful behavior; (2) parental anxiety management skills; and (3) communication and problem-solving skills training for the parent. Sessions were structured such that the first portion of each meeting involved the child and therapist and the latter portion involved the parent, child, and therapist. In their first trial, Barrett et al. (1996) found that outcomes were better when parents were involved in this way. However, subsequent studies have not offered the same clear support for the superiority of the family approach over the individual (e.g., Barrett, Duffy, Dadds, & Rapee, 2001; Cobham, 1998; Mendlowitz et al., 1999; Nauta, Scholing, Emmelkamp, & Minderaa, 2003). Barrett and colleagues have modified the treatment program from their first RCT (i.e., Barrett et al., 1996). Now referred to as the FRIENDS program, the treatment is designed as both an early intervention and a primary prevention program. We return to the evidence for the prevention program shortly.

Silverman, Kurtines, Ginsburg, Weems, Lumpkin, and colleagues' (1999) study provides a good illustration of a group CBT approach. Based on the notion of "transfer of control" (e.g., Silverman & Kurtines, 1996), the model depicts the therapist as an expert consultant to each family who provides knowledge to the youth and a parent, typically in the form of skills development. The knowledge is tailored to effect change in the youth, and the change is accomplished by transferring control from the therapist to the parent to the child. The key to treatment of anxiety in this model involves control of the occurrence, and successful implementation, of child exposure and approach behavior. The goal is accomplished through contingency management (for the parent) and self-control training (for the youth). The group treatment involves ten 80-minute sessions, 70 minutes of which are spent in two separate groups—children in one, and parents of the children in the other. In the final 10 minutes of each session, parents and children come together. The program addresses contingency contracting, group social skills training, self-control (cognitive) training, and exposure tasks. Parents are trained in the anxiety processes of their children, as well as the ways in which parental responses reinforce anxious behavior. In the RCT, Silverman, Kurtines, Ginsburg, Weems, Lumpkin, and colleagues found that the intervention was superior to a wait-list control group at posttreatment.

Overall, CBT has very strong empirical support in its individual, parent/family, and group formats. Although direct comparisons among these variants are few, we offer two tentative conclusions. First, support is only just emerging for the notion that parent involvement enhances treatment outcomes beyond those obtained by working with children alone. This is despite the great appeal of involving parents, based largely on research indicating that parental behavior correlates with childhood anxiety, suggesting that changes in parental behavior could help reduce children's anxiety (e.g., Chorpita & Barlow, 1998; Ginsburg, Silverman, & Kurtines, 1995). Second, there is no evidence that group CBT produces outcomes superior to those for individual CBT.

CBT for OCD

Literature on the treatment of pediatric OCD has only recently begun to accumulate, and investigations of psychosocial treatments have lagged behind those of pharmacological treatments (e.g., Henin & Kendall, 1997; March, 1995). Recent efforts to develop and test psychosocial treatments for OCD have showed considerable (albeit tentative) promise, with CBT playing a dominant role. To date, however, only a single RCT has been published; the rest of the evidence for CBT is limited to multiple-baseline studies, case reports, and open trials (e.g., Knox et al., 1996). In the one RCT, Barrett, Healy-Farrell, and March (2004) compared two CBT packages with a wait-list control condition. Both CBT programs specified parent involvement in sessions; one was delivered in an individual format (i.e., one child and a parent and sibling), and the other was delivered in a group format. Based on March and Mulle's (1996) CBT program "How I Ran OCD Off My Land," Barrett and colleagues' (2004) FOCUS program includes several strategies: (1) psychoeducation, (2) anxiety management skills (e.g., relaxation), (3) cognitive strategies, and (4) exposure and response prevention (ERP). ERP is an exposure variant specifically designed for the compulsions found in clients with OCD. In ERP, children are exposed to the feared stimuli about which they obsess (e.g., germs, violent thoughts). After such exposure, the compulsive response is prevented. ERP is a common technique in CBT approaches for adult and youth OCD (Abramowitz, 1996; Foa, Steketee, Grayson,

Turner, & Latimer, 1984; March & Leonard, 1996). One novel aspect of the Barrett and colleagues (2004) manual is its involvement of the parent and sibling. Each session included time with (1) an individual child (or, in the group condition, a group of children), (2) a parent and sibling, and (3) the whole family (i.e., parent, child, and sibling). Parallel content is covered in the individual and parent–sibling sessions. The findings from the trial suggested that the individual and group variants both produced significant change in youths beyond that experienced in the wait-list control group.

Overall, the paucity of the literature belies firm conclusions about the efficacy of CBT for OCD, particularly because only one RCT has been published. More RCTs are clearly needed to determine the efficacy of CBT for OCD. Comparisons of CBT to pharmacological approaches would be particularly helpful, as the evidence in support of pharmacology for OCD is also growing (Coghill, 2002; see below for more information on medications with OCD and other anxiety disorders). In addition, as suggested in some open trials (e.g., Franklin et al., 1998), the necessity of anxiety management techniques to bolster the impact of the exposure and response prevention paradigm requires further study.

CBT for PTSD

A growing literature offers suggestions regarding how professionals might help children cope after disasters (e.g., LaGreca, Silverman, Vernberg, & Roberts, 2002). However, the treatment outcome literature on PTSD in youths is limited, despite the relatively high rates of chronic stressors in childhood (physical and sexual abuse, family or neighborhood violence, etc.), not to mention natural disasters and other potentially traumatic single events such as motor vehicle accidents (e.g., March, Amaya-Jackson, Murray, & Schulte, 1998). Nevertheless, in the last several years, several RCTs have been reported with positive findings for CBT. Almost all of this research has focused on children who experienced sexual abuse (though one recent RCT examined a CBT approach for children who experienced a disaster; Goenjian et al., 1997). We review for illustration the CBT approach for abused children that has the most empirical support to date.

Deblinger and colleagues have developed and tested a CBT program that has to date received empirical support across one open trial, two RCTs, and a follow-up study (Cohen, Deblinger, Mannarino, & Steer, 2004; Deblinger & Heflin, 1996; Deblinger, McLeer, & Henry, 1990; Deblinger, Steer, & Lippmann, 1999). In the most recent RCT, trauma-focused CBT (TF-CBT) was found to be superior to a child-centered therapy approach for 8- to 14-year-old sexually abused youths. The TF-CBT model involves three treatment phases, the first two of which run in parallel: (1) individual child sessions, (2) groups for nonoffending caregivers, and (3) caregiver–child joint sessions. The child sessions include three treatment "modules": (1) skills training (including emotion recognition and expression skills, cognitive restructuring skills, relaxation training skills, and problem-solving skills); (2) exposure therapy; and (3) psychoeducation on maltreatment and its effects. The parallel group therapy for nonoffending caregivers focuses on skill development (e.g., parenting skills, assisting the child's coping skills development), exposure therapy, and psychoeducation. Finally, the model includes a module of conjoint caregiver–child sessions that involve a continuation of the gradual exposure process, with a focus on facilitating conversation between caregiver and child about the maltreatment.

In sum, CBT for PTSD appears promising, with several RCTs supporting its use with sexually abused children. Still, the evidence base leaves many unresolved questions regarding such treatments. For example, the role or necessity of an exposure component to treatment is not known. In addition, it is not known to what extent the treatment approach might differ, depending on the nature (i.e., sexual abuse, physical abuse, natural disaster) and chronicity (i.e., prolonged exposure vs. single incident) of the trauma or stressor.

Overall, CBT has shown great promise for the treatment of a variety of childhood anxiety disorders. However, evidence remains relatively limited to a few moderately sized RCTs that applied stringent inclusion criteria. In addition, there are very few comparative studies that involve non-CBT active treatments, and none that compare CBT to medication. Furthermore, the evidence is weak for OCD (only one RCT) and for PTSD when the focus of the trauma is something other than sexual abuse (only one RCT). We return to these gaps later in the chapter.

Other Psychosocial Treatments

Several other treatment approaches other than those reviewed above have emerged as having good or moderate empirical support; these can be seen in Table 4.4 and Appendix 4.4. They include tutoring, at the level of "good support" (i.e., tutoring was better than an alternative treatment in two different clinical trials; Genshaft, 1982; Genshaft & Hirt, 1980); and education, elaborative rehearsal, group play therapy, parent training, and study skills training, at the level of "moderate support" (i.e., each with a single demonstration of superiority to an active treatment or placebo; Clement & Milne, 1967; Heyne et al., 2002; Jones, Ollendick, McLaughlin, & Williams, 1989; Williams & Jones, 1989; Wilson & Rotter, 1986).

The targets of these interventions included test anxiety, shyness, fear of fire, and school refusal; therefore, none of these interventions was designed formally to target phobias or other anxiety disorders, per se. Given the limited number of trials (usually a single study) across which information can be aggregated about each intervention, the effectiveness parameters (Table 4.3) and any corresponding inferences about generalizability should be viewed with caution.

Prevention of Anxiety Disorders

Formal, manualized, and dedicated prevention programs for anxiety disorders have only recently begun being developed (Donovan & Spence, 2000). As evidence on risk factors for anxiety disorders has increased, the ability of prevention researchers to identify youths at risk has expanded. Some of the studies reviewed above could be construed as "prevention," insofar as these studies did not recruit children with diagnosable conditions. As an example, several of the trials conducted about dental fears were conducted with dental-naive but nonfearful children; hence such studies could be construed as prevention. In this section, we provide a brief overview to some recent developments in the anxiety prevention literature. In terms of *dedicated* prevention programs (i.e., programs developed to target children with subclinical but notable levels of anxiety) for anxiety disorders, two different age groups have been addressed: school-age and preschool. We review a representative program for each group.

The FRIENDS approach discussed earlier was developed for school-age children. Based on the Coping Koala program (Barrett et al., 1996), the program involved 10 weekly sessions for groups of 5–12 youths, with three parent sessions conducted concurrently with the child sessions. In the child sessions, the therapists taught youths an anxiety management plan, the FEAR steps (Kendall, 1994; see above) and used group processes to reinforce positive strategies and individual efforts to overcome fears. The parent sessions focused on child anxiety management skills; the FEAR plan and how parents could encourage/model coping with fears; and parental anxiety management skills. Dadds, Spence, Holland, and Barrett (1997) reported on an RCT of the intervention. Families of youths who passed several screening levels were randomly assigned to the intervention group or the monitoring group. At postintervention, differences were not consistently in evidence between the two groups; however, at a 6-month follow-up, a significant advantage for the intervention group emerged. More recently, Dadds and colleagues (1999) reported on 1- and 2-year follow-ups of the program that strongly supported the utility of the program.

LaFreniere and Capuano (1997) developed an early intervention for preschoolers who were identified as anxious/withdrawn by teachers. The intervention involved 20 sessions designed to teach parenting and attachment-promoting skills. For example, sessions focused on child-directed play; behavior modification of problematic behavior; and education on developmental needs of children. The intervention was found to increase children's social competence and parental use of appropriate control, compared to a no-treatment control group. However, differences were not found across all outcome areas. Though the intervention shows promise, further investigations are needed, especially ones focusing on subsequent rates of disorder and symptomatology across time in the two groups. Rapee and Jacobs (2002) reported similar findings for their open trial of a prevention program designed for preschoolers with inhibited temperamental style (Kagan et al., 1994).

The development of preventive interventions for childhood anxiety disorders has only just begun. Given the accretion of findings suggesting poor outcomes for youths with anxiety disorders as they grow older (e.g.,

Pine et al., 1998), the need for a continued focus on prevention is clear. In addition, the preliminary findings of LaFreniere and Capuano (1997) and of Rapee and Jacobs (2002) are heartening, insofar as they indicate that we can intervene with very young children, potentially increasing the chance of promoting more adaptive development earlier in life.

Psychopharmacological Treatments

Although this chapter (like this book as a whole) focuses primarily on psychosocial treatments for children and adolescents, there is ample reason to provide a brief review of psychopharmacological treatments for childhood anxiety. As recent reviews indicate, child mental health treatment increasingly involves medications (e.g., Goodwin, Gould, Blanco, & Olfson, 2001; Olfson, Marcus, Weissmann, & Jensen, 2002; Zito et al., 2003). In fact, an estimated 6% of youths receive some form of psychotropic medication (e.g., Zito et al., 2003). Furthermore, medication use has been rising rapidly in recent years: The number of children under age 18 receiving medication therapy for mental health problems has increased almost threefold from 1987 to 1996 (Olfson et al., 2002), and the number of children receiving multiple psychotropic medications is also increasing (e.g., Martin, Van Hoof, Stubbe, Sherwin, & Scahill, 2003; Olfson et al., 2002). We briefly review the evidence for use of medications for child anxiety disorders; we first examine treatments for GAD, SAD, and social phobia, and then the more substantial body of work on OCD.

Medications for GAD, SAD, and Social Phobia

Evidence before the mid-1990s was mixed for the use of various medications (e.g., tricyclic antidepressants, benzodiazepines) for most childhood anxiety disorders (e.g., Bernstein & Kinlan, 1997; Coghill, 2002; Kearney & Silverman, 1998; Velosa & Riddle, 2000), leading some reviewers to conclude that "psychological therapies [are] . . . the mainstay for child and adolescent anxiety disorder" (Coghill, 2002, p. 363; see also Kearney & Silverman, 1998). However, recent evidence has suggested that some medications, particularly selective serotonin reuptake inhibitors (SSRIs), may be an effective treatment for some anxiety disorders; the evidence is strongest for OCD (see below), but GAD, SAD, and social phobia have been examined as well (e.g., Birmaher et al., 2003; Coghill, 2002; March, Biederman, et al., 1998; Pine et al., 2001; Riddle et al., 2001). For example, Pine and colleagues (2001) found the SSRI fluvoxamine superior to placebo in a sample of 74 youths ages 7 to 17; response rate beyond the placebo was 47% on Clinical Global Impression (CGI) Improvement scores (response equal to CGI scores below 4). In a somewhat smaller sample, Birmaher and colleagues (2003) found that another SSRI, fluoxetine was superior to placebo, with a response rate 26% better than placebo on the CGI (CGI ≤ 2). A third SSRI, sertraline, has shown promise for social anxiety disorder (i.e., social phobia) in a small open trial (Compton et al., 2001).

The two RCTs represent the only recent controlled evidence for medication treatments for childhood anxiety disorders other than OCD. Although both trials suggest that medication treatment has great promise, caution is needed, because there are no studies yet that compare any medication to another active treatment. As an example, the treatment literatures on attention-deficit/hyperactivity disorder and depression each contain at least one trial comparing a medication treatment to another active treatment (e.g., MTA Cooperative Group, 1999; Treatment for Adolescent Depression Study, 2004).

Medications for OCD

Consistent with the strong literature on adult pharmacotherapy for treatment of OCD (e.g., Ackerman & Greenland, 2002; Dougherty, Rauch, & Jenike, 2004; Stein, Spadaccini, & Hollander, 1995), evidence for medication treatment of OCD in childhood and adolescence is more plentiful than that for the other anxiety disorders. Before the late 1990s, most of the evidence in the child/adolescent literature supported the efficacy of clomipramine (e.g., March & Leonard, 1996). However, because clomipramine has a relatively unfavorable side effect profile, other medications have been investigated more recently. Furthermore, there is some evidence that behavior therapy produced superior effects to those of clomipramine on some indices, though the study had a small sample (*n* = 22; De Haan, Hoogduin, Buitelaar, & Keijsers, 1998).

Several recent RCTs have found that SSRIs are more effective than pill placebo. At least three trials have supported the efficacy of fluoxetine (Geller et al., 2001; Liebowitz et al., 2002; Riddle et al., 1992); these trials represent almost 100 treated youths. Response rates ranged from 16% to 30% beyond the response rate of placebo (the primary outcome measure was the child version of the Yale–Brown Obsessive–Compulsive Scale). Evidence for sertraline and fluvoxamine has also been reported, with response rates beyond placebo of 16% for sertraline (March, Biederman, et al., 1998) and 16% for fluvoxamine (Riddle et al., 2001)

Geller and colleagues (2003) reported a meta-analysis that included these RCTs as well as some earlier trials. They concluded that (1) clomipramine produced better outcomes than any of the SSRIs; (2) no SSRI was significantly better than another; and (3) despite the outcome superiority of clomipramine, SSRIs represent a viable treatment choice because of their more favorable side effect profile. Similar to the medication trials for other anxiety disorders, the next generation of studies in this area should apply designs comparing two active medications, medications versus psychotherapy, and combination therapies.

INTERVENTION COMPONENTS

To return to the issue of psychosocial treatments, one notable issue regarding their clinical utility is the great diversity of treatment manuals representing theoretically similar approaches. For example, the review above of CBT and its variants represents over a dozen different treatment manuals. The decision to consider each of these as an independent intervention or to consider them variants of a single intervention is a decision with significant consequences for their evaluation (Chambless & Hollon, 1998; Chorpita et al., 2002). One the one hand, one could credit each intervention with only its fraction of empirical support for the group (e.g., Coping Cat has two clinical trials among the many for CBT). At the other extreme, one could consider all CBT manuals collectively as having multiple successful demonstrations in a variety of forms and contexts.

The implications of this issue are discussed in greater detail elsewhere (Chorpita et al., 2002), but they raise here the fundamental issue of when to consider interventions the same or different. Chorpita, Daleiden, and Weisz (2005a) have recently developed a structured approach to this issue, which involves the identification and coding of individual clinical strategies or "practice elements" within each protocol. Those interventions sharing a common set of practice elements could more reasonably be considered a variant of a common approach. A particular advantage of this exer-

cise is that it highlights the common therapeutic elements across the different areas of intervention, helping to define intervention boundaries, and pointing to the possibility of important or universal ingredients.

Figure 4.3 represents the relative frequency of practice elements across a subset of anxiety interventions (i.e., we selected 39 treatments whose protocols were available for coding from the full list of efficacious treatments out-

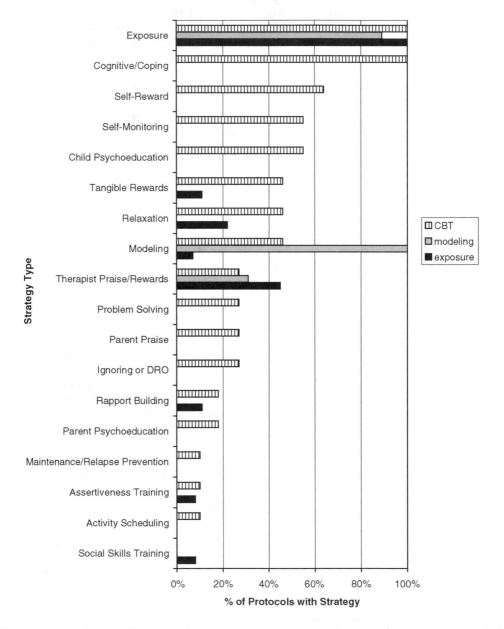

FIGURE 4.3. Practice elements for selected anxiety treatments. DRO, direct reinforcement of other behavior.

lined in the appendices). As shown in Figure 4.3, CBT appears to be characterized by the universal presence of both cognitive and exposure approaches, with relatively frequent use of self-reward, self-monitoring, child psychoeducation, tangible rewards, relaxation, and modeling. Less frequent components of CBT include therapist use of praise; problem-solving training for youths; instruction in parental use of praise; differential reinforcement of other behavior or ignoring; rapport building; parent psychoeducation; maintenance strategies; assertiveness training; and activity scheduling. Generally, this pattern suggests that CBT protocols appear to be defined by the presence of cognitive and exposure-based techniques, along with a variety of additional techniques.

Those protocols considered exposure therapies appear to be defined (not surprisingly) by the universal presence of exposure, along with the occasional structured use of therapist praise. Additional techniques in a minority of exposure protocols include relaxation (e.g., as with systematic desensitization), tangible rewards, rapport building, assertiveness training, and social skills training. Exposure therapies can thus be reasonably well defined by the presence of exposure, along with the absence of cognitive or modeling strategies. One exception to this was noted in an exposure protocol in which the therapist first explicitly modeled contact with the stimulus (Öst, 1989); arguably, such a protocol could be classified as a modeling treatment instead of an exposure treatment.

Finally, the modeling protocols were (as expected) universally characterized by the presence of modeling, and in the majority of cases included some exposure to the stimulus. The structured use of therapist praise or rewards was the only other strategy observed in these protocols. In general, this use of relatively few techniques with modeling protocols appears in part to be an artifact of the older literature on modeling, as the number of practice elements used in a single protocol has increased steadily over the past 40 years across all areas of the fear and anxiety literature.

COMMENTS AND FUTURE DIRECTIONS

Overall, the literature on treatment of childhood fears and anxieties reflects considerable support for at least the following three approaches: exposure, modeling, and CBT. A cause for optimism is that there are a host of other interventions "knocking at the door" of achieving solid empirical support for their efficacy. That said, the remainder of this chapter is intended to raise some of the issues that might warrant further consideration as the future of childhood anxiety intervention research takes shape.

Effectiveness Research

Despite the summary of evidence supporting the use of psychosocial interventions for childhood anxiety disorders, the collective findings do not fully address many of the "real-world" issues, given that the supportive data emanate largely from traditional laboratory-based research. It is widely believed that even those manuals with strongest support for their efficacy cannot simply be "installed" in service settings without attention to system issues and obstacles (Hoagwood, Burns, Kiser, Ringeisen, & Schoenwald, 2001; Schoenwald & Hoagwood, 2001b; Weisz, 2004). To understand some of the obstacles regarding transportability of these approaches, it is first necessary to examine these larger system operations more closely.

In addressing issues related to dissemination of these interventions into practice settings, Chorpita (2003) has argued that different research questions are appropriate for addressing the multiple layers of influence involved in service delivery. Central to this argument is the notion that the effects in practice settings often flow from supervisor to therapist to child, and that these effects can ultimately be measured in clinical outcomes. In this paradigm, traditional efficacy research (and nearly every study to date on the treatment of anxiety falls into this category) answers the question of whether an intervention is successful when most or all of the "upstream" elements in therapy are highly controlled (i.e., careful screening of the youth, high allegiance of the therapist, expert investigator serving as clinical supervisor). It is possible to relax these controls in such a way as to allow greater approximation of the true service settings to which treatments must ultimately be delivered. For example, in some research the referral stream can be part of a true service setting or community mental health system, and no special exclusionary criteria apply, but all other conditions are otherwise maximized (e.g., university-based therapists and supervisors). Schoenwald and Hoagwood (2001b) have termed this type of effectiveness research "transportability" research, as it allows for inferences about whether a particular intervention might be transported into a true practice setting. Moving to the next level, some research can use system employees (e.g., school counselors, private practitioners) as therapists. Schoenwald and Hoagwood have termed such research "deployment" research, in that it studies the performance of a treatment once it is deployed in a system. This research is what is most commonly referred to as "effectiveness" research, and it allows for inferences about the performance of a treatment under naturalistic conditions. Perhaps the strategy that allows for the broadest inferences to be made are those that evaluate intervention programs in the context of naturally occurring systems, internally managed and supervised. Studies focusing more on effectiveness are only recently beginning, and the field will certainly benefit from evaluating which of the interventions reviewed above will prove robust in more naturalistic settings and contexts.

Evolution of Interventions

As this chapter attests, we have accumulated solid evidence in support of the efficacy of treatments for childhood anxiety disorders tested in research settings. Unfortunately, these therapies are not the ones typically used in "real-world" settings such as community mental health clinics (e.g., Weisz, Hawley, Pilkonis, Woody, & Follette, 2000; Weisz, Weiss, & Donenberg, 1992), and only recently have efforts been made to deploy evidence-based approaches in such settings (e.g., Chorpita et al., 2002; Weisz, Southam-Gerow, Gordis, & Connor-Smith, 2003). This gap between science and practice represents a critical public health issue, as indicated by the U.S. National Institute of Mental Health's (NIMH's) various initiatives and workgroups examining the gap and how to close it (e.g., Hoagwood & Olin, 2002; Street, Niederehe, & Lebowitz, 2000).

Although scholarly and policy-based explanations of the genesis of this discrepancy are both thoughtful and plentiful, we briefly discuss two such explanations. First, most evidence-based treatments for anxiety disorders have been developed to focus on children with only anxiety disorders. This is despite a large body of evidence indicating that many children with anxiety disorders referred to clinics have multiple comorbid disorders (Angold, Costello, & Erkanli, 1999; National Advisory Mental Health Council Workgroup, 2001; Southam-Gerow, Chorpita, Taylor, & Miller, 2004; Southam-Gerow, Weisz, & Kendall, 2003). Although some evidence suggests that comorbidity may not be relevant to outcome (e.g., Kendall, Brady, & Verduin, 2001; Southam-Gerow, Kendall, & Weersing, 2001), the levels of comorbidity in the samples of these studies are different from those found in typical service clinics (Southam-Gerow et al., 2003). Thus, for example, the robustness of CBT for anxiety disorders outside of university-based clinical settings is unknown (Chorpita et al., 2002).

A second and perhaps more vexing issue is that there are several other potentially important groups of variables to consider in disseminating interventions for anxiety to service settings, and we know very little about some of these variables. A model outlined by Schoenwald and Hoagwood (2001b) depicts several types of variables that should be considered in treatment development and adaptation, including (1) client, (2) provider, (3) agency, and (4) service system variables (see Figure 4.4; cf. Hoagwood, Burns, & Weisz, 2002). Although the importance of these variables may seem obvious, the fact remains that when treatments are developed, treatment developers rarely go beyond considering some (but probably not all) of the relevant client variables. In other words, a treatment developer's central focus is commonly on targeting a specific disorder or problem without considering other aspects of the child or family (e.g., family living situation, family preference for treatment modality). Historically, there has been comparatively little consideration of the provider, agency, or system in which that treatment might ultimately be expected to work.

In its defense, this treatment development approach has yielded much in the way of well-controlled empirical evidence on the effects of treatments in specific contexts with specific children/families. However, it is not without problems. For example, by focusing on a child's disorder only, one can ignore other potentially relevant variables at the client level. Comorbidity is one obvious example, as discussed above; other variables might include age, gender, and socioeconomic status. Another example might be client decision-making processes, including

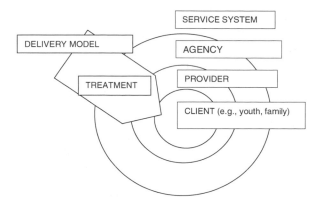

FIGURE 4.4. Framework for treatment development and adaptation, depicting the types of variables that need to be considered. From Schoenwald and Hoagwood (2001a). Copyright 2001 by Civic Research Institute. Adapted by permission.

consideration of client preference. Although the literature is only just emerging, there is some indication that the client decision-making processes and client preference may influence how well treatments will work (e.g., Lavori et al., 2001; Sherbourne, Sturm, & Wells, 1999). As a result, in some settings clinical researchers have developed decision-making aids to guide patients in their decisions, although so far this has been done only with adult samples (e.g., Rothert et al., 1997). Such components could be added to treatments for anxiety and may be particularly important for exposure treatments because of how fear-provoking they are.

In addition, as is reflected in Table 4.4, there is very little research that involves ethnic minority youths; Safren and colleagues (2000) have recently discussed this issue. Fortunately, most studies now report the ethnicity of the participants. Still, though, the vast majority of studies we reviewed involved solely or primarily European American participants. Although some work suggests that minority status is not related to treatment outcome (e.g., Silverman, Kurtines, Ginsburg, Weems, et al., 1999; Southam-Gerow et al., 2001), whether this finding will hold up outside research settings is unclear. This is particularly a concern, given that the percentage of ethnic minorities participating in the evidence base is generally lower than the percentage utilizing the service clinics (e.g., Southam-Gerow et al., 2003).

There are some reasons to suspect that consideration of ethnicity will be important in bringing treatments to scale in the community. As Safren and colleagues (2000) note in their review, minority families may be less likely to seek mental health services for a variety of reasons, including discomfort about sharing concerns with individuals outside their cultural group. Another issue relates back to client preference. Some research suggests that minority individuals have less favorable views about treatment, both medication and psychotherapy, than European Americans do (e.g., Chavira, Stein, Bailey, & Stein, 2003; McMiller & Weisz, 1996)—a fact that may explain the relative underutilization of mental health services by minority groups (e.g., Leslie et al., 2003; Paulose-Ram, Jonas, Orwig, & Safran, 2004). Some good recent progress has been made in testing assessment and treatments with diverse samples (e.g., Boyd, Ginsburg, Lambert, Cooley, & Campbell, 2003; Ginsburg & Drake, 2002; Lambert, Cooley, Campbell, Benoit, & Stansbury, 2004; Pina & Silverman, 2004), and more work along these lines is clearly needed.

In addition to these various client variables, myriad provider, agency, and service system variables may have an impact treatment outcome but are rarely studied in the context of childhood anxiety treatment. For example, at the provider level, we know from surveys that many clinicians find manualized treatments unattractive (e.g., Addis & Krasnow, 2000), and that exposure therapy in particular is viewed with resistance by many providers (e.g., Becker, Zayfert, & Anderson, 2004). One approach to bridge the science–practice gap would be to obtain feedback from these consumers of mental health treatment, make changes to treatment based on that input, and then test the outcome of those changes. Such a collaborative approach may increase the likelihood that an evidence-based treatment will have "staying power" in an agency after a researcher has left at the end of a study (e.g., Hoagwood et al., 2002).

Agency and systemic factors may also have an impact on a treatment, despite the fact that they are rarely considered in the development and adaptation of mental health interventions. In fact, most of our interventions were developed in settings with almost none of the same contextual influences that are found in most service settings, such as financial considerations (e.g., clients must pay fees, the clinic must pay rent and its employees), issues of employee retention, and issues of third-party oversight (e.g., insurance company auditors must review claims for treatment). In addition, Glisson and colleagues have spent more than a decade documenting the importance of organizational culture and climate for mental health services outcomes (Glisson, 2002; Glisson & Hemmelgarn, 1998; Hohmann & Shear, 2002; Schoenwald & Hoagwood, 2001b). Because a potentially powerful intervention could be rendered ineffective in the wrong culture or climate, treatment researchers ignore these variables at their peril.

Flexibility and Prescription

Weisz (2004) has recently outlined a model suggesting that optimum intervention design requires evolution of a protocol, based on the interplay between the intervention program and the context in which it is to be deployed. Consistent with the comments above, Weisz makes a case for the idea that adaptation of psychological interventions is critical to their uptake and effectiveness in clinical contexts. However, minimal research exists to date to suggest what types of adaptations are needed, and which adaptations might threaten the efficacy of a protocol.

Nevertheless, one model for adaptation has emerged, based on the model of matching intervention components to specific aspects of a child's problem. Such efforts, referred to as "prescriptive" treatment approaches, have been examined among children diagnosed with GAD (Eisen & Silverman, 1998) and among children exhibiting school refusal behaviors (Kearney & Silverman, 1990).

In one investigation examining the utility of prescribing or matching treatment approaches to children's presenting diagnostic features, Eisen and Silverman (1998) applied one of two treatment approaches to children diagnosed with GAD. For those children presenting with primarily cognitive features of GAD, a cognitive response class treatment was provided; for those children presenting with primarily somatic symptoms of GAD, a somatic response class treatment was implemented. Results indicated that although both prescriptive and nonprescriptive treatments yielded improvements in symptomatic presentation across several outcome measures, treatments that were prescribed for or matched with client characteristics resulted in greater improvements over a shorter period of time (Eisen & Silverman, 1998). These findings suggest the importance of prescribing treatments targeting specific symptom areas, rather than providing a standardized treatment package on the basis of a child's diagnosis alone. Given that all of the treatment components applied by Eisen and Silverman for both cognitive and somatic aspects of GAD were active treatments, it is not surprising that both types of treatment yielded beneficial effects, even when they were not explicitly prescribed. However, it is of note that the children in this study demonstrated improvements when administered only one prescribed treatment component, and did not appear to suffer consequences as a result of the omission of the nonprescriptive treatment component.

Similar findings were obtained in a related examination of the application of prescriptive treatments on the basis of specific client characteristics, conducted by Kearney and Silverman (1990) with anxious children demonstrating school refusal behavior. The prescription of treatment approaches designed to target each client's specific reasons for not attending school were found to result in meaningful improvements in school attendance, anxiety, depression, and overall distress levels in those children investigated (Kearney & Silverman, 1993). More recent research has lent support to this model—in particular, by showing that anxiety is particularly correlated with functional profiles involving negative reinforcement (e.g., Higa, Daleiden, & Chorpita, 2002).

Thus, although more research needs to be done, at least one possible adaptation that could characterize future developments in anxiety interventions involves this property of flexibility and prescription. At the same time, although some of the literature is quite positive regarding prescriptive strategies (e.g., Eisen & Silverman, 1998), there is some evidence that flexibility in interventions implicitly harbors possible risks (e.g., Schulte, Kunzel, Pepping, & Schute-Bahrenberg, 1992), and debates on both sides of the flexibility controversy (e.g., Jacobson et al., 1989; Persons, 1991; Wilson, 1996) cause us to ponder the challenges associated with prescription at the level of specific individuals. Given the implications for appeal to clinicians and for addressing comorbidity, we hope that future research will provide clearer answers regarding this issue.

Modularity in Design

In an effort to provide a more generalized model of adaptability for different contexts, Chorpita, Daleiden, and Weisz (2005b) have outlined concepts related to the "modular design" of psychotherapy. In short, this term refers to the notion that strategies within protocols can be packaged in such a way that they can be rearranged, omitted, extended, or selectively combined. Thus, with a modular intervention, it is possible to adjust or scale the content (i.e., which modules are used), the treatment duration, and the pace. For example, one youth might receive 16 sessions of exposure; another might receive 5 sessions. One youth might be administered a time-out program in the context of the anxiety treatment; others might not. Although one advantage of modularity is its suitability to adaptation and scaling for applied contexts, a detailed understanding of how to arrange and select modules to form a suitable intervention awaits considerable additional research. Nevertheless, early tests of this approach using simplified, rational rules for module selection show early promise (Chorpita, Daleiden, et al., 2005b).

Important Components of CBT

Yet another issue that warrants investigation regarding the treatment of childhood anxiety involves improved understanding of the important components of interventions. Although it appears that phobias are more commonly treated with streamlined interventions (exposure, modeling, perhaps one more technique),

generalized, social, and other anxiety areas have typically been treated with a larger number of clinical strategies.

Some evidence points to the idea that exposure may be a rather critical component in these interventions. For example, in an investigation of the additive effects of treatment components implemented with two children exhibiting nighttime fears, Ollendick, Hagopian, and Huntzinger (1991) utilized a multiple-baseline design across subjects, in which two different treatment components were sequentially applied. Subsequent to the introduction of a combination of cognitive techniques, including self-induced relaxation, self-monitoring, and verbal self-instruction, reinforcement contingencies were implemented for an increase in exposure to the feared situation. Treatment effects were observed to commence upon the introduction of reinforcement contingencies for heightened levels of exposure to the targeted situation (Ollendick et al., 1991). Another source of support for exposure as a critical component in anxiety interventions can be ascertained from an RCT of CBT (Kendall et al., 1997). In this investigation, children were treated sequentially with two treatment components: a cognitive–educational treatment component, followed by an enactive exposure treatment component. Analyses of midtreatment data revealed no significant treatment effects across child or parent indicators, suggesting that the cognitive–educational treatment component, in isolation, was not responsible for any observed differences between the treatment and the waitlist control groups. Differences between groups only emerged after the onset of exposure in the CBT protocol.

Neither of these examples represents the type of prospective dismantling study that would be required to address questions regarding active treatment components, nor was either study intended to do so. Such inferences are indeed challenging, given that some components of treatment (e.g., cognitive therapy) might exert later effects on other parts of therapy (e.g., exposure). Aside from interaction among treatment components, other possibilities—such as client–treatment interaction (Kiesler, 1966) and component order effects (Hayes, Barlow, & Nelson-Gray, 1999)—offer a multiplicity of confounds. At this time, we appear to know a lot more about what works for childhood fears and anxieties than we know about why those interventions work, as has been the case in the treatment outcome literature more generally (e.g., Kazdin, 2003).

Interestingly, the tradition of treating fear and anxiety in youths began with a rather unitary approach to the constructs, offering one or two strategies for treating all manifestations of anxiety. As the field grew, and the nosology of anxiety and its disorders diversified, interventions became increasingly complex and differentiated. Given some of the recent integration noted at the beginning of this chapter, and the advent of a hierarchical understanding of anxiety disorders in youths (i.e., multiple specific syndromes influenced by a general higher-order risk factor), one wonders whether there might be a return to more focused or simplified interventions. Barlow, Allen, and Choate (2004) have very recently proposed a compelling argument along these lines, in which streamlined interventions of the future might target an underlying "negative affect syndrome." In the context of some of the dissemination issues raised above, perhaps simpler interventions that can address many targets, while requiring the learning of only a few skills, will be a central part of the next generation of treatments. Then again, perhaps more complex, flexible, or prescriptive interventions that can adapt to client and setting characteristics will rule the day. Fortunately, thanks to over a generation of dedicated anxiety researchers, there is already an enormous empirical platform upon which to build. It will be interesting to see how treatment development in this area continues to unfold, and to see what new promises it brings.

ACKNOWLEDGMENTS

Preparation of this chapter was supported in part through a grant from the Hawaii Department of Health and through the Research Network on Youth Mental Health, sponsored by the John D. and Catherine T. MacArthur Foundation. We would like to thank Susan Bush, Alicia Emerson, Candice Lau, Kathryn Taylor, and John Young for their assistance with materials for this chapter.

REFERENCES

Abramowitz, J. S. (1996). Variants of exposure and response prevention in the treatment of obsessive–compulsive disorder. *Behavior Therapy, 27,* 583–600.

Achenbach, T. M., & Rescorla, L. A. (2001). *Manual for the ASEBA school-age forms and profiles.* Burlington: University of Vermont, Research Center for Children, Youth, and Families.

Ackerman, D. L., & Greenland, S. (2002). Multivariate meta-analysis of controlled drug studies for obsessive–compulsive disorder. *Journal of Clinical Psychopharmacology, 22,* 309–317.

Addis, M. E., & Krasnow, A. D. (2000). A national survey of practicing psychologists' attitudes toward psychotherapy treatment manuals. *Journal of Consulting and Clinical Psychology, 68,* 331–339.

Albano, A. M., Chorpita, B. F., & Barlow, D. H. (2003). Childhood anxiety disorders. In E. J. Mash & R. A. Barkley (Eds.), *Child psychopathology* (2nd ed., pp. 279–329). New York: Guilford Press.

American Psychiatric Association. (2000). *Diagnostic and statistical manual of mental disorders* (4th ed., text rev.). Washington, DC: Author.

American Psychological Association(APA) Task Force on Psychological Intervention Guidelines. (1995). *Template for developing guidelines: Interventions for mental disorders and psychosocial aspects of physical disorders.* Washington, DC: APA.

Anastasi, A., & Urbina, S. (1997). *Psychological testing* (7th ed.). Upper Saddle River, NJ: Prentice Hall.

Anderson, J. C. (1994). Epidemiology. In T. H. Ollendick, N. J. King, & W. Yule (Eds.), *International handbook of phobic and anxiety disorders in children and adolescents* (pp. 293–315). New York: Plenum Press.

Andrews, W. R. (1971). Behavioral and client-centered counseling of high school underachievers. *Journal of Counseling Psychology, 18,* 93–96.

Angold, A., Costello, E. J., & Erkanli, A. (1999). Comorbidity. *Journal of Child Psychology and Psychiatry, 40,* 57–87.

Bandura, A. (1969). *Principles of behavior modification.* New York: Holt, Rinehart & Winston.

Bandura, A. (1977). *Social learning theory.* Englewood Cliffs, NJ: Prentice-Hall.

Bandura, A. (1978). Reflections on self-efficacy. *Advances in Behaviour Research and Therapy, 1,* 237–269.

Bandura, A. (1982). Self-efficacy mechanism in human agency. *American Psychologist, 37,* 122–147.

Bandura, A., Blanchard, E. B., & Ritter, B. (1969). Relative efficacy of desensitization and modeling approaches for inducing behavioral, affective, and attitudinal changes. *Journal of Personality and Social Psychology, 13,* 173–199.

Bandura, A., Grusec, J. E., & Menlove, F. L. (1967). Vicarious extinction of avoidance behavior. *Journal of Personality and Social Psychology, 5,* 16–23.

Bandura, A., & Menlove, F. L. (1968). Factors determining vicarious extinction of avoidance behavior through symbolic modeling. *Journal of Personality and Social Psychology, 3,* 99–108.

Barabasz, A. F. (1973). Group desensitization of test anxiety in elementary school. *Journal of Psychology, 83,* 295–301.

Barkley, R. A. (1997). *Defiant children: A clinician's manual for assessment and parent training* (2nd ed.). New York: Guilford Press.

Barlow, D. H. (1988). *Anxiety and its disorders: The nature and treatment of anxiety and panic.* New York: Guilford Press.

Barlow, D. H. (2002). *Anxiety and its disorders: The nature and treatment of anxiety and panic* (2nd ed.). New York: Guilford Press.

Barlow, D. H., Allen, L. B., & Choate, M. L. (2004). Toward a unified treatment for emotional disorders. *Behavior Therapy, 35,* 205–230.

Barlow, D. H., Chorpita, B. F., & Turovsky, J. (1996). Fear, panic, anxiety, and the disorders of emotion. In D. A. Hope (Ed.), *Nebraska Symposium on Motivation: Vol. 43. Perspectives on anxiety, panic, and fear* (pp. 251–328). Lincoln: University of Nebraska Press.

Barrett, P. M. (1998). Evaluation of cognitive-behavioral group treatments for childhood anxiety disorders. *Journal of Clinical Child Psychology, 27,* 459–468.

Barrett, P. M., Dadds, M. R., & Rapee, R. M. (1996). Family treatment of childhood anxiety: A controlled trial. *Journal of Consulting and Clinical Psychology, 64,* 333–342.

Barrett, P. M., Duffy, A. L., Dadds, M. R., & Rapee, R. M. (2001). Cognitive-behavioral treatment of anxiety disorders in children: Long-term (6-year) follow-up. *Journal of Consulting and Clinical Psychology, 69,* 135–141.

Barrett, P. M., Healy-Farrell, L., & March, J. S. (2004). Cognitive-behavioral family treatment of childhood obsessive–compulsive disorder: A controlled trial. *Journal of the American Academy of Child and Adolescent Psychiatry, 43,* 46–62.

Barrios, B. A., & O'Dell, S. L. (1998). Fears and anxieties. In E. J. Mash & R. A. Barkley (Eds.), *Treatment of childhood disorders* (2nd ed., pp. 249–337). New York: Guilford Press.

Beck, A. T., & Emery, G., with Greenberg, R. L. (1985). *Anxiety disorders and phobias: A cognitive perspective.* New York: Basic Books.

Beck, A. T., Rush, A. J., Shaw, B. F., & Emery, G. (1979). *Cognitive therapy of depression.* New York: Guilford Press.

Becker, C. B., Zayfert, C., & Anderson, E. (2004). A survey of psychologists' attitudes towards and utilization of exposure therapy for PTSD. *Behaviour Research and Therapy, 42,* 277–292.

Beidel, D. C., Turner, S. M., & Morris, T. L. (2000). Behavioral treatment of childhood social phobia. *Journal of Consulting and Clinical Psychology, 68,* 1072–1080.

Bell-Dolan, D. J. (1995). Social cue interpretation of anxious children. *Journal of Clinical Child Psychology, 24,* 2–10.

Bell-Dolan, D. J., Last, C. G., & Strauss, C. C. (1990). Symptoms of anxiety disorders in normal children. *Journal of the American Academy of Child and Adolescent Psychiatry, 29,* 759–765.

Bell-Dolan, D. J., & Wessler, A. E. (1994). Attributional style of anxious children: Extensions from cognitive theory and research on adult anxiety. *Journal of Anxiety Disorders, 8,* 79–96.

Bentler, P. M. (1962). An infant's phobia treated with reciprocal inhibition therapy. *Journal of Child Psychology and Psychiatry, 3,* 185–189.

Bernstein, G. A., & Borchardt, C. M. (1991). Anxiety disorders of childhood and adolescence: A critical review. *Journal of the American Academy of Child and Adolescent Psychiatry, 30,* 519–532.

Bernstein, G. A., & Kinlan, J. (1997). Summary of the practice parameters for the assessment and treatment of children and adolescents with anxiety disorders. *Journal of the American Academy of Child and Adolescent Psychiatry, 36,* 1639–1641.

Biglan, A. (1987). A behavior-analytic critique of Bandura's self-efficacy theory. *Behavior Analyst, 10,* 1–15.

Bird, H. R., Gould, M. S., & Staghezza, B. M. (1993). Patterns of diagnostic comorbidity in a community sample of children aged 9 through 16 years. *Journal of the American Academy of Child and Adolescent Psychiatry, 32,* 361–368.

Birmaher, B., Axelson, D. A., Monk, K., Kalas, C., Clark, D. B., Ehmann, M., et al. (2003). Fluoxetine for the treatment of childhood anxiety disorders. *Journal of the American Academy of Child and Adolescent Psychiatry, 42*(4), 415–423.

Birmaher, B., Khetarpal, S., Brent, D., Cully, M., Balach, L., Kaufman, J., et al. (1997). The Screen for Child Anxiety Related Emotional Disorders (SCARED): Scale construction and psychometric characteristics. *Journal of American Academy of Child and Adolescent Psychiatry, 36,* 545–553.

Blanchard, E. B. (1970). Relative contributions of modeling, informational influences, and physical contact in extinction of phobic behavior. *Journal of Abnormal Psychology, 76,* 55–61.

Borkovec, T. S., Shadick, R., & Hopkins, M. (1991). The nature of normal and pathological worry. In R. M. Rapee & D. H. Barlow (Eds.), *Chronic anxiety: Generalized anxiety disorder and mixed anxiety–depression.* New York: Guilford Press.

Bornstein, P. H., & Knapp, M. (1981). Self-control desensitization with a multi-phobic boy: A multiple baseline design. *Journal of Behavior Therapy and Experimental Psychiatry, 12,* 281–285.

Boyd, R. C., Ginsburg, G. S., Lambert, S. F., Cooley, M. R., & Campbell, K. D. M. (2003). Screen for Child Anxiety Related Emotional Disorders (SCARED): Psychometric Properties in an African-American parochial high school sample. *Journal of the American Academy of Child and Adolescent Psychiatry, 42,* 1188–1196.

Brooks, V. B. (1986). How does the limbic system assist motor learning?: A limbic comparator hypothesis. *Brain, Behavior, and Evolution, 29,* 29–53.

Brown, T. A., Chorpita, B. F., & Barlow, D. H. (1998). Structural relationships among dimensions of the

DSM-IV anxiety and mood disorders and dimensions of negative affect, positive affect, and autonomic arousal. *Journal of Abnormal Psychology, 107,* 179–192.

Caspi, A., Elder, G. H., & Bem, D. J. (1988). Moving away from the world: Life-course patterns of shy children. *Developmental Psychology, 24,* 824–831.

Chambless, D. L., & Hollon, S. D. (1998). Defining empirically supported therapies. *Journal of Consulting and Clinical Psychology, 66,* 7–18.

Chavira, D. A., Stein, M. B., Bailey, K., & Stein, M. T. (2003). Parental opinions regarding treatment for social anxiety disorder in youth. *Journal of Developmental and Behavioral Pediatrics, 24,* 315–322.

Chorpita, B. F. (2001). Control and the development of negative emotions. In M. W. Vasey & M. R. Dadds (Eds.), *The developmental psychopathology of anxiety* (pp. 112–142). New York: Oxford University Press.

Chorpita, B. F. (2003). The frontier of evidence-based practice. In A. E. Kazdin & J. R. Weisz (Eds.), *Evidence-based psychotherapies for children and adolescents* (pp. 42–59). New York: Guilford Press.

Chorpita, B. F., Albano, A. M., & Barlow, D. H. (1996). Cognitive processing in children: Relationship to anxiety and family influences. *Journal of Clinical Child Psychology, 25,* 170–176.

Chorpita, B. F., Albano, A. M., & Barlow, D. H. (1998). The structure of negative emotions in a clinical sample of children and adolescents. *Journal of Abnormal Psychology, 107,* 74–85.

Chorpita, B. F., & Barlow, D. H. (1998). The development of anxiety: The role of control in the early environment. *Psychological Bulletin, 117,* 3–19.

Chorpita, B. F., & Daleiden, E. L. (2002). Tripartite dimensions of emotion in a child clinical sample: Measurement strategies and implications for clinical utility. *Journal of Consulting and Clinical Psychology, 70,* 1150–1160.

Chorpita, B. F., Daleiden, E., & Weisz, J. R. (2005a). Identifying and selecting the common elements of evidence based interventions: A distillation and matching model. *Mental Health Services Research, 7,* 5–20.

Chorpita, B. F., Daleiden, E., & Weisz, J. R. (2005b). Modularity in the design and application of therapeutic interventions. *Applied and Preventive Psychology, 11,* 141–156.

Chorpita, B. F., & Lilienfeld, S. O. (1999). Clinical assessment of anxiety sensitivity in children: Where do we go from here? *Psychological Assessment, 11,* 212–224.

Chorpita, B. F., Moffitt, C. E., & Gray, J. A. (2005). Psychometric properties of the Revised Child Anxiety and Depression Scale in a clinical sample. *Behaviour Research and Therapy, 43,* 309–322.

Chorpita, B. F., Plummer, C. M., & Moffitt, C. E. (2000). Relations of tripartite dimensions of emotion to childhood anxiety and mood disorders. *Journal of Abnormal Child Psychology, 28,* 299–310.

Chorpita, B. F., Taylor, A. A., Francis, S. E., Moffitt, C. E., & Austin, A. A. (2004). Efficacy of modular cog-nitive behavior therapy for childhood anxiety disorders. *Behavior Therapy, 35,* 263–287.

Chorpita, B. F., Vitali, A. E., & Barlow, D. H. (1997). Behavioral treatment of choking phobia in an adolescent: An experimental analysis. *Journal of Behavior Therapy and Experimental Psychiatry, 28,* 307–315.

Chorpita, B. F., Yim, L. M., Donkervoet, J. C., Arensdorf, A., Amundsen, M. J., McGee, C., et al. (2002). Toward large-scale implementation of empirically supported treatments for children: A review and observations by the Hawaii Empirical Basis to Services Task Force. *Clinical Psychology: Science and Practice, 9,* 165–190.

Chorpita, B. F., Yim, L. M., Moffitt, C. E., Umemoto, L. A., & Francis, S. E. (2000). Assessment of symptoms of DSM-IV anxiety and depression in children: A Revised Child Anxiety and Depression Scale. *Behaviour Research and Therapy, 38,* 835–855.

Clark, D. A., Sugrin, I., & Bolton, D. (1982). Primary obsessional slowness: A nursing treatment programme with a 13-year-old male adolescent. *Behaviour Research and Therapy, 20,* 289–292.

Clark, L. A. (1989). Depressive and anxiety disorders: Descriptive psychopathology and differential diagnosis. In P. C. Kendall & D. Watson (Eds.), *Anxiety and depression: Distinctive and overlapping features* (pp. 83–129). New York: Academic Press.

Clark, L. A., & Watson, D. (1991). A tripartite model of anxiety and depression: Psychometric evidence and taxonomic implications. *Journal of Abnormal Psychology, 100,* 316–336.

Clark, L. A., Watson, D., & Mineka, S. (1994). Temperament, personality, and the mood and anxiety disorders. *Journal of Abnormal Psychology, 103,* 103–116.

Clement, P. W., & Milne, D. C. (1967). Group play therapy and tangible reinforcers used to modify the behavior of 8-year-old boys. *Behaviour Research and Therapy, 5,* 301–312.

Cobham, V. E., Dadds, M. R., & Spence, S. H. (1998). The role of parental anxiety in the treatment of childhood anxiety. *Journal of Consulting and Clinical Psychology, 66,* 893–905.

Coghill, D. (2002). Evidence-based psychopharmacology for children and adolescents. *Child and Adolescent Psychiatry, 15*(4), 361–368.

Cohen, J. A., Deblinger, E., Mannarino, A. P., & Steer, R. A. (2004). A multisite, randomized controlled trial for children with sexual abuse-related PTSD symptoms. *Journal of the American Academy of Child and Adolescent Psychiatry, 43*(4), 393–402.

Cohen, J. A., & Mannarino, A. P. (1996). A treatment outcome study for sexually abused preschool children: Initial findings. *Journal of the American Academy of Child and Adolescent Psychiatry, 35,* 42–50.

Cole, D. A., Martin, J. M., Peeke, L. A., Seroczynski, A. D., & Fier, J. (1999). Children's over- and underestimation of academic competence: A longitudinal study of gender differences, depression, and anxiety. *Child Development, 70,* 459–473.

Compton, S. N., Grant, P. J., Chrisman, A. K., Gammon, P. J., Brown, V. L., & March, J. S. (2001). Sertraline in children and adolescents with social anxiety disorder: An open trial. *Journal of the American Academy of Child and Adolescent Psychiatry, 40*(5), 564–571.

Cornwall, E., Spence, S. H., & Schotte, D. (1996). The effectiveness of emotive imagery in the treatment of darkness phobia in children. *Behaviour Change, 13,* 223–229.

Costello, E. J., Angold, A., & Keeler, G. P. (1999). Adolescent outcomes of childhood disorders: The consequences of severity and impairment. *Journal of the American Academy of Child and Adolescent Psychiatry, 38,* 121–128.

Cradock, C., Cotler, S., & Jason, L. A. (1978). Primary prevention: Immunization of children for speech anxiety. *Cognitive Therapy and Research, 2,* 289–296.

Craske, M. G. (1999). *Anxiety disorders: Psychological approaches to theory and treatment.* Boulder, CO: Westview Press.

Dadds, M. R., Holland, D. E., Laurens, K. R., Mullins, M., Barrett, P. M., & Spence, S. H. (1999). Early intervention and prevention of anxiety disorders in children: Results at 2-year follow-up. *Journal of Consulting and Clinical Psychology, 67,* 145–150.

Dadds, M. R., Spence, S. H., Holland, D. E., & Barrett, P. M. (1997). Prevention and early intervention for anxiety disorders: A controlled trial. *Journal of Consulting and Clinical Psychology, 65,* 627–635.

Dahlquist, L. M., Gil, K. M., Armstrong, F. D., Ginsberg, A., & Jones B. (1985). Behavioral management of children's distress during chemotherapy. *Journal of Behavior Therapy and Experimental Psychiatry, 16,* 325–329.

Dalgleish, T., Taghavi, R., Neshat-Doost, H., Moradi, A., Canterbury, R., & Yule, W. (2003). Patterns of processing bias for emotional information across clinical disorders: A comparison of attention, memory, and prospective cognition in children and adolescents with depression, generalized anxiety, and posttraumatic stress disorder. *Journal of Clinical Child and Adolescent Psychology, 32*(1), 10–21.

D'Amato, M. R. (1970). *Experimental psychology: Methodology, psychophysics, and learning.* New York: McGraw-Hill.

Davis, A. F., Rosenthal, T. L., & Kelley, J. E. (1981). Actual fear cues, prompt therapy, and rationale enhance participant modeling with adolescents. *Behavior Therapy, 12,* 536–542.

Deblinger, E., & Heflin, A. H. (1996). *Treating sexually abused children and their nonoffending parents: A cognitive behavioral approach.* Thousand Oaks, CA: Sage.

Deblinger, E., McLeer, S. V., & Henry, D. (1990). Cognitive behavioral treatment for sexually abused children suffering post-traumatic stress: Preliminary findings. *Journal of the American Academy of Child and Adolescent Psychiatry, 29,* 747–752.

Deblinger, E., Steer, R. A., & Lippmann, J. (1999). Two-year follow-up study of cognitive behavioral therapy for sexually abused children suffering post-traumatic stress symptoms. *Child Abuse and Neglect, 23*(12), 1371–1378.

Deffenbacher, J. L., & Kemper, C. C. (1974). Counseling test-anxious sixth graders. *Elementary School Guidance and Counseling, 21,* 23–29.

De Haan, E., Hoogduin, K., Buitelaar, J. K., & Keijsers, G. P. J. (1998). Behavior therapy versus clomipramine for the treatment of obsessive–compulsive disorder in children and adolescents. *Journal of the American Academy of Child and Adolescent Psychiatry, 37,* 1022–1029.

Delprato, D. J., & McGlynn, F. D. (1984). Behavioral theories of anxiety disorders. In S. M. Turner (Ed.), *Behavioral theories and treatment of anxiety* (pp. 1–49). New York: Plenum Press.

De Rosier, M. E. (2004). Building relationships and combating bullying: Effectiveness of a school-based social skills group intervention. *Journal of Clinical Child and Adolescent Psychology, 33,* 196–201.

deRoss, R., Chorpita, B. F., & Gullone, E. (2002). The Revised Child Anxiety and Depression Scale: A psychometric investigation with Australian youth. *Behaviour Change, 19,* 90–101.

Donovan C. L., & Spence S. H. (2000). Prevention of childhood anxiety disorders. *Clinical Psychology Review, 20,* 509–531.

Dougherty, D. D., Rauch, S. L., & Jenike, M. A. (2004). Pharmacotherapy for obsessive–compulsive disorder. *Journal of Clinical Psychology, 60,* 1195–1202.

Eastman, C., & Marzillier, J. S. (1984). Theoretical and methodological difficulties in Bandura's self-efficacy theory. *Cognitive Therapy and Research, 8,* 213–229.

Eisen, A. R., & Silverman, W. K. (1998). Prescriptive treatment for generalized anxiety disorder in children. *Behavior Therapy, 29,* 105–121.

Eysenck, H. J. (1979). The conditioning model of neurosis. *Behavioral and Brain Sciences, 2*(2), 155–199.

Farrell, S. P., Hains, A. A., & Davies, W. H. (1998). Cognitive behavioral interventions for sexually abused children exhibiting PTSD symptomatology. *Behavior Therapy, 29,* 241–255.

Faust, J., & Melamed, B. G. (1984). Influence of arousal, previous experience, and age on surgery preparation of same day of surgery and in-hospital pediatric patients. *Journal of Consulting and Clinical Psychology, 52,* 359–365.

Faust, J., Olson, R., & Rodriguez, H. (1991). Same-day surgery preparation: Reduction of pediatric patient arousal and distress through participant modeling. *Journal of Consulting and Clinical Psychology, 59,* 475–478.

Fergusson, D. M., Horwood, L. J., & Lynskey, M. T. (1993) Prevalence and comorbidity of DSM-III-R diagnoses in a birth cohort of 15 year olds. *Journal of the American Academy of Child and Adolescent Psychiatry, 32,* 1127–1134.

Flannery-Schroeder, E. C., & Kendall, P. C. (2000). Group and individual cognitive-behavioral treatments for youth with anxiety disorders: A randomized clinical trial. *Cognitive Therapy and Research, 24,* 251–278.

Foa, E. B., & Kozak, M. J. (1986). Emotional processing of fear: Exposure to corrective information. *Psychological Bulletin, 99,* 20–35.

Foa, E. B., Steketee, G., Grayson, B., Turner, M., & Latimer, P. (1984). Deliberate exposure and blocking of obsessive–compulsive rituals: Immediate and longterm effects. *Behavior Therapy, 15,* 450–472.

Francis, S. E., Gray, J. A., & Chorpita, B. F. (2000, November). *Measurement of functional impairment in children with internalizing and externalizing disorders.* Paper presented at the annual meeting of the Association for Advancement of Behavior Therapy, New Orleans, LA.

Franklin, M. E., Kozak, M. J., Cashman, L. A., Coles, M. E., Rheingold, A. A., & Foa, E. B. (1998). Cognitive-behavioral treatment of pediatric obsessive–compulsive disorder: An open clinical trial. *Journal of the American Academy of Child and Adolescent Psychiatry, 37*(4), 412–419.

Freud, S. (1955). Two case studies. In J. Strachey (Ed. & Trans.), *The standard edition of the complete works of Sigmund Freud* (Vol. 10, pp. 5–318). London: Hogarth Press. (Original work published 1909)

Gallagher, H. M., Rabian, B. A., & McCloskey, M. S. (2004). A brief group cognitive-behavioral intervention for social phobia in childhood. *Journal of Anxiety Disorders, 18,* 459–479.

Geer, J. H., Davison, G. C., & Gatchel, R. I. (1970). Reduction of stress in humans through nonveridical perceived control of aversive stimulation. *Journal of Personality and Social Psychology, 16,* 731–738.

Geller, D. A., Biederman, J., Stewart, S. E., Mullin, B., Martin, A., Spencer, T., et al. (2003). Which SSRI?: A meta-analysis of pharmacotherapy trials in pediatric obsessive–compulsive disorder. *American Journal of Psychiatry, 160,* 1919–1928.

Geller, D. A., Hoog, S., Heiligenstein, J. H., Ricardi, R. K., Tamura, R., Kluszynski, S., et al. (2001). Fluoxetine treatment for obsessive–compulsive disorder in children and adolescents: A placebo-controlled clinical trial. *Journal of the American Academy of Child and Adolescent Psychiatry, 40*(7), 773–779.

Genshaft, J. L. (1982). The use of cognitive behavior therapy for reducing math anxiety. *School Psychology Review, 11,* 32–34.

Genshaft, J. L., & Hirt, M. L. (1980). The effectiveness of self-instructional training to enhance math achievement in women. *Cognitive Therapy and Research, 4,* 91–97.

Gilbert, B. O., Johnson, S. B., Spillar, R., McCallum, M., Silverstein, J. H., & Rosenbloom, A. (1982). The effects of a peer modeling film on children learning to self-inject insulin. *Behavior Therapy, 13,* 186–193.

Gillett, E. (2001). Signal anxiety from the adaptive point of view. *Psychoanalytic Psychology, 18,* 268–286.

Ginsburg, G. S., & Drake, K. L. (2002). School-based treatment for anxious African-American adolescents: A controlled pilot study. *Journal of the American Academy of Child and Adolescent Psychiatry, 41,* 768–775.

Ginsburg, G. S., Silverman, W. K., & Kurtines, W. M. (1995). Family involvement in treating children with phobic and anxiety disorders: A look ahead. *Clinical Psychology Review, 15,* 457–473.

Gladstone, T. R. G., & Kaslow, N. J. (1995). Depression and attributions in children and adolescents: A metaanalytic review. *Journal of Abnormal Child Psychology, 3,* 597–606.

Glisson, C. (2002). The organizational context of children's mental health services. *Clinical Child and Family Psychology Review, 5,* 233–253.

Glisson, C., & Hemmelgarn, A. (1998). The effects of organizational climate and interorganizational coordination on the quality and outcomes of children's service systems. *Child Abuse and Neglect, 22,* 401–421.

Goenjian, A. K., Karayan, I., Pynoos, R. S., Minassian, D., Najarian, L. M., Steinberg, A. M., et al. (1997). Outcome of psychotherapy among early adolescents after trauma. *American Journal of Psychiatry, 154,* 536–542.

Goodwin, R., Gould, M. S., Blanco, C., & Olfson, M. (2001). Prescription of psychotropic medications to youths in office-based practice. *Psychiatric Services, 52,* 1081–1087.

Gray, J. A. (1982). *The neuropsychology of anxiety.* New York: Oxford University Press.

Gray, J. A. (1987). *The psychology of fear and stress* (2nd ed.). Cambridge, UK: Cambridge University Press.

Gray, J. A., & McNaughton, N. (1996). The neuropsychology of anxiety: Reprise. In D. A. Hope (Ed.), *Nebraska Symposium on Motivation, 1995: Perspectives on anxiety, panic, and fear* (pp. 61–134). Lincoln: University of Nebraska Press.

Graziano, A. M., & Mooney, K. C. (1980). Family self-control instruction for children's nighttime fear reduction. *Journal of Consulting and Clinical Psychology, 48,* 206–213.

Gresham, F. M., & Nagle, R. J. (1980). Social skills training with children: Responsiveness to modeling and coaching as a function of peer orientation. *Journal of Consulting and Clinical Psychology, 48,* 718–729.

Harris, K. R., & Brown, R. D. (1982). Cognitive behavior modification and informed teacher treatments for shy children. *Journal of Experimental Education, 50,* 137–143.

Hayes, S. C., Barlow, D. H., & Nelson-Gray, R. O. (1999). *The scientist practitioner: Research and accountability in the age of managed care.* Boston: Allyn & Bacon.

Henin, A., & Kendall, P. C. (1997). Obsessive–compulsive disorder in childhood and adolescence. *Advances in Clinical Child Psychology, 19,* 75–131.

Heyne, D., King, N. J., Tonge, B. J., Rollings, S., Young, D., Pritchard, M., et al. (2002). Evaluation of child therapy and caregiver training in the treatment of school refusal. *Journal of the American Academy of Child and Adolescent Psychiatry, 41,* 687–695.

Higa, C. K., Daleiden, E. L., & Chorpita, B. F. (2002).

Assessing school refusal behavior: Psychometric properties and clinical utility of the School Refusal Assessment Scale (SRAS). *Journal of Psychopathology and Behavior Assessment, 24,* 247–258.

Hill, J. H., Liebert, R. M., & Mott, D. E. W. (1968). Vicarious extinction of avoidance behavior through films: An initial test. *Psychological Reports, 22,* 192.

Hoagwood, K., Burns, B. J., Kiser, L., Ringeisen, H., & Schoenwald, S. K. (2001). Evidence-based practice in child and adolescent mental health services. *Psychiatric Services, 52,* 1179–1189.

Hoagwood, K., Burns, B. J., & Weisz, J. R. (2002). A profitable conjunction: From science to service in children's mental health. In B. J. Burns & K. Hoagwood (Eds.), *Community treatment for youth: Evidence-based interventions for severe emotional and behavioral disorders* (pp. 327–338). New York: Oxford University Press.

Hoagwood, K., & Olin, S. (2002). The NIMH Blueprint for Change Report: Research priorities in child and adolescent mental health. *Journal of the American Academy of Child and Adolescent Psychiatry, 41,* 760–767.

Hodges, K., & Wong, M. M. (1996). Psychometric characteristics of a multidimensional measure to assess impairment: The Child and Adolescent Functional Assessment Scale. *Journal of Child and Family Studies, 5,* 445–467.

Hohmann, A. A., & Shear, M. K. (2002). Community-based intervention research: Coping with the "noise" of real life in study design. *American Journal of Psychiatry, 159,* 201–207.

Howard, B. L., & Kendall, P. C. (1996). Cognitive-behavioral family therapy for anxiety-disordered children: A multiple-baseline evaluation. *Cognitive Therapy and Research, 20,* 423–443.

Jacobson, N. S., Schmaling, K. B., Holtzworth-Munroe, A., Katt, J. L., Wood, L. E., & Follette, V. M. (1989). Research-structured versus clinically flexible versions of social learning-based marital therapy. *Behaviour Research and Therapy, 27,* 173–180.

Jersild, A. T., & Holmes, F. (Eds.). (1935). *Children's fears* (Child Development Monograph No. 20). New York: Columbia University Press.

Johnson, T., Tyler, V., Thompson, R., & Jones, E. (1971). Systematic desensitization and assertive training in the treatment of speech anxiety in middle-school students. *Psychology in the Schools, 8,* 263–267.

Joiner, T. E., Jr., Catanzaro, S. J., & Laurent, J. (1996). Tripartite structure of positive and negative affect, depression, and anxiety, in child psychiatric inpatients. *Journal of Abnormal Psychology, 105,* 401–409.

Jones, M. C. (1924a). The elimination of children's fears. *Journal of Experimental Psychology, 1,* 383–390.

Jones, M. C. (1924b). A laboratory study of fear: The case of Peter. *Pedagogical Seminar, 31,* 308–315.

Jones, R. T., Ollendick, T. H., McLaughlin, K. J., & Williams, C. E. (1989). Elaborative and behavioral rehearsal in the acquisition of fire emergency skills and the reduction of fear of fire. *Behavior Therapy, 20,* 93–101.

Kagan, J. (1997). Temperament and the reactions to unfamiliarity. *Child Development, 68,* 139–143.

Kagan, J., Snidman, N., Arcus, D., & Reznick, S. (1994). *Galen's prophecy: Temperament in human nature.* New York: Basic Books.

Kandel, H. J., Ayllon, T., & Rosenbaum, M. S. (1977). Flooding or systematic exposure in the treatment of extreme social withdrawal in children. *Journal of Behavior Therapy and Experimental Psychiatry, 8,* 75–81.

Kane, M. T., & Kendall, P. C. (1989). Anxiety disorders in children: A multiple-baseline evaluation of a cognitive-behavioral treatment. *Behavior Therapy, 20,* 499–508.

Kanfer, F. H., Karoly, P., & Newman, A. (1975). Reduction of children's fear of the dark by competence-related and situational threat-related verbal cues. *Journal of Consulting and Clinical Psychology, 43,* 251–258.

Kazdin, A. E. (2003). Psychotherapy for children and adolescents. *Annual Review of Psychology, 54,* 253–276.

Kazdin, A. E., & Bass, D. (1989). Power to detect differences between alternative treatments in comparative psychotherapy outcome research. *Journal of Consulting and Clinical Psychology, 57,* 138–147.

Kearney, C. A., & Silverman, W. K. (1990). A preliminary analysis of a functional model of assessment and treatment for school refusal behavior. *Behavior Modification, 14,* 340–366.

Kearney, C. A., & Silverman, W. K. (1993). Measuring the function of school refusal behavior: The School Refusal Assessment Scale. *Journal of Clinical Child Psychology, 22,* 85–96.

Kearney, C. A., & Silverman, W. K. (1998). A critical review of pharmacotherapy for youth with anxiety disorders: Things are not as they seem. *Journal of Anxiety Disorders, 12,* 83–102.

Keller, M. B., Lavori, P., Wunder, J., Beardslee, W. R., Schwartz, C. E., & Roth, J. (1992). Chronic course of anxiety disorders in children and adolescents. *Journal of the American Academy of Child and Adolescent Psychiatry, 31,* 595–599.

Keller, M. F., & Carlson, P. M. (1974). The use of symbolic modeling to promote social skills in preschool children with low levels of social responsiveness. *Child Development, 45,* 912–919.

Kendall, P. C. (1992). Childhood coping: Avoiding a lifetime of anxiety. *Behavioural Change, 9,* 1–8.

Kendall, P. C. (1994). Treating anxiety disorders in children: Results of a randomized clinical trial. *Journal of Consulting and Clinical Psychology, 62,* 100–110.

Kendall, P. C. (2002). *Coping Cat therapist manual.* Ardmore, PA: Workbook.

Kendall, P. C., Brady, E. U., & Verduin, T. L. (2001). Comorbidity in childhood anxiety disorders and treatment outcome. *Journal of the American Academy of Child and Adolescent Psychiatry, 40*(7), 787–794.

Kendall, P. C., Chansky, T. E., Kane, M. T., Kim, R., Kortlander, E., Ronan, K. R., et al. (1992). *Anxiety disorders in youth: Cognitive behavioral interventions.* Needham Heights, MA: Allyn & Bacon.

Kendall, P. C., Choudhury, M., Hudson, J., & Webb, A. (2002). *The C.A.T. Project workbook for the cognitive behavioral treatment of anxious adolescents.* Ardmore, PA: Workbook.

Kendall, P. C., Flannery-Schroeder, E., Panichelli-Mindel, S. M., Southam-Gerow, M., Henin, A., & Warman, M. (1997). Therapy for youths with anxiety disorders: A second randomized clinical trial. *Journal of Consulting and Clinical Psychology, 65,* 366–380.

Kendall, P. C., Kane, M., Howard, B., & Siqueland, L. (1990). *Cognitive-behavioral treatment of anxious children: Treatment manual.* Ardmore, PA: Workbook.

Kendall, P. C., & MacDonald, J. P. (1993). Cognition in the psychopathology of youth and implications for treatment. In K. S. Dobson & P. C. Kendall (Eds.), *Psychopathology and cognition* (pp. 387–427). San Diego, CA: Academic Press.

Kendall, P. C., Safford, S., Flannery-Schroeder, E., & Webb, A. (2004). Child anxiety treatment: Outcomes in adolescence and impact on substance use and depression at 7.4-year follow-up. *Journal of Consulting and Clinical Psychology, 72,* 276–287.

Kendall, P. C., & Southam-Gerow, M. A. (1996). Long-term follow-up of cognitive-behavioral therapy for anxiety-disordered youth. *Journal of Consulting and Clinical Psychology, 64,* 724–730.

Kendall, P. C., Stark, K. D., & Adam, T. (1990). Cognitive deficit or cognitive distortion of childhood depression. *Journal of Abnormal Child Psychology, 18*(3), 255–270.

Kiesler, D. J. (1966). Some myths of psychotherapy research and the search for a paradigm. *Psychological Bulletin, 65,* 110–136.

King, N. J., Cranston, F., & Josephs, A. (1989). Emotive imagery in children's nighttime fears: A multiple baseline design evaluation. *Journal of Behavior Therapy and Experimental Psychiatry, 20,* 125–135.

King, N. J., Gullone, E., Tonge, B. J., & Ollendick, T. H. (1993). Self-reports of panic attacks and manifest anxiety in adolescents. *Behaviour Research and Therapy, 31,* 111–116.

King, N. J., Hamilton, D., & Ollendick, T. H. (1988). *Children's phobias: A behavioral perspective.* Chichester, UK: Wiley.

King, N. J., Tonge, B. J., Heyne, D., Pritchard, M., Rollings, S., Young, D., et al. (1998). Cognitive-behavioral treatment of school-refusing children: A controlled evaluation. *Journal of the American Academy of Child and Adolescent Psychiatry, 37*(4), 395–403.

King, N. J., Tonge, B. J., Mullen, R., Myerson, N., Heyne, D., Rollings, S., et al. (2000). Treating sexually abused children with posttraumatic-stress symptoms: A randomized clinical trial. *Journal of the American Academy of Child and Adolescent Psychiatry, 39,* 1347–1355.

Klingman, A., Melamed, B. G., Cuthbert, M. I., & Hermecz, D. A. (1984). Effects of participant modeling on information acquisition and skill utilization. *Journal of Consulting and Clinical Psychology, 52,* 414–422.

Klorman, R., Hilpert, P. L., Michael, R., LaGana, C., & Sveen, O. B. (1980). Effects of coping and mastery modeling on experienced and inexperienced pedodontic patients' disruptiveness. *Behavior Therapy, 11,* 156–168.

Knox, L. S., Albano, A.M., & Barlow, D. H. (1996). Parental involvement in the treatment of childhood obsessive compulsive disorder: A multiple-baseline examination incorporating parents. *Behavior Therapy, 27,* 93–115.

Kondas, O. (1967). Reduction of examination anxiety and "stage fright" by group desensitization and relaxation. *Behaviour Research and Therapy, 5,* 275–281.

Kornhaber, R. C., & Schroeder, H. E. (1975). Importance of model similarity on extinction of avoidance behavior in children. *Journal of Consulting and Clinical Psychology, 43,* 601–607.

Kuroda, J. (1969). Elimination of children's fears of animals by the method of experimental desensitization: An application of learning theory to child psychology. *Psychologia, 12,* 161–165.

LaFreniere, P. J., & Capuano, F. (1997). Preventive intervention as means of clarifying direction of effects in socialization: Anxious–withdrawn preschoolers case. *Development and Psychopathology, 9,* 551–564.

LaGreca, A. M., Silverman, W. K., Vernberg, E. M., & Roberts, M. C. (Eds.). (2002). *Helping children cope with disasters and terrorism.* Washington, DC: American Psychological Association.

Lambert, S. F., Cooley, M. R., Campbell, K. D., Benoit, M. Z., & Stansbury, R. (2004). Assessing anxiety sensitivity in inner-city African American children: Psychometric properties of the Childhood Anxiety Sensitivity Index. *Journal of Clinical Child and Adolescent Psychology, 33,* 248–259.

Lang, P. J. (1977). Fear imagery: An information processing analysis. *Behavior Therapy, 8,* 862–886.

Lang, P. J. (1979). A bio-informational theory of emotional imagery. *Psychophysiology, 16,* 495–512.

Langley, A. K., Bergman, L., McCracken, J., & Piacentini, J. C. (2004). Impairment in childhood anxiety disorders: Preliminary examination of the Child Anxiety Impact Scale–Parent Version. *Journal of Child and Adolescent Psychopharmacology, 14*(1), 105–114.

Last, C. G., Hansen, C., & Franco, N. (1998). Cognitive-behavioral treatment of school phobia. *Journal of the American Academy of Child and Adolescent Psychiatry, 37,* 404–411.

Lavori, P. W., Rush, A. J., Wisniewski, S. R., Alpert, J. E., Fava, M., Kupfer, D. J., et al. (2001). Strengthening clinical effectiveness trials: Equipoise-stratified randomization. *Biological Psychiatry, 50,* 792–801.

Laxer, R. M., Quarter, J., & Walker, K. (1969). Systematic desensitization and relaxation of high-test-anxious secondary school students. *Journal of Counseling Psychology, 16*, 446–451.

Laxer, R. M., & Walker, K. (1970). Counterconditioning versus relaxation in the desensitization of test anxiety. *Journal of Counseling Psychology, 17*, 431–436.

Lazarus, A. A., & Abramovitz, A. (1962). The use of "emotive imagery" in the treatment of children's phobias. *Journal of Mental Science, 108*, 191–195.

Leal, L. L., Baxter, E. G., Martin, J., & Marx, R. W. (1981). Cognitive modification and systematic desensitization with test anxious high school students. *Journal of Counseling Psychology, 28*, 525–258.

Lee, V. (1989). Comments about the isolation of behavior analysis. *Behavior Analyst, 12*, 85–87.

Leitenberg, H., & Callahan, E. J. (1973). Reinforced practice and reduction of different kinds of fears in adults and children. *Behaviour Research and Therapy, 11*, 19–30.

Leslie, L. K., Weckerly, J., Landsverk, J., Hough, R. L., Hurlburt, M. S., & Wood, P. A. (2003). Racial/ethnic differences in the use of psychotropic medication in high-risk children and adolescents. *Journal of the American Academy of Child and Adolescent Psychiatry, 42*, 1433–1442.

Levis, D. J., & Brewer, K. E. (2001). The neurotic paradox: Attempts by two-factor fear theory and alternative avoidance models to resolve the issues associated with sustained avoidance responding in extinction. In R. R. Mowrer & S. B. Klein (Eds.), *Handbook of contemporary learning theories* (pp. 561–597). Mahwah, NJ: Erlbaum.

Lewis, S. (1974). A comparison of behavior therapy techniques in the reduction of fearful avoidance behavior. *Behavior Therapy, 5*, 648–655.

Liebowitz, M. R., Turner, S. M., Piacentini, J., Beidel, D. C., Clarvit, S. R., Davies, S. O., et al. (2002). Fluoxetine in children and adolescents with OCD: A placebo-controlled trial. *Journal of the American Academy of Child and Adolescent Psychiatry, 41*, 1431–1438.

Little, S., & Jackson, B. (1974). The treatment of test anxiety through attentional and relaxation training. *Psychotherapy: Theory, Research, and Practice, 11*, 175–178.

Lochman, J. E., & Wells, K. C. (2002). Contextual social-cognitive mediators and child outcome: A test of the theoretical model in the Coping Power program. *Development and Psychopathology, 14*, 945–967.

Lonigan, C. J., Hooe, E. S., David, C. F., & Kistner, J. A. (1999). Positive and negative affectivity in children: Confirmatory factor analysis of a two-factor model and its relation to symptoms of anxiety and depression. *Journal of Consulting and Clinical Psychology, 67*, 374–386.

Lovibond, P. F., Siddle, D. A., & Bond, N. W. (1993). Resistance to extinction of fear-relevant stimuli: Preparedness or selective sensitization? *Journal of Experimental Psychology: General, 122*, 449–461.

Lumpkin, P. W., Silverman, W. K., Weems, C. F., Markham, M. R., & Kurtines, W. M. (2002). Treating a heterogeneous set of anxiety disorders in youths with group cognitive behavioral therapy: A partially nonconcurrent multiple-baseline evaluation. *Behavior Therapy, 33*, 163–177.

Manassis, K., Mendlowitz, S. L., Scapillato, D., Avery, D., Fiksenbaum, L., Freire, M., et al. (2002). Group and individual cognitive-behavioral therapy for childhood anxiety disorders: A randomized trial. *Journal of the American Academy of Child and Adolescent Psychiatry, 41*, 1423–1430.

Mann, J., & Rosenthal, T. L. (1969). Vicarious and direct counter-conditioning of test anxiety through individual and group desensitization. *Behaviour Research and Therapy, 31*, 9–15.

March, J. S. (1995). Cognitive behavioral psychotherapy for children and adolescents with OCD: A review and recommendations for treatment. *Journal of the American Academy of Child and Adolescent Psychiatry, 34*, 7–18.

March, J. S., Amaya-Jackson, L., Murray, M. C., & Schulte, A. (1998). Cognitive-behavioral psychotherapy for children and adolescents with posttraumatic stress disorder after a single-incident stressor. *Journal of the American Academy of Child and Adolescent Psychiatry, 37*, 585–593.

March, J. S., Biederman, J., Wolkow, R., Safferman, A., Mardekian, J., Cook, E. H., et al. (1998). Sertraline in children and adolescents with obsessive-compulsive disorder: A multicenter randomized controlled trial. *Journal of the American Medical Association, 280*, 1752–1756.

March, J. S., & Leonard, H. (1996). Obsessive-compulsive disorder in children and adolescents: A review of the past 10 years. *Journal of the American Academy of Child and Adolescent Psychiatry, 35*, 1265–1273.

March, J. S., & Mulle, K. (1996). Banishing OCD: Psychotherapy for cognitive-behavioral obsessive-compulsive disorders. In E. D. Hibbs & P. S. Jensen (Eds.), *Psychosocial treatments for child and adolescent disorders: Empirically based strategies* (pp. 83–102). Washington, DC: American Psychological Association.

March, J. S., & Mulle, K. (1998). *OCD in children and adolescents: A cognitive-behavioral treatment manual.* New York: Guilford Press.

March, J. S., Parker, J. D. A., Sullivan, K., Stallings, P., & Conners, C. K. (1997). The Multidimensional Anxiety Scale for Children (MASC): Factor structure, reliability, and validity. *Journal of the American Academy of Child and Adolescent Psychiatry, 36*, 554–565.

Marks, I. M. (1969). *Fears and phobias.* New York: Academic Press.

Martin, A., Van Hoof, T., Stubbe, D., Sherwin, T., & Scahill, L. (2003). Multiple psychotropic pharmacotherapy among child and adolescent enrollees in Connecticut Medicaid managed care. *Psychiatric Services, 54*(1), 72–77.

Matson, J. L. (1981). Assessment and treatment of clinical fears in mentally retarded children. *Journal of Applied Behavior Analysis, 14*, 287–294.

Matson, J. L. (1983). Exploration of phobic behavior in
a small child. *Journal of Behavior Therapy and Experimental Psychiatry, 14*, 257–259.

McMahon, R. J., & Forehand, R. L. (2003). *Helping
the noncompliant child: Family-based treatment for
oppositional behavior* (2nd ed.). New York: Guilford
Press.

McMiller, W. P., & Weisz, J. R. (1996). Help-seeking
preceding mental health clinic intake among African-
American, Latino, and Caucasian youths. *Journal of
the American Academy of Child and Adolescent Psychiatry, 35*, 1086–1094.

McNally, R. J. (1987). Preparedness and phobias: A review. *Psychological Bulletin, 101*, 283–303.

McNally, R. J., & Foa, E. B. (1986). Preparedness and
resistance to extinction to fear-relevant stimuli: A
failure to replicate. *Behaviour Research and Therapy,
24*, 529–535.

McNally, R. J., & Reiss, S. (1985). The preparedness
theory of phobias: The effects of initial fear level on
safety-signal conditioning to fear-relevant stimuli.
Psychophysiology, 21, 647–652.

Melamed, B. G., Meyer, R., Gee, C., & Soule, L. (1976).
The influence of time and type of preparation on children's adjustment to hospitalization. *Journal of Pediatric Psychology, 1*, 31–37.

Melamed, B. G., & Siegel, L. J. (1975). Reduction of
anxiety in children facing hospitalization and surgery
by use of filmed modeling. *Journal of Consulting and
Clinical Psychology, 43*, 511–521.

Melamed, B. G., Yurcheson, R., Fleece, E. L.,
Hutcherson, S., & Hawes, R. (1978). Effects of film
modeling on the reduction of anxiety-related behaviors in individuals varying in level of previous experience in the stress situation. *Journal of Consulting and
Clinical Psychology, 46*, 1357–1367.

Mendlowitz, S. L., Manassis, K., Bradley, S., Scapillato,
D., Miezitis, S., & Shaw, B. F. (1999). Cognitive-
behavioral group treatments in childhood anxiety
disorders: The role of parental involvement. *Journal
of the American Academy of Child and Adolescent
Psychiatry, 38*, 1223–1229.

Menzies, R. G., & Clarke, J. C. (1993). A comparison
of *in vivo* and vicarious exposure in the treatment of
childhood water phobia. *Behaviour Research and
Therapy, 31*, 9–15.

Mineka, S., & Öhman, A. (2002). Phobias and preparedness: The selective, automatic, and encapsulated nature of fear. *Biological Psychiatry, 52*, 927–937.

Mineka, S., Watson, D., & Clark, L. A. (1998). Comorbidity of anxiety and unipolar mood disorders. *Annual Review of Psychology, 49*, 377–412.

Mowrer, O. H. (1939). A stimulus–response analysis of
anxiety and its role as a reinforcing agent. *Psychological Review, 46*, 553–565.

Mowrer, O. H. (1947). On the dual nature of learning: A
reinterpretation of "conditioning" and "problem
solving." *Harvard Educational Review, 17*, 102–148.

Mowrer, O. H. (1960). *Learning theory and behavior.*
New York: Wiley.

MTA Cooperative Group. (1999). A 14-month randomized clinical trial of treatment strategies for attention-
deficit/hyperactivity disorder. *Archives of General
Psychiatry, 56*, 1073–1086.

Muller, S. D., & Madsen, C. H. (1970). Group desensitization for "anxious" children with reading problems. *Psychology in the Schools, 7*, 184–189.

Muris, P., Meesters, C., & van Melick, M. (2002).
Treatment of childhood anxiety disorders: A preliminary comparison between cognitive-behavioral
group therapy and a psychological placebo intervention. *Journal of Behavior Therapy and Experimental
Psychiatry, 33*, 143–158.

Muris, P., Merckelbach, H., Holdrinet, I., & Sijsenaar,
M. (1998). Treating phobic children: Effects of
EMDR versus exposure. *Journal of Consulting and
Clinical Psychology, 66*, 193–198.

Murphy, C. M., & Bootzin, R. R. (1973). Active and passive participation in the contact desensitization of
snake fear in children. *Behavior Therapy, 4*, 203–211.

National Advisory Mental Health Council Workgroup
on Child and Adolescent Mental Health Intervention
Development and Deployment. (2001). *Blueprint for
change: Research on child and adolescent mental
health*. Rockville, MD: U.S. Public Health Service.

Nauta, M. H., Scholing, A., Emmelkamp, P. M. G., &
Minderaa, R. B. (2003). Cognitive-behavioral therapy for children with anxiety disorders in a clinical
setting: No additional effect of a cognitive parent
training. *Journal of the American Academy of Child
and Adolescent Psychiatry, 42*, 1270–1278.

Nocella, J., & Kaplan, R. M. (1982). Training children
to cope with dental treatment. *Journal of Pediatric
Psychology, 7*, 175–178.

Obler, M., & Terwilliger, R. F. (1970). Pilot study on the
effectiveness of systematic desensitization with neurologically impaired children with phobic disorders.
Journal of Consulting and Clinical Psychology, 34,
314–318.

O'Connor, R. D. (1972). Relative efficacy of modeling,
shaping, and the combined procedures for modification of social withdrawal. *Journal of Abnormal Psychology, 79*, 327–334.

Öhman, A., & Mineka, S. (2001). Fears, phobias, and
preparedness: Toward an evolved module of fear
and fear learning. *Psychological Review, 108*, 483–
522.

Olfson, M., Marcus, S. C., Weissman, M. M., & Jensen,
P. S. (2002). National trends in the use of
psychotropic medications by children. *Journal of the
American Academy of Child and Adolescent Psychiatry, 41*(5), 514–521.

Ollendick, T. H. (1983). Reliability and validity of the
Revised Fear Survey Schedule for Children (FSSC-R).
Behaviour Research and Therapy, 21, 685–692.

Ollendick, T. H. (1995). Cognitive behavioral treatment
of panic disorder with agoraphobia in adolescents: A
multiple baseline design analysis. *Behavior Therapy,
26*, 517–531.

Ollendick, T. H., Hagopian, L. P., & Huntzinger, R. M. (1991). Cognitive-behavior therapy with nighttime fearful children. *Journal of Behavior Therapy and Experimental Psychiatry, 22,* 113–121.

Ollendick, T. H., & King, N. J. (1994). Diagnosis, assessment, and treatment of internalizing problems in children: The role of longitudinal data. *Journal of Consulting and Clinical Psychology, 62,* 918–927.

Ollendick, T. H., & King, N. J. (1998). Empirically supported treatments for children with phobic and anxiety disorders. *Journal of Clinical Child Psychology, 27,* 156–167.

Ollendick, T. H., King, N. J., & Frary, R. B. (1989). Fears in children and adolescents: Reliability and generalizability across gender, age, and nationality. *Behaviour Research and Therapy, 27,* 19–26.

Ollendick, T. H., Matson, J. L., & Helsel, W. J. (1985). Fears in children and adolescents: Normative data. *Behaviour Research and Therapy, 23,* 465–467.

Öst, L. (1989). One-session treatment for specific phobias. *Behavior Research and Therapy, 27,* 1–7.

Öst, L. G., Alm, T., Brandberg, M., & Breitholtz, E. (2001). One vs. five sessions of exposure and five sessions of cognitive therapy in the treatment of claustrophobia. *Behaviour Research and Therapy, 39,* 167–183.

Parish, T. S., Buntman, A. D., & Buntman, S. R. (1976). Effect of counterconditioning on test anxiety as indicated by digit span performance. *Journal of Educational Psychology, 68,* 297–299.

Paulose-Ram, R., Jonas, B. S., Orwig, D., & Safran, M. A. (2004). Prescription psychotropic medication use among the U.S. adult population: Results from the third National Health and Nutrition Examination Survey, 1988–1994. *Journal of Clinical Epidemiology, 57,* 309–317.

Pavlov, I. (1927). *Conditioned reflexes* (G. V. Anrep, Trans.). New York: Oxford University Press.

Persons, J. B. (1991). Psychotherapy outcome studies do not accurately represent current models of psychotherapy: A proposed remedy. *American Psychologist, 46,* 99–106.

Peterson, L., Schultheis, K., Ridley-Johnson, R., Miller, D. J., & Tracy, K. (1984). Comparison of three modeling procedures for the presurgical and postsurgical reactions of children. *Behavior Therapy, 15,* 197–203.

Pina, A. A., & Silverman, W. K. (2004). Clinical phenomenology, somatic symptoms, and distress in Hispanic/Latino and Euro-American youths with anxiety disorders. *Journal of Clinical Child and Adolescent Psychology, 33,* 227–236.

Pine, D. S., Cohen, P., Gurley, D., Brook, J., & Ma, Y. (1998). The risk for early-adulthood anxiety and depressive disorders in adolescents with anxiety and depressive disorders. *Archives of General Psychiatry, 55,* 56–64.

Pine, D. S., Walkup, J. T., Labellarte, M. J., Riddle, M. A., Greenhill, L., Klein, R., et al.. (2001). Fluvoxamine for the treatment of anxiety disorders in children and adolescents. *New England Journal of Medicine, 344,* 1279–1285.

Pintner, R., & Lev, J. (1940). The intelligence of the hard of hearing school child. *Journal of Genetic Psychology, 55,* 31–48.

Rabian, B., Peterson, R. A., Richters, J., & Jensen, P. S. (1993). Anxiety sensitivity among anxious children. *Journal of Clinical Child Psychology, 22,* 441–446.

Rachman, S. (1977). The conditioning theory of fear-acquisition: A critical examination. *Behaviour Research and Therapy, 15,* 375–387.

Rachman, S. (1990). The determinations and treatment of simple phobias. *Advances in Behaviour Research and Therapy, 12,* 1–30.

Rachman, S. (1991). Neoconditioning and the classical theory of fear acquisition. *Clinical Psychology Review, 11,* 115–173.

Rapee, R. M., & Jacobs, D. (2002). The reduction of temperamental risk for anxiety in withdrawn preschoolers: A pilot study. *Behavioural and Cognitive Psychotherapy, 30,* 211–216.

Reynolds, C. R., & Richmond, B. O. (1978). What I Think and Feel: A revised measure of children's manifest anxiety. *Journal of Abnormal Child Psychology, 6,* 271–280.

Riddle, M. A., Reeve, E. A., Yaryura-Tobias, J. A., Yang, H. M., Claghorn, J. L., Gaffney, G., et al. (2001). Fluvoxamine for children and adolescents with obsessive–compulsive disorder: A randomized, controlled, multicenter trial. *Journal of the American Academy of Child and Adolescent Psychiatry, 40,* 222–229.

Riddle, M. A., Scahill, L., King, R. A., Hardin, M. T., Anderson, G. M., Ort, S. I., et al. (1992). Double-blind, crossover trial of fluoxetine and placebo in children and adolescents with obsessive–compulsive disorder. *Journal of the American Academy of Child and Adolescent Psychiatry, 31,* 1062–1069.

Ritter, B. (1968). The group desensitization of children's snake phobias using vicarious and contact desensitization procedures. *Behaviour Research and Therapy, 6,* 1–6.

Roberts, M. C., Wurtle, S. K., Boone, R. R., Gither, L. J., & Elkins, P. D. (1981). Reductions of medical fears by use of modeling: A preventive application in a general population of children. *Journal of Pediatric Psychology, 6,* 293–300.

Rosenfarb, I., & Hayes, S. C. (1984). Social standard setting: The Achilles heel of informational accounts of therapeutic change. *Behavior Therapy, 15,* 515–528.

Rothert, M. L., Holmes-Rovner, M., Rovner, D., Kroll, J., Breer, L., Talarczyk, G., et al. (1997). An educational intervention as decision support for menopausal women. *Research in Nursing and Health, 20,* 377–387.

Safren, S. A., Gonzalez, R. E., Horner, K. J., Leung, A. W., Heimberg, R. G., & Juster, H. R. (2000). Anxiety in ethnic minority youth: Methodological and conceptual issues and review of the literature. *Behavior Modification, 24,* 147–183.

Saigh, P. A. (1986). *In vitro* flooding in the treatment of a six-year-old boy's posttraumatic stress disorder. *Behaviour Research and Therapy, 24,* 685–688.

Saigh, P. A. (1987). *In vitro* flooding of a posttraumatic stress disorder. *School Psychology Review, 16,* 203–211.

Sanderson, W. C., Rapee, R. M., & Barlow, D. H. (1989). The influence of an illusion of control on panic attacks induced via the inhalation of 5.5% carbon dioxide enriched air. *Archives of General Psychiatry, 46,* 157–164.

Schmidt, N. B., Woolaway-Bickel, K., Trakowski, J., Santiago, H., Storey, J., Koselka, M., et al. (2000). Dismantling cognitive-behavioral treatment for panic disorder: Questioning the utility of breathing retraining. *Journal of Consulting and Clinical Psychology, 68,* 417–424.

Schoenwald, S. K., & Hoagwood, K. (2001a, Winter). Effectiveness and dissemination research: Their mutual roles in improving mental health services for children and adolescents. *Report on Emotional and Behavioral Disorders in Youth, 2,* 3–4, 18–20.

Schoenwald, S. K., & Hoagwood, K. (2001b). Effectiveness, transportability, and dissemination of interventions: What matters when. *Psychiatric Services, 52,* 1190–1197.

Schulte, D., Kuenzel, R., Pepping, G., & Schulte-Bahrenberg, T. (1992). Tailor-made versus standardized therapy of phobic patients. *Advances in Behaviour Research and Therapy, 14,* 67–92.

Seligman, M. E. P. (1970). On the generality of the laws of learning. *Psychological Review, 77,* 406–418.

Seligman, M. E. P. (1971). Phobias and preparedness. *Behavior Therapy, 2,* 307–320.

Sherbourne, C. D., Sturm, R., & Wells, K. B. (1999). What outcomes matter to patients? *Journal of General Internal Medicine, 14,* 357–363.

Sheslow, D. V., Bondy, A. S., & Nelson, R. O. (1982). A comparison of graduated exposure, verbal coping skills, and their combination in the treatment of children's fear of the dark. *Child and Family Behavior Therapy, 4,* 33–45.

Shortt, A. L., Barrett, P. M., & Fox, T. L. (2001). Evaluating the FRIENDS Program: A cognitive-behavioral group treatment for anxious children and their parents. *Journal of Clinical Child Psychology, 30,* 525–535.

Silverman, W. K., & Ginsburg, G. S. (1998). Anxiety disorders. In T. H. Ollendick & M. Hersen (Eds.), *Handbook of child psychopathology* (pp. 239–268). New York: Plenum Press.

Silverman, W. K., & Kurtines, W. M. (1996). *Anxiety and phobic disorders: A pragmatic approach.* New York: Plenum Press.

Silverman, W. K., Kurtines, W. M., Ginsburg, G. S., Weems, C. F., Lumpkin, P. W., & Carmichael, D. H. (1999). Treating anxiety disorders in children with group cognitive-behavioral therapy: A randomized clinical trial. *Journal of Consulting and Clinical Psychology, 67*(6), 995–1003.

Silverman, W. K., Kurtines, W. M., Ginsburg, G. S., Weems, C. F., Rabian, B., & Serafini, L. T. (1999). Contingency management, self-control, and education support in the treatment of childhood phobic disorders: A randomized clinical trial. *Journal of Consulting and Clinical Psychology, 67*(5), 675–687.

Silverman, W. K., & Weems, C. F. (1999). Anxiety sensitivity in children. In S. Taylor (Ed.), *Anxiety sensitivity: Theory, research, and treatment of the fear of anxiety* (pp. 239–268). Mahwah, NJ: Erlbaum.

Southam-Gerow, M. A., Chorpita, B. F., Miller, L. M., & Taylor, A. A. (2005). *Differences in characteristics of child and adolescent referrals to a specialty mental health clinic versus a community mental health program.* Manuscript under review.

Southam-Gerow, M. A., & Kendall, P. C. (2000). A preliminary study of the emotion understanding of youths referred for treatment of anxiety disorders. *Journal of Clinical Child Psychology, 29,* 319–327.

Southam-Gerow, M. A., Kendall, P. C., & Weersing, V. R. (2001). Examining outcome variability: Correlates of treatment response in a child and adolescent anxiety clinic. *Journal of Clinical Child Psychology, 30,* 422–436.

Southam-Gerow, M. A., Weisz, J. R., & Kendall, P. C. (2003). Youth with anxiety disorders in research and service clinics: Examining client differences and similarities. *Journal of Clinical Child and Adolescent Psychology, 32,* 375–385.

Spence, S. H. (1997). Structure of anxiety symptoms among children: A confirmatory factor-analytic study. *Journal of Abnormal Psychology, 106,* 280–297.

Spence, S. H. (1998). A measure of anxiety symptoms among children. *Behaviour Research and Therapy, 36,* 545–566.

Spence, S. H., Barrett, P. M., & Turner, C. M. (2003). Psychometric properties of the Spence Children's Anxiety Scale with young adolescents. *Journal of Anxiety Disorders, 17*(6), 605–625.

Spence, S. H., Donovan, C., & Brechman-Toussaint, M. (2000). The treatment of childhood social phobia: The effectiveness of a social skills training-based, cognitive-behavioural intervention, with and without parental involvement. *Journal of Child Psychology and Psychiatry and Allied Disciplines, 41,* 713–726.

Stein, B. D., Jaycox, L. H., Kataoka, S. H., Wong, M., Tu, W., Elliott, M. N., et al. (2003). A mental health intervention for schoolchildren exposed to violence: A randomized controlled trial. *Journal of the American Medical Association, 290,* 603–611.

Stein, D. J., Spadaccini, E., & Hollander, E. (1995). Meta-analysis of pharmacotherapy trials for obsessive–compulsive disorder. *International Clinical Psychopharmacology, 10,* 11–18.

Street, L. L., Niederehe, G., & Lebowitz, B. D. (2000). Toward greater public health relevance for psychotherapeutic intervention research: An NIMH workshop report. *Clinical Psychology: Science and Practice, 7*(2), 127–137.

Suarez, L., & Bell-Dolan, D. (2001). The relationship of child worry to cognitive biases: Threat interpretation and likelihood of event occurrence. *Behavior Therapy, 32,* 425–442.

Task Force on Promotion and Dissemination of Psychological Procedures, Division of Clinical Psychology,

American Psychological Association. (1995). Training in and dissemination of empirically-validated psychological treatments: Report and recommendations. *The Clinical Psychologist, 48*, 3–23.

Taylor, A. A., Francis, S. E., Chorpita, B. F., Southam-Gerow, M. A., & Lam, C. (2003, November). *Examining differences between publicly and privately referred youth at a university-based clinic.* Poster presented at the annual meeting of the Association for the Advancement of Behavior Therapy, Boston.

Treatment for Adolescents with Depression Study. (2004). Fluoxetine, cognitive-behavioral therapy, and their combination for adolescents with depression: Treatment for Adolescents with Depression Study (TADS) randomized controlled trial. *Journal of the American Medical Association, 292*, 807–820.

U.S. Department of Health and Human Services. (1999). *Mental health: A Report of the Surgeon General.* Rockville, MD: National Institutes of Health, National Institute of Mental Health.

Ultee, C. A., Griffioen, D., & Schellekens, J. (1982). The reduction of anxiety in children: A comparison of the effects of "systematic desensitization *in vitro*" and systematic desensitization *in vivo.*" *Behaviour Research and Therapy, 20*, 61–67.

van der Ploege-Stapart, J. D., & van der Ploege, H. M. (1986). Behavioral group treatment of test anxiety: An evaluation study. *Journal of Behavior Therapy and Experimental Psychiatry, 17*, 255–259.

Van Hasselt, V. B., Hersen, M., Bellack, A. S., Rosenblum, N. D., & Lamparski, D. (1979). Tripartite assessment to the effects of systematic desensitization in a multi-phobic child: An experimental analysis. *Journal of Behavior Therapy and Experimental Psychiatry, 10*, 51–55.

Vasey, M. W. (1993). Development and cognition in childhood anxiety: The example of worry. *Advances in Clinical Child Psychology, 15*, 1–39.

Vasey, M. W., & Dadds, M. R. (Eds.). (2001). *The developmental psychopathology of anxiety.* London: Oxford University Press.

Vasey, M. W., Daleiden, E. L., Williams, L. L., & Brown, L. M. (1995). Biased attention in childhood anxiety disorders: A preliminary study. *Journal of Abnormal Child Psychology, 23*, 267–279.

Vasey, M. W., & MacLeod, C. (2001). Information-processing factors in childhood anxiety: A review and developmental perspective. In M. W. Vasey & M. R. Dadds (Eds.), *The developmental psychopathology of anxiety* (pp. 253–277). London: Oxford University Press.

Velosa, J. F., & Riddle, M. A. (2000). Pharmacologic treatment of anxiety disorders in children and adolescents. *Child and Adolescent Psychiatric Clinics of North America, 9*, 119–133.

Watson, J. B., & Morgan, J. J. B. (1917). Emotional reactions and psychological experimentation. *American Journal of Psychology, 28*, 163–174.

Watson, J. B., & Rayner, R. (1920). Conditioned and emotional reactions. *Journal of Experimental Psychology, 3*, 1–14.

Weissbrod, C. W., & Bryan, J. H. (1973). Filmed treatment as an effective fear-reduction technique. *Journal of Abnormal Child Psychology, 1*, 196–201.

Weisz, J. R. (2004). *Psychotherapy for children and adolescents: Evidence-based treatments and case examples.* Cambridge, UK: Cambridge University Press.

Weisz, J. R., & Hawley, K. M. (1998). Finding, evaluating, refining, and applying empirically supported treatments for children and adolescents. *Journal of Clinical Child Psychology, 27*, 206–216.

Weisz, J. R., Hawley, K. M., Pilkonis, P. A., Woody, S. R., & Follette, W. C. (2000). Stressing the (other) three Rs in the search for empirically supported treatments: Review procedures, research quality, relevance to practice and the public interest. *Clinical Psychology: Science and Practice, 7*, 243–258.

Weisz, J. R., Southam-Gerow, M. A., Gordis, E. B., & Connor-Smith, J. K. (2003). Primary and secondary control enhancement training for youth depression: Applying the deployment-focused model of treatment development and testing. In A. E. Kazdin & J. R. Weisz (Eds.), *Evidence-based psychotherapies for children and adolescents* (pp. 165–183). New York: Guilford Press.

Weisz, J. R., Weiss, B., & Donenberg, G. R. (1992). The lab versus the clinic: Effects of child and adolescent psychotherapy. *American Psychologist, 47*(12), 1578–1585.

Williams, C. E., & Jones, R. T. (1989). Impact of self-instructions on response maintenance and children's fear of fire. *Journal of Clinical Child Psychology, 18*, 84–89.

Wilson, G. T. (1996). Manual-based treatments: The clinical application of research findings. *Behaviour Research and Therapy, 34*, 295–314.

Wilson, N. H., & Rotter, J. C. (1986). Anxiety management training and study skills counseling for students on self-esteem and test anxiety and performance. *School Counselor, 34*, 18–31.

Wolpe, J. (1958). *Psychotherapy by reciprocal inhibition.* Stanford, CA: Stanford University Press.

Wolpe, J., & Rowan, V. C. (1988). Panic disorder: A product of classical conditioning. *Behaviour Research and Therapy, 26*, 441–450.

Zinbarg, R. E., & Mineka, S. (2001). Understanding, treating, and preventing anxiety, phobias, and anxiety disorders. In M. E. Carroll & J. B. Overmier (Eds.), *Animal research and human health: Advancing human welfare through behavioral science* (pp. 19–28). Washington, DC: American Psychological Association.

Zito, J. M., Safer, D. J., dosReis, S., Gardner, J. F., Magder, L., Soeken, K., et al. (2003). Psychotropic practice patterns for youth: A 10-year perspective. *Archives of Pediatric and Adolescent Medicine, 157*, 17–25.

Zoccolillo, M. (1992). Co-occurrence of conduct disorder and its adult outcomes with depressive and anxiety disorders: A review. *Journal of the American Academy of Child and Adolescent Psychiatry, 31*, 547–556.

APPENDIX 4.1. Efficacious Treatments for Fears and Anxieties in Youths: Exposure and Its Variants

Reference	Entry criterion	Design	Treatment	Controls/comparisons	Results
Andrews (1971)	High anxiety	RCT	Relaxation plus exposure	Client-centered therapy, wait list	Exposure plus relaxation was superior to client-centered therapy and wait list.
Bandura, Blanchard, & Ritter (1969)	Fear of snakes	RCT	Systematic desensitization	No treatment	Systematic desensitization was superior to no treatment for approach behavior.
Barabasz (1973)	Test anxiety	RCT	Imaginal desensitization	No treatment	Imaginal desensitization was superior to no treatment on galvanic skin response.
Bornstein & Knapp (1981)	Fear of separation, travel, illness	Multiple-baseline	Imaginal exposure		Exposure led to positive improvements.
Chorpita, Vitali, & Barlow (1997)	Fear of choking	Multiple-baseline	Reinforced practice		Intervention led to systematic reduction in anxiety ratings across a variety of foods.
Cornwall, Spence, & Schotte (1996)	Fear of dark	RCT	Exposure	Wait list	Exposure was superior to wait list
Deffenbacher & Kemper (1974)	Test anxiety	RCT	Imaginal exposure	No treatment	Imaginal exposure was superior to no treatment.
Johnson, Tyler, Thompson, & Jones (1971)	Fear of public speaking	RCT	Reinforced practice	Imaginal exposure; no treatment	Reinforced practice was superior to no treatment.
			Imaginal exposure	Reinforced practice; no treatment	Exposure was superior to no treatment.
Kandel, Ayllon, & Rosenbaum (1977)	Social anxiety	Multiple-baseline	Systematic desensitization		Youths showed increased social interaction as a function of the treatment.
King, Cranston, & Josephs (1989)	Nighttime fears	Multiple-baseline	Emotive imagery		Emotive imagery led to improvements for nighttime fears.
Kondas (1967)	Fear of public speaking	RCT	Imaginal exposure plus relaxation	Relaxation; imaginal exposure; no treatment	Imaginal exposure plus relaxation was superior to either treatment alone and to no treatment.
Laxer, Quarter, & Walker (1969)	Test anxiety	RCT	Desensitization plus relaxation	No treatment	Desensitization plus relaxation was superior to no treatment.
Laxer & Walker (1970)	Test anxiety	RCT	Systematic desensitization	Relaxation; simulation (exposure) alone; relaxation plus simulation (exposure); attention control; no treatment	Systematic desensitization was superior to no treatment.
Leal, Baxter, Martin, & Marx (1981)	Test anxiety	RCT	Exposure	Cognitive modification; wait list	Exposure was superior to cognitive and wait list regarding performance.
Leitenberg & Callahan (1973)	Fear of dark	RCT	Exposure	No treatment	Exposure was superior to no treatment on time spent in dark room.
Lewis (1974)	Fear of swimming	RCT	Participation	Modeling; modeling plus participation; no treatment	Modeling plus participation was superior to modeling and no treatment.
Mann & Rosenthal (1969)	Test anxiety	RCT	Group direct desensitization	Individual vicarious desensitization; individual desensitization; group vicarious desensitization, observing single model; group vicarious desensitization, observing group of models; no treatment	Treatment was better than no treatment on a measure of test anxiety, and no different from other active treatments.

Compliance	Gender	Age	Ethnicity	Therapist	Frequency	Duration	Contacts	Dose	Setting	Format
100%	Boys	14–17	N/R	BA	Weekly	10 weeks	10	45 minutes	School	Individual
83%	Both	13–59	N/R	N/R	Twice weekly	2.5 weeks	5	N/R	Clinic	Individual
100%	Both	11–12	Caucasian, African American	N/R	Daily	5 days	5	N/R	School	Individual
100%	Boys	12	Caucasian	PhD	N/R	8 weeks	N/R	N/R	N/R	Individual
100%	Girl	13	Caucasian	MA	Weekly	16 weeks	14	50 minutes	Clinic	Individual
100%	Both	7–10	N/R	MA	Weekly	6 weeks	4	40 minutes	Clinic	Individual
100%	Both	11–12	N/R	N/R	Weekly	1 day	7	45 minutes	N/R	Group
80%	N/R	12–14	N/R	N/R	Twice weekly	5 weeks	9	50 minutes	School	Group
80%	N/R	12–14	N/R	N/R	Twice weekly	5 weeks	9	50 minutes	School	Group
100%	Boys	8	N/R	N/R	3/week	16–20 weeks	17	31 minutes	School	Individual
100%	Both	6–11	N/R	MA	Weekly	1 day	6–13	30 minutes	Home	Individual
100%	Both	11–15	N/R	PhD	Weekly	4 weeks	15	N/R	N/R	Group
100%	Both	18	N/R	BA	Daily or twice daily	6 weeks	30	20 minutes	School	Group
92%	Both	N/R	N/R	BA	2–3/week	8 weeks	20	20 minutes	School	Group
100%	N/R	15–17	N/R	MA	Weekly	6 weeks	6	1 hour	N/R	Group
100%	Both	6	N/R	N/R	Twice weekly	1 day	8	N/R	Clinic	Individual
100%	Both	5–12	African American	N/R	Once	60 days	1	18 minutes	Community	Individual
100%	Both	12–13	N/R	MA, PhD	Weekly	8 weeks	8	50 minutes	Clinic	Group

(continued)

Reference	Entry criterion	Design	Treatment	Controls/comparisons	Results
Mann & Rosenthal (1969) *(cont.)*			Individual desensitization	Group vicarious desensitization, observing single model; group vicarious desensitization, observing group of models; group direct desensitization; individual vicarious desensitization; no treatment	Treatment was better than no treatment on a measure of test anxiety, and no different from other active treatments.
Menzies & Clarke (1993)	Fear of swimming	RCT	*In vivo* exposure	*In vivo* exposure plus vicarious exposure; vicarious exposure; no treatment	*In vivo* exposure was superior to vicarious exposure and no treatment.
			In vivo exposure plus vicarious exposure	Vicarious exposure; *in vivo* exposure; no treatment	*In vivo* exposure plus vicarious exposure was superior to vicarious exposure and no treatment.
Muris, Merckelbach, Holdrinet, & Sijsenaar (1998)	Spider phobia	Crossover	*In vivo* exposure	EMDR	Both led to improvements; exposure was superior to EMDR on a behavior test.
Murphy & Bootzin (1973)	Fear of snakes	RCT	Contact desensitization	No treatment	Treatment was superior to no treatment.
Obler & Terwillinger (1970)	Phobia of bus or dog	RCT	Exposure	No treatment	Treatment was superior to no treatment.
Öst, Alm, Brandberg, & Breitholtz (2001)	Mixed phobias	RCT	Exposure with child alone	Exposure with parent present; wait list	Exposure with child alone was superior to wait list on a behavioral approach test.
			Exposure with parent present	Exposure with child alone; wait list	Exposure with parent present was superior to wait list on a behavioral approach test.
Parish, Buntman, & Buntman (1976)	Test anxiety	RCT	*In vitro* (imaginal) desensitization using slide show and positive statements	Attention placebo; no treatment	Experimental treatment was superior to attention placebo and no treatment.
Ritter (1968)	Fear of snakes	RCT	Contact desensitization	Vicarious desensitization; no treatment	Contact group was superior to vicarious group and no treatment.
Saigh (1986)	Trauma	Multiple-baseline	*In vitro* (imaginal) flooding		Flooding led to decreased subjective anxiety across a variety of traumatic scenes.
Saigh (1987)	Trauma	Multiple-baseline	*In vitro* (imaginal) flooding		Flooding led to decreased subjective anxiety across a variety of traumatic scenes.
Sheslow, Bondy, & Nelson (1982)	Fear of dark	RCT	Graduated exposure	Coping skills/graduated exposure; verbal coping skills; contact control	Exposure was superior to coping skills alone and a placebo control.
Ultee, Griffioen, & Schellekens (1982)	Fear of swimming	RCT	*In vivo* exposure	*In vitro* (imaginal) exposure plus *in vivo* exposure; no treatment	*In vivo* exposure was superior to control treatment condition and to no treatment.
Van Hasselt, Hersen, Bellack, Rosenblum, & Lamparski (1979)	Fears of blood, heights, or test taking	Multiple-baseline	Relaxation; systematic desensitization		Desensitization showed the most consistent and systematic effects in the reduction of cognitive measures of anxiety.
Wilson & Rotter (1986)	Test anxiety	RCT	Exposure plus relaxation	Study habits; exposure plus relaxation plus study habits; attention placebo; no treatment	Treatment was superior to attention placebo and no treatment.
			Exposure plus relaxation plus study habits	Attention placebo; exposure plus relaxation; study habits; no treatment	Treatment was superior to attention placebo and no treatment.

Note. RCT, randomized controlled trial; N/R, not recorded; EMDR, eye movement desensitization and reprocessing.

Compliance	Gender	Age	Ethnicity	Therapist	Frequency	Duration	Contacts	Dose	Setting	Format
100%	Both	12–13	N/R	MA, PhD	Weekly	18 weeks	8	50 minutes	Clinic	Individual
100%	Both	3–8	N/R	Under-graduates	Weekly	3 weeks	3	30 minutes	Community	Individual
100%	Both	3–8	N/R	Under-graduates	Weekly	3 weeks	3	30 minutes	Community	Individual
100%	Girls	8–17	Caucasian	N/R	Once	4 days	1	90 minutes	Clinic	Individual
100%	Both	9–11	N/R	N/R	Daily	12 weeks	4	8 minutes	Clinic	Individual
100%	Both	7–11	N/R	BA	Weekly	1 day	10	300 minutes	Community, clinic	Individual
88%	Both	7–17	N/R	PhD	Weekly	8 days	2	180 minutes	Clinic	Individual
88%	Both	7–17	N/R	PhD	Weekly	2 weeks	2	180 minutes	Clinic	Parent–child
100%	Both	9–13	N/R	N/R	Every other day	15 minutes	4	10 minutes	School	Group
100%	Both	5–11	N/R	PhD	Daily	2 days	2	35 minutes	Clinic	Group
100%	Boys	6	N/R (Lebanese national)	N/R	N/R	4 weeks	10	60 minutes	Clinic	Individual
100%	Girls	14	N/R (Lebanese national)	N/R	2/week	3 days	8	75 minutes	Clinic	Individual
100%	Both	4–5	N/R	MA	Daily	3 days	3	30 minutes	School	Individual
100%	Both	5–10	N/R	BA	2/week	4 weeks	8	30 minutes	Community	Individual
100%	Boys	11	Caucasian	N/R	N/R	1 day	N/R	N/R	Clinic	Individual
83%	Both	11–13	African American, Caucasian	PhD	Twice weekly	3 weeks	6	45 minutes	N/R	Group
100%	Both	11–13	African American, Caucasian	PhD	Twice weekly	3 weeks	6	45 minutes	N/R	Group

APPENDIX 4.2. Efficacious Treatments for Fears and Anxieties in Youths: Modeling and Its Variants

Reference	Entry criterion	Design	Treatment	Controls/comparisons	Results
Bandura, Blanchard, & Ritter (1969)	Fear of snakes	RCT	Live modeling with guided participation	Symbolic modeling; systematic desensitization; no treatment	Live modeling with guided participation was superior to all other conditions for approach behavior.
			Symbolic modeling	Systematic desensitization; live modeling with guided participation; no treatment	Symbolic modeling was superior to no treatment for approach behavior.
Bandura, Grusec, & Menlove (1967)	Fear of dogs	RCT	Modeling with neutral context	Exposure in positive context; modeling with positive context; positive context alone	Both modeling conditions were superior to exposure and positive context alone on measures of approach.
			Modeling with positive context	Modeling with neutral context; exposure in positive context; positive context alone	Both modeling conditions were superior to exposure and positive context alone on measures of approach.
Bandura & Menlove (1968)	Fear of dogs	RCT	Modeling (multiple filmed models)	Attention placebo (neutral film); modeling (single filmed model)	Both modeling conditions were superior to the control group.
			Modeling (single filmed model)	Modeling (multiple filmed models); attention placebo (neutral film)	Both modeling conditions were superior to the control group.
Clark, Sugrin, & Bolton (1982)	Fear of making mistakes	Multiple-baseline	Modeling plus reinforcement		Improvement on 3 of 4 behaviors, but relapse when treatment was discontinued.
Davis, Rosenthal, & Kelley (1981)	Fear of spiders	RCT	Modeling plus exposure to analogue—delayed	Modeling plus exposure—delayed; modeling plus exposure to analogue—spaced; modeling plus exposure—spaced; modeling plus exposure to analogue—immediate; modeling plus exposure—immediate	Immediate exposure to real stimuli led to best outcomes.
			Modeling plus exposure to analogue—immediate	Modeling plus exposure—immediate; modeling plus exposure to analogue—delayed; modeling plus exposure—delayed; modeling plus exposure to analogue—spaced; modeling plus exposure—spaced	Immediate exposure to real stimuli led to best outcomes.
			Modeling plus exposure to analogue—spaced	Modeling plus exposure—spaced; modeling plus exposure to analogue—immediate; modeling plus exposure—immediate; modeling plus exposure to analogue—delayed; modeling plus exposure—delayed	Immediate exposure to real stimuli led to best outcomes.
			Modeling plus exposure—delayed	Modeling plus exposure to analogue—spaced; modeling plus exposure—spaced; modeling plus exposure to analogue—immediate; modeling plus exposure—immediate; modeling plus exposure to analogue—delayed	Immediate exposure to real stimuli led to best outcomes.
			Modeling plus exposure—immediate	Modeling plus exposure to analogue—delayed; modeling plus exposure—delayed; modeling plus exposure to analogue—spaced; modeling plus exposure—spaced; modeling plus exposure to analogue—immediate	Immediate exposure to real stimuli led to best outcomes.
			Modeling plus exposure—spaced	Modeling plus exposure to analog—immediate; modeling plus exposure—immediate; modeling plus exposure to analogue—delayed; modeling plus exposure—delayed; modeling plus exposure to analogue—spaced	Immediate exposure to real stimuli led to best outcomes.

Compliance	Gender	Age	Ethnicity	Therapist	Frequency	Duration	Contacts	Dose	Setting	Format
100%	Both	13–59	N/R	N/R	Twice weekly	2.5 weeks	5	N/R	Clinic	Individual
100%	Both	13–59	N/R	N/R	Twice weekly	2.5 weeks	5	N/R	Clinic	Individual
100%	Both	3–5	N/R	N/R	2/day	4 days	8	10 minutes	Clinic	Group
100%	Both	3–5	N/R	N/R	2/day	4 days	8	10 minutes	Clinic	Group
100%	Both	3–5	N/R	N/R	2/day	4 days	8	N/R	Clinic	Group
100%	Both	3–5	N/R	N/R	2/day	4 days	8	N/R	Clinic	Group
100%	Boys	13	N/R	MA	Variable	14 weeks	Variable	Variable	Hospital	Individual
100%	Girls	13–18	N/R	MA	Once	1 day	1	3 hours	N/R	Individual
100%	Girls	13–18	N/R	MA	Once	1 day	1	3 hours	N/R	Individual
100%	Girls	13–18	N/R	MA	Weekly	3 weeks	3	1 hour	N/R	Individual
100%	Girls	13–18	N/R	MA	Once	1 day	1	3 hours	N/R	Individual
100%	Girls	13–18	N/R	MA	Once	12 weeks	1	3 hours	N/R	Individual
100%	Girls	13–18	N/R	MA	Weekly	3 weeks	3	1 hour	N/R	Individual

(continued)

Reference	Entry criterion	Design	Treatment	Controls/comparisons	Results
Faust & Melamed (1984), Study 1	Surgery in hospital	RCT	Modeling with slide show	Attention placebo	Modeling slide show was superior to control at reducing fears.
Faust, Olson, & Rodriguez (1991)	Fear of medical procedures	RCT	Modeling alone	Modeling with mother; standard preparatory procedure	Both modeling interventions were superior to control.
			Modeling with mother	Modeling alone; standard preparatory procedure	Both modeling interventions were superior to control.
Gilbert et al. (1982)	Fear of injections	RCT	Modeling film	Placebo film	Modeling film had no impact beyond the placebo film on anxiety.
Gresham & Nagle (1980)	Social isolation	RCT	Coaching with video	Modeling and coaching with video; modeling with video; no treatment	Active treatments were all more effective than no treatment.
			Modeling and coaching with video	Modeling with video; coaching with video; no treatment	Active treatments were all more effective than no treatment.
			Modeling with video	Coaching with video; modeling and coaching with video; no treatment	Active treatments were all more effective than no treatment.
Hill, Liebert, & Mott (1968)	Animal fears	RCT	Modeling with film	No treatment	Modeling film was superior to no treatment.
Keller & Carlson (1974)	Social isolation	RCT	Modeling video	Placebo control video	Modeling led to increases in social behavior compared with placebo.
Klingman, Melamed, Cuthbert, & Hermecz (1984)	Dental fear	RCT	Participant modeling	Symbolic modeling	Participant modeling was superior to symbolic modeling on measures of dental fears.
Klorman, Hilpert, Michael, LaGana, & Sveen (1980), Study 3	Dental-naive	RCT	Coping model—video	Mastery model—video; placebo	Both modeling approaches led to better outcomes for youth naïve to dental procedures, compared with placebo.
			Mastery model—video	Coping model—video; placebo	Both modeling approaches led to better outcomes for youth naïve to dental procedures, compared with placebo.
Kornhaber & Schroeder (1975)	Fear of snakes	RCT	Fearful adult model—video	Fearless child model—video; fearful child model—video; fearless adult model—video; no treatment	Child modeling was superior to adult modeling and control; fearful/fearless model was not relevant.
			Fearful child model—video	Fearless adult model—video; fearful adult model—video; fearless child model—video; no treatment	Child modeling was superior to adult modeling and control; fearful/fearless model was not relevant.
			Fearless adult model—video	Fearful adult model—video; fearless child model—video; fearful child model—video; no treatment	Child modeling was superior to adult modeling and control; fearful/fearless model was not relevant.
			Fearless child model—video	Fearful child model—video; fearless adult model—video; fearful adult model—video; no treatment	Child modeling was superior to adult modeling and control; fearful/fearless model was not relevant.
Lewis (1974)	Fear of swimming	RCT	Modeling	Modeling plus participation; participation; no treatment	Modeling was superior to no treatment.
			Modeling plus participation	Participation; modeling; no treatment	Modeling plus participation was superior to all other conditions.
Mann & Rosenthal (1969)	Test anxiety	RCT	Group vicarious desensitization, observing group of models	Group direct desensitization; individual vicarious desensitization; individual desensitization; group vicarious desensitization, observing single model; no treatment	Treatment was better than no treatment on a measure of test anxiety, and no different from other active treatments.

Compliance	Gender	Age	Ethnicity	Therapist	Frequency	Duration	Contacts	Dose	Setting	Format
100%	Both	4–17	N/R	N/R	Once	1 day	1	10 minutes	Hospital	Individual
100%	N/R	4–10	N/R	N/R	Once	1 day	1	10 minutes	Hospital	Individual
100%	N/R	4–10	N/R	N/R	Once	18 weeks	1	10 minutes	Hospital	Individual
100%	Both	6–9	Caucasian, African American	N/R	Once	1 day	1	7–8 minutes	Summer camp	Individual
100%	Both	8–10	N/R	N/R	Twice weekly	3 weeks	6	20 minutes	School	Group
100%	Both	8–10	N/R	N/R	Twice weekly	4 weeks	6	20 minutes	School	Group
100%	Both	8–10	N/R	N/R	Twice weekly	3 weeks	6	20 minutes	School	Group
100%	Boys	Preschool	N/R	N/R	Once	16–20 weeks	1	11 minutes	N/R	N/R
100%	Both	3–5	N/R	N/R	Daily	4 days	4	5 minutes	Preschool	Individual
100%	Both	8–13	N/R	None	Once	1 day	1	20 minutes	Dental office	Individual
100%l	Both	5–10	Caucasian	N/R	Once	16 weeks	1	10 minutes	Dental office	Individual
100%	Both	4–11	Caucasian	N/R	Once	1 day	1	10 minutes	Dental office	Individual
100%	Girls	7–9	N/R	N/R	Once	1 day	1	6–7 minutes	Mobile laboratory	Individual
100%	Girls	7–9	N/R	N/R	Once	1 day	1	6–7 minutes	Mobile laboratory	Individual
100%	Girls	7–9	N/R	N/R	Once	5 days	1	6–7 minutes	Mobile laboratory	Individual
100%	Girls	7–9	N/R	N/R	Once	1 day	1	6–7 minutes	Mobile laboratory	Individual
100%	Both	5–12	African American	N/R	Once	1 day	1	18 minutes	Community	Individual
100%	Both	5–12	African American	N/R	Once	1 day	1	18 minutes	Community	Individual
100%	Both	12–13	N/R	MA, PhD	Weekly	8 weeks	8	50 minutes	Clinic	Group

(continued)

Reference	Entry criterion	Design	Treatment	Controls/comparisons	Results
Mann & Rosenthal (1969) *(cont.)*			Group vicarious desensitization, observing single model	Group vicarious desensitization, observing group of models; group direct desensitization; individual vicarious desensitization; individual direct desensitization; no treatment	Treatment was better than no treatment on a measure of test anxiety, and no different from other active treatments.
			Individual vicarious desensitization	Individual direct desensitization; group vicarious desensitization, observing single model; group vicarious desensitization, observing group of models; group direct desensitization; no treatment	Treatment was better than no treatment on a measure of test anxiety, and no different from other active treatments.
Matson (1981)	Fear of talking to adults	Multiple-baseline	Participant modeling (mother as model)		Treatment led to gains and were maintained at 6-month follow-up
Matson (1983)	Animal fears	Multiple-baseline	Modeling (mother as model)		Fear of dog decreased.
Melamed & Siegel (1975)	Fear of medical procedures	RCT	Modeling film	Placebo film	Modeling film was superior to control film for postoperation behavior problems.
Melamed, Yurcheson, Fleece, Hutcherson, & Hawes (1978)	Dental fear	RCT	Modeling plus information, long—video	Modeling plus information, short—video; information, long—video; information, short—video	Modeling treatments were superior to information approaches.
			Modeling plus information, short—video	Information, long—video; information, short—video; modeling plus information, long—video	Modeling treatments were superior to information approaches.
O'Connor (1972)	Social isolation	RCT	Modeling—video	Modeling—video, plus reinforcement; reinforcement; no treatment	Modeling with or without reinforcement led to better outcomes than reinforcement or no treatment.
			Modeling—video, plus reinforcement	Reinforcement; modeling—video; no treatment	Modeling with or without reinforcement led to better outcomes than reinforcement or no treatment.
Peterson, Schultheis, Ridley-Johnson, Miller, & Tracy (1984)	Fear of medical procedures	RCT	Puppet modeling	Video modeling; video modeling—inaccurate, contact placebo	All modeling treatments were better than placebo.
			Video modeling	Video modeling—inaccurate; contact placebo; puppet modeling	All modeling treatments were better than placebo.
			Video modeling—inaccurate	Contact placebo; puppet modeling; video modeling	All modeling treatments were better than placebo.
Ritter (1968)	Fear of snakes	RCT	Vicarious desensitization	Contact desensitization; no treatment	Modeling group was superior to no treatment.
Roberts, Wurtele, Boone, Gither, & Elkins (1981)	Fear of medical procedures	RCT	Modeling—slide show/exposure	Attention placebo	Modeling slide show was superior to control in reducing hospital fears.
Rosenfarb & Hayes (1984)	Fear of Dark	RCT	Modeling—tape (private)	Self-statement (public); self-statement (private); modeling—tape (public); no treatment	Modeling and cognitive therapies were better if child was told experimenter knew which tape child heard.
			Modeling—tape (public)	Modeling—tape (private); self-statement (public); self-statement (private); no treatment	Modeling and cognitive therapies were better if child was told experimenter knew which tape child heard.

Compliance	Gender	Age	Ethnicity	Therapist	Frequency	Duration	Contacts	Dose	Setting	Format
100%	Both	12–13	N/R	MA, PhD	Weekly	8 weeks	8	50 minutes	Clinic	Group
100%	Both	12–13	N/R	MA, PhD	Weekly	8 weeks	8	50 minutes	Clinic	Individual
100%	Girls	8–10	Caucasian	PhD	Variable	N/R	Variable	Variable	Clinic	Parent–child
100%	Girl	3	N/R	PhD	N/R	N/R	23	15–25 minutes	Home	Individual
100%	Both	4–12	Caucasian, African American	N/R	Once	1 day	1	15 minutes	Hospital	Individual
100%	Both	4–11	African American, Caucasian	N/R	Once	1 day	1	10 minutes	Dental office	Individual
100%	Both	4–11	African American, Caucasian	N/R	Once	12 weeks	1	4 minutes	Dental office	Individual
100%	N/R	Preschool	N/R	MA	Once	1 day	1	23 minutes	Preschool	Individual
100%	N/R	Preschool	N/R	MA	Daily	2 weeks	11	323 minutes	Preschool	Individual plus milieu
100%	Both	2–11	N/R	MA	Once	1 day	1	50 minutes	Hospital	Individual
100%	Both	2–11	N/R	MA	Once	1 day	1	50 minutes	Hospital	Individual
100%l	Both	2–11	N/R	MA	Once	1 day	1	50 minutes	Hospital	Individual
100%	Both	5–11	N/R	PhD	Daily	2 days	2	35 minutes	Clinic	Group
100%	Both	7–12	N/R	N/R	Once	1 day	1	30 minutes	School	Group
100%	Both	5–6	N/R	N/R	Once	1 day	1	9 minutes	School	Individual
100%	Both	5–6	N/R	N/R	Once	1 day	1	9 minutes	School	Individual

(continued)

Reference	Entry criterion	Design	Treatment	Controls/comparisons	Results
Weissbrod & Bryan (1973)	Fear of snakes	RCT	Modeling— younger age, opposite sex	Modeling—same age and sex; modeling—same age, opposite sex; modeling—younger age, same sex; modeling with replica	All modeling treatments with real stimulus were better than modeling with replica.
			Modeling— same age and sex	Modeling—same age, opposite sex; modeling—younger age, same sex; modeling—younger age, opposite sex; modeling with replica	All modeling treatments with real stimulus were better than modeling with replica.
			Modeling— same age, opposite sex	Modeling—younger age, same sex; modeling—younger age, opposite sex; modeling—same age and sex; modeling with replica	All modeling treatments with real stimulus were better than modeling with replica.
			Modeling— younger age, same sex	Modeling—younger age, opposite sex; modeling—same age and sex; modeling—same age, opposite sex; modeling with replica	All modeling treatments with real stimulus were better than modeling with replica.

Note. Abbreviations as in Appendix 4.1.

Compliance	Gender	Age	Ethnicity	Therapist	Frequency	Duration	Contacts	Dose	Setting	Format
100%	Boys	9–11	N/R	N/R	Once	1 day	1	5 minutes	Research trailer	Individual
100%	Boys	9–11	N/R	N/R	Once	1 day	1	5 minutes	Research trailer	Individual
100%	Boys	9–11	N/R	N/R	Once	1 day	1	5 minutes	Research trailer	Individual
100%	Boys	9–11	N/R	N/R	Once	1 day	1	5 minutes	Research trailer	Individual

APPENDIX 4.3. Efficacious Treatments for Fears and Anxieties in Youths: Cognitive–Behavioral Therapy (CBT) and Its Variants

Reference	Entry criterion	Design	Treatment	Controls/comparisons	Results
Barrett (1998)	OAD, SAD, SOP	RCT	CBT	CBT plus family anxiety management; wait list	CBT was superior to wait list on measures of anxiety and diagnoses.
			CBT plus family anxiety management	CBT; wait list	CBT plus family anxiety management was superior to wait list on measures of anxiety and diagnoses, with marginally larger effects on anxiety measures at 12-month follow-up relative to CBT alone.
Barrett, Dadds, & Rapee (1996)	OAD, SAD, SOP	RCT	CBT	CBT plus family anxiety management; wait list	CBT was superior to no treatment on measures of anxiety and diagnoses.
			CBT plus family anxiety management	CBT; wait list	CBT plus family anxiety management was superior to no treatment on measures of anxiety and diagnoses. Some benefits for younger children and girls were noted for CBT plus family anxiety management relative to CBT alone.
Barrett, Healy-Farrell, & March (2004)	OCD	RCT	Group CBT plus parent	CBT plus parent; wait list	Both forms of CBT were better than control, but not different from each other.
		RCT	CBT (parent & child)	Group CBT plus parent; wait list	Both forms of CBT were better than control, but not different from each other.
Beidel, Turner, & Morris (2000)	SOP	RCT	CBT	Attention placebo	CBT was superior to attention placebo.
Chorpita, Taylor, Francis, Moffitt, & Austin (2004)	GAD, SAD, PDA, SP, SOP, Anx NOS	Multiple-baseline	CBT	Self-monitoring	All participants were free of primary diagnosis at posttreatment and 6-month follow-up.
Cobham, Dadds, & Spence (1998)	SAD, OAD, GAD, SOP, SP	RCT	CBT plus parent anxiety management	CBT alone	Both groups improved; CBT plus parent anxiety management was superior for youths with anxious parents.
Cohen, Deblinger, Mannarino, & Steer (2004)	PTSD (sexual abuse)	RCT	Trauma-focused CBT	Child-centered therapy	Trauma-focused CBT was superior to alternative therapy.
Cohen & Mannarino (1996)	Sexual abuse	RCT	CBT for sexually abused preschoolers	Nondirective supportive therapy	CBT was superior to nondirective supportive therapy.
Cradock, Cotler, & Jason (1978)	Fear of public speaking	RCT	Cognitive rehearsal	Exposure; wait list	Cognitive rehearsal was superior to wait list on confidence only; no other differences.
Dahlquist, Gil, Armstrong, Ginsberg, & Jones (1985)	Fear of medical procedures	Multiple-baseline	CBT		Improvements were noted on most measures.

Compliance	Gender	Age	Ethnicity	Therapist	Frequency	Duration	Contacts	Dose	Setting	Format
83%	Both	7–14	Caucasian, Asian American	PhD	Weekly	12 weeks	12	120 minutes	Clinic	Group
88%	Both	7–14	Caucasian, Asian American	PhD	Weekly	12 weeks	12	120 minutes	Clinic	Group plus parent
89%	Both	7–14	N/R	PhD	Weekly	12 weeks	12	70 minutes	Clinic	Individual
92%	Both	7–14	N/R	PhD	Weekly	12 weeks	12	60–80 minutes	Clinic	Individual
100%	Both	7–17	N/R	N/R	Weekly	14 weeks; boosters at 1 & 3 months	16	90 minutes	Clinic	Group, parent–sibling, and sibling–parent–child
92%	Both	7–17	N/R	N/R	Weekly	14 weeks; boosters at 1 & 3 months	16	90 minutes	Clinic	Individual, parent–sibling, and sibling–parent–child
86%	Both	8–12	Caucasian, African American, Hispanic	N/R	Twice weekly	12 weeks	24	60–90 minutes	Clinic	Group and individual
64%	Both	7–12	Caucasian, Asian American, Pacific Islander	MA	Weekly	14 weeks	5–17	60 minutes	Community, clinic, school	Individual
91%	Both	7–14	N/R	N/R	Weekly	14 weeks	14	60 minutes	Clinic	Group
78%	Both	8–14	Caucasian, African American	MA, PhD	Weekly	12 weeks	12	45 minutes (parent), 45 minutes (child)	Clinic	Individual, parent, and parent–child
100%	Both	2–7	Caucasian, African American	MA	Weekly	12 weeks	12	50 minutes (parent), 40 minutes (child)	Clinic	Individual, parent, and parent–child
85%	Girls	14–15	N/R	MA	Daily	6 days	6	1 hour	School	Group
100%	Both	11–13	N/R	MA	N/R	3 weeks	N/R	N/R	Hospital	Individual

(continued)

Reference	Entry criterion	Design	Treatment	Controls/comparisons	Results
Deblinger & Heflin (1996)	PTSD (sexual abuse)	RCT	CBT (individual)	CBT (parent); CBT (parent & child); community control	All forms of CBT were superior to community control.
			CBT (parent & child)	Community control; CBT (individual); CBT (parent)	All forms of CBT were superior to community control.
			CBT (parent)	CBT (parent & child); community control; CBT (individual)	All forms of CBT were superior to community control.
De Rosier (2004)	Peer dislike, bullying, or social anxiety	RCT	CBT	No treatment	CBT was better than no treatment.
Farrell, Hains, & Davies (1998)	Sexual abuse	Multiple-baseline	CBT (individual)		Treatment led to reductions in PTSD symptoms.
Flannery-Schroeder & Kendall (2000)	SP, SAD, SOP, GAD, OCD	RCT	CBT (individual)	Group CBT; wait list	Both forms of CBT were superior to wait list, with individual CBT showing slightly better effects for diagnosis.
			Group CBT	CBT (individual); wait list	Both forms of CBT were superior to wait list, with individual CBT showing slightly better effects for diagnosis.
Gallagher, Rabian, & McCloskey (2004)	SOP	RCT	Group CBT	Wait list	Group CBT was superior to wait list.
Goenjian et al. (1997)	PTSD (disaster)	RCT	CBT	No treatment	Participants in brief CBT fared better on measures of PTSD symptoms.
Graziano & Mooney (1980)	Fear of dark	RCT	Family self-control instruction	No treatment	Participants in brief CBT fared better on measures of nighttime fears.
Harris & Brown (1982)	Shyness	RCT	CBT	Informed teachers; no treatment	CBT was better than control and no treatment.
Heyne et al. (2002)	School refusal	RCT	CBT plus parent and teacher training	Parent and teacher training; CBT	Combined intervention was superior at posttreatment to CBT (individual), but no differences at follow-up.
Howard & Kendall (1996)	SAD, GAD, SOP	Multiple-baseline	Family CBT		Treatment produced gains on standardized measures and diagnostic status.
Kane & Kendall (1989)	OAD	Multiple-baseline	CBT		Treatment produced gains on standardized measures and diagnostic status.
Kanfer, Karoly, & Newman (1975)	Fear of dark	RCT	Competence self-talk	Stimulus self-talk; neutral self-talk	Children making coping statements (e.g., "I am brave") fared better than those making stimulus statements (e.g., "The dark is fun") and those making neutral statements (e.g., "Mary had a little lamb").
Kendall (1994)	OAD, SAD, AD	RCT	CBT	Wait list	CBT resulted in greater improvements on measures of anxiety than no treatment.

Compliance	Gender	Age	Ethnicity	Therapist	Frequency	Duration	Contacts	Dose	Setting	Format
90%	Both	7–13	Caucasian, African American, Hispanic	MA	Weekly	12 weeks	12	45 minutes	Clinic	Individual
90%	Both	7–13	Caucasian, African American, Hispanic	MA	Weekly	12 weeks	12	90 minutes	Clinic	Individual and parent
90%	Both	7–13	Caucasian, African American, Hispanic	MA	Weekly	12 weeks	12	45 minutes	Clinic	Parent
100%	Both	7–10	Caucasian, African American, Hispanic, Asian American	BA, MA	Weekly	12 weeks	8	50 minutes	School	Group
100%	Both	8–10	African American, Caucasian, Hispanic	MA	Weekly	1 day	10	60 minutes	Clinic	Individual
82%	Both	8–14	Caucasian	MA	Weekly	1 day	18	50 minutes	Clinic	Individual
82%	Both	8–14	Caucasian	MA	Weekly	18 weeks	18	90 minutes	Clinic	Group
100%	Both	8–11	Caucasian, African American	MA	Weekly	8 weeks	3	3 hours	Clinic	Group
100%	Both	12–13	N/R (Armenian national)	N/R	Twice weekly	3 weeks	6	30 minutes (group), 60 minutes (individual)	School	Group and individual
100%	Both	6–12	N/R	Under-graduates	Weekly	3 weeks	3	N/R	Clinic	Group
100%	Both	9–12	N/R	N/R	Twice weekly	N/R	10	45 minutes	School	Group
95%	Both	7–14	N/R (Australian national)	MA	Twice weekly	4 weeks	8	50 minutes	Clinic and school	Individual, and parent and school consults
100%	Both	9–13	N/R	MA	Weekly	5 weeks	16–20	50 minutes	Clinic	Parent–child
100%	Both	9–13	N/R	MA	Twice weekly	1 day	16–20	1 hour	Clinic	Individual
100%	Both	5–6	N/R	Under-graduates	Once	1 day	1	N/R	School	Individual
74%	Both	9–13	Caucasian, African American	MA	Weekly	16 weeks	16	50 minutes	Clinic	Individual

(continued)

Reference	Entry criterion	Design	Treatment	Controls/comparisons	Results
Kendall et al. (1997)	OAD, SAD, AD	RCT	CBT	Wait list	CBT resulted in greater improvements on measures of anxiety than wait list.
King et al. (1998)	School refusal, primarily with anxiety disorder as well	RCT	CBT	Wait list	CBT resulted in better school attendance than wait list.
King et al. (2000)	Sexual abuse with PTSD symptoms	RCT	CBT (individual)	CBT (family); wait list	CBT was better than wait list on measures of anxiety symptoms and global functioning.
		RCT	CBT (family)	CBT (individual); wait list	CBT (family) was better than wait list on measures of anxiety symptoms and global functioning.
Knox, Albano, & Barlow (1996)	OCD	Multiple-baseline	CBT		CBT with parent involvement showed positive results for the 4 participants.
Leal et al. (1981)	Test anxiety	RCT	Cognitive modification	Exposure; wait list	Cognitive superior to exposure and wait list re: anxiety.
Lumpkin, Silverman, Weems, Markham, & Kurtines (2002)	SP, SAD, SOP, GAD, OCD	Multiple-baseline	Group CBT		CBT reduced anxiety symptoms in participants.
Manassis et al. (2002)	GAD, SAD, SP, SOP, PD[A]	RCT	Group CBT plus parent	CBT plus parent	CBT (individual and group) both produced improvement (*n*'s sufficiently large for equivalence).
			CBT plus parent	Group CBT plus parent	CBT (individual and group) both produced improvement (*n*'s sufficiently large for equivalence).
March, Amaya-Jackson, Murray, & Schulte (1998)	PTSD	Multiple-baseline	CBT		All participants improved on study measures; 57% of completers were diagnosis-free at posttreatment.
Muris, Meesters, & van Melick (2002)	GAD, SAD, SOP	RCT	Group CBT	Group education support; no treatment	CBT was superior to education support and control.
Nauta, Scholing, Emmelkamp, & Minderaa (2003)	SAD, GAD, SOP, PD[A]	RCT	CBT plus parent	CBT; wait list	CBT plus parent was superior to wait list only.
			CBT	CBT plus parent; wait list	CBT was superior to wait list only.
Nocella & Kaplan (1982)	Dental fear	RCT	Stress inoculation	Attention placebo; no treatment	Stress inoculation was superior to placebo and no treatment for dental procedures.
Ollendick (1995)	PDA	Multiple-baseline	CBT		CBT reduced panic symptoms systematically across 4 participants.
Rosenfarb & Hayes (1984)	Fear of dark	RCT	Self-statement (public)	Self-statement (private); modeling—tape (public); modeling—tape (private); no treatment	Self-statement worked better if child was told experimenter knew which tape child heard.

Compliance	Gender	Age	Ethnicity	Therapist	Frequency	Duration	Contacts	Dose	Setting	Format
75%	Both	9–13	Caucasian, African American, Hispanic	MA	Weekly	16 weeks	16	50 minutes	Clinic	Individual
100%	Both	5–15	N/R	PhD	1.5/week	20 weeks	6	50 minutes	Clinic	Individual
75%	Both	5–17	N/R	PhD	Weekly	20 weeks	20	50 minutes	Clinic	Individual
75%	Both	5–17	N/R	PhD	Weekly	6–13 weeks	20 (plus 20 with parent)	50 minutes	Clinic	Individual and parent
100%	Both	8–13	Caucasian	MA	3/week, weekly, every other week	15 weeks	30	90 minutes	Clinic	Individual
100%	N/R	15–17	N/R	MA	Weekly	6 weeks	6	1 hour	N/R	Group
67%	Both	6–16	N/R	MA	Weekly	12 weeks	12	90 minutes	Clinic	Group
100%	Both	8–12	Caucasian, African American, Asian American	MA	Weekly	12 weeks	12	90 minutes	Clinic	Group child and group parent
100%	Both	8–12	Caucasian, African American, Asian American	MA	Weekly	8 weeks	12	90 minutes	Clinic	Individual and parent
82%	Both	10–15	Caucasian, African American, Native American, Asian American	N/R	Weekly	Variable	18	N/R	Clinic	Group
100%	Both	9–12	Caucasian	MA	Twice weekly	6 weeks	12	30 minutes	School	Group
100%	Both	7–18	Caucasian	MA	Weekly	1 day	12 (plus 7 with parent)	N/R	Clinic	Individual and parent
100%	Both	7–18	Caucasian	MA	Weekly	12 weeks	12	N/R	Clinic	Individual
100%	Both	5–13	N/R	N/R	Once	10 weeks	1	15 minutes	Dental office	Individual
100%	Both	13–17	Caucasian	PhD	Weekly	2 weeks	8	N/R	Clinic	Individual
100%	Both	5–6	N/R	N/R	Once	N/R	1	9 minutes	School	Individual

(continued)

Reference	Entry criterion	Design	Treatment	Controls/comparisons	Results
Sheslow, Bondy, & Nelson (1982)	Fear of dark	RCT	Coping skills/ graduated exposure	Verbal coping skills; graduated exposure; contact control	Exposure plus coping skills was superior to coping skills alone and a placebo control.
Shortt, Barrett, & Fox (2001)	SAD, GAD, SOP	RCT	Family-based group CBT	No treatment	The group CBT program was superior to no treatment on measures of anxiety, and 69% were diagnosis-free at posttreatment.
Silverman, Kurtines, Ginsburg, Weems, Lumpkin, et al. (1999)	GAD, SOP, OAD	RCT	Group CBT	Wait list	Treatment was superior to no treatment on main study variables; 64% no longer had primary diagnosis at posttreatment.
Spence, Donovan, & Brechman-Toussaint (2000)	SOP	RCT	CBT (parent & child)	CBT without parents; wait list	CBT with parents was superior to wait list; no difference between active treatments.
			CBT (individual)	CBT with parents; wait list	CBT without parents was superior to wait list; no difference between active treatments.
Stein et al. (2003)	Trauma with PTSD symptoms	RCT	CBT	Wait list	CBT was superior to wait list.
van der Ploege-Stapart & van der Ploege (1986)	Test anxiety	RCT	CBT	Wait list	CBT was superior to wait list.

Compliance	Gender	Age	Ethnicity	Therapist	Frequency	Duration	Contacts	Dose	Setting	Format
100%	Both	4–5	N/R	MA	Daily	10–14 weeks	3	30 minutes	School	Individual
92%	Both	6–10	Caucasian	MA	Weekly	10–14 weeks	12 (plus 10 parent)	70 minutes (group), 40 minutes (parent)	Clinic	Group with parent
68%	Both	6–16	Caucasian, Hispanic	MA, PhD	Weekly	10 weeks	N/R	55 minutes	Clinic	Group
94%	Both	7–14	N/R	PhD	Weekly plus boosters	12 weeks plus boosters at 2 and 6 months	14	60 minutes	Clinic	Group plus parent
79%	Both	7–14	N/R	PhD	Weekly plus boosters	12 weeks plus boosters at 2 and 6 months	14	60 minutes	Clinic	Group
89%	Both	10–13	N/R	MA	Weekly	10 weeks	10	40 minutes (estimated from length of one class)	School	Group
100%	Both	12–20	N/R	N/R	Weekly	N/R	9	90 minutes	School	Group (plus one parent)

Note. OAD, overanxious disorder; SAD, separation anxiety disorder; SOP, social phobia; OCD, obsessive–compulsive disorder; GAD, generalized anxiety disorder; PDA, panic disorder with agoraphobia; SP, specific phobia; Anx NOS, anxiety disorder not otherwise specified; PTSD, posttraumatic stress disorder; AD, avoidant disorder. Other abbreviations as in Appendix 4.1.

APPENDIX 4.4. Efficacious Treatments for Fears and Anxieties in Youths: Other Interventions

Reference	Entry criterion	Design	Treatment	Controls/comparisons	Results
Clement & Milne (1967)	Shyness	RCT	Group play therapy (Ginott), no tokens	No-therapist play; group play therapy (Ginott), plus tokens	Play group without tokens was superior to play group without a therapist.
			Group play therapy (Ginott), plus tokens	Group play therapy (Ginott), no tokens; no-therapist play	Play group including tokens was superior to play group without tokens and play group without a therapist.
Genshaft (1982)	Math anxiety	RCT	Tutoring plus self-instruction	Tutoring; no treatment	Tutoring plus self-instruction was superior to tutoring only and no treatment.
Genshaft & Hirt (1980)	Math anxiety	RCT	Tutoring plus self-instruction	Tutoring; no treatment	Tutoring plus self-instruction was superior to tutoring only and no treatment.
Heyne et al. (2002)	School refusal	RCT	Parent and teacher training	CBT plus parent and teacher training; CBT	Parent and teacher training was superior to CBT alone, but no differences at follow-up.
Jones, Ollendick, McLaughlin, & Williams (1989)	Fear of fire	RCT	Elaborative rehearsal	Behavioral rehearsal; no treatment	Elaborative rehearsal of fire safety skills produced reductions in fear of fire, relative to brief behavioral rehearsal or no treatment.
Williams & Jones (1989)	Fear of fire	RCT	Education	Education plus self-instruction training; placebo; wait list	Education was better than placebo and wait list.
			Education plus self-instruction training	Education; placebo; wait list	Education plus self-instruction training was better than placebo and wait list; it was also superior to education alone on some measures.
Wilson & Rotter (1986)	Test anxiety	RCT	Study habits training	Exposure plus relaxation plus study habits; attention placebo; exposure plus relaxation; no treatment	Training in study habits was superior to attention placebo and no treatment.

Note. Abbreviations as in earlier appendices.

Compliance	Gender	Age	Ethnicity	Therapist	Frequency	Duration	Contacts	Dose	Setting	Format
100%	Boys	8–9	Caucasian	N/R	Weekly	14 weeks	14	N/R	N/R	Child group and parent group
100%	Boys	8–9	Caucasian	N/R	Weekly	14 weeks	14	N/R	N/R	Child group and parent group
100%	Girls	13	N/R	N/R	Twice weekly	3 weeks	16	40 minutes	School	Group
100%	Girls	12–13	N/R	MA	Twice weekly	3 weeks	6	40 minutes	School	Group
90%	Both	7–14	N/R (Australian national)	MA	Twice weekly	4 weeks	9	50 minutes	Clinic and school	Individual, and parent and school consults
100%	Both	9	N/R	Undergraduates	Daily	3 days	3	60 minutes	School	Group
100%	Both	7–10	N/R	BA, MA	Once	1 day	1	50–60 minutes	School	Group
100%	Both	7–10	N/R	BA, MA	Once	1 day	1	50–60 minutes	School	Group
100%	Both	11–13	African American, Caucasian	PhD	Twice weekly	3 weeks	6	45 minutes	N/R	Group

5

Depressive Disorders
during Childhood and Adolescence

Kevin D. Stark, Janay Sander, Michelle Hauser, Jane Simpson,
Sarah Schnoebelen, Rand Glenn, and Johanna Molnar

Depression among children and adolescents is a relatively common, enduring, and recurrent disorder (Kovacs, Feinberg, Crouse-Novak, Paulauskas, & Finkelstein, 1984) that has an adverse impact on a youngster's psychosocial development (Lewinsohn, Rohde, Seeley, Klein, & Gotlib, 2003) and in some cases is associated with self-destructive and life-threatening behaviors (Weissman et al., 1999). Depressive disorders during childhood and adolescence may be more virulent and of longer duration than depressive disorders in adults (Jensen, Ryan, & Prien, 1992). Depressive disorders during childhood are a risk factor for the development of additional psychological disturbances (Kovacs et al., 1984) and for the development of depressive disorders later in life (Pine, Cohen, Gurley, Brook, & Ma, 1998). The number of youths who are experiencing depressive disorders is increasing at the same time that the age of onset is decreasing (Burke, Burke, Regier, & Rae, 1991).

Over the past decade, a great deal of research into depressive disorders during childhood and adolescence has been completed. The primary focus of this chapter is on the treatment of depressive disorders. Perhaps the most exciting research in this area is being conducted and reported at the time of writing this chapter. Preliminary reports are appearing in the literature on a large-scale efficacy study of cognitive-behavioral therapy (CBT), fluoxetine, and the

combination of CBT and fluoxetine for depressed adolescents (March, 2004). Another large-scale study evaluating the efficacy of CBT with and without parent training is being conducted with depressed girls between the ages of 9 and 13 years by our research group. Prior to reviewing this research and describing our treatment program, we describe basic research on youth depression.

PRIMARY SYMPTOMS AND DIAGNOSTIC CRITERIA

Diagnostic Criteria

The *Diagnostic and Statistical Manual of Mental Disorders,* fourth edition, text revision (DSM-IV-TR; American Psychiatric Association [APA], 2000) groups mood disorders into two categories: depressive disorders and bipolar disorders. Both types of disorders are characterized by depressive episodes. However, bipolar disorders include the presence of a manic episode. The focus of this chapter is on depressive disorders, which are divided into three diagnostic categories based on symptom expression, severity, and duration. Major depressive disorder (MDD) is characterized by a severe presentation of multiple symptoms for at least a 2-week period of time; dysthymic disorder (DD) is less severe, but of protracted duration; and depressive disorder not otherwise specified (DDNOS) has a disturbance in mood as its central characteristic, but does not meet diagnostic criteria for MDD or DD.

For a diagnosis of MDD, the child must be experiencing a mood disturbance (either dysphoria, irritability, or anhedonia) for a period of at least 2 weeks, and the symptoms must be present more often than not. At least four of the following symptoms must be present during the same period: (1) significant, unintentional weight gain or loss (or, in children, failure to gain weight as would be expected); (2) insomnia or hypersomnia; (3) psychomotor retardation or agitation; (4) fatigue or loss of energy; (5) feelings of worthlessness or extreme guilt; (6) diminished concentration or ability to make decisions; and/or (7) recurring thoughts of death, suicidality, or suicide attempt. These symptoms must be present nearly every day; must represent a change from previous functioning; and must cause impairment or distress in social, academic, occupational, or other areas of functioning. In order to meet criteria for MDD, these symptoms may not have been caused by the physiological effects of a substance or medical condition, and may not be due to bereavement. They must also not be better explained by schizoaffective disorder or superimosed on another psychotic disorder, and there must never have been a manic, hypomanic, or mixed disorder (APA, 2000).

DD is often described as a chronic, low-grade depression. The depressed or irritable mood must be present for more days than not, and in youths must last for at least 1 year. In addition to dysphoria or irritability, at least two of the following symptoms must be present: (1) overeating or poor appetite; (2) insomnia or hypersomnia; (3) fatigue or low energy; (4) poor self-esteem; (5) poor concentration or trouble making decisions; and/or (6) feelings of hopelessness (APA, 2000).

When an individual exhibits some of the symptoms of MDD or DD but does not meet the diagnostic criteria, a diagnosis of DDNOS may be appropriate. For example, if a youngster is reporting a mood disturbance along with a number of additional symptoms, but the disturbance has lasted for less than 1 year, then a diagnosis of DDNOS may be appropriate (APA, 2000).

Developmental Considerations

The general consensus of the field is that the basic expression of childhood depression is similar to that of adult depression. Thus it is believed that the adult criteria, with modifications that reflect the developmental expression of symptoms, can be used to diagnose depressive disorders during childhood (e.g., Carlson & Kashani, 1988; Kovacs, 1996b; Luby et al., 2002). Within the DSM-IV-TR (APA, 2000), there are few distinctions between the diagnostic criteria for depressive disorders in children and those in adults. The single difference for MDD in children, compared to adults, is the possible presence of irritable mood rather than dysphoric mood. For DD, children need only suffer with the pattern of depressive symptoms for 1 year rather than 2 years to meet diagnostic criteria (APA, 2000). However, research suggests that there are additional differences by developmental level in symptom presentation.

Because their moods are more sensitive to environmental events, young children may not experience a prolonged mood disturbance that is devoid of periods of elevated mood. Rather, they are more likely to experience variation in mood from day to day, characterized by a pattern of more frequent and longer-lasting periods of irritability, sadness, and anhedonia that are broken up by periods of elevated mood. Thus it may be necessary to alter the duration requirements for a diagnosis of a depressive disorder in very young children (Luby et al., 2003). In addition, young children may experience irritability or flat affect rather than dysphoria as the dominant mood disturbance. For example, depressed preschoolers experience irritability (Kashani, Allan, Beck, Bledsoe, & Reid, 1997) and anhedonia (Luby et al., 2002, 2003) as their primary mood disturbance. Weiss and Garber (2003) hypothesize that anger and dysphoria may be developmental anomalies of the same underlying symptom. Luby and colleagues hypothesize that anhedonia expressed as having "no fun" is an early marker of MDD. However, it is important to note that the preschoolers who were experiencing DD in the Kashani and colleagues (1997) study did not report anhedonia; rather, they reported irritability as their primary mood disturbance. Thus it is possible that anhedonia characterizes the mood disturbance of preschoolers who are experiencing MDD, whereas irritability is the dominant mood disturbance among preschoolers who are experiencing DD.

In addition to developmental differences in the expression of the primary mood disturbance, other symptoms may be expressed in a developmentally sensitive fashion. For example, preoccupation with death or suicidal ideation may be expressed through themes in play, rather than directly in response to queries (Luby et al., 2003). Lack of energy may be expressed through a pattern of engaging in more passive play activities versus activities that require more energy. Similarly, a child may complain that he or she doesn't have the energy necessary to complete schoolwork. Due to limited verbal and cognitive abilities, a depressed child may express the distress through aggressive behavior (e.g., Kashani et al., 1997). Social withdrawal may appear to be shyness or a preference for solitary play. Several investigators have reported that older depressed individuals are more likely than younger ones to endorse neurovegetative symptoms (Carlson & Kashani, 1988; Kovacs, Obrosky, & Sherrill, 2003; Ryan et al., 1987; Weiss & Garber, 2003). However, contradictory findings have been reported by Luby and colleagues (2002, 2003), who reported that preschool-age children who were experiencing MDD commonly experienced vegetative symptoms, including appetite changes and sleep disturbance. They were also more likely to experience psychomotor agitation rather than retardation. Impaired concentration, however, is reportedly consistent across developmental levels (Biederman, Newcorn, & Sprich, 1991; Carlson & Kashani, 1988).

Cognitive development may contribute to some differences between children's expression of depressive symptoms and that of adolescents or adults. In support of the cognitive limitation hypothesis, prepubertal children endorse hopelessness less frequently than adolescents (Carlson & Kashani, 1988; Luby et al., 2002; Kashani et al., 1997; Ryan et al., 1987). Hopelessness requires a level of generalization and concept formation that young children may not yet possess. It has been suggested that children lack the capacity for the abstract reasoning and formal operational thinking required to produce the internal, global, and stable explanatory style associated with depression (Turner & Cole, 1994). In depressed preadolescents and adolescents, a lack of perceived personal competence was associated with depression; however, in adolescents, the more abstract concept of contingencies (whether an outcome actually depends on an individual's behavior in general) is also related to depression (Weisz, Southam-Gerow, & McCarty, 2002). Negative life events

are better predictors of depression in 8-year-olds, while a pessimistic attributional style predicted depression in 11- and 12-year-olds (Nolen-Hoeksema, Girgus, & Seligman, 1991). Therefore, at younger ages, it is possible that environmental conditions are greater contributors to the depressed state than cognitive factors are (Weiss & Garber, 2003). Children and adolescents endorse higher levels of guilt and low self-esteem than adults do (Mitchell, McCauley, Burke, & Moss, 1988), and this may reflect the developmental tendency toward egocentricity. Later childhood and adolescence bring an increase in reports of the cognitive correlates of depression, including hopelessness and low self-esteem; adolescents have also been noted to begin to display a greater number of neurovegetative symptoms, such as sleep and appetite disturbance, although not at the same level as adults (Birmaher et al., 2000; Borchardt & Meller, 1996).

Another developmental difference may be in the way that severity of symptoms is expressed in depressed youths or in the actual severity of the experience and expression of depressive symptoms. Applying adult symptom severity criteria may not capture the symptomatic experience of children with MDD, as they may display symptoms to a less severe degree than adults (Ryan et al., 1987). Thus some depressed youths may go undiagnosed if the adult criteria are used. It appears as though the adult criteria are effective for diagnosing more severe forms of depressive disorders during childhood, but these criteria may be too stringent for less severe cases.

In addition to the diagnostic developmental patterns described above, researchers have indicated that prepubertal children have higher rates of depressed appearance (Ryan et al., 1987), comorbid separation anxiety (Mitchell et al., 1988; Ryan et al., 1987), temper tantrums and behavioral problems (Borchardt & Meller, 1996) and auditory hallucinations (Chambers, Puig-Antich, Tabrizi, & Davies, 1982; Mitchell et al., 1988; Ryan et al., 1987). Adolescents are more likely to have suicidal ideation, as well as a history of suicide attempts and delusional thinking (Birmaher et al., 2000; Carlson & Kashani, 1988). When an inpatient sample was considered, there was no significant difference between children and adolescents in prevalence or presentation of psychotic symptoms (Borchardt & Meller, 1996). Other symptoms that increase with age include diurnal variation (depression worse in the morning) and psychomotor retardation (Borchardt & Meller, 1996; Carlson & Kashani, 1988). Irritability may continue to be a dominant component of the mood disturbance into adolescence (Birmaher et al., 2000).

How do the symptoms of depression affect children and adolescents? Depression can have a significant negative impact on the life of any youth. Depressive symptoms can impair functioning and quality of life as much as, or more than, chronic medical conditions such as diabetes, angina, pulmonary problems, and arthritis (Wells et al., 1989). Symptoms such as depressed mood, irritability, and diminished interest in activities can lead to cognitive, familial, and social problems (Hammen & Rudolph, 1996). There is also an increased likelihood of suicidality and suicidal ideation in depressed adolescents. In general, prepubertal onset of depression is associated with an increased risk for developing a bipolar disorder, as well as the potential for recurrent depressive episodes (Kovacs, 1996a). MDD is also accompanied by poor psychosocial outcome, comorbid conditions, and high risk of substance abuse (Kovacs, Goldston, & Gatsonis, 1993). Thus acute treatment and prevention are critical.

PREVALENCE AND SEX RATIO

Prevalence

Prevalence rates progressively increase with age until the time of late childhood and early adolescence, when the rate jumps and then continues to increase through late adolescence, when it reaches adult levels (Burke et al., 1991; Costello, Mustillo, Erkanli, Keeler, & Angold, 2003). Depressive disorders have been reported among children between the ages of 3 and 6 years, although they are relatively rare and associated with extreme abuse or neglect (Kashani & Carlson, 1987). Kashani and Carlson (1987) reported that 0.9% of preschool-age children were experiencing MDD, although in an earlier study of preschoolers, Kashani, Ray, and Carlson (1984) did not find any cases of MDD. In another investigation of 2- to 6-year-olds referred to a child development unit, Kashani and colleagues (1997) reported that 2.7% of these preschoolers were experiencing DD.

The prevalence rates for school-age children appear to be substantially higher; they progres-

sively increase between 9 and 11 years of age, and then they may decline slightly at age 12 (Costello et al., 2003). Kashani and colleagues (1983) reported rates of 1.85% for MDD and 3–4% for DD among 9-year-olds. In a study of 8- and 12-year-olds (Kashani, Orvaschel, Rosenberg, & Reid, 1989), a rate of 1.4% was reported for MDD. Costello and colleagues (1988) reported lower rates of 0.4% for MDD and 0.6% for DD among 7- to 11-year-olds. Anderson, Williams, McGee, and Silva (1987) reported prevalence rates of 0.5% for MDD and 1.7% for DD among 11-year-olds. Similar prevalence rates for MDD (1.8%), but higher rates for DD (6.4%), have been reported for 8- to 11-year-old children in Spain (Polaino-Lorente & Domenech, 1993). In general, it appears as though 1.5–2.5% of elementary-age children will be experiencing either MDD or DD.

Existing research indicates that prevalence rates for adolescents are higher than those reported for children. In a study conducted by Costello and colleagues (2003), the 3-month prevalence rate for 13-year-olds was 2.6%; for 14-year-olds it was 2.7%; for 15-year-olds it was 3.7%; and for 16-year-olds it was 3.1%. In an investigation of 13-year-olds (McGee & Williams, 1988), rates of 0.4% for MDD and 1.6% for DD were reported. In a study of 15-year-olds, 1.2% were found to have current MDD; an additional 1.9% had had an episode in the past, and 1.1% were experiencing DD (McGee et al., 1990). Results from a large high school population indicated that the prevalence rate for unipolar depression was 2.9% (Lewinsohn, Hops, Roberts, Seeley, & Andrews, 1993). This 2.9% figure is very similar to the 3% reported by Rohde, Lewinsohn, and Seeley (1991). However, it is significantly lower than the 5.3% reported by Haarasilta, Marttunen, Kaprio, and Aro (2001); the 8% reported by Kashani and colleagues (1987); the 9.2% reported by Rushton, Forcier, and Shectman (2003); and the 12% reported by Andrews, Garrison, Jackson, Addy, and McKeown (1993). Researchers estimate that by the age of 14 years 7.2% of adolescents have experienced an episode of MDD, and that by the end of adolescence between 16.8% (Newman et al., 1996) and 18.5% (Lewinsohn, Hops, et al., 1993) of youths will have experienced an episode of depression.

It appears that higher prevalence rates are found among youths from a variety of special populations. Children who are referred for educational problems appear to suffer from higher rates of depression. Weinberg, Rutman, Sullivan, Penick, and Dietz (1973) reported that 49% of the children from an educational diagnostic clinic were depressed. Investigators have reported prevalence rates ranging from 20% to 50% for adolescents enrolled in special education programs (e.g., Mattison, Humphrey, Kales, Hernit, & Finkenbinder, 1986). Lobovits and Handal (1985) reported a prevalence rate of 34% for youngsters who were referred to a psychiatric clinic for behavioral and academic problems. As would be expected, the prevalence rates are high for youths who are receiving mental health services (e.g., Brady & Kendall, 1992). The prevalence rate of depression among elementary-age children from psychiatric clinics ranges in the literature from 2.1% (Christ, Adler, Isacoff, & Gershansky, 1981) to 61% (Weinberg et al., 1973). Studies of inpatient children have reported a range from 26% (Asarnow & Bates, 1988) to 58% (Carlson & Cantwell, 1980) or 59% (Kashani, Venzke, & Millar, 1981). Hodges and Siegel (1985) noted that prevalence rates for adolescent psychiatric patients have ranged from 13% to 60%, while Petersen and colleagues (1993) reported that depression rates averaged 42% across studies of clinic samples. Children with a variety of medical problems, including headaches (40%) (Ling, Oftedal, & Weinberg, 1970); orthopedic patients (23%) (Kashani, Barbero, & Bolander, 1981); patients with cancer (17%) (Kashani & Hakami, 1982); and general medical patients (Kashani, Barbero, et al., 1981) all experience higher rates of depression than children in the general population.

Sex Ratio

Before adolescence, approximately equal numbers of boys and girls experience depression (Speier, Sherak, Hirsch, & Cantwell, 1995). However, after puberty, females are twice as likely as boys to experience depression (Birmaher et al., 1996; Poznanski & Mokros, 1994; Rushton et al., 2003). Girls begin to show higher rates of depression between 13 and 15 years of age (e.g., Ge, Conger, & Elder, 2001; Twenge & Nolen-Hoeksema, 2002; Wade, Cairney, & Pevalin, 2002), and they are more likely to experience their first episode between the ages of 15 and 18 (Hankin,

Abramson, Silva, McGee, & Angell, 1998). In adolescence, females consistently score higher on measures of emotional distress, particularly depression (e.g., Casper, Belanoff, & Offer, 1996).

Findings are mixed with regard to gender differences in the course and severity of depression. Some literature has reported that females experience more severe symptoms (Kandel & Davies, 1986), more persistent symptoms (Rushton et al., 2003), and a different pattern of symptoms (Casper et al., 1996 Ostrov, Offer, & Howard, 1989) than males, and that the difference in symptom pattern is not due to response style (Nolen-Hoeksema et al., 1991). Other studies using diagnostic interviews have found no gender differences in severity of depressive symptoms or likelihood of having recurrent episodes (Hankin et al., 1998).

Gender has a unique effect on adult psychosocial outcomes of individuals with adolescent-onset depression. For women, depression in adolescence is associated with hospitalization, abuse of tranquilizers, school dropout, and marital distress (Kandel & Davies, 1986). In a clinically referred sample, Kovacs (2001) did not find gender differences in terms of age of onset for initial or recurrent episodes, rate of recovery, comorbid disorders, or specific symptom profiles. Although findings have been mixed with regard to gender differences in depression, the consistent finding that girls report more depressive symptoms in early adolescence signals a need to target interventions toward preadolescent and early adolescent girls.

VULNERABILITY, STRESS, AND GENDER

Vulnerability

Some authors suggest that there are gender-specific pathways to depression in adolescence with respect to family variables (Compton, Snyder, Schrepferman, Bank, & Shortt, 2003); specifically, boys become more aggressive and girls become more passive in response to coercive family patterns. Although the mechanisms through which the gender difference in depression emerges are still unknown, several models have been proposed. The models that appear to be supported by the most evidence are diathesis–stress models that discuss vulnerabilities and stressors unique to girls (e.g., Hankin & Abramson, 2001; Nolen-Hoeksema &

Girgus, 1994). These models provide evidence that girls have more cognitive, biological, and interpersonal vulnerability factors prior to adolescence and face more stressful events during the transition to adolescence, leading to higher rates of depression.

A ruminative style of coping with stressors is both linked to depression and more often present in females than males (Nolen-Hoeksema, 1987). Females, when faced with stress, are more likely to ruminate about their depressed mood and its cause than to attempt actively to solve the problem. Nolen-Hoeksema (1987) argues that women are socialized to use this coping style because of gender role stereotypes associated with emotionality. This hypothesis may explain the tendency for adolescent girls to rate negative events as more stressful than boys (Rudolph & Hammen, 1999). A more negative attributional style about stressful events, and more negative thoughts about the self in response to a negative event, have also been found in females, and this difference in cognitive style mediates the gender difference in depressive symptoms (Hankin & Abramson, 2002).

Stereotypical female gender role characteristics, primarily expressivity and a lack of instrumentality, have been proposed as vulnerability factors in depression (Marcotte, Alain, & Gosselin, 1999; Nolen-Hoeksema & Girgus, 1994). Puberty is hypothesized to be associated with an increased focus on the significance of gender and identification with stereotypical gender roles (Hill & Lynch, 1983). As youths move from childhood to adolescence, girls become less instrumental and more expressive, and boys become more instrumental and less expressive. It appears that for both genders, depression is more associated with a decrease in instrumentality than with an increase in expressivity (Marcotte et al., 1999; Petersen, Sarigiani, & Kennedy, 1991); this finding suggests that treatment should focus on building a sense of agency and control over one's mood and thoughts, while maintaining a focus on awareness and expression of one's emotions and thoughts.

The greater need for affiliation that is present in females has also been conceptualized as a vulnerability factor in depression (Hankin & Abramson, 2001). A loss of interpersonal connectedness with others through interpersonal rejection and conflict can be considered both a vulnerability factor and a stressor. Depressive symptoms can occur in response to negative social interactions, especially for those individuals who put a particular importance on relationships with others (Hammen, 1999). Girls are more likely than boys to base their self-esteem and self-worth on relationships with others and on others' judgments of appearance and behavior, making them more likely to be depressed when rejected by peers (Nolen-Hoeksema & Girgus, 1994).

Stress

Females report more stress in general (Wagner & Compas, 1990), report more interpersonal stress specifically (Hammen, 1991; Rudolph & Hammen, 1999), and are more upset by stressors (Rudolph & Hammen, 1999); moreover, stress is a stronger predictor of depressive symptoms for girls than for boys (Rudolph & Hammen, 1999; Schraedley, Gotlib, & Hayward, 1999). Hankin and Abramson (2001) suggest that females encode negative events in more detail, and they note that this may derive from parent socialization of females to talk more about emotions, especially sadness. Interpersonal stress is associated with higher depression and lower self-esteem for female adolescents, but not males (Moran & Eckenrode, 1991; Rudolph et al., 2000). Depressed female adolescents (Rudolph & Hammen, 1999; Rudolph et al., 2000) and adults (Hammen, 1991) experience interpersonal, dependent stress at a higher level and report being more distressed by interpersonal conflict.

When faced with interpersonal stress, females ruminate and blame themselves for their perceived incompetence (Rudolph & Hammen, 1999). Adolescent girls are especially aware of conflict in relationships, and they experience stress indirectly through friendships. They report "network events," or instances when members of their peer group are experiencing stress, as upsetting (Compas & Wagner, 1991). This tendency reflects the increased interconnectedness between female relationships in adolescence. Adolescent females place a higher value on friendships as a source of emotional support, and thus are more upset when friendships are threatened or broken. Attachment to peers appears to be a significant variable in depression for adolescent girls; this factor accounts for a significant variation in suicidal ideation in female psychiatric inpatients (DiFilippo & Overholser, 2000).

A growing body of literature has also linked depression to "relational aggression," a form of aggression common in females that seeks to harm others by damaging interpersonal relationships (Crick & Grotpeter, 1995). The tendency for females to use interpersonal relationships as a medium for hurting peers (Crick & Grotpeter, 1995) seems fitting, given that adolescents, and especially female adolescents, have a stronger need for closeness and affiliation. This type of behavior can be conceptualized as a considerable source of interpersonal stress in adolescence for both victims and perpetrators of relational aggression. Targets of relational aggression are denied the opportunity to satisfy needs for closeness and affiliation. Individuals who engage in relational aggression are rejected by peers and romantic partners for their aggressive behavior (Hankin & Abramson, 2001). Depression, peer rejection, and relational aggression have been linked with one another. Both bullies and victims of relational aggression are more likely to be depressed and rejected by peers (Crick & Grotpeter, 1995; Prinstein, Boergers, & Vernberg, 2001; Slee, 1995), and girls who are rejected by their peers are more likely to be depressed (Bell-Dolan, Foster, & Smith Christopher, 1995). There seems to be a reciprocal relationship between internalizing symptoms and rejection by peers (Hodges & Perry, 1999). Girls who are depressed are easy targets for rejection because of their socially unskilled behavior, depressed appearance, and withdrawal. Conversely, rejection, or even a perception of rejection, leads to negative thoughts about the self and depressive symptoms.

Puberty and Body Dissatisfaction

Girls reach puberty earlier than boys and in general are less satisfied with the changes associated with puberty. Girls who mature early or experience menarche at an earlier age than their peers are more likely to experience psychopathology, particularly depression (Ge et al., 2001; Graber, Lewinsohn, Seeley, & Brooks-Gunn, 1997; Petersen et al., 1991; Stice, Presnell, & Bearman, 2001). In a study using diagnostic interviews, girls who matured early were more likely to have lower self-esteem, a history of a suicide attempt, and a lifetime history of eating and disruptive behavior disorders (Graber et al., 1997). Late-maturing boys were more likely to have inter-nalizing problems. According to self-report, being "on time" with regard to puberty is more important to girls than to boys (Siegal, Yancey, Aneshensel, & Schuler, 1999). In a longitudinal study, Petersen and colleagues (1991) found that a higher prevalence of depression in adolescent girls is related to the simultaneous onset of puberty and school change—an experience that most boys do not have.

Body dissatisfaction becomes prevalent in early adolescence, particularly for girls, and is strongly linked to depression. For girls, confidence in appearance is the most important contributor to self-worth, whereas for boys, confidence in abilities is most important (American Association of University Women, 1992). Some studies have found that the relationship between gender and depression is much less significant when body image is controlled for (Hankin & Abramson, 2001; Siegal, 2002; Siegal et al., 1999). It has also been found that the relationship between early menarche and depression is smaller when body mass, body dissatisfaction, and dieting behavior are controlled for (Stice et al., 2001). In regard to gender differences in body dissatisfaction, Kostanski and Gullone (1998) reported that while there were no gender differences in actual body mass, Australian girls rated their bodies as two or more sizes bigger than their ideal size and scored higher than boys on a measure of body dissatisfaction and drive for thinness, while boys rated their bodies as within two sizes of their ideal. Other studies have found that as girls go through adolescence, they feel more negative about their bodies, while boys feel more positive about their bodies (Allgood-Merten, Lewinsohn, & Hops, 1990; Richards, Boxer, Petersen, & Albrecht, 1990). Body dissatisfaction has been found both to correlate with depression in males and females (Kostanski & Gullone, 1998) and to predict depression in girls (Stice & Bearman, 2001); however, the same relationship has not been found for actual body mass and depressive symptoms (Kostanski & Gullone, 1998; Stice & Bearman, 2001). Thus dissatisfaction with perceived body size is more important than actual body size and weight in depression. Pressure to be thin, and an internalization of a thin body as an ideal body are related to later body dissatisfaction in early adolescent girls (Stice & Bearman, 2001). It is unclear whether the weight gain associated with puberty is a risk factor for depression in girls who mature early, but it appears that girls who mature early are at increased risk for depression, especially if they have experienced pressure to be thin or have internalized a thin ideal body and are gaining weight while their on-time peers are not.

Family Variables

Healthy relationships between parents and children, both boys and girls, serve as protective factors on adjustment (Petersen et al., 1991). Warm, supportive relationships between parents and their children are associated with psychosocial coping resources and positive self-esteem among adolescents (Sheeber & Sorensen, 1998). It appears as though parent–child relationships may affect symptoms of depression through the mediating experiences of self-esteem (Avison & Mcalpine, 1992). Furthermore, it appears as though the family plays a different role in the psychosocial development of boys and girls. In adolescence, the family plays a greater role in girls' social and emotional adjustment, while peers play a greater role in boys' adjustment (Kavanagh & Hops, 1994). Fathers' behavior appears to have a stronger impact on the adjustment of girls than of boys. Positive relationships with their fathers protect early adolescent girls from stress and the development of a depressive disorder (Petersen et al., 1991), and negative behavior from fathers creates a non-nurturing home context for girls but not boys (Kavanagh & Hops, 1994). Perceived messages about the self, the world, and the future (the "cognitive triad") from parents are related to children's own cognitive triad, as well as the severity of their depressive symptoms. Whereas messages from mothers predicted the cognitive triad and severity of depressive symptoms for both boys and girls, messages from fathers only predicted the cognitive triad and severity of symptoms for girls. Moreover, the perceived messages from fathers accounted for a greater percentage of variance in the cognitive triad of girls than did messages from mothers (Stark, Schmidt, & Joiner, 1996). Fathers had a greater impact on how girls think about themselves, others, and the future than did mothers. Thus, in treating depressed girls, it may be important to make a greater effort to involve fathers in treatment and to encourage fathers to send positive messages about the self, the world, and the future.

In general, then, the literature on gender and depression in youths suggests that girls and boys experience depression differently in terms of vulnerability, prevalence, and symptoms; experience different types of stressors; and react differently to family variables. Thus it is important to address gender issues in the conceptualization and treatment of depression in children and adolescents.

ETHNICITY

Ethnicity is another important issue to consider in the conceptualization and treatment of depression. The literature on ethnicity and depression suggests that some racial groups experience more severe depression, experience different symptoms, and are less likely to receive help from mental health professionals. Minority students have been found to report higher rates of depression in many studies (Cuffe, Waller, Cuccaro, Pumariega, & Garrison, 1995; Roberts, Roberts, & Chen, 1997; Rushton et al., 2003). Female African American students report higher rates of depression than European American students do (Garrison, Jackson, Marsteller, McKeown, & Addy, 1990). In another study, Emslie, Weinberg, Rush, Adams, and Rintelmann (1990) reported that Hispanic females had the highest depression scores, while non-Hispanic white males had the lowest scores. Hispanic and mixed-ancestry middle school students were found to report more suicidal ideation, but not total depressive symptoms, in one study (Olvera, 2001), although in a meta-analysis of studies using the Children's Depression Inventory (CDI; Kovacs, 1981), Hispanic children scored higher (Twenge & Nolen-Hoeksema, 2002). Interestingly, this study did not find any differences with respect to socioeconomic status.

In a study looking at the Center for Epidemiologic Studies Depression Scale (CES-D)—a measure that is used in many studies looking at racial group differences in depression and service utilization—Iwata, Turner, and Lloyd (2002) found that black, U.S.-born Hispanic, non-U.S.-born Hispanic, and non-Hispanic white adolescents and young adults responded differently to the items and scales on the CES-D. The African American participants were more likely to score high on the somatic items, but low on the depression scale. The U.S.-born Hispanic participants scored low on the interpersonal item but high on the low positive affect scale. Thus there may be differences in the way that different ethnic groups respond to self-report measures of depressive symptoms, an important point to be mindful of when conceptualizing treatment for psychosocial concerns in minority youths. It may be important to assess minority children, adolescents, and parents' beliefs about "depression"; the meaning that symptoms of depression hold for them; and how they are experiencing their symptoms emotionally, physically, and cognitively.

Ethnicity's Interactions with Vulnerability, Stress, and Gender

Vulnerability

There is evidence that Hispanic and African American adolescents utilize religious and spiritual resources to a greater extent than European American adolescents, and that utilization of these resources is inversely related to depressive symptoms (Miller & Gur, 2002), thus suggesting that European American adolescents use these social support and coping resources to a lesser degree. These resources include internal resources such as personal devotion and a sense of connection with a divine spirit, and external resources such as participation in the religious community. However, one study found that Hispanic students use less social coping than their non-Hispanic white peers (Olvera, 2001). Roberts and colleagues (1997) theorized that the higher prevalence of depression in Mexican American children may result from a greater belief in fatalism, which leads to an external locus of control and lack of coping. In treating minority children and adolescents for depression, it is important to assess the coping resources that they have available to them, and the degree to which they perceive control over their futures. It may be important to increase their use of active coping, while being sensitive to their religious beliefs, family values, and cultural traditions.

Puberty and Body Dissatisfaction

Hispanic and African American girls have been found to be more likely than European American girls to experience early menarche (Stice et al., 2001). Ge and colleagues (2003) explored the effects of pubertal transition on a sample of African American youths and found that while gender differences in depression were not significant in fifth grade, they were significant

in seventh grade (after most girls had gone through puberty). In this sample, children who matured early reported more symptoms; although the symptoms went away after pubertal change for boys, they remained higher for girls who matured early. Taken together with the finding that girls were more likely than boys to stay depressed if they were depressed at baseline (Rushton et al., 2003), the finding that girls are more likely to remain depressed if they reach puberty early suggests that girls who mature early are at increased risk for depression. It is possible that early-maturing girls are experiencing more depression because they develop secondary characteristics that make them appear older, which may lead them to be pressured to engage in activities that they are not cognitively or emotionally mature enough to manage (Ge, Conger, & Elder, 1996; Graber et al., 1997). It is possible that this combination of increased stressors with insufficient cognitive and emotional coping strategies to deal with such stressors leads to more suicide attempts in this population (Graber et al., 1997).

In studies looking at body image and depression in diverse samples, findings have been mixed for African American youths. One study (Siegal, 2002) found that while as a whole African American youths appeared to feel more positively about their bodies, the relationship between negative body image and depression was *stronger* for African American girls than for European American girls. This finding was also not consistent with an earlier study that reported that African American girls feel more positively about their bodies than European American, Asian, or Hispanic girls (Siegal et al., 1999). In this study, body image accounted for a large portion of gender differences, but not ethnic differences, in depressive symptoms.

Family Variables

Mothers' behavior also seems to play a large role in the adjustment of adolescent girls, particularly for Hispanic children and adolescents. In a study of Mexican preadolescent children, girls who experienced their mothers as controlling reported more depressive symptoms after puberty, whereas girls who perceived that their mothers were supportive of their autonomy did not experience as many symptoms immediately after puberty (Benjet & Hernandez-Guzman, 2002).

Ethnicity and Service Utilization

Investigators have reported differences in service utilization between racial groups. In one study, although African American adolescents scored higher on a measure of depressive symptoms, they were less likely than European American adolescents to receive outpatient services for any disorder, and were more likely to drop out of outpatient services early (Cuffe et al., 1995). Possible reasons for underutilization are that African American adolescents tolerate a higher level of symptoms, or have lower expectations that treatment will be helpful. In a study of racial group differences in the use of psychotropic medication, African American youths with Medicaid insurance were half as likely to have been prescribed medication as European American youths with Medicaid insurance—a difference that remained constant across geographic region (rural, suburban, and urban) (Zito, Safer, DosReis, & Riddle, 1998). Hypotheses proposed by the authors of these studies include unfamiliarity with and uncertainty about the mental health system; utilization of nonprofessional resources, such as the church, extended family, and community; and a lack of behavioral pediatricians and psychiatrists practicing in poor inner-city neighborhoods. Contrary to these hypotheses, African American adults reported in one study that they were *more* likely to seek mental health services for a serious emotional problem, and would feel comfortable and not embarrassed about talking to a mental health professional (Diala et al., 2001). Other hypotheses include possible cultural bias of rating scales or cultural differences in perceptions of how severe symptoms need to be before help is sought (Cuffe et al., 1995; Zito et al., 1998).

ONSET, COURSE, AND OUTCOME

Onset

The age of onset for a depressive disorder may be related to the type of depressive disorder that a child is experiencing. As noted earlier, depressive disorders can develop at any time prior to adulthood; however, sometime between 15 and 19 years appears to be the most common time for onset of MDD (Burke et al., 1991; Haarasilta et al., 2001). In contrast, DD may have an earlier age of onset, with a number of investigators reporting that it first appears at the age of 11 years (Kovacs et al., 1984; Lewinsohn, Hoberman, & Rosenbaum, 1988; Lewinsohn, Hops, et al., 1993). Age of onset has been found to be a predictor of severity of the disorder, but studies differ on the nature of its effect; some researchers report that an earlier age of onset is associated with a more severe episode (Kovacs et al., 1984; McGee & Williams, 1988), while others report that a later age of onset is associated with a more severe episode (Harrington, Fudge, Rutter, Pickles, & Hill, 1990).

Course

Longitudinal research indicates that MDD and DD follow different courses. The average duration of an episode of MDD is reported to be between 32 and 36 weeks (Kovacs et al., 1984; Kovacs, Obrosky, Gatsonis, & Richards, 1997; McCauley et al., 1993; Olsson & von Knorring, 1999; Strober, Lampert, Schmidt, & Morrell, 1993). The rate of recovery tends to be slow, with the greatest improvement starting between the 24th and 36th weeks (Strober et al., 1993). Within 6 months of the onset of an episode of MDD, the episode has remitted for 40% of the children. At 1 year, 80% of the children are no longer experiencing a depressive episode (Kovacs et al., 1997; McCauley et al., 1993). The natural course of DD is more protracted, with the average length of an episode ranging from 3 years (Kovacs et al., 1984) to almost 4 years (Kovacs et al., 1997). A chronic course is reported for a significant percentage of depressed children. Over a 2-year period, approximately 5–10% of these youths remain depressed (Keller et al., 1988; McCauley et al., 1993; McGee & Williams, 1988; Strober et al., 1993), although it is not clear whether these figures vary between the diagnostic groups (MDD and DD).

Predictors of Duration of an Episode

A few variables have been identified that appear to predict the duration of a depressive episode. Severity is one such predictor of duration, with more severe episodes having a more protracted course (McCauley et al., 1993). Severity is also a predictor of the recurrence of episodes (Emslie et al., 1997). Another predictor, family dysfunction, is associated with a more protracted course (McCauley et al., 1993). Finally, gender has been associated with the overall severity and course of a depressive disorder, with females experiencing more severe and protracted episodes (Kovacs et al., 1984). Kovacs and colleagues (1997) noted that treatment had no impact on the duration of a first episode of MDD or DD.

Some youngsters who are depressed will later develop bipolar disorder (Kovacs et al., 1984). Identification of variables that can be used to identify youngsters who will later develop bipolar disorder is critical. These youngsters may not respond to a psychosocial treatment program and may benefit from a pharmacological regimen that differs from those typically used for youngsters who have unipolar depression. It appears as though an episode of psychotic depression (Strober et al., 1993) or comorbid attention-deficit/hyperactivity disorder (ADHD) may be risk factors for the later occurrence of bipolar disorder (Carlson & Kashani, 1988).

Recurrence

Longitudinal research addresses another important characteristic of depressive disorders: They are recurrent. Kovacs and colleagues (1984) reported that 72% of their population of depressed youths experienced an additional depressive episode within 5 years. McCauley and colleagues (1993) reported that 54% of their sample experienced a second depressive episode within a 3-year period. In a unique study, Emslie and colleagues (1997) followed youngsters who had been successfully treated as inpatients for depression for up to 3 years following treatment. These investigators reported that 61% experienced a recurrence of another episode of MDD with most of the recurrences occurring within two years of the index episode. The first year following recovery appeared to be the time of highest risk, as almost half the youngsters who experienced a recurrence did so during the first year following recovery. A few variables predicted recurrence, including older age, psychotic subtype, and more severe initial episode. Thus it appears as though depressed youths are at serious risk for experiencing additional depressive episodes.

Outcome

Without treatment, most depressed youths are likely to become depressed adults (Newman et al., 1996; Pine et al., 1998). Unfortunately, most such youths do not receive treatment (Lewinsohn, Rohde, Klein, & Seeley, 1999). Consequently, they are at heightened risk for a variety of undesirable psychosocial outcomes. More specifically, they are at heightened risk for school dropout, teen pregnancy, and substance abuse (Lewinsohn et al., 1999; Weissman et al., 1999). In addition, experience of a depressive disorder during adolescence is a risk factor for suicide (Gould et al., 1998). Children who experience their first depressive disorder prior to adolescence have a fourfold lifetime increased risk of suicide attempts (Weissman et al., 1999). Young adults with a history of MDD during adolescence experience a variety of functional impairments, including poorer global functioning, lower quality of relationships with family, a smaller social network, greater major and minor adversity, lower life satisfaction, and greater mental health treatment utilization; however, it is not clear whether this relationship is due to the depressive episode, psychiatric comorbidity, depression recurrence, prior functioning, or current depressive symptoms (Lewinsohn et al., 2003). Children who experience a depressive episode experience significantly higher rates of bipolar I disorder, alcohol abuse/dependence, and conduct disorder as young adults. They are also more likely to have a history of outpatient treatment and psychiatric hospitalizations during the early adult years (Weissman et al., 1999).

COMORBIDITY

Fewer than one-third of children who are diagnosed with a depressive disorder are solely experiencing depression. Most depressed children are also experiencing another psychological disorder (Hammen & Rudolph, 2003). Depressive disorders are most frequently comorbid with anxiety disorders and disruptive behavior disorders (Kovacs, 1990). Comorbid conditions represent more severe disturbances that create a more complex clinical picture (Rohde et al., 1991). These youngsters may have a poorer prognosis than children who present with a single diagnosis (Cole & Carpentieri, 1990); comorbidity also may increase the likelihood that a youngster will attempt suicide (Kovacs et al., 1993). Due to the co-occurrence of depression with other disorders, the accurate identification and successful treatment of depressive disorders is a complex task. A comorbid condition may be so severe, or its symptoms may be so upsetting to the adults in a youngster's life, that it dominates the diagnostic picture and the depressive disorder goes unidentified. For example, the depressive symptoms of an adolescent with conduct disorder may go unnoticed because of the immediate concerns about the youngster breaking laws and family rules, and because the conflict between the youngster and his or her caregivers is so upsetting that it is the primary focus of the family. As noted in a later section of this chapter, different and/or additional treatments may be needed when comorbid conditions are present along with depression.

The most common disorders that are comorbid with depression among children are anxiety disorders (Brady & Kendall, 1992; Kovacs, 1990). The frequency of co-occurring depressive and anxiety disorders has led some investigators to suggest that they are the same disorders (Finch, Lipovsky, & Casat, 1989) expressed differently over the evolution of the disturbance, with anxiety disorders predating the depressive disorders (Kendall & Ingram, 1987; Kovacs, Gatsonis, Paulaskas, & Richards, 1989). However, positive affect is useful in distinguishing between the two types of disorders. Whereas both anxiety and depressive disorders involve high negative affect, low positive affect appears to be more characteristic of depressive disorders. Depressive disorders also commonly co-occur with conduct disorder (Kovacs et al., 1989; Petersen et al., 1993). In adolescence, depressive disorders are also comorbid with substance abuse and eating disorders (Lewinsohn, Hops, et al., 1993; Petersen et al.,1993).

ETIOLOGY: WITHIN-CHILD FACTORS

There are multiple etiological pathways to the development of depressive disorders during childhood, and the paths differ among children. As noted earlier, the predominant etiological models are diathesis–stress models, in which stress is hypothesized to interact with a vulnerability within a child to produce a depressive disorder. The stressors may take any of many forms, and may be chronic or acute. The diathesis or pathway also varies across theories and probably across youngsters, and includes several different types of variables (Stark,

Laurent, Livingston, Boswell, & Swearer, 1999). In this section, a cognitive–interpersonal pathway is described, along with possible biological pathways. It is believed that a combination of biological, cognitive, behavioral, and familial/environmental variables reciprocally interact with one another and with stress to produce and maintain a depressive disorder (Stark et al., 1999). First, current biological models of the etiology of depressive disorders are described.

Biological Factors in Depression

Despite the frequency with which depressive disorders are noted in children and adolescents, there is a relative lack of research examining the neurological abnormalities underlying juvenile depression. As indicated earlier, developmental differences in the symptomatology of depression have been found. Furthermore, researchers studying the neurobiological correlates of depression have noted that depressed children who have suffered early life stress, such as abuse or neglect, do not necessarily display the same pattern of stress hormone abnormalities as adults suffering trauma or significant stress (for a review, see Kaufman & Charney, 2001). In addition, children and adults have exhibited differential responses to antidepressant medication; for example, the inefficacy of tricyclic antidepressants in youth samples has been noted (Hazell, O'Connell, Heathcote, Robertson, & Henry, 1995; see Wagner & Ambrosini, 2001, for a review). Therefore, it is reckless to assume that the neurological manifestations of depression are precisely the same in adults and in youths. On the other hand, in the absence of a body of literature to describe the neurobiological correlates of child and adolescent depression, the adult literature serves as a useful starting point in understanding the potential chemical and neurofunctional mechanisms of depression and subsequent recovery.

Neurochemical Correlates of Depression

MONOAMINE HYPOTHESIS OF DEPRESSION

The emergence of the "monoamine hypothesis" of depression and antidepressant drug action can be traced back to the 1950s, when it was discovered that reserpine, a chemical that depletes the storage of monoamines (a group of neurotransmitters sharing chemical characteristics), induced depressive symptoms (Delgado, 2000). The majority of research attention has focused on the roles of serotonin and norepinephrine (and, to a lesser extent, dopamine) in depression. Simplistically, the theory suggests that reduced monoamine availability contributes to depression. This hypothesis has been compelling, since drugs that act to increase the level of these neurotransmitters—the best known being the selective serotonin reuptake inhibitors (SSRIs)—have been shown to relieve depressive symptoms. As outlined by Leonard (2000), reductions in central nervous system monoamine supply may result from dysfunction in the process of synthesis, storage, or release of these neurotransmitters, or through abnormalities in postsynaptic receptor or subcellular messenger activity.

Another means of testing the monoamine hypothesis has been through neurotransmitter depletion paradigms, which have provided some intriguing information regarding the biological basis of depression and the therapeutic effects of antidepressant drugs. Tryptophan, an amino acid present in the human diet, is necessary for the production of serotonin, and therefore can be removed from the diet to study the resulting effect on neurotransmission. Similarly, the production of norepinephrine can be manipulated through the administration of a-methyl-p-tyrosine (AMPT), which inhibits its production. An increase in depressive symptoms after tryptophan depletion has been exhibited in patients with remitted depression (Delgado et al., 1990, 1999; Moreno et al., 1999; Smith, Fairburn, & Cowen, 1997; Spillmann et al., 2001), although not in patients responding to desipramine (Delgado et al., 1999). Furthermore, the effect has been noted in healthy subjects with a family history of depression (Benkelfat, Ellengogen, Dean, Palmour, & Young, 1994; Klaassen, Riedel, van Someren, Honig, & van Praag, 1999) and bipolar disorder (Quintin, Benkelfat, & Launay, 2001), but not in healthy controls with no family history of depression (Benkelfat et al., 1994; Klaassen et al., 1999; Moreno et al., 1999). Some studies, however, have not replicated these findings (e.g., Moore et al., 1998). A recent meta-analysis by Booij and colleagues (2002) has indicated that individual differences moderate the response to the tryptophan challenge, with recurrent depressive episodes, female gender, prior SSRI treatment, and previous suicidality associated with a higher level of symptom onset.

Therefore, many agree that a simplistic monoamine hypothesis that accounts only for a shortage of neurotransmitters in the central nervous system does not fully describe the presentation of depression (e.g., Booij et al., 2002; Delgado, 2000; Hirschfeld, 2000). Furthermore, Hirschfeld (2000) has outlined several other difficulties with the monoamine hypothesis, including the fact that the effects of antidepressant medications are not specific to depression (as these drugs also reduce symptoms of obsessive–compulsive disorder [OCD] and panic disorder), and that not all drugs affecting the noradrenergic and serotonergic systems result in the remission of symptoms. A more recent hypothesis regarding the biological etiology of depression conceptualizes depression as a neurochemical stress reaction.

DEPRESSION AS RELATED TO A NEUROCHEMICAL STRESS REACTION

Research attention has focused on depression as an overreaction of the neurochemical stress system (Barden, Reul, & Holsboer, 1995; Chrousos & Gold, 1992; Gold, Goodwin, & Chrousos, 1988a, 1988b), and particular emphasis has been placed on hypothalamic–pituitary–adrenal (HPA) axis dysfunction (Nemeroff, 1996, 1998). The HPA axis is a neuroendocrine system that plays a key role in the stress response. When either a physical or psychological threat is present, the hypothalamus increases production of corticotropin-releasing factor (CRF). CRF causes a secretion of adrenocorticotropic hormone (ACTH) in the pituitary, which results in cortisol release in the adrenal gland (Nemeroff, 1998). The body is now ready for either "flight or flight." The dexamethasone suppression test (DST) has been frequently used to test functioning of this axis. In healthy individuals, administration of dexamethasone initiates an inhibitory feedback system and signals the pituitary to decrease ACTH production, and subsequently cortisol levels drop. A frequent finding in depressed adult patients has been increased levels of cortisol in bodily fluid at baseline and after the DST (for a review, see Parker, Schatzberg, & Lyons, 2003). Shelton (2000) has outlined the potential relationship between adaptive elements of the stress response system and depressive symptoms. He characterizes agitation, loss of appetite, anxiety, insomnia, and reduced sexual interest as self-preservation behavior (hyperarousal), whereas the adaptive mechanism of energy conservation may be seen in symptoms such as fatigue, hypersomnia, psychomotor retardation, and overeating. Shelton labels the third mechanism as "behavioral disengagement" or "adaptive learning," which may present in depression as anhedonia, low motivation, or memory and concentration difficulties.

Although compelling in many ways, such a conceptualization of depression has been less consistently supported by studies in samples of depressed youths. Research with child populations has failed to show consistent HPA abnormalities in children and adolescents, with many studies showing no difference in cortisol or ACTH levels between depressed and nondepressed youngsters (Birmaher, Dahl, et al., 1992; Birmaher, Ryan, et al., 1992; Dorn et al., 1996; Kutcher et al., 1991; Puig-Antich et al., 1989). Although HPA axis dysfunction has not been commonly noted in general studies of childhood depression, some research has suggested that this hormonal disturbance may be present only in depressed children with abuse histories (Heim & Nemeroff, 2001; Kaufman et al., 1998), although a blunted rather than an augmented ACTH response was found in at least one study (De Bellis et al., 1994). In the De Bellis and colleagues (1994) study, typical cortisol levels persisted despite blunted ACTH, suggesting the possibility of hyperresponsiveness of the adrenal glands. However, finer analyses have suggested that only depressed children who were being currently maltreated (such as emotional abuse or exposure to domestic violence) showed an augmented ACTH response (Kaufman et al., 1997). Considering the high rates of depression in children who have been abused or otherwise maltreated (Kaufman, 1991), researchers have argued that such life experiences create a biological vulnerability to maladaptive stress reactions later in life (Heim & Nemeroff, 2001). Heim and Nemeroff (2001) argue that youths with this biological subtype of depression may be at greater risk for comorbid anxiety disorders, including posttraumatic stress disorder (PTSD).

Growth hormone tests provide a mechanism through which to examine the integrity of the pituitary gland. Blunted secretion of growth hormone after pharmacological challenges with substances such as growth-hormone-releasing hormone, or after insulin-induced hypoglycemia, have been noted in youths with depression (e.g., Jensen & Garfinkel, 1990; Ryan et al., 1994). Although the cause of the dysregulation of the growth hormone secretion after such challenges is not completely known, it has been hypothesized to be associated with other changes in brain chemistry (Ryan et al., 1994). Hypersecretion of growth hormone at night without pharmacological challenges has received some support in youth samples (Kutcher et al., 1988, 1991), but not consistently (Dahl et al., 1992), although Dahl and colleagues (1992) found that a subgroup of suicidal depressed adolescents had nocturnal hyposecretion of growth hormone. Furthermore, it has been suggested that stressful life events are related to elevated levels of growth hormone secretion in depressed children (Williamson, Birmaher, Dahl, Al-Shabbout, & Ryan, 1996).

Therefore, it appears that the process of mapping out the neurochemical development of early-onset depression may be a complex task. Considering the possibilities presented above of differing HPA axis profiles between children and adults suffering from depression, developmentally sensitive research on these and other biological contributors to depression is extremely important (Kaufman & Charney, 2001). It is also likely that the biological underpinnings of depression may vary depending on the etiology of the mood disturbance or presence of comorbid conditions, as suggested by the research on biochemical changes resulting from early life stress.

The concept of brain plasticity suggests that dysregulation of neurochemistry results in alteration of brain structure or function. An understanding of the neurobiology of depression has also emerged from imaging studies, although again these studies are generally limited to adult samples. It remains to be determined whether many of the findings reported below are reflective of the neurobiological correlates of childhood depression.

Neuroanatomical and Neurofunctional Underpinnings of Depression

Neuroanatomical differences have been noted in adults with depression. Comprehensive reviews of the literature exist (see, e.g., Drevets, 2001), but these are only briefly described here. Perhaps the most frequently reported finding has been a reduction in hippocampal volume

(Bremner et al., 2000; Frodl et al., 2002, Mervalla et al., 2000; Shah, Ebmeier, Glabus, & Goodwin, 1998; Sheline, Gado, Kraemer, 2003; Sheline, Sanghavi, Mintun, & Gado, 1999; Sheline, Wang, Gado, Csernansky, & Vannier, 1996), although this has not been found consistently (Axelson et al., 1993; Posener et al., 2003; Vakali et al., 2000), with Posener and colleagues reporting a difference in hippocampal shape but not size. The hippocampus is thought to play a role in learning and memory, and its apparent abnormalities in depression are thought to be involved in the cognitive symptoms of depression. In one of the few neuroimaging studies done in a pediatric population, it was found that depressed adolescents exhibited larger amygdala–hippocampal volume ratios than controls, although increased ratios were associated with severity of anxious symptoms rather than severity of depressive symptoms (MacMillan et al., 2003). Other research with adult samples has indicated volumetric reductions in areas of the prefrontal cortex, thought to be responsible for higher-order reasoning and goal-directed behavior (e.g., Drevets et al., 1997, Ongur, Drevets, & Price, 1998), and a study of young women (ages 17–23) with adolescent onset of depression revealed similar prefrontal reductions (Botteron, Raichle, Drevets, Heath, & Todd, 2002). However, the failure to find volumetric reductions in the prefrontal regions in mildly depressed patients has also been noted (Brambilla et al., 2002). The few studies that have examined depressed adolescents have also reported reduced volume in the frontal lobes (Steingard et al., 2002)—in particular, smaller white matter volumes, which the authors suggest may reflect an abnormality in the myelination process.

Functional neuroimaging techniques, which look at metabolism patterns of the brain at rest or when performing a task, have frequently reported reduced functioning in the dorsolateral prefrontal cortex (an area generally implicated in cognitive processing) and increased activation in limbic and paralimbic regions (regions thought to be responsible for emotional processing and modulation) (e.g., Cohen et al., 1992; Drevets, Bogers, & Raichle, 2002; Ebert, Feistel, & Barocka, 1991). Other brain areas implicated in depression include the basal ganglia (e.g., Baxter et al., 1985; Buchsbaum et al., 1986; Kennedy et al., 2001), the anterior cingulate cortex (e.g., Drevets, Spitznagel, &

Raichle, 1995; Mayberg et al., 1999), and the amygdala (e.g., Abercrombie et al., 1998; Drevets et al., 1995, 2002; Sheline et al., 2001). The most compelling integrated neurobiological model of depression describes disturbance in the reciprocal relationship between the cognitive/attentional networks in the brain and the regions responsible for processing emotion; this is termed the "limbic–cortical network" model (Mayberg, 2003).

As the understanding of the neurobiology of depression increases, possibilities for better diagnosis and prediction of treatment outcomes should follow. In particular, the ability to predict which subjects will respond to a given treatment is an especially intriguing prospect and is beginning to receive research attention (Brody et al., 2001; Davidson, Irwin, Anderle, & Kalin, 2003; Ketter et al., 1999; Mayberg et al., 1997; Pizzagalli et al., 2001). Considering that mental health services are costly to provide and often in short supply, a biologically informed understanding of which treatments are most likely to benefit a particular patient would radically change the efficiency and efficacy of service delivery.

Cognitive–Interpersonal Pathway

An emerging paradigm is the integration of cognitive and interpersonal theories as a means of describing a pathway for the development of depressive disorders (Rudolph, Hammen, & Burge, 1995; Shirk, 1998). Within this theoretical perspective, a cognitive theory of depression—either Beck's cognitive theory (e.g., Beck, 1967) or Abramson's learned hopelessness theory of depression (e.g., Abramson, 1999; Abramson, Metalsky, & Alloy, 1989; Flynn & Garber, 1999)—is integrated with interpersonal theories. Our own work has concentrated on an integration of Beck's cognitive theory of depression with attachment theory (Stark et al., 1999) and is described in the following paragraphs.

Depressive disorders are characterized by a disturbance in cognition that is activated by specific vulnerabilities to stressful events (Hammen & Goodman-Brown, 1990). Once activated, the disturbance in cognition produces a negative distortion in perceptions about the self, the world, and the future (the cognitive triad; Beck, 1967). Driving the cognitive disturbance are dysfunctional core "schemas" that are hierarchically linked to other less central but related schemas. Schemas are hypothesized to serve as filters that guide what is attended to, how it is perceived, and what meaning is derived from stimuli. Schemas combine with environmental events to produce an individual's conscious thoughts. The most central or core schema is the "self-schema." The self-schema consists of the individual's most central rules for life, and it facilitates the encoding, storage, and retrieval of self-relevant information (Prieto, Cole, & Tageson, 1992). The self-schema of depressed children is unrealistically negative, characterized by a sense of loss, unlovability, worthlessness, or helplessness; it may account for such symptoms as selective attention to, and personalization of, salient events (Beck, Rush, Shaw, & Emery, 1979).

Research with children has indicated that children without a psychological disturbance possess a positive self-schema that is lacking in depressed youngsters (Hammen & Zupan, 1984; Jaenicke et al., 1987; Zupan, Hammen, & Jaenicke, 1987). However, in one study, Zupan and colleagues (1987) found evidence of a stronger negative self-schema among the depressed youngsters. It is possible that the lack of a positive self-schema is a developmental precursor to a negative self-schema. The absence of an adaptive self-schema may lead to an imbalance in information processing, in which fewer instances of positive self-relevant information are processed and internalized into the self-schema. This leads to a negative bias in information processing that serves to confirm the depressed individual's less positive—or actively negative—sense of self, world, and future.

Cole and Turner's (1993) research indicates that the schematic functioning of depressed youths is not as structuralized as that of depressed adults. A child's self-schema affects his or her perceptions of experiences and is simultaneously shaped by these experiences. Thus, if the youngster's life experiences are chronically stressful or in other ways unhealthy, they will be integrated into and shape the sense of self, which will become structuralized over time through repeated learning experiences. Once structuralized, the self-schema guides information processing, and the youngster begins selectively attending to information that confirms the sense of self and ignoring schema-inconsistent information. However, if the youngster's environment changes, or if the youngster is exposed to other corrective experiences, the overall development of the self-schema may change as these alternative experiences become internalized through repeated learning experiences and form an adaptive self-schema or a less potent negative self-schema (Stark et al., 1999).

How does the self-schema develop? Beck (e.g., Beck et al., 1979) and other cognitive theorists (e.g., Young & Lindemann, 1992) hypothesize that depressive schemas are formed through early learning experiences, especially those within the family. Young (1991) hypothesizes that maladaptive schemas could be the result of inadequate parenting or ongoing aversive experiences within the family milieu, such as repeated criticism or rejection. Mahoney (1982) hypothesizes that schemas are hierarchically organized according to the time at which they develop with those developing earliest influencing the subsequent development of other schemas. The first schema to develop is the self-schema, and as the first, it influences the development of other schemas. Attachment theory offers some direction for understanding how the family may contribute to the earliest development of schematic functioning.

"Attachment" is defined as a set of behaviors that characterize the style of interaction between the child and his or her caretakers, particularly during stressful situations. Attachment behaviors are hypothesized to reflect the youngster's "internal working model." The internal working model (Bowlby, 1980) is a cognitive representation of the self, of others in the relational world (especially the primary caretaker), and of the relationship between the child and the primary caregiver (Berman & Sperling, 1994). As such, the cognitive representations that constitute the internal working model are analogous to the core schema. Thus, from the cognitive perspective, the internal working model consists of the self-schema, a schema that represents an amalgam of significant others, and a schema about the relationship between the child and his or her primary caretaker. The internal working model, like the core schema, is hypothesized to provide the framework for expectations that guide interactions with others in new and existing relationships. To borrow from cognitive-behavioral theory—more specifically, Bandura's (1978) concept of "reciprocal determinism"—the child's interpersonal behavior leads to reactions from others that then influence the child and his or her perceptions of the interaction as well as expectations for future relationships. In addition, the outcome of the interaction provides the child with information about the self. In a similar fashion, the cognitive representations of relationships appear to guide information processing that is related to the youngster's view of self (Rudolph et al., 1995).

Both cognitive theory and attachment theory are concerned with the child's developing sense of self. Beck postulated that the sense of self is formed within an interpersonal context, and yet the self-schema is the central variable in information processing. From the cognitive perspective, the self-schema is shaped by experiences within an interpersonal context at the same time that it filters and constructs perceptions about these experiences. Attachment theory is concerned with the developing sense of self, but greater emphasis is placed on the relationship schema and the schema about others. These schemas are hypothesized to influence the development of the self-schema. Thus, although there is agreement across the cognitive and interpersonal perspectives that the self-schema interacts with the schemas about relationships and others, the difference is in the hypotheses about which schemas are prepotent and influence the development of other schemas.

Like the cognitive theorists, the interpersonal theorists have suggested mechanisms through which a child's internal working model is developed. It has been hypothesized that consistency in interactions in the caregiving environment leads to internalization of the attachment relationship (Colin, 1996). The internal working model is formed through communications between the child and caregiver (Bretherton, 1990). Although the interpersonal theorists hypothesize that the internal working model is internalized through interactions with significant others, the actual process that leads to internalization is not stated. This is a point where cognitive theory may be integrated, as cognitive theorists hypothesize that the internalization process results from repeated learning experiences.

The coherence and organization of the relationship between the child and the primary caregiver determine whether an attachment is secure or insecure. Kobak, Sudler, and Gamble (1991) suggest that an insecure–anxious attachment, which is often linked to a psychologically unavailable or rejecting caregiver, fosters an internal working model of the self as unlovable. The child interprets the mother's rejection or unavailability as evidence that he or she is unworthy of attention and is unlovable. Priel and Shamai (1995) hypothesize that an insecure–ambivalent attachment style, characterized by hypervigilance to the caregiver by the youngster and high dependence on others, is related to expectations that the primary caregiver as well as significant others will not support the youngster in stressful situations. Thus attachment theorists hypothesize that the nature of the attachment style determines the child's schemas of relationships with the primary caregiver, others, and the self, and that these schemas interact and influence each other.

Although several studies have linked insecure attachment to depression (e.g., Cowan, Cohn, Cowan, & Pearson, 1996; Rosenstein & Horowitz, 1996), it should be noted that attachment behaviors are internalized through repeated learning experiences and become schemas. The schemas guide information processing, which is hypothesized to lead to the development of a depressive disorder. In addition, attachment behaviors influence the development of the child's emotion regulation skills and expectations for social support. Thus an insecure attachment style may be a risk factor for the development of a depressive style of thinking, a deficit in emotion regulation skills, and failure to use social support (which stems from the expectation that others are not going to help eliminate stress); all of these characteristics increase the risk for depression. In contrast, secure attachment may act as a protective factor that leads to the development of an adaptive information-processing style and of healthy emotion regulation and coping skills. Insecure attachment is the context in which a negative sense of self, world, and future begins to develop. Thus it represents a cognitive–interpersonal pathway to the development of depression.

Cognitive and interpersonal theorists suggest that schemas are formed through early childhood experiences within the family, yet no research has directly tested this hypothesis with very young children. However, research is emerging with youngsters in middle childhood. Children are active information processors who derive meaning from day-to-day interactions, and the self-schema, as the most basic core schema, develops first through learning experiences within the family. Each interaction with the world represents a learning experience that provides the developing child with information about the self. As the self-schema develops, it becomes more structuralized and guides information processing in a fashion that confirms the developing sense of self. Furthermore, the child begins to construct an environment that confirms this sense of self through his or her perceptions and actions. Thus, from the cognitive perspective, the diathesis for a depressive disorder is a negative sense of self (or, as research with children indicates, a lack of a positive sense of self), which is formed through early interactions with caregivers and maintained by interactions within the family and with peers, as well as through other day-to-day experiences.

BEYOND THE CHILD: THE SYSTEM'S ROLES IN ETIOLOGY

In work with a minor, it is necessary to include any relevant relationship or setting that could be affecting the maintenance of, or has potential to assist in recovery from, depression. It has long been recognized that children are embedded within an environmental context, and that they interact and transact with their environment to maintain depression. Bronfenbrenner's (1979) model of ecology suggests that the child's context includes the concepts of "ontogenic development," or those internal factors of a child that influence his or her development; the "microsystem," or the immediate environment, particularly the family; the "exosystem," or community elements; and the "macrosystem," the beliefs and values of the culture. These various layers affect the child in a differential manner, based on their proximity (Bronfenbrenner, 1979). Most research describing the development of depression has focused on the two most proximal areas to the child—his or her internal developmental characteristics and the microsystem (Cicchetti & Toth, 1998)—and, to a lesser extent, on exosystemic factors. Perhaps because the treatment for juvenile depression has historically been child-centered, there is limited research on the manner through which contextual factors may influence the degree of success achieved by a particular intervention. However, with greater emphasis in the field on the system, the primary contextual variables that are most important for most minors are reviewed below: the family, the school, and peer relationships.

Family Environment

Clinical observation and research have indicated that many depressed children experience a disturbed family environment (Stark & Brookman, 1992). Families of depressed children are characterized by greater chaos, abuse and neglect (Kashani, Ray, & Carlson, 1984); high conflict (Forehand et al., 1988; Jewell & Stark, 2003); low levels of cohesion (Jewell & Stark, 2003); a critical, punitive, and belittling or shaming parenting style (e.g., Arieti & Bemporad, 1980); communication difficulties (Puig-Antich et al., 1985a, 1985b); and lower activity level (Stark, Humphrey, Crook, & Lewis, 1990). Lack of support and approval from within the family is a consistently reported finding in studies of the families of depressed children (Sheeber & Sorensen, 1998). Families of depressed children also tend to be characterized by parental rejection, hostility, inattention, low involvement, and lack of affection (Orvaschel, Weissman, & Kidd, 1980); however, some research suggests a higher degree of enmeshment in the families of depressed children, leading to inappropriate boundaries and greater reactivity (Jewell & Stark, 2003). Interactions between parents and depressed youngsters have been observed to include more negative and fewer positive exchanges than interactions between nondisordered children and their parents (Messer & Gross, 1995). Family environmental factors were found to be related to psychosocial functioning 3 years after initial assessment (McCauley et al., 1993).

Disturbed family functioning has also been found to have a prospective relationship with both the development of depressive symptoms (Sheeber, Hops, Alpert, Davis, & Andrews, 1997) and the recurrence of depressive episodes during adolescence (Sanford et al., 1995), as well as being related to the maintenance of major depressive episodes in children (Goodyer, Hebert, Secher, & Pearson, 1997). Furthermore, parent–child conflict appears to be an important predictor of child and adolescent suicidal behavior (Brent et al., 1993; Husain, 1990). Difficulties in the sibling relationship have also been noted in children experiencing depressive symptoms (Puig-Antich et al., 1985a). Even in remission, the relationships between previously depressed children and both their parents and siblings continue to be impaired (Puig-Antich et al., 1985b).

Furthermore, parental pathology has been frequently noted to be associated with childhood depression (Beardslee, Versage, & Gladstone, 1998). This association is characterized by greater risk for depression (Warner, Weissman, Fendrick, Wickramaratne, & Moreau, 1992; Weissman et al., 1987), longer and more severe episodes (Weissman et al., 1987), a higher likelihood of comorbid disorders (Hammen & Brennan, 2001), and poorer interpersonal adjustment (Hammen & Brennan, 2001; Weissman et al., 1987). The majority of the literature has focused on maternal depression and the specific interactional patterns between depressed mothers and their children. For example, depressed mothers have been noted to be more critical, off-task, and unproductive in their encounters with their children (Gordon et al., 1989). Paternal psychopathology has received significantly less research attention, with one recent study suggesting that paternal psychopathology was related only to children's externalizing diagnoses, whereas maternal depression was associated with all diagnoses (Brennan, Hammen, Katz, & Le Brocque, 2002).

It is important to note that family characteristics can also serve as a source of support and a buffer against stress. Healthy parent–child relationships have been documented as protective factors for adjustment (Petersen et al., 1991) and are associated with greater psychosocial coping resources among adolescents, as well as positive self-esteem (Sheeber & Sorenson, 1998). Furthermore, positive parenting practices such as high levels of warmth, low psychological control, and appropriate involvement also serve as protective factors (Brennan, Le Brocque, & Hammen, 2003). It appears as though the family generally plays an increasingly important role in adolescent girls' adjustment, whereas peers play a greater role in boys' adjustment (Kavanagh & Hops, 1994).

Several mechanisms through which family disturbances contribute to the development of depressive disorders have been hypothesized. First, it has been suggested that the parents' cognitive style shapes the messages sent to a child about the self, world, and future, which in turn influence the child's cognitive style (Stark et al., 1996). Negative messages about the self, world, and future adversely affect the child's cognitive triad and may lead to greater vulnerability to a depressive disorder. One study found that messages from the parents about the self, world, and future predicted the severity of depressive symptoms in children, and that this severity was completely mediated by a child's cognitive triad (Stark et al., 1996). A similar relationship between negative parental messages, a child's negative cognitive triad, and the presence and severity of comorbid depressive symptoms among children diagnosed with ADHD has been reported (Schmidt, Stark, Carlson, & Anthony, 1998).

A second mechanism through which family dysfunction influences the development of depressive disorders has been discussed by Alloy and colleagues (2001), who have described this as a social learning mechanism of cognitive vulnerability to depression. One of the risk factors their study empirically supported was negative parenting practices as reported by undergraduates and their parents, including emotional rejection, particularly from fathers. Emotional rejection was also conceptualized as a lack of acceptance and warmth, which is also a hallmark feature of insecure attachment. Conversely, secure attachment relationships are characterized by comfort and acceptance (Solomon & George, 1999). In the families of depressed children, the tone of the mother–child (and, to a somewhat lesser extent, the father–child) relationship has been characterized as cold, hostile, tense, and even rejecting (Puig-Antich et al., 1985a). Expressed affection is contingent on behavior consistent with parental expectations (Cole & Rehm, 1986). Perhaps the parenting practices described by Alloy and colleagues inadvertently addressed the underlying felt attachment insecurity, which could be related to the schemas that individuals maintain with regard to what comfort, support, and acceptance they expect from others in general. In other words, perhaps the parenting practices *defined* the cognitive expectations, which shaped the self-schemas. As described by Whisman and Friedman (1998), "cognitive and interpersonal styles are likely to mutually reinforce and sustain one another" (p. 150). Perhaps the self-schema is truly indistinguishable from interpersonal behavior because they are so interrelated, and underlying scripts, schemas, and expectations may indeed be so reciprocal that they cannot be separated into cognitive and interpersonal factors at all.

In children, who are in the process of forming their personal identities and defining their cognitive and interpersonal styles, depression may have a dramatic influence on this process. It is accepted that depression has an impact on social functioning. What is not yet known is how well a child can recover from depression in terms of interpersonal expectations and schemas, which presumably guide interactions with others, according to cognitive theory (Clarke et al., 1999). Furthermore, more information about treatment options, such as those incorporating interpersonal skills and family therapy components, could reinforce adaptive, and correct maladaptive, cognitive–interpersonal styles to buffer against future depressive episodes (Sander, 2001).

School Environment

Youths spend much of their waking time in school, and school provides the social and academic environment for children and adolescents to learn new skills, try out alternative ways of relating, and experience competency and mastery. The school environment, particularly perceived classroom belonging and teacher support, have been related to academic motivation, especially for females (Goodenow, 1993; Midgley, Feldlaufer, & Eccles, 1989). Furthermore, school factors are clearly related to the emotional well-being of students. For example, students in one study reported a reduction in teacher support and self-esteem between sixth and eighth grades, and they reported an increase in depressive symptoms during this same period (Reddy, Rhodes, & Mulhall, 2003). The reverse was also true: Increased teacher support was associated with increases in self-esteem and decreases in depression. Furthermore, students generally perceived decreasing teacher support through middle school, although girls perceived higher initial support than boys (Reddy et al., 2003). Previous research has also shown that positive teacher–student relationships promote positive school-related emotions, self-esteem, and a sense of belonging across age levels (Hoge, Smith, & Hanson, 1990; Murray & Greenberg, 2000; Pianta, 1994; Roeser, Midgley, & Urdan, 1996). Importantly, students with low perceptions of belonging are more likely to experience depression, social rejection, and school problems (Anderman, 2002). Interestingly, the relationship between depression and school belonging is moderated by the overall sense of belonging across students in the school

(Anderman, 2002). Finally, student self-esteem has been enhanced by other school climate factors, such as an autonomy-supporting environment (Ryan & Grolnick, 1986).

Peer Relationships

Peer relationships have been found to influence the maintenance of depressed mood. Children who had difficulties with friendships at presentation and after onset of depression were more likely to experience persistent symptoms of depression than were those who did not report peer difficulties (Goodyer, Germany, Gowrusankur, & Altham, 1991; Goodyer et al., 1997; Sanford et al., 1995). Greater social impairment is associated with a greater recurrence of depression (Warner et al., 1992). Depressed children were less likely to report having a best friend and experiencing more difficulty in making and keeping relationships than either healthy or anxious children (Puig-Antich et al., 1985a). In addition, parents of depressed children reported that their children were exposed to higher levels of teasing (Puig-Antich et al., 1985a). Peer rejection and withdrawal have been linked with depressed mood and with self-reported loneliness, which mediated depressed mood (Boivin, Hymel, & Bukowski, 1995). Furthermore, research suggests that the length of the depressive episode is associated with peer relationship difficulties (Puig-Antich et al., 1985a). Adolescents begin to draw environmental information increasingly from their peers, and in turn begin to experience a higher level of peer-related interpersonal stressors (Rudolph & Hammen, 1999; Wagner & Compas, 1990). Furthermore, the increased cognitive perspective-taking ability that begins to emerge in middle childhood (Cole, Jacquez, & Maschman, 2001) becomes more refined into adolescence, making social comparisons a powerful vehicle in appraising self-worth.

CONSIDERING CONTEXT IN TREATMENT DELIVERY

In moving toward a consideration of how systemic features play a role in obtaining favorable treatment outcomes, we can think of contextual factors in terms of both moderational and mediational effects. These more sophisticated systems of analysis are receiving greater attention (Kraemer, Wilson, Fairburn, & Agras, 2002; Weersing & Weisz, 2002). However, to date, there exists a limited body of research from which to make generalizations about the contextual variables moderating and mediating outcomes.

Moderational Perspective

Several authors have argued that both developmental and contextual variables moderate the efficacy of treatment for children and adolescents (Cicchetti & Toth, 1998; Weisz & Hawley, 2002). As outlined by Kolko, Brent, Baugher, Bridge, and Birmaher (2000), though, many studies of treatment efficacy have not studied moderators of treatment outcome. Furthermore, much of the existing moderational research is focused on child-specific internal variables, rather than providing information about the contextual factors that determine the degree to which children benefit from intervention. For example, one meta-analysis suggested that the relationship between psychotherapeutic outcome and child characteristics was moderated by level of cognitive development (Durlak, Fuhrman, & Lampman, 1991). Similarly, age and degree of social impairment have been shown to serve as moderators, with younger patients and those with less social impairment exhibiting greater symptom reduction (Jayson, Wood, Kroll, Fraser & Harrington, 1998). Predictors of poorer response to CBT have included greater severity of depression at pretreatment, higher levels of cognitive distortion (Brent et al., 1998; Clarke et al., 1992), and greater hopelessness (Brent et al., 1998). However, these data provide little information about the contextual features moderating treatment effectiveness.

Mediational Perspective

Although numerous cognitive variables have been hypothesized to mediate improvement in depressive symptoms after CBT, there has been little research evaluating these propositions (Reinecke, Ryan, & DuBois, 1998). One study directly assessing mediators of treatment outcome found that CBT produced a treatment-specific effect of improvement in cognitive distortion (Kolko et al., 2000), but changes in cognitive processes have not been found to mediate overall outcome (Durlak et al., 1991; Kolko et al., 2000). Adding to the confusion, CBT was also found to be as effective as family therapy in creating changes in adaptive family functioning; therefore, as Weersing and Weisz (2002) stated, "it also produced nonspecific change in 'mediators' belonging to another theoretical model of intervention" (p. 13). Certainly, the argument that nonspecific therapeutic factors may be just as important as, or more important than, orientation-specific factors in producing change appears to be true (Hubble, Duncan, & Miller, 1999; Imber, Pilknois, & Sotsky, 1990).

It is also of interest to consider how intervening in multiple contexts may lead to adaptive change. Such a systemic perspective certainly makes the study of mediational variables more complicated. In integrated treatments that include work with the child, teachers, and parents, it may be difficult to determine which interventions or what underlying processes are facilitating the change. Unfortunately, as Weersing and Weisz (2002) point out, although many studies include the measurement of process variables that could conceivably mediate treatment outcome, these variables are generally utilized as outcome measures rather than tested as mediators. However, it is important to recognize that even these potential mediating variables involved cognitive and behavioral processes, such as cognitive distortion, hopelessness, and engagement in pleasant events (Weersing & Weisz, 2002); therefore, they do not provide information about the contextual variables reviewed earlier that, if mobilized, may serve as mechanisms of change. Let us hope that the call for more direct investigation of the mechanisms of therapeutic change in clinical treatment studies will provide a greater understanding regarding the means by which intervention in the environment effects change.

APPROACHES TO TREATING THE DEPRESSED CHILD OR ADOLESCENT

The two treatment models that have been the most widely studied are CBT and interpersonal therapy for adolescents (IPT-A). The models of depression that form the theoretical basis for the treatments differ more than the treatments themselves do. In fact, as we have noted elsewhere (Stark et al., 1999), the treatments share more components than they have different ones. In fact, artistically delivered CBT will target change in interpersonal relationships as well as the distorted thoughts and beliefs surrounding dysfunctional relationships when they underlie the youngster's depression. Thus the common treatment components may be the reasons why both interventions are effective at treating depressed youths. The treatment models are briefly described below, followed by a more detailed description of our CBT program for depressed 9- to 13-year-old girls. In the description of this intervention, the emphasis on building, strengthening, and changing interpersonal relationships will become apparent. Thus, when the parent training component is included, the intervention is better described as CBT within the interpersonal context.

Cognitive-Behavioral Therapy

There is no single model of CBT for youths; rather, a variety of different treatment components and combinations of components fall under the general rubric of "CBT." For example, Durlak and colleagues (1991) reported that seven separate core components and an eighth less common component are combined into 42 different treatment packages. Similarly, there is no single model of CBT for depression. In general, the goals of CBT for depression are improving youngsters' coping, emotion regulation, problem-solving, and social skills. At the same time, a primary goal is changing the youngsters' negatively distorted automatic thoughts and the beliefs underlying them. The interventions vary in the degree to which they target for change the skills deficits and the underlying structures that lead to the depressive thinking. The therapeutic relationship is characterized by collaboration, in which a child and therapist work together as a team. Sessions are highly structured and follow a specific sequence.

Treatment typically begins with a few sessions of psychoeducation about the nature of depression and the cognitive-behavioral model of depression. Children are taught that their symptoms stem from skills deficits and from their negative thinking. An additional objective of the psychoeducation is to sensitize the youngsters to the changes they experience in their emotions and other depressive symptoms. These changes then serve as a cue to engage in coping, emotion regulation, or problem-solving skills. After the psychoeducational phase, treatment shifts to a skills acquisition phase in which the youngsters are taught coping, emotion regulation, problem-solving, and social skills. Typically, youngsters are taught to

engage in more and a wider variety of pleasant activities. These skills help to activate the children and provide some relief from depressive symptoms. During the final phase of treatment, the youngsters are taught to identify their negative thoughts and to replace them with more realistic and positive thoughts. Negative thoughts about the self, life in general, interpersonal relationships, and the future are all targets for change. Ultimately, the targets of change are the children's schemas that underlie negative thinking. Children are given structured therapeutic homework assignments to apply the skills and cognitive restructuring strategies to their daily lives. Typically, the treatment is completed in 16 sessions lasting 1 hour each.

Interpersonal Therapy for Adolescents

Over the past few years, Mufson and colleagues (1994) have adapted basic interpersonal therapy to the treatment of depressed adolescents (IPT-A). The primary therapeutic goals of IPT-A are to decrease depressive symptoms and to improve interpersonal functioning. To accomplish these goals, the youngster and the therapist identify one or two problem areas from among the following: (1) grief, (2) interpersonal role disputes, (3) role transitions, (4) interpersonal deficits, and (5) living in a single-parent family.

Treatment is divided into three phases, each of which consists of four sessions. During the initial phase, problem areas are identified; a rationale for treatment is provided; a formal therapeutic contract is written and signed; and the adolescent's role in therapy is defined. Some psychoeducation about the nature and impact of depression is provided to the youngster and his or her parent(s). The therapist works with the youngster and the parent(s) to ensure that the youth is socially engaged in the family, in the school, and with friends. Family members are asked to encourage the youth to engage in as many age-appropriate pleasant activities as possible.

During the middle phase of treatment, the nature of each previously identified problem is clarified; effective strategies for attacking the problems are identified; and relevant plans are developed and implemented. In the development of plans, an overarching goal is the desire to improve interpersonal functioning. Youngsters are taught to monitor the experience of depressive symptoms and their emotional experiences.

To achieve these therapeutic objectives, the therapist utilizes exploratory questioning, encouragement of affect, linkage of affect with events, clarification of conflicts, communication analysis, and behavior change techniques such as role playing. Throughout these sessions, the therapist provides the youngster with feedback about symptom change in an attempt to enhance self-esteem. The therapist and youngster work together as a team. They assess the accuracy of the initial formulation of problem areas and evaluate the impact of ongoing events occurring outside sessions for their impact on depressive symptoms. The therapist evaluates the youngster's interpersonal style through their within-session interactions. With the youngster's informed permission, the family is encouraged to support the treatment goals.

The final phase of treatment (sessions 9–12) is the termination phase. The primary objectives of this phase are to prepare the youngster for termination and to establish a sense of personal competence for dealing with future problems. The youngster's feelings about termination are discussed, and feelings of competence are engendered.

THE ACTION TREATMENT PROGRAM: AN EXAMPLE OF CBT FOR DEPRESSION

In this section, the intervention for depressed girls that we are evaluating as part of a 5-year investigation funded by the National Institute of Mental Health (NIMH) is described. The intervention is prototypical of CBT for depressed youths. The primary components are appropriate for males and females, and for children, adolescents, and adults. However, by design, the delivery format, treatment activities, specific coping skills, emphasis on interpersonal relationships, and the illustrations on the treatment materials are all specific to girls within the 9–13 age range. In addition, the treatment manual is designed so that the examples used within the meetings and the material that the girls bring to the meetings are specific to this age range. The examples used to illustrate the application of the treatment are based on our experiences with girls who have completed treatment.

During development of the intervention, we included both male and female therapists. However, it became evident during this piloting that different dynamics exist between girls and male therapists versus female therapists. This is due to multiple variables, including the large percentage of depressed girls who have estranged or unknown fathers, and the number of girls who have been victims of abuse perpetrated by males in their lives. It also may stem from the differences in ways that girls interact with adult males and females. Thus all of the therapists participating in the treatment outcome study are female graduate students. The language in the following discussion reflects the gender composition of the therapists and participants in the study.

Overview of Treatment

Girls who are experiencing a depressive disorder are identified through a multiple-gate assessment procedure (e.g., Kendall, Cantwell, & Kazdin, 1989). After parental consent and child assent are secured, girls complete the CDI (Kovacs, 1981) in large groups. As girls complete the questionnaire, research staff check the suicidal ideation item (#9) and immediately interview any child who indicates a desire to end her life. In addition, the questionnaires are scored immediately after they are completed. Girls who score in excess of 1 standard deviation above the mean are interviewed with a DSM symptom interview that assesses the presence of depressive symptoms. This relatively brief interview is used to eliminate the relatively large number of false positives. If a girl reports the presence of depressive symptoms during the DSM interview, her parent (or other primary caregiver) receives a phone call from the interviewer inviting the child and parent to complete a diagnostic interview, and a permission letter is sent home. If parental consent and child assent are received, then she passes through the screening gates and is interviewed with the Schedule for Affective Disorders and Schizophrenia for School-Age Children (K-SADS; Orvaschel & Puig-Antich, 1994). In addition, the parent is interviewed with the K-SADS. If the youngster receives a diagnosis of MDD or DD, she is invited to participate in the evaluation of the treatment program. The participants are severely depressed; to date, 71% have had MDD as their primary disorder, and over 60% have had additional comorbid conditions.

The ACTION treatment is a gender-specific, developmentally sensitive group treatment program for depressed girls that follows a structured therapist's manual (Stark, Simpson, et al., 2004) and workbook (Stark, Schnoebelen, et al., 2004). The treatment is conducted in the schools in groups of four to six girls. Each of the 20 group and 2 individual meetings lasts approximately 60 minutes and is conducted twice a week for 11 weeks. The children's treatment is designed to be fun and engaging, while teaching the youngsters a variety of skills that are applied to their depressive symptoms, interpersonal difficulties, and other stressors. The skills are taught to the children through didactic presentations and activities; they are rehearsed during in-session activities; and they are applied through therapeutic homework. Skill application is monitored and recorded through completion of workbook activities, and completion of the therapeutic homework is encouraged through an in-session reward system.

The treatment program is based on a self-control model in which youngsters use skills to achieve and maintain a pleasant mood, or they use a change in mood, negative thoughts, or another depressive symptom as a sign that they need to engage in the coping, problem-solving, and/or cognitive restructuring strategies taught within the program. By paying attention to their experiences in these three realms, the youngsters become better aware of their own emotions and thus can use progressively smaller changes as a cue to engage in coping, problem solving, or cognitive restructuring. A variety of activities completed within the meetings and as homework help the participants to become more aware of their personal experiences.

Participants are taught coping skills for managing their unpleasant emotions and other depressive symptoms. The skills are taught to the youngsters within sessions through activities that demonstrate the impact of the coping skills on their unpleasant moods. Depressed youths often experience undesirable situations that are not within their control and thus cannot be changed by the youngsters. In such situations, the children can take action to improve their mood and other depressive symptoms through using the coping skills that are taught and applied during the first nine meetings.

Problem solving is taught to depressed youths to help them change undesirable situations that are within their control and can be changed. The youths are taught a five-step problem-solving process: (1) problem definition, (2) goal definition, (3) solution generation, (4) consequential thinking, and (5) self-evaluation. The steps are defined in a developmentally sensitive way. The steps are modeled by the therapist and then applied to hypothetical situations. Once again, activities are used to illustrate the meaning and purpose of each step. Over time, the therapist helps the youngsters to apply problem solving to their own real-life problems. The workbook has problem-solving worksheets that guide the youngsters through the process as they apply it outside meetings. By the middle of treatment, the youngsters are typically proficient at using coping and problem-solving skills. Use of these skills provides them with symptom relief, including an improvement in mood. This improvement allows them to enter the next phase of treatment, which focuses on identifying and changing negative thoughts.

Depressed youths commonly view themselves, their daily experiences, and the future in an unrealistically negative way. To counter this, depressed youths are taught to recognize their negative thoughts. Often, they have a very difficult time pulling themselves out of the quagmire of negative thinking. We refer to this as getting "stuck in the negative muck." The youngsters are taught to recognize their negative thoughts and then to counter them by using a number of cognitive restructuring strategies. Once again, a variety of within-session activities and therapeutic homework exercises are used to teach youngsters to be "thought judges," who use two questions to evaluate the validity of their negative thoughts: (1) What's another way of looking at it? and (2) What's the evidence? If a negative thought is realistic and reflects a situation that can be changed, then a youngster is encouraged to use problem solving to develop and follow a plan that produces improvement. If the situation is real but cannot be changed, then the youngster is taught to use a coping strategy to manage her reaction to the situation.

A more complete description of each treatment component is provided later. In general, the first nine sessions focus primarily on affective education, and on teaching coping and problem-solving skills. Sessions 10 through 19 focus primarily on learning and applying cognitive restructuring, as well as continued use of previously learned strategies. Beginning with the 11th meeting and continuing through the 20th meeting, children work to improve their sense of self. Prior to describing the intervention strategies, however, we discuss the format, group size, duration, spacing of meetings, and structure of meetings. These are less obvious but important ingredients in the treatment program.

Implementation Issues

Format of Treatment

In the majority of treatment outcome studies, the treatment is delivered in a group format, while most youths seen on an outpatient basis receive individual therapy. For research purposes, we have used a group format, due to the need to treat approximately 150 girls in 3 years. However, an important question has not been addressed in the literature: Is one format more effective than the other? Based on clinical experience, there are some advantages to both formats, and at times a hybrid model that includes both has appeared to be ideal (although practically unrealistic). What are the advantages of group CBT for depression?

ADVANTAGES OF GROUP CBT

There are a number of very obvious and some subtle advantages to conducting group CBT for depression. Perhaps the greatest advantage of group CBT is that it is more economical, as up to six youths can participate in the same 60- to 90-minute meeting. Thus it is possible to provide more youngsters with treatment. Another obvious advantage is that children can see that they are not the only ones who experience depression. Sometimes this helps to counter secondary depressive thoughts, such as "I'm such a loser; I'm the only one in the world who can't do this."

The group members can also be sources of emotional and interpersonal support. For example, one of the participants who felt especially rejected was invited to eat lunch with two group members and their other friends. The group members can provide encouragement for each other as well. For example, a girl who had comorbid social anxiety disorder became less anxious about being around peers as a result of the support that she received from the group. The other group members encouraged her to join them in the activities and to talk to other students.

Moreover, the group format is ideal for helping participants overcome interpersonal difficulties as interpersonal issues are enacted in the group. This enables the therapist to observe difficulties, teach alternative appropriate behaviors, and assess and restructure the automatic thoughts or beliefs that underlie maladaptive behaviors.

The group experience itself can help counter some negative beliefs and automatic thoughts. In a cohesive group, participants are supportive. This helps them feel supported, listened to, and understood, and it counters negative beliefs such as "No one likes me" or "No one cares about me." In some groups, the intimacy of interactions leads to the development of friendships, and the girls socialize outside of group meetings. Once again, these interactions can restructure the depressive belief that "I don't have any friends" or "I can't trust anyone." One group of girls had regular sleepovers on the weekends, which led to an increase in their engagement in pleasant activities, caused a corresponding decrease in time spent thinking about unpleasant things, and countered the aforementioned negative beliefs. When friendships form, they can be therapeutic for the youngsters. However, the therapist has to ensure that no one is left out, as that would support the depressive belief "No one likes me." This has not proven to be difficult, as participants have been sensitive to this issue and have tried not to leave anyone out of their interactions.

Since each group is made up of same-age and same-gender peers, the participants' statements to one another are especially powerful. Over time, participants adopt the therapist's questions and other therapeutic statements. Thus participants say to each other many of the same things that the therapist has said. They also can be very helpful with restructuring the negative thoughts of other participants. They may know a participant well enough to give her evidence that contradicts a negative belief. For example, one girl stated that none of the boys liked her. One of the other girls stated, "That's not true. At the last dance, there was a group of boys around you all of the time, and they all wanted to dance with you." The other girls in the group were able to provide her with additional contradictory evidence.

We maximize these advantages of conducting group CBT. In order to restructure negative thoughts, participants have to be able to identify their own negative thoughts. It is easier for children to recognize and restructure the negative thoughts of others relative to their own. One way to help them learn to identify negative thoughts is to play a game of "Catch the Negative Thought." When a participant or therapist (the therapist purposely makes some negative statements) expresses a negative thought, other group members try to be the first to identify it by saying "Negative thought." This sensitizes the girls to their own negative thoughts. As treatment progresses to cognitive restructuring, it is easier to restructure someone else's thoughts. Thus the participants first learn how to restructure the negative thoughts of others, which prepares them for restructuring their own negative thoughts and beliefs.

DISADVANTAGES OF GROUP CBT

The primary limitation of group CBT for depression is that it is less intense: There isn't as much time spent on any one child as there is in individual treatment. Time has to be distributed across participants, or they get bored and don't benefit from treatment. It is difficult to keep a group of youths engaged in treatment every meeting. When the focus of the group's attention is on one child, the other children get bored if the topic is not personally relevant. If a child has a particularly complex problem that is brought to the group's attention, and it is so complex that the other members cannot help with it, then the therapist's attention may become focused on that one child for so long that other participants disengage. When this happens, group therapy becomes individual therapy one group member at a time.

Group CBT is also very taxing for the therapist, as she has to be cognizant of so many things at once. For example, the therapist has an agenda. Each agenda item may or may not be appropriate for the children's current concerns; thus a judgment about how to proceed has to be made. The therapist has to determine whether the participants are engaged in the activity or procedure that is being used to help them acquire the therapeutic skills. The therapist has to watch for opportunities to make the skill real for the children. In other words, the

therapist has to watch for opportunities to show the children how they can apply that skill to a real-life situation. The therapist has to be alert for negative thoughts and schema-consistent thoughts, and then make a decision about whether to restructure them or to note them for future meetings. The therapist also has to watch for and encourage prosocial behavior and she has to try to manage group behavior. Since CBT for depression is driven by both an idiosyncratic case conceptualization and research with depressed children, the therapist is trying to evaluate the validity of the conceptualization for each child during the interactions within the meeting. The conceptualization typically evolves over the course of treatment. Then the therapist has to integrate each conceptualization with the meeting as described in the treatment manual.

As noted earlier, cognitive restructuring is difficult to do in the group because of the amount of time and attention that has to be focused on one child. Typically, to restructure a thought or belief effectively, a series of increasingly intimate and specific questions must be asked. If the other participants can't relate to the questions, then they disengage during this time. The target child also may become self-conscious with all of the attention and then give vague or elusive responses in an attempt to keep things private. This makes cognitive restructuring itself less effective.

Another disadvantage of groups is that participants may not get along with each other, or they may have a history of conflict. Children who are interpersonally aggressive or have a history of interpersonal conflict may not be appropriate to have in the same group, as their history may prevent them from feeling that the group environment is safe enough to be comfortable with self-disclosure. During the early phases of treatment, this can be very difficult to manage, and the group members are typically not at a skill level where they can take these conflicts and intervene in a constructive way that facilitates the growth of both bullies and victims.

Group Size

Although groups enable the therapist to see multiple children at once, there is a point at which a group becomes too large to be of therapeutic value. In a group that is working well (e.g., no interpersonal conflicts, participants are actively engaged in treatment, etc.), the maximum number of children appears to be six. The primary problem of having more participants is that there isn't enough time to attend to each person's concerns. The more children in the group, the less time there is for each member to talk about the topic of the day or her individual concerns. At the simplest level, this slows treatment down, as each child is only getting 10–15 minutes of therapy time directly focused on her. More participants may want to talk about a particular concern than the remaining time in the meeting permits, resulting in a participant having to wait until the next meeting. That concern may or may not be relevant at the next meeting, or the child may forget what she wanted to discuss. In addition, failure to attend to a participant's concerns can lead to activation of depressive beliefs such as "The therapist doesn't care about me," "I am not important to other people," "No one cares about me," and the like. This can have a serious adverse impact on the therapeutic relationship and may reinforce the participant's negative beliefs. With other children, it can draw out their passive–aggressive, defiant, or other undesirable attention-getting behaviors. These behaviors can be very destructive, as other group members either become annoyed or see that these behaviors can be an effective tool for getting attention and also use them; or they can create an interpersonal wedge between participants, and sometimes between a participant and the therapist. We are finding that four is a good size for a group of depressed 9- to 13-year-old girls. With four participants, a group feels and works like a group, but is small enough that there is more time for each participant.

Duration

How many meetings are necessary and sufficient for treatment to be maximally effective? This question has yet to be empirically addressed in the literature. The answer is not simple, as it is idiosyncratic to each client. Currently, our treatment participants are completing 20 group meetings plus 2 individual meetings over 11 weeks. Additional individual meetings are completed during this period on an as-needed basis. In our research, symptom severity is assessed every other week, and the majority of girls have significantly improved by the 18th meeting. A few of the youngsters

(12%) continue to need additional meetings, including a few who appear to need long-term therapy due to the complexity of their problems. For example, a participant may be experiencing a combination of depression and PTSD that results from a history of sexual abuse. If the abuse has not been treated in the past, then it takes a number of meetings to address these issues. In other instances, the child may be experiencing symptoms related to the emergence of a personality disorder. Or a child may be living within a chaotic environment, where the primary caregiver is experiencing a psychiatric disorder and/or the other caregiver may be intermittently involved in the youngster's life; the parents may be experiencing couple difficulties; the caregiver may introduce and then break up with a series of partners; a caregiver may be incarcerated; or still other family problems may exist.

The duration of each meeting is developmentally dependent: The meetings are scheduled for more time for older youths and for less time with younger children, as their attention span is shorter. We prefer 1-hour meetings with groups of 9- and 10-year-olds, and 90-minute meetings with children 11 and older.

Spacing of Meetings

Traditionally, in cognitive therapy for depression (e.g., Beck et al., 1979), meetings are held more frequently at the beginning of treatment and then are spaced out as termination is approached. Twice-weekly meetings are completed for the first few weeks in an attempt to achieve more rapid reduction in symptom severity. Subsequently, meetings are held weekly until symptom reduction has been achieved. Meetings are then held every other week and eventually monthly, until the client has recovered, has acquired the therapeutic strategies, and can independently apply them to her own depressive symptoms, stressors, problems, and negative thinking.

During the pilot phase of our research protocol, we planned to follow this traditional schedule. However, the numerous advantages of twice-weekly meetings soon became evident. They helped participants build rapport and trust with the therapist and each other. The short time between meetings also reduced the amount of material they forgot; since they remembered more, less time was needed to help them remember or understand therapeutic concepts. The therapist could also thread together material from one meeting to the next more easily. Participants were more likely to remember and thus complete their therapeutic homework as well. Finally, the greater frequency of meetings also caused children's consciousness to be filled with the therapeutic dialogue from previous meetings.

Another important advantage to the twice-weekly meeting schedule is that there is less time between occurrence of a critical event and meeting with the therapist. Thus a participant is more likely to remember the event and the thoughts and emotions associated with it. In addition, since less time passes between an event and the next meeting, the destructive impact of undesirable events can be minimized, as the group can process, problem-solve, devise effective coping plans, and restructure maladaptive perceptions of the event's meaning before it has a chance to become part of the youngster's meaning structures. Similarly, if a therapeutic homework assignment has an unwanted outcome, it can be processed, problem-solved, and restructured before it has too much of an adverse impact.

Still other advantages of the schedule involve desirable outcomes. For example, a participant may be given a homework assignment to use a coping strategy, such as doing something fun and distracting when she first experiences a decline in mood. The youngster notices the mood shift and starts to dance in a goofy way to her favorite music, and this produces an improvement in mood. She recognizes the improvement and is eager to tell the group about it. Because she is able to report this experience and receive rewarding feedback promptly, she is encouraged to continue to cope with depressed mood, and it helps build the belief that she can influence her mood. This shift in her belief system is crucial, as this underlying sense of self-efficacy is what we strive to create during treatment.

During the pilot protocol, when treatment meetings switched from twice weekly to once a week, we immediately noticed that participants were not remembering as much from previous meetings; they were not completing their therapeutic homework as often; and they were less engaged in treatment. Consequently, we decided to maintain the twice-weekly schedule for the entire treatment. Perhaps the benefits of the twice-weekly meetings reflect the developmental differences between children and adults.

Structure of Meetings

The therapy sessions in CBT are structured, and each meeting follows a sequence of events. We have modified this sequence to be developmentally appropriate. The sequence of events in each meeting is listed in Table 5.1. Following a consistent sequence provides participants with a sense of security, as they know what to expect.

RAPPORT BUILDING

Meetings begin with a few minutes of unstructured "chat time" to reestablish rapport and to ease youngsters into more personal discussions. Participants determine what is discussed during this time, and typically they want to talk about what has happened between meetings. Children like to use this time to get to know each other in a less formal way, to get to know the therapist better, or just to talk informally about things as a means of building trust and interpersonal relationships. These discussions may be completely irrelevant to treatment, or they may be relevant and allow the therapist to identify possible agenda items. If the discussion becomes therapeutically relevant, then the therapist uses the discussion to teach skills or concepts. For example, a child may bring up an interpersonal problem that she has faced between meetings, and the therapist may decide to use the situation as an opportunity to demonstrate how to use problem solving (it is a situation that the child can change). When the situation is therapeutically relevant, but doesn't fit with the skill that was scheduled to be taught, the therapist may teach the situationally relevant skill instead of the skill that was going to be taught from the treatment manual. This unstructured "chat time" appears to be most important to preadolescents and young teens, as they have a greater need to talk with peers as a means of gaining trust.

TABLE 5.1. Outline of the Structure of Treatment Meetings

- Rapport building ("chat time")
- Agenda setting
- Goal attainment check-in
- Review of previous meeting and homework
- Skill building/coping skill activity
- Review of main points
- Positive behavior review
- Assignment of therapeutic homework

AGENDA SETTING

Since CBT is structured and time-limited, a good deal of between-meeting planning must be completed, and time has to be used wisely. The therapist plans for each meeting by developing and updating the case conceptualizations and then integrating the conceptualizations with the session as described in the treatment manual. Thus the therapist enters each meeting with a plan that becomes the agenda. It is also important for children to take ownership for the content of the meetings, so they are asked to contribute to the agenda. Most children are not used to doing this, so the therapist has to teach them to add to the agenda.

GOAL ATTAINMENT CHECK-IN

After the third treatment meeting, all of the assessment data are combined with observations of the participants' behavior and comments to create an initial case conceptualization for each child. Based on this conceptualization, the therapist identifies treatment-relevant goals for each client. The child is encouraged to add to the list of goals so that it is a collaborative process. The goals are stated in positive, developmentally sensitive terms. The therapist's goals are shared with the children to ensure that the goals also are consistent with each girl's personal goals for treatment. For example, a child's goal may be "To feel happier more often." Each goal is written down, along with the corresponding coping, problem-solving, or cognitive restructuring procedure(s) that will be used to achieve the goal.

During every meeting, the therapist asks the children how they are progressing in their plans for achieving treatment goals. Each girl is asked whether she has made any progress: Has she taken any actions? Does she have any questions about the plan or how to implement it? Did she try to do something, but experienced a problem that interfered with progress? If so, what was it? Problem solving is used to overcome impediments. The children are also asked whether they have identified any new goals. As a girl reports success, the other group members applaud, or shower her with the soft, spongy, smiley-faced balls that are used in the "Catch the Positive" activity (see below).

In some cases, children have difficulty making progress toward goal attainment. The group may problem-solve to help such a youngster develop new plans, or the therapist may meet individually with the child to see whether the primary roadblock is negative thinking or something that she doesn't want to discuss in the group. If the problem is a negatively distorted thought, the therapist will restructure the negative thought. In some cases, the child may need additional encouragement through an in-session or home reward system. Sometimes, the goals are too ambitious and have to be broken down into subgoals, and plans have to be revised.

REVIEW OF PREVIOUS MEETING AND HOMEWORK

Clients who think about the sessions outside of meetings are going to make the most movement in the shortest amount of time. The therapist leads a review of important points from the previous meeting and asks about each child's experiences with the therapeutic homework. The objective of this review is to thread together material covered in each meeting, because the meetings build on each other. Thus the review helps each child to remember the material covered in the previous meeting and sets the stage for the new material. It is also designed to support the directive to think about and remember what is covered during each meeting.

SKILL BUILDING

Skill building is the therapeutic heart of the intervention. During each meeting, either a new skill is taught; the group is taught more about a previously learned skill; or the members are given practice in applying the skill. Typically this involves some didactic teaching, although we always strive to use activities that enable the children to experience the impact of the skill at the moment within the session. The skills are taught in an additive fashion, in which one skill serves as the base for the next. This segment of the meeting represents the largest investment in time.

Three primary intervention strategies are taught to the youngsters: coping skills, problem solving, and cognitive restructuring (each is described in more detail below). They are all used to reduce stress, improve interpersonal relationships, enhance self-efficacy, and improve the youngsters' sense of self,

Applying the skills to their immediate symptoms and other concerns is as important as learning new skills. Meeting time is spent demonstrating how to apply the skill to existing concerns. It is most effective if the concern can be brought into the room and the skill can be directly applied to the concern in the moment so that the child can experience the benefits of applying the skill. For example, a child may describe an experience during chat time, and the therapist may choose to introduce the skill at that moment. Applying the skill during the meeting allows the therapist to observe the child's attempts to apply the skill and to provide corrective feedback.

COPING SKILLS ACTIVITY

The most powerful way to teach youngsters coping skills is to demonstrate their effectiveness within the meeting. Typically, this can be accomplished with a brief (5- to 10-minute) activity. These activities and the specific skills are described later in this chapter. The activity can be enacted at any point during the meeting, and the therapist is free to choose the coping skill that she thinks would be most beneficial for the group. For example, if the group seems especially lethargic or "down," it is helpful to use an activity that is energizing so that it invigorates the group. There is one requirement: All five categories of coping strategies have to be demonstrated by the ninth meeting. This ensures that the youngsters have experienced and know how to use each strategy by the midpoint of treatment.

REVIEW OF MAIN POINTS

Prior to ending a meeting, the therapist leads the children through a review of the main points. Typically, this involves asking for a description of what they think are the main points. During this discussion, the therapist assesses the group's understanding and recall. Misunderstandings and failures to acquire a skill are corrected.

POSITIVE BEHAVIOR REVIEW

Positive behavior review is referred to as the "Catch the Positive" activity. Child clients do not know how to derive the most from their therapy experience. Thus it is important to teach them how to be effective clients. Before the end of each meeting, the therapist tells the children what they did that was especially helpful. In other words, the therapist verbally reinforces the children for behaviors that maximize their therapy experiences. As the thera-

pist compliments each child with a specifically worded statement that describes the desirable behavior, she tosses a soft, spongy, smiley-faced ball to the child, who catches it. Initially, the behaviors that are reinforced include good client behaviors (e.g., listening, contributing to the discussion, discussing how something applies to themselves, being supportive of other group members, etc.). After the children are behaving in a way that maximizes their therapy experience, desirable interpersonal behaviors are reinforced by the therapist. Over the course of treatment, the person giving the compliments is not only the therapist; the children begin to take turns giving each other compliments. Over the last six meetings, the children are also asked to notice what they have done well during the meeting and to give *themselves* compliments.

ASSIGNMENT OF THERAPEUTIC HOMEWORK

Each meeting ends with the assignment of therapeutic homework. The homework is designed to help participants apply the skills they have learned in treatment. Therapeutic homework is a critical part of the intervention. It is imperative that the clients apply their skills to depressive symptoms and other concerns outside of the meeting time. To structure this, and to increase the probability that the clients will complete their therapeutic homework, it is helpful to use a workbook (Stark, Schnoebelen, et al., 2004). Further discussion of therapeutic homework appears in a later section.

Core Therapeutic Components

Affective Education

"Affective education" refers to the educational component of treatment that teaches participants about depression and how to manage it. It is the portion of treatment that helps the participants to become more aware of their own experiences of depression—including their thoughts, emotions, and behavior, and the relationship among thoughts, emotions, and behavior. In essence, the participants are taught the CBT model of depression, how to personalize the model, and how to manage depression. In addition, this is the portion of treatment that helps clients become increasingly self-aware, particularly of therapeutically relevant experiences such as their depressive thoughts, unpleasant emotions, and other depressive symptoms. Clients are then taught to use these experiences as cues to engage in a variety of cognitive strategies and therapeutic skills. Affective education is threaded throughout the treatment program and is especially evident during the first few meetings.

Due to developmental limitations, children are taught a simplified model of depression in which sadness is caused by negative thoughts and undesirable outcomes. In order to manage depression, the children learn three basic strategies: (1) If the undesirable situation can't be changed, use a coping strategy; (2) if the undesirable situation can be changed, use problem solving to improve it; and (3) catch negative thoughts and change them to more realistic and positive thoughts. In order to use these three strategies, the youngsters have to recognize their unpleasant emotions, realize that they are experiencing a problem, and perceive that they are experiencing negative thoughts. We help the youngsters to identify their emotions by acting like "emotion detectives" who investigate their own experience of the emotion in the "3 B's": Body, Brain, and Behavior. In other words, we teach them to become more aware of their emotional experiences by tuning in to how their bodies are reacting, what they are thinking, and how they are acting. During the meetings, when a child states that she is experiencing a particular emotion, the therapist asks her to describe what is happening in her body, what she is thinking, and how she is behaving. Simultaneously, the therapist will use a simple cookie-cutout drawing of a person to illustrate what was happening in the girl's body, brain, and behavior that served as the clues that she was experiencing a particular emotion. As the sessions progress and the girls become more proficient at the process, they complete the drawings themselves. The girls also complete therapeutic homework assignments in which they catch their emotional experiences and independently illustrate a drawing using the 3 B's.

A critical component of the treatment program is teaching the youngsters the relationship between negative thoughts and undesirable emotions and behaviors. To help children understand this relationship, the therapist links thoughts to emotions by asking, "What were you thinking when . . . ?" or "What was going through your head when . . . ?" Activities and homework assignments also are used to help the children to become aware of the link be-

tween their thoughts and emotions. For example, participants may take turns pulling the name of an emotion out of a bag and then describing the thoughts that would lead to that emotion. Or they may pull a thought bubble out of a bag and then state the emotion that would result from that thought. As treatment progresses, the participants engage in a number of activities that help them become proficient at identifying their negative thoughts.

Goal Setting

CBT is a collaborative approach to psychological treatment, in which the child is fully informed of the objectives of treatment and the methods that are going to be employed to achieve these objectives. Central to this collaborative process is helping the client to identify his or her goals for therapy. In the case of treating a child, it also may involve helping the child's parents to identify their goals for their child's treatment, as well as their goals for changing their family or parenting practices.

CASE CONCEPTUALIZATION AND THE GOAL-SETTING MEETING

In the ACTION program, the therapist begins the goal-setting process by reviewing the plethora of assessment tools that each youngster completes prior to treatment (see Table 5.2). The information provided by these tools is used

---

TABLE 5.2. List of Assessment Tools Completed by Participants in the ACTION Treatment Study

Child-completed measures

Beck Youth Inventory
Children's Depression Inventory
Schedule for Affective Disorders and Schizophrenia for School-Age Children
Cognitive Triad Inventory for Children
Children's Cognitive Style Questionnaire
Self-Report Measure of Family Functioning
Family Messages Measure
Thematic Apperception Test
Life Events Checklist

Parent-completed measures

Schedule for Affective Disorders and Schizophrenia for School-Age Children
Child Behavior Checklist
Cognitive Triad Inventory
Symptom Checklist 90—R
Self-Report Measure of Family Functioning

to complete an initial case conceptualization of the child. The conceptualization is then translated into treatment goals—positively worded statements about desired outcomes. From the CBT perspective, case conceptualization is a fluid process that changes as more is learned about the client (e.g., Beck, 1995). The initial conceptualization evolves as new information is gleaned from the first three group meetings. The therapist meets individually with each participant between the third and fourth group meetings, and works with each participant to identify her greatest concerns and to collaboratively identify three or four goals for treatment. Thus the therapist merges the goals that she has generated during case conceptualization with the child's goals and concerns to develop a set of mutually agreed-upon goals for treatment. In addition, the therapist describes the treatment procedures that will be used to help the youngster achieve her goals. Before the end of the goal-setting meeting, the therapist asks the child if she would be willing to share her goals with the group. If the child prefers to keep any goal confidential, then this request is respected. During the fourth group meeting, participants share goals with each other and brainstorm how each group member can help the others to obtain their goals. The strategies for helping each other are recorded on their goal sheets, so that they can refer to them as needed.

As noted earlier, at the beginning of every subsequent meeting there is a "goal attainment check-in" time, to report progress toward goal attainment and to celebrate progress. As goals are achieved, participants identify new goals they want to work toward.

MAINTAINING PROGRESS TOWARD GOALS

Progress toward goal attainment can be documented visually for each child (see Figure 5.1). Individual charts are used, because a group chart might create competition and reinforce negative thoughts about the self when other group members make more progress toward goal attainment. Problem solving is used to generate new plans if original plans don't work. Stickers (for younger children) or check marks (for older children and adolescents) are used to recognize and reinforce progress toward a goal. Examples of participants' goals appear in Table 5.3.

Coping Skills Training

The ACTION treatment is based on several underlying assumptions that are rooted in research: (1) Depressed youths experience a deficit in coping skills (for a review, see Stark, Sander, Yancy, Bronik, & Hoke, 2000), but they can learn these skills; (2) learning and applying coping skills will produce an improvement in depressive symptoms; (3) depressed youngsters experience a variety of emotions, and the intensity of these emotions vary over the course of a day; (4) children can be taught to recognize a decline in mood and to use this as a cue to engage in coping; and (5) similarly, they can be taught to recognize an improvement in mood and to record the events that are associated with the improvement. Thus coping

Goal	Coping	Problem-Solving	Change Thinking	I'm making progress!

FIGURE 5.1. Chart for monitoring progress toward goal attainment.

TABLE 5.3. Examples of Goals from Current and Past Group Members

- To feel better
- To feel less lonely/sad
- To sleep better
- To get along better with people (i.e., friends, parents, teachers, siblings)
- To make more friends
- To change/talk back to negative thoughts in general, or specific thoughts such as "I hate myself"
- To feel better about myself
- To do better in school
- To share problems with the group
- To avoid fights/control my temper
- To express feelings/open up to other people
- Feel happier
- Learn to get myself out of a bad mood by myself

skills represent a foundational component of the intervention.

Depressed youths appear to experience greater mood lability than depressed adults. This may be a developmental phenomenon, related to their greater exposure to mood-enhancing events and other distractions that occur naturally throughout their day. Even youths who are more severely depressed experience some temporary lessening of their sadness at varying times of the day. The greater likelihood of experiencing an improvement in mood may be due to children being less capable of withdrawing and isolating themselves from others and the outside world. It may also be due to their exposure to many nondepressed peers who engage them in various social, recreational, and academic activities.

Due to the central role of coping skills in CBT for the treatment of childhood disorders and the typically greater reactivity of depressed youths, we attempted to identify coping skills to include in the ACTION treatment program. The treatment outcome literature and the literature on the development of emotion regulation were reviewed to identify coping skills that could be incorporated into the treatment program. Both literature bases were too general in their descriptions of emotion regulation strategies to help direct the choice of skills to be taught. Consequently, we completed a pilot study to identify developmentally appropriate coping strategies.

Teachers were provided with a definition of "resilience" and an example of a resilient child.

After receiving parental permission and child assent, teachers nominated especially resilient students; from this pool of potential participants, we randomly selected 10 boys and 10 girls from the fourth, fifth, sixth, and seventh grades from each of two school districts (both school districts are participating in our ongoing treatment study). These students participated in focus groups (each group consisted of five same-sex, same-grade students) in which the students were asked to discuss their strategies for managing sadness, anger, and anxiety. Five general categories of coping strategies consistently emerged from their discussions: (1) Do something fun and distracting; (2) do something soothing and relaxing; (3) do something that expends energy; (4) talk to someone; and (5) change the way you think about it. Coping skills from these five general categories were used to manage all three unpleasant emotions. Based on these results, the emotion regulation literature, and existing interventions for depression, we included training in skills from these five categories of coping skills in the intervention program.

Coping skills are taught both as general strategies for enhancing mood and more specifically as strategies that can be used when a child is experiencing an unfortunate or stressful situation that she cannot change. Thus clients are taught emotion-focused coping. Coping skills are specifically taught to the participants and practiced during meetings 2–9. Coping skills training is emphasized at the beginning of treatment, because these skills help the youngsters produce an immediate improvement in mood. This mood improvement makes it easier for the youngsters to learn and benefit from problem solving and cognitive restructuring, which are taught later. There is some flexibility built into the program, as the therapist chooses the skills to be taught and applied during each session—with, however, the constraint that examples from all five of the categories have to be taught within the first nine meetings. As long as this constraint is heeded, the therapist chooses the coping skills that she believes are most needed by the group each meeting. It is important to note that the therapist may include coping skills training at any point during treatment when it may be helpful to a client or to the larger group. For example, students in Texas have to complete "high-stakes testing" that determines whether they pass to the next grade. This is a stressful time for the entire school, as funding and individuals' jobs are dependent on the results. This testing occurs over 3 days. For some of our earlier groups, the testing was completed during the later part of treatment, and for other groups it was completed during the meetings that focused on coping skills training. Regardless, the therapists incorporated the testing and the associated stress into the treatment meetings planned for those days. They taught the youngsters soothing and relaxing coping skills and applied them to the stress they were feeling about the tests. In addition, problem solving was used to help the children to develop plans for reducing stress and preparing for the anxiety during the actual testing.

Simply talking about coping skills and how they work is not adequate, as it becomes nothing more than an intellectual exercise for children. Depressed children, and perhaps children with other disorders, have to experience the benefits of coping skills before they will actually try to use them. When one of the five coping strategies is first taught to the participants, the therapist begins by asking the girls to rate their moods at the moment. Or they may be asked to complete a brief imagery activity in which they imagine experiencing a personally relevant stressful event; then they are asked to rate their mood. After the mood rating, the therapist asks the girls to participate in an activity in which they actually use one of the coping skills. For example, the girls may be asked to play with hula hoops for 5 minutes along with the therapist (fun and distracting); they may be asked to play freeze tag (exerting energy); they may wiggle their toes in sand while imaging a relaxing beach scene (soothing and relaxing); they may talk with one another about a stressor; or they may be asked to talk back to their negative thoughts (see the section on cognitive restructuring). After completing the activity, they stop and re-rate their moods. Inevitably, their moods improve dramatically, and this improvement is discussed along with ideas for how to maintain it. The group generates a list of examples of things they can do, or already do, from this general category of coping strategies. In addition, they discuss the mechanism that makes each coping strategy work. The girls then brainstorm situations where they could use the coping strategies, and they are instructed to try to use one of these coping skills the next time they experience similar situations.

Although it is apparent that the youngsters

can learn and benefit from using coping skills, therapeutic improvement is dependent on their applying the skills outside of group meetings. To facilitate this, therapeutic homework is assigned. This homework progresses from identifying changes in emotion and the accompanying thoughts, to noting a change in emotions, the context of the emotional change, and the coping skill used to improve mood. In general, participants have a relatively easy time learning coping skills and applying them to their depressive symptoms. By the midpoint of treatment, they give examples of how they use coping skills to improve their moods. In fact, they like the skills so much that it is difficult to get them to use other skills.

Initially, the participants are taught to use mood-enhancing activities as general coping strategies and methods for improving mood. Engagement in more pleasant activities is used as a method for elevating the children's overall mood. To accomplish this, the group is asked to generate a list of "fun activities" that are within their control. Each participant is asked to identify the activities from which she derives the most pleasure, and to use activities from this list to create a pleasant events schedule that the children refer to as a "Catch the Positive" List (CPL). These lists consist of mood-enhancing activities and events, with spaces for indicating their occurrence or nonoccurrence each day of the week. At the bottom of the page is a mood meter where the child rates her mood for the day. The child is instructed to engage in as many of the pleasant activities as possible, and to indicate her involvement through placing a check mark in the appropriate box. Mood is enhanced through increased engagement in pleasant activities and through restructuring the youngster's belief that nothing good ever happens in her life.

Problem-Solving Training

As participants acquire a better understanding of their emotions, accurately identify them, recognize their impact on behavior and thinking, and understand that they can take action to moderate the intensity and impact of their emotions, we teach the girls that some undesirable situations that lead to unpleasant affect can be changed. Problem solving is the strategy that they can use to change undesirable situations. The five-step problem-solving sequence is introduced during the fifth meeting. During this meeting, the group members also create a comprehensive list of the problems that girls their age typically face. Without identifying any child, the therapist also contributes examples of problems that the girls experience or have experienced. Then the members go through the list and determine whether each problem can be changed or whether it is a problem that they can't change. If they can't change the problem, then they use emotion-focused coping. Problem solving counters rigidity and hopelessness, as the youngsters see that there may be some options of which they were previously unaware. The children also gain a sense of self-efficacy as they experience success and mastery over the environment.

The problem-solving procedure that we use is a modification of the one described by Kendall (e.g., Kendall & Braswell, 1993). Children are taught to break problem solving down into five component steps through education, modeling, coaching, rehearsal, and feedback. To simplify the process and to help the girls remember the five steps, girls are taught the "5 P's."

The first step in the process is problem identification and definition. Children refer to this step as "Problem." This may be the most difficult step for depressed children to learn, as they often view a problem as a personal threat. To a depressed child, the existence of a problem means that there is something wrong with her, or the problem represents an impending loss. In addition, depressed children feel overwhelmed by problems; they believe that they cannot solve them, and that even if they did solve an existing problem, it would be replaced by another one. Thus, their sense of hopelessness has to be combated through concrete evidence in their life experiences that they can in fact overcome problems.

The second step is goal identification and definition, which children refer to as "Purpose." In order to define possible solutions and to evaluate plans, it is necessary to know the desired outcome of the solutions to the problems. The therapist asks participants whether their plans will achieve their purpose. For example, commonly a participant will choose to respond to rumors by retaliating through spreading rumors about the bully. This will not achieve the child's goal of retaining friends while stopping the rumors.

The third step is generation of alternative so-

lutions: Children are taught to brainstorm as many possible solutions as they can without evaluating them. The children refer to this step as "Plans." This is difficult for depressed youngsters, since they typically come up with more reasons for why a plan won't work than for why it might work. Even when they can't identify specific reasons why it won't work, they base their prediction on how they are feeling (emotional reasoning). Thus it is important to improve mood through coping skills training. When children are first learning to generate solutions, the range and number of possibilities that they can generate are often limited. Consequently, they have to be taught additional possibilities. It is important to teach them not to evaluate the alternatives while they are trying to generate them, since depressed youths have a tendency to believe that nothing will work. Thus the youngsters may once again short-circuit the process and think that they can't solve the problem.

The ACTION program includes a game that teaches brainstorming. The group is divided into two teams. A player picks a problem out of a bag. Each team has 2 minutes to generate as many solutions as possible. If players stop to evaluate solutions, they lose time and thus don't generate as many solutions, so the game pulls for brainstorming.

The fourth step involves predicting likely outcomes for each possible solution and then picking the plan that best matches a child's goal. Children refer to this step as "Predict and Pick." As the youngsters progress into real-life problems, the therapist often has to help them recognize potential positive outcomes, as well as limitations and self-defeating consequences of other possibilities. Once again, it is necessary at this step to combat the youngsters' pessimism.

The fifth step involves enacting a plan and evaluating its effectiveness. If the plan is working, the youngster congratulates herself with a symbolic "Pat on the back." If the outcome is undesirable, the youngster reconsiders possible solutions, chooses an alternative one, and enacts it. Nevertheless, the child will give herself a symbolic "Pat on the back" for trying. Coping statements for unsuccessful plans have to be included in the treatment.

Initially, the therapist provides the participants with "hypothetical" problems that give them practice at using the five steps during group meetings. However, the therapist actually provides them with practice problems that are similar to the ones they have reported facing in real life. In addition, during each of the subsequent meetings, the participants solve a problem that is common to girls their age (e.g., interpersonal conflicts and teasing), as well as problems that are identified through completion of therapeutic homework. As treatment progresses, the girls are given the homework assignment to use problem solving to solve at least one problem between meetings.

Teaching children the problem-solving steps is the easy part of the training. The difficult part is getting them to *use* problem solving to change the situations that cause stress and distress. The participants are specifically taught the five steps during meetings 5–9. In addition, during these meetings they complete homework assignments that help them apply problem solving. At first, the homework assignments facilitate recognition of problems. Then the homework forms guide the participants through the application of the steps to the real-life problems that they experience during meetings 10–19.

Participants are encouraged to bring their problems to the meetings. A problem may come up during a discussion; someone may remember a problem and add it to the agenda for the group to discuss; or a problem may be recorded on a homework form. Since the therapist collects and reviews the homework forms, she becomes aware of the problems the girls face. The therapist and group members help each youngster with a problem to develop a plan for solving it. Then the therapist monitors the child's success at applying the plan to her problem. The plan is altered as necessary.

Cognitive Restructuring

A primary objective of the ACTION treatment for depressed children is to change their negative distorted thinking to more positive and realistic thinking. Children are taught various strategies for identifying and altering their maladaptive cognitions. Cognitive restructuring is introduced during coping skills training in a more general fashion as "changing the way you are thinking." The children learn to think more positively in general as they generate self-statements that they can think when they are feeling upset or are faced with a particular stressor.

Negative thoughts are restructured directly and indirectly throughout treatment. Direct restructuring of negative thoughts is completed through teaching the youngsters to identify their negative thoughts, question them, and then replace them with more realistic and positive thoughts. Formal training in cognitive restructuring appears later in therapy (meetings 10–20), due to the fact that it requires the youngsters to become more self-focused, which can exacerbate depressive symptoms. Providing the youngsters with coping and problem-solving skills earlier in treatment helps them to manage the upset that comes with increased self-focus. It also appears as though the improvement in mood and symptoms that results from other treatment components provides the youngsters with some personal distance from their maladaptive thoughts and beliefs, which seems to open them to cognitive restructuring.

Restructuring of negative thoughts is also completed indirectly through guided learning experiences that are incorporated into treatment. Specific homework assignments provide each child with learning that contradict existing negative beliefs and build new, more adaptive beliefs. The CPL is used to help the girls restructure their negative thoughts. For example, a girl may believe that she is unlovable and that no one expresses any love toward her. With the help of the group, a list of parental behaviors that express love is generated, and the girl adds these behaviors to her CPL and monitors their occurrence between meetings. As they occur, she fills in the check marks each day. This assignment only restructures the child's belief if it is a reflection of a distortion in her thinking. It will not work if the parents actually do not express their love for her.

Another indirect method for teaching children to think more positively is to model more adaptive thoughts. The therapist verbalizes her thoughts, or verbalizes more adaptive thoughts that the children might use to replace negative thoughts. Typically, the procedure involves modeling more adaptive thoughts and asking children to put them into their own words and then rehearse them. In addition to using cognitive modeling when specific thoughts are being targeted, the therapist thinks aloud whenever she confronts a problem or some other situation that enables her to model adaptive thoughts for a child. This is done throughout treatment as a means of planting the seeds of more adaptive thinking.

The first step in directly restructuring negative thoughts is helping children recognize and be aware of the tendency to think negatively. This is accomplished through affective education, as noted earlier. The next step is helping the children to be able to "catch" their negative thoughts. This is accomplished first through catching negative thoughts that are expressed through any group member's statements, and then through catching their own negative thoughts within group meetings. Subsequently, the girls are asked to catch and record their negative thoughts on homework forms. Then the girls bring the negative thoughts to the group for help in restructuring them.

Once a negative thought has been identified, the child asks one of the two "What" questions as a means of evaluating its validity and for developing adaptive thoughts to replace the negative ones. As noted earlier, these two questions are (1) What's another way to think about it? and (2) What's the evidence? The children learn to use the question that is better suited for different negative thoughts. "What's another way to think about it?" is the easier of the two questions for the children to learn. They use this question to generate alternative, plausible, and positive thoughts for the situation. "What's the evidence?" is used when the objective facts do not support the child's negative thought.

The standard cognitive restructuring procedure is difficult to teach children to use (once again, this reflects a developmental difference between children and adults). A powerful tool that is part of the ACTION program is an activity that the girls refer to as "talking back to the muck monster." When the participants are having difficulty changing, or letting go of, negative thinking, we refer to this as being "stuck in the negative muck." The girls like and understand this metaphor. When they are stuck in the negative muck, it is the "muck monster" that is filling them with negative thoughts and holding them back from extricating themselves from the muck. To help the girls learn how to apply cognitive restructuring independently during the ACTION treatment, girls are asked to use the two "What" questions to talk back to the muck monster. To accomplish this, an extra chair is brought to the group meetings. The chair is for the muck mon-

ster. The therapist prepares a list of the most common negative thoughts for each group member. The list comes from thoughts that have been verbalized during group meetings, thoughts that were endorsed on the pretreatment measures, and thoughts that have been recorded on the homework forms. The therapist then projects the thoughts that are coming from the muck monster in the empty chair, and each girl uses the two questions to guide her talking back to the negative thoughts. She can get help from the other group members in doing this. The girl may be encouraged to talk back to the muck monster very forcefully by yelling at it. The other group members often assist and cheer her on as she strongly disputes the negative thoughts and then replaces them with more realistic positive thoughts. It is also possible to switch roles and have the target girl provide the thoughts for the muck monster while the therapist forcefully talks back to the muck monster. The girls enjoy this activity, and it really seems to help them learn how to use cognitive restructuring. Since they enjoy it, this activity can be used multiple times with any participant.

The workbook contains a number of forms that guide the children through the process of catching, countering, and replacing negative thoughts. During meetings 10–20, the girls complete these forms as homework assignments. In addition to the group meetings that focus on teaching cognitive restructuring, the second individual session is completed between the 10th and 11th group meetings. The primary objective of this meeting is to help each participant to identify her most common negative thoughts and beliefs and to practice restructuring them. This extra individual help seems to be necessary, as the cognitive restructuring process is idiosyncratic and focuses on one child at a time.

One of the ultimate goals of treatment is changing dysfunctional schemas that are hypothesized to give rise to errors in information processing, depressogenic automatic thoughts, dysfunctional emotions, and behaviors associated with depressive disorders in children. Cognitive restructuring procedures are designed to modify clients' thinking and premises, assumptions, and attitudes underlying their thoughts (Meichenbaum, 1977). Through using the two "What" questions, using the CPL, and completing specific homework assignments, children are able to tear down old negative beliefs and build new, more positive beliefs.

Building a Positive Sense of Self

The last eight meetings focus on changing the depressed youngsters' negative beliefs about the self. This component appears last, because all of the other skills are brought to bear on the process of working toward and recognizing self-improvement, and changing the negative beliefs about the self. Depressed children evaluate their performances, possessions, and personal qualities more negatively than nondepressed youths, and their self-evaluations tend to be negatively distorted (Kendall, Stark, & Adam, 1990). In other words, they tend to be unrealistically and unreasonably negative in their self-evaluations. Children can be taught to evaluate themselves more reasonably and positively when it is realistic to do so. During this process, they learn to recognize their positive attributes, outcomes, and possessions.

One of the tools that is used to help youngsters develop a more positive sense of themselves is the "self-map" (see Figure 5.2). Each circle within the map represents an area of a child's life and an aspect of self-definition. The self-map helps children to broaden their self-definition and to recognize more strengths than they were previously aware they had. Partici-

pants are asked to fill in each bubble with relevant strengths. In addition, parents and teachers are interviewed by the therapist to identify their perceptions of a child's strengths in each of the domains. We have found that this information can be very powerful, as the children enjoy receiving the compliments.

The CPL is used as the children are asked to self-monitor evidence that supports the positive description that is outlined on the self-map. For example, a child may place a lot of self-worth on her musical talent. She will be instructed to self-monitor her successes during class, individual instruction, practice, and concerts. In addition, emphasis will be placed on her making efforts toward becoming a better musician rather than comparing herself to others. Furthermore, emphasis will be placed on the personal pleasure she derives from playing her instrument.

In some instances, children's negative self-evaluations are accurate, and they can benefit from change. In such instances, the goal of treatment is to help the youngsters to translate personal standards into realistic goals, and then to develop and carry out plans for attaining their goals. Following the translation process, children prioritize the areas where they are working toward self-improvement.

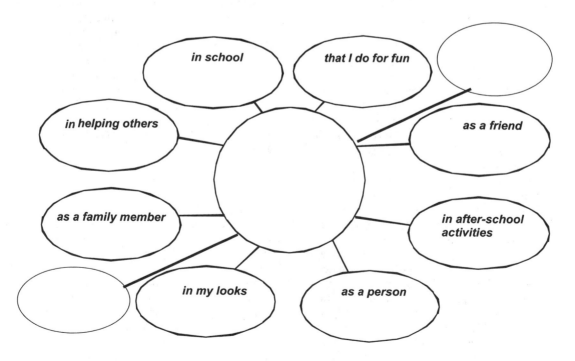

FIGURE 5.2. Self-map.

Initially, a plan is formulated for producing improvement in an area where success is probable. The long-term goal is broken down into subgoals, and problem solving is used to develop plans that will lead to subgoal attainment and eventually goal attainment. Prior to enacting plans, children try to identify possible impediments to carrying out the plans. Once again, problem solving is used to develop contingency plans for overcoming the impediments. Once the plans (including contingency plans) have been developed, children self-monitor their progress toward change. Alterations in plans are made along the way as necessary.

ACTION Kits

One of the developmental differences between conducting CBT with depressed children and conducting it with depressed adults is that the children are less likely to remember what they have discussed in the meetings. To help them remember the central therapeutic concepts, we have constructed "ACTION kits." The kits consist of a set of five color-coded cards. On these cards are the following: (1) a simple schematic depicting when to use coping skills, problem solving, and cognitive restructuring; (2) a visual depiction of how to use the "3 B's" to identify emotions; (3) a visual depiction of the five categories of coping skills; (4) the five problem-solving steps ("5 P's"); and (5) the two primary questions that guide cognitive restructuring. In addition, each kit includes one of the smiley-faced "Catch the Positive" balls, and a personalized goal form including plans for achieving goals. These kits are given to the girls between the sixth and seventh meetings, after all of the major treatment strategies have been introduced.

The therapist uses her own kit during the group meetings to model its use. For example, when a participant's homework reveals that she was feeling angry between meetings, the therapist pulls out the card that depicts when to use each of the three primary treatment strategies. Since it was a situation with a classmate that could be changed, the group decides to use problem solving, and the therapist uses the problem-solving card to guide the development of a plan. However, the therapist notes that it can be difficult to develop constructive plans when a person is feeling angry, so she also pulls out the coping skills card, and the child chooses

coping skills that will help her reduce anger so that she can think more clearly. Thus the therapist introduces the idea that it is helpful to combine the three primary treatment strategies. For example, a child may have to apply coping skills to improve dysphoric mood before she can effectively restructure a negative thought. It is common for children to have to use multiple skills at once to improve their mood and other depressive symptoms. The therapist uses the group members' therapeutic homework and concerns that they bring to the group to help them learn how to do this.

Homework

Therapeutic homework is an integral part of treatment. Homework assignments are designed to help children *apply* skills that they have learned within the meetings to real-life situations that occur outside treatment. The workbook (Stark, Schnoebelen, et al., 2004) structures therapeutic homework. Each assignment is designed to support application of the skill that was taught during that meeting. Examples of a coping skills form, a problem-solving form, and a cognitive restructuring homework form are provided in Figures 5.3, 5.4, and 5.5, respectively.

Many children don't like to complete therapeutic homework. To encourage them to do it, we include a within-session reward system. Children who complete the assignment can choose a reward from the preferred prize bag, and children who do not complete the assignment are given the opportunity to choose from the less desirable bag for attending the meeting. In addition, the therapists use more desirable rewards randomly for completion of homework.

When a child fails to complete a homework assignment, she is asked to complete it to the best of her recollection at the start of the meeting. If a child consistently has problems completing homework, the therapist will meet individually with the child, and they will problem-solve to help her develop a plan for completing her therapeutic homework. If a participant continues to have difficulty completing her homework, we have used a number of additional strategies (including e-mail and telephone call reminders, and stopping in the school counselor's office prior to school). Ideally, with a younger child, we would like the primary caregiver to encourage her to complete

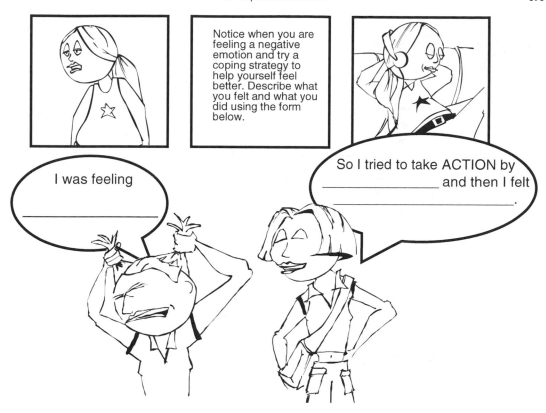

FIGURE 5.3. Coping skills worksheet.

PSYCHOSOCIAL TREATMENT OUTCOME RESEARCH

Treatment as Usual

it. With an older child or adolescent, parental involvement in homework is less desirable.

Although depressive disorders occur at a relatively high rate among adolescents (Rushton et al., 2003), only about 1% of youths receive either psychosocial or pharmacological outpatient treatment for depression in a year. Racial minority youth, especially African Americans, are the least likely to receive treatment, and youths who are uninsured are less likely to receive treatment than those who have insurance are (Olfson, Gameroff, Marcus, & Waslick, 2003). Thus the majority of depressed youths do not participate in treatment.

Information about the treatment of depressed youths from the general U.S. population is beginning to appear. Olfson and colleagues (2003) have found that most depressed youths (79%) who participate in treatment complete one or more sessions of psychotherapy and almost two thirds (59.8%) are treated with medication. About one in five youths (21%) are solely treated with medication, and almost half of treated youths (47.1%) receive a combination of psychotherapy and medication. Among youths who receive psychotherapy, approximately one-third (33.5%) attend one or two sessions, and 75% complete fewer than eight sessions per year. A minimal dose of psychotherapy is considered to be eight sessions (Howard, Kopta, Krause, & Orlinsky, 1986). Thus it appears as though even the majority of depressed youngsters who are fortunate enough to participate in treatment don't receive adequate treatment. Most depressed youths are treated by a physician (76.7%), one-third are treated by a psychologist, 6.3% are treated by a social worker, and 18.2% are treated by another type of provider (the previously noted percentages exceed 100%, because some youths receive services from more than one provider from more than one profession) (Olfson et al., 2003). Thus the training and ex-

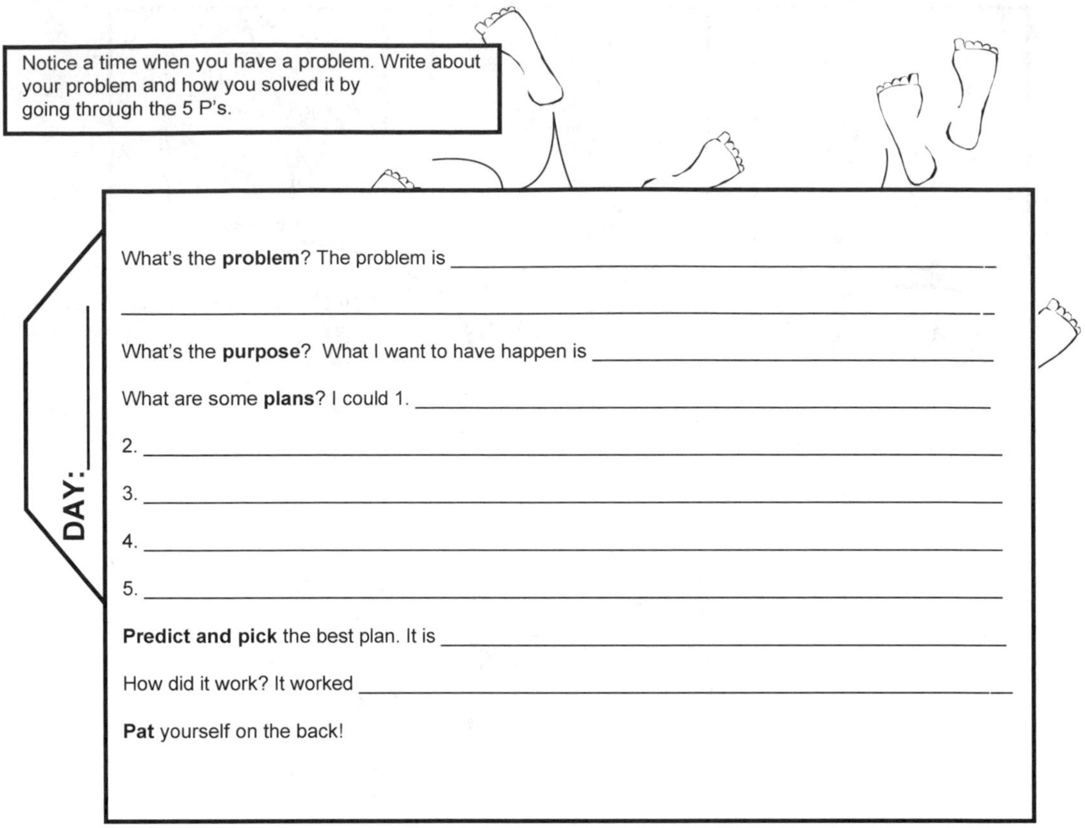

Notice a time when you have a problem. Write about your problem and how you solved it by going through the 5 P's.

DAY: _____

What's the **problem**? The problem is _____

_____

What's the **purpose**? What I want to have happen is _____

What are some **plans**? I could 1. _____

2. _____

3. _____

4. _____

5. _____

Predict and pick the best plan. It is _____

How did it work? It worked _____

Pat yourself on the back!

FIGURE 5.4. Problem-solving worksheet.

pertise of the providers are going to vary greatly, and it is very unlikely that the individuals providing psychotherapy are going to have training and experience with evidence-based interventions.

Although a small percentage of depressed youths participate in treatment, the majority of those who seek psychotherapy go to a community mental health center (CMHC), private practitioner, or therapist in another setting, rather than a university clinic that provides state-of-the-art evidence-based interventions. In general, child psychotherapists in the community do not use evidence-based interventions; rather, they use an eclectic mix of treatment procedures (Addis & Krasnow, 2000). Weisz (2000, p. 837) states that "most of the 2.5 million American children seen in clinical practice each year receive interventions that have never been tested in a clinical trial." There is no evidence to support the efficacy of this approach to child psychotherapy with children who experience psychological disorders in gen-

eral (Bickman, Noser, & Summerfelt, 1999). Furthermore, it appears as though this form of child psychotherapy is no more effective than no treatment at all (Andrade, Lambert, & Bickman, 2000). Weersing and Weisz (2002) reported that the standard of care for depressed youths who received services through a CMHC was also an eclectic mix of primarily psychodynamic procedures, with some cognitive and behavioral techniques delivered in a median of 11 sessions. Although, again, a minimal dose of psychotherapy is eight sessions (which assumes that the treatment is efficacious) (Howard et al., 1986), 35.8% of the patients completed fewer than this minimally acceptable number of sessions (Weersing & Weisz, 2002).

Therefore, though there is great variability in the services that depressed youths receive in terms of type, dose, and providers' professional training, it is clear that the majority of depressed youths do not receive adequate mental health care. Given this variability in the quality of services and usage, it is not surprising that treatment as usual in the community does not appear to be as effective as the treatment delivered within a research protocol. Weersing and Weisz (2002), for example, reported that the median number of sessions in a research protocol for depressed youths was 12; that depressed youths who received treatment through a research protocol improved much more quickly than those who received treatment in a CMHC; and that their scores were significantly better than those for the CMHC sample immediately following treatment. Furthermore, at posttreatment, depressed youths who received CBT reported enough improvement in depressive symptoms that their scores fell near those of a normative sample. This significant difference between the youths who received CBT and those who received treatment as usual through the CMHC was maintained through 1- and 3-month follow-up assessments. In comparison to youths who received CBT, youths who received the eclectic treatment through the CMHC showed a trajectory of change similar to that of participants in the research protocols who had been randomly assigned to a wait-list condition. For youths in the CMHC group, change occurred at a slow rate. In fact, their rate of improvement was much slower than that for the youths who received CBT, and it was twice as slow as that for youths who did not receive treatment. It took the CMHC sample a year to catch up to the youths who received CBT. It appears as though the eclectic treatment produced no more improvement in depressive symptoms than that which occurred through the natural passing of time.

Perhaps the failure to find any evidence for the effectiveness of traditional child therapy was attributable to the limited number of sessions that the youngsters received in the CMHC, and/or to a failure to assess the change likely to accrue over longer periods of time from more insight-oriented treatments. Weiss, Catron, Harris, and Phung (1999) addressed this issue in a study of the effectiveness of traditional child therapy that included an open-ended treatment protocol; this protocol allowed the therapists to work with children for

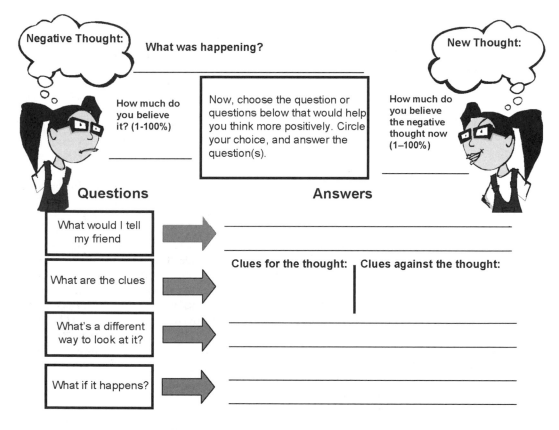

FIGURE 5.5. Cognitive restruscturing worksheet.

up to 18 months and did not place any limits on the type of treatment or number of meetings completed over this period of time. In addition, the investigators tracked the youngsters' internalizing and externalizing symptoms over a 2-year follow-up period, which should have been enough time for "sleeper" effects to appear. Overall, the results provided little to no support for the effectiveness of traditional child psychotherapy. Children who were experiencing elevated symptoms of internalizing or externalizing disorders self-reported no more change than did students who received tutoring over this same period of time. Parents also did not report any significant improvement in their children's internalizing or externalizing symptoms; however, teachers did report some improvement in internalizing symptoms over this period. Nevertheless, while improvement was reported, the youngsters were rated as experiencing higher-than-average rates of internalizing symptoms. Thus they did not approach a typical level of functioning following treatment. Overall, there does not appear to be evidence to support the effectiveness of traditional child therapy for the treatment of youths with either elevated levels of depressive symptoms or depressive disorders. How do these disappointing results compare to the results of interventions that are delivered as part of a research protocol?

Research-Based Treatments

Cognitive-Behavioral Therapy

CBT has been labeled "possibly efficacious" for depressed children and "probably efficacious" for depressed adolescents (Kazdin & Weisz, 1998), according to the criteria for empirically supported treatments (Chambless & Hollon, 1998). Although several different research teams have reported that CBT is effective at producing significant improvements in depressive symptoms and that an average of 60% of the youngsters are no longer depressed following treatment, the label of "well-established" has not been applied to CBT for depressive disorders in youths. This may be due in part to the methodological limitations of existing research, as well as the paucity of treatment outcome studies. Furthermore, significant improvements were not reported in all of the investigations. In the most methodologi-

cally rigorous study with the largest sample of clinically depressed youths, the Treatment of Adolescent Depression Study (TADS; March, 2004), the efficacy of CBT is clearly brought into question as a stand-alone intervention, and its continued status as "probably efficacious" is in question.

Lewinsohn, Clarke, and colleagues have adapted and tested their Coping with Depression course as both a prevention and treatment program for depressed adolescents (Clarke et al., 1995; Clarke, Hornbrook, et al., 2001; Clarke, Rohde, Lewinsohn, Hops, & Seeley, 1999; Lewinsohn, Clarke, Hops, & Andrews, 1990). The course, which included standard delivery of intervention plus booster sessions, was effective in treating depression when used either with adolescents alone or with adolescents and their parents (Clarke et al., 1999; Lewinsohn et al., 1990). Booster sessions did not prevent recurrence of depressive episodes. However, adolescents who were depressed at the time of posttreatment assessments had quicker recovery rates if they received booster sessions (Clarke et al., 1999). Other researchers have also indicated that continuation of CBT is effective in preventing relapse (Kroll, Harrington, Jayson, Fraser, & Gowers, 1996).

Trials of CBT with children and younger adolescents have shown generally positive results in comparison to no treatment (Butler, Mietzitis, Friedman, & Cole, 1980; Stark, Reynolds, & Kaslow, 1987; Weisz, Thurber, Sweeney, Proffitt, & LeGagnoux, 1997), an attention placebo (Butler et al., 1980), and traditional school counseling groups (Stark, 1990). Yet several studies have found no difference between CBT and other treatments. Most of these included a comparison treatment to CBT and determined that both were effective in reducing symptoms.

In a study with 7- to 12-year-old children (Liddle & Spence, 1990), an eight-session CBT intervention that incorporated social skills, cognitive restructuring, and interpersonal problem solving was not found to be superior to no treatment or an attention placebo. However, it is not possible to draw conclusions from this study, because its small sample size limited the power to find significant between-group differences. A closer review of the results indicated that participants in CBT reported a standard deviation's reduction in symptoms, whereas participants in the other two conditions reported about half as much change. Furthermore, the mean score of participants in the active treatment moved to within the "normal" range, while children in the other two conditions continued to report levels of depressive symptoms that exceeded the "normal" range of functioning.

Comprehensive CBT interventions have been compared to relaxation training (one component of CBT for depressive and anxiety disorders). Kahn, Kehle, Jenson, and Clark (1990) reported that CBT, relaxation, and self-modeling were equally effective at decreasing depressive symptoms and producing clinically significant change in a sample of depressed middle school students, and CBT and relaxation were superior to a wait-list control. Two other studies compared CBT to relaxation training (Reynolds & Coats, 1986; Wood, Harrington, & Moore, 1996) in depressed adolescents, with similar findings. Reynolds and Coats (1986) found that participants in both CBT and relaxation training reported fewer depressive symptoms and a higher academic self-concept at posttreatment than did participants in a wait-list control group. Wood and colleagues (1996) provided brief CBT (six sessions) in an individual therapy format. They reported greater change in depressive symptoms, more patient satisfaction, greater self-esteem, and better global functioning for participants who received the comprehensive CBT treatment than for those who completed relaxation training. The investigators noted that this was not surprising, since the treatment was so short and it was designed to treat acute symptoms.

During the 3 months following successful treatment of depression, youths are at risk for a relapse. Kroll and colleagues (1996) provided youths who had been successfully treated with CBT (Wood et al., 1996) an additional 6 months of CBT; results indicated that youngsters who received the additional treatment were significantly less likely to relapse. However, between-group differences in severity of depressive symptoms were reduced at follow-up assessment. It appeared that participants in the relaxation group continued to recover after treatment terminated, while those in CBT maintained their gains. However, it is important to note that participants from the relaxation condition were more likely to participate in other treatments between posttreatment and follow-up, while the CBT participants were less

likely to seek additional treatment after the original trial of brief therapy.

CBT has been compared to other treatments. Brent and colleagues (Birmaher et al., 2000; Brent, Holder, & Kolko, 1997) compared individual CBT, systematic behavioral family therapy, and nondirective supportive therapy for 107 depressed adolescents. They found that participants receiving CBT demonstrated more change than those in the other treatment conditions in terms of rate of improvement, remission rate, and parent-rated treatment credibility at posttreatment. However, the mean differences between conditions on those variables at long-term follow-up were not significantly different. Vostanis, Feehan, Grattan, and Bickerton (1996) investigated outcomes for brief CBT (six to nine sessions) compared to nonfocused supportive therapy in children and adolescents. Participation in either treatment was associated with decreases in depressive symptoms at posttreatment and a 9-month follow-up. Vostanis and colleagues noted, however, that the participants were not exposed to the cognitive restructuring component of treatment, which is considered a central component of CBT (Beck et al., 1979).

In the TADS, March (2004) evaluated the relative efficacy of fluoxetine, CBT, the combination of fluoxetine and CBT, and placebo for the treatment of 351 adolescents who received primary diagnoses of moderate to severe MDD. Participants received 12 weeks of treatment. The CBT included both "required" skill-building sessions and optional or "modular" sessions, and thus allowed flexible, developmentally sensitive, and individual tailoring of the treatment to address each adolescent's needs. The required skill-building sessions were completed over the first six meetings and included psychoeducation about depression and its causes, goal setting with each adolescent, mood monitoring, increasing engagement in pleasant activities, social problem solving, and cognitive restructuring. In the subsequent optional modules (meetings 7–12), each teen and therapist collaboratively chose the teen's relevant social skills deficits and worked on the development of these skills (e.g., social engagement, communication, negotiation, compromise, or assertion). Additional family sessions could be completed; these included psychoeducation for parents about depression and conjoint sessions that focused on addressing identified parent–adolescent concerns. Participants completed a mean of 11 sessions.

Results of the investigation indicated that the combination of fluoxetine and CBT produced the greatest improvement in symptoms of MDD. Fluoxetine alone was effective, but not as effective as the combination. CBT alone was less effective than fluoxetine and not significantly more effective than placebo. Examination of the clinical significance of the improvements indicated that a positive response to treatment was reported for 71% of the participants who participated in the combined treatment, 60.6% of the youngsters who received fluoxetine, 43.2% of the youngsters who received CBT, and 34.8% of the youngsters who received a placebo.

A major issue in the treatment of depressed youths is the apparent increase in suicidal ideation and behavior that has been associated with taking an SSRI. In a later section of this chapter, this issue is discussed in greater depth. It is important to note here that a trend toward more suicidal behavior, but not suicidal ideation, was found in the fluoxetine-only group. Of greatest relevance to this section of the chapter is that CBT appeared to have a protective effect on both suicidal ideation and behavior. This protective effect was found in both the CBT-only condition and in the combined treatment condition.

Interpersonal Psychotherapy for Adolescents

In a review of psychotherapies for children and adolescents, Curry (2001) noted that "IPT-A has considerable promise as a treatment for adolescents" (p. 1093). Several studies have looked at the effectiveness of IPT-A for depressed adolescents (Mufson & Fairbanks, 1996; Mufson et al., 1994; Mufson, Moreau, Weissman, & Garfinkel, 1999; Rossello & Bernal, 1999; Santor & Kusumakar, 2001). A pilot study of IPT-A conducted with 14 depressed adolescents (Mufson & Fairbanks, 1996; Mufson et al., 1994) provided initial support for the treatment; at a 1-year follow-up, only one adolescent met criteria for a mood disorder. A controlled trial with 48 depressed adolescents (Mufson et al., 1999) demonstrated that participants who received IPT-A experienced a greater decrease in depressive symptoms, were more likely to meet recovery criteria, and experienced greater improvement in social functioning and social problem solv-

ing than participants in the control group. In their most recent investigation, Mufson and colleagues (2004) evaluated the effectiveness of IPT-A with 63 adolescents who received diagnoses of MDD, DD, adjustment disorder with depressed mood, or DDNOS. The treatment was delivered in an urban school clinic in eight consecutive 35-minute sessions followed by four sessions completed over the next 4–8 weeks. Adolescents in the control condition received treatment as usual; it is also important to note that they completed an average of 7.9 sessions. Participants who received IPT-A reported significantly fewer depressive symptoms on the Hamilton Rating Scale for Depression, and more of the youths who received IPT-A had recovered (50% vs. 34%). One month later, the participants who received IPT-A continued to do significantly better than the youths who received treatment as usual. IPT-A has also been demonstrated to be effective in other laboratories with novice therapists (Santor & Kusumaker, 2001), although not in a controlled trial.

In a study comparing CBT and IPT-A, Rossello and Bernal (1999) reported that both active treatments were effective in decreasing depressive symptoms in Puerto Rican adolescents, relative to a wait-list condition. However, several significant methodological limitations of this study limit the conclusions that can be drawn from it, including the small sample size, sole reliance on self-report measures, and a unique and nonstandardized version of CBT. More specifically, the CBT began with targeting cognition for four sessions, followed by pleasant events scheduling, and finally focusing on social skills. Typically, CBT begins with behavioral interventions such as pleasant events scheduling that produce more immediate symptom relief, which helps open the participant to cognitive restructuring.

As noted elsewhere (Blagys & Hilsenroth, 2002; Stark et al., 1999), the fact that CBT and IPT-A are efficacious may be due to the overlap in treatment components. In practice, the interventions have more in common than they differ. In fact, an artful cognitive-behavioral therapist is likely to apply the treatment strategies to interpersonal difficulties when they are the source of distress for a youngster; this makes the distinction between the two interventions even more minute. The primary difference between the two treatments is that CBT includes cognitive restructuring and IPT-A does not.

However, as we have noted earlier, changing interactions between children and their parents is a powerful way to change the children's thinking about relationships that are important to them, as well as their self-perception of lovability. The primary difference between CBT and IPT-A is in their theoretical underpinnings rather than in their application.

The Broader Context of Outcome Research

It is important to place the treatment outcome literature on depressed youths into the context of the limitations of the field. A series of articles (Kazdin, 2000; Kendall, 2000; Weisz, 2000) appeared in the *Archives of General Psychiatry*, in which the authors outlined a research agenda for treatment outcome research with children experiencing psychological disorders. The major points that can be drawn from this series ring true for the literature on the treatment of depressed youths. However, the literature on the treatment of depressed youths suffers from an even more fundamental problem: a paucity of treatment outcome studies. The volume of treatment outcome research with clinically depressed youths is less than that for other childhood disorders.

Kazdin (2000) noted that children in most of the outcome studies are less seriously impaired, are experiencing less comorbidity, are exposed to less parental psychopathology, and are less disadvantaged in general. It would appear as though this concern holds true for most of the investigations into the efficacy of various treatments for depressed youths. In the vast majority of studies noted in the preceding section, participants did not receive diagnoses of a depressive disorder; rather, they reported elevated symptoms of depression. Thus they are likely to be less seriously impaired, and they are much less likely to be experiencing comorbid disorders.

The lower rate of effectiveness of CBT in the TADS cannot be based solely on differences in the severity of depression experienced by participants in the majority of studies relative to the TADS. Participants in both the Brent and colleagues (1997) and March (2004) studies were clinic-referred youths who were experiencing MDD and a multiplicity of comorbid conditions. Despite the similarity of the samples in the severity of their depressive disorders, the results for the two forms of CBT used in these investigations were very different, despite the fact that they were similar in terms of the number of sessions that participants completed in each study. In the Brent and colleagues investigation, a treatment that was more true to cognitive therapy (Beck et al., 1979) was used. It emphasized collaborative empiricism; socialization to the cognitive therapy model; monitoring and modification of automatic thoughts, assumptions, and beliefs; and acquisition of problem-solving, affect regulation, and social skills. As noted earlier, therapists in the TADS (March, 2004) did not adhere to traditional cognitive therapy. Rather, the participants learned six skills (including identification and changing of automatic thoughts) in the first six meetings, followed by six sessions of social skills training. Perhaps this dramatic difference in the two treatments was the reason why very different results were found. In the Brent and colleagues investigation, the depressive episodes of 60% of the youths who participated in CBT were in remission at posttreatment, versus 43% of the youths who participated in CBT in the TADS.

Another concern about the samples that have participated in the research-based intervention studies relative to those in the general population is that the samples consisted primarily of middle-class youths of European descent (Kazdin, 2000). However, it is important to note that some investigators are to be commended (e.g., Mufson et al., 2004) for conducting research with youths who come from economically disadvantaged and environmentally stressed backgrounds. Nonetheless, given the aforementioned limitations in the samples, it is not clear whether the results of studies that used youths who were experiencing subclinical levels of depression can be applied to youths who present at clinics; the latter youths may have a more complex and severe clinical picture, which may be more difficult to treat.

Weisz (2000) is more optimistic about the generalizability of the results of the existing research and about the efficacy of the interventions with depressed youths. He believes that the most basic issue in the treatment outcome research is this: Although effective interventions have been found, virtually none of the empirically tested treatments have made their way into regular practice in the United States. He believes that we must evaluate treatments within the milieus where they are going to be implemented, so that we can see whether they can be successfully applied. One method for promoting the transportability of research-based treatments is to manualize them, so that others can follow the same protocol. However, as Kendall (2000) notes, it is necessary to recognize the individuality of each child and each therapist—but manuals don't do this. They try to "even the playing field" in terms of the therapists, and they treat all children as if they were the same. In reality, the great variability in therapists' training, theoretical orientation, experience, skills, interpersonal abilities, and other personal characteristics makes it impossible to truly "even the playing field" among them. Furthermore, each child client is unique, which makes it difficult to apply a manualized treatment without having expert training in its use. Moreover, as Kazdin (2000) and Kendall (2000) both note, the numerous developmental differences across youngsters cannot be addressed within a manualized treatment.

To implement a manualized treatment effectively, a therapist must possess at the very least the ability to conceptualize a youngster's problems from the theoretical perspective of the manual's author, thus enabling the therapist to apply the intervention more flexibly and realistically to the child's day-to-day life, symptoms, and difficulties. Although the ACTION program is manualized, the therapists conceptualize the case of each child participant and plan ahead for ways that they can apply the skills covered in a particular session to the child's unique cognitive, behavioral, environmental, and emotional difficulties. Second, the therapist must truly understand the "big picture" of the manual and the endpoint to which the manualized treatment is taking the child, in order to be able to implement the treatment effectively. This way, as the child discusses his or her between-session difficulties, the therapist can recognize that an opportunity exists to apply a treatment strategy that will help the youngster to achieve the long-term goals of treatment. Without these most basic understandings of the treatment, the manual cannot be implemented in an effective fashion. Instead, it is very likely to be implemented in a stilted and irrelevant fashion that is not adapted to the needs of the particular child client. A related question is this: How much and what type of training is necessary to be able to effectively implement a manualized treatment? Furthermore, how much ongoing supervision is necessary for a therapist to be able to implement the intervention effectively? The answer to both questions

is the same: A lot. The exact amount remains a question to be addressed in future research.

Although the primary objective of a treatment for depressed youths is symptom reduction that produces recovery from a depressive episode, an effective intervention should also produce significant practical improvements in a child's life. It is important to include a broader set of outcome variables, such as functional impairment, academic functioning, parent and family functioning, and social functioning (Kazdin, 2000), in the evaluation of a treatment. This has been done to a very limited extent in the relevant depression literature through completion of the Children's Functional Assessment Scale (e.g., March, 2004).

Kazdin (2000) notes that it is important to assess the impact of treatment on comorbid conditions. To date, this has been done to a very limited extent. For example, in the Stark and colleagues (1987) study, symptoms of anxiety (the most common comorbid condition with depression) were also assessed at pre- and posttreatment, and the results indicated that participants also reported a decline in symptoms of anxiety. However, it is not possible to generalize from this to a reduction in anxiety disorders. For example, a pattern is beginning to emerge in our current NIMH-funded evaluation of the ACTION program: Girls who have a history of sexual or physical abuse that has resulted in comorbid PTSD report improvements in their depression but not their PTSD. During follow-up treatment with CBT specifically for PTSD, the girls experience rapid improvement of the PTSD, as they are able to apply their coping and cognitive restructuring skills to the upset and unrealistic thinking associated with the traumatic events and the meanings they derived from them. We have also found that it is necessary to teach the participants directly how to apply the skills they are learning to their experiences of anxiety as well as depression. A related question that needs to be addressed, but wasn't raised in the 2000 issue of the *Archives of General Psychiatry*, is this: Does the presence of comorbid conditions have a negative impact on treatment when depression is the focus of treatment? The results of research addressing this question are mixed. Weersing and Weisz (2002) did not find that any of their comorbidity predictors were significant. Comorbid disruptive behavior disorders did not appear in one study to affect the treatment of the depressive disorder (Clarke et al.,

1995), whereas they were predictive of poor treatment response in another study (Rohde, Clarke, & Lewinsohn, 2001). Similarly, comorbid anxiety has been found to predict poor treatment response (Clarke et al., 1995), good treatment response (Rohde et al., 2001), and superior response to CBT relative to other alternative treatments (Brent et al., 1997).

Prior to the TADS, there was an emerging consensus in the results of relevant studies that on average, 60% of depressed youths treated with CBT reported clinically significant improvements in depression. This raised another question: What variables predicted who would improve and who wouldn't improve through completion of a trial of CBT? It appears as though a less severe depressive disorder prior to initiation of treatment, lower rates of parent–child conflict, lower levels of cognitive distortion, lower hopelessness, and greater general functioning predict a better treatment outcome (Birmaher et al., 2000).

Kazdin (2000) and Kendall (2000) emphasize the importance of determining whether the interventions produce changes in the targets of treatment (e.g., depressive cognition), and whether changes in these variables predict improvement in depression. There is some evidence that CBT targeting change in automatic thoughts and cognitive distortions among depressed adolescents produced changes in depressive cognition. However, there also were some changes in family functioning that were not targeted by the CBT (Kolko et al., 2000). In a meta-analysis of CBT interventions for children with a variety of disturbances, including depression, the effectiveness of CBT was moderated by cognitive–developmental level; this finding suggests that CBT is affecting child functioning through changes in cognition (Durlak et al., 1991). However, these same investigators did not find that changes in cognitive processes were related to improvements in behavior.

Is there a dosage effect for psychosocial treatments of depression in youths? In other words, do children who complete more treatment sessions report greater improvement than those who complete fewer sessions? Again, the results of relevant research are mixed. A dosage effect was found in one study (Weersing & Weisz, 2002), but not in another study (Mufson et al., 2004).

In the adult treatment literature, there is a phenomenon of "sudden gains," in which a participant reports significant improvement between one session and the next. This one-session change can occur at any time during treatment. Gaynor and colleagues (2003) evaluated this phenomenon with depressed youths. Similar to research with adults, sudden gains were found for depressed adolescents who were participating in individual treatment (either CBT or nonspecific supportive therapy). Sudden gains were not found among participants who were receiving systemic family therapy. It is thought that sudden gains stem from some kind of cognitive "click" that occurs during treatment. However, the reason for this phenomenon is unknown and remains a question to be addressed in future research.

Meta-Analytic Research

As discussed by Michael and Crowley (2002), it appears overall that children and adolescents, regardless of level of severity of depressive symptoms, may benefit from *any* intervention—including CBT and several other modalities. However, developmental consideration of the treatment studies included by Michael and Crowley suggests that adolescents may fare better than children do; they may show greater improvement as a result of being more suited to CBT interventions (the bulk of the literature includes such interventions), which target the thinking skills more typical of adolescents. Children appeared to benefit less overall from both psychosocial and pharmacological interventions in the studies included in that meta-analysis. Reinecke and colleagues (1998) reported findings indicating that CBT was useful for reducing depressive symptoms in youths, and that the treatment gains were maintained over time. The effect sizes observed at posttesting fell in the moderate to large range.

PSYCHOPHARMACOLOGY OF DEPRESSION IN CHILDREN AND ADOLESCENTS

History

Psychiatrists have a number of medication choices for treating depressive disorders (Table 5.4), but most medications have not been thoroughly studied in the child and adolescent population. This lack of research into their efficacy and safety has become a point of great controversy.

TABLE 5.4. Generic and Brand Names of Current Antidepressant Medications

Generic name	Brand name
SSRIs	
Fluoxetine	Prozac
Sertraline	Zoloft
Citalopram	Celexa
Escitalopram	Lexapro
Paroxetine	Paxil
Fluvoxamine	Luvox
Atypical antidepressants	
Bupropion	Wellbutrin
Venlafaxine	Effexor
Mirtazapine	Remeron
Nefazodone	Serzone
TCAs	
Imipramine	Tofranil
Desipramine	Norpramin
Nortriptyline	Pamelor, Aventyl
Amytriptyline	Elavil
Clomipramine	Anafranil
MAOIs	
Phenelzine	Nardil
Tranylcypromine	Parnate
Isocarboxazid	Marplan

Tricyclic antidepressants (TCAs) were formerly the mainstay for treating depression in children and adolescents. TCAs are named for their three-ring structure with attached amines. They include the tertiary amines imipramine, amitriptyline, and clomipramine, and the secondary amines desipramine and nortriptyline. TCAs have been used in adults since the 1950s. In the 1960s, they were first used in children to treat ADHD in place of stimulants (Gunderson & Geller, 2003). Subsequently, TCAs began to be used to treat child and adolescent depression. TCAs act primarily on the norandrenergic system, but also exert some activity on the serotonergic systems. They also have muscarinic and histaminic activity. TCAs are associated with a variety of side effects and safety issues, including cardiac conduction delays that are thought to have caused death in at least 10 pediatric patients.

After the introduction of the SSRIs in 1986, their popularity soared in treating depressed adults because of their low side effect profile and relative safety. In particular, the SSRIs did not cause the cardiac conduction delays observed with some of the TCAs. SSRIs increase the amount of serotonin signaling between neurons by preventing reuptake of serotonin. SSRIs differ in their selectivity to the serotonin receptor and in their active metabolites. These chemical differences, along with the individual's genetics, lead to variations in efficacy and side effect profiles. The SSRIs include fluoxetine (Prozac), sertraline (Zoloft), paroxetine (Paxil), fluvoxamine (Luvox), citalopram (Celexa), and escitalopram (Lexapro). Simultaneously, a new wave of medications that affect other neurotransmitters emerged, including bupropion (Wellbutrin), mirtazapine (Remeron), nefazodone (Serzone), and venlafaxine (Effexor).

SSRIs began to be used gradually in the adolescent population and eventually in children. Physicians initially used these medications with youths without U.S. Food and Drug Administration (FDA) approval; this approval was not given to the SSRI at first because their efficacy and safety had not been studied with children and adolescents. The SSRIs proved clinically effective, but no studies corroborated these observations until the 1990s. SSRIs are now first-line agents for treating child and adolescent depression (Birmaher & Brent, 2003). The newer antidepressants, such as bupropion and mirtazapine, do not have an adequate empirical base with children; however, they are sometimes used as second-line treatments for those youths who do not respond to SSRIs.

Thus far, none of the SSRIs has produced irreversible damage in children and adolescents. However, as the SSRIs gained wide use with depressed adolescents, concerns emerged about the safety of this class of medications: Reports suggested that they were responsible for increased suicidal ideation and behavior among youths. In 2003, the British Medicines and Healthcare products Regulatory Agency (MHRA) (www.mhra.gov.uk) concluded that most of the SSRIs do not show benefits exceeding their risks of suicidal ideation, and thus should not be prescribed in the child and adolescent population. As of December 2003, only fluoxetine had two controlled studies showing efficacy, and therefore was the only agent deemed acceptable to the MHRA. In response to the MHRA report, the FDA recommended that paroxetine not be used to treat depression in youths under age 18; the FDA subsequently advised that sertraline, citalopram, escitalopram, bupropion, nefazodone, and mirtazapine should be used in juveniles cautiously, and that families should be warned of possible suicidality concerns, particularly early in treatment.

Adding to the controversy was the subsequent release of the preliminary results of the TADS (March, 2004), indicating that fluoxetine did not increase the occurrence of suicidal ideation and indeed had somewhat of a protective effect. However, there was a higher rate of suicidal behavior among adolescents who were treated with fluoxetine only. Thus, while fluoxetine had a protective effect on suicidal *ideation*, it may have had an adverse effect on suicidal *behavior*. This further suggests that a complex relationship may exist among treatment with an SSRI, suicidal ideation, and suicidal behavior.

Most child and adolescent psychiatrists in the United States continue to prescribe SSRIs to children and adolescents, based on their experience of both safety and effectiveness in patients. However, the standard of care is to address possible suicidal or homicidal ideation with the youngster and his or her caregivers when these agents are initiated.

Considerations in Treating Depressed Youths with an SSRI

Most physicians extrapolate from adult studies, or consider their colleagues' experiences with antidepressants, in order to prescribe medications for depressed youths. As for an adult, choosing an antidepressant for a child or adolescent is based on safety, efficacy, side effects, and family history. Safety concerns in children relate to both the developing body and developing brain. The Texas Children's Medication Algorithm Project (Hughes et al., 1999) provides a stepwise approach to treating MDD in children and adolescents who meet DSM-IV-TR criteria and who warrant medication. This algorithm (periodically updated and available at www.dshs.state.tx.us/mhservices) recommends that treatment proceed from simple monotherapy to more complex combinations to achieve remission of depression (see Figure 5.6).

Side effects may differ in the child and adolescent population from those found in adults. Nevertheless, physicians attempt to choose the SSRI that they believe will produce maximum effects while minimizing the discomfort and safety concerns associated with various side ef-

Stage 1. SSRI.

Stage 2. Alternative SSRI.

Stage 3. Drug from an alternative class (bupropion [Bup], mirtazapine, nefazodone [Nef], TCA, or venlafaxine).

Stage 4. Combination of two antidepressants (TCA + SSRI, Bup* + SSRI, Nef** + SSRI, Bup + Nef) *or* lithium + antidepressant.

Stage 5. Combination of two antidepressants or lithium + antidepressant.

Stage 6. MAOI.

FIGURE 5.6. The Texas Children's Medication Algorithm. From Hughes et al. (1999). Copyright 1999 by the American Academy of Child and Adolescent Psychiatry. Adapted by permission.

fects. Since psychiatric illnesses appear to have heritable components, often parents may have tried or responded to particular psychotropic agents. Family members may respond similarly to medications, so this variable can sometimes help clinicians narrow the choices for a particular agent. Common side effects of SSRIs in children and adolescents include akathisia (restlessness), decreased appetite, upset stomach, headache, and insomnia. A more problematic side effect is increased aggression/disinhibition, which occurs in a small percentage of patients. This may lead to behavioral problems, especially in adolescents, whose judgment and decision-making skills may be immature. Increased activation may also cause increased anxiety in those patients with comorbid anxiety symptoms. Serum levels of fluoxetine in children have been found to be twice those of adolescents and adults in pharmacokinetic studies (Wilens et al., 2002). Starting with very low doses of medication may help to prevent side effects and maintain a youngster's compliance. Drug half-life and active metabolites may affect how often the drug is taken and lead to "discontinuation syndrome" when doses are missed. Discontinuation syndrome is characterized by dizziness, nausea, headache, paresthesias (tingling, etc.), and dysphoria. These symptoms may last from days to weeks and may not begin until a few days or weeks after the drug is stopped. Paroxetine has the shortest half-life among the SSRIs, and is sometimes associated with a more severe discontinuation syndrome. These drugs should be tapered gradually over weeks to minimize discontinuation symptoms. Only fluoxetine has an active metabolite with a long half-life that remains in the body for an extended period (4–6 weeks), so it may be stopped abruptly without severe discontinuation symptoms occurring.

It is important for parents to supervise administration of psychotropic medication in children and adolescents. Medication adherence is a common problem in all patients, but presents a particular challenge in the child and adolescent population. Psychoeducation is important to emphasize the use of antidepressant medication on a daily basis for an extended period of time. Adolescents will frequently be allowed by parents to self-administer their antidepressant medication. This not only can be dangerous in suicidal patients, but can cause adherence problems. Adolescents will frequently discontinue their medication when they begin to feel better, which leads to a relapse of symptoms within a matter of weeks.

Efficacy is ultimately determined by remission of depressive symptoms. A medication trial should be maintained for at least 4–8 weeks at a therapeutic dose before switching to another medication due to nonresponse (Hughes et al., 1999), although side effects that cannot be managed may require switching earlier. When a medication is effective, it should be continued for at least 6–12 months after initiation of the drug (Pine, 2002). After this period of time, a gradual taper over weeks to months can be attempted, although patients should continue to be seen to monitor symptoms suggestive of relapse. Parents should be advised that the patient should be watched closely for signs of a relapse or recurrence of depression after medication has been discontinued.

Efficacy of TCAs

TCAs have not shown efficacy in children for the treatment of MDD despite their positive results in adults. The two largest studies of TCAs were stopped because of the poor observed response (Geller, 1992; Puig-Antich & Gittleman, 1982). Bostic, Prince, Frazier, DeJong, and Wilens (2003) found that the younger the patient, the less likely TCAs were to improve depressive symptoms. A meta-analysis in 2000 and 2001 by the Cochrane Group found no benefit of TCAs in juvenile depression.

Efficacy of SSRIs

Research has supported the efficacy of SSRIs for the treatment of depression in children and adolescents. Emslie and colleagues (1997) published the first large-scale evaluation of an SSRI (fluoxetine) with depressed youths between the ages of 7 and 17. Fluoxetine was significantly more effective than a placebo in the reduction of depression. Additional support for the efficacy of fluoxetine has been reported by March (2004) in the TADS, where fluoxetine alone or in combination with CBT produced greater improvements in depression than did CBT alone or a pill placebo. Sertraline has also demonstrated efficacy for the treatment of MDD in children and adolescents (Wagner & Ambrosini, 2003). Outcome studies with paroxetine have produced mixed results. Wagner and Ambrosini (2001) found citalopram to be superior to placebo in one controlled study. Escitalopram is currently being studied for use in pediatric depression in a multisite, controlled trial (Wagner & Ambrosini, 2003).

Alternative Antidepressants

It is important to note that none of the alternative agents described here are FDA-approved for the treatment of juvenile depression. Thus they are used off-label.

Bupropion

Bupropion, an aminoketone, was released in the United States in 1989 for use as an antidepressant in adults. In children and adolescents, it has been studied as a treatment for ADHD. It has been shown to be superior to placebo for ADHD in open studies (Conners et al., 1996). Side effects include decreased appetite, headaches, activation, insomnia, and nausea. Initial studies demonstrated an increase in seizure activity that appeared dose-related and led to a reformulation of the drug in an extended-release form (bupropion SR). Studies of bupropion for depression in children and adolescents are limited to case reports and open trials. An open trial of bupropion SR for MDD in 11 adolescents indicated that the medication produced marked improvement in symptoms (Glod, Lynch, Flynn, Berkowitz, & Baldessarini, 2003). In a study of 24 adolescents with comorbid ADHD and depression, bupropion

SR was well tolerated and effective in reducing symptoms of both disorders in 58% of the participants (Daviss et al., 2001).

Mirtazapine

Mirtazapine has atypical effects on serotonin; that is, it does not block the reuptake of serotonin as the traditional SSRIs do. It has been used for adult MDD in the United States since 1996. Common side effects include somnolence, increased appetite, and weight gain. Mirtazapine did not differ from placebo in a controlled study of juveniles with depression (Emslie, 2001).

Nefazodone

In 1995, another atypical serotonergic antidepressant, nefazodone, was released in the United States for treatment of adult depression. A case report series by Wilens, Spencer, Biederman, and Schleifer (1997) of seven juveniles indicated that nefazodone was well tolerated and improved MDD in juveniles. A pharmacokinetic trial of nefazodone in 28 depressed children and adolescents was associated with significant reductions in depressive symptoms (Findling et al., 2000). In January 2002, the FDA required a "black box" warning to be added to the product information, due to nefazodone's association with liver abnormalities, liver failure, and death. Future clinical use of nefazodone is unclear because of this possibility of liver problems.

Venlafaxine

Venlafaxine exerts predominantly serotonergic activity, but at larger doses also exerts noradrenergic activity. Venlafaxine was released in the United States in 1994. It has been studied in the pediatric population in one placebo-controlled trial for the treatment of MDD and failed to show a benefit over placebo (Madoki, Tapia, Tapia, & Sumner, 1997). The study used low doses of venlafaxine (75 mg/day), which may have been subtherapeutic.

Monoamine Oxidase Inhibitors

The efficacy of the monoamine oxidase inhibitors (MAOIs) for the treatment of depression was discovered in the 1950s, and three MAOI agents have been approved in the United States for the treatment of MDD in adults. Despite their efficacy for treatment of depression in adults, the significant side effect profile of MAOIs has limited their usefulness. MAOIs cannot be combined with drugs that have monoamine agonist activity or with foods containing tyramine, such as aged meats, cheeses, wine, and some legumes (Blackwell, 1963). The three agents—phenelzine (Nardil), tranylcypromine (Parnate), and isocarboxazid (Marplan)—inhibit monoamine oxidase, which results in elevated levels of neurotransmitters. A few open studies of MAOIs have been completed with children and adolescents, to evaluate their impact on both depression and ADHD. Although the MAOIs are effective in treating both conditions, a life-threatening hypertensive crisis may occur if dietary restrictions are not followed. These dietary concerns in children and adolescents cause the risks of these agents to exceed their benefits, so only in very unusual circumstances (e.g., incapacitating recurrent depressive episodes unresponsive to SSRIs, atypical antidepressants, or TCAs) should MAOIs be considered.

IMPACT OF COMORBIDITY ON TREATMENT

Since the majority of depressed youths will be experiencing additional psychological disorders, it is important to discuss the implications of comorbidity for treatment. At the most basic level, the combination of disorders is likely to produce a more severe disturbance (Mitchell, McCauley, Burke, & Moss, 1988). This means that mental health professionals, the client, and the child's parents can expect a more protracted course of treatment—one that is going to include multiple modes of intervention. Pharmacotherapy is more likely to be needed, and the parents and family are more likely to become involved in treatment through either parent training, family therapy, or their own treatment.

As noted earlier in this chapter, anxiety disorders are the most common co-occurring disorders with depression. Treatment of these comorbid conditions may include a combination of pharmacological treatment and psychosocial treatments. Most anxiety disorders have been treated successfully with SSRIs in the adult population, and the SSRIs can be effective treatments for anxiety disorders in the pediatric population as well. When children are experiencing MDD and an anxiety disorder, an SSRI may be used to treat both disorders. Generalized anxiety disorder (GAD) is generally treated with buspirone in adults. Studies with buspirone in the pediatric population are limited. When GAD is combined with MDD, an SSRI may be sufficient to treat both disorders. If symptoms of GAD continue after a patient is placed on an SSRI, then buspirone may be added. Benzodiazepines are successful in treating adult anxiety disorders, but they have not been as successful for pediatric patients. They may cause behavioral disinhibition that creates more problems than the benzodiazepines solve. Accordingly, benzodiazepines are more frequently used in juveniles for brief intervals (2–4 weeks) until an SSRI exerts useful clinical effects.

When anxiety co-occurs with MDD, it is often associated with maternal unavailability and inconsistency, which may threaten the child's sense of stable attachment (Kovacs et al., 1989). Thus the therapist will need to assess the mother–child relationship and determine whether this pattern exists. If so, then treatment will also target the cause of the unavailability and inconsistency, including parental psychopathology or other serious health concerns, marital/couple conflict, parental substance abuse, or poor parenting behaviors. Consequently, the parent may be referred for treatment (psychosocial and/or pharmacological); the family may be referred for therapy; the parents may be referred for couple therapy; or the parent(s) may be referred for parent training. In addition to these interventions, the child treatment is likely to be altered to address both depression and anxiety. The typical CBT interventions for the two types of disorders have some overlap in treatment components and many differences in how they are directed. Both treatments include affective education, coping skills training, problem-solving training, and cognitive restructuring. The primary difference is that the treatment for anxiety is directed toward applying the aforementioned skills to graded exposure activities, reducing stress, and countering the expectation that something bad is going to happen (the theme of anxious thinking). For depression, in contrast, the aforementioned skills are applied to improving mood, changing negative thinking about the self and significant relationships, and

reducing stress. The parents of an anxious child are taught to coach their child through attacking his or her fears. In contrast, the parents of a depressed child are taught to use positive behavior management strategies, family problem solving, conflict resolution skills, and techniques for altering interaction patterns that support depressive thinking.

Besides GAD, another anxiety disorder commonly co-occurring with depressive disorders is PTSD. When this occurs, the traditional treatment for depression has to be integrated with CBT for PTSD (e.g., Deblinger & Heflin, 1996). The coping and problem-solving skills are used to treat both the mood disorder and the symptoms of PTSD. In addition, the coping skills can be used to manage the distress experienced during exposure exercises. The cognitive restructuring strategies are used to change not only depressive thinking, but also the maladaptive thoughts that stem from the abuse experience (e.g., "I caused it to happen," "I ruined our family," "People just want to hurt you"). The child's nonoffending parent or parents are involved in treatment to help them overcome the anxiety and guilt they feel about their child's trauma experiences, and to open communication between the parent(s) and child about the trauma experience.

If the comorbid anxiety disorder is OCD, then the treatment will once again be complicated by the combination of disorders and require a more complex treatment. OCD and MDD are an especially insidious combination of disorders. The depressed youth is going to be flooded by negative thoughts about the self, life in general, relationships with significant others, and the future. All of these thoughts can be viewed as threatening and thus more likely to become obsessions. The child may thus become even more internally focused and may get stuck in depressive thoughts that are going to drive the depressive disorder to a more severe level. A related consideration is that at least one of the child's parents will probably also be experiencing a depressive and/or anxiety disorder. Since fluoxetine has been found to be effective for both OCD (for a review, see March, Leonard, & Swedo, 1995) and depression (see the relevant section of this chapter), it may be most efficacious to initiate a trial of fluoxetine upon diagnosis of the combination of disorders. The medication is likely to affect the depressive disorder first and then the OCD a few weeks later. Whereas the medication is likely to have a moderate impact on the OCD, it may have a more dramatic impact on the depressive disorder. Regardless, the reduction in the severity of both disorders will increase the probability of successfully treating them with a psychosocial intervention. The psychosocial intervention would combine standard CBT for depression with exposure and response prevention (ERP) treatment for OCD (March & Mulle, 1998). The obsessive–compulsive complexes will be targeted for treatment first as weakening of the disorder will enable the treatment of the depressive disorder. The youngster who is experiencing OCD cannot objectively evaluate or change his or her obsessions. They are held to be true, regardless of how irrational or nonsensical they are. They are true "because they feel that way." The child will not be able to use cognitive restructuring strategies to objectively evaluate and change his or her depressive thoughts as long as the OCD is rigidly ruling thinking. Since changing depressive cognitions is at the core of CBT for depression, then the depressive disorder cannot be effectively treated until after the OCD has been addressed. It also is important to note that ERP is a very powerful and effective treatment for OCD. The improvement that the youngster experiences through treatment of obsessive–compulsive complexes leads to a heightened sense of self-efficacy that can have a positive impact on the depressive disorder. Parents are taught how to create appropriate ERP and how to coach their child through ERP.

When a child is experiencing a depressive disorder and ADHD, this comorbid condition is treated pharmacologically. The first-line treatments for ADHD, psychostimulants, have been used safely and effectively in combination with SSRIs to treat comorbid ADHD and MDD (Gammon & Brown, 1991). The TCAs are second-line treatments for ADHD and have been shown to treat ADHD with comorbid depression or anxiety in a number of studies (Biederman, Baldessarini, Wright, Keenan, & Faraone, 1993; Cox, 1982; Wilens, Biederman, Geist, Steingard, & Spencer, 1993; Wilens, Biederman, & Spencer, 1995). Bupropion also appears useful in treating combined MDD and ADHD (Daviss et al., 2001). Atomoxetine, a norepinephrine reuptake inhibitor, was released in 2003 as a nonstimulant medication for the treatment of ADHD. Early experience suggests that it can safely be combined with some SSRIs to treat MDD and ADHD. (See also Smith, Barkley, & Shapiro, Chapter 2, this volume.)

Another very insidious comorbid condition is the combination of a depressive disorder with conduct disorder or oppositional defiant disorder. The depressed youngster's negative sense of self is supported through his or her antisocial behavior and the resulting reactions from parents and the community. The antisocial behavior results in lots of punishment and verbal berating, which further confirm the negative self-schema. At the same time, the antisocial behavior may be thrilling; as such, it may provide the child with temporary relief from dysphoria and with supportive reactions from peers. Similarly, for a youngster who is experiencing elevated levels of irritability, the antisocial behavior may seem like a justifiable reaction to the perceived mistreatment. The antisocial acts may have a cathartic effect on anger and thus also reinforce the aberrant behavior.

When depression co-occurs with conduct disorder, it is difficult to determine which disorder should be treated first. The conduct disorder tends to continue after the depression is treated, and vice versa. When the conduct disorder is accompanied by substance abuse, treatment of the substance abuse should take precedence. When substance abuse does not accompany the conduct disorder, the two disorders may have to be treated simultaneously. A combination of parent training/family therapy directed at the coercive family system and pharmacological treatment for the depressive disorder may be the focus of the initial intervention efforts. As progress is made with the family and the youngster's behavior comes under control, CBT for depression may be initiated. The intervention is aimed at changing the child's negative self-schema, teaching problem solving for dealing with the remnants of the antisocial behavior (e.g., ongoing conflicts with peers, restitution to the community), social skills training to assist with changing peer groups, and teaching the youngster how to derive thrills and pleasure from socially acceptable behaviors.

Children who are experiencing comorbid depression and an externalizing disorder (either ADHD or conduct disorder) are at increased risk for developing bipolar I disorder. Thus these youngsters must be monitored for the appearance of a manic episode. They also create a dilemma for the prescribing physician, as treatment of the depression with an SSRI could induce an irreversible manic episode. However, initial treatment with a mood-stabilizing agent is less desirable because of the unwanted side effect profile. Close monitoring, and coordination among the psychologist, psychiatrist, and parents, are warranted as they work together to identify the most effective medication regimen.

WORKING WITHIN CONTEXT: THE ACTION PROGRAM AS AN EXAMPLE

Considering the importance of contextual factors in the development and maintenance of depressive disorders and their potential to act as significant mediators and moderators of treatment outcome, it is important for practitioners not only to be aware of the contextual influences experienced by their clients, but also to intervene with systems whenever possible. An illustration of intervention in multiple domains of context for treating depressive disorders in youths can be found within the ACTION treatment program. Although the cornerstone of the ACTION program is CBT, parent training and teacher consultation are also important.

The process of conducting the intervention within one of the schools during school hours has the advantage of operating within children's major systems. Participants come directly from classes and bring real-life problems or concerns into the meeting. These concerns can be discussed, and the therapeutic skills the children learn can be immediately applied. Being situated within the school offers the additional advantage of access to school personnel for consultative services. Therapists can meet directly with teachers to gain their observations of children's behavior. Furthermore, teachers can be taught to encourage the girls to apply the skills in the classroom. For example, depressed children are often socially withdrawn because of core beliefs such as "I'm unlovable" or "I'm unlikable." However, many of these youngsters desire social contact. Teachers can implement reinforcement programs for approach-related behavior. This environmental support facilitates the development of new skills and, in turn, helps provide experience contradictory to negative core beliefs.

When a therapist and teacher meet, they discuss the major presenting concerns in the classroom and tailor teacher-implemented interventions to support therapeutic goals. To continue the example from above, a teacher and student may establish two times during the day in which the student reports to the teacher social contacts she has initiated (smiling and saying "hello," inviting a partner to work, etc.). Especially when the teacher and child have a good relationship, this established time together can be reinforcing in and of itself. In addition to strengthening the teacher–student relationship—which, as described earlier, has been shown to be important in student well-being—this also serves to establish the teacher as a resource to help the student problem-solve challenging social situations.

Currently, the efficacy of a parent training component to the ACTION program is being evaluated. The parent training creates change in a child's most immediate environmental context. One of the primary objectives of the parent training component is to provide parents with ways to reinforce and support the skills the children are learning. Again, it is stressed that since children only meet as part of the group for a relatively short period of time, practice outside the group is essential. Furthermore, parents are taught to identify and change the behaviors that send negative messages to their children and thus support the children's maladaptive thinking. The ACTION program also teaches parents empathic listening, effective communication, positive behavior management, and conflict resolution. Since the daughters attend half the parent training meetings, there are many opportunities to practice these skills during the meetings. Finally, many of the activities included in the parent training component revolve around strengthening the parent–child relationship, including scheduling pleasant family events and learning to use effective praise.

PREVENTION OF DEPRESSION

Due to the chronicity, severity, long-term adverse effects, and high recurrence rate of depressive disorders (Hammen & Rudolph, 1996), interventions designed to prevent initial onset and/or relapse are needed. As noted earlier in the chapter, findings from a study by Wells and colleagues (1989) suggest that depression can impair functioning and quality of life as much as, or more than, chronic medical conditions such as diabetes, angina, pulmonary problems, or arthritis. Consequently, there is interest in identifying predictors of a possible depressive disorder. Although researchers have studied a variety of factors that may contribute to the development of depression in youths, no single risk factor has come to the fore; this suggests that multiple pathways may lead to the development of depressive disorders.

Preventive interventions can occur at three levels: They can target the general public, subgroups identified as at higher risk than the general population, or high-risk individuals who are experiencing symptoms predictive of a future disorder (Mrazek & Haggerty, 1994). Gillham, Shatte, and Freres (2000) suggest that CBT can prevent initial onset of MDD in at-risk individuals. However, further research is needed to determine the preventive effect of CBT. The current prevention literature calls for either the development of new preventive interventions or the enhancement of existing programs' efficacy and dissemination. Hollon and colleagues (2002) name three priorities in future innovation in prevention programs: the development of new and more effective interventions that address both symptom change and functional capacity; the development of interventions that prevent onset and recurrence of clinical episodes in at-risk populations; and the development of user-friendly interventions and nontraditional delivery methods to increase access to evidence-based interventions. Lochman (2001) has called for continual empirical refinement of interventions, even after initial efficacy studies have been completed. He has further emphasized the importance of developmental theory as a basis for guiding the development of preventive interventions.

The Penn Resiliency Program is a school-based depression prevention program. It focuses on teaching cognitive and social problem-solving skills to groups of middle school students who have been identified as at risk for developing depressive disorders due to the chronic stress of poverty (Cardemil, Reivich, & Seligman, 2002). The preventive intervention produced a significant reduction in depressive symptoms among Hispanic and Chinese samples, but not for the African American sample (Muñoz, Penilla, Urizar, 2002). These results are interesting and raise important questions about the importance of developing culturally sensitive interventions.

ETHICAL AND LEGAL CONSIDERATIONS

Therapists working with depressed youths must consider all the same general legal and ethical points that apply to all nonemancipated minors in treatment. In most cases, the legal guardian must consent to the provision of services, except in emergency or safety-related situations. It is also important for the client to provide informed assent to treatment, as well as to understand the limited legal rights of minors in treatment, to the extent that a child can do so. Essentially, it is the legal guardian who holds the confidentiality privilege, not the youth in treatment, except in special circumstances (e.g., related to abuse). The exceptional circumstances under which a minor can consent to treatment by law will vary somewhat by state. Such points are important to cover in the informed consent and assent process at the beginning of treatment.

However, clinicians can make arrangements during the time of getting informed consent for services, with whoever the legal guardian is, about how information from treatment will be shared. Most parents and legal guardians will see the advantage of allowing the clinician to decide what is or is not in young clients' best interest to share with parent figures, and most parents of adolescents do recognize that teens prefer to be free to discuss personal thoughts without parents' knowing everything discussed. At the same time, it is usually wise to involve the parents and keep the parents informed about treatment and its progress. However, in order to preserve the trust of an adolescent client in particular, it is also important to include the client in the process of sharing information that is not urgent. Urgent matters, such as safety-related concerns and suicide risk, must always be shared with the caregiver, who is essential in carrying out any safety plan or monitoring. If there is an opportunity to involve the young client in sharing suicidal plans and creating a safety plan, that is preferred. However, the safety of the client is of utmost importance, even if the client begs the therapist not to share information about suicidality with the legal guardian. In the very rare circumstance where a parent or guardian is informed of high suicide risk and does not agree to follow a safety plan recommended by mental health professionals, or actively disregards the child's claim of self-harm intent, the clinician still has the responsibility to ensure the child's safety. This may entail a report to child protective services for the parent's or guardian's lack of action to keep the child safe.

TREATMENT AND MANAGED CARE

It would be ideal for managed care companies to support a combination of psychiatric and psychological treatment for depressive disorders. Requiring separate medical and mental health deductibles may be an unfair burden on the insured, as both are required and the distinction between the two types of services is likely to be an artificial one, since both forms of treatment are directed at the same underlying "disease." When depression is comorbid with another disorder, then a more protracted course of treatment that includes additional ancillary interventions is likely to be necessary for a successful outcome. Though most plans limit the number of sessions covered by insurance, it appears as though the minimum necessary for successful treatment may be in the 18–20 range, and the spacing of those meetings may need to be closer together than the traditionally sanctioned weekly meetings. Twice-a-week meetings may be more effective with children. Of course, this schedule has to be weighed against the burden that it places on parents in terms of transportation and expense (copayment, amount of the deductible) associated with this regimen.

Although acute treatment of a depressive disorder is likely to be effective, the long-term maintenance of the treatment's effects is unknown. If the parents and child decide to discontinue an antidepressant after a year and the child is no longer in therapy, the child continues to be at risk for experiencing another depressive episode. Is it possible to prevent this through booster sessions, even though the child may not be experiencing depressive symptoms at the time of the booster meetings? This continues to be an issue that needs to be empirically addressed, but regularly scheduled booster meetings may have a prophylactic effect that saves the insurance company money in the long run and prevents the child from experiencing another depressive episode.

Another issue for managed care is supporting the safety of the depressed child and his or her significant others. This may mean supporting hospitalization of the youngster for a long enough period that the child is no longer at risk of harming him- or herself or significant others. Given the very real risk of suicide among depressed youths, it is important to make hospitalization an obtainable reality when necessary. Furthermore, when a child is experiencing comorbid conditions such as severe MDD and OCD or conduct disorder, then longer-term hospitalization may be necessary to ensure successful treatment, as well as safety of the youngster and the broader community.

FINAL THOUGHTS

In many ways, the research that has been completed since the previous edition of this book has helped the field to understand better how to identify, assess, and treat children who are experiencing depressive disorders. At the same time that our understanding of the disorder has improved, however, psychologists have been slow to incorporate these findings into psychosocial treatments. Although CBT has demonstrated efficacy in some studies, the preliminary results of the TADS suggest that it is of limited efficacy with depressed adolescents. Preliminary data show that the ACTION treatment, a gender-specific and developmentally sensitive intervention, has demonstrated efficacy relative to a minimal-contact control condition for depressed 9- to 13-year-old girls. Empirical support has been established for some of the antidepressants with depressed adolescents; fluoxetine, one of the SSRIs, has received the most support. It also appears as though the combination of fluoxetine and CBT is more effective than either intervention alone for depressed adolescents. Why is the combination of fluoxetine and CBT more effective than either intervention alone? Perhaps the medication potentiates the changes in thinking that are the target of treatment for the CBT. That is, an improvement in mood may enable a depressed youngster to use the skills taught in CBT. It also may loosen the youngster's thinking, so that he or she can gain enough distance to be able to rationally evaluate and counter the negative thinking.

Another important line of research will be determining the relative efficacy of different types of psychosocial interventions. Perhaps CBT is not the most efficacious intervention for depressive disorders. Is IPT-A more efficacious? Are interventions that simply build personal competence, such as academic and social skills training, equally or more efficacious? There are a myriad of approaches to treating psychological disorders, any of which may be more efficacious than existing treatments.

Although existing research has focused on treating children's depressive disorders, children do not grow up within a vacuum: They are affected by their parents, siblings, and other family members. Parental psychopathology may be a predictor of treatment outcome. For example, having a parent with a bipolar disorder may be a stressor in a depressed child's life. It may contribute to the child's concerns about being "unlovable," as the parent's excessive irritability communicates this message during manic episodes, and the emotional unavailability of the parent during depressive episodes communicates a similar message. Family disturbances, marital/couple discord, family chaos, loss of a parent due to divorce, or pregnancy out of wedlock can all represent stressors and potential predictors of treatment outcome. Determining whether these variables have an impact on the efficacy of child treatment is important. If they do, then it may be necessary to determine what ancillary forms of treatment are necessary to create an efficacious intervention.

Related to issues about efficacy are issues of effectiveness. The "effectiveness" of an intervention can be defined as how well the intervention works when it is transported out of the "ivory tower" to practitioners in the field. In other words, when CBT is implemented by psychologists in practice, is it effective? The current large-scale treatment outcome studies include manualized treatments. Thus a treatment program could be disseminated to practitioners who, theoretically, could use the manual as a guide to providing treatment. However, to date, such effectiveness research has not been conducted. Experience suggests that interventions are not as portable as they may appear. There are many subtle aspects to the effective implementation of a manualized treatment that are not described in the manual because they are difficult to put into words, and because including that level of minutiae would create an unwieldy manual. A treatment manual is based on the conceptualizations of depression held by its authors. This conceptualization may have come from years of research and studying literature in the field. To implement the treatment effectively and artfully requires a similar expert

understanding of the conceptual model of the manual's authors. A description of the model is typically not included in the manual for a variety of reasons. Perhaps one of them is that it takes an extensive amount of teaching for therapists to understand the model and to translate it into something that guides practice.

How much conceptual training is necessary for a therapist to be an effective delivery agent for a manualized treatment? Most psychologists have not had extensive training in CBT during graduate school. Thus they not only won't have a solid grasp of the conceptual model underlying the treatment of depressed youths; they may not have adequate experience in using CBT techniques to implement them masterfully. Thus an overarching effectiveness question that has not been addressed is this: How much training of therapists is necessary for them to become effective at implementing the treatment programs for depression? Based on current experience, it takes at least 6–12 months of training (including intense supervision) to become effective at implementing a manualized CBT intervention program for depressed youths. Thus, although we may be advancing the field by moving toward the use of empirically proven interventions, this is now the real question for researchers and practitioners alike: What kind of training, and how much training, are necessary to enable a therapist to become an effective delivery agent for the efficacious interventions? In a related vein, if a combination of an SSRI and CBT is going to be the most efficacious intervention for the most youngsters, then psychologists and psychiatrists are going to have to receive training in how to work together to maximize the effectiveness of the intervention. Furthermore, both fields are going to have to become more effective at helping parents to understand the benefits and potential disadvantages of treatment with an SSRI. Currently, parents tend to be afraid of the potential harm that taking medications could cause their children; thus they are resistant to initiating a trial of an antidepressant.

An entirely different but important line of investigation is research into the psychological and brain-based changes that occur as a result of treatment. For example, the ACTION treatment program targets changes in coping skills, problem solving, and the child's cognitive triad. Although the intervention appears to be efficacious, it is not yet possible to determine whether the improvements are due to changes in these specific variables, or whether some other variable has changed. Thus it is important for future researchers to determine the mechanism of change. A promising line of research would parallel the research that uses neuroimaging to evaluate the changes in brain functioning among pediatric patients with OCD who are successfully treated with ERP therapy (Schwartz, Stoessel, Baxter, Martin, & Phelps, 1996). Does CBT, for example, lead to an improvement in brain functioning when the intervention is effective?

REFERENCES

Abercrombie, H. C., Schaefer, S. M., Larson, C. L., Oakes, T. R., Lindgren, K. A., Holden, J. E., et al. (1998). Metabolic rate in the right amygdala predicts negative affect in depressed patients. *NeuroReport, 9*, 3301–3307.

Abramson, L. Y. (1999). *Developmental maltreatment and cognitive vulnerability to depression.* Paper presented at the biennial meeting of the Society for Research in Child Development, Albuquerque, NM.

Abramson, L. Y., Metalsky, G. I., & Alloy, L. B. (1989). Hopelessness depression: A theory-based subtype of depression. *Psychological Review, 96*, 358–372.

Addis, M. E., & Krasnow, A. D. (2000). A national survey of practicing psychologists' attitudes toward psychotherapy treatment manuals. *Journal of Consulting and Clinical Psychology, 68*, 331–339.

Allgood-Merten, B., Lewinsohn, P. M., & Hops, H. (1990). Sex differences and adolescent depression. *Journal of Abnormal Psychology, 99*, 55–63.

Alloy, L. B., Abramson, L. Y., Tashman, N. A., Berrebbi, D. S., Hogan, M. E., Whitehouse, W. G., et al. (2001). Developmental origins of cognitive vulnerability to depression: Parenting, cognitive, and inferential feedback styles of the parents of individuals at high and low cognitive risk for depression. *Cognitive Therapy and Research, 25*, 397–423.

American Association of University Women. (1992). *How schools shortchange girls: The AAUW report: A study of major findings on girls in education.* Washington, DC: American Association of University Women Educational Foundation.

American Psychiatric Association. (2000). *Diagnostic and statistical manual of mental disorders* (4th ed., text rev.). Washington, DC: Author.

Anderman, E. M. (2002). School effects on psychological outcomes during adolescence. *Journal of Educational Psychology, 94*, 795–809.

Anderson, J. C., Williams, S., McGee, R., & Silva, P. A. (1987). DSM-III disorders in preadolescent children: Prevalence in a large sample from the general population. *Archives of General Psychiatry, 44, 69*–76.

Andrade, A., Lambert, W., & Bickman, L. (2000). Dose effect in child psychotherapy: Outcomes associated with negligible treatment. *Journal of the American Academy of Child and Adolescent Psychiatry, 39*, 161–168.

Andrews, V. C., Garrison, C. Z., Jackson, K. L., Addy, C. L., & McKeown, R. E. (1993). Mother–adolescent agreement on the symptoms of and diagnoses of adolescent depression and conduct disorders. *Journal of the American Academy of Child and Adolescent Psychiatry, 32*, 731–738.

Arieti, S., & Bemporad, J. R. (1980). The psychological organization of depression. *American Journal of Psychiatry, 137*, 1360–1365.

Asarnow, J. R., & Bates, S. (1988). Depression in child psychiatric inpatients: Cognitive and attributional patterns. *Journal of Abnormal Child Psychology, 16*, 601–615.

Avison, W. R., & Mcalpine, D. D. (1992). Gender differences in symptoms of depression among adolescents. *Journal of Health and Social Behavior, 33*, 77–96.

Axelson, D. A., Doraiswamy, P. M., McDonald, W. M., Boyko, O. B., Tupler, L. A., Patterson, L. J., et al. (1993). Hypercoritsolemia and hippocampal changes in depression. *Psychiatry Research, 47*, 163–173.

Bandura, A. (1978). The self system in reciprocal determinism. *American Psychologist, 33*, 344–358.

Barden, N., Reul, J. M. H. M., & Holsboer, F. (1995). Do antidepressants stabilize mood through actions on the hypothalamic–pituitary–adrenocortical system? *Trends in Neurosciences, 18*, 6–11.

Baxter, L. R., Phelps, M. E., Mazziotta, J. C., Schwartz, J. M., Gerner, R. H., Selin, C. E., et al. (1985). Cerebral metabolic rates for glucose in mood disorders: Studies with positron emission tomography and fluorodeoxyglucose F 18. *Archives of General Psychiatry, 42*, 441–447.

Beardslee, W. R., Versage, E. M., & Gladstone, T. R. (1998). Children of affectively ill parents: A review of the past 10 years. *Journal of the American Academy of Child and Adolescent Psychiatry, 37*, 1134–1141.

Beck, A. T. (1967). *Depression: Clinical, experimental, and theoretical aspects.* New York: Harper & Row.

Beck, A. T., Rush, J., Shaw, B. F., & Emery, G. (1979). *Cognitive therapy of depression.* New York: Guilford Press.

Beck, J. S. (1995). *Cognitive therapy: Basics and beyond.* New York: Guilford Press.

Bell-Dolan, D., Foster, S., & Smith Christopher, J. (1995). Girls' peer relations and internalizing problems: Are socially neglected, rejected, and withdrawn girls at risk? *Journal of Clinical Child Psychology, 24*, 463–473.

Benjet, C., & Hernandez-Guzman, L. (2002). A short-term longitudinal study of pubertal change, gender, and psychological well-being of Mexican early adolescents. *Journal of Youth and Adolescence, 31*, 429–442.

Benkelfat, C., Ellenbogen, M. A., Dean, P., Palmour, R. M., & Young, S. N. (1994). Mood-lowering effect of tryptophan depletion: Enhanced susceptibility in young men at genetic risk for major affective disorders. *Archives of General Psychiatry, 51,* 687–697.

Berman, W. H., & Sperling, M. B. (1994). The structure and function of adult attachment. In M. B. Sperling & W. H. Berman (Eds.), *Attachment in adults* (pp. 1–30). New York: Guilford Press.

Bickman, L., Noser, K., & Summerfelt. W. T. (1999). Long-term effects of a system of care on children and adolescents. *Journal of Behavioral Health Services Research, 26,* 185–202.

Biederman, J., Baldessarini R. J., Wright, V., Keenan, K., & Faraone, S. (1993). A double-blind placebo controlled study of desipramine in the treatment of attention deficit disorder: III. Lack of impact of comorbidity and family history factors on clinical response. *Journal of the American Academy of Child and Adolescent Psychiatry, 32,* 199–204.

Biederman, J., Newcorn, J., & Sprich, S. (1991). Comorbidity of attention deficit hyperactivity disorder with conduct, depressive, anxiety, and other disorders. *American Journal of Psychiatry, 148*(5), 564–577.

Birmaher, B., & Brent, D. A. (2003). Antidepressants: II. Tricyclic agents. In A. Martin, L. Scahill, D. S. Chaney, & J. F. Leckman (Eds.), *Pediatric psychopharmacology: Principles and practice* (pp. 466–483). New York: Oxford University Press.

Birmaher, B., Brent, D. A., Kolko, D., Baugher, M., Bridge, J., Holder, D., et al. (2000). Clinical outcome after short-term psychotherapy for adolescents with major depressive disorder. *Archives of General Psychiatry, 57,* 29–36.

Birmaher, B., Dahl, R. E., Ryan, N. D., Rabinovich, H., Ambrosini, P., Al-Shahbout, M., et al. (1992). The dexamethasone suppression test in adolescent outpatients with major depressive disorder. *American Journal of Psychiatry, 149,* 1040–1045.

Birmaher, B., Ryan, N. D., Dahl, R. E., Rabinovich, H., Ambrosini, P., Williamson, D. E., et al. (1992). Dexamethasone suppression test in children with major depressive disorder. *Journal of the American Academy of Child and Adolescent Psychiatry, 31,* 291–297.

Birmaher, B., Ryan, N., Williamson, D. E., Brent, D. A., Kaufman, J., Dahl, R. E., et al. (1996). Childhood and adolescent depression: A review of the past 10 years. Part I. *Journal of the American Academy of Child and Adolescent Psychiatry, 35,* 1427–1439.

Blackwell, B. (1963). Hypertensive crisis due to monoamine-oxidase inhibition. *Lancet, ii,* 849–851.

Blagys, M. D., & Hilsenroth, M. J. (2002). Distinctive activities of cognitive-behavioral therapy: A review of the comparative psychotherapy process literature. *Clinical Psychology Review, 22,* 671–706.

Boivin, M., Hymel, S., & Bukowski, W. M. (1995). The roles of social withdrawal, peer rejection, and victimization by peers in predicting loneliness and depressed mood in childhood. *Development and Psychopathology, 7,* 765–785.

Booij, L., Van der Does, W., Benkelfat, C., Bremner, J. D., Cowen, P. J., Fava, M., et al. (2002). Predictors of mood response to acute tryptophan depletion: A reanalysis. *Neuropsychopharmacology, 27,* 852–861.

Borchardt, C. M., & Meller, W. H. (1996). Symptoms of affective disorder in pre-adolescent vs. adolescent inpatients. *Journal of Adolescence, 19,* 155–161.

Bostic, J. Q., Prince, J., Frazier, J., DeJong, S., & Wilens, T. E. (2003). Pediatric psychopharmacology update. *Psychiatric Times, 20,* 9.

Botteron, K. N., Raichle, M. E., Drevets, W. C., Heath, A. C., & Todd, R. D. (2002). Volumetric reduction in left subgenual prefrontal cortex in early onset depression. *Biological Psychiatry, 51,* 342–344.

Bowlby, J. (1980). *Attachment and loss: Vol. 3. Loss, sadness and depression.* New York: Basic Books.

Brady, E. U., & Kendall, P. C. (1992). Comorbidity of anxiety and depression in children and adolescents. *Psychological Bulletin, 111,* 244–255.

Brambilla, P., Nicoletti, M. A., Harenski, K., Sassi, R. B., Mallinger, A. G., Frank, E., et al. (2002). Anatomical MRI study of subgenual prefrontal cortex in bipolar and unipolar subjects. *Neuropsychopharmacology, 27,* 792–799.

Bremner, J. D., Narayan, M., Anderson, E. R., Staib, L. H., Miller, H., & Charney, D. S. (2000). Hippocampal volume reduction in major depression. *American Journal of Psychiatry, 157,* 115–117.

Brennan, P. A., Hammen, C., Katz, A. R., & Le Brocque, R. M. (2002). Maternal depression, paternal psychopathology, and adolescent diagnostic outcome. *Journal of Consulting and Clinical Psychology, 70,* 1075–1085.

Brennan, P. A., Le Brocque, R., & Hammen, C. (2003). Maternal depression, parent–child relationships, and resilient outcomes in adolescence. *Journal of the American Academy of Child and Adolescent Psychiatry, 42,* 1469–1477.

Brent, D. A., Holder, D., & Kolko, D. (1997). A clinical psychotherapy trial for adolescent depression comparing cognitive, family, and supportive therapy. *Archives of General Psychiatry, 54,* 877–885.

Brent, D. A., Kolko, D. J., & Birmaher, B. (1998). Predictors of treatment efficacy in a clinical trial of three psychosocial treatments for adolescent depression. *Journal of the American Academy of Child and Adolescent Psychiatry, 37,* 906–914.

Brent, D. A., Perper, J. A., Mortiz, G., Allman, C., Friend, A., Roth, C., et al. (1993). Psychiatric risk factors for adolescent suicide: A case–control study. *Journal of the American Academy of Child and Adolescent Psychiatry, 32,* 521–529.

Bretherton, I. (1990). Communication patterns, internal working models, and the intergenerational transmission of attachment relationship. *Infant Mental Health Journal, 11,* 237–252.

Brody, A. L., Saxena, S., Mandelkern, M. A., Fairbanks, L. A., Ho, M. L., & Baxter, L. R. (2001). Brain metabolic change associated with symptom factor improvement in major depressive disorder. *Biological Psychiatry, 50,* 171–178.

Bronfenbrenner, U. (1979). *The ecology of human development.* Cambridge, MA: Harvard University Press.

Buchsbaum, M. S., Wu, J., DeLisi, L. E., Holcomb, H., Kessler, R., Johnson, J., et al. (1986). Frontal cortex and basal ganglia metabolic rates assessed by positron emission tomography with [^{18}F]2–deoxyglucose in affective illness. *Journal of Affective Disorders, 10,* 137–152.

Burke, K. D., Burke, J. D., Regier, D. A., & Rae, D. S. (1991). Age at onset of selected mental disorders in five community populations. *Archives of General Psychiatry, 47,* 511–517.

Butler, L., Mietzitis, S., Friedman, R., & Cole, E. (1980). The effect of two school-based intervention programs on depressive symptoms in preadolescents. *American Educational Research Journal, 17,* 111–119.

Cardemil, E. V., Reivich, K. J., & Seligman, M. E. P. (2002). The prevention of depressive symptoms in low-income minority middle school students. *Prevention and Treatment, 5,* Article 0008. Retrieved from http://journals.apa.org/prevention/volume5/pre0050008.html

Carlson, G. A., & Cantwell, D. P. (1980). A survey of depressive symptoms, syndrome and disorder in a child psychiatric population. *Journal of Child Psychology and Psychiatry, 21,* 19–25.

Carlson, G. A., & Kashani, J. H. (1988). Phenomenology of major depression from childhood through adulthood: Analysis of three studies. *American Journal of Psychiatry, 145,* 1222–1225.

Casper, R. C., Belanoff, J., & Offer, D. (1996). Gender differences, but no racial group differences, in self-reported psychiatric symptoms in adolescents. *Journal of the American Academy of Child and Adolescent Psychiatry, 35,* 500–508.

Chambers, W. J., Puig-Antich, J., Tabrizi, M. A., & Davies, M. (1982). Psychotic symptoms in prepubertal major depressive disorder. *Archives of General Psychiatry, 39,* 921–928.

Chambless, D. L., & Hollon, S. D. (1998). Defining empirically supported therapies. *Journal of Consulting and Clinical Psychology, 66,* 7–18.

Christ, A. E., Adler, A. G., Isacoff, M., & Gershansky, I. S. (1981) Depression: Symptoms versus diagnosis in 10, 412 hospitalized children and adolescents (1957–1977). *American Journal of Psychotherapy, 35,* 400–412.

Chrousos, G. P., & Gold, P. W. (1992). The concepts of stress and stress disorders: Overview of physical and behavioral homeostasis. *Journal of the American Medical Association, 267,* 1244–1252.

Cicchetti, D., & Toth, S. L. (1998). The development of depression in children and adolescents. *American Psychologist, 55,* 221–241.

Clarke, G. N., Hawkins, W., Murphy, M., & Sheeber, L. B. (1995). Targeted prevention of unipolar depressive disorder in an at-risk sample of high school adolescents: A randomized trial of group cognitive intervention. *Journal of Child and Adolescent Psychiatry, 32,* 312–321.

Clarke, G. N., Hops, H., & Lewinsohn, P. M. (1992). Cognitive-behavioral group treatment of adolescent depression: Prediction of outcome. *Behavior Therapy, 23,* 341–354.

Clarke, G. N., Hornbrook, M., Lynch, F., Plen, M., Gale, J., Beardslee, W., et al. (2001). A randomized trial of a group cognitive intervention for preventing depression in adolescent offspring of depressed parents. *Archives of General Psychiatry, 58,* 1127–1134.

Clarke, G. N., Rohde, P., & Lewinsohn, P. M. (1999). Cognitive-behavioral treatment of adolescent depression: Efficacy of acute group treatment and booster sessions. *Journal of the American Academy of Child and Adolescent Psychiatry, 38,* 272–279.

Clarke, G. N., Rohde, P., Lewinsohn, P. M., Hops, H., & Seeley, J. R. (1999). Cognitive-behavioral treatment of adolescent depression: Efficacy of acute group treatment and booster sessions. *Journal of the American Academy of Child and Adolescent Psychiatry, 38,* 272–279.

Cohen, R. M., Gross, M., Nordahl, T. E., Semple, W. E., Oren, D. A., & Rosenthal, N. (1992). Preliminary data on the metabolic brain pattern of patients with winter seasonal affective disorder. *Archives of General Psychiatry, 49,* 545–552.

Cole, D. A., & Carpentieri, S. (1990). Social status and the comorbidity of child depression and conduct disorder. *Journal of Consulting and Clinical Psychology, 58,* 748–757.

Cole, D. A., Jacquez, F. M., & Maschman, T. L. (2001). Social origins of depressive cognitions: A longitudinal study of self-perceived competence in children. *Cognitive Therapy and Research, 25,* 377–395.

Cole, D. A., & Rehm, L. P. (1986). Family interaction patterns and childhood depression. *Journal of Abnormal Child Psychology, 14,* 297–314.

Cole, D. A., & Turner, J., Jr. (1993). Models of cognitive mediation and moderation in child depression. *Journal of Abnormal Psychology, 102,* 271–281.

Colin, V. L. (1996). *Human attachment.* Philadelphia: Temple University Press.

Compas, B. E., & Wagner, B. M. (1991). Psychosocial stress during adolescence: Intrapersonal and interpersonal processes. In M. E. Colten & S. Gore (Eds.), *Adolescent stress: Causes and consequences* (pp. 67–85). New York: de Gruyter.

Compton, K., Snyder, J., Schrepferman, L., Bank, L., & Shortt, J. W. (2003). The contribution of parents and siblings to antisocial and depressive behavior in adolescents: A double jeopardy coercion model. *Development and Psychopathology, 15,* 163–182.

Conners, C. K., Casat, C. D., Gualtieri, C. T., Weller, E., Reader, M., Reiss, A., et al. (1996). Bupropion hydrochloride in attention deficit disorder with hyperactivity. *Journal of the American Academy of Child and Adolescent Psychiatry, 35,* 1314–1321.

Costello, E. J., Costello, A. J., Edelbrock, C., Burns, B. J., Dulcan, M. K., Brent, D., et al. (1988). Psychiatric disorders in pediatric primary care. *Archives of General Psychiatry, 45,* 1107–1116.

Costello, E. J., Mustillo, S., Erkanli, A., Keeler, G., & Angold, A. (2003). Prevalence and development of psychiatric disorders in childhood and adolescence. *Archives of General Psychiatry, 60,* 837–844.

Cowan, P. A., Cohn, D. A., Cowan, C. P., & Pearson, J. L. (1996). Parents' attachment histories and children's externalizing and internalizing behaviors: Exploring family systems models of linkage. *Journal of Consulting and Clinical Psychology, 64,* 53–63.

Cox, W. (1982). An indication for the use of imipramine in attention deficit disorder. *American Journal of Psychiatry, 139,* 1059–1060.

Crick, N. R., & Grotpeter, J. K. (1995). Relational aggression, gender, and social psychological adjustment. *Child Development, 66,* 710–722.

Cuffe, S. P., Waller, J. L., Cuccaro, M. L., Pumariega, A. J., & Garrison, C. Z. (1995). Race and gender differences in the treatment of psychiatric disorders in young adolescents. *Journal of the American Academy of Child and Adolescent Psychiatry, 34,* 1536–1543.

Curry, J. F. (2001). Specific psychotherapies for childhood and adolescent depression. *Biological Psychiatry, 49,* 1091–1100.

Dahl, R. E., Kaufman, J., Ryan, N., Perel, J., al-Shabbout, M., D., Birmaher, B., et al. (1992). The dexamethasone suppression test in children and adolescents: A review and a controlled study. *Biological Psychiatry, 32,* 109–126.

Davidson, R. J., Irwin, W., Anderle, M. J., & Kalin, N. H. (2003). The neural substrates of affective processing in depressed patients treated with venlafaxine. *American Journal of Psychiatry, 160,* 64–75.

Daviss, W. B., Bentivoglio, P., Racusin, R., Brown, K., Bostic, J., & Wiley, L. (2001). Bupropion sustained release in adolescents with comorbid attention-deficit/hyperactivity and depression. *Journal of the American Academy of Child and Adolescent Psychiatry, 40,* 307–314.

De Bellis, M. D., Chrousos, G. P., Dorn, L. D., Burke, L., Helmers, K., Kling, M. A., et al. (1994). Hypothalamic–pituitary–adrenal axis dysregulation in sexually abused girls. *Journal of Clinical Endocrinology and Metabolism, 78,* 249–255.

Deblinger, E., & Heflin, A. H. (1996). *Treating sexually abused children and their nonoffending parents: A cognitive behavioral approach.* Thousand Oaks, CA: Sage.

Delgado, P. L. (2000). Depression: The case for a monoamine deficiency. *Journal of Clinical Psychiatry, 51*(Suppl. 6), 7–11.

Delgado, P. L., Charney, D. S., Price, L. H., Aghajanian, G. K., Landis, H., & Heninger, G. R. (1990). Serotonin function and the mechanism of antidepressant action: Reversal of antidepressant-induced remission by rapid depletion of plasma tryptophan. *Archives of General Psychiatry, 47,* 411–418.

Delgado, P. L., Miller, H. L., Salomon, R. M., Licinio, J., Krystal, J. H., Moreno, F. A., et al. (1999). Tryptophan-depletion challenge in depressed patients treated with desipramine or fluoxetine: Implications for the role of serotonin in the mechanism of antidepressant action. *Biological Psychiatry, 46,* 212–220.

Diala, C. C., Muntaner, C., Walrath, C., Nickerson, K., LaVeist, T., & Leaf, P. (2001). Racial/ethnic differences in attitudes toward seeking professional mental health services. *American Journal of Public Health, 91,* 805–807.

DiFilippo, J. M., & Overholser, J. C. (2000). Suicidal ideation in adolescent psychiatric inpatients as associated with depression and attachment relationships. *Journal of Clinical Child Psychology, 29,* 155–166.

Dorn, L. D., Burgess, E. S., Susman, E. J., von Eye, A., De Bellis, M. D., Gold, P. W., et al. (1996). Response to CRH in depressed and nondepressed adolescents: Does gender make a difference? *Journal of the American Academy of Child and Adolescent Psychiatry, 35,* 764–773.

Drevets, W. C. (2001). Neuroimaging and neuropathological studies of depression: Implications for the cognitive-emotional features of mood disorders. *Current Opinion in Neurobiology, 11,* 240–249.

Drevets, W. C., Bogers, W., & Raichle, M. E. (2002). Functional anatomical correlates of antidepressant drug treatment assessed using PET measures of regional glucose metabolism. *European Neuropsychopharmacology, 12,* 527–544.

Drevets, W. C., Price, J. L., Simpson, J. R., Todd, R. D., Reich, T., Vannier, M., et al. (1997). Subgenual prefrontal cortex abnormalities in mood disorders. *Nature, 386,* 824–827.

Drevets, W. C., Spitznagel, E., & Raichle, M. E. (1995). Functional anatomical differences between major depressive subtypes. *Journal of Cerebral Blood Flow and Metabolism, 15*(Suppl. 1), S93.

Durlak, J. A., Fuhrman, T., & Lampman, C. (1991). Effectiveness of cognitive-behavior therapy for maladapting children: A meta-analysis. *Psychological Bulletin, 110,* 204–214.

Ebert, D., Feistel, H., & Barocka, A. (1991). Effects of sleep deprivation on the limbic system and the frontal lobes in affective disorders. *Psychiatry Research: Neuroimaging, 40,* 247–251.

Emslie, G. J. (2001). *Treatment of major depressive disorder in children and adolescents.* Paper presented at the 48th annual meeting of the American Academy of Child and Adolescent Psychiatry, Honolulu, HI.

Emslie, G. J., Rush, A. J., Weinberg, W. A., Gullion, C.

M., Rintelmann, J., & Hughes, C. W. (1997). Recurrence of major depressive disorder in hospitalized children and adolescents. *Journal of the American Academy of Child and Adolescent Psychiatry, 36,* 785–792.

Emslie, G. J., Weinberg, W. A., Rush, A. J., Adams, R. M., & Rintelmann, J. W. (1990). Depressive symptoms by self-report in adolescence: Phase I of the development of a questionnaire for depression by self-report. *Journal of Child Neurology, 5,* 114–121.

Finch, A. J. Jr., Lipovsky, J. A., & Casat, C. D. (1989). Anxiety and depression in children and adolescents: Negative affectivity or separate constructs? In P. C. Kendall & D. Watson (Eds.), *Anxiety and depression: Distinctive and overlapping features* (pp. 171–202). San Diego, CA: Academic Press.

Findling, R. L., Preskorn, S. H., Marcus, R. N., Magnus, R. D., D'Amico, F., Marathe, P., et al. (2000). Nefazodone pharmacokinetics in depressed children and adolescents. *Journal of the American Academy of Child and Adolescent Psychiatry, 39,* 1008–1016.

Flynn, C., & Garber, J. (1999). *Predictors of depressive cognitions in young adolescents.* Paper presented at the biennial meeting of the Society for Research in Child Development, Albuquerque, NM.

Forehand, R., Body, G., Slotkin, J., Gauber, R., McCombs, A., & Long, N. (1988). Young adolescents and maternal depression: Assessment, interrelations and family predictors. *Journal of Consulting and Clinical Psychology, 56,* 422–426.

Frodl, T., Meisenzahl, E. M., Zetzsche, T., Born, C., Grooll, C., Jager, M., et al. (2002). Hippocampal changes in patients with a first episode of major depression. *American Journal of Psychiatry, 159,* 1112–1118.

Gammon, G. D., & Brown, T. E. (1993). Fluoxetine and methylphenidate in combination for treatment of attention deficit disorder and comorbid depressive disorder. *Journal of Child and Adolescent Psychopharmacology, 3,* 1.

Garrison, C. Z., Jackson, K. L., Marsteller, F., McKeown, R., & Addy, C. (1990). A longitudinal study of depressive symptomatology in young adolescents. *Journal of the American Academy of Child and Adolescent Psychiatry, 29,* 580–585.

Gaynor, S. T., Weersin, V. R., Kolko, D. J., Birmaher, B., Heo, J., & Brent, D. A. (2003). The prevalence and impact of large sudden improvements during adolescent therapy for depression: A comparison across cognitive-behavioral, family and supportive therapy. *Journal of Consulting and Clinical Psychology, 71,* 386–393.

Ge, X., Conger, R. D., & Elder, G. H. (1996). Coming of age too early: Pubertal influences on girls' vulnerability to psychological distress. *Child Development, 67,* 3386–3400.

Ge, X., Conger, R. D., & Elder, G. H. (2001). Pubertal transition, stressful life events, and the emergence of gender differences in adolescent depressive symptoms. *Developmental Psychology, 37,* 404–417.

Ge, X, Kim, I. J., Brody, G. H., Conger, R. D., Simons, R. L., Gibbons, F. X., et al. (2003). It's about timing and change: Pubertal transition effects on symptoms of major depression among African American youths. *Developmental Psychology, 39,* 430–439.

Geller, B., Cooper, T. B., Graham, D. L., Fetner, H. H., Marsteller, F. A., & Wells J. M. (1992). Pharmacokinetically double-blind placebo-controlled study of nortriptyline in 6- to 12-year-olds with major depressive disorder. *Journal of the American Academy of Child and Adolescent Psychiatry, 31,* 34–44.

Gillham, J. E., Shatte, A. J., & Freres, D. R. (2000). Preventing depression: A review of cognitive-behavioral and family interventions. *Applied and Preventive Psychology, 9,* 63–88.

Glod, C. A., Lynch, A., Flynn, E., Berkowitz, C., & Baldessarini, R. J. (2003). Open trial of bupropion SR in adolescent major depression. *Journal of Child and Adolescent Psychiatric Nursing, 16,* 123–130.

Gold, P. W., Goodwin, F. K., & Chrousos, G. P. (1988a). Clinical and biochemical manifestations of depression: Relations to the neurobiology of stress: I. *New England Journal of Medicine, 319,* 348–353.

Gold, P. W., Goodwin, F. K., & Chrousos, C. P. (1988b). Clinical and biochemical manifestations of depression: Relations to the neurobiology of stress: II. *New England Journal of Medicine, 319,* 413–420.

Goodenow, C. (1993). Classroom belonging among early adolescent students: Relationships to motivation and achievement. *Journal of Early Adolescence, 13,* 21–43.

Goodyer, I. M., Germany, E., Gowrusankur, J., & Altham, P. (1991). Social influences on the course of anxious and depressive disorders in school-age children. *British Journal of Psychiatry, 158,* 676–684.

Goodyer, I. M., Herbert, J., Secher, S. M., & Pearson, J. (1997). Short-term outcome of major depression: I. Comorbidity and severity at presentation as predictors of persistent disorder. *Journal of the American Academy of Child and Adolescent Psychiatry, 36,* 179–187.

Gordon, D., Burge, D., Hammen, C. Adrian, C., Jaenicke, C., & Hiroto, D. (1989). Observations of interactions of depressed women with their children. *American Journal of Psychiatry, 146,* 50–55.

Gould, M. S., King, R., Greenwald, S., Fisher, P., Schwab-Stone, M., & Kramer, R. (1998). Psychopathology associated with suicidal ideation and attempts among children and adolescents. *Journal of the American Academy of Child and Adolescent Psychiatry, 37,* 915–923.

Graber, J. A., Lewinsohn, P. M., Seeley, J. R., & Brooks-Gunn, J. (1997). Is psychopathology associated with the timing of pubertal development? *Journal of the American Academy of Child and Adolescent Psychiatry, 36,* 1768–1776.

Gundersen, K., & Geller, B. (2003). Antidepressants: II. Tricyclic agents. In A. Martin, L. Scahill, D. S. Charney, & J. F. Leckman (Eds.), *Pediatric psychopharmacology: Principles and practice* (pp. 284–294). New York: Oxford University Press.

Haarasilta, L., Marttunen, M., Kaprio, J., & Aro, H. (2001). The 12–month prevalence and characteristics of major depressive episode in a representative nationwide sample of adolescents and young adults. *Psychological Medicine, 31,* 1169–1179.

Hammen, C. (1991). Generation of stress in the course of unipolar depression. *Journal of Abnormal Psychology, 100,* 555–561.

Hammen, C. (1999). The emergence of an interpersonal approach to depression. In T. Joiner & J. C. Coyne (Eds.), *The interactional nature of depression* (pp. 21–35). Washington, DC: American Psychological Association.

Hammen, C., & Brennan, P. A. (2001). Depressed adolescents of depressed and nondepressed mothers: Tests of an interpersonal impairment hypothesis. *Journal of Consulting and Clinical Psychology, 69,* 284–294.

Hammen, C., & Goodman-Brown, T. (1990). Self-schemas and vulnerability to specific life stress in children at risk for depression. *Cognitive Therapy and Research, 14,* 215–227.

Hammen, C., & Rudolph, K. D. (1996). Childhood depression. In E. J. Mash & R. A. Barkley (Eds.), *Child psychopathology* (pp. 153–195). New York: Guilford Press.

Hammen, C., & Rudolph, K. D. (2003). Childhood mood disorders. In E. J. Mash & R. A Barkley (Eds.), *Child psychopathology* (2nd ed., pp. 233–278). New York: Guilford Press.

Hammen, C., & Zupan, B. A. (1984). Self-schemas, depression, and the processing of personal information in children. *Journal of Experimental Child Psychology, 37,* 598–608.

Hankin, B. L., & Abramson, L. Y. (2001). Development of gender differences in depression: An elaborated cognitive vulnerability-transactional stress theory. *Psychological Bulletin, 127*(6), 773–796.

Hankin, B. L., & Abramson, L. Y. (2002). Measuring cognitive vulnerability to depression in adolescence: Reliability, validity, and gender differences. *Journal of Clinical Child and Adolescent Psychology, 31*(4), 491–504.

Hankin, B. L., Abramson, L. Y., Silva, P. A., McGee, R., & Angell, K. E. (1998). Development of depression from preadolescence to young adulthood: Emerging gender differences in a 10-year longitudinal study. *Journal of Abnormal Psychology, 107,* 128–140.

Harrington, R., Fudge, H., Rutter, M., Pickles, A., & Hill, J. (1990). Adult outcome of childhood and adolescent depression: I. Psychiatric status. *Archives of General Psychiatry, 47,* 465–473.

Hazell, P., O'Connell, D., Heathcote, D., Robertson, J., & Henry, D. (1995). Efficacy of tricyclic drugs in treating child and adolescent depression. *British Medical Journal, 310,* 897–901.

Heim, C., & Nemeroff, C. B. (2001). The role of childhood trauma in the neurobiology of mood and anxiety disorders: Preclinical and clinical studies. *Biological Psychiatry, 49,* 1023–1039.

Hill, J. P., & Lynch, M. E. (1983). The intensification of gender-related role expectations during early adolescence. In J. Brooks-Gunn & A. C. Peterson (Eds.), *Girls at puberty* (pp. 201–228). New York: Plenum Press.

Hirschfeld, R. M. A. (2000). History and evolution of the monoamine hypothesis of depression. *Journal of Clinical Psychiatry, 61*(Suppl. 6), 4–12.

Hodges, E. V. E., & Perry, D. G. (1999). Personal and interpersonal antecedents and consequences of victimization by peers. *Journal of Personality and Social Psychology, 76,* 677–685.

Hodges, K. K., & Siegel, L. J. (1985). Depression in children and adolescents. In E. E. Beckham & W. R. Leber (Eds.), *Handbook of depression: Treatment, assessment, and research* (pp. 517–555). Homewood, IL: Dorsey.

Hoge, D. R., Smith, E. K., & Hanson, S. L. (1990). School experiences predicting changes in self-esteem of sixth and seventh-grade students. *Journal of Educational Psychology, 82,* 117–127.

Hollon, S. D., Muñoz, R. F., Barlow, D. H., Beardslee, W. R., Bell, C. C., & Bernal, G. (2002). Psychosocial intervention development for the prevention and treatment of depression: Promoting innovation and increasing access. *Biological Psychiatry, 52,* 610–630.

Howard, K. I., Kopta, S. M., Krause, M. S., & Orlinsky, D. E. (1986). The dose–effect relationship in psychotherapy. *American Psychologist, 41,* 159–164.

Hubble, M. A., Duncan, B. L., & Miller, S. D. (1999). Directing attention to what works. In M. A. Hubble & B. L. Duncan (Eds.), *Heart and soul of change: What works in therapy* (pp. 407–447). Washington, DC: American Psychological Association.

Hughes, C., Emslie, G., Crimson, M. L., Wagner, K., Birmaher, B., Geller, B., et al. (1999) The Texas Children's Medication Algorithm Project: Report of the Texas Consensus Conference Panel on Medication Treatment of Childhood Major Depressive Disorder. *Journal of the American Academy of Child and Adolescent Psychiatry, 38,* 1442–1454.

Husain, S. A. (1990). Current perspective on the role of psychosocial factors in adolescent suicide. *Psychiatric Annals, 20*(3), 122–124.

Imber, S. D., Pilkonis, P. A., & Sotsky, S. M. (1990). Mode-specific effects among three treatments for depression. *Journal of Consulting and Clinical Psychology, 58,* 352–359.

Iwata, N., Turner, R. J., & Lloyd, D. A. (2002). Race/ethnicity and depressive symptoms in community-dwelling young adults: A differential item functioning analysis. *Psychiatry Research, 110,* 281–289.

Jaenicke, C., Hammen, C., Zupan, B., Hiroto, D.,

Gordon, D., Adrian, C., et al. (1987). Cognitive vulnerability in children at risk for depression. *Journal of Abnormal Child Psychology, 15,* 559–572.

Jayson, D., Wood, A., Kroll, L., Fraser, J., & Harrington, R. (1998). Which depressed patients respond to cognitive behavioral treatment? *Journal of the American Academy of Child and Adolescent Psychiatry, 37,* 35–39.

Jensen, J. B., & Garfinkel, B. G. (1990). Growth hormone dysregulation in children with major depressive disorder. *Journal of the American Academy of Child and Adolescent Psychiatry, 29*(2), 295–301.

Jensen, P. S., Ryan, N. D., & Prien, R. (1992). Psychopharmacology of child and adolescent major depression: Present status and future directions. *Journal of Child and Adolescent Psychopharmacology, 2,* 31–45.

Jewell, J., & Stark, K. D. (2003). Comparing the family environments of adolescent with conduct disorder or depression. *Journal of Child and Family Studies, 12,* 77–89.

Kahn, J. S., Kehle, T. J., Jenson, W. R., & Clark, E. (1990). Comparison of cognitive-behavioral relaxation, and self-modeling interventions for depression among middle-school students. *School Psychology Review, 19,* 196–212.

Kandel, D. B., & Davies, M. (1986). Adult sequelae of adolescent depressive symptoms. *Archives of General Psychiatry, 43,* 255–262.

Kashani, J. H., Allan, W. D., Beck, N. C., Bledsoe, Y., & Reid, J. C. (1997). Dysthymic disorder in clinically referred preschool children. *Journal of the American Academy of Child and Adolescent Psychiatry, 36,* 1426–1433.

Kashani, J. H., Barbero, G. J., & Bolander, F. D. (1981). Depression in hospitalized pediatric patients. *Journal of the American Academy of Child Psychiatry, 20,* 123–134.

Kashani, J. H., & Carlson, G. A. (1987). Seriously depressed preschoolers. *American Journal of Psychiatry, 144,* 348–350.

Kashani, J. H., Carlson, G. A., Beck, N. C., Hoeber, E. W., Corcoran, C. M., McAllister, J. A., et al. (1987). Depression, depressive symptoms, and depressed mood among a community sample of adolescents. *American Journal of Psychiatry, 144,* 931–934.

Kashani, J. H., & Hakami, N. (1982). Depression in children and adolescents with malignancy. *Canadian Journal of Psychiatry, 27,* 474–477.

Kashani, J. H., McGee, R., O., Clarkson, S. E., Anderson, J. C., Walton, L. A., Williams, S., et al. (1983). Depression in a sample of 9-year-old children: Prevalence and associated characteristics. *Archives of General Psychiatry, 40,* 1217–1223.

Kashani, J. H., Orvaschel, H., Rosenberg, T. K., & Reid, J. C. (1989). Psychopathology in a community sample of children and adolescents: A developmental perspective. *Journal of the American Academy of Child and Adolescent Psychiatry, 28,* 701–706.

Kashani, J. H., & Ray, J. S. (1983). Depressive related symptoms among preschool-age children. *Child Psychiatry and Human Development, 13,* 233–238.

Kashani, J. H., Ray, J. S., & Carlson, G. A. (1984). Depression and depressive-like states in preschool-age children in a child development unit. *American Journal of Psychiatry, 141,* 1397–1402.

Kashani, J. H., Venzke, R., & Millar, E. A. (1981). Depression in children admitted to hospital for orthopaedic procedures. *British Journal of Psychiatry, 138,* 21–25.

Kaufman, J. (1991). Depressive disorders in maltreated children. *Journal of the American Academy of Child and Adolescent Psychiatry, 30,* 257–265.

Kaufman, J., Birmaher, B., Perel, J., Dahl, R. E., Moreci, P., Nelson, B., et al. (1997). The corticotrophin-releasing hormone challenge in depressed abused, depressed nonabused, and normal control children. *Biological Psychiatry, 42,* 669–679.

Kaufman, J., Birmaher, B., Perel, J., Dahl, R. E., Stull, S., Brent, D., et al. (1998). Sertonergic functioning in depressed abused children: Clinical and familial correlates. *Biological Psychiatry, 44,* 973–981.

Kaufman, J., & Charney, D. (2001). Effects of early stress on brain structure and function: Implications for understanding the relationship between child maltreatment and depression. *Development and Psychopathology, 13,* 451–471.

Kavanagh, K., & Hops, H. (1994). Good girls? Bad boys?: Gender and development as contexts for diagnosis and treatment. *Advances in Clinical Child Psychology, 16,* 45–79.

Kazdin, A. (2000). Developing a research agenda for child and adolescent psychotherapy. *Archives of General Psychiatry, 57,* 829 835.

Kazdin, A. E., & Weisz, J. R. (1998). Identifying and developing empirically supported child and adolescent treatments. *Journal of Consulting and Clinical Psychology, 66,* 19–36.

Keller, M. B., Beardslee, W., Lavori, P. W., Wunder, J., Dorer, D. L., & Samuelson, H. (1988). Course of major depression in non-referred adolescents: A retrospective study. *Journal of Affective Disorders, 15,* 235–243.

Kendall, P. C. (2000). Round of applause for an agenda and regular report cards for child and adolescent psychotherapy research. *Archives of General Psychiatry, 57,* 839–840.

Kendall, P. C., & Braswell, L. (1993). *Cognitive-behavioral therapy for impulsive children* (2nd ed.). New York: Guilford Press.

Kendall, P. C., Cantwell, D. P., & Kazdin, A. E. (1989). Depression in children and adolescents: Assessment issues and recommendations. *Cognitive Therapy and Research, 13,* 109–146.

Kendall, P. C., & Ingram, R. (1987). The future for cognitive assessment of anxiety: Let's get specific. In L. Michelson & L. M. Ascher (Eds.), *Anxiety and stress disorders: Cognitive-behavioral assessment and treatment* (pp. 89–104). New York: Guilford Press.

Kendall, P. C., Stark, K. D., & Adam, T. (1990). Cognitive deficit or cognitive distortion in childhood depression. *Journal of Abnormal Child Psychology, 18,* 255–270.

Kennedy, S. H., Evans, K. R., Kruger, S., Mayberg, H. S., Meyer, J. H., McCann, S., et al. (2001). Changes in regional brain glucose metabolism measured with positron emission tomography after paroxetine treatment of major depression. *American Journal of Psychiatry, 158,* 899–905.

Ketter, T. A., Kimbrell, T. A., George, M. S., Willis, M. W., Benson, B. E., Danielson, A., et al. (1999). Baseline cerebral hypermetabolism associated with carbamazepine response, and hypometabolism with nimodipine response in mood disorders. *Biological Psychiatry, 46,* 1346–1374.

Klaassen, T., Riedel, W. J., van Someren, A., Honig, A., & van Praag, H. M. (1999). Mood effects of 24-hour tryptophan depletion in healthy first-degree relatives of patients with affective disorders. *Biological Psychiatry, 46,* 489–497.

Kobak, R., Sudler, N., & Gamble, W. (1991). Attachment and depressive symptoms during adolescence: A developmental pathways analysis. *Development and Psychopathology, 3,* 461–474.

Kolko, D. J., Brent, D. A., Baugher, M., Bridge, J., & Birmaher, B. (2000). Cognitive and family therapies for adolescent depression: Treatment specificity, mediation, and moderation. *Journal of Consulting and Clinical Psychology, 68,* 603–614.

Kostanski, M., & Gullone, E. (1998). Adolescent body image dissatisfaction: Relationships with self-esteem, anxiety, and depression controlling for body mass. *Journal of Child Psychology and Psychiatry, 39,* 255–262.

Kovacs, M. (1981). Rating scales to assess depression in school aged children. *Acta Paedopsychiatrica, 46,* 305–315.

Kovacs, M. (1990). Comorbid anxiety disorders in childhood-onset depressions. In J. D. Maser & R. C. Cloninger (Eds.), *Comorbidity of mood and anxiety disorders* (pp. 271–281). Washington, DC: American Psychiatric Association.

Kovacs, M. (1996a). The course of childhood onset depressive disorder. *Psychiatric Annals, 26,* 326–330.

Kovacs, M. (1996b). Presentation and course of major depressive disorder during childhood and later years of the life span. *Journal of the American Academy of Child and Adolescent Psychiatry, 35,* 705–715.

Kovacs, M. (2001). Gender and the course of major depressive disorder through adolescence in clinically referred youngsters. *Journal of the American Academy of Child and Adolescent Psychiatry, 40,* 1079–1085.

Kovacs, M., Feinberg, T. L., Crouse-Novak, M. A., Paulauskas, S. L., & Finkelstein, R. (1984). Depressive disorders in childhood: I. A longitudinal prospective study of characteristics and recovery. *Archives of General Psychiatry, 41,* 229–237.

Kovacs, M., Gatsonis, C., Paulauskas, S. L., & Richards, C. (1989). Depressive disorders in childhood: IV. A longitudinal study of comorbidity with and risk

for anxiety disorders. *Archives of General Psychiatry, 46,* 776–782.

Kovacs, M., Goldston, D., & Gatsonis, C. (1993). Suicidal behaviors and childhood-onset depressive disorders: A longitudinal investigation. *Journal of the American Academy of Child and Adolescent Psychiatry, 32,* 8–20.

Kovacs, M., Obrosky, D. S., & Sherrill, J. (2003). Developmental changes in the phenomenology of depression in girls compared to boys from childhood onward. *Journal of Affective Disorders, 74,* 33–48.

Kovacs, M., Obrosky, S. Gatsonis, C., & Richards, C. (1997). First-episode major depressive and dysthymic disorder in childhood: Clinical and sociodemographic factors in recovery. *Journal of the American Academy of Child and Adolescent Psychiatry, 36,* 777–785.

Kraemer, H. C., Wilson, G. T., Fairburn, C. G., & Agras, W. S. (2002). Mediators and moderators of treatment effects in randomized clinical trials. *Archives of General Psychiatry, 59,* 877–883.

Kroll, L., Harrington, R., Jayson, D., Fraser, J., & Gowers, S. (1996). Pilot study of continuation cognitive-behavioral therapy for major depression in adolescent psychiatric patients. *Journal of the American Academy of Child and Adolescent Psychiatry, 35,* 1156–1161.

Kutcher, S. P., Malkin, D., Silverberg, J., Marton, P., Williamson, P., Malkin, A., et al. (1991). Nocturnal cortisol, thyroid stimulating hormone, and growth hormone secretory profiles in depressed adolescents. *Journal of the American Academy of Child and Adolescent Psychiatry, 30,* 407–414.

Kutcher, S. P., Williamson, P., Silverberg, J., Marton, P., Malkin, D., & Malkin, A. (1988). Nocturnal growth hormone secretion in depressed older adolescents. *Journal of the American Academy of Child and Adolescent Psychiatry, 27,* 751–754.

Leonard, B. E. (2000). Evidence for a biochemical lesion in depression. *Journal of Clinical Psychiatry, 61*(Suppl. 6), 12–17.

Lewinsohn, P. M., Clarke, G. N., Hops, H., & Andrews, J. (1990). Cognitive-behavioral treatment for depressed adolescents. *Behavior Therapy, 21,* 385–401.

Lewinsohn, P. M., Hoberman, H. M., & Rosenbaum, M. (1988). A prospective study of risk factors for unipolar depression. *Journal of Abnormal Psychology, 97,* 251–264.

Lewinsohn, P. M., Hops, H., Roberts, R. E., Seeley, J. R., & Andrews, J. A. (1993). Adolescent psychopathology: I. Prevalence and incidence of depression and other DSM-III-R disorders in high school students. *Journal of Abnormal Psychology, 102,* 133–144.

Lewinsohn, P. M., Rohde, P., Klein, D. N., & Seeley, J. R. (1999). Natural course of adolescent major depressive disorder: I. Continuity into young adulthood. *Journal of the American Academy of Child and Adolescent Psychiatry, 38,* 56–63.

Lewinsohn, P. M., Rohde, P., Seeley, J. R., & Fischer, S. A. (1993). Age-cohort changes in the lifetime occurrence of depression and other mental disorders. *Journal of Abnormal Psychology, 102,* 110–120.

Lewinsohn, P. M., Rohde, P., Seeley, J. R., Klein, D. N., & Gotlib, I. H. (2003). Psychosocial functioning of young adults who have experienced and recovered from major depressive disorder during adolescence. *Journal of Abnormal Psychology, 112,* 353–363.

Liddle, B., & Spence, S. H. (1990). Cognitive-behaviour therapy with depressed primary school children: A cautionary note. *Behavioural Psychotherapy, 18,* 85–102.

Ling, W., Oftedal, G., & Weinberg, W. (1970). Depressive illness in childhood presenting as severe headache. *American Journal of Diseases of Children, 120,* 122–124.

Lobovits, D. A., & Handal, P. J. (1985). Childhood depression: Prevalence using DSM-III criteria and validity of parent and child depression scales. *Journal of Pediatric Psychology, 10,* 45–54.

Lochman, J. E. (2001). Issues in prevention with school-aged children: Ongoing intervention refinement, developmental theory, prediction and moderation, and implementation and dissemination. *Prevention and Treatment, 4.*

Luby, J. L., Heffelfinger, A. K., Mrakotsky, C., Brown, K. M., Hessler, M. J., Wallis, J. M., et al. (2003). The clinical picture of depression in preschool children. *Journal of the American Academy of Child and Adolescent Psychiatry, 42,* 340–349.

Luby, J. L., Heffelfinger, A. K., Mrakotsky, C., Hessler, M. J., Brown, K., & Heldebrand, T. (2002). Preschool major depressive disorder (MDD): Preliminary validation for developmentally modified DSM-IV criteria. *Journal of the American Academy of Child and Adolescent Psychiatry, 41,* 928–937.

MacMillan, S., Szeszko, P. R., Moore, G. J., Madden, R., Lorch, E., Ivey, J., et al. (2003). Increased amygdala: Hippocampal volume ratios associated with severity of anxiety in pediatric major depression. *Journal of Child and Adolescent Psychopharmacology, 13,* 65–73.

Madoki, M. W., Tapia, M. R., Tapia, M. A., & Sumner, G. S. (1997). Venlafaxine in the treatment of children and adolescents with major depression. *Psychopharmacology Bulletin, 33,* 149–154.

Mahoney, M. J. (1982). *Cognition and behavior modification.* Cambridge, MA: Ballinger.

March, J. S. (2004). The Treatment for Adolescents with Depression Study (TADS): Short-term effectiveness and safety outcomes. *Journal of the American Medical Association, 292,* 807–820.

March, J. S., Leonard, H. L., & Swedo, S. E. (1995). Pharmacotherapy of obsessive–compulsive disorder. *Child and Adolescent Psychiatric Clinics of North America, 4,* 217–236.

March, J. S., & Mulle, K. (1998). *OCD in children and adolescents: A cognitive-behavioral treatment manual.* New York: Guilford Press.

Marcotte, D., Alain, M., & Gosselin, M. (1999). Gender differences in adolescent depression: Gender-typed characteristics or problem-solving skills deficits? *Sex Roles, 41,* 31–48.

Mattison, R. E., Humphrey, J., Kales, S., Hernit, R., & Finkenbinder, R. (1986). Psychiatric background of diagnosis of children evaluated for special class placement. *Journal of Child Psychiatry, 46,* 1142–1147.

Mayberg, H. S. (2003). Modulating dysfunctional limbic–cortical circuits in depression: Towards development of brain-based algorithms for diagnosis and optimized treatment. *British Medical Bulletin, 54,* 193–207.

Mayberg, H. S., Brannan, S. K., Mahurin, R. K., Jerabek, P. A., Brickman, J. S., Tekell, J. L., et al. (1997). Cingulate function in depression: A potential predictor of treatment response. *NeuroReport, 8,* 1057–1061.

Mayberg, H. S., Liotti, M., Brannan, S. K., McGinnis, S., Mahurin, R. K., Jerabek, P. A., et al. (1999). Reciprocal limbic–cortical function and negative mood: Converging PET findings in depression and normal sadness. *American Journal of Psychiatry, 156,* 675–682.

McCauley, E., Myers, K., Mitchell, J., Calderon, R., Schloredt, K., & Treder, R. (1993). Depression in young people: Initial presentation and clinical course. *Journal of the American Academy of Child and Adolescent Psychiatry, 29,* 611–619.

McGee, R., Feehan, M., Williams, S., Partridge, F., Silva, P. A., & Kelly, J. (1990). DSM-III disorders in a large sample of adolescents. *Journal of the American Academy of Child and Adolescent Psychiatry, 29,* 611–619.

McGee, R., & Williams, S. (1988). A longitudinal study of depression in nine year old children. *Journal of the American Academy of Child and Adolescent Psychiatry, 27,* 12–20.

Meichenbaum, D. (1977). *Cognitive behavior modification.* New York: Plenum Press.

Mervalla, E., Fohr, J., Kononen, M., Valkonen-Korhonen, M., Vainio, P., Partanen, K., et al. (2000). Quantitative MRI of the hippocampus and amygdale in severe depression. *Psychological Medicine, 30,* 117–125.

Messer, S. C., & Gross, A. M. (1995). Childhood depression and family interaction: A naturalistic observation study. *Journal of Clinical Child Psychology, 24,* 77–88.

Michael, K. D., & Crowley, S. L. (2002). How effective are treatments for child and adolescent depression?: A meta-analytic review. *Clinical Psychology Review, 22,* 247–269.

Midgley, C., Feldlaufer, H., & Eccles, J. S. (1989). Student/teacher relations and attitudes toward mathematics before and after the transition to junior high school. *Child Development, 60,* 981–992.

Miller, L., & Gur, M. (2002). Religiosity, depression, and physical maturation in adolescent girls. *Journal of the American Academy of Child and Adolescent Psychiatry, 41,* 206–214.

Mitchell, J., McCauley, E., Burke, P. M., & Moss, S. J. (1988). Phenomenology of depression in children and adolescents. *Journal of the American Academy of Child and Adolescent Psychiatry, 27,* 12–20.

Moore, P., Gillin, C., Bhatti, T., DeModena, A., Seifritz, E., Clark, C., et al. (1998). Rapid tryptophan depletion, sleep electrocephalogram, and mood in men with remitted depression on serotonin reuptake inhibitors. *Archives of General Psychiatry, 55,* 534–539.

Moran, P. B., & Eckenrode, J. (1991). Gender differences in the costs and benefits of peer relationships during adolescence. *Journal of Adolescent Research, 6,* 396–409.

Moreno, F. A., Gelenberg, A. J., Heninger, G. R., Potter, R. L., McKnight, K. M., Allen, J., et al. (1999). Tryptophan depletion and depressive vulnerability. *Biological Psychiatry, 46,* 498–505.

Mrazek, P., & Haggerty, R. (Eds.). (1994). *Reducing risks for mental disorders: Frontiers for preventive intervention research.* Washington, DC: National Academy Press.

Mufson, L., & Fairbanks, J. (1996). Interpersonal psychotherapy for depressed adolescents: a one-year naturalistic follow-up study. *Journal of the American Academy of Child and Adolescent Psychiatry, 35,* 1145–1155.

Mufson, L., Moreau, D., Weissman, M. M., & Garfinkel, R. (1999). Efficacy of interpersonal psychotherapy for depressed adolescents. *Archives of General Psychiatry, 56,* 573–579.

Mufson, L., Moreau, D., Weissman, M. M., Wickramartne, P., Martin, J., & Samoilov, A. (1994). Modification of interpersonal psychotherapy with depressed adolescents (IPT-A): Phase I and II studies. *Journal of the American Academy of Child and Adolescent Psychiatry, 33,* 695–705.

Mufson, L., Pollack Dorta, K., Wickramaratne, P., Nomura, Y., Olfson, M., & Weissman, M. (2004). A randomized effectiveness trial of interpersonal psychotherapy for depressed adolescents. *Archives of General Psychiatry, 61,* 577–584.

Munoz, R. F., Penilla, C., & Urizar, G. (2002). Expanding depression prevention research with children of diverse cultures. *Prevention and Treatment, 5,* Article 13. Retrieved from http://journals.apa.org/prevention/volume5/pre0050013c.html

Murray, C., & Greenberg, M. T. (2000). Children's relationship with teachers and bonds with school: An investigation of patterns and correlates in middle childhood. *Journal of School Psychology, 38,* 423–445.

Nemeroff, C. B. (1996). The corticotrophin-releasing factor (CRF) hypothesis of depression: New findings and new directions. *Molecular Psychiatry, 1,* 336–342.

Nemeroff, C. B. (1998). The neurobiology of depression. *Scientific American, 278,* 42–49.

Newman, D. L., Moffitt, T. E., Caspi, A., Magdol, L., Silva, P. A., & Stanton, W. R. (1996). Psychiatric disorder in a birth cohort of young adults: Prevalence, comorbidity, clinical significance, and new case incidence from ages 11 to 21. *Journal of Consulting and Clinical Psychology, 64,* 552–562.

Nolen-Hoeksema, S. (1987). Sex differences in unipolar depression: Evidence and theory. *Psychological Bulletin, 101,* 259–282.

Nolen-Hoeksema, S., & Girgus, J. S. (1994). The emergence of gender differences in depression during adolescence. *Psychological Bulletin, 115,* 424–443.

Nolen-Hoeksema, S., Girgus, J. S., & Seligman, M. E. P. (1991). Sex differences in depression and explanatory style in children. *Journal of Youth and Adolescence, 20,* 233–245.

Olfson, M., Gameroff, M. J., Marcus, S. C., & Waslick, B. D. (2003). Outpatient treatment of child and adolescent depression in the United States. *Archives of General Psychiatry, 60,* 1236–1242.

Olsson, G. I., & von Knorring, A. L. (1999). Adolescent depression: prevalence in Swedish high-school students. *Acta Psychiatrica Scandinavica, 99,* 324–331.

Olvera, R. L. (2001). Suicidal ideation in Hispanic and mixed-ancestry adolescents. *Suicide and Life-Threatening Behavior, 31,* 416–427.

Ongur, D., Drevets, W. C., & Price, J. L. (1998). Glial reduction in the subgenual prefrontal cortex in mood disorders. *Proceedings of the National Academy of Sciences USA, 95,* 13290–13295.

Orvaschel, H., & Puig-Antich, J. H. (1994). *Schedule for Affective Disorders and Schizophrenia for School-Age Children (Epidemiologic version)* (5th ed.). Pittsburgh, PA: Western Psychiatric Institute and Clinic.

Orvaschel, H., Weissman, M. M., & Kidd, K. K. (1980). Children and depression. *Journal of Affective Disorders, 2,* 1–16.

Ostrov, E., Offer, D., & Howard, K. I. (1989). Gender differences in adolescent symptomatology: A normative study. *Journal of the American Academy of Child and Adolescent Psychiatry, 28,* 394–398.

Parker, K. J., Schatzberg, A. F., & Lyons, D. M. (2003). Neuroendocrine aspects of hypercortisolism in major depression. *Hormones and Behavior, 43,* 60–66.

Petersen, A. C., Compas, B. E., Brooks-Gunn, J., Stemmler, M., Ey, S., & Grant, K. E. (1993). Depression in adolescence. *American Psychologist, 48,* 155–168.

Petersen, A. C., Sarigiani, P. A., & Kennedy, R. E. (1991). Adolescent depression: Why more girls? *Journal of Youth and Adolescence, 20,* 247–271.

Pianta, R. C. (1994). Patterns of relationships between children and kindergarten teachers. *Journal of School Psychology, 32,* 15–31.

Pine, D. S. (2002) Treating children and adolescents with selective serotonin reuptake inhibitors: How long is appropriate? *Journal of Child and Adolescent Psychopharmacology, 12,* 189–203.

Pine, D. S., Cohen, P., Gurley, D., Brook, J., & Ma, Y. (1998). The risk for early-adulthood anxiety and depressive disorders in adolescents with anxiety and depressive disorders. *Archives of General Psychiatry, 55,* 56–64.

Pizzagalli, D., Pascual-Marqui, R., Nitschke, J. B., Oakes, T. R., Larson, C. L., Abercrombie, H. C., et al. (2001). Anterior cingulate activity as a predictor of degree of treatment response in major depression: Evidence from brain electrical tomography analysis. *American Journal of Psychiatry, 158,* 405–415.

Polaino-Lorente, A., & Domenech, E. (1993). Prevalence of childhood depression: Results of the first study in Spain. *Journal of Child Psychology and Psychiatry, 34,* 1007–1017.

Posener, J., Wang, L., Price, J. L., Gado, M. H., Provin, M. A., Miller, M. I., et al. (2003). High-dimensional mapping of the hippocampus in depression. *American Journal of Psychiatry, 160,* 83–89.

Poznanski, E. O., & Mokros, H. B. (1994). Phenomenology and epidemiology of mood disorders in children and adolescents. In W. M. Reynolds & H. F. Johnston (Eds.), *Handbook of depression in children and adolescents* (pp. 19–39). New York: Plenum Press.

Priel, B., & Shamai, D. (1995). Attachment style and perceived social support: Effects on affect regulation. *Personality and Individual Differences, 19,* 235–241.

Prieto, S. L., Cole, D. A., & Tageson, C. W. (1992). Depressive self-schemas in clinic and nonclinic children. *Cognitive Therapy and Research, 16,* 521–534.

Prinstein, M., Boergers, J., & Vernberg, E. (2001). Overt and relational aggression in adolescents: Social-psychological adjustment of aggressors and victims. *Journal of Clinical Child Psychology, 30,* 479–491.

Puig-Antich, J., Dahl, R. E., Ryan, N., Novacenko, H., Goetz, D., Goetz, R., et al. (1989). Cortisol secretion in prepubertal children with major depressive disorder: Episode and recovery. *Archives of General Psychiatry, 46,* 801–808.

Puig-Antich, J., & Gittleman, R. (1982). Depression in childhood and adolescence. In E. Paykel (Ed.), *Handbook of affective disorders* (pp. 379–392). New York: Guilford Press.

Puig-Antich, J., Lukens, E., Davies, M., Goetz, D., Brennan-Quattrock, J., & Todak, G. (1985a). Psychosocial functioning in prepubertal major depressive disorders: I. Interpersonal relationships during the depressive episode. *Archives of General Psychiatry, 42,* 500–507.

Puig-Antich, J., Lukens, E., Davies, M., Goetz, D., Brennan-Quattrock, J., & Todak, G. (1985b). Psychosocial functioning in prepubertal major depressive disorders: II. Interpersonal relationships after sustained recovery from affective episode. *Archives of General Psychiatry, 42,* 511–517.

Quintin, P., Benkelfat, C., & Launay, J. M. (2001). Clinical and neurochemical effect of acute tryptophan depletion in unaffected relatives of patients with bipolar affective disorder. *Biological Psychiatry, 50,* 184–190.

Reddy, R., Rhodes, J. E., & Mulhall, P. (2003). The influence of teacher support on student adjustment in the middle school years: A latent growth curve study. *Development and Psychopathology, 15,* 119–138.

Reinecke, M. A., Ryan, N. E., & DuBois, D. L. (1998). Cognitive-behavioral therapy of depression and depressive symptoms during adolescence: A review and meta-analysis. *Journal of the American Academy of Child and Adolescent Psychiatry, 37,* 26–34.

Reynolds, W. M., & Coats, K. I. (1986). A comparison of cognitive-behavioral therapy and relaxation training for the treatment of depression in adolescents. *Journal of Consulting and Clinical Psychology, 54,* 653–660.

Richards, M. H., Boxer, A. M., Petersen, A. C., & Albrecht, R. (1990). Relation of weight to body image in pubertal girls and boys from two communities. *Developmental Psychology, 26,* 313–321.

Roberts, R. E., Roberts, C. R., & Chen, Y. R. (1997). Ethnocultural differences in prevalence of adolescent depression. *American Journal of Community Psychology, 25,* 95–110.

Roeser, R. W., Midgley, C., & Urdan, T. C. (1996). Perceptions of the school psychological environment and early adolescents' psychological and behavioral functioning in school: The mediating role of goals and belonging. *Journal of Educational Psychology, 88,* 408–422.

Rohde, P., Clarke, G. N., & Lewinsohn, P. M. (2001). Impact of comorbidity on a cognitive-behavioral group treatment for adolescent depression. *Journal of the American Academy of Child and Adolescent Psychiatry, 40,* 795–802.

Rohde, P., Lewinsohn, P. M., & Seeley, J. R. (1991). Comorbidity of unipolar depression: II. Comorbidity with other mental disorders in adolescents and adults. *Journal of Abnormal Psychology, 100,* 214–222.

Rosenstein, D. S., & Horowitz, H. A. (1996). Adolescent attachment and psychopathology. *Journal of Consulting and Clinical Psychology, 64,* 244–253.

Rossello, J., & Bernal, G. (1999). The efficacy of cognitive-behavioral and interpersonal treatments for depression in Puerto Rican adolescents. *Journal of Consulting and Clinical Psychology, 67,* 734–745.

Rudolph, K. D., & Hammen, C. (1999). Age and gender as determinants of stress exposure, generation, and reactions in youngsters: A transactional perspective. *Child Development, 70,* 660–677.

Rudolph, K. D., Hammen, C., & Burge, D. (1995). Cognitive representations of self, family, and peers in school-age children: Links with social competence and sociometric status. *Child Development, 66,* 1385–1402.

Rudolph, K. D., Hammen, C., Burge, D., Lindberg, N., Herzberg, D., & Daley, S. E. (2000). Toward an interpersonal life-stress model of depression: The developmental context of stress generation. *Development and Psychopathology, 12,* 215–234.

Rushton, J. L., Forcier, M., & Schectman, R. M. (2003). Epidemiology of depressive symptoms in the national longitudinal study of adolescent health. *Journal of the American Academy of Child and Adolescent Psychiatry, 41,* 199–205.

Ryan, N. D., Dahl, R. E., Birmaher, B., Williamson, D. E., Iyengar, S., Nelson, B., et al. (1994). Stimulatory tests of growth hormone secretion in prepubertal major depression: Depressed versus normal children. *American Journal of Child and Adolescent Psychiatry, 33,* 824–833.

Ryan, N. D., Puig-Antich, J., Ambrosinin, P., Rabinovich, H., Robinson, D., Nelson, B., et al. (1987). The clinical picture of major depression in children and adolescents. *Archives of General Psychology, 44,* 854–861.

Ryan, R. M., & Grolnick, W. S. (1986). Personality processes and individual differences. *Journal of Personality and Social Psychology, 50,* 550–558.

Sander, A. J. B. (2001). Toward an integration of Beck's cognitive theory and Bowlby's attachment theory: Self-schema and adult attachment classification in relation to depressive symptoms (Doctoral dissertation, University of Texas at Austin, 2001). *Dissertation Abstracts International, 62,* 4060B.

Sanford, M., Szatmari, P., Spinner, M., Munroe-Blum, H., Jamieson, E., Walsh, C., et al. (1995). Predicting the one-year course of adolescent major depression. *Journal of the American Academy of Child and Adolescent Psychiatry, 34,* 1618–1628.

Santor, D. A., & Kusumakar, V. (2001). Open trial of interpersonal therapy in adolescents with moderate to severe major depression: Effectiveness of novice IPT therapists. *Journal of the American Academy of Child and Adolescent Psychiatry, 40,* 236–240.

Schmidt, K. L., Stark, K. D., Carlson, C. L., & Anthony, B. J. (1998). Cognitive factors differentiating attention-deficit-hyperactivity disorder with and without a co-morbid mood disorder. *Journal of Consulting and Clinical Psychology, 66,* 673–679.

Schraedley, P. K., Gotlib, I. H., & Hayward, C. (1999). Gender differences in the correlates of depressive symptoms in adolescents. *Journal of Adolescent Health, 25,* 98–108.

Schwartz, J. M., Stoessel, P. W., Baxter, L. R., Martin, K. M., & Phelps, M. E., (1996). Systematic changes in cerebral glucose metabolic rate after successful behavior modification treatment of obsessive–compulsive disorder. *Archives of General Psychiatry, 53,* 109–113.

Shah, P., Ebmeier, K. P., Glabus, M. F., & Goodwin, G. M. (1998). Cortical grey matter reduction associated with treatment-resistant chronic unipolar depression. *British Journal of Psychiatry, 172,* 527–532.

Sheeber, L., Hops, H., Alpert, A., Davis, B., & Andrews, J. (1997). Family support and conflict: Prospective relations to adolescent depression. *Journal of Abnormal Child Psychology, 25,* 333–344.

Sheeber, L., & Sorensen, E. (1998). Family relationships of depressed adolescents: A multimethod assessment. *Journal of Clinical Child Psychology, 27,* 268–277.

Sheline, Y., Barch, D. M., Donnelly, J. M., Ollinger, J.

M., Synder, A. Z., & Mintun, M. A. (2001). Increased amygdala response to masked emotional faces in depressed subjects resolves with antidepressant treatment: An fMRI study. *Biological Psychiatry, 50,* 651–658.

Sheline, Y., Gado, M. H., & Kraemer, H. C. (2003). Untreated depression and hippocampal volume loss. *American Journal of Psychiatry, 160,* 1–3.

Sheline, Y., Sanghavi, M., Mintun, M. A., & Gado, M. H. (1999). Depression duration but not age predicts hippocampal volume loss in medically healthy women with recurrent major depression. *Journal of Neuroscience, 19,* 5034–5043.

Sheline, Y., Wang, P., Gado, M., Csernansky, J., & Vannier, M. (1996). Hippocampal atrophy in major depression. *Proceedings of the National Academy of Sciences USA, 93,* 3908–3913.

Shelton, R. C. (2000). Cellular mechanisms in the vulnerability to depression and response to antidepressants. *Psychiatric Clinics of North America, 23,* 713–729.

Shirk, S. R. (1998). Interpersonal schemata in child psychotherapy: A cognitive-interpersonal perspective. *Journal of Clinical Child Psychology, 27,* 4–16.

Siegal, J. M. (2002). Body image change and adolescent depressive symptoms. *Journal of Adolescent Research, 17,* 27–41.

Siegal, J. M., Yancey, A. K., Aneshensel, C. S., & Schuler, R. (1999). Body image, perceived pubertal timing, and adolescent mental health. *Journal of Adolescent Health, 25,* 155–165.

Slee, P. T. (1995). Peer victimization and its relationship to depression among Australian primary school students. *Personality and Individual Differences, 18,* 57–62.

Smith, K. A., Fairburn, C. G., & Cowen, P. J. (1997). Relapse of depression after rapid depletion of tryptophan. *Lancet, 349,* 915–919.

Solomon, J., & George, C. (1999). The measurement of attachment security in infancy and childhood. In J. Cassidy & P. R. Shaver (Eds.), *Handbook of attachment: Theory, research, and clinical applications* (pp. 287–318). New York: Guilford Press.

Speier, P. L., Sherak, D. L., Hirsch, S., & Cantwell, D. P. (1995). Depression in children and adolescents. In E. E. Beckham & W. R. Leber (Eds.), *Handbook of depression* (2nd ed., pp. 467–481). New York: Guilford Press.

Spillmann, M. K., Van der Does, A. J. W., Rankin, M. A., Vuolo, R. D., Alpert, J. E., Nierenberg, A. A., et al. (2001). Tryptophan depletion in SSRI-recovered depressed outpatients. *Psychopharmacology, 155,* 123–127.

Stark, K. D. (1990). *Childhood depression: School-based intervention.* New York: Guilford Press.

Stark, K. D., & Brookman, C. (1992). Childhood depression: Theory and family–school intervention. In M. J. Fine & C. Carlson (Eds.), *Family–school intervention: A systems perspective* (pp. 247–271). Needham Heights, MA: Allyn & Bacon.

Stark, K. D., Humphrey, L. L., Crook, K., & Lewis, K. (1990). Perceived family environments of depressed and anxious children: Child's and maternal figure's perspectives. *Journal of Abnormal Child Psychology, 18, 527–547.*

Stark, K. D., Laurent, J., Livingston, R., Boswell, J., & Swearer, S. (1999). Implications of research for the treatment of depressive disorders during childhood. *Applied and Preventive Psychology, 8, 79–102.*

Stark, K. D., Reynolds, W. M., & Kaslow, N. J. (1987). A comparison of the relative efficacy of self-control therapy and a behavioral problem-solving therapy for depression in children. *Journal of Abnormal Child Psychology, 15, 91–113.*

Stark, K. D., Sander, J. B., Yancy, M. G., Bronik, M. D., & Hoke, J. A. (2000). Treatment of depression in childhood and adolescence: Cognitive-behavioral procedures for the individual and family. In P. C. Kendall (Ed.), *Child and adolescent therapy: Cognitive behavioral procedures* (2nd ed., pp. 173–234). New York: Guilford Press.

Stark, K. D., Schmidt, K., & Joiner, T. E. (1996). Depressive cognitive triad: Relationship to severity of depressive symptoms in children, parents' cognitive triad, and perceived parental messages about the child him or herself, the world, and the future. *Journal of Abnormal Child Psychology, 24, 615–625.*

Stark, K. D., Schnoebelen, S., Simpson, J., Hargrave, J., Glenn, R., & Molnar, J. (2004). *Children's workbook for ACTION.* Broadmore, PA: Workbook.

Stark, K. D., Simpson, J., Schnoebelen, S., Hargrave, J., Glenn, R., & Molnar, J. (2004). *Therapist's manual for ACTION.* Broadmore, PA: Workbook.

Steingard, R. J., Renshaw, P. F., Hennen, J., Lenox, M., Cintron, C. B., Young, A. D., et al. (2002). Smaller frontal lobe white matter volumes in depressed adolescents. *Biological Psychiatry, 52, 413–417.*

Stice, E., & Bearman, S. K. (2001). Body-image and eating disturbances prospectively predict increases in depressive symptoms in adolescent girls: A growth curve analysis. *Developmental Psychology, 37, 597–607.*

Stice, E., Presnell, K., & Bearman, S. K. (2001). Relation of early menarche to depression, eating disorders, substance abuse, and comorbid psychopathology among adolescent girls. *Developmental Psychology, 37, 608–619.*

Strober, M., Lampert, C., Schmidt, S., & Morrell, W. (1993) The course of major depressive disorder in adolescents: I. Recovery and risk of manic switching in a follow-up of psychotic and nonpsychotic subtypes. *Journal of the American Academy of Child and Adolescent Psychiatry, 32, 34–42.*

Turner, J. E., & Cole, D. A. (1994). Developmental differences in cognitive diatheses for child depression. *Journal of Abnormal Child Psychology, 22, 15–32.*

Twenge, J. M., & Nolen-Hoeksema, S. (2002). Age, gender, race, sociometric status, and birth cohort differences on the Children's Depression Inventory: A meta-analysis. *Journal of Abnormal Psychology, 111, 578–588.*

Vakali, K., Pillay, S. S., Lafer, B., Fava, M., Renshaw, P. F., Bonello-Cintron, C. M., et al. (2000). Hippocampal volume in primary unipolar major depression: A mangnetic resonance imaging study. *Biological Psychiatry, 47, 1087–1090.*

Vostanis, P., Feehan, C., Grattan, E., & Bickerton, W. (1996). Treatment for children and adolescents with depression: Lessons from a controlled trial. *Clinical Child Psychology and Psychiatry, 1, 199–212.*

Wade, T. J., Cairney, J., & Pevalin, D. J. (2002). Emergence of gender differences in depression during adolescence: National panel results from three countries. *Journal of the American Academy of Child and Adolescent Psychiatry, 41(2), 190–198.*

Wagner, B. M., & Compas, B. E. (1990). Gender, instrumentality, and expressivity: Moderators of the relation between stress and psychological symptoms during adolescence. *American Journal of Community Psychology, 18, 383–406.*

Wagner, K. D., & Ambrosini, P. J. (2001). Childhood depression: Pharmacological therapy/treatment (Pharmacotherapy of childhood depression). *Journal of Clinical Psychology, 30, 88–97.*

Wagner, K. D., & Ambrosini, P. J. (2003) Efficacy of sertraline in the treatment of children and adolescents with major depressive disorder: Two randomized controlled trials. *Journal of the American Medical Association, 290, 1033–1041.*

Warner, V., Weissman, M. M., Fendrick, M., Wickramaratne, P., & Moreau, D. (1992). The course of major depression in the offspring of depressed parents. *Archives of General Psychiatry, 49, 795–801.*

Weersing, V. R., & Weisz, J. R. (2002). Community clinic treatment of depressed youth: Benchmarking usual care against CBT clinical trials. *Journal of Consulting and Clinical Psychology, 43, 3–29.*

Weinberg, W. A., Rutman, J., Sullivan, L., Penick, E. C., & Dietz, S. G. (1973). Depression in children referred to an educational diagnostic center: Diagnosis and treatment. *Journal of Pediatrics, 83, 1065–1072.*

Weiss, B., Catron, T., Harris, V., & Phung, T. M. (1999). The effectiveness of traditional child psychotherapy. *Journal of Consulting and Clinical Psychology, 67, 82–94.*

Weiss, B., & Garber, J. (2003). Developmental differences in the phenomenology of depression. *Development and Psychopathology, 15, 403–430.*

Weissman, M. M., Gammon, G. D., John, K., Merikangas, K. R., Warner, V., Prusoff, B. A., & Sholomskas, D. (1987). Children of depressed parents: Increased psychopathology and early onset of major depression. *Archives of General Psychiatry, 44, 847–853.*

Weissman, M. M., Wolk, S., Goldstein, R. B., Moreau, D., Adams, P., Greenwald, S., et al. (1999). Depressed adolescents grown-up. *Journal of the American Medical Association, 281*, 1707–1713.

Weisz, J. R. (2000). Agenda for child and adolescent psychotherapy research: On the need to put science into practice. *Archives of General Psychiatry, 57*, 837–838.

Weisz, J. R., & Hawley, K. M. (2002). Developmental factors in the treatment of adolescents. *Journal of Consulting and Clinical Psychology, 70*, 21–43.

Weisz, J. R., Southam-Gerow, M. A., & McCarty, C. A. (2002). Control-related beliefs and depressive symptoms in clinic-referred children and adolescents: Developmental differences and model specificity. *Journal of Abnormal Psychology, 110*, 97–109.

Weisz, J. R., Thurber, C. A., Sweeney, L., Proffitt, V. D., & LeGagnoux, G. L. (1997). Brief treatment of mild-to-moderate child depression using primary and secondary control enhancement training. *Journal of Consulting and Clinical Psychology, 65*, 703–707.

Wells, K. B., Stewart, A., Hays, R. D., Burnam, M. A., Rogers, W., & Daniels, M. (1989). The functioning and well-being of depressed patients: Results from the Medical Outcomes Study. *Journal of the American Medical Association, 262*, 914–919.

Whisman, M. A., & Friedman, M. A. (1998). Interpersonal problem behaviors associated with dysfunctional attitudes. *Cognitive Therapy and Research, 22*, 149–160.

Wilens, T. E., Biederman, J., Geist, D. E., Steingard, R., & Spencer, T. (1993). Nortriptyline in the treatment of attention deficit hyperactivity disorder: A chart review of 58 cases. *Journal of the American Academy of Child and Adolescent Psychiatry, 32*, 343–349.

Wilens, T. E., Biederman, J. B., & Spencer, T. (1995). A systematic assessment of tricyclic antidepressants in the treatment of adult attention-deficit hyperactivity

disorder. *Journal of Nervous and Mental Disease, 183*, 48–50.

Wilens, T. E., Cohen, L., Biederman, J., Abrams, A., Neft, D., Faird, N., et al. (2002). Fluoxetine pharmacokinetics in pediatric patients. *Journal of Clinical Psychopharmacology, 22*, 569–575.

Wilens, T. E., Spencer, T. J., Biederman, J., & Schleifer, D. (1997). Cases study: Nefazodone for juvenile mood disorders. *Journal of the American Academy of Child and Adolescent Psychiatry, 36*, 481–485.

Williamson, D. E., Birmaher, B., Dahl, R. E., Al-Shabbout, M., & Ryan, N. D. (1996). Stressful life events influence nocturnal growth hormone secretion in depressed children. *Biological Psychiatry, 40*, 1176–1180.

Wood, A., Harrington, R., & Moore, A. (1996). Controlled trial of a brief cognitive-behavioural intervention in adolescent patients with depressive disorders. *Journal of Child Psychiatry, 37*, 737–746.

Young, J. E. (1991). *Cognitive therapy for personality disorders: A schema-focused approach.* Sarasota, FL: Professional Resource Exchange.

Young, J. E., & Lindemann, M. D. (1992). An integrative schema-focused model for personality disorders. *Journal of Cognitive Psychotherapy: An International Quarterly, 6*, 11–23.

Zito, J. M., Safer, D. J., DosReis, S., & Riddle, M. A. (1998). Racial disparity in psychotropic medications prescribed for youths with Medicaid insurance in Maryland. *Journal of the American Academy of Child and Adolescent Psychiatry, 37*, 179–184.

Zupan, B. A., Hammen, C., & Jaenicke, C. (1987). The effects of current mood and prior depressive history on self-schematic processing in children. *Journal of Experimental Child Psychology, 43*, 149–158.

IV

DEVELOPMENTAL DISORDERS

Mental Retardation

Benjamin L. Handen and Richard H. Gilchrist

Efforts to provide educational and psychological treatment for children and adults with mental retardation have an extensive history. In modern times, such attempts can be dated back to the work of Edouard Seguin in 19th-century France, who led a movement emphasizing that individuals with a variety of disabling conditions could be taught if provided appropriate training. By the middle of the 19th century, this movement had taken root in the United States and led to the establishment of a number of schools for children and adults with mental retardation. These early institutions were based on the principle of "moral education"—that is, the assumption that through appropriate education, individuals with mental retardation could be elevated to a level of "normal" human existence. Yet by the turn of the century it became apparent that this experiment had been a failure, and that only a small percentage of individuals with mental retardation were able to return successfully to society and independent living situations. Gradually, institutions began to change in character, serving less of an educational and more of a custodial role. Rather than educating individuals with mental retardation, the institutions served to protect individuals with mental retardation from society (Wolfensberger, 1969).

Over a century later, we once again find ourselves in a period when there is considerable optimism regarding treatment options for individuals with mental retardation. The deinstitutionalization movement of the 1960s, several court cases, and the passing of state and federal mandates for the provision of services to pre-schoolers and school-age children with mental retardation in the 1970s and 1980s all brought about considerable change in the service delivery system for this population. This spurred the growth of the inclusion movement of the 1990s, which renewed the promise of full participation for individuals with mental retardation in our schools and communities.

As we enter the early part of the 21st century, treatment efforts have been focused in a wide range of areas. Many interventions have been directed toward children with mental retardation, while others have emphasized the provision of services to families or teachers of such children. Some novel efforts have been directed toward changing communities themselves. The present chapter addresses several specific types of child-focused interventions, including educational efforts and the management of behavior problems (including specific behavioral interventions and treatment of behavioral disorders that are more often seen in children with mental retardation than in the general population). In addition, parent training and community-based interventions are covered. Finally, the chapter examines psychopharmacological interventions and future directions.

DEFINITION AND CLASSIFICATION OF MENTAL RETARDATION

The definition of "mental retardation" has been revised a number of times during the past five decades, most recently in 2002. The

411

American Association on Mental Retardation (AAMR) currently defines the term as follows: "Mental retardation is a disability characterized by significant limitations both in intellectual functioning and in adaptive behavior as expressed in conceptual, social, and practical adaptive skills. This disability originates before age 18" (2002, p. 1). The refinements to this definition have been made in direct response to our changing understanding of the disorder and to various consumer, professional, political, and social forces.

For example, in 1959 the American Association on Mental Deficiency (AAMD), as the AAMR was then called, specified that individuals with IQ scores 1 standard deviation or more below the mean of 100 were to be considered to have mental retardation (Heber, 1959). Because most IQ tests had a mean of 100 and a standard deviation of 15–16 points, this affected a significant portion of the U.S. adult and child population (up to 16%, or 32 million people). In 1973, the cutoff point was changed to 2 standard deviations below the mean (IQ below 70), thereby lowering the incidence of mental retardation to about 3%, or 6 million individuals (Grossman, 1973). A further revision of the definition in 1983 provided greater clarity for clinicians working in the field: "Mental retardation refers to significantly subaverage intellectual functioning resulting in or associated with impairments in adaptive behavior and manifested during the developmental period" (Grossman, 1983, p. 11). Three specific factors were involved in this definition: (1) IQ score below 70, (2) associated adaptive deficits, and (3) the occurrence of deficits prior to age 18. Even this definition was not without some controversy, however, due to disagreement among professionals regarding both the definition of adaptive behavior as well as how to assess it (Zigler & Hodapp, 1986).

The 1992 AAMR Definition

In 1992, the AAMR proposed and adopted a new definition of mental retardation, which read as follows:

> Mental retardation refers to substantial limitations in present functioning. It is characterized by significantly subaverage intellectual functioning, existing concurrently with related limitations in two or more of the following applicable adaptive skills areas: communication, self-care, home liv-

ing, social skills, community use, self-direction, health and safety, functional academics, leisure, and work. Mental retardation manifests before age 18. (AAMR, 1992, p. 5)

Three aspects of this new definition were especially controversial. First, the IQ range had once again been changed to include individuals with an IQ standard score of approximately 70–75 or below. Second, there was a requirement that up to 10 areas of adaptive functioning be assessed; however, there continued to be no agreed-upon parameters for assessing adaptive behavior in a number of these areas (MacMillan, Gresham, & Siperstein, 1995). Finally, the AAMR eliminated the previously used classification system that divided individuals with mental retardation into four categories, based on level of cognitive functioning. These changes are discussed in greater detail below.

Classification Systems

Various classification systems have been developed for individuals with mental retardation during the past several decades. Such systems are needed because of the heterogeneity of this population. They serve as means of distinguishing among subgroups, which enable clinicians to determine the level and intensity of required services and to examine long-term prognosis and treatment outcome. The two most common types of classification systems involve division by either functional ability or etiology.

There are three commonly used classification systems based on functional ability. One is based on the 1973 and 1983 AAMD definitions of mental retardation, which divided severity of disability into four categories ("mild," "moderate," "severe," and "profound"). This classification system continues to be widely accepted and used. For example, the American Psychiatric Association (APA) has retained these four categories of cognitive functioning to categorize individuals with mental retardation in the most recent version (fourth edition, text revision) of the *Diagnostic and Statistical Manual of Mental Disorders* (DSM-IV-TR; APA, 2000). According to DSM-IV-TR, individuals who function within the mild range of mental retardation constitute approximately 85% of those diagnosed with mental retardation. Those with moderate mental retardation account for approximately 10% of those with mental retardation. Individuals with severe mental retardation make up approximately 3–

4% of the population of children and adults with mental retardation. Finally, about 1–2% of children and adults with mental retardation fall in the category of profound mental retardation.

In both the 1992 and 2002 revisions of its classification system, the AAMR has placed individuals with mental retardation along a continuum of needed levels of support (i.e., "intermittent," "limited," "extensive," and "pervasive"). For example, an individual with mental retardation can be described as "a 10-year-old female with mental retardation who requires limited supports in self-care and extensive supports in communication." Although some might assume that a child diagnosed with mild mental retardation would require intermittent supports in most areas, this is not necessarily true. For example, a child with an IQ of 65 may require no assistance in self-care and only intermittent supports in social skills, but because of a severe expressive language disorder may require extensive supports in communication. Such functional descriptions are designed to assist clinicians and educators to plan for an individual's service needs.

Finally, educators have developed their own classification system for purposes of program placement. Terms such as "educable mentally retarded" (EMR, referring to children functioning in the mild range of mental retardation) or "trainable mentally retarded" (TMR, referring to children functioning within the moderate range of mental retardation) have been used for a number of years. Yet, with the growing trend of inclusion practices, these labels provide little guidance for classroom placement. Instead, some districts have moved toward more functional descriptors of a child's needs as placement becomes less often based on level of cognitive functioning. Instead, appropriate services follow the child, who may be served in any number of settings (including regular education classrooms). It is important that clinicians who assess and treat children with mental retardation understand the different classification systems, in order to communicate with professionals from a range of disciplines.

Recently, some states have moved away from EMR and TMR as placement terms. For example, the state of Pennsylvania now serves students with learning disabilities (but without mental retardation) and students with mild mental retardation in a combined placement called "learning support." Most students attend a learning support classroom for only a portion of their school day. Students with moderate mental retardation are served in a placement called "life skills support." Several other states have also changed the names of their special education placement programs in recent years.

An alternative type of classification system divides individuals into categories based on etiology. It has been generally accepted that between 40% and 60% of individuals with mental retardation have an organic etiology for their cognitive and adaptive skills deficits (Curry et al., 1997). The remaining individuals are assumed to have mental retardation stemming from psychosocial or familial factors. However, the AAMR (1992) publication on the definition and classification of mental retardation suggested that this two-factor classification system is no longer appropriate (a position raffirmed in the 2002 revision). First, as Masland (1988) has argued, the fact that there is no known cause for the presence of mental retardation in a particular individual does not necessarily mean that an organic etiological explanation does not exist. It may be that our knowledge and technology are not yet advanced enough to detect many of the causes of mental retardation. For example, it was not until 1969 that fragile X syndrome was discovered (Lubbs, 1969). This syndrome may account for a considerable number of males with mental retardation and is caused by what appears to be a pinching of the tips of the long arm of the X chromosome. Other genetic disorders, such as Smith–Magenis syndrome (Smith et al., 1986) and velocardiofacial syndrome (Shprintzen et al., 1978), have also been identified during over the past several decades. There has also been a greater appreciation of the potential adverse effects of lead poisoning, even at subclinical levels, on IQ (Canfield et al., 2003). Second, multiple possible causal factors may have an impact on the person with mental retardation; some of these may be considered familial, and others organic. Therefore, the AAMR (2002, pp. 126–127) has proposed a multifactorial approach to etiology involving the following four categories of risk factors:

1. *Biomedical*: factors that relate to biologic processes, such as genetic disorders, prematurity, malnutrition, seizure disorders, and traumatic brain injury.
2. *Social*: factors that relate to social and family interaction, such as poor prenatal care, lack of stimulation, and family poverty.

3. *Behavioral*: factors that relate to potentially causal behaviors, such as maternal substance abuse, child abuse, and domestic violence.
4. *Educational*: factors that affect the availability of educational supports that promote mental development and the development of adaptive skills (e.g., parental cognitive disability, limited early intervention services, inadequate family support).

The 2002 AAMR Definition

Although the etiological categories listed above have been retained in the most recent (AAMR, 2002) definition of mental retardation, other areas have been revised and are worth noting. The 2002 revision has resulted in a return to the 2-standard-deviation IQ test cutoff for mental retardation (i.e., the cutoff has been lowered from a standard score of 75 back to 70). In addition, IQ range has once again been deemed appropriate for use in describing individuals with mental retardation (i.e., individuals may be described as having mild, moderate, severe, or profound levels of mental retardation). A revision in adaptive behavior deficits has also been made. Whereas the 1992 AAMR definition required specific deficits in at least 2 of 10 specific skills areas, the 2002 definition requires significant limitations in "adaptive behavior as expressed in conceptual, social, and practical adaptive skills" (AAMR, 2002, p. 1). These three broader domains are felt to be more consistent with available research on adaptive behavior. The support intensity needs have been retained, however. Feedback obtained since the 1992 definition indicated that many families and individuals with mental retardation preferred the shift away from a focus on impairment to one describing the supports necessary for an individual (Polloway, 1997). The focus on supports was also felt to provide better guidance regarding the types of services needed (Polloway, 1997, p. 176).

There were a number of difficulties with the 1992 definition (AAMR, 2002). First, there remained few standardized tools for assessing adaptive functioning and no standardized means of assessing strengths or limitations. With the elimination of IQ as a means of describing individuals' levels of functioning, there was no clear substitute terminology. Many researchers, educators, and service providers criticized the elimination of the severity levels (mild, moderate, severe, and profound), be-

cause it was no longer possible to classify individuals with mental retardation. The elimination of severity levels even affected teacher certification requirements in some states (where teachers were specifically certified in teaching students with severe/profound or mild/moderate mental retardation). The use of support intensity levels was criticized as well, because these had no psychometric properties, making them subjective and unreliable; at the same time, they were felt to be cumbersome. Although proponents argued that the intensity levels were not meant to be psychometrically sound, these levels were often used as if they were. A further area of concern was that the number of individuals diagnosed with mental retardation would increase when the IQ cutoff was raised from 70 to the 70–75 range. It was feared that this would result in an overrepresentation of minorities diagnosed with mental retardation. Finally, there were issues related to the imprecision of the 10 adaptive behavior domains, as these had not been determined empirically.

As discussed in the newest AAMR (2002) publication, there was also some controversy regarding the names for the various subtypes of mental retardation, as well as pressure to explore an alternative to the term "mental retardation" itself. MacMillan, Siperstein, and Gresham (1996) have proposed using the term "cognitive impairment" or "general learning disability" for individuals with mild mental retardation. This same group has recommended that the term "mental retardation" be reserved for individuals with organicity (excluding individuals with mild mental retardation). In fact, the term "intellectual disability" has been adopted by many European and international groups. Some self-advocacy groups of individuals with mental retardation have also suggested that a new term be found to replace "mental retardation." In response, AAMR's board of directors has begun to explore options for such a change (AAMR, 2002).

PSYCHIATRIC DISORDERS IN CHILDREN WITH MENTAL RETARDATION

Although children with mental retardation can experience the entire range of psychiatric disorders, establishing a diagnosis in this population is often challenging (Reiss, 1994). Benson and Aman (1999) cite a number of reasons for this:

(1) Language deficits often make it difficult for a child with mental retardation to report internal and feeling states; (2) some behaviors may be maladaptive, yet developmentally appropriate (e.g., an adolescent with mental retardation takes an item from a peer, but has no concept of "stealing"); (3) few available assessment instruments have been normed for this population; (4) sensory and/or physical impairments may complicate diagnosis; and (5) some clinicians are influenced by "diagnostic overshadowing" (i.e., they fail to look for or consider mental disorders in a person with mental retardation). Diagnosis of psychiatric disorders in children and adolescents with mental retardation often requires that the clinician rely on observable behavior rather than self-report (MacLean, 1993). As with typically developing children who require mental health treatment, parent and teacher reports are also of considerable value. It is generally accepted that conventional diagnostic criteria for psychiatric disorders, such as those found in DSM-IV-TR (APA, 2000), can be reasonably applied to children and adolescents functioning in the mild range of mental retardation (IQs above 50). However, these criteria may be less appropriate or useful for those functioning below that range (MacLean, 1993).

The presence of behavior and/or comorbid psychiatric disorders in children with mental retardation may present the most significant obstacle to inclusion in both educational settings and community settings (Johnson, 2002). Such disorders can affect the level of restrictiveness of educational placements (Singer & Irwin, 1987). There is considerable evidence that both children and adults with mental retardation are at greater risk than the general population for developing psychiatric disorders (Emerson, 2003; Quay & Hogan, 1999). Historically, many professionals in the field questioned whether certain disorders (especially internalizing disorders, such as depression or anxiety) could co-occur with mental retardation. Yet it is now well established that individuals with mental retardation can be diagnosed with any comorbid psychiatric disorder (Reiss, 1994).

Recent prevalence studies have documented that between 30% and 50% of children with mental retardation have psychiatric diagnoses or behavior problems (Emerson, 2003; Linna, Piha, Kumpulainen, Tamminen, & Almqvist, 1999; Stromme & Diseth, 2000). Rates of psy-chiatric disorders in this population have been found to be up to three times those of typically developing children and adolescents (Linna et al., 1999). Such rates are consistent with those reported by Rutter, Tizard, Yule, Graham, and Whitmore (1976) in the Isle of Wight study. Although boys (Stromme & Diseth, 2000) and older children (Emerson, 2003) with mental retardation appear to be at greatest risk, level of mental retardation does not appear to increase an individual's risk of a psychiatric diagnosis (Stromme & Diseth, 2000).

Among the most common behavioral disorders in children with mental retardation are attention-deficit/hyperactivity disorder (ADHD) and conduct problems (Emerson, 2003). ADHD is three to five times more prevalent among children with mental retardation than among typically developing children. Recent surveys indicate that between 9% and 16% of children with mental retardation meet diagnostic criteria for ADHD (Emerson, 2003; Stromme & Diseth, 2000). Outcome studies have found that the majority of children with mental retardation and ADHD continue to exhibit symptoms 2–4 years after treatment (Aman, Pejeau, Osborne, Rojahn, & Handen, 1996; Handen, Janosky, & McAuliffe, 1997).

Emerson (2003) found 25% of a random sample of 438 children with mental retardation in Great Britain to have conduct problems. The most common concern was oppositional defiant disorder, reported in 13% of the group. Although considerable research has been conducted with externalizing disorders, such as ADHD and conduct problems, less is known about the rate of internalizing disorders among children and adolescents with mental retardation. Recent surveys indicate that the rate of anxiety disorders among children with mental retardation ranges from 3% to 8.7%, while depression affects only about 1.5% of this population (Emerson, 2003; Linna et al., 1999).

Several syndromes or disorders are often associated with mental retardation and specific maladaptive behaviors. For example, children with fragile X syndrome typically function in the mild to moderate range of mental retardation and often exhibit attentional deficits, hyperactivity, hand flapping, hand biting, perseverative speech, preoccupation with inanimate objects, shyness, and poor social interaction (AAMR, 2002; Hagerman & Sobesky, 1989). Lesch–Nyhan syndrome is often associated with severe self-injury (Nyhan, 1976), while children with Prader–Willi syndrome have an abnormality in the hypothalamic region of the brain, resulting in insatiable overeating and impulse control problems (AAMR, 2002; Reber, 1994). Rett's disorder is generally characterized by regression in skills following a typical early course of development, and the subsequent appearance of stereotyped hand movements (APA, 2000). Angelman syndrome is often associated with unprovoked laughter, hyperactivity, and sleep disorders, while children with Williams syndrome often have short attention spans but are quite social and often have strong musical skills (AAMR, 2002; Einfeld & Aman, 1995). Children with Smith–Magenis syndrome are often impulsive, have sleep disorders, and engage in stereotypic and self-injurious behaviors (AAMR, 2002). Children with autistic disorder often engage in a range of maladaptive behaviors, such as stereotyped and repetitive motor mannerisms (e.g., hand or finger flapping), impairments in social interactions, and deficits in communication (e.g., delayed expressive language development, stereotyped and repetitive use of language)(APA, 2000). The presence of specific maladaptive behaviors during an assessment may suggest that a particular disorder or syndrome should be considered. In addition, knowledge of such disorders and any associated behavioral deficits and excesses can greatly inform the development of an appropriate treatment plan.

PREVENTION

Prevention efforts are typically categorized as "primary," "secondary," and "tertiary" (Kasten & Coury, 1991). Primary interventions focus on preventing health problems that can lead to mental retardation; such interventions include providing good prenatal care, providing routine health care, preventing accidents, preventing maternal drug and alcohol use during pregnancy, removing lead paint from houses, and so forth. Secondary interventions are attempts to correct situations that are likely to lead to mental retardation. These efforts include amniocentesis, chorion villus sampling, genetic counseling, newborn screening for phenylketonuria (PKU) and subsequent treatment if required, surgical placement of a shunt to treat hydrocephaly, treatment for congenital hypothyroidism, and the development of an ef-

fective rubella vaccine. In addition, the provision of services such as Head Start or other efforts to prevent developmental delays falls under the category of secondary prevention. Finally, tertiary prevention involves treatment of already existing mental retardation. This might include chelation therapy for a child with lead poisoning, or corrective surgery for a congenital heart defect for a child with Down syndrome (which could prevent functional impairment later in life).

Many past research efforts have had significant effects on preventing mental retardation. For example, almost half of children whose mothers contracted rubella (German measles) during the first trimester of pregnancy experienced serious abnormalities, including mental retardation, blindness, and/or deafness (Baroff & Olley, 1999). The development of an effective rubella vaccine in 1969 eliminated this risk for children whose mothers were vaccinated prior to their pregnancy. Another cause of mental retardation was identified in children who inherited PKU. Individuals with PKU are unable to break down the amino acid phenylalanine, which is found in many foods. Over time, this leads to mental retardation. A simple test of a newborn's blood plasma can detect this condition. Placed on a special, phenylalanine-free diet, children with PKU will develop normally.

There are ongoing research efforts to identify additional genetic causes for mental retardation, some of which were previously thought to be familial (e.g., fragile X syndrome). We can expect to see additional discoveries in the future. It is estimated that the prevalence of severe and profound mental retardation could be decreased by 20% simply through using currently available prevention strategies (Stevenson, Massey, Schroer, McDermott, & Richter, 1996). Similarly, we are learning more about the potential adverse affects of environmental toxins (e.g., lead, asbestos). As states enact laws to promote the use of seat belts, bicycle helmets, and other safety devices, we should also witness a decrease in the number of traumatic head injuries and associated cognitive impairments in children. Although it might be thought that the advent of neonatal intensive care units and ventilators in the 1970s would have resulted in a reduction of mental retardation secondary to prematurity or birth complications, follow-up studies of low-birthweight infants suggest an incidence of mental retardation ranging from 4% to 8% (Aziz et al., 1995; Victorian Infant Collaborative Study Group, 1991, 1995).

EDUCATIONAL SERVICES

Relevant Laws and Court Decisions

The most common treatment interventions offered to children with mental retardation are school-based educational services. Toward this end, an important group of laws has been enacted guaranteeing education for these children. Perhaps the most important piece of legislation has been the Individuals with Disabilities Education Act (IDEA) of 1990. The IDEA (P.L. 101-476) was originally called the Education for All Handicapped Children Act (P.L. 94-142), which was first passed by Congress in 1975. This landmark piece of legislation has resulted over the years in significant changes in how children with mental retardation (and other disabilities) are educated. The initial purpose of the IDEA was to

> assure that all children with disabilities have available to them . . . a free appropriate pubic education which emphasizes special education and related services designed to meet their unique needs, to assure that the rights of children with disabilities and their parents or guardians are protected, to assist states and localities to provide for the education of all children with disabilities, and to assess and assure the effectiveness of efforts to educate children with disabilities. (20 U.S.C. 1400[c])

The IDEA encompasses six major principles:

1. *Zero rejection.* Schools must educate all children with disabilities from ages 6 through 17 years (states that provide educational services for children 3–5 and 18–21 years of age are also required to provide educational services to children with disabilities in those age groups).

2. *Nondiscriminatory identification and evaluation.* All testing must be conducted in a student's native language, and students cannot be discriminated against on the basis of their race, culture, or native language. In addition, placement decisions cannot be based on a single test score.

3. *Free, appropriate public education.* All children, regardless of disability, are entitled to a free, appropriate public education. An indi-

vidualized education program (IEP) must be developed for each child with special needs.

4. *Least restrictive environment.* Students must be educated in the least restrictive school environment. School districts must specifically justify why a student cannot participate with typically peers in academic classes and nonacademic activities (e.g., lunch, gym, transportation). School districts must provide a continuum of placement options in order to meet the least restrictive environment needs of each student.

5. *Due process safeguards.* Parents who disagree with the results of an evaluation or a placement decision can obtain a due process hearing.

6. *Parent and student participation and shared decision making.* Both parents and the identified student must be involved in decisions regarding the design and implementation of services.

In addition to these six principles, the IDEA requires that a student be provided related services and assistive technology if the student's disability prevents him or her from fully participating in educational activities. Such services have included special transportation, speech and language therapy, physical and occupational therapy, and counseling. The IDEA was reauthorized in 1997 (P.L. 105-17) and again in 2004 as the Individuals with Disabilities Education Improvement Act of 2004 (P.L. 108-446). While most of the original provisions have been retained, the reauthorized bill includes a number of new provisions. For example, paperwork has been reduced, thereby increasing teacher instruction time. School districts will be allowed to use funds to provide early intervening services (i.e., services for students who have not yet been identified with disabilities but are in need of academic and/or behavioral support). Additionally, the definition of a learning disability has been revised (allowing for greater flexibility in identifying students with learning problems) and changes have been made in the process for amending IEPs. Furthermore, the bill provides funds for the training of school staff in effective teaching strategies and outlines steps to be taken to prevent the overidentification of minority students (Council for Exceptional Children, 2005). Additional updates on the reauthorized bill can be found on websites hosted by advocacy groups such as the Council for Exceptional Children (2005).

A number of subsequent laws and legal decisions have followed during the 30-plus years since P.L. 94-142 was initially signed into law. Many of these laws and decisions have had an impact on services and treatment of children with mental retardation. For example, the Education of the Handicapped Act Amendments of 1986 (P.L. 99-457) required school districts to serve preschoolers with disabilities (between 3 and 5 years of age), beginning in the 1990–1991 school year. In 1979, a group of parents (*Armstrong v. Kline*) won a case against their school district requiring that children with severe disabilities be offered year-round educational services. Some states now have a mechanism to provide extended-school-year services to students with disabilities. However, such services are not uniformly offered in all states and school districts.

Issues relating to the disciplining and suspending of students with disabilities have also been addressed by the courts and by amendments to the IDEA. For example, in 1988 the U.S. Supreme Court heard *Honig v. Doe* and ruled that a student with disabilities could not be expelled from school for disciplinary reasons. The maximum a child with disabilities could be suspended from school was 10 days (as long as the reason for suspension was not related to the student's disability). The 1997 IDEA amendments allow school districts to discipline students with and without disabilities in the same manner. However, a suspension/expulsion of greater than 10 days, or a proposed change in placement, requires that the IEP team meet. At this meeting, a review (called a "manifestation determination") is conducted to determine whether the suspension is related to the student's disability. Only if this is not found to be the case can the district continue to impose the same disciplinary procedures used with typical students.

Early Intervention

Children with mental retardation generally follow a developmental pattern similar to that of their typically developing peers. However, the rate and limits of development will be based on a range of factors, including the severity of the disabling condition, family support, and the type of programming offered (Guralnick & Bricker, 1987). Early intervention is designed to "provide early identification and provision of services to reduce or eliminate the effects of disabilities or to prevent the development of other problems, so that the need for subsequent special services is reduced" (McConnell, 1994, pp.78).

A small group of early studies documented that the provision of educational services prior to age 6 might have a significant impact on both the rate and limits of development in children with mental retardation. For example, Skeels (1966) reported the results of a 30-year follow-up of two groups of institutionalized infants. One group was removed from an orphanage at 18 months of age and transferred to an institution where they were cared for by a group of women with mental retardation, and the other group remained in the orphanage, where they received little stimulation. The children in the two groups were comparable, with cognitive functioning ranging from mental retardation to the low-average range of intelligence. At a 2-year follow-up, the children raised in the institution had gained an average of 28 IQ points, while those remaining in the orphanage had lost an average of 26 IQ points (Skodak & Skeels, 1949). At the 30-year follow-up, the 13 individuals in the "treatment" group were all self-supporting and living in the community, with a 12th-grade median educational level. Of the 12 "control" children, 8 remained institutionalized (1 had died), with a 3rd-grade median educational level. Although this study has significant methodological weaknesses, such as the comparability of the two groups and the extent to which the significant differences between them could be attributed to early experiences (Ramey & Baker-Ward, 1982), it provided compelling documentation of the ability to affect the rate of development positively.

A subsequent study by Kirk (1958) compared the progress of 81 preschoolers with mental retardation (IQs = 45–80) who were assigned to one of four interventions: a community-based preschool program, an institutional preschool program, community living with no services, and institutionalization with no services. Both groups of children who attended preschool programs outperformed their peers on a range of developmental measures. However, these differences failed to be observed at a 1-year follow-up after the first year of elementary school.

The typical early intervention program uses a developmental model to guide educational objectives, in conjunction with a behavioral teaching technology. The service delivery models typically fall into three categories: home-based, center-based, or a combination of the two. Often, services are provided by multiple agencies, requiring the coordination of efforts across programs. Harbin, McWilliam, and Gallagher (2000) describe four key elements of early intervention service delivery:

1. *Family-centered approach*: responding to family priorities, empowering family members, using a holistic approach with the family, and being insightful and sensitive to the family.
2. *Integration of therapies*: integrating therapy into a child's natural environment by consulting with all individuals who spend time with the child.
3. *Inclusion*: providing services in natural environments that include both typically and nontypically developing children.
4. *Transition*: anticipating problems and improving the transition from early intervention to preschool programs.

Although these elements are considered best practices, many programs struggle to implement these concepts. Service providers often lack the training and knowledge of community resources to offer a family-centered approach to service provision (Gallagher, 1997b; McWilliam & Lang, 1994). In addition, the majority of therapies continue to utilize a traditional pull-out model (Gallagher, 1997a). Although progress has been made in providing services in natural environments, the majority of early intervention programs continue to serve children in noninclusive settings (Kochanek & Buka, 1995). Finally, despite federal law requirements regarding the need to facilitate the transition from early intervention to preschool, families have continued to express complaints about this process (Gallagher, 1997c).

Documenting the efficacy of early intervention services has also been challenging, due in large part to difficulties in conducting well-controlled research in this area. Such problems include selecting reliable outcome measures; comparing results across different populations; comparing a wide variety of programs (each with different treatment intensities, teaching strategies, and focuses); and dealing with the ethical issues of withholding services so as to provide a comparison group (Heward, 2000).

Hence the interpretation of the findings of this literature must be tempered with an understanding of these methodological limitations.

A review of the early childhood research from 1975 to 1990 found "a consistent pattern of modest, short-term, program-favoring effects on selected outcome measures" (Halpern, 2000, p. 375). Gains were most often seen in areas associated with a given program's treatment emphasis, such as maternal praise, children's language, and parental coping. Services provided directly to children were associated with the greatest gains. This literature included programs serving not only children with mental retardation, but disadvantaged children and other groups felt to be at risk for the development of learning problems.

A brief examination of the early intervention literature in Down syndrome offers an example of the efficacy of such services in a group of children with mental retardation. The findings of the research on preschoolers with Down syndrome are hopeful, especially in view of earlier work clearly documenting that while gradual improvement in cognitive development occurs, the rate of development among children with Down syndrome slows progressively over time (Guralnick & Bricker, 1987). Consequently, infants with Down syndrome evidence a considerable overlap in developmental functioning with typically developing infants, but experience a general decline on measures of cognitive functioning through early childhood (Carr, 1975; Morgan, 1979).

The results of work evaluating the efficacy of early intervention in children with Down syndrome suggests that this decline in cognitive functioning can be reduced, especially in the short term. Such results have been obtained not only in less well-controlled studies (e.g., Kysela, Hillyard, McDonald, & Ahlsten-Taylor, 1981) in which only pre- and post-treatment measures were used, but also in a number of studies in which control groups were utilized (e.g., Aronson & Fallstrom, 1977; Connolly, Morgan, Russell, & Richardson, 1980; Rynders & Horrobin, 1980). However, there remains a paucity of literature regarding the effects of program duration and intensity, the impact of individual differences (e.g., presence of cardiac defects or hearing loss), and the potential effects of inclusion on outcome (Spiker & Hopmann, 1997). In addition, there has been some disagreement regarding the long-term effects of early intervention in this population. For example, a 1988 review of research from 21 early intervention programs concluded that there was no strong evidence to suggest that early intervention for children with Down syndrome enhanced subsequent school performance (Gibson & Harris, 1988). However, other researchers cited the poor methodological quality of many of the long-term follow-up studies (Harris, 1988). In addition, a few subsequent follow-up studies have documented some gains attributable to early intervention (e.g., Connolly, Morgan, Russell, & Rulliton, 1993; Fewell & Oelwein, 1991). There has not been substantial growth in the literature in this area since the early to mid-1990s.

Some proponents of early intervention for children at risk (e.g., children with developmental delays, children with low birthweight) have felt that changes on curriculum-based measures or general cognitive assessment tools often fail to provide a thorough picture of the positive effects of early intervention efforts. This is illustrated by controversy over data from the Infant Health and Development Program (IHDP) for low-birthweight children, indicating few long-term program effects on IQ (Brooks-Gunn et al., 1994; McCarton et al., 1997). These findings, however, were felt to be at odds with a large body of evidence documenting the effects of environmental variables, such as early intervention, on mental development (Blair & Wahlsten, 2002). Ramey and Ramey (1998) point out that early intervention is often designed to *prevent* developmental decline due to a variety of risk factors (e.g., low birthweight, low maternal IQ), rather than to focus on *raising* a child's IQ. In fact, a number of well-controlled, randomized studies have documented long-term gains in a range of areas following early intervention. For example, the Abecedarian Project found significantly fewer grade retentions and special education placements, along with higher performance on achievement tests, for children with developmental delays receiving early intervention in comparison to controls at follow-up assessments through 15 years of age (Campbell & Ramey, 1995). However, IQ differences between groups had decreased to only 5 points (vs. much larger differences in the preschool years) at age 15 (Martin, Ramey, & Ramey, 1990). Similar results have been documented in other studies, along with reduced crime rates, decreased teenage pregnancy, and increased

high school graduation rates (Burchinal, Campbell, Bryant, Wasik, & Ramey, 1997; Schweinhart, Barnes, & Weikart, 1993). More recent research—such as work by Reynolds, Temple, and Ou (2003), who followed 1,539 children from the Chicago Longitudinal Study—found participation in preschool to be associated with significantly higher levels of school readiness, achievement, and educational attainment, along with lower rates of child maltreatment, juvenile delinquency, special education placement, and grade retention. Finally, Hill, Brooks-Gunn, and Waldfogel (2003) recently reexamined data from the IHDP, using a "control group" of children with low participation rates in their full-day early intervention program. At follow-up at 8 years of age, high-participation-rate children evidenced significantly higher IQs than the controls. In addition to program intensity, other variables that have been hypothesized to affect the long-term outcome of early intervention included a child's length of time in the program (some programs' efforts, such as those of the IHDP, stopped at age 3), as well as the quality of subsequent educational services.

Primary and Secondary School Education

Once children with mental retardation reach school age, various placement options are often available. The most restrictive settings include residential treatment, private programs, and center-based programs (entire schools devoted to serving children with special needs). Less restrictive options begin with special education classes, which are located within a regular school but provide few or no opportunities for children with mental retardation to interact with typically developing peers. In many settings, children with special needs are integrated (or mainstreamed) into nonacademic classes such as gym, art, music, and homeroom, where academic demands are at a minimum. More recently, the inclusion movement's emphasis on placing children with special needs in a regular classroom for all subject areas has gained support. Any required ancillary services are provided in the classroom, and the classroom teacher is provided consultation in adapting the curriculum for each child with special needs.

Prior to the signing of P.L. 94-142 in 1975, most children with mental retardation were educated in segregated classrooms. Since that time, there has been considerable debate regarding the best setting for educating children with disabilities. "Inclusion" involves the full integration of children with disabilities into heterogeneous classrooms for the entire school day. Any special services a child needs are provided to the child in that same setting (Scruggs & Mastropieri, 1996). Advocates for inclusion cite a number of advantages of educating children with typical peers: (1) Research indicates that children with disabilities perform as well in inclusive as in segregated classrooms; (2) with proper support, many students with disabilities can function within a regular classroom setting; (3) inclusion increases interactions between children with disabilities and their typical peers; and (4) children with disabilities benefit from their interactions with typical peers, and typical classmates get to know children with disabilities (Taylor, 1999). Opponents of inclusion for all children with disabilities cite research indicating that children with more serious problems perform better in segregated classes (Borthwick-Duffy, Palmer, & Lane, 1996; Fuchs & Fuchs, 1995). In addition, opponents of inclusion are concerned that the presence of disabled students in regular classrooms may interfere with the learning of typical students; that regular students may start to mimic inappropriate behaviors of disabled students; and that fewer services will be available for students placed in inclusive settings (Taylor & Harrington, 2003). However, such concerns have not been well supported (e.g., Sharpe, York, & Knight, 1994). Recent research suggests that preschool teachers are more supportive of inclusion for less involved children, and that parents are "very satisfied" with their children's inclusion experiences (Rafferty & Boettcher, 2000).

Much of the research on inclusion has focused on the entire population of students with disabilities—including children with learning disabilities (without mental retardation), speech/language impairments, physical disabilities, visual/hearing impairments, and emotional disturbances, as well as those with mental retardation. The ability of a given student to benefit from inclusion may depend in part upon the child's needs. Opponents of full inclusion would argue that children with mental retardation may have different needs as they become older. For example, it may be more appropriate for an adolescent with moderate mental retardation to devote a class period to

community skills than to join classmates in a history lesson. Many schools use a combination of inclusion and pull-out services for children with mental retardation. Much of the prior research on the benefits of inclusion (vs. noninclusive education) had significant methodological problems (e.g., small sample sizes, nonrandom assignment, inappropriate dependent measures; Hocutt, 1996), making it difficult to draw firm conclusions. Despite such controversies, there continues to be a gradual move toward greater inclusion of students with mental retardation. Recent data from the National Center for Education Statistics (2002) indicate that 14.1% of students with mental retardation were placed full-time in regular education classrooms in the 1999–2000 school year, up from 13.4% during the 1998–1999 school year.

BEHAVIOR PROBLEM MANAGEMENT

Addressing behavior problems has historically been a primary treatment focus in the field of mental retardation, with applied behavior analysis (ABA) among the most well-researched treatment approaches. In fact, the American Psychological Association Division of Clinical Psychology's Task Force on Promotion and Dissemination of Psychological Procedures (1995) identified "behavior modification" (a term that is often interchangeable with "ABA") as an empirically validated treatment for individuals with developmental disabilities. ABA includes the treatment of a range of maladaptive behaviors (such as aggression, self-injury, and feeding problems), as well as assistance in the development of desirable behaviors (such as work completion, remaining in seat, and using alternative forms of communication). Behavior modification interventions have also been considered to be empirically supported treatments for addressing the behavioral concerns of individuals with autism, as well as those with hyperactivity and oppositionality (behaviors that are often concerns for individuals with mental retardation) (Chambless & Ollendick, 2001).

The field of ABA has changed considerably over time. Whereas many of the early interventions in the 1960s and 1970s focused on the effect of reinforcement and other consequences on maladaptive behavior, the field has more recently emphasized concepts such as positive behavior support (PBS) functional analysis, functional communication (FC), establishing operations, and behavioral momentum. The field has also matured to the point that a national certification program in ABA is now available. A discussion of these newer concepts, as well as a review of some of the well-established ABA intervention strategies, follows.

Positive Behavior Support

During the past 15 years, the use of PBS has gained considerable acceptance. PBS followed the success of functional behavior assessment (FBA) in guiding the development of behavioral interventions. Although a number of treatment interventions developed in the 1960s and 1970s were shown to be successful in reducing maladaptive behaviors in individuals with mental retardation, these interventions were often based on the use of consequences alone. Many of these treatments were not easily implemented within integrated school and community settings (Horner et al., 1990; Ruef, Poston, & Humphrey, 1999). "The goal of positive behavior support (PBS) is to apply behavioral principles in the community in order to reduce problem behaviors and build appropriate behaviors that result in durable change and a rich lifestyle" (Carr et al., 1999, p. 3). PBS is seen as proactive in nature. It starts with the completion of an FBA; the results of the FBA inform the development of the PBS plan. The use of PBS has been supported by recent mandates, including the 1997 amendments to the IDEA, which call for the use of FBA and positive supports and strategies (Tilly et al., 1998).

The FBA seeks to determine the communicative intent of the behavior, setting events, antecedents, and current consequences. From this information, a testable hypothesis is developed regarding the predictors and consequences maintaining the behavior. This hypothesis should directly inform the PBS plan (Crone & Horner, 2003). The PBS plan typically emphasizes the use of specific environmental modifications and supports. In addition, the plan focuses on the development of alternative skills and behaviors for the individual. The PBS plan then seeks to manipulate consequences that have been found to inadvertently reinforce inappropriate behavior. A crisis plan may need to be put into place (e.g., requiring the use of time out), should the individual

engage in behavior that is considered dangerous to him- or herself or others. Finally, the plan is implemented, data are collected, and progress is assessed on a regular basis. The PBS plan is then modified as necessary.

FBA and Functional Analysis of Behavior

The best way to understand the relationship between a target behavior and the environment (as well as the possible communicative intent of the behavior) is to conduct an FBA or a functional behavior analysis. Either of these types of assessment should directly inform the development of a PBS plan.

FUNCTIONAL BEHAVIOR ASSESSMENT

An FBA can take many forms, depending on the complexity of the behavior. According to Crone and Horner (2003), a clinician can conduct either a "simple FBA" or a "full FBA." A simple FBA consists of an interview with the student's teacher to obtain the following information: (1) description of the behavior problem, (2) identification of times of day the behavior is most likely to be observed, (3) identification of antecedents (predictors) and setting events for the behavior, and (4) identification of consequences that affect the recurrence of the behavior. Crone and Horner (2003) provide a number of questionnaires that can be used to guide the teacher interview. Conversely, a full FBA builds upon information gathered from the simple FBA and includes interviews with additional staff and family members, as well as a behavioral observation of the student in a natural setting. Figure 6.1 is a Functional Assessment Observation Form that seeks to identify the following:

1. *Behavior*: An indication of which behavior was observed.
2. *Predictors*: A description of the elements in the situation (also referred to as the antecedents) that may have triggered the behavior.
3. *Consequences*: A description of the consequences that followed the behavior.
4. *Function of behavior*: A guess as to the communicative intent or function of the behavior. Research has demonstrated that functions can be divided into two categories: "get/obtain" and "escape/avoid." Within these two categories are subsumed

Behavior								
Antecedents								
• Attending to another student								
• Made demand								
• Ended activity								
• Transition								
• Student by self								
• Told "no"								
• Other								
Consequences								
• Ignored								
• Ended demand								
• Insisted that student comply								
• Placed student in time out								
• Gave in to student								
• Removed student from area								
• Sent to principal								
• Talked to student								
• Other								
Possible Function								
• To obtain attention								
• To avoid a demand								
• To get something								
• Self-stimulation								
• Other								

FIGURE 6.1. Functional Assessment Observation Form. Data from Iwata (1995) and O'Neill et al. (1997).

the desire for attention, anger at being denied an item that was requested, self-stimulatory functions, and escaping a demand.

FUNCTIONAL ANALYSIS OF BEHAVIOR

A functional analysis of behavior (unlike an FBA) involves the *direct manipulation of variables* to test the various functional relationships. The typical functional analysis is based on that originally described by Iwata, Dorsey, Slifer, Bauman, and Richman (1982), but with some variations. Commonly, four different conditions are used: (1) no demand/control (e.g., a no-demand play situation or child

alone); (2) demand/escape (during which demands are made of the child and removed contingent upon the appearance of the target behavior—e.g., head banging, aggression); (3) attention (during which attention is given to the child contingent upon the occurrence of the target behavior); and (4) tangible (during which tangible items, such as food or favorite toys, are provided contingent upon the occurrence of the target behavior).

A recent example of the use of functional analysis is provided by Piazza, Patel, Gulotta, Sevin, and Layer (2003), who evaluated 15 children with feeding disorders (typically involving food refusal). Child behavior was observed under four different feeding conditions: (1) baseline (simply talking to the child throughout the meal and leaving a spoonful of food near the child's mouth); (2) attention (coaxing and other forms of adult attention following food refusal); (3) escape (removing the food following refusal to eat); and (4) tangible (providing tangible items—e.g., favorite toys, foods, or drinks—when the child refused to eat). Results showed increased food refusal for 10 of the 15 children during one or more of the conditions; this suggested that environmental variables played a role in the feeding problem, and it provided guidance regarding possible treatment interventions that could be individualized for each child.

Changing Behaviors

Once an FBA or a functional analysis has been conducted and baseline data obtained, the clinician is ready to design and implement a PBS plan. PBS plans typically focus on three areas: (1) modifying antecedents; (2) teaching alternative behaviors; and (3) arranging specific consequences to reduce maladaptive behaviors.

TECHNIQUES FOR MODIFYING ANTECEDENTS

One aspect of a PBS plan is to identify possible antecedents to the behavior problem. Some antecedents may be altered so as to prevent the occurrence of the behavior. The following suggestions for altering antecedents are adapted from a parent training manual developed by the National Institute of Mental Health Autism Research Unit on Pediatric Psychopharmacology (2002).

1. *Avoid situations.* Sometimes certain situations are stressful to a child and can lead to disruptive behavior. For example, a child may find eating lunch in the cafeteria noisy and overstimulating (resulting in agitation). Behavior problems can be prevented by having the child eat in a quieter area.

2. *Control the environment.* Some teachers control their classroom environment by seating certain children away from others or in desks with partitions that limit distractions. A parent with a child who engages in pica (ingesting inedible objects) may need to keep all small objects locked up or out of reach.

3. *Do things in small doses or steps.* Some children can handle situations for only short periods of time. Rather than avoiding these situations entirely, a child can spend limited time in such settings (while staff members work to gradually build the child's ability to tolerate the setting).

4. *Change the order of events.* This can be especially helpful for a child who has difficulty stopping an enjoyable activity in order to complete a task. For example, a young boy may become angry and aggressive when his mother asks him to turn off the TV to get dressed for school. The mother decides to have the child get dressed *before* being allowed to watch TV (using TV as the reinforcer for getting dressed).

There has also been much recent interest in the use of "establishing operations" as a preventive strategy as well. An establishing operation is any change in the environment that momentarily alters the effectiveness of reinforcement (or punishment) (Pierce & Chaney, 2004). A common example is food deprivation (or being hungry) and its effect on the reinforcement value of food. Hence a special education teacher may find using food to reinforce appropriate behavior to be less effective immediately after the students have had lunch. Another example of the effect of establishing operations on behavior is described by O'Reilly, Lacey, and Lancioni (2000), who demonstrated that background noise (an establishing operation) increased noncompliance in a child with Williams syndrome (a disorder in which individuals often have hypersensitivity to sound).

Finally, "behavioral momentum" has been increasingly used as an antecedent strategy to increase compliance (Ducharme & Drain, 2004; Romano & Roll, 2000). This typically involves increasing compliance by using a short sequence of high probability (or easy) commands prior to making requests that are less likely to be followed by compliance. Ducharme and Drain (2004) used behavioral momentum to increase compliance to parental requests in four children with autism and developmental delays. A hierarchy of academic and nonacademic requests was developed for each child (using four levels from "high compliance" to "low compliance"). Parents began with high-compliance requests, followed by praise for appropriate responding. Over several weeks, the lower-compliance demands were gradually introduced while the children continued to display high rates of compliance. Generalization to untrained requests and maintenance of treatment effects at 6-month follow-up were noted.

TECHNIQUES FOR TEACHING ALTERNATIVE BEHAVIORS

The second aspect of a PBS plan is to teach alternative skills and behaviors. Crone and Horner (2003) describe alternative or competing behaviors as those that are mutually exclusive. In other words, an individual cannot engage in both the behavior problem and competing behavior simultaneously. For example, a competing behavior for a child who does not comply with teacher requests would be to complete given assignments. Once alternative behaviors are identified, they need to be taught and/or strengthened.

Positive Reinforcement. The most effective means to strengthen or increase appropriate competing behaviors is positive reinforcement. This involves the presentation of a stimulus (e.g., praise, food) contingent upon the occurrence of the target behavior, which results in an increase in the rate of that behavior. Identifying appropriate reinforcers for children with mental retardation can often be challenging. This is because many naturally occurring reinforcers (e.g., positive feedback from others, smiles, or pleasure felt from completing a challenging task) are not necessarily motivating to all children with mental retardation. In addition, some children with mental retardation have not been exposed to a wide range of potential reinforcers, due to limited experiences in the community or with peers.

Several researchers have developed systems for identifying potential reinforcers for children with mental retardation. Hagopian, Long, and Rush (2004) divide such strategies into two categories: (1) indirect measures, where parents or staff members who are familiar with the individual complete reinforcer checklists and provide a relative ranking (e.g., Fisher, Piazza, Bowman, & Amari, 1996; Matson et al., 1999); and (2) direct measures, in which individuals are presented with a single reinforcer, paired reinforcers, or an array of potential reinforcers, and preferences are assessed (e.g., Hagopian, Rush, Lewin, & Long, 2001; Roscoe, Iwata, & Kahng, 1999). For example, individuals functioning within the severe to profound range of mental retardation may be presented with such items as hugs, verbal interactions, liquids, vibrating toys, music, and toys

that light up. A final method of identifying potential reinforcers is simply to observe a child for a period of time to identify his or her high-probability behaviors. Premack (1959) demonstrated that behaviors in which an individual freely engaged might be effectively used to reinforce low-rate behaviors. Using the "Premack principle," one may find that some seemingly unlikely options—such as being allowed to engage in self-stimulatory behaviors or simply being left alone—may serve as potential reinforcers for a child.

Reinforcers are either unconditioned/primary or conditioned/secondary reinforcers. Primary reinforcers, such as food or liquids, are naturally effective reinforcers. Secondary reinforcers require an individual to learn that a given stimulus has reinforcing properties. This typically occurs as the child interacts with his or her environment. However, for children with mental retardation, the clinician may need to start with a primary reinforcer (e.g., food) in order to begin to increase desired behaviors. When the primary reinforcers are paired frequently with other stimuli (e.g., praise, hugs), the latter assume reinforcing properties as well.

Reinforcers are often divided into a number of categories: edible reinforcers (food, liquids); social reinforcers (praise, hugs); material/tangible reinforcers (toys, prizes); activity reinforcers (playing a game, listening to music); and generalized reinforcers (tokens, money)(Hall & Hall, 1998). Generalized reinforcers, such as tokens, can be extremely effective for children with mental retardation. As described above, these conditioned reinforcers are developed by their frequent pairing with other, established reinforcers. Tokens are effective because they allow a child both to delay reinforcement and to choose from a range of potential reinforcers. For example, it may not be feasible for a child to earn time playing a computer game after completing a single task. However, awarding the child a token serves to reinforce task completion and allows the child to delay exchanging the token for a reinforcer until later in the day (e.g., when a total of 10 tokens have been earned). The use of generalized reinforcers also eliminates problems with satiation (a child tiring of a particular reinforcer), in that a wide variety of reinforcing items can be purchased.

Following a few guidelines may help to increase reinforcement effectiveness. The first guideline is that the reinforcer should be appropriate. In other words, one should establish that the chosen consequence is reinforcing to the child and that it matches the behavioral requirement. For example, a child may find breaks reinforcing, but providing a 15-minute break following only 5 minutes of work is probably not an appropriate match between the behavior required and the reinforcer. Second, the reinforcer should always be paired with other naturally occurring events or stimuli to develop other secondary or learned reinforcers (e.g., pairing edible reinforcers with praise). Third, when a new behavior is being taught, reinforcement should initially be provided immediately following the behavior. For example, if a child is being taught to look at staff members when prompted, "Look at me," reinforcement should immediately follow the making of eye contact. This serves to strengthen the association between the desired behavior and the reinforcer, and it also prevents nontarget behaviors from being inadvertently reinforced. Naturally occurring reinforcers should also be used whenever possible. For example, if a child is being taught to ask for juice, juice should be the reinforcer. Finally, a continuous reinforcement schedule (reinforcing every occurrence of the target behavior) should be used initially to establish a new behavior. For example, if a child is being taught to hang up his or her coat upon arrival in the classroom, this should be praised each time the behavior occurs. Once a behavior is established, an intermittent reinforcement schedule can be introduced.

It has been suggested that the use of extrinsic reinforcement tends to reduce task interest and creativity, as well as to undermine intrinsic motivation (Eisenberger & Cameron, 1996). Consequently, some teacher training materials and business publications specifically recommend against the use of reward or incentive systems (e.g., Kohn, 1993; Tagano, Moran, & Sawyer, 1991). Yet, in a review of this issue by Eisenberger and Cameron (1996), the detrimental effects of reinforcement were found to occur only under specific conditions that could easily be remedied. Their analysis of the literature on reinforcement suggests that it is important for reinforcement to be based on task completion or the meeting of a certain level of quality. Conversely, studies in which reinforcement has had decremental effects on subsequent performance have typically involved a single presentation of reinforcement (independent of performance), followed by a period of time in which reinforcement is withheld. Subsequent performance is then found to decrease, relative to that of individuals who had not been reinforced initially for their performance. However, such situations are not typical of true-life learning experiences, in which individuals often perform tasks repeatedly and are reinforced repeatedly prior to the termination of reward. In such cases, little if any decrement in performance is noted. Similar results have been noted in research on creativity, where such behavior can either be enhanced or thwarted, depending on how reinforcement is administered (see Eisenberger & Selbst, 1994).

Negative Reinforcement. The use of negative reinforcement can also result in an increase in behavior. Whereas positive reinforcement is a process in which a behavior is strengthened by the presentation of a stimulus (e.g., an object or event) that follows the behavior, negative reinforcement strengthens a behavior by removing an unpleasant stimulus (e.g., a task demand) as a consequence of the behavior. The use of negative reinforcement is different from punishment. In punishment, an aversive or unpleasant event follows the occurrence of the target behavior and results in a *decrease* in the rate of that behavior. Conversely, negative reinforcement results in an *increase* in the occurrence of a target behavior. For example, Iwata, Dorsey, Slifer, Bauman, and Richman (1994) found that some children with mental retardation engage in self-injurious behavior (SIB) to avoid or escape from adult demands. The demand is reduced or terminated when SIB occurs, thereby negatively reinforcing this behavior (i.e., increasing the rate of SIB). Carr, Newsom, and Binkoff (1980) demonstrated that two children with mental retardation were able to decrease demands placed upon them by engaging in aggressive behavior (staff members had negatively reinforced aggression). A parent who nags her daughter until she cleans her room is also using negative reinforcement. Another example of the everyday use of negative reinforcement is the teacher who requires her students to sit quietly in their seats before allowing them out for recess (where the unpleasant stimulus of having to remain seated is removed once the desired behavior of seating quietly is exhibited).

Functional Communication. FC involves teaching an individual a more appropriate and functional alternative to a maladaptive behavior to communicate. For example, if a child frequently talks out in class to obtain teacher attention, the child can be taught to raise his or her hand as a functional alternative. Carr and Durand (1985) demonstrated the power of teaching FC skills to a group of adolescents who exhibited aggression and SIB. A functional analysis of the behavior found that aggression and SIB served to communicate the desire to terminate or avoid tasks, and that they occurred most often during periods of low adult attention and high task difficulty. The adolescents were taught to say "I don't understand" if an error was made during a difficult task, or to ask "Am I doing good work?" during easier tasks. The rates of aggression and SIB were functionally related to the use of these new communicative skills.

A more recent example of an FC intervention was described by Tarbox, Wallace, Tarbox, Landaburu, and Williams (2004), involving the teaching of FC skills to two adults with mental retardation who engaged in aggressive behavior in response to staff demands. The individuals were taught either to sign "Break" or to say "Go away" if they didn't want to comply with a work demand (in which case a staff member would provide a 30-second break before reinstating the demand). Subsequent rates of aggression decreased from about two times per minute to almost zero per minute. A return to baseline conditions resulted in a subsequent return to higher rates of aggression.

TECHNIQUES FOR USING CONSEQUENCES TO REDUCE MALADAPTIVE BEHAVIORS

The final aspect of a PBS plan involves the use of consequences for reducing target maladaptive behaviors. As Crone and Horner (2003) suggest, one should first rearrange any currently used consequences that may be inadvertently maintaining maladaptive behavior. For example, staff members who send a child home from school every time he or she misbehaves may actually be reinforcing disruptive behavior if the child prefers being home to remaining in school. Hence the PBS plan will need to change this contingency.

PBS plans may also include providing specific consequences to reduce or eliminate maladaptive behaviors. During the past 15–20 years, local, state, and federal guidelines have been developed to provide rules and regulations regarding how such techniques are to be implemented. Most guidelines specifically allow the use of the majority of behavioral interventions described below. However, programs both to increase and to decrease specific behaviors must often be submitted to and approved by an internal review committee, and ongoing documentation and periodic review are required. For example, the state of Pennsylvania, as most states do, provides specific guidelines for the use of restrictive interventions in settings such as sheltered workshops and community residences (e.g., Department of Public Welfare, Office of Mental Retardation, Commonwealth of Pennsylvania, 1995). Such guidelines promote the use of least restrictive interventions prior to more restrictive programs. Any program that restricts clients' access to reinforcers, whether it be a complex token economy system or the use of a simple contingency (e.g., telling clients that they must finish their dinner to watch TV), may require a written protocol and committee approval under some guidelines.

There has also been a strong movement to promote only positive interventions in work with children with mental retardation (e.g., Donnellan, LaVigna, Negri-Shoeltz, & Fassbender, 1988; Horner et al., 1990). However, there may be some situations where specific consequences will need to be put into place following the occurrence of maladaptive behaviors. The interventions described below are presented in what is generally considered to be the order from least to most restrictive (Pierce & Cheney, 2004). Although these interventions have changed little over the past two decades, they remain important components of many PBS plans.

Differential Reinforcement. Differential reinforcement involves reinforcing a range of alternative behaviors, such as incompatible behaviors (DRI) or other behaviors (DRO). Implementing DRI requires the clinician to identify a behavior or class of behaviors incompatible with the target behavior he or she is attempting to decrease. For example, Miltenberger, Handen, and Capriotti (1987) used a range of interventions, including DRI, to treat hand stereotypies in a child with mental retardation. In this study, behaviors incompatible with the stereotypies (e.g., keeping hands down, using hands to play with toys) were specifically reinforced.

DRO has also been called "differential reinforcement of *zero* rates of behavior." This differs somewhat from DRI, in that reinforcement is given following a period of time in which a specific behavior has not occurred. Reinforcement is not based on the occurrence of a specific behavior, as in DRI. DRO can be useful in decreasing disruptive or interfering behaviors. For example, Conyers and colleagues (2004) used DRO to successfully reduce disruptive behavior in 25 children in a preschool classroom. Children earned tokens at 10-minute intervals in which there was an absence of disruptive behavior.

The advantages of differential reinforcement procedures are that they are constructive, benign, and acceptable, and that they can result in lasting change (Sulzer-Azaroff & Mayer, 1991). It is best to select behaviors to reinforce that are already well established in a child's repertoire, that are likely to be supported in the natural environment (e.g., talking nicely will be more likely to result in attention from others), and that serve equivalent functions to those of the maladaptive behaviors. For example, Durand (1999) used FC training to teach five students with severe disabilities and behavior problems (e.g., aggression, SIB, tantrums) to use assistive communication devices in school to request objects and activities that were presumed to maintain their maladaptive behaviors. Following training, behavior rates not only decreased in school, but generalized to the community with untrained community members (who were able to understand the requests the students made with the assistive communication devices). DRO effectiveness can be enhanced by maximizing the opportunities for reinforcement (e.g., if self-stimulatory behaviors occur every 3 minutes, the DRO schedule should start at about 2 minutes) and only gradually adjusting the schedule of reinforcement once gains are made (Sulzer-Azaroff & Mayer, 1991).

Differential reinforcement procedures also have a number of potential disadvantages. First, the effects may be delayed, requiring that other interventions be used in combination with DRI/DRO to deal with occurrences of the targeted undesirable behavior. For example, reinforcing appropriate use of hands for a child who is aggressive may also require that time out be used following incidents of hitting. DRO requires that those implementing the program continue to watch for maladaptive behaviors, and it is also possible that other maladaptive behaviors will be inadvertently reinforced.

Extinction. Extinction involves withholding reinforcement following a behavior that was previously reinforced (Pierce & Cheney, 2004). To implement an extinction program, the most important step is to identify what is presently maintaining the target behavior. For example, Reed and colleagues (2004) demonstrated that if inappropriate behaviors during feeding (e.g., pushing the food away, turning the head away) resulted in termination of demands to eat, such behaviors were likely to be negatively reinforced and would persist. Similarly, Iwata and colleagues (1994) found that some children who exhibit SIB do so to gain adult attention. Consequently, when an adult attempts to leave the child, SIB increases and is reinforced when the adult returns and attends to the child.

Extinction results in a gradual reduction in behavior, but a reduction that is often long-lasting. It is most effective when used in combination with positive reinforcement. For example, Piazza and colleagues (2003) compared the effects of positive reinforcement alone, escape extinction alone (not terminating food presentation contingent upon maladaptive behavior), and positive reinforcement with escape extinction in the treatment of food and fluid refusal for children with feeding disorders. Consumption only increased when escape extinction was implemented. Although the presence of positive reinforcement had little effect on intake, it was associated with other beneficial effects (e.g., greater decreases in negative vocalizations and inappropriate behavior) for some subjects.

In clinical settings, "extinction" is often referred to as "planned ignoring." However, planned ignoring can only be an effective form of extinction if adult attention is determined to be the source of reinforcement for the target behavior. Sulzer-Azaroff and Mayer (1991) cite a number of potential disadvantages to the use of extinction. The first involves its delayed effects; because of these, extinction could be an inappropriate intervention for such behaviors as running into the street or exposing oneself in public. The second potential disadvantage is the frequent appearance of an "extinction burst." In other words, when a behavior is initially placed on extinction, it typically becomes worse (e.g., a child who whines when not getting his or her way will probably whine more when parents first stop responding to this behavior). Again, this property makes extinction an inappropriate intervention for behaviors that may reach dangerous levels. There is also some evidence that the use of extinction can induce aggression (Skinner, 1953). Finally, extinction may be difficult to implement in situations in which the clinician cannot control the source of reinforcement. For example, adults may ignore a child who swears, but peers may continue to respond, thereby helping to reinforce and maintain the behavior.

Response Cost. Response cost involves making the loss of a reinforcer contingent upon the target response. Because it is an aversive procedure, such a program must be consistent with regulatory law and may need to be approved by an institutional review committee. Response cost is different from punishment because it involves removal of a reinforcer following the target behavior, rather than presentation of an aversive consequence contingent upon a specific behavior. For example, loss of a privilege (e.g., watching television) due to an episode of aggression involves response cost. Response cost can also be used as part of a token economy system, where a child is fined points or tokens contingent upon a target behavior. For instance, Conyers and colleagues (2004) implemented a token economy in a classroom of 25 preschoolers with disruptive behaviors. An alternating-treatments design was used, in which behavior was reduced either when the children earned tokens for the absence of disruptive behavior (DRO) or when they lost tokens following the occurrence of disruptive behavior (response cost). Although DRO was initially the more successful treatment, response cost proved over time to be more effective.

The advantages of response cost, according to Sulzer-Azaroff and Mayer (1991), are a strong and rapid reduction in behavior, convenience, and possible long-lasting effects. Despite such advantages, response cost also has a number of potential problems. First, the very ease of its use makes abuse of response cost more likely. For example, it can be used too often and/or penalties can be too harsh if the program is not well monitored. Once a child loses too many points or privileges, there may be little incentive to try to earn points or privileges back. In addition, as with any aversive intervention, such programs may result in aggression or escape. For instance, a child may increase levels of maladaptive behavior in response to being fined, or may avoid situations in which a fine might be levied. It is also

important when response cost is implemented to combine the intervention with a reinforcement program. For example, Leblanc, Hagopian, and Maglieri (2000) successfully used a token economy in combination with response cost to decrease inappropriate social behavior in an adult male with mental retardation. DRO was used to reinforce the absence of inappropriate behaviors (e.g., placing his face close to others, attempting to kiss others, swearing, touching his genital area). The subject began each session with a "bank" of five tokens. The occurrence of any of the target behaviors resulted in a one-token fine and a resetting of the DRO time interval. Finally, Sulzer-Azaroff and Mayer suggest that children have a reserve of points before fines are implemented, and that the magnitude of the fines be determined empirically. In other words, the behavior should be monitored under different cost magnitudes until the desired reduction in behavior is obtained.

Time Out. Time out involves limiting access to sources of reinforcement for a specified period of time contingent upon a target behavior (Sulzer-Azaroff & Mayer, 1991). Unlike response cost, removal of reinforcement occurs for a period of time rather than by a specified amount (e.g., two tokens). For time out to be used effectively, the clinician must control all potential sources of reinforcement. For example, time out would be inappropriate for a child who engages in high rates of self-stimulation or SIB. Such a child would be less likely to find removal from an activity and/or attention to be aversive. Similarly, adult attention should be limited during the time-out period. Sulzer-Azaroff and Mayer (1991) suggest that the duration of time out be kept relatively short. Studies that have compared different durations of time out have found periods of 5 minutes or less to be as effective for most children as 15- to 30-minute periods (Kendall, Nay, & Jeffers, 1975; White, Nielsen, & Johnson, 1972). In addition, a study by Mace, Page, Ivancic, and O'Brien (1986) found time out to be just as effective whether children were required to sit quietly at the end of the time-out period or were simply allowed to return to the group at the conclusion of time out, regardless of their behavior. As with all other procedures designed to reduce behavior, time out is most effective when combined with other reinforcement interventions.

Time out has been most often associated with the removal of a child from the group to a time-out room or area. However, many variations of time out can be just as effective. Nelson and Rutherford (1983) describe the use of planned ignoring, in which an adult simply drops his or her head and remains motionless for a few seconds following a maladaptive response. For example, a teacher might use a 10-second planned ignoring response whenever a student starts to engage in inappropriate speech (e.g., laughing, swearing). Another variation is contingent observation, which involves removing the child only a few feet from the area for time out, so that he or she can observe activities but not participate. Foxx and Shapiro (1978) describe the use of time-out ribbons in a group of students with severe mental retardation. Students lost their ribbons for a few minutes following the occurrence of specific maladaptive behaviors. Reinforcers such as treats and praise were only given to students who were wearing their ribbons. More restrictive forms of time out involve removing a child to either a specific time-out area within a room or a separate time-out room. Time out is designed to occur for relatively short periods of time, such as 5–10 minutes. One common rule of thumb is to use 1 minute for each year of age (e.g., a 5-year-old would be in time out for 5 minutes).

Hall and Hall (1998) suggest that the main advantage of time out is its ability to reduce behavior. Another advantage for families is its utility (i.e., a child can be placed in a time-out chair in most settings—at home, at a relative's house, in a store). However, there are also several disadvantages to the use of time out. Sulzer-Azaroff and Mayer (1991) suggest that time out has the potential for abuse and may lead to the suppression of other, appropriate behaviors. In addition, when a child is in time out, there is a loss of learning time (especially opportunities to be reinforced for engaging in appropriate behaviors). Time out is also not universally effective. For example, Doleys, Wells, Hobbs, Roberts, and Cartelli (1976) found time out to be less effective in improving rates of compliance in a group of children with mental retardation than social punishment (i.e., scolding) was. Similarly, Solnick, Rincover, and Peterson (1977) found time out to be ineffective at eliminating tantrums in a 6-year-old girl with autism, because the child simply engaged in stereotypic behaviors during

the time-out period. In the same study, time out failed to decrease spitting and SIB in a 16-year-old adolescent with mental retardation until the non-time-out environment was "enriched" (i.e., highly desirable activities were placed in the classroom so that time out resulted in a loss of access to these materials). One might hypothesize that time out for noncompliance might also be ineffective because one might actually reinforce noncompliant behavior by allowing a child to escape from a demand situation. However, Handen, Parrish, McClung, Kerwin, and Evans (1992) compared time out and guided compliance (i.e., physically assisting a child to comply with a request) as treatments for noncompliance in preschoolers with developmental disabilities. Time out was found to be the more effective intervention, as long as a child was returned to the demand situation immediately after the time-out period.

The most significant disadvantages of time out are the legal restrictions and public concerns regarding its use. For example, the *Wyatt v. Stickney* (1972) decision specifically prohibits the use of seclusion for individuals with mental retardation, but allows for professionally supervised time out as part of a behavior-shaping program. Various settings and jurisdictions have specific policies regarding the use of time out. As with all behavioral interventions, a clinician will need to be aware of the regulations that apply to his or her particular region and facility.

Common Behavior Problems in Mental Retardation

Several behavioral concerns either tend to be specific to individuals with mental retardation or are seen at high rates in this population. SIB and stereotypy are two classes of behavior that are frequently reported among children and adults with mental retardation.

Self-Injurious Behavior

The ability to assess and treat SIB is extremely important for any clinician working with children with mental retardation. SIB is defined as a response that produces physical injury to the individual's own body (Tate & Baroff, 1966). Such behaviors often include head banging, self-biting, self-hitting, hair pulling, eye poking, pica, and chronic rumination. Estimates of the incidence of SIB range from 7% to 23%, with most surveys reporting about 15% (Kahng, Iwata, & Lewin, 2002). For example, a survey of approximately 10,000 individuals in 13 residential facilities in Texas documented that 13.6% of this population displayed some form of SIB (Griffin, Williams, Stark, Altmeyer, & Mason, 1986). Kahng and colleagues (2002) reviewed 396 papers on SIB published between 1964 and 2000. They found that most research subjects were male (57% of the sample), and that the majority of individuals (71%) functioned within the severe to profound range of mental retardation, indicating that SIB is related to cognitive functioning levels. The most common forms of SIB were head banging/hitting (49% of the sample) and biting (30% of the sample). However, 27.6% of the sample displayed multiple topographies of SIB.

Much has been written on the etiology and treatment of SIB. A few known syndromes are specifically associated with a high incidence of SIB. For example, Lesch–Nyhan syndrome (Lesch & Nyhan, 1964) is a sex-linked disorder of purine metabolism in which individuals engage in severe self-mutilation (e.g., self-biting). The extent of SIB in this syndrome appears to be unrelated to cognitive functioning levels (Nyhan, 1976). This relationship between SIB and a biochemical defect is of considerable importance in furthering our understanding of both SIB and neurobiology. SIB has also been noted in a number of other genetic disorders, although at rates significantly lower than that seen in Lesch–Nyhan syndrome. These include Cornelia de Lange syndrome, Rett syndrome, Tourette syndrome, and fragile X syndrome. However, no causal links between these disorders and SIB has been found. SIB is also frequently reported to occur in children with autism.

Neurobiological studies, most of which have been conducted with animals, have suggested some possible models for the occurrence of SIB. For example, preliminary results suggest that dopamine depletion in the basal ganglia or an imbalance in neurotransmitter function in brain dopamine pathways due to aberrant perinatal development may lead to SIB in children with Lesch–Nyhan syndrome (see review by Schroeder, Breese, & Mueller, 1989). Other work has been conducted to investigate the endogenous opioid peptide hypothesis (Sandman et al., 1983), in which beta-endorphin levels increase with the occurrence of SIB; consequently, the pain threshold is elevated, and tol-

erance for SIB is raised. This hypothesis has resulted in the conceptualization of SIB as an addictive behavior. The implications of such neurobiological research might lead to pharmacological interventions directly based on neurobiological theory (see the section on psychopharmacological treatment).

The recent use of functional analysis for the assessment of SIB has led to specific treatment interventions and has resulted in the greater selection of reinforcement-based interventions (vs. punishment) during the past 10–15 years (Pelios, Morren, Tesch, & Axelrod, 1999). Functional analysis posits that SIB is maintained (and possibly developed) by environmental contingencies. One example is illustrated by Iwata and colleagues (1982), who used this model to better understand variables associated with SIB in nine children with developmental disabilities. During an extended baseline period, children were repeatedly observed for 15-minute blocks of time. Each child was exposed to four different experimental conditions: social disapproval for SIB; academic demands in which the clinician turned away for 30 seconds following SIB (with praise given for task completion); a no-demand play situation (with SIB ignored); and an alone condition. Six of nine subjects exhibited higher levels of SIB under specific stimulus conditions, suggesting that within-subject variability was a function of environmental features. Figure 6.2 illustrates the percentage of 10-second intervals in which SIB was observed for four subjects. These findings have implications for the selection of appropriate treatment interventions. For example, Child 1, who displayed self-injury only during the academic (i.e., demand) condition, might successfully be treated with interventions such as (1) behavioral momentum (starting with demands with a high probability of compliance before introducing academic demands); (2) FC (teaching the child an appropriate signal for the desire to stop working); or (3) guided compliance/escape extinction (blocking SIB and guiding the child through the demand in order to prevent escape).

Although many different interventions have been used to treat SIB, the available treatment procedures have changed little during the past decade. In their recent review of the SIB literature, Kahng and colleagues (2002) divided behavioral treatment into seven categories: antecedent manipulation, extinction, reinforce-

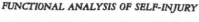

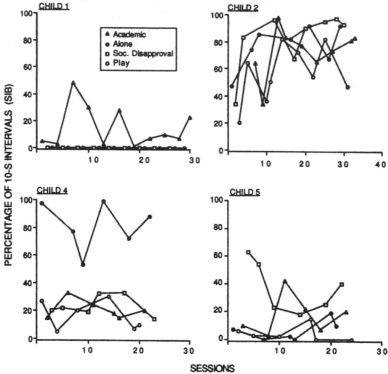

FIGURE 6.2. Percentage of intervals of self-injury for subjects 1, 2, 4, and 5 across sessions and experimental conditions. From Iwata, Dorsey, Slifer, Bauman, and Richman (1982, p. 14). Copyright 1982 by Elsevier. Reprinted by permission.

ment (e.g., DRO and DRA), punishment (e.g., time out, facial screening, overcorrection), restraint, response blocking, and other. (An eighth category, pharmacological treatment, is addressed later in this chapter.) Antecedent manipulation interventions are described in detail by Carr, Taylor, Carlson, and Robinson (1989) and involve making changes in the range of possible stimuli associated with SIB. For example, one might reduce the difficulty of work tasks or reduce transitions or noise levels, if these are associated with increased rates of SIB. Either response blocking or the use of protective equipment (e.g., helmet, mitts, arm splints) prevents an individual from engaging in SIB and disrupts the response–reinforcer relationship (this disruption is also referred to as "sensory extinction") (Kuhn, DeLeon, Fisher, & Wilke, 1999). Many of the studies reviewed by Kahng and colleagues combined treatment interventions (e.g., reinforcement with extinc-

tion), but others assessed single treatment modalities. For example, Pace, Iwata, Edwards, and McCosh (1986) combined treatments by using inflatable air splints to prevent a 15-year-old adolescent with mental retardation from scratching skin from behind his ears. During treatment sessions, adult praise and touch were provided for playing with toys (reinforcement). Over time, the air pressure in the splints was gradually decreased (a fading procedure) while the absence of SIB was maintained.

With the increased (and sometimes state-mandated) use of functional analysis, the choice of treatment for SIB should be based on the assessment results. For example, if a child is found to engage in SIB primarily as a means to avoid or escape task demands, interventions might include adjusting the difficulty of task demands, along with guided compliance (Van Houten, Rolider, & Houlihan, 1992). Kahng and colleagues (2002) found most published treatments to be successful in significantly reducing SIB by at least 80%. Reinforcement alone or in combination with response blocking proved to be slightly less effective (with mean reductions in SIB rates across studies of 72–73%), while reinforcement in combination with antecedent manipulation was the most effective (100% decrease in SIB rates in four published studies). However, these results should be interpreted with some caution, as researchers and editors tend only to report their successes (Johnson & Baumeister, 1978). Despite almost 400 studies of SIB during a 35-year time span, only 13% of studies provided follow-up data (mean of 15.7 months), and only 11% assessed generalization.

Stereotypic Behavior

The terms "SIB" and "stereotypic behavior" are often confused and have frequently been interchanged (Schroeder, 1991). However, they refer to two separate classes of behavior, which may well have their basis in different biological mechanisms (Schroeder, 1991). Stereotypic behaviors often include body rocking, mouthing, finger and hand movements, and object manipulation (such as spinning toys). DSM-IV-TR (APA, 2000) includes both SIB and stereotypic behavior in the diagnostic criteria for stereotypic movement disorder, although it adds the qualifier "with self-injurious behavior" for individuals with SIB. (Stereotypies are also among the criteria for several other DSM-IV-TR diagnoses, such as autistic disorder and other pervasive developmental disorders.) Wehmeyer (1994) found that close to 15% of young children with mental retardation displayed stereotypic behavior. Stremme and Diseth (2000), in their survey of Norwegian children with mental retardation, found 5.5% of their sample to display stereotypic behavior.

Schroeder (1991) divides the theories of the etiology of stereotypic behavior into those depicting it as driven by endogenous or internal factors and those proposing more environmental variables. Although these two types of theories are not necessarily mutually exclusive, the former suggest that such behaviors are highly resistant to change by modification of external stimuli. Behavioral models propose that some individuals may have learned to engage in stereotypic behavior to escape demands, to avoid undesired situations, or to attain attention. For other individuals, such behavior appear to be maintained by automatic reinforcement (not controlled by social events). As with SIB, a functional analysis should provide the best means of determining the true function of a given individual's stereotypic behavior.

Examples of successful treatment interventions to treat various forms of stereotypic behavior include Haring and Kennedy's (1990) use of tokens to reinforce on-task behavior and omission of stereotypic behavior (DRO) in severely disturbed children, as well as Foxx, McMorrow, Bittle, and Ness's (1986) reinforcement of alternative behavior to replace public masturbation by a 16-year-old male with severe mental retardation. More recently, Ringdahl, Wacker, Berg, and Harding (2001) describe the case of a 2-year-old with developmental disabilities who engaged in stereotypic behavior (mouthing carpet fibers and hair from a hairbrush). A functional analysis indicated that the automatic reinforcement was probably maintaining the behavior. A subsequent assessment, in which the child was given the choice of access to toys and adult attention versus access to a hairbrush, found the former to be preferred (during which time mouthing did not occur). Consequently, the recommended treatment was to provide ready access to preferred items. As with SIB, there has been little in the way of new treatment strategies for stereotypic behavior during the past decade. The main emphasis has been on connecting the findings of the functional analysis with the recommended treatment.

Documenting Progress

Data Collection

In addition to conducting an FBA or functional analysis, it is important to collect baseline data regarding the rate and/or duration of the behavior. This information will be needed to determine whether the behavior treatment plan is working. Various methods are available for collecting such data. The easiest method involves simply recording the frequency of the target behavior (i.e., counting the number of occurrences of the event). For example, Hagopian, van Stone, and Crockett (2003) conducted a functional analysis to assess the relationship between falling to the ground and various situations (e.g., providing attention for falling, making demands, ignoring the behavior, and a no-demand play condition) in an adolescent with profound mental retardation. The dependent measure was simply the number of times the subject was observed to fall to the ground during each 10-minute observation. Other examples include recording the number of aggressive acts during the school day or the number of times a student uses inappropriate language (e.g., swore).

A second option involves recording the duration of an event (when the length of time a behavior occurs is of importance). This may be useful for observing behaviors such as remaining in seat, playing appropriately, or crying. The clinician simply records the total time a child engages in the target behavior during the observation period. Some behaviors occur at an extremely high rate or are continuous, making it difficult to record either frequency or duration (especially if the data are being taken by a member of the classroom staff). In such a case, interval time sampling can be used. The day is divided into an equal number of time intervals (e.g., 10-minute intervals). One common method of coding is to use partial-interval time sampling. For example, Figure 6.3 depicts (fictional) partial-interval time-sampling data on Susie's swearing during the first 2 hours of school. Any time Susie swears during a 10-minute interval, the appropriate interval is marked. Once an interval has been scored, no data are recorded until the next time interval starts.

Other methods of time sampling include whole-interval recording (where the behavior must persist for the entire interval before it is recorded) and momentary time sampling (recording whatever behavior is observed precisely at the end of the time interval).

Single-Subject Designs

Every behavior treatment plan can be considered a single-subject experimental design. For example, once a PBS plan has been implemented, it will be important to continue to obtain data on the frequency or duration of the target behavior in order to assess the plan's efficacy. At the very least, such data involves an "A-B" design, which allows the clinician to examine behavior both prior to and following the intervention. However, several alternative and more powerful single-subject designs are available; these allow the clinician to demonstrate a functional relationship between the intervention and target behavior.

Pierce and Cheney (2004) describe a number of single-subject designs that can be used when implementing a behavior change program. The most basic design is a "reversal" or "A-B-A-B" design. This simply involves returning to baseline conditions (A) after implementing a behavioral procedure (B). Experimental control of the procedure is demonstrated when the behav-

Name: Susie

Date: 12/4/03

Behavior: Swearing

Hour/Minute	1–10	11–20	21–30	31–40	41–50	51–60
9:00 A.M.	X			X	X	X
10:00 A.M.		X	X			
11:00 A.M.						
12:00 noon						
1:00 P.M.						
2:00 P.M.						
3:00 P.M.						

Total Number of Intervals Rated: _____

Percentage of Intervals Behavior Rated: _____

FIGURE 6.3. Partial-Interval Time-Sampling Form.

ior returns to baseline levels and changes again when the behavioral procedure is reinstituted. One disadvantage of such a design is that a clinician may not wish to return to baseline conditions after obtaining a significant decrease in behaviors such as SIB or aggression. A second design option is a "multiple-baseline" design. This can be conducted across behaviors, settings, or individuals. For example, data are obtained on a target behavior across a number of individuals. A behavioral program is implemented for only a single child while data continue to be collected on the others. Experimental control is demonstrated if the behavior changes for the targeted child but not for the remaining individuals (The intervention is subsequently implemented for each succeeding child, while baseline conditions remain in effect for the others.). Finally, an "alternating-treatment" design allows experimental control to be demonstrated by altering two or more different interventions in succession with the same child. For example, a teacher may compare the relative effectiveness of two different treatment programs for a girl who talks without raising her hand in class. In the morning, a point system is implemented in which a point is awarded every 30 minutes if the child has been following the classroom rule of raising her hand and being called upon before talking. Conversely, in the afternoon, the student is verbally reprimanded by the teacher every time she talks out and is then reminded that she must raise her hand instead. After 2–3 weeks of treatment, the data on the two interventions can be compared.

OTHER TYPES OF TREATMENT PROGRAMS

Parent Training

There has been considerable empirical support for the efficacy of behavioral parent training among typically developing children with disorders or problem behaviors such as ADHD, aggression, and noncompliance (Forehand & Kotchick, 2002). In fact, a number of parent training manuals have been deemed empirically supported treatments (Woody & Sanderson, 1998). Parent training has become a well-accepted component in treatment plans for children with mental retardation and other developmental disabilities (Breiner & Beck, 1984; Callias, 1987; Harris, Alessandri, & Gill, 1991), with a number of studies demonstrating

that parent-based treatment interventions can be superior to clinic-based treatment alone (e.g., Koegel, Schreibman, Britten, Burke, & O'Neill, 1982). Parent training models have been successfully used in a number of educational and clinic settings, such as the LEAP Preschool Program (Strain & Cordisco, 1994), the Individualized Support Program at the University of South Florida (Dunlap, 1999), the Pivotal Response Training Model (Koegel, Koegel, Shoshan, & McNerney, 1999), and the Douglas Developmental Center Program (Harris, Handleman, Arnold, & Gordan, 2000). Yet most of these programs primarily serve children with autism (many of whom have developmental delays and/or mental retardation, however).

Parent training programs for children with developmental disabilities may differ in emphasis, but most are based on the principles of ABA as described earlier (Baker, 1996). Programs typically include a functional analysis of behavior, training parents to record the child's response, modification of the child's behavior through environmental manipulation (antecedent management), differential reinforcement of appropriate behaviors, and the systematic introduction of new skills and behaviors. Parent instruction typically involves didactic information, readings, practice with feedback, home visits for consultation and demonstration of interventions, telephone consultation, and follow-up contact (see Newsom & Hovanitz, Chapter 7, this volume). Most also include the use of homework assignments tailored to a particular family's needs (Baker, 1996).

Researchers in the field have demonstrated that parents can be trained in a wide range of behavioral interventions, including time out, positive reinforcement, token economies, and skill acquisition (see review by Harris et al., 1991). Several different approaches to parent training are available to the clinician. One option is to teach parents to manage behavior problems specific to their child's individual needs. Conversely, parents can be instructed in a general course or curriculum that covers a range of basic topics relevant to most families with children with mental retardation (e.g., reinforcement principles, behavior problem management, skills teaching). Finally, the option of providing individual or group instruction must also be considered. For example, there is some available literature documenting the efficacy of parent training within a group setting (e.g., Harris, 1983). However, in some cases, individualized instruction may be more appropriate. Clark and Baker (1983) identified a number of risk factors for parents who tended to do poorly with group instruction, including lower socioeconomic status, less experience with behavior modification techniques, and anticipation of greater problems in teaching their children. Conversely, parents who were in intact marriages and who had made prior efforts to teach their children were more likely to complete the parent training course and to report successful outcomes.

Most programs use parent training to supplement other services, making moderate demands on parents' time and effort. For example, the Project for Developmental Disabilities used a group training curriculum that involved parents in 10 weekly 2-hour sessions, along with a home teaching requirement of about 5 minutes per day (Baker, 1989). Working with a similar population, Feldman and Werner (2002) conducted weekly in-home parent training sessions (over a 3- to 6-month period). Results indicated significantly fewer child behavior problems and family stress in these families than in families not receiving such services. Although outcome results suggest that children with more severe mental retardation tend to show fewer gains, parent outcomes (e.g., acquisition of behavioral skills, follow-through) have been unrelated to a child's age, sex, diagnosis, or level of mental retardation (Baker, Landen, & Kashima, 1991; Clark & Baker, 1983). Follow-up studies have found that parents of children with developmental disabilities continue to use their newly acquired behavioral skills long after training has been completed (Baker, Heifetz, & Murphy, 1980; Feldman & Werner, 2002).

Despite a long tradition of research in this area, there has been relatively little recent work on parent training and children with mental retardation. One of the few available structured parent training books focusing exclusively on children with mental retardation is the *Steps to Independence* manual for children with special needs (Baker & Brightman, 1997); it covers such areas as teaching self-help skills, enhancing language skills, toilet training, and behavior problem management. Consequently, many gaps remain in our understanding of how best to provide parent training for families of children with mental retardation.

Psychotherapy

There has been little empirical research on the efficacy of psychotherapy for individuals with mental retardation. Typically, mental retardation has been used as an exclusionary criterion for psychotherapy efficacy studies (Matson, 1984). Many clinicians continue to assume that intellectual deficits often account for emotional and behavioral symptomatology in this population, that individuals with mental retardation do not have mental health disorders, that such individuals cannot understand therapeutic concepts, or that they become overly dependent (Butz, Bowling, & Bliss, 2000).

An analogue study of mental health professionals found that clinicians were more likely to offer behaviorally oriented recommendations than individual counseling and psychotherapy to individuals with mental retardation (Alford & Locke, 1984). A national survey conducted by Dorn and Prout (1993) found that adults with mild mental retardation were significantly less likely than adults without mental retardation to be offered psychotherapeutic services. There has been a recent push for increased psychotherapy research in the area of mental retardation. Prout, Chard, Nowak-Drabik, and Johnson (2000) have called for improved rigor in research, including better descriptions of subjects (including age and IQ), the use of reliable and valid dependent measures, better description of treatment procedures, and the assessment of both clinical and statistical significance of outcome.

Prout and Nowak-Drabik (2003) recently reviewed 92 psychotherapy studies from 1968 to 1998 involving individuals with mental retardation. "Psychotherapy" was defined as face-to-face meetings involving counseling or skill training (e.g., social skills, assertiveness). Behavior modification, classroom interventions, and consultative treatments were not included, although papers describing psychotherapy that was "behavioral" in orientation were included in the review (it was not clear how this was defined). A consensus panel rated each paper in regard to the type of research and outcome; ratings were made on a 5-point scale from "no effect" (1) to "marked effect" (5). Results of the review of 83 studies found a moderate level of effectiveness (mean rating of 2.72) across age, level of mental retardation, technique, and theoretical approach. Other trends noted were significantly higher outcome ratings for studies that involved clinic-based treatment, individual treatment, and treatments that were behavioral in orientation. The most striking finding was the poor quality of this literature, which was dominated by case studies or single-subject designs, vague outcome data (often marginally related to the treatment), poor descriptions of treatments, and minimal information regarding subject characteristics. Although Prout and Nowak-Drabik have concluded that psychotherapy should be considered as part of the treatment plan for individuals with mental retardation, the field remains far from being able to match a specific psychotherapy intervention to particular client characteristics or presenting problems.

Social Skills Training

Social skills deficits are often identified as important target areas for children with mental retardation. The development of appropriate social skills is necessary both for fostering friendships within the community and, later on, for succeeding in competitive or semi-competitive employment. Social skills cover a wide range—from maintaining eye contact when speaking with others, using language, and sharing toys, to more complex skills such as problem solving and entering groups. Although one of the goals of inclusion is the development of social relationships, studies have found that simply placing a student with mental retardation in a classroom of typically developing peers does not necessarily lead to increased social interactions or to the development of social skills (Staub, Spalding, Peck, Gallucci, & Schwartz, 1996). Instead, specific efforts must be made to foster the development of friendships and to teach social skills. Strategies typically fall into three categories: (1) teaching specific social skills to the student with mental retardation; (2) teaching typically developing peers to initiate social interactions, engage in peer tutoring activities, and the like with classmates who have developmental disabilities; and (3) working with teachers (especially those in general education) to promote interactions and adapt lesson plans to promote interactions between typically developing peers and students with disabilities.

Prompting and various reinforcement procedures have been used to teach play and social interaction skills to children with mental retar-

dation as well as other disabilities (e.g., Coe, Matson, Fee, Manikam, & Linarello, 1990; Zanolli, Daggett, & Adams, 1996). Jolly, Test, and Spooner (1993) taught children with severe disabilities to use badges to initiate play interactions with typically developing peers. Several curricula are also available to teach social skills to individuals with mental retardation and other developmental disorders (e.g., McAfee, 2002).

Typically developing peers have been successfully used to reinforce, prompt, or initiate social interactions with children with disabilities (e.g., McGee, Almeida, Sulzer-Azaroff, & Feldman, 1992; Odom, Chandler, Ostrosky, McConnell, & Reaney, 1992). Various educational interventions have also shown some promise in helping to increase social interactions between children with mental retardation and their peers. These include a "circle of friends" (O'Brien, Forest, Snow, & Hasbury, 1989), cooperative learning programs (Piercy, Wilton, & Townsend, 2002), and peer tutoring and buddy programs (Cooke, Heron, Heward, & Test, 1982; Staub et al., 1996).

Finally, teachers are often paramount to encouraging and promoting social interactions among all children in their classrooms. Ferguson, Meyer, Jeanchild, Juniper, and Zingo (1992) describe three specific roles for teachers: (1) locating resources and matching them to students' needs, (2) modifying lesson plans to include children with disabilities, and (3) working with other professionals in the school to collaborate in meeting the needs of students with disabilities.

Community-Based Interventions

Family-centered assessment and intervention (Dunst, Trivette, & Deal, 1994) have come to be recognized as playing an important role in serving the needs of children with special needs and their families. This assessment and treatment model encompasses three goals: (1) identifying family needs, priorities, or concerns; (2) locating formal and informal resources for meeting the needs; and (3) helping families identify and use their strengths and capabilities to procure resources in ways that strengthen family functioning (Hobbs et al., 1984). Family-centered or community-based resources offer a direct contrast to a service-based resources model, which has historically been provided by agencies and school systems. The latter model is defined as "a specific or particular activity employed by a professional or professional agency for rendering help or assistance to an individual or group, such as occupational therapy or special instruction" (Trivette, Dunst, & Deal, 1997, p. 75). Conversely, community-based resources are defined as "the full range of possible types of community help or assistance that might be mobilized and used to meet the needs of an individual or group" (Trivette et al., p. 76). Such an approach emphasizes utilizing multiple sources of informal and formal community resources to address the needs of a child and his or her family, rather than relying on professional assistance.

According to Trivette and colleagues (1997), the service-based resources model has a number of inherent weaknesses. For example, this model tends to be self-limiting, because it is defined by what professionals do and is professionally centered. A second weakness is that the service-based model is based on providing limited resources only to the most needy families, as determined by professionals. Finally, this model often limits the use of richer and more diverse informal services and support networks that are available in the community.

The community-based resources model is supported by a growing body of empirical evidence that documents the benefits of community-based practices over service-based interventions in terms of their impact on families. For example, Dunst, Trivette, Starnes, Hamby, and Gordon (1993) conducted extensive case studies of the characteristics and effects of various types of practices employed by human service agencies in their work with a group of 22 families. The families were asked to rate their reactions or feelings to various practices, as well as to rate the treatment outcome (on a 5-point scale) for both service-based and community-based practices. Findings indicated that practices deemed as community-based were associated with significantly more positive outcomes than were service-based models. A second study compared service-based (formalized respite care) and community-based (collaborative effort to identify a range of community-based child care options) early intervention programming with 30 families that had been randomly assigned to one of these two possible treatments. Results indicated that resource-based approaches demonstrated significantly greater change than

community-based models on measures of the number of individuals who provided child care, successful attempts to obtain child care, perceived control over obtaining child care, and overall satisfaction with child care (Dunst, 1991). Finally, 1,300 parents of children participating in early intervention programs were requested to rate the extent to which service practices emphasized community resources, the level of progress their children had made, and the extent to which parents felt in control over the kinds or services and activities that were provided (Trivette et al., 1997). Results indicated significantly higher ratings of child progress and parental control when practices were community-based rather than service-based.

Another aspect of community-based interventions is to ensure that children with mental retardation are provided with full participation in everyday activities. Several developmental models emphasize the importance of involvement in everyday activities toward enhancing learning and development (Dunst, Hamby, Trivette, Raab, & Bruder, 2002). Such activities include daily routines (e.g., food shopping, bedtime routines), play activities (e.g., playgrounds, video games), and community involvement (e.g., sports, church). Research on everyday experiences of preschoolers and early elementary school-age children with developmental delays has found that families' efforts to provide such experiences for their children with disabilities are similar to those made by families of young children without delays (Gallimore, Weisner, Bernheimer, Guthrie, & Nihira, 1993). Surprisingly, the research in this area suggests that children with developmental disabilities are involved in a greater number of daily activities than had been previously thought (Dunst et al., 2002). Hence additional research is needed to gain a better understanding of how daily experiences affect development (Gauvain, 1999).

Twelve specific categories of community-based resources are listed below (Dunst, Trivette, & Deal, 1988):

1. Economic resources
2. Physical and environmental resources
3. Food and clothing resources
4. Medical and dental care resources
5. Employment and vocational resources
6. Transportation and communication resources
7. Adult education and enrichment resources

8. Child education and intervention resources
9. Child care resources
10. Recreational resources
11. Emotional resources
12. Cultural and social resources

For instance, specific examples of recreational resources include story times at a local library, classes at the YMCA/YWCA or community center, play groups, and children's programs offered at churches.

Trivette and colleagues (1997) describe a number of steps for assessing community-based resources. The first is to identify a family's needs, concerns, and priorities. Next, one must help the family members identify resources for meeting each of these needs. This can best be accomplished through the development of a community network map, which identifies individuals and institutions that come in contact with the family and resources that might be tapped to address family concerns. Trivette and colleagues recommend that resources available to address each concern be mapped separately, so as to keep this process focused.

PSYCHOPHARMACOLOGICAL TREATMENT

Children and adults with mental retardation have a long history of being prescribed psychotropic medications. As with individuals who do not have mental retardation, such medications are used to treat specific symptoms; they are not prescribed to treat mental retardation per se. A review of prevalence studies of psychotropic drug use among individuals with mental retardation from 1986 to 1995 found medication rates in institutions to range from 12% to 40%, while community medication rates ranged from 19% to 29% (exclusive of data on anticonvulsant drugs)(Singh, Ellis, & Wechsler, 1997). Stolker, Koedoot, Heerdink, Leufkens, and Nolen (2002) documented that 22.8% of individuals with mental retardation residing in group homes in the Netherlands were prescribed psychotropics—a rate generally consistent with the findings of Singh and colleagues (1997). Several variables appear to affect prescribing rates, including restrictiveness of setting (i.e., greater medication use in institutions than in community settings), age (i.e., adults receive psychotropic medication at higher rates

than children), and severity of mental retardation (i.e., individuals with lower IQs are more likely to receive psychotropic medication) (Singh et al., 1997).

Table 6.1 provides a summary of five general drug classes (psychostimulants, antidepressants, neuroleptics, mood stabilizers, and other drugs), along with their indications for use in children.

Psychostimulants

Stimulant medications are prescribed for the treatment of ADHD, which (as noted earlier in the chapter) affects 9–16% of children with mental retardation (Emerson, 2003; Stromme & Diseth, 2000). Methylphenidate is the most thoroughly studied agent in children with mental retardation, with at least 20 well-controlled group studies (e.g., Aman, Buican, & Arnold, 2003; Aman et al., 1997; Handen, Feldman, Lurier, & Murray, 1999; Pearson et al., 2003). Examination of this research indicates response rates to range from 45% to 66% (Aman, Armstrong, Buican, & Sillick, 2002)—a rate considerably lower than the 77% average response rate among typically developing children (Greenhill et al., 2001). Gains have been noted on measures of inattention, on-task behavior, task completion, and play behavior. Predictors of positive response include IQ above 50 (Aman, Kern, McGhee, & Arnold, 1993; Aman, Marks, Turbott, Wilsher, & Merry, 1991; Aman et al., 1993) and higher baseline scores on parent/teacher ratings of inattention and activity level (Handen, Janosky, McAuliffe, Breaux, & Feldman, 1994). This population also appears to be at greater risk for the development of adverse events (in comparison to typically developing children), such as motor tics and social withdrawal, especially at moderate doses (Handen, Feldman, Gosling, Breaux, & McAuliffe, 1991). There are no contemporary studies of other psychostimulant agents—including dextroamphetamine, mixed amphetamine salts (Adderall), and pemoline (Cylert)—in children with ADHD and mental retardation.

Antidepressants

The use of antidepressants has changed greatly over the past decade, with selective serotonin reuptake inhibitors (SSRIs) becoming the treatment of choice (over tricyclic antidepressants)

TABLE 6.1. Selected Psychopharmacological Agents

Drug class	Examples	Indications
Short-acting stimulants	Methylphenidate (Ritalin, Methylin[a]), dexmethylphenidate (Focalin), dextroamphetamine (Dexedrine), amphetamine	ADHD and sleep disorders
Long-acting stimulants	Methylphenidate (Concerta, Metadate SR, Metadate CD, Ritalin LA, Ritalin SR), mixed amphetamine salts (Adderall, Adderall XR)	ADHD
Antidepressants	Fluoxetine (Prozac)	Depression (children and adults), obsessive–compulsive disorder (children), generalized anxiety disorder,[b] aggression[b]
	Sertraline (Zoloft)	Depression (adults), generalized anxiety disorder, posttraumatic stress disorder, obsessive–compulsive disorder (children), aggression[b]
	Paroxetine (Paxil)	Depression (adults), generalized anxiety disorder, obsessive–compulsive disorder (adults), posttraumatic stress disorder, aggression[b]
	Fluvoxamine (Luvox)	Obsessive–compulsive disorder (children and adults)
	Vitalopram (Celexa)	Depression (adults), generalized anxiety disorder,[b] obsessive–compulsive disorder,[b] aggression[b]
	Escitalopram (Lexapro)	Depression (adults), generalized anxiety disorder (adults), obsessive–compulsive disorder,[b] aggression[b]
	Venlafaxine (Effexor, Effexor XR)	Depression (adults), generalized anxiety disorder,[b] obsessive–compulsive disorder,[b] aggression[b]
	Nefazodone (Serzone)	Depression (adults)
	Duloxetine (Cymbalta)	Depression (adults), diabetic neuropathy
	Mirtazapine (Remeron)	Depression (adults), insomnia[b]
	Bupropion (Wellbutrin, Wellbutrin SR, Wellbutrin XL)	Depression (adults), smoking cessation, ADHD,[b] generalized anxiety disorder,[b] obsessive–compulsive disorder,[b] aggression[b]
Atypical antipsychotics	Risperidone (Risperdal), olanzapine (Zyprexa), quetiapine (Seroquel), ziprasidone (Geodon), aripiprazole (Abilify)	Schizophrenia, other psychosis, aggression,[b] self-injurious behavior[b]
Mood stabilizers	Lithium (Lithobid, Eskalith)	Bipolar disorder, aggression,[b] depression[b]
	Oxcarbazepine (Trileptal)	Seizures, bipolar disorder,[b] self-injurious behavior,[b] aggression[b]
	Valproic acid (Depakene), divalproex sodium (Depakote, Depakote ER)	Seizures, bipolar disorder, aggression,[b] self-injurious behavior[b]
	Carbamazepine (Tegretol)	Seizures, bipolar disorder,[b] aggression,[b] self-injurious behavior[b]
	Lamotrigine (Lamictal)	Seizures, bipolar disorder (adults), aggression,[b] self-injurious behavior[b]
	Topiramate (Topamax)	Seizures, bipolar disorder,[b] aggression,[b] self-injurious behavior[b]
Other medications	Clonidine (Catapres), guanfacine (Tenex)	High blood pressure, generalized anxiety disorder,[b] aggression,[b] self-injurious behavior[b]
	Atomoxetine (Strattera)	ADHD

[a]New oral solution and chewable tablets.
[b]Not approved by the FDA for this use.

in children, with and without mental retardation (Antochi, Stavrakaki, & Emery, 2003; Green, 2001). SSRIs have also been used for treatment of disorders other than depression, including obsessive–compulsive disorder and other anxiety disorders, agitation, and SIB. In fact, some researchers believe that repetitive behaviors, such as stereotypies and SIB, may be manifestations of obsessions and compulsions. Consequently, such symptoms may possibly respond to treatment with serotonergic medications, such as SSRIs (Aman, Arnold, & Armstrong, 1999; Hellings, Kelley, Gabrielli, Kilgore, & Shah, 1996).

A primary reason for this shift is that SSRIs have a much better safety profile than tricyclics. Although the prescribing of SSRIs has reduced many side effects, the U.S. Food and Drug Administration (FDA) (2004) has recently issued an order that all antidepressant medicines must carry a "black box" warning. This was due to an increased risk of suicidal thinking and behavior in children and adolescents. SSRIs have also been reported to lead to activation among patients with bipolar disorder in some cases, and this may increase suicidal ideation. Additional side effects that have been associated with the use of SSRIs include excitement or anxiety, drowsiness, dry mouth, upset stomach, insomnia, and changes in appetite and weight (Golden, 2004). Below is a brief summary of SSRI treatment studies among individuals with mental retardation.

Sertraline (Zoloft) has been approved to treat children older than 6 years of age for obsessive–compulsive disorder (Green, 2001). No studies could be identified that specifically examined the use of sertraline in children with mental retardation. However, in studies in adults with mental retardation, this agent has been found to be effective in the treatment of SIB and aggression (Hellings, Zarcone, Crandall, Wallace, & Schroeder, 2001; Luiselli, Blew, & Thibadeau, 2001). An open-label trial of sertraline in nine children with pervasive developmental disorders (many of whom had mental retardation) reported similar success in decreasing perseverative and compulsive behaviors, as well as outbursts (Steingard, Zimnitzky, DeMaso, Bauman, & Bucci, 1997).

Fluvoxamine (Luvox) has been approved in children at least 8 years of age for the treatment of obsessive–compulsive disorder (Green, 2001). We are unaware of any studies that have been conducted involving fluvoxamine and

children with mental retardation. Among adults with mental retardation, fluvoxamine has been shown to reduce aggression (La Malfa, Bertelli, & Conte, 2001). In one study involving children with autistic spectrum disorders, significant side effects and minimal clinical efficacy were noted (McDougle, 1998).

Fluoxetine (Prozac) has been approved for use in adults and children (at least 8 years of age) to treat major depressive disorder. Limited research is available on the use of fluoxetine in children with mental retardation. In a review of 15 case reports and 4 prospective open-label trials of fluoxetine in children and adults with mental retardation and/or pervasive developmental disorders, Aman and colleagues (1999) found that the majority reported decreased irritability, self-injury, or depressive symptoms. A primary concern with the use of fluoxetine is that there are conflicting data on whether this agent decreases aggression or whether aggression is a significant side effect (Troisi, 1997).

Citalopram (Celexa) and its active isomer escitalopram (Lexapro) are the newest and most selective SSRIs to be marketed. No studies could be identified looking specifically at citalopram and escitalopram's use in children with mental retardation. Verhoeven, Veendrik-Meekes, Jacobs, van den Berg, and Tuinier (2001), in a study of adults with mental retardation, reported efficacy in the treatment of atypical depressive symptoms.

Paroxetine (Paxil) has been approved only for use in adults. A few case reports and open-label studies have shown mixed results in the population of adolescents and adults with mental retardation to treat aggression, SIB, and symptoms of depression (Branford, Bhaumik, & Naik, 1998; Davanzo, Belin, Widawski, & King, 1998; Masi, Marcheschi, & Pfanner, 1997; Snead, Boon, & Presberg, 1994).

Neuroleptics

Neuroleptics have a long history of use for the management of aggression, hyperactivity, SIB, stereotypies, and antisocial behaviors. During the past decade, the typical antipsychotics (e.g., thioridazine, haloperidol) have been replaced by atypical antipsychotics (e.g., risperidone, olanzapine), which appear to have a safer side effect profile (Madrid, State, & King, 2000). Despite this, children prescribed atypical antipsychotics remain at risk for a number of side effects, including some that can be potentially life-threatening.

Individuals with mental retardation are at higher risk for extrapyramidal side effects, including akathisia, pseudo-parkinsonism, and acute dystonic reactions (Van Bellinghen & De Troch, 2001). Weight gain has been a particular concern for children (with and without mental retardation) who are prescribed risperidone and olanzapine (Posey & McDougle, 2003). All atypical antipsychotics can cause tiredness and tardive dyskinesia; they can also increase the risk for a number of conditions, including heart disease, diabetes mellitus Type II, ischemic stroke, and hypertension (Hellings et al., 2001). Risperidone use (even at low doses) can cause an increase in prolactin, which may lead to gynecomastia, galactorrhea, and amenorrhea (Hellings, 1999). Neuroleptic malignant syndrome (which can be life-threatening) is a known risk factor for individuals with developmental delay and mental retardation (Marriage, 2002). With the exception of risperidone, which is approved for adolescents 15 years of age and older, none of the atypicals are approved for use in children. Consequently, they are prescribed as "off-label" medications.

The first atypical antipsychotic, clozapine, was developed in the 1960s and is rarely prescribed as an initial for children with mental retardation, due to the possibility of agranulocytosis (which can be life-threatening) and seizures (Posey & McDougle, 2003). Risperidone was the second atypical antipsychotic to be developed and has become the best-studied of these medications in the treatment of children with mental retardation and comorbid psychiatric symptoms. It has been found helpful in individuals with mental retardation in controlling symptoms of hyperactivity, obsessive–compulsive and repetitive behaviors, irritability, explosive aggressive behavior, and SIB (Aman & Madrid, 1999; Hellings, 1999; Turgay, Binder, Snyder, & Fisman, 2002; Van Bellinghen & De Troch, 2001).

Olanzapine has only recently been the subject of study in individuals with mental retardation, and only open-label studies are available as yet. In an open study of adults for the treatment of SIB, 57% showed improvement and 14% showed worsening effects (McDonough, Hillery, & Kennedy, 2000). In studies of children (unlike adults), a high percentage of subjects (21%) treated with olanzapine have developed acute dystonic reactions (Friedlander,

Lazar, & Klancnik, 2001). In a study of five children without mental retardation, all five children were removed from olanzapine due to adverse side effects, despite favorable effects on aggression and psychosis (Krishnamoorthy & King, 1998). The studies in typically developing children are in stark contrast to the studies in adults with mental retardation, which show that olanzapine was well tolerated (by 66.7% of the study sample) (Williams, Clarke, Bouras, Martin, & Holt, 2000). None of the adults needed to be removed from olanzapine due to side effects.

Quetiapine, the fourth atypical antipsychotic to be marketed in the United States, has also not been subjected to any controlled trials among individuals with mental retardation. Only one open-label study and one retrospective chart review could be identified dealing with children with developmental disabilities. In an open-label study of boys with autism, quetiapine was found to be poorly tolerated (Martin, Koenig, Scahill, & Bregman, 1999). In a retrospective chart review, quetiapine led to statistically significant gains in the treatment of conduct problems, inattention, and hyperactivity (Hardan, Roger, & Handen, 2003).

Ziprasidone is one of the newer atypical antipsychotics to be marketed. We know of no studies of ziprasidone in children with developmental delays, except for one study of youths with autistic disorder, which showed promising results in the control of aggression, agitation, and irritability (McDougle, Kem, & Posey, 2002). In this study, weight gain was not an observed finding; this is consistent with adult studies of ziprasidone. However, ziprasidone has been noted to increase the QT_c interval (which has been associated with sudden death in other drugs known to prolong this interval). Aripiprazole is the newest antipsychotic to be marketed. Only a single case study of aripiprazole in children with pervasive developmental disorders has been published (in which two out of five children had mental retardation). Aripiprazole was found to be helpful in treating aggression, SIB, and agitation (Stigler, Posey, & McDougle, 2004).

Mood Stabilizers

The mood stabilizers include lithium and certain antiepileptic medications, as well as both typical and atypical antipsychotic medications (see above). Mood stabilizers were originally found to be helpful in the treatment of bipolar disorder. From their initial use in bipolar disorder, the role of mood stabilizers has expanded to treatment of various problems and disorders, including SIB, aggressive behavior, depression (lithium only), impulsivity, and conduct disorder (Aman, Collier-Crespin, & Lindsay, 2000; Green, 2001; Santosh & Baird, 1999).

Lithium, an alkali metal, is a naturally found element that has been used since the 1880s for the treatment of psychiatric disorders (Kaplan & Sadock, 1993; Schou, 2001). Lithium has been approved for children over the age of 12 for the treatment of bipolar disorder; its use in children younger than 12 years of age is not recommended (Green, 2001).

In populations of people with developmental disabilities, lithium has been found to be beneficial for mood lability, aggression, and SIB (Antochi et al., 2003). Lithium has also become the treatment of choice in cycloid psychosis, a psychotic disorder occurring mainly in Prader–Willi syndrome (a chromosomal microdeletion at 15q11 resulting in intellectual defect, pathological overeating, and hypotonia) (Antochi et al., 2003; Jorde, Carey, & White, 1995).

Individuals with mental retardation may be at higher risk for lithium's side effects, including weight gain, hypothyroidism, tremor, polydipsia, polyuria, nephrogenic diabetes insipidus, severe acne, electrocardiogram changes, and muscle weakness (Antochi et al., 2003; Green, 2001). Besides these serious side effects, lithium is also associated with higher risk for toxicity. Signs of toxicity include gastrointestinal disturbance, slurred speech, ataxia (difficulty walking), blurred vision, seizures, delirium, coma, and death. It has been associated with birth defects as well.

The antiepileptic medications have been increasingly used for a range of psychiatric problems, including mood fluctuations, aggression, and anxiety. Despite a high rate of usage for seizure disorders in the population of children with mental retardation, there are limited data on the use of antiepileptics to control behavior problems in this population (Madrid et al., 2000). No antiepileptic medication has been approved for use in children in the treatment of psychiatric disorders. However, three antiepileptic medications are used most commonly: valproic acid/divalproex sodium, carbamazepine, and oxcarbazepine. Valproate has been found useful in the treatment of adults and children with mental retardation who show aggression and SIB (Antochi et al., 2003; Kowatch & Bucci, 1998). This usefulness is tempered by potential side effects, including idiosyncratic fulminant hepatic failure and idiosyncratic hemorrhagic pancreatitis (both of which can be life-threatening) (*Physicians' Desk Reference*, 2004). The hepatic failure is most common in children with developmental disabilities under the age of 2 years (Fenichel, 1997).

Studies of carbamazepine use in adults with mental retardation have yielded mixed results (Aman et al., 2000), and little data exist regarding its use in children with mental retardation for treatment of psychiatric disorders. Finally, oxcarbazepine, a relatively new antiepileptic, has been found effective in the treatment of bipolar disorder (Centorrino et al., 2003; Ketter, Wang, Becker, Nowakowska, & Yang, 2003), but no data were found on its use in children with mental retardation.

Other Medications

Other medications that may be considered include alpha agonists and atomoxetine. Alpha agonists (clonidine and guanfacine) are approved for treatment of hypertension, but have also been used (off-label) to treat symptoms associated with ADHD (overactivity, impulsivity), Tourette syndrome, other tic disorders, and sleep problems (Antochi et al., 2003). Although we are unaware of any studies of these agents in children with mental retardation, studies of children with pervasive developmental disorders have documented decreased hyperactivity and inattention with their use (Fankhauser, Karumanchi, German, Yates, & Karumanchi, 1992; Jaselskis, Cook, & Fletcher, 1992; Posey et al., 2004).

Recently, atomoxetine (Strattera) was approved by the FDA for treatment of ADHD. Preliminary studies have suggested that atomoxetine, a nonstimulant, may be as efficacious as methylphenidate and have fewer side effects (Spencer et al., 2002). The use of atomoxetine in children with mental retardation is also of interest, because this agent has less potential than stimulants to increase seizures, which occur more often among individuals with mental retardation (Eli Lilly & Company, 2002). Additional advantages of atomoxetine include the ability to dose once daily, clinical effects lasting as long as 24 hours, and minimal potential for abuse. There are no available studies of atomoxetine among children with mental retardation.

FUTURE DIRECTIONS

A number of compelling issues face the field of mental retardation during the new millennium. Hodapp and Dykens (1996) discuss five current issues and future directions: definitional issues, improving service delivery, joining the cultures of behavioral research, dual diagnosis, and the changing nature of populations with mental retardation. Heward (2000) emphasizes three key areas where progress has been made but where much work remains: (1) rights of persons with mental retardation, (2) prevention of mental retardation, and (3) "normalization" and self-determination. To these lists should probably be added issues related to psychopharmacology. It will be important that professionals within the field be aware of the impact each of these issues may have on their work. Some of these issues are presented below.

Definition of Mental Retardation

The field of mental retardation is continuing to struggle with issues relating to the very definition of "mental retardation." The 2002 revision of the AAMR definition lowered the IQ range for mental retardation from "below 70 or 75" to "below 70," along with a revision in the requirement for deficits in adaptive behavior. Many of these revisions were the result of feedback within the field. However, it is too early to determine whether this new definition will be accepted by all professional associations, school districts, or states. In addition, there is a movement among self-advocacy groups of individuals with mental retardation to replace the term "mental retardation." In fact, as noted earlier, AAMR's board of directors has begun to explore options for such a change (AAMR, 2002).

Trends in Service Delivery Systems and Funding

Perhaps the most important future direction involves service delivery systems themselves. The trend toward inclusion of students with mental retardation in classrooms with typically developing peers will continue to grow. A greater number of special education teachers will work within an itinerant model—providing services to students in their regular classrooms, team-teaching with regular education colleagues, and offering consultation. In fact, several universities (e.g., Duquesne University) have begun to require that students in training for regular education also be trained as special education teachers. This reflects the need for all teachers to be skilled at instructing children with a wide range of abilities. We may soon see state teacher certification requirements reflecting this philosophy of inclusion. Inclusion efforts that have shown growing promise among preschool and elementary school classrooms will need to be expanded to serve adolescents of middle and high school age. Despite the move toward inclusion for students with mental retardation, fewer than 15% of this population are currently educated in general education classrooms (National Center for Education Statistics, 2002).

Other issues that may affect services and service delivery involve funding. In many states, funding of special education services has increasingly fallen to the local school district. This has become more of a concern as federal mandates have required additional services for this population. Funds for respite care, in-home care, after-school programs, and extended-school-year services have become scarcer with the economic recession of the past few years.

Changing Nature of the Population

Hodapp and Dykens (1996) provide data on the growing numbers of children with developmental disabilities as a result of alcohol and/or drug use among pregnant mothers; increased cases of lead poisoning in children; the rise in the pediatric population with AIDS; maternal undernutrition during the prenatal period; inadequate prenatal care; and maternal hepatitis or sexually transmitted diseases other than HIV/AIDS (Conlon, 1992). Research indicates that all these factors may be related to low birthweights, microcephaly, cognitive problems, and/or learning deficits (Conlon, 1992; Needleman, Schell, Bellinger, Leviton, & Alfred, 1990). It remains unclear to what extent these groups of children will come to represent a greater proportion of individuals with mental retardation, as interventions such as improved *in utero* genetic diagnosis and gene therapies cure or lessen the effects of various other conditions presently associated with mental retardation. In addition, with improved medical services and technology, we are seeing increased life expectancy for individuals with mental retardation and a growing subspecialization in the area of geriatric services.

Prevention

It is likely that continuing gains will be made in the area of prevention. Research is identifying additional genetic causes for mental retardation, as well as a growing list of potential environmental toxins (e.g., lead, asbestos, mercury). There continues to be improvement in our ability to diagnose (and sometimes treat) disorders *in utero* that may be associated with mental retardation. State and federal laws have also increased the use of safety devices (e.g., car seat restraints for infants and toddlers, car airbags, helmet laws for children), which should decrease the number of head injuries and resulting cognitive impairments in children.

Medication Efficacy

As we have discussed earlier, relatively little is known about many of the medications used to treat both children and adults with mental retardation. This is due both to many professionals' mistaken assumption that individuals with mental retardation are less likely to have psychiatric disorders, and to the fact that children and adults with mental retardation have tended to be excluded in many medication efficacy studies. With the growing acceptance that individuals with mental retardation can have the full range of psychiatric disorders and may actually be at greater risk than the general population for behavioral/emotional problems, there has been an increase in drug studies with this population.

CONCLUSION

The field of mental retardation has witnessed significant change in a range of areas during the past few decades. From the initial passage of P.L. 94-142 and its subsequent reenactment as the IDEA, to the discovery of a wide variety of methods for the prevention of mental retardation, the field is active and vibrant. The past

few decades have witnessed historic changes in the ways in which children with mental retardation are educated. The efforts of early intervention and the increasing use of inclusion have clearly had a major impact on special education and the ability of students with mental retardation to become more fully integrated into society. Gains in our ability to teach adaptive, communication, social, and academic skills as well as to address behavioral/emotional disorders, have also allowed students with mental retardation to function much more independently in school, at home, and in the community.

This chapter has presented information on a range of child-focused interventions (e.g., educational efforts, behavior problem management, psychopharmacological interventions), as well as parent training and community-based interventions. Our approach to the treatment of behavior problems in children with mental retardation has been to address the development of appropriate communication and social skills, along with the reinforcement of alternative appropriate behaviors. The needs to conduct a thorough functional assessment prior to treatment, to implement empirically supported interventions, to use single-subject designs to demonstrate clinical efficacy, and to program for generalization have also been emphasized. Finally, the appropriateness of adjunctive treatments, such as pharmacotherapy, has been discussed. Only through a carefully considered combination of a range of resources and interventions can the needs of children with mental retardation and their families be met.

REFERENCES

Alford, J. D., & Locke, B. L. (1984). Clinical responses to psychopathology of mentally retarded persons. *American Journal of Mental Deficiency, 89,* 195–197.

Aman, M. G., Armstrong, S., Buican, B., & Sillick, T. (2002). Four-year follow-up of children with low intelligence and ADHD: A replication. *Research in Developmental Disabilities, 23,* 119–134.

Aman, M. G., Arnold, L. E., & Armstrong, S. C. (1999). Review of serotonergic agents and perseverative behavior in patients with developmental disabilities. *Mental Retardation and Developmental Disabilities, 5,* 279–289.

Aman, M. G., Buican, B., & Arnold, L. E. (2003). Methylphenidate treatment in children with borderline IQ and mental retardation: Analysis of three aggregated studies. *Journal of Child and Adolescent Psychopharmacology, 13,* 29–40.

Aman, M. G., Collier-Crespin, A., & Lindsay, R. L. (2000). Pharmacotherapy of disorders in mental retardation. *European Child and Adolescent Psychiatry, 9*(Suppl. 1), I98–I107.

Aman, M. G., Kern, R. A., McGhee, D. E., & Arnold, L. E. (1993). Fenfluramine and methylphenidate in children with mental retardation and ADHD: Clinical and side effects. *Journal of the American Academy of Child and Adolescent Psychiatry, 32,* 851–859.

Aman, M. G., Kern, R. A., Osborne, P., Tumuluru, R., Rojahn, J., & del Medico, V. (1997). Fenfluramine and methylphenidate in children with mental retardation and borderline IQ: Clinical effects. *American Journal on Mental Retardation, 101,* 521–534.

Aman, M. G., & Madrid, A. (1999). Atypical antipsychotics in persons with developmental disabilities. *Mental Retardation and Developmental Disabilities, 5,* 253–263.

Aman, M. G., Marks, R. E., Turbott, S. H., Wilsher, C. P., & Merry, S. N. (1991). Clinical effects of methylphenidate and thioridazine in intellectually subaverage children. *Journal of the American Academy of Child and Adolescent Psychiatry, 30,* 246–256.

Aman, M. G., Pejeau, C., Osborne, P., Rojahn, J., & Handen, B. (1996). Four-year follow-up of children with low intelligence and ADHD. *Research in Developmental Disabilities, 17,* 417–432.

American Association on Mental Retardation (AAMR). (1992). *Mental retardation: Definition, classification, and systems of supports* (9th ed.). Washington, DC: Author.

American Association on Mental Retardation (AAMR). (2002). *Mental retardation: Definition, classification, and systems of support* (10th ed.). Washington, DC: Author.

American Psychiatric Association (APA). (2000). *Diagnostic and statistical manual of mental disorders* (4th ed., text rev.). Washington, DC: Author.

Antochi, R., Stavrakaki, C., & Emery, P. C. (2003). Psychopharmacological treatments in persons with dual diagnosis of psychiatric disorders and developmental disabilities. *Postgraduate Medicine, 9,* 139–146.

Armstrong v. Kline, 476 F. Supp. 583 (E.D. Pa. 1979).

Aronson, M., & Fallstrom, K. (1977). Immediate and long-term effects of developmental training in children with Down's syndrome. *Developmental Medicine and Child Neurology, 19,* 489–494.

Aziz, K., Vickar, D., Sauve, R., Etches, P., Pain, K., & Robertson, C. P. (1995). Province-based study of neurologic disability of children weighing 500 through 1249 grams at birth in relation to neonatal cerebral ultrasound findings. *Pediatrics, 95,* 837–844.

Baker, B. L. (1989). *Parent training and developmental disabilities.* Washington, DC: American Association on Mental Retardation.

Baker, B. L. (1996). Parent training. In J. W. Jacobson & J. A. Mulick (Eds.), *Manual of diagnosis and profes-sional practice in mental retardation* (pp. 289–300). Washington, DC: American Psychological Association.

Baker, B. L., & Brightman, A. J. (1997). *Steps to independence: Teaching everyday skills to children with special needs* (3rd ed.). Baltimore: Brookes.

Baker, B. L., Heifetz, L., & Murphy, D. (1980). Behavioral training for parents of mentally retarded children: One-year follow-up. *American Journal of Mental Deficiency, 85,* 31–38.

Baker, B. L., Landen, S. J., & Kashima, K. J. (1991). Effects of parent training on families of children with mental retardation: Increased burden or neutralized benefit? *American Journal on Mental Retardation, 96,* 127–136.

Baroff, G. S., & Olley, J. (1999). *Mental retardation: Nature, cause, and management* (3rd ed.). Philadelphia: Brunner/Mazel.

Benson, B. A., & Aman, M. G. (1999). Disruptive behavior disorders in children with mental retardation. In H. C. Quay & A. E. Hogan (Eds.), *Handbook of disruptive behavior disorders* (pp. 559–578). New York: Plenum Press.

Blair, C., & Wahlsten, D. (2002). Why early intervention works: A reply to Baumeister and Bacharach. *Intelligence, 30,* 129–140.

Borthwick-Duffy, S. A., Palmer, D. S., & Lane, K. L. (1996). One size doesn't fit all: Full inclusion and individual differences. *Journal of Behavioral Education, 6,* 311–329.

Branford, D., Bhaumik, S., & Naik, B. (1998). Selective serotonin re-uptake inhibitors for the treatment of perseverative and maladaptive behaviours of people with intellectual disability. *Journal of Intellectual Disability Research, 42,* 301–306.

Breiner, J., & Beck, S. (1984). Parents as change agents in the management of their developmentally delayed children's noncompliant behaviors: A critical review. *Applied Research in Mental Retardation, 5,* 259–278.

Brooks-Gunn, J., McCarton, C. M., Casey, P. H., McCormick, M. C., Bauer, C. R., Bernbaum, J. C., et al. (1994). Early intervention in low-birth-weight premature infants: Results through age 5 years from the Infant Health and Development Program. *Journal of the American Medical Association, 272,* 1257–1262.

Burchinal, M. R., Campbell, F. A., Bryant, D. M., Wasik, B. H., & Ramey, C. T. (1997). Early intervention and mediating processes in cognitive performance of children of low-income African American families. *Child Development, 68,* 935–954.

Butz, M. R., Bowling, J. B., & Bliss, C. A. (2000). Psychotherapy with the mentally retarded: A review of the literature and its implication. *Professional Psychology: Research and Practice, 31,* 42–47.

Callias, M. (1987). Teaching parents, teachers and nurses. In W. Yule & J. Carr (Eds.), *Behavior modification for people with mental handicaps* (2nd ed., pp. 211–244). London: Croom Helm.

Campbell, F. A., & Ramey, C. T. (1995). Cognitive and

school outcomes for high risk African-American students at middle adolescence: Positive effects of early intervention. *American Educational Research Journal, 32,* 743–772.

Canfield, R. L., Henderson, C. R., Cory-Slechta, D. A., Cox, C., Jusko, T. A., & Lanphear, B. P. (2003). Intellectual impairment in children with blood lead concentrations below 10 mug per deciliter. *New England Journal of Medicine, 348,* 1517–1526.

Carr, E. G., & Durand, M. (1985). Reducing behavior problems through functional communication training. *Journal of Applied Behavior Analysis, 18,* 111–126.

Carr, E. G., Horner, R. H., Turnbull, A. P., Marquis, J. G., McLaughlin, D., McAtee, M., et al. (1999). *Positive behavior support for people with developmental disabilities.* Washington, DC: American Association on Mental Retardation.

Carr, E. G., Newsom, C. D., & Binkoff, J. A. (1980). Escape as a factor in the aggressive behavior of two retarded children. *Journal of Applied Behavior Analysis, 13,* 101–117.

Carr, E. G., Taylor, J. C., Carlson, J. I., & Robinson, S. (1989, September). *Reinforcement and stimulus-based treatments for severe behavior problems in developmental disabilities.* Paper presented at the Consensus Development Conference on Destructive Behavior, National Institutes of Health, Bethesda, MD.

Carr, J. (1975). *Young children with Down's syndrome.* London: Butterworth.

Centorrino, F., Albert, M. J., Berry, J. M., Kelleher, J. P., Fellman, V., Line, G., et al. (2003). Oxcarbazepine: Clinical experience with hospitalized psychiatric patients. *Bipolar Disorder, 5,* 370–374.

Chambless, D. L., & Ollendick, T. H. (2001). Empirically supported psychological interventions: Controversies and evidence. *Annual Review of Psychology, 52,* 685–716.

Clark, D. B., & Baker, B. L. (1983). Predicting outcome in parent training. *Journal of Consulting and Clinical Psychology, 51,* 309–311.

Coe, D., Matson, J., Fee, V., Manikam, R., & Linarello, C. (1990). Training nonverbal and verbal play skills to mentally retarded and autistic children. *Journal of Autism and Developmental Disorders, 20,* 177–187.

Conlon, C. J. (1992). New threats to development: Alcohol, cocaine, and AIDS. In M. L. Batshaw & Y. M. Perret (Eds.), *Children with disabilities: A medical primer* (pp. 111–136). Baltimore: Brookes.

Connolly, B., Morgan, S., Russell, F. F., & Rulliton, W. L. (1993). A longitudinal study of children with Down syndrome who experienced early intervention programming. *Physical Therapy, 73,* 170–181.

Connolly, B., Morgan, S., Russell, F. F., & Richardson, B. (1980). Early intervention with Down syndrome children: Follow-up report. *Physical Therapy, 60,* 1405–1408.

Conyers, C., Miltenberger, R., Maki, A., Barenz, R., Jurgens, M., Sailer, A., et al. (2004). A comparison of response cost and differential reinforcement of other behavior to reduce disruptive behavior in a preschool classroom. *Journal of Applied Behavior Analysis, 37,* 411–415.

Cooke, N. L., Heron, T. E., Heward, W. L., & Test, D. W. (1982). Integrating a Down syndrome student into a classwide peer tutoring system. *Mental Retardation, 20,* 22–25.

Council for Exceptional Children. (2005). *IDEA Law and Resources.* Retrieved from http://www.cec.sped.org

Crone, D. A., & Horner, R. H. (2003). *Building positive behavior support systems in schools.* New York: Guilford Press.

Curry, C. J., Stevenson, R. E., Aughton, D., Byrne, J., Carey, J., Cassidy, S., et al. (1997). Evaluation of mental retardation: Recommendations of a consensus conference. *American Journal of Medical Genetics, 72,* 468–477.

Davanzo, P. A., Belin, T. R., Widawski, M. H., & King, B. H. (1998). Paroxetine treatment of aggression and self-injury in persons with mental retardation. *American Journal on Mental Retardation, 102,* 427–437.

Department of Public Welfare, Office of Mental Retardation, Commonwealth of Pennsylvania. (1995). *Licensing inspection instrument for community homes for individuals with mental retardation regulations.* Harrisburg: Author.

Doleys, D. M., Wells, K. C., Hobbs, S. A., Roberts, M. W., & Cartelli, L. M. (1976). The effects of social punishment on noncompliance: A comparison with timeout and positive practice. *Journal of Applied Behavior Analysis, 9,* 471–482.

Donnellan, A. M., LaVigna, G. G., Negri-Shoeltz, N., & Fassbender, L. L. (1988). *Progress without punishment: Effective approaches for learners with behavior problems.* New York: Teachers College Press.

Dorn, T. A., & Prout, H. T. (1993). Service delivery patterns for adults with mild mental retardation at community mental health centers. *Mental Retardation, 31,* 292–296.

Ducharme, J. M., & Drain, T. (2004). Errorless academic compliance training: Improving generalized cooperation with parental requests in children with autism. *Journal of the American Academy of Child and Adolescent Psychiatry, 43,* 163–171.

Dunlap, G. F. L. (1999). A demonstration of behavior support for young children with autism. *Journal of Positive Behavioral Interventions, 2,* 77–87.

Dunst, C. J. (1991, February). *Empowering families: Principles and outcomes.* Paper presented at the 4th Annual Research Conference, "A System of Care of Children's Mental Health: Expanding the Research Base," Tampa, FL.

Dunst, C. J., Hamby, D., Trivette, C. M., Raab, M., & Bruder, M. B. (2002). Young children's participation in everyday family and community activity. *Psychological Reports, 91,* 875–897.

Dunst, C. J., Trivette, C. M., & Deal, A. G. (1988). *Enabling and empowering families: Principles and guidelines for practice.* Cambridge, MA: Brookline Books.

Dunst, C. J., Trivette, C. M., & Deal, A. G. (1994). *Supporting and strengthening families: Methods, strategies and practices* (Vol. 1). Cambridge, MA: Brookline Books.

Dunst, C. J., Trivette, C. M., Starnes, A. L., Hamby, D. W., & Gordon, N. J. (1993). *Building and evaluating family support initiatives: A national study of programs for persons with developmental disabilities.* Baltimore: Brookes.

Durand, V. M. (1999). Functional communication training using assistive devices: Recruiting natural communities of reinforcement. *Journal of Applied Behavior Analysis, 32,* 247–267.

Education for All Handicapped Children Act of 1975, P.L. 94-142, 20 U.S.C. 1400 et seq. (1975).

Education of the Handicapped Act Amendments of 1986, P.L. 99-457, 20 U.S.C. 1400 et seq. (1986).

Einfeld, S. L., & Aman, M. G. (1995). Issues in the taxonomy of psychopathology in children and adolescents with mental retardation. *Journal of Autism and Developmental Disorders, 25,* 143–167.

Eisenberger, R., & Cameron, J. (1996). Detrimental effects of reward: Reality or myth? *American Psychologist, 51,* 1153–1166.

Eisenberger, R., & Selbst, M. (1994). Does reward increase or decrease creativity? *Journal of Personality and Social Psychology, 49,* 520–528.

Eli Lilly & Company. (2002). *Data on file.* Indianapolis, IN: Author.

Emerson, E. (2003). Prevalence of psychiatric disorders in children and adolescents with and without intellectual disability. *Journal of Intellectual Disability Research, 47,* 51–58.

Fankhauser, M., Karumanchi, V., German, M., Yates, A., & Karumanchi, S. (1992). A double-blind, placebo-controlled study of the efficacy of transdermal clonidine in autism. *Journal of Clinical Psychiatry, 53,* 77–82.

Feldman, M. A., & Werner, S. E. (2002). Collateral effects of behavioral parent training on families of children with developmental disabilities and behavior disorders. *Behavioral Interventions, 17,* 75–83.

Fenichel, G. M. (1997). *Clinical pediatric neurology: A signs and symptoms approach.* Philadelphia: Saunders.

Ferguson, D. L., Meyer, G., Jeanchild, L., Juniper, L., & Zingo, J. (1992). Figuring out what to do with grownups: How teachers make inclusion "work" for students with disabilities. *Journal of the Association for Persons with Severe Handicaps, 17,* 218–226.

Fewell, R. R., & Oelwein, P. L. (1991). Effective early intervention: Results from the Model Preschool Program for Children with Down Syndrome and Other Developmental Delays. *Topics in Early Childhood Special Education, 11,* 56–68.

Fisher, W. W., Piazza, C. C., Bowman, L., & Amari, A. (1996). Integrating caregiver report with a systematic choice assessment. *American Journal on Mental Retardation, 101,* 15–25.

Forehand, R., & Kotchick, B. A. (2002). Behavioral

parent training: Current challenges and potential solutions. *Journal of Child and Family Studies, 11,* 377–384.

Foxx, R. M., McMorrow, M., Bittle, R., & Ness, J. (1986). An analysis of social skills generalization in two natural settings. *Journal of Applied Behavior Analysis, 19,* 299–305.

Foxx, R. M., & Shapiro, S. T. (1978). The timeout ribbon: A nonexclusionary timeout procedure. *Journal of Applied Behavior Analysis, 11,* 125–136.

Friedlander, R., Lazar, S., & Klancnik, J. (2001). Atypical antipsychotic use in treating adolescents and young adults with developmental disabilities. *Canadian Journal of Psychiatry, 46,* 741–745.

Fuchs, D., & Fuchs, L. (1995). Sometimes separate is better. *Educational Leadership, 50,* 22–26.

Gallagher, J. (1997a). *The million dollar question: Unmet service needs for young children with disabilities.* Chapel Hill: Early Childhood Research Institute on Service Utilization, Frank Porter Graham Child Development Center, University of North Carolina at Chapel Hill.

Gallagher, J. (1997b). The role of the professional working with children with disabilities and their families. In *Services for young children with disabilities: An ecological perspective.* Chapel Hill: Early Childhood Research Institute on Service Utilization, Frank Porter Graham Child Development Center, University of North Carolina at Chapel Hill.

Gallagher, J. (1997c). Service delivery for young children with disabilities: Focus group data from parents and providers. In *Services for young children with disabilities: An ecological perspective.* Chapel Hill: Early Childhood Research Institute on Service Utilization, Rank Porter Graham Child Development Center, University of North Carolina at Chapel Hill.

Gallimore, R., Weisner, T. S., Bernheimer, L. P., Guthrie, D., & Nihira, K. (1993). Family responses to young children with developmental delays: Accommodation activity in ecological and cultural context. *American Journal on Mental Retardation, 98,* 185–206.

Gauvain, M. (1999). Everyday opportunities for the development of planning skills: Sociocultural and family influences. In A. Goncu (Ed.), *Children's engagement in the work: Sociocultural perspectives* (pp. 173–201). Cambridge, UK: Cambridge University Press.

Gibson, D., & Harris, A. (1988). Aggregated early intervention effects for Down's syndrome persons: Patterning and longevity of benefits. *Journal of Mental Deficiency Research, 32,* 1–17.

Golden, R. N. (2004). Making advances where it matters: Improving outcomes in mood and anxiety disorders. *CNS Spectrums, 9*(Suppl. 4), 14–22.

Green, W. H. (2001). *Child and adolescent clinical psychopharmacology.* Philadelphia: Lippincott Williams & Wilkins.

Greenhill, L. L., Swanson, J. M., Vitiello, B., Davies, M., Clevenger, W., Wu, M., et al. (2001). Impairment and deportment responses to different methylphenidate doses in children with ADHD: The MTA titration trial. *Journal of the American Academy of Child and Adolescent Psychiatry, 40,* 180–187.

Griffin, J. C., Williams, D. E., Stark, M. T., Altmeyer, B. K., & Mason, M. (1986). Self-injurious behaviour: A state-wide prevalence survey of the extent and circumstances. *Applied Research in Mental Retardation, 7,* 105–116.

Grossman, J. J. (Ed.). (1973). *Manual on terminology and classification in mental retardation.* Washington, DC: American Association on Mental Deficiency.

Grossman, J. J. (Ed.). (1983). *Classification in mental retardation.* Washington, DC: American Association on Mental Deficiency.

Guralnick, M. J., & Bricker, D. (1987). Cognitive and general developmental delays. In M. J. Guralnick & F. C. Bennett (Eds.), *The effectiveness of early intervention for at-risk and handicapped children* (pp. 115–168). Orlando, FL: Academic Press, Inc.

Hagerman, R. J., & Sobesky, W. E. (1989). Psychopathology in fragile X syndrome. *American Journal of Orthopsychiatry, 59,* 142–152.

Hagopian, L. P., Long, E. S., & Rush, K. (2004). Preference assessment procedures for individuals with developmental disabilities. *Behavior Modification, 28,* 668–677.

Hagopian, L. P., Rush, K., Lewin, A. B., & Long, E. S. (2001). Evaluating the predictive validity of a single stimulus engagement preference assessment. *Journal of Applied Behavior Analysis, 34,* 475–486.

Hagopian, L. P., van Stone, M., & Crockett, J. L. (2003). Establishing schedule control over dropping to the floor. *Behavioral Interventions, 18,* 291–297.

Hall, R. V., & Hall, M. L. (1998). *How to select reinforcers* (2nd ed.), Austin, TX: Pro-Ed.

Halpern, R. (2000). Early childhood intervention for low-income children and families. In J. P. Shonkoff and S. J. Meisels (Eds.), *Handbook of early childhood intervention* (2nd ed., pp. 361–386). New York: Cambridge University Press.

Handen, B. L., Feldman, H., Gosling, A., Breaux, A. M., & McAuliffe, S. (1991). Adverse side effects of Ritalin among mentally retarded children with ADHD. *Journal of the American Academy of Child and Adolescent Psychiatry, 30,* 241–245.

Handen, B. L., Feldman, H. M., Lurier, A., & Murray, P. J. (1999). Efficacy of methylphenidate among preschool children with developmental disabilities and ADHD. *Journal of the American Academy of Child and Adolescent Psychiatry, 38,* 805–812.

Handen, B. L., Janosky, J., & McAuliffe, S. (1997). Long-term follow-up of children with mental retardation and ADHD. *Journal of Abnormal Child Psychology, 25,* 287–295.

Handen, B. L., Janosky, J., McAuliffe, S., Breaux, A. M., & Feldman, H. (1994). Prediction of response to methylphenidate among children with ADHD and mental retardation. *Journal of the American Academy of Child and Adolescent Psychiatry, 33,* 1185–1193.

Handen, B. L., Parrish, J. M., McClung, T. J., Kerwin, M. E., & Evans, L. D. (1992). Using guided compliance versus time out to promote child compliance: A preliminary comparative analysis in an analogue context. *Research in Developmental Disabilities, 13,* 159–170.

Harbin, G. L., McWilliam, R. A., & Gallagher, J. J. (2000). Services for young children with disabilities and their families. In J. P. Shonkoff & S. J. Meisels (Eds.), *Handbook of early childhood intervention* (2nd ed., pp. 387–415). New York: Cambridge University Press.

Hardan, A., Roger, J., & Handen, B. (2003). *Quetiapine open-label trial in children and adolescents with developmental disorder.* Paper presented at the 156th annual meeting of the American Psychiatric Association, San Francisco.

Haring, T. G., & Kennedy, C. H. (1990). Contextual control of problem behavior in students with severe disabilities. *Journal of Applied Behavior Analysis, 23,* 235–243.

Harris, S. L. (1983). *Families of the developmentally disabled: A guide to behavioral intervention.* New York: Pergamon Press.

Harris, S. L. (1988). Early intervention: Does developmental therapy make a difference? *Topics in Early Childhood Special Education, 7,* 20–32.

Harris, S. L., Alessandri, M., & Gill, M. J. (1991). Training parents of developmentally disabled children. In J. L. Matson & J. A. Mulick (Eds.), *Handbook of mental retardation* (2nd ed., pp. 373–381). New York: Pergamon Press.

Harris, S., Handleman, J., Arnold, M. S., & Gordan, R. F. (2000). The Douglas Developmental Disabilities Center: Two models of service delivery. In J. S. Handleman & S. L. Harris (Eds.), *Preschool education programs for children with autism* (2nd ed., pp. 233–260). Austin, TX: Pro-Ed.

Heber, R. (1959). A manual on terminology and classification in mental retardation (rev.). *American Journal of Mental Deficiency, 56*(Monograph Suppl.).

Hellings, J. A. (1999). Psychopharmacology of mood disorders in persons with mental retardation and autism. *Mental Retardation and Developmental Disabilities Research Reviews, 5,* 270–78.

Hellings, J. A., Kelley, L. A., Gabrielli, W. F., Kilgore, E., & Shah, P. (1996). Sertraline response in adults with mental retardation and autistic disorder. *Journal of Clinical Psychiatry, 57,* 333–336.

Hellings, J. A., Zarcone, J. R., Crandall, K., Wallace, D., & Schroeder, S. R. (2001). Weight gain in a controlled study of risperidone in children, adolescents and adults with mental retardation and autism. *Journal of Child and Adolescent Psychopharmacology, 11,* 229–238.

Heward, W. L. (2006). *Exceptional children* (8th ed.). Upper Saddle River, NJ: Merrill.

Hill, J. L., Brooks-Gunn, J., & Waldfogel, J. (2003). Sustained effects of high participation in an early intervention for low-birth-weight premature infants. *Developmental Psychology, 39,* 730–744.

Hobbs, N., Dokecki, P., Hoover-Dempsey, K., Moroney, R., Shayne, M., & Weeks, K. (1984). *Strengthening families.* San Francisco: Jossey Bass.

Hocutt, A. M. (1996). Effectiveness of special education: Is placement the critical factor? *The Future of Children, 6,* 77–102.

Hodapp, R. M., & Dykens, E. M. (1996). Mental retardation's two cultures of behavioral research. *American Journal on Mental Retardation, 98,* 675–687.

Honig v. Doe, 484 U.S. 305 (1988).

Horner, R. H., Dunlap, G., Koegel, R. L., Carr, E. G., Sailor, W., Anderson, J., et al. (1990). Toward a technology of "nonaversive" behavioral support. *Journal of the Association for Persons with Severe Handicaps, 15,* 125–132.

Individuals with Disabilities Education Act (IDEA), P.L. 101-476, 20 U.S.C. 1400 et seq. (1990).

Individuals with Disabilities Education Act (IDEA) Amendments of 1997, P.L. 105-17, 20 U.S.C. 1400 et seq. (1997).

Iwata, B. (1995). *Structured ABC Analysis Form.* Tallahasee: The Florida Center on Self-Injury.

Iwata, B., Dorsey, M., Slifer, K., Bauman, K., & Richman, G. (1982). Toward a functional analysis of self-injury. *Analysis and Intervention in Developmental Disabilities, 3,* 1–20.

Iwata, B., Dorsey, M., Slifer, K., Bauman, K., & Richman, G. (1994). Toward a functional analysis of self-injury. *Journal of Applied Behavior Analysis, 27,* 197–210.

Jaselskis, C. A., Cook, E. H., & Fletcher, K. E. (1992). Clonidine treatment of hyperactive and impulsive children with autistic disorder. *Journal of Clinical Psychopharmacology, 12,* 322–237.

Johnson, C. R. (2002). Mental retardation. In M. Hersen (Ed.), *Clinical behavior therapy: Adults and children* (pp. 420–433). Hoboken, NJ: Wiley.

Johnson, W. L., & Baumeister, A. A. (1978). Self-injurious behavior: A review and analysis of methodological details of published studies. *Behavior Modification, 2,* 465–487.

Jolly, A. C., Test, D. W., & Spooner, F. (1993). Using badges to increase initiations of children with severe disabilities in a play setting. *Journal of the Association for Persons with Severe Handicaps, 18,* 46–51.

Jorde, L. B., Carey, J. C., White, R. L. (1995). *Medical genetics.* St. Louis, MO: Mosby.

Kahng, S., Iwata, B. A., & Lewin, A. B. (2002). Behavioral treatment of self-injury, 1964–2000. *American Journal on Mental Retardation, 107,* 212–221.

Kaplan, H. I., Sadock, B. J. (1993). *Psychiatric drug treatment.* Baltimore: Williams & Wilkins.

Kasten, E. F., & Coury, D. L. (1991). Health policy and prevention of mental retardation. In J. L. Matson & J. A. Mulick (Eds.), *Handbook of mental retardation* (2nd ed., pp. 336–344). New York: Pergamon Press.

Kendall, P. C., Nay, W. R., & Jeffers, J. (1975). Timeout duration and contrast effects: A systematic evalua-

tion of a successive treatments design. *Behavior Therapy, 6,* 609–615.

Ketter, T. A., Wang, P. W., Becker, O. V., Nowakowska, C., & Yang, Y. S. (2003). The diverse roles of anticonvulsants in bipolar disorders. *Annals of Clinical Psychiatry, 15,* 95–108.

Kirk, S. A. (1958). *Early education of the mentally retarded.* Urbana: University of Illinois Press.

Kochanek, T. T., & Buka, S. L. (1995). *The Early Childhood Research Institute on Service Utilization: Study environments and a portrait of children, families and service providers within them.* Providence: Early Childhood Research Institute on Service Utilization, Rhode Island College.

Koegel, L. K., Koegel, R. L., Shoshan, Y., & McNerney, E. (1999). Pivotal response intervention: II. Preliminary long-term outcome data. *Journal of the Association for Persons with Severe Handicaps, 24,* 186–198.

Koegel, R. L., Schreibman, L., Britten, K., Burke, J., & O'Neill, R. (1982). A comparison of parent training to direct child treatment. In R. L. Koegel, A. Rincover, & A. L. Egel (Eds.), *Educating and understanding the autistic child* (pp. 260–279). San Diego, CA: College Hill Press.

Kohn, A. (1993). *Punished by rewards.* Boston: Houghton Mifflin.

Kowatch, R. A., & Bucci, J. P. (1998). Mood stabilizers and anticonvulsants. *Pediatric Clinics of North America, 45,* 1173–1186.

Krishnamoorthy, J., & King, B. H.(1998). Open-label olanzapine treatment in five preadolescent children. *Journal of Child and Adolescent Psychopharmacology, 8,* 7–13.

Kuhn, D., DeLeon, I., Fisher, W., & Wilke, A. (1999). Clarifying an ambiguous functional analysis with matched and mismatched extinction procedures. *Journal of Applied Behavior Analysis, 32,* 99–102.

Kysela, G., Hillyard, A., McDonald, L., & Ahlsten-Taylor, J. (1981). Early intervention: Design and evaluation. In R. L. Schiefelbusch & D. D. Bricker (Eds.), *Language intervention series: Vol. 6. Early language: Acquisition and intervention* (pp. 341–388). Baltimore: University Park Press.

La Malfa, G., Bertelli, M., & Conte, M. (2001). Fluvoxamine and aggression in mental retardation. *Psychiatric Services, 52,* 1105.

Leblanc, L., Hagopian, L., & Maglieri, K. (2000). Use of a token economy to eliminate excessive inappropriate social behavior in an adult with developmental disabilities. *Behavioral Interventions, 15,* 135–143.

Linna, S. L., Piha, J., Kumpulainen, K., Tamminen, T., & Almqvist, F. (1999). Psychiatric symptoms in children with intellectual disability. *European Child and Adolescent Psychiatry, 8*(Suppl. 4), 77–82.

Lesch, M., & Nyhan, W. (1964). A familial disorder of uric acid metabolism and central nervous system function. *American Journal of Medicine, 36,* 561–570.

Lubbs, H. A. (1969). A marker-X chromosome. *American Journal of Human Genetics, 21,* 231–244.

Luiselli, J. K., Blew, P., & Thibadeau, S. (2001). Therapeutic effects and long-term efficacy of antidepressant medication for persons with developmental disabilities: Behavioral assessment in two cases of treatment-resistant aggression and self-injury. *Behavior Modification, 25,* 62–78.

Mace, F. C., Page, T. J., Ivancic, M. T., & O'Brien, S. (1986). Effectiveness of brief time-out with and without contingent delay: A comparative analysis. *Journal of Applied Behavior Analysis, 19,* 79–86.

MacLean, W. E., Jr. (1993). Overview. In J. L. Matson & R. P. Barrett (Eds.), *Psychopathology in the mentally retarded* (2nd ed., pp. 1–14). Boston: Allyn & Bacon.

MacMillan, D. L., Gresham, F. M., & Siperstein, G. N. (1995). Heightened concerns over the 1992 AAMR definition: Advocacy versus precision. *American Journal on Mental Retardation, 100,* 87–97.

MacMillan, D. L., Siperstein, G. N., & Gresham, F. M. (1996). A challenge to the viability of mild mental retardation as a diagnostic category. *Exceptional Children, 62,* 356–371.

Madrid, A. L., State, M. W., & King, B. H. (2000). Pharmacologic management of psychiatric and behavioral symptoms in mental retardation. *Child and Adolescent Psychiatric Clinics of North America, 9,* 225–243.

Marriage, K. (2002). Schizophrenia and related psychoses. In S. P. Kutcher (Ed.), *Practical child and adolescent psychopharmacology* (pp. 134–158). Cambridge, UK: *Cambridge University Press.*

Martin, A., Koenig, K., Scahill, L., & Bregman, J. (1999). Open-label quetiapine in the treatment of children and adolescents with autistic disorder. *Journal of Child and Adolescent Psychopharmacology, 9,* 99–107.

Martin, S. L., Ramey, C. T., & Ramey, S. L. (1990). The prevention of intellectual impairment in children of impoverished families: Findings of a randomized trial of educational day care. *American Journal of Public Health, 80,* 844–847.

Masi, G., Marcheschi, M., & Pfanner, P. (1997). Paroxetine in depressed adolescents with intellectual disability: An open label study. *Journal of Intellectual Disability Research, 41,* 268–272.

Masland, R. H. (1988). *Career research award address.* Paper presented at the annual meeting of the American Association of Mental Retardation, Washington, DC.

Matson, J. L. (1984). Psychotherapy with persons who are mentally retarded. *Mental Retardation, 22,* 170–175.

Matson, J. L., Bielecki, J., Mayville, E., Smalls, Y., Bamburg, J., & Baglio, C. (1999). The development of a reinforcer choice assessment scale for persons with severe and profound mental retardation. *Research in Developmental Disabilities, 20,* 379–384.

McAfee, J. (2002). *Navigating the social world.* Arlington, TX: Future Horizons.

McCarton, C. M., Brooks-Gunn, J., Wallace, I. F., Bauer, C. R., Bennett, F. C., Bernbaum, J. C., et al. (1997). Results at age 8 years of early intervention for low-birth-weight premature infants: The Infant Health and Development Program. *Journal of the American Medical Association, 277,* 126–132.

McConnell, S. R. (1994). Social context, social validity, and program outcome in early intervention. In R. Gardner III, D. M. Sainato, J. O. Cooper, T. E. Heron, W. L. Heward, J. Eshleman, et al. (Eds.), *Behavior analysis in education: Focus on measurably superior instruction* (pp. 75–85). Pacific Grove, CA: Brooks/Cole.

McDonough, M., Hillery, J., & Kennedy, N. (2000). Olanzapine for chronic, stereotypic self-injurious behaviour: A pilot study in seven adults with intellectual disability. *Journal of Intellectual Disability Research, 44,* 677–684.

McDougle, C. J. (1998). *Efficacy of fluvoxamine in children with autistic disorder.* Unpublished manuscript.

McDougle, C. J., Kem, D. L., & Posey, D. J.(2002). Case series: Use of ziprasidone for maladaptive symptoms in youths with autism. *Journal of the American Academy of Child and Adolescent Psychiatry, 41,* 921–927.

McGee, G. G., Almeida, M. C., Sulzer-Azaroff, B., & Feldman, R. S. (1992). Promoting reciprocal interactions via peer incidental teaching. *Journal of Applied Behavior Analysis, 25,* 515–524.

McWilliam, R. A., & Lang, L. L. (1994). *What North Carolina professionals think of early intervention services.* Report for the Children and Families Committee of the North Carolina Interagency Coordinating Council for Children with Disabilities Ages Birth to 5 and Their Families.

Miltenberger, R. G., Handen, B., & Capriotti, R. (1987). Physical restraint, visual screening and DRI in the treatment of stereotypy. *Scandinavian Journal of Behavior Therapy, 16,* 51–57.

Morgan, S. B. (1979). Development and distribution of intellectual and adaptive skills in Down syndrome children: Implications for early intervention. *Mental Retardation, 17,* 247–249.

National Center for Education Statistics. (2002). *Digest of education statistics.* Washington, DC: Author.

National Institute of Mental Health Autism Research Unit on Pediatric Psychopharmacology. (2002). *Parent management training manual.* Washington, DC: Author.

Needleman, H. L., Schell, A., Bellinger, D., Leviton, L., & Alfred, E. D. (1990). The long-term effects of exposure to low doses of lead in childhood: An 11-year follow-up report. *New England Journal of Medicine, 322,* 83–88.

Nelson, C. M., & Rutherford, R. B. (1983). Timeout revisited: Guidelines for its use in special education. *Exceptional Education Quarterly, 3,* 56–67.

Nyhan, W. (1976). Behavior in the Lesch–Nyhan syndrome. *Journal of Autism and Childhood Schizophrenia, 6,* 235–252.

O'Brien, J., Forest, M., Snow, J., & Hasbury, D. (1989). *Action for inclusion.* Toronto: Frontier College Press.

Odom, S. L., Chandler, L. K., Ostrosky, M., McConnell,

S. R., & Reaney, S. (1992). Fading teacher prompts from peer initiation interventions for young children with disabilities. *Journal of Applied Behavior Analysis, 25,* 307–317.

O'Neill, R. E., Horner, R. H., Albin, R. W., Storey, K., & Sprague, J. R. (1997). *Functional assessment and program development for problem behavior: A practical handbook.* Baltimore: Brookes.

O'Reilly, M. F., Lacey, C., & Lancioni, G. E. (2000). Assessment of the influence of background noise on escape-maintained problem behavior and pain behavior in a child with Williams syndrome. *Journal of Applied Behavior Analysis, 33,* 511–514.

Pace, G. M., Iwata, B. A., Edwards, G. L., & McCosh, K. C. (1986). Stimulus fading and transfer in treatment of self-restraint and self-injurious behavior. *Journal of Applied Behavior Analysis, 19,* 381–389.

Pearson, D. A., Santos, C., Roache, J., Casat, C., Loveland, K. A., Lachar, D., et al. (2003). Treatment effects of methylphenidate on behavioral adjustment in children with mental retardation and ADHD. *Journal of the American Academy of Child and Adolescent Psychiatry, 42,* 209–216.

Pelios, L., Morren, J., Tesch, D., & Axelrod, S. (1999). The impact of functional analysis methodology on treatment choice for self-injurious and aggressive behavior. *Journal of Applied Behavior Analysis, 32,* 185–195.

Physicians' Desk Reference (58th ed.). (2004). Oradell, NJ: Medical Economics.

Piazza, C. C., Patel, M. R., Gulotta, C. S., Sevin, B. M., & Layer, S. A. (2003). On the relative contributions of positive reinforcement and escape extinction in the treatment of food refusal. *Journal of Applied Behavior Analysis, 36,* 309–324.

Pierce, W. D., & Cheney, C. D. (2004). *Behavior analysis and learning* (3rd ed.). Mahwah, NJ: Erlbaum.

Piercy, M., Wilton, K., & Townsend, M. (2002). Promoting the social acceptance of young children with moderate–severe intellectual disabilities using cooperative-learning techniques. *American Journal on Mental Retardation, 107,* 352–360.

Polloway, E. (1997). Developmental principles of the Luckasson et al. (1992) AAMR definition of mental retardation. *Education and Training in Mental Retardation and Developmental Disabilities, 32,* 174–178.

Posey, D. J., & McDougle, C. J. (2003). Use of atypical antipsychotics in autism. In E. Hollander (Ed.), *Autism spectrum disorders* (pp. 247–264). New York: Dekker.

Posey, D. J., Puntney, J. I., Sasher, T. M., Kem, D. L., Kohn, A., & McDougle, C. J. (2004). Guanfacine treatment of hyperactivity and inattention in pervasive developmental disorders: A retrospective analysis of 80 cases. *Journal of Child and Adolescent Psychopharmacology, 14,* 233–242.

Premack, D. (1959). Toward empirical behavior laws: I. Positive reinforcement. *Psychological Review, 66,* 219–233.

Prout, H. T., Chard, K. M., Nowak-Drabik, K. M., & Johnson, D. M. (2000). Determining the effectiveness of psychotherapy with persons with mental retardation: The need to move toward empirically based research. *NADD Bulletin, 6,* 83–86.

Prout, H. T., & Nowak-Drabik, K. M. (2003). Psychotherapy with persons who have mental retardation: An evaluation of effectiveness. *American Journal on Mental Retardation, 108,* 82–93.

Quay, H., & Hogan, A. (1999). *Handbook of disruptive behavior disorders.* New York: Plenum Press.

Rafferty, Y., & Boettcher, C. (2000, July–August). *Inclusive education for preschoolers with disabilities: Comparative views of parents and practitioners.* Paper presented at the Fifth Annual Head Start National Research Conference, Washington, DC.

Ramey, C., & Baker-Ward, L. (1982). Psychosocial intervention for infants with Down syndrome: A controlled trial. *Pediatrics, 65,* 463–468.

Ramey, C. T., & Ramey, S. L. (1998). Early intervention and early experience. *American Psychologist, 53,* 109–120.

Reber, M. (1994). Dual diagnosis: Psychiatric disorders and mental retardation. In M. L. Batshaw & Y. M. Perret (Eds.), *Children with disabilities: A medical primer* (3rd ed., pp. 421–440). Baltimore: Brookes.

Reed, G., Piazza, C., Patel, M., Layer, S., Bachmeyer, M., Bethke, S., et al. (2004). On the relative contributions of noncontingent reinforcement and escape extinction in the treatment of food refusal. *Journal of Applied Behavior Analysis, 37,* 27–41.

Reiss, A. (1994). *Handbook of challenging behaviors: Mental health aspects of mental retardation.* Worthington, OH: International Diagnostic Systems.

Reynolds, A. J., Temple, J. A., & Ou, S. R. (2003). School-based early intervention and child well-being in the Chicago Longitudinal Study. *Child Welfare, 82,* 633–656.

Ringdahl, J., Wacker, D., Berg, W., & Harding, J. (2001). Repetitive behavior disorders in persons with developmental disabilities. In D. Woods & R. Miltenberger (Eds.), *Tic disorders, trichotillomania, and other repetitive behavior disorders: Behavioral approaches to analysis and treatment* (pp. 297–314). Norwell, MA: Kluwer Academic.

Romano, J. P., & Roll, D. (2000). Expanding the utility of behavioral momentum for youth with developmental disabilities. *Behavioral Interventions, 15,* 99–111.

Roscoe, E. M., Iwata, B. A., & Kahng, S. W. (1999). Relative versus absolute reinforcement effects: Implications for preference assessments. *Journal of Applied Behavior Analysis, 32,* 479–493.

Ruef, M., Posten, D., & Humphrey, K. (1999). *PBS: Putting the "positive" into behavioral support. An introductory training packet.* Lawrence: University of Kansas, Beach Center on Families and Disability.

Rutter, M., Tizard, J., Yule, W., Graham, P., & Whitmore, K. (1976). Research report: Isle of Wight studies, 1964–1974. *Psychological Medicine, 6,* 313–332.

Rynders, J. E., & Horrobin, J. M. (1980). Educational provisions for young children with Down's syndrome. In J. Gottlieb (Ed.), *Educating mentally retarded persons in the mainstream* (pp. 109–147). Baltimore: University Park Press.

Sandman, C. A., Datta, P., Barron-Quinn, J., Hoehler, F., Williams, C., & Swanson, J. (1983). Naloxone attenuates self-abusive behavior in developmentally disabled clients. *Applied Research in Mental Retardation, 3,* 5–11.

Santosh, P. J., & Baird, G. (1999). Psychopharmacotherapy in children and adults with intellectual disability. *Lancet, 354,* 233–242.

Schou, M. (2001). Lithium treatment at 52. *Journal of Affective Disorders, 67,* 21–32.

Schroeder, S. R. (1991). Self-injury and stereotypy. In J. L. Matson & J. A. Mulick (Eds.), *Handbook of mental retardation* (2nd ed., pp. 382–396). Elmsford, NY: Pergamon Press.

Schroeder, S. R., Breese, G. R., & Mueller, R. A. (1989). Dopaminergic mechanisms in self-injurious behavior. In D. K. Routh & M. Wolraich (Eds.), *Advances in developmental and behavioral pediatrics* (Vol. 9, pp. 181–198). Greenwich, CT: JAI Press.

Schweinhart, L. J., Barnes, H. V., & Weikart, D. P. (1993). *Significant benefits: The High Scope/Perry preschool study through age 27* (Monographs of the High Scope Educational Research Foundation, No. 10). Ypsilanti, MI: High Scope Press.

Scruggs, T. E., & Mastropieri, M. A. (1996). Teachers' perceptions of mainstreaming/inclusion: A research synthesis. *Exception Children, 63,* 59–74.

Sharpe, M. N., York, J. L, & Knight, J. (1994). Effects of inclusion on the academic performance of classmates without disabilities: A preliminary study. *Remedial and Special Education, 15,* 281–287.

Shprintzen, R. J., Goldberg, R. B., Lewin, M. L., Sidoti, E. J., Berkman, M. D., Argamaso, R. V., et al. (1978). A new syndrome involving cleft palate, cardiac anomalies, typical facies, and learning disabilities: Velo-cardio-facial syndrome. *Cleft Palate Journal, 15,* 56–62.

Singer, G., & Irwin, L. (1987). Human rights review of intrusive behaviors for students with severe handicaps. *Exceptional Children, 54,* 46–52.

Singh, N., Ellis, C., & Wechsler, H. (1997). Psychopharmacoepidemiology of mental retardation: 1966 to 1995. *Journal of Child and Adolescent Psychopharmacology, 7,* 255–266.

Skeels, H. M. (1966). Adult status of children with contrasting early life experiences: A follow-up study. *Monographs of the Society for Research in Child Development, 31*(3, Serial No. 105).

Skinner, B. F. (1953). *Science and human behavior.* New York: Macmillan.

Skodak, M., & Skeels, H. (1949). A final follow-up study of one hundred adopted children. *Journal of Genetic Psychology, 74,* 84–125.

Smith, A. C. M., McGavran, L., Robinson, J., Waldstein, G., Macfarlane, J., Zonana, J., et al. (1986). Interstitial deletion of (17)(p11.2p11.2) in nine patients. *American Journal of Medical Genetics, 24,* 393–414.

Snead, B. W., Boon, F., & Presberg, J. (1994). Paroxetine for self-injurious behavior. *Journal of the American Academy of Child and Adolescent Psychiatry, 33,* 909–910.

Solnick, J. V., Rincover, A., & Peterson, C. R. (1977). Some determinants of the reinforcing and punishing effects of time-out. *Journal of Applied Behavior Analysis, 10,* 415–424.

Spencer, T., Heiligenstein, J., Biederman, J., Faries, D., Kratochvil, C., Conners, K., & Potter, N. (2002). Results from 2 proof-of-concept, placebo-controlled studies of atomoxetine in children with attention-deficit/hyperactivity disorder. *Journal of Clinical Psychiatry, 63,* 1140–1147.

Spiker, D., & Hopmann, M. R. (1997). The effectiveness of early intervention for children with Down syndrome. In M. J Guralnick (Ed.), *The effectiveness of early intervention* (pp. 271–305). Baltimore: Brookes.

Staub, D., Spaulding, M., Peck, C. A., Gallucci, C., & Schwartz, I. S. (1996). Using nondisabled peers to support the inclusion of students with disabilities at the junior high school level. *Journal of the Association for Persons with Severe Handicaps, 21,* 194–205.

Steingard, R. J., Zimnitzky, B., DeMaso, D. R., Bauman, M. L., & Bucci, J. P. (1997). Sertraline treatment of transition-associated anxiety and agitation in children with autistic disorder. *Journal of Child and Adolescent Psychopharmacology, 7,* 9–15.

Stevenson, R. E., Massey, P. S., Schroer, R., McDermott, S., & Richter, B. (1996). Preventable fraction of mental retardation: Analysis based on individuals with severe mental retardation. *Mental Retardation, 34,* 182–188.

Stigler, K. A., Posey, D. J., & McDougle, C. J. (2004). Aripiprazole for maladaptive behavior in pervasive developmental disorders. *Journal of Child and Adolescent Psychopharmacology, 14,* 455–463.

Stolker, J. J., Koedoot, P. J., Heerdink, E. R., Leufkens, H. G., & Nolen, W. A. (2002). Psychotropic drug use in intellectually disabled group-home residents with behavioural problems. *Pharmacopsychiatry, 35,* 9–23.

Strain, P. S., & Cordisco, L. K. (1994). LEAP Preschool. In S. L. Harris & J. S. Handleman (Eds.), *Preschool education programs for children with autism* (pp. 225–244). Austin, TX: Pro-Ed.

Stromme, P., & Diseth, T. H. (2000). Prevalence of psychiatric diagnoses in children with mental retardation: Data from a population-based study. *Developmental Medicine and Child Neurology, 42,* 266–270.

Sulzer-Azaroff, B., & Mayer, R. G. (1991). *Behavior analysis for lasting change.* Fort Worth, TX: Holt, Rinehart & Winston.

Tagano, D. W., Moran, D. J., III, & Sawyer, J. K. (1991). *Creativity in early childhood classrooms.* Washington, DC: National Education Association.

Tarbox, J., Wallace, M. D., Tarbox, R., Landaburu, H., & Williams, W. L. (2004). Functional analysis and treatment of low rate problem behavior in individuals with developmental disabilities. *Behavioral Interventions, 19,* 187–204.

Task Force on Promotion and Dissemination of Psychological Procedures, Division of Clinical Psychology, American Psychological Association. (1995). Training in and dissemination of empirically validated psychological treatments: Report and recommendations. *The Clinical Psychologist, 48,* 3–23.

Tate, B. G., & Baroff, G. S. (1966). Aversive control of self-injurious behaviour in a psychotic boy. *Behaviour Research and Therapy, 4,* 499–501.

Taylor, G. R. (1999). *Curriculums models and strategies for educating individuals with disabilities in inclusive classrooms.* Springfield, IL: Thomas.

Taylor, G. R., & Harrington, F. T. (2003). *Educating the disabled: Enabling learners in inclusive setting.* Lenham, MD: Scarecrow Press.

Tilly, W. D., Knoster, T. K., Kovaleski, J., Bambara, L., Dunlap, G., & Kincaid, D. (1998). *Functional behavioral assessment: Policy development in light of emerging research and practice.* Alexandria, VA: National Association of State Directors of Special Education.

Trivette, C. M., Dunst, C. J., & Deal, A. G. (1997). Resource-based early intervention practices. In S. K. Thurman, J. R. Cronwell, & S. R. Gottwald (Eds.), *The contexts of early intervention: Systems and settings* (pp. 73–92). Baltimore: Brookes.

Troisi, A. (1997). Fluoxetine and aggression. *Neuropsychopharmacology, 16,* 373–374.

Turgay, A., Binder, C., Snyder, R., & Fisman, S.(2002). Long-term safety and efficacy of risperidone for the treatment of disruptive behavior disorders in children with subaverage IQs. *Pediatrics, 110,* e34.

U.S. Food and Drug Administration (FDA). (2004, October 15). *Public health advisory.* Rockville, MD: Author.

Van Bellinghen, M., & De Troch, C. (2001). Risperidone in the treatment of behavioral disturbances in children and adolescents with borderline intellectual functioning: A double-blind, placebo-controlled pilot trial. *Journal of Child and Adolescent Psychopharmacology, 11,* 5–13.

Van Houten, R., Rolider, A., & Houlihan, M. (1992). Treatments of self-injury based on teaching compliance and/or brief physical restraint. In J. K. Luiselli, J. L. Matson, & N. N. Singh (Eds.), *Self-injurious behavior: Analysis, assessment, and treatment* (pp. 181–199). New York: Springer-Verlag.

Verhoeven, W. M., Veendrik-Meekes, M. J., Jacobs, G. A., van den Berg, Y. W., & Tuinier, S.(2001). Citalopram in mentally retarded patients with depression: A long-term clinical investigation. *European Psychiatry, 16,* 104–108.

Victorian Infant Collaborative Study Group. (1991). Eight-year outcome in infants with birth weight of 500 to 999 grams: Continuing regional study of 1979 and 1980 births. *Journal of Pediatrics, 118,* 761–767.

Victorian Infant Collaborative Study Group. (1995). Neurosensory outcome at 5 years and extremely low birthweight. *Archives of Disease in Childhood, 73,* F143–F146.

Wehmeyer, M. L. (1994). Factors related to the expression of typical and atypical repetitive movements of young children with intellectual disability. *International Journal of Disability, Development and Education, 41,* 33–49.

White, G. D., Nielsen, G., & Johnson, S. M. (1972). Timeout duration and the suppression of deviant behavior in children. *Journal of Applied Behavior Analysis, 5,* 111–120.

Williams, H., Clarke, R., Bouras, N., Martin, J., & Holt, G. (2000). Use of the atypical antipsychotics olanzapine and risperidone in adults with intellectual disability. *Journal of Intellectual Disability Research, 44,* 164–169.

Wolfensberger, W. (1969). The origin and nature of our institutional models. In R. B. Kugel & W. Wolfensberger (Eds.), *Changing patterns in residential services for the mentally retarded* (pp. 59–171). Washington, DC: U.S. Government Printing Office.

Woody, S. R., & Sanderson W. C. (1998). *Manuals for empirically supported treatments: 1998 update.* Niwot, CO: Division 12 Central Office.

Wyatt v. Stickney, 344 F. Supp. 373, 387 (M.D. Ala. 1972).

Zanolli, K., Daggett, J., & Adams, T. (1996). Teaching preschool age autistic children to make spontaneous initiations to peers using priming. *Journal of Autism and Developmental Disorders, 26,* 407–422.

Zigler, E., & Hodapp, R. (1986). *Understanding mental retardation.* Cambridge, UK: Cambridge University Press.

7

Autistic Spectrum Disorders

Crighton Newsom and Christine A. Hovanitz

The autistic spectrum disorders (ASDs) are a group of neurodevelopmental disorders whose characteristic features are usually evident by early childhood. The most definitive characteristic is a significant failure in socialization. Children with severe ASDs show little interest in other people, often including their own families. Even the most mildly affected youngsters have interactions with others that are markedly odd and inept. A second area of obvious deficiency is language. Up to half of such children are delayed in their acquisition of words; they may be mute or minimally verbal before treatment, and they fail to compensate by using gestures. The other half have some meaningful speech, but also frequently echo the words or phrases of others without understanding them. Third, children with ASDs exhibit a very limited repertoire of behaviors, interests, and activities, dominated by stereotyped routines and by toy play that is solitary, repetitive, and unimaginative. Higher-functioning children and adolescents often show extensive, highly idiosyncratic preoccupations with topics of interest only to them. Many children show intense disruptive, aggressive, and self-injurious behaviors that place great stress on their families and challenge the most experienced professionals.

The majority of children with ASDs are found to have mental retardation when assessed with intelligence tests and adaptive behavior scales, although they show considerable scatter across cognitive and developmental domains. A few children show some advanced "splinter" skills within a circumscribed area, such as music, numbers, or reading. Not surprisingly, children with ASDs have proved sufficiently challenging, both clinically and theoretically, to attract considerable attention from researchers and practitioners in all the helping professions.

HISTORY

There are a few scattered reports of children who apparently had some type of ASD in the 19th century (Maudsley, 1867), including the famous case of the Wild Boy of Aveyron, a feral child brought to the care and tutelage of the young physician Jean-Marc-Gaspard Itard (Itard, 1801/1962; Shattuck, 1994). However, such children were usually not distinguished from children with mental retardation. In the early decades of the 20th century, investigators began to make finer discriminations among children with severe deviations in development, identifying and describing children who regressed after a period of typical development (Heller, 1908/1954) and children who seemed to have childhood-onset schizophrenia (Potter, 1933). During the 1940s and 1950s, various syndromes thought to be related to schizophrenia but with strong early determinants were described. Kanner's "early infantile autism" (Kanner, 1943/1973) attracted sustained attention and endured, and interest in Heller's "dementia" and especially in Asperger's "autistic psychopathy" (Asperger, 1944/1991) has become more prominent over the past decade.

The endurance of Kanner's syndrome can be attributed to several factors, primarily the fact

455

that his description of his first 11 patients with autistic disorder was unusually detailed and observant. Perhaps most important, the disorder itself is inherently compelling not only to scientists and clinicians but also to the general public, as evidenced in frequent mass media presentations. The main features of Kanner's syndrome included extreme self-isolation; obsessive insistence on the "preservation of sameness"; muteness or noncommunicative speech with echolalia, pronoun reversal, and idiosyncratic usages of words and phrases; excellent rote memory; very literal thinking; typical physical development; and apparently average intellectual potential (Kanner, 1943/1973). Kanner attributed the condition to some innate inability to establish social relationships that was present from birth or shortly thereafter; accordingly, he named the syndrome "early infantile autism."

Infantile autism soon became a popular and widely used diagnosis during the 1950s, when it was believed to be a mental illness due to faulty parenting. During the 1960s, several lines of research and treatment that changed that view were established. Early epidemiological and medical studies showed that most autistic children also presented with mental retardation, that they came from all socioeconomic levels, and that a small but significant percentage had signs of frank neurological impairment (Rutter & Lockyer, 1967; Schain & Yannet, 1960). Other research began to identify deficits in basic perceptual, cognitive, and linguistic processes, again indicating the likelihood of neurological dysfunction (Hermelin & O'Connor, 1964; Pronovost, Wakstein, & Wakstein, 1966; Tubbs, 1966). Behavioral clinical researchers found that some of the core problems of autistic children, such as social deficits, language abnormalities, and maladaptive behaviors, were amenable to procedures derived from operant learning theory (Hewett, 1965; Lovaas, Berberich, Perloff, & Schaeffer, 1966; Lovaas, Freitag, Gold, & Kassorla, 1965; Risley & Wolf, 1967). The data emerging from these and many other studies forced a reconceptualization of autism as a neurodevelopmental disorder rather than a mental illness. Rutter (1988) summarized the shift to a developmental perspective by stating, "Autistic children have not withdrawn from reality because of mental illness; rather, they have failed fully to enter reality because of a widespread and serious disturbance in the developmental process" (p. 265).

Accompanying this shift in perspective to ASDs as pervasive developmental disorders (PDDs) has been an acceleration of research on virtually every topic that is or might be relevant to understanding and treating children with ASDs, in fields ranging from genetics to national educational policy. Most recently, the creation of "centers of excellence" in autism research in the United States and greatly increased funding for basic research in biomedical factors have led to an explosion of knowledge. New technologies for unraveling the human genome and conducting advanced functional brain imaging may lead to major breakthroughs in understanding the etiologies and effects of this group of disorders. Rutter and Schopler's (1987) observation nearly 20 years ago that autism is probably the most studied of all childhood disorders remains true today. Consequently, this chapter can only sample a very large literature; however, detailed consideration is given to several areas of current interest, including the apparent rise in the prevalence of autism, the possible role of vaccines in its etiology, and recent progress in early intensive behavioral intervention.

NATURE AND DIAGNOSIS

This chapter follows current usage in using "ASDs" (Wing & Attwood, 1987) as synonymous with "PDDs" as described in the *Diagnostic and Statistical Manual of Mental Disorders*, fourth edition, text revision (DSM-IV-TR; American Psychiatric Association [APA], 2000). Children with developmental disabilities can be located within a hypothetical continuum of pervasiveness and severity of disability (Cohen, Paul, & Volkmar, 1986). At the most pervasive end of the continuum fall children with profound mental retardation and multiple other handicaps, who exhibit a fairly uniform pattern of profound impairments across the domains of intellectual, adaptive, social, language, and motor functioning. At the least pervasive end of the continuum lie children with specific developmental disorders, typically showing impairments in only one domain. Children classified as having ASDs fall at various points between these two extremes, showing uneven patterns of impairments across several domains, but are generally closer to the most pervasive end. Within the group with ASDs, there are at least two large, overlapping subgroups differing on developmental status. One group has generally higher intelligence, speech that is generally communicative but with bizarre features and unusual prosody, and relentlessly perseverative behaviors. The second group has lower intelligence, prominent motor stereotypies, sensory abnormalities, and seriously impaired language and imitation skills (Stevens et al., 2000; Waterhouse et al., 1996). It is essential to bear in mind that the point of the "autistic spectrum" concept is that each of the impairments can occur in widely varying degrees of severity and take many different forms (Wing & Potter, 2002).

The current diagnostic criteria for ASDs/ PDDs in DSM-IV-TR and in the *International Classification of Diseases*, 10th revision (ICD-10; World Health Organization, 1992), used in Europe, follow Rutter's (1978) and Wing and Gould's (1979) concepts of autism as a "triad of impairments"—impairments in socialization, in communication, and in range of behaviors, interests, and activities. The social impairment is the most salient impairment and perhaps the most important. Thus Gillberg (1992) has proposed that the ASDs can be subsumed under a broader spectrum of "disorders of empathy," and investigators have long theorized that the social impairment may underlie the communication and behavior repertoire impairments (Klin, Jones, Schultz, Volkmar, & Cohen, 2002a). However, the diagnosis definitely requires that all three be apparent in the child's clinical presentation to a marked degree. The child's symptoms must always be evaluated in the context of his or her developmental level. For example, a lack of interactive play in a 4-year-old with a low-average IQ is far more ominous than it would be in a 2-year-old with a developmental age of 6 months. Stereotyped, repetitive behaviors may not be obvious in a 2-year-old, but when present along with social and communication delays, they are highly indicative of an ASD. Flexibility in applying diagnostic criteria and interpreting the results of standardized tests is essential (Charman & Baird, 2002).

Autistic Disorder

In making diagnostic distinctions between children with autistic disorder and children with other disabilities, the initial focus is on the quality and extent of the child's social functioning. The diagnosis requires an obvious, qualitative impairment in social interaction that is below the child's overall developmental level, as manifested by at least two of the following patterns of behavior (APA, 2000):

1. Notable impairment in using nonverbal behaviors to initiate and maintain social contact, such as eye-to-eye gaze, facial expression, body orientation, and gestures.
2. Failure to develop relationships appropriate to the child's developmental level with siblings and peers.
3. Absence of spontaneous seeking to share enjoyment, interests, or achievements with other people, indicated by the absence of bringing, showing, or pointing out objects of interest.
4. Absence of social or emotional reciprocity, indicated by little or no interest in the give-and-take of social interaction and absent or diminished empathy.

The social impairments are among the earliest heralds of autistic disorder. Delayed orienting to name, aversion to touch, poor visual orientation, and mouthing of objects differentiate children with autistic disorder from those with Down syndrome and from typical infants by 8–12 months (Baranek, 1999; Werner, Dawson, Osterling, & Dinno, 2000). By 12 months, infants with autistic disorder are less likely to look at others, to show an object or point to objects, and to orient to their names than are typically developing infants (Osterling & Dawson, 1994).

Differential diagnosis is most difficult at the developmental extremes. At the low end of the developmental continuum, the social deficits of children with autistic disorder can be difficult to distinguish from those of children with severe or profound mental retardation. Usually, however, even a child with profound mental retardation will show simple social behaviors such as eye contact, smiling, and social approach that are commensurate with his or her developmental level (Wing, 1981b). The Checklist for Autism in Toddlers (Baron-Cohen, Allen, & Gillberg, 1992), a brief screening tool addressing critical early social behaviors, can be used with 2- to 3-year-old children to help distinguish those with autistic disorder from those with other developmental delays (Scambler, Rogers, & Wehner, 2001). In formal assessments that have included the Vineland Adaptive Behavior Scales (Sparrow,

Balla, & Cicchetti, 1984), children with autism score at a significantly lower level in the Socialization domain than their overall mental ages would predict (Klin, Volkmar, & Sparrow, 1992; Volkmar et al., 1987). Delays in social behaviors on the Socialization domain are more strongly related to the autistic disorder diagnosis than are delays in Communication, Daily Living Skills, and Maladaptive Behaviors, accounting for 48% of the variance in diagnosis (Gillham, Carter, Volkmar, & Sparrow, 2000).

Among children with average intelligence or mild mental retardation, it can be difficult to distinguish autistic disorder from Asperger's disorder (Wing, 1991), schizoid and schizotypal personality disorders (Wolff, 1995), or schizophrenia in childhood (Asarnow, 1994; Asarnow, Tompson, & McGrath, 2004; Konstantareas & Hewitt, 2001). In general, children with autistic disorder differ from such children by (1) having a lower overall level of cognitive functioning, academic achievement, and language development (Sparrow et al., 1986; Wing, 1981a, 1981b); (2) showing somewhat better motor coordination (Sparrow et al., 1986; Wing, 1981a); and (3) showing earlier onset and more severe social and language deficits (Asarnow, 1994). However, it is still not clear where and how sharply the lines should be drawn between these groups (Frith, 1991; Petty, Ornitz, Michelman, & Zimmerman, 1984; Wolff, 1995).

The second criterion that must be satisfied for the autistic disorder diagnosis is a qualitative impairment in communication, shown by at least one of the following (APA, 2000):

1. Absence or delay in the development of speech, together with failure to compensate through other means of communication (such as gesture or mime).
2. In a child with adequate speech, notable impairment in initiating or sustaining a conversation that is commensurate with the child's developmental level.
3. Repetitive and stereotyped use of language, or frequent use of words or phrases with idiosyncratic meanings.
4. Absence of spontaneous, varied pretend play or interactive play appropriate to the child's developmental level.

Assessments in early childhood find that verbal skills are typically lower than nonverbal

skills (Carpentieri & Morgan, 1994). In children with phrase speech, comprehension is usually more impaired than expression; this is the reverse of what is seen in typical development and in developmental language disorders (Fein, Lucci, Braverman, & Waterhouse, 1992). Higher-functioning children with fluent speech have difficulty using language as a tool for social interaction, showing various pragmatic communication deficits. They may fail to make a relevant response to a comment, expand on comments, recognize the connotations of words (Happe, 1991), use mental state verbs (Tager-Flusberg, 1992), make inferences (Dennis, Lazenby, & Lockyer, 2001), or understand how a speaker's attitude modifies literal meaning (Happe, 1993). As a result, they often fail to use or to understand irony, jokes, *faux pas*, lies, and metaphors.

The third criterion for autistic disorder addresses a highly restricted range of interests and repetitive, stereotyped behaviors, as manifested by at least one of the following (APA, 2000):

1. Preoccupation with one or a few restricted interests that is atypical in either intensity or focus.
2. Rigid adherence to specific, nonfunctional rituals or routines.
3. Repetitive and stereotyped motor mannerisms, such as hand or finger flapping, object manipulation, body rocking, or bizarre-looking whole-body movements.
4. Persisting preoccupation with parts of objects.

Young children with autistic disorder frequently show minimal play skills that are both delayed and deviant. Symbolic (pretend) play may never develop. A child may perseverate in repetitive, stereotyped behaviors (stereotypies) such as flapping one or both hands in front of the eyes while staring at a light, spinning the wheels of a toy car instead of rolling it along the floor, or lining up objects in a particular order over and over again (Lovaas, Newsom, & Hickman, 1987; Turner, 1999). Guess and Carr (1991) have offered a multistage theory of stereotypies. In typical infants and in children who have profound mental retardation, stereotypies are largely biologically determined (Lewis et al., 1996). At a somewhat higher level of development, stereotypies are homeostatic responses to environmental under- or over-stimulation, serving to regulate arousal at an optimal level (Thelen, 1979). At a still higher level, stereotypies and repetitive self-injurious behaviors are operant behaviors, controlled by positive and negative reinforcers (Carr, 1977; Durand & Carr, 1987).

In the most capable children, there may be an obsessive interest in numbers, letters, timetables, dinosaurs, or almost any other topic. The perseveration on circumscribed topics of interest seen in high-functioning children has been little studied, but is known to emerge from developmentally lower stereotyped behaviors as treatment progresses and the children advance developmentally (Epstein, Taubman, & Lovaas, 1985). Deficits in shifting attention may predispose a child to develop perseverative behaviors (Ozonoff, 1997).

Although what has come to be known as "regressive autism" is not an official subcategory of the PDDs in DSM-IV-TR, it affects 20–49% of all children with ASDs. It typically begins between 15 and 30 months of age and may or may not have been preceded by delays in developmental milestones (Davidovitch, Glick, Holtzman, Tirosh, & Safir, 2000). The most commonly reported symptoms of regression are loss of meaningful word use, of receptive language, of nonverbal communication skills, and of eye contact and other social skills, but not loss of motor skills. No specific physical, neurological, or environmental events have yet been linked to regressive autism (Davidovitch et al., 2000), although the possible role of subclinical epilepsy has been suggested (Tuchman & Rapin, 1997).

DSM-IV-TR does not require that the autistic disorder criteria in each of the three main areas (social interaction, communication, and range of behaviors) must all be exhibited by a certain age, but it does require that symptoms in at least one of the areas be present prior to 3 years of age. The final diagnostic criterion requires that the clinical presentation must not be better accounted for by Rett's disorder or childhood disintegrative disorder (CDD). However, autistic disorder is diagnosed instead of Asperger's disorder if the child meets the criteria for both.

The most commonly used special instruments for diagnosing autistic disorder are the Childhood Autism Rating Scale (Schopler, Reichler, & Renner, 1988), the Autism Diagnostic Interview—Revised (ADI-R; Lord, Rutter, & Le Couteur, 1994), and the Autism Diagnostic Observation Schedule (Lord et al., 2000). A recent review of these scales appears in Ozonoff, Goodlin-Jones, and Solomon (2005).

Asperger's Disorder

Asperger's disorder applies to children with autistic features at the upper levels of intelligence. Such children show the social impairments and restricted, stereotyped interests characteristic of children with autistic disorder, but not the severe language impairments (APA, 2000). Indeed, there is still controversy over the need for thinking of these children as having anything but autistic disorder with average or near-average intelligence and language, exhibiting "high-functioning autism" (Gillberg, 2001; Howlin, 2003; Prior et al., 1998). Comprehensive neuropsychological assessment may fail to reveal any differences in Wechsler profiles, brain hemispheric strengths and weaknesses, or executive functioning (Manjiviona & Prior, 1999; Szatmari, Tuff, Finlayson, & Bartolucci, 1990). However, some investigators have found higher Verbal than Performance IQs and poorer spatial abilities in children with Asperger's disorder—findings opposite to those usually seen in autistic disorder (Gilchrist et al., 2001; Ozonoff, Rogers, & Pennington, 1991). In clinical practice, the diagnosis of Asperger's disorder tends to be applied more often than autistic disorder to the children on the spectrum with the highest IQs and no history of language delay (Manjiviona & Prior, 1999).

Children with Asperger's disorder are usually of average or high intelligence, but often have specific learning disabilities. They tend to be extremely egocentric, socially inept, and preoccupied with some highly circumscribed interest. Social attachment to family members is often well established, but social overtures to peers are often very inappropriate. They give the impression of social naiveté and behavioral rigidity, because they compensate for their lack of intuitive, spontaneous social skills by interacting according to formal rules of behavior and rigid social conventions (Klin & Volkmar, 1995). Their speech is grammatically correct, often with large vocabularies, but noticeably odd in intonation, volume, and rhythm. Speech is often tangential and circumstantial, indicative of a thought disorder (Dykens, Volkmar, & Glick, 1991). Children with Asperger's disorder are markedly loquacious: They typically ramble on at great length about topics of interest only to themselves, oblivious to any social cues from the listener showing boredom or exasperation. Such children also tend to be physically clumsy in both fine and gross motor skills (Frith, 1991; Green, Gilchrist, Burton, & Cox, 2000), though this does not distinguish them from children with high-functioning autism (Ghaziuddin & Butler, 1998; Manjiviona & Prior, 1995). Very young children may show hyperlexia (the ability to read many words with little or no comprehension). There are no well-established diagnostic instruments for Asperger's disorder, although the relatively new Asperger's Syndrome Diagnostic Interview (Gillberg, Gillberg, Rastam, & Wentz, 2001) and the Gilliam Asperger's Disorder Scale (Gilliam, 2003) have psychometric properties adequate to deserve consideration as part of a comprehensive assessment.

Rett's Disorder

The placement of Rett's disorder and CDD in the same category as autistic disorder and Asperger's disorder has been questioned, because the first two are neurodegenerative diseases with apparently different causes and courses from those of the latter two (Malhotra & Gupta, 2002). Rett's disorder is a disorder of neurological arrest in early childhood (Bauman, Kemper, & Arin, 1995). It occurs mostly in girls, who begin to exhibit several specific deficits after 6–12 months of typical development. Head growth decelerates, gross motor skills deteriorate, and a loss of interest in the environment and increasingly severe mental retardation are seen. Between 12 and 36 months, rapid developmental regression and a loss of purposeful hand use occur. These children also develop characteristic, stereotypical hand wringing, twisting, or tapping; bruxism; gait dyspraxia; and episodic hyperventilation (Hagberg, 1995). Rett's disorder occurs almost exclusively in females, because the gene most often involved in its causation lies on the paternally derived X chromosome (Amir et al., 1999). Only a few male variants have been reported (Leonard et al., 2001). Aside from the classic presentation described above, phenotypic expression is highly variable, depending on the type of genetic mutation, and there is even a "preserved speech variant" in which phrase speech is spared and some improvement occurs by early adolescence (De Bona et al., 2000). When Rett characteristics appear in a child initially suspected of regressive autism, genetic testing should definitely be pursued.

Childhood Disintegrative Disorder

CDD (originally known as Heller's dementia) is a very rare disorder involving a profound regression in cognitive, language, motor, social, and self-care skills, along with the development of prominent stereotypies, following at least 2 years of typical development. The child's clinical presentation may closely resemble autistic disorder, although the mean age of onset of noticeable symptoms is typically much later for CDD (35 months vs. 12 months; Volkmar & Rutter, 1995). Cases of CDD show a high rate of electroencephalographic (EEG) abnormalities (Mouridsen, Rich, & Isager, 2000), and the regression can sometimes be traced to an identifiable neurological degenerative process (Rutter, 1985).

PDD Not Otherwise Specified

PDD Not Otherwise Specified (PDD NOS) is a remainder category for children who show autistic features but do not fully meet the criteria for one of the other PDD diagnoses. In making this diagnosis, the examiner needs to rule out schizophrenia and schizoid personality disorder; schizotypal, avoidant, and obsessive–compulsive personality disorders; and attention-deficit/hyperactivity disorder (ADHD). The PDD NOS diagnosis is also used for cases of "atypical autism"—individuals who do not meet the criteria for autistic disorder because of late age of onset, atypical symptomatology, or subthreshold symptomatology (Frances, First, & Pincus, 1995). In one comparative study, about one quarter of children with PDD NOS resembled children with Asperger's disorder but had a transient language delay or mild cognitive impairment; another quarter resembled children with autistic disorder but had a late onset, exhibited severe cognitive delay, or were too young to be clearly diagnosable as autistic; and half failed to warrant an autistic disorder diagnosis because of fewer stereotyped and repetitive behaviors (Walker et al., 2004). An instrument that can help distinguish children with PDD NOS and average intelligence from children with autistic disorder and those with ADHD is the Children's Social Behavior Questionnaire (Luteijn, Luteijn, Jackson, Volkmar, & Minderaa, 2000).

Differential Diagnosis

Complicating the differential diagnosis are a number of syndromes resembling ASDs. Medical evaluation is a necessary and often decisive step in making decisions about these syndromes. First, there are genetic disorders whose clinical presentation sometimes also warrants an ASD diagnosis. These include children with fragile X syndrome, tuberous sclerosis (Lauritsen & Ewald, 2001), and untreated phenylketonuria (Baieli, Pavone, Meli, Fiumara, & Coleman, 2003). Down syndrome, Angelman syndrome, and neurofibromatosis have also been found to present with ASD symptomatology (Gillberg & Forsell, 1984; Rasmussen, Borjesson, Wentz, & Gillberg, 2001; Steffenburg, Gillberg, Steffenburg, & Kyllerman, 1996).

Several other disorders resemble ASDs in their clinical presentation, but include features that have caused them to be classified differently. In Landau–Kleffner syndrome, typically developing children gradually or suddenly lose first receptive, then expressive language at 3–7 years of age (acquired epileptiform aphasia). They develop a characteristic form of epilepsy, with seizures mainly while asleep; the EEG shows spike-and-wave discharges in the auditory–speech areas of the temporal cortex. The epilepsy usually subsides at puberty, but the communication and memory impairments often persist into adulthood (Robinson, Baird, Robinson, & Simonoff, 2001; Stefanatos, Kinsbourne, & Wasserstein, 2002). Landau–Kleffner syndrome may be confused with regressive autism. In regressive autism, however, a child loses social, play, and cognitive behaviors as well as language, and when seizures are present, they tend to be more subtle (often subclinical) and to involve more brain regions than are seen in Landau–Kleffner syndrome (Lewine et al., 1999).

Children with Asperger's disorder may have neuropsychological profiles similar to those of children with the nonverbal learning disability (NLD) syndrome (Gunter, Ghaziuddin, & Ellis, 2002; Klin, Volkmar, Sparrow, Cicchetti, & Rourke, 1995). The NLD syndrome consists of deficits in tactile perception, psychomotor coordination, visual–spatial organization, nonverbal problem solving, and appreciation of humor. Such children also exhibit good verbal memory skills, difficulty in adapting to novel situations, better reading than arithmetic skills, and obvious deficits in social judgment and social interaction. The extent to which NLD syndrome overlaps with Asperger's disorder remains to be determined; they may be essentially the same disorder viewed from different perspectives.

Comorbid Conditions

The most common coexisting condition in the ASDs is mental retardation, which affects about 75% of children with autistic disorder (Bailey, Phillips, & Rutter, 1996); fewer than 5% of children with Asperger's disorder (Gillberg & Gillberg, 1989); and, by definition, all children with Rett's disorder and CDD.

Anxiety, mood, and personality disorders are very common in adolescents and adults with high-functioning autism and Asperger's disorder (Ghaziuddin, Ghaziuddin, & Greden, 2002; Gillberg & Billstedt, 2000). Anxiety disorders, especially social phobia, and Cluster C personality disorders, especially obsessive–compulsive personality disorder, are frequently seen in adults with Asperger's disorder (Soderstrom, Rastam, & Gillberg, 2002; Tani et al., 2003). Dysthymia and sometimes major depression may be present (Green et al., 2000).

Sensory and perceptual abnormalities are seen in various manifestations, such as hyper- or hyposensitivity to sounds, lights, textures, touch, or odors; elevated pain threshold; overselective attention; impaired shifting of attention; and inadequate cross-modal integration (Courchesne et al., 1994). These phenomena are so common that many in the field believe that sensory and attention deficits should be considered cardinal symptoms (e.g., Courchesne et al., 1994; Wainwright-Sharp & Bryson, 1993; Waterhouse, 1988). Suspected hearing loss is often the first concern raised by parents when their child does not respond to the sound of his or her name and fails to acquire language. However, only about 3.5% of children with autistic disorder are found to have a severe to profound hearing loss. The problem is usually inattention: Event-related brain potentials show that children with ASDs orient normally to simple and complex tones, but not to speech sounds (Ceponiene et al., 2003). Many more children (about 18%) show hyperacusis, an oversensitivity to loud sounds (Rosenhall, Nordin, Sandstrom, Ahlsen, & Gillberg, 1999).

The most well-documented attention deficit in children with ASDs is overselective attention, a tendency to respond to only a small fraction of complex stimuli. In early studies this was described as "stimulus overselectivity" (Lovaas, Koegel, & Schreibman, 1979), and it seemed to vary inversely with developmental level (Schover & Newsom, 1976). More recent studies with children of average intelligence who have ASDs have found evidence suggesting the presence of a high-level cognitive processing style termed "weak central coherence," which involves better attention to parts than wholes and a failure to appreciate context and meaning (Frith, 1989; Happe, 1996, 1997).

Associated Problems

Severe problem behaviors are frequently associated with ASDs, including tantrums, self-injurious behaviors, property destruction, and physical aggression. Also common are gastrointestinal complaints, most often diarrhea and constipation, affecting 24% of children in one recent survey (Molloy & Manning-Courtney, 2003). Sleep disorders are even more common, occurring in a majority of children with ASDs under 8 years of age (Richdale, 1999; Schreck & Mulick, 2000). Over 90% of adults with Asperger's disorder report some type of insomnia associated with significant anxiety and mood disorders (Tani et al., 2003). From one-quarter to one-third of children with ASDs will develop a seizure disorder (Volkmar & Nelson, 1990). Epilepsy tends to be more prevalent among adolescents and adults, in individuals with moderate to severe mental retardation and/or motor deficits, and in those with severe receptive language deficits (Tuchman & Rapin, 2002).

PREVALENCE

Rising Rates

For several decades, epidemiological studies typically reported rates of autistic disorder in the range of 4–5 per 10,000 children, and rates of all ASDs at about 20 per 10,000 (Wing, 1993). In the late 1980s, substantially higher rates began to be reported in studies from Canada (Bryson, Clark, & Smith, 1988), Japan (Matsuishi et al., 1987), and Europe (Gillberg, Steffenburg, & Schaumann, 1991). The most recent large study in North America was conducted in metropolitan Atlanta by the Centers for Disease Control and Prevention (CDC) of the U.S. Department of Health and Human Services. It found the prevalence of three ASDs (autistic disorder, Asperger's disorder, and PDD NOS) to be 34 per 10,000 among children ages 3–10 years in 1996 (Yeargin-Allsopp et al., 2003). Ninety-one percent of the children met the DSM-IV criteria for autistic disorder, for a prevalence rate of 31 per 10,000. Some other recent studies reported similar rates of children with ASDs in the United Kingdom (Webb et al., 2003), Sweden (Arvidsson et al., 1997), and Japan (Honda, Shimizu, Misumi, Niimi, & Ohashi, 1996). Others have found much higher rates, including 58–63 per 10,000 in the United Kingdom (Baird et al., 2000; Chakrabarti & Fombonne, 2001) and 67 per 10,000 in Brick Township, New Jersey (Bertrand et al., 2001). Taking into account all the epidemiological studies, the CDC now suspects that the true prevalence of all ASDs is about 60 per 10,000 (Yeargin-Allsopp, 2003).

Other evidence of the increase in ASDs comes from studies of incidence (new cases per year). Kaye, Melero-Montes, and Jick (2001) found that newly diagnosed autistic disorder in children under 13 increased sevenfold in the United Kingdom from 1988 to 1999, from 0.3 per 10,000 to 2.1 per 10,000 per year. Increases of 18% per year in autistic disorder and 55% per year for other ASDs from 1991 to 1996 were found in one region of the United Kingdom by Powell and colleagues (2000). In the United States, a number of states are now conducting incidence studies under grants from the CDC, as mandated by the Children's Health Act of 2000 (Yeargin-Allsopp, 2003).

There is some evidence that the rates of ASDs may have reached a plateau, at least in some locations (Chakrabarti & Fombonne, 2005; Lingam et al., 2003). Lingam and colleagues (2003) found that the prevalence of autistic disorder in northeast London increased from 1979 to 1992 and then stabilized from 1992 to 1996 at a rate of 26 per 10,000. However, other recent studies suggest that the rates of ASDs continues to increase each year (California Department of Developmental Services, 2003; Chakrabarti & Fombonne, 2001; Gurney et al., 2003).

The prevalence rates for ASDs besides autistic disorder have seldom been studied. Prevalence estimates of Asperger's disorder range from 26 to 71 per 10,000 (Gillberg, 2001). The rate of Rett's disorder is about 1–4 per 10,000, and that of CDD is 0.2 per 10,000 (Fombonne, Simmons, Ford, Meltzer, & Goodman, 2003).

The male-to-female ratio in autistic disorder varies across studies, but boys always outnumber girls. Since 1996, reported ratios have ranged from 1.8:1 (Fombonne, du Mazaubrun, Cans, & Grandjean, 1997) to 15.7:1 (Baird et al., 2000), with a median across seven studies of 4.3:1. The male-to-female ratio is inversely related to intelligence level. For example, Yeargin-Allsopp and colleagues (2003) found that the ratio was 6.7:1 for children with ASD and intelligence in the average range, but that this declined steadily to 1.3:1 for children with profound mental retardation.

Why Is the Prevalence of ASDs Increasing?

Much work remains to be done to elucidate whether recent high prevalence rates reflect a true increase in ASD since the 1980s— constituting an epidemic due to some yet-to-be-discovered environmental exposure *in utero* or soon after birth—or are the results of factors that have simply led to more children receiving an ASD diagnosis than in the past. Although the possibility is seldom mentioned, it is certainly possible that both trends—a true increase, along with more frequent use of ASD diagnoses—are interacting to drive up prevalence rates. Debate about these questions is still ongoing, and no firm conclusion is possible at present, but the arguments for the two main alternatives can be summarized.

The main evidence for the position that the increased prevalence rates index an actual increase in the number of children with ASDs since the mid-1980s comes from a study of children with autistic disorder enrolled in the California Department of Developmental Services regional centers (M.I.N.D. Institute, 2002). Researchers at the M.I.N.D. Institute were asked to examine the validity of a report by the California Department of Developmental Services (1999) of a 273% increase in children with autistic disorder from 1987 to 1998. In the M.I.N.D. Institute study, information on two birth cohorts, one born in 1983–1985 and one in 1993–1995, was obtained from the parents of children with autistic disorder. The accuracy of each child's diagnosis was evaluated by administering a structured interview including the ADI-R, which can be scored to determine whether the child meets DSM-IV crite-

ria for autistic disorder. The main finding was that nearly 90% of the children in both cohorts met the DSM-IV diagnostic criteria for autistic disorder, indicating that the broadening of diagnostic criteria over the years could not account for the tripling of cases from 1987 to 1998 of children with autistic disorder during a time when the general population grew by only 20%. The study ruled out the misclassification of children with mental retardation (without autism) as having autistic disorder in more recent years as a factor that may have artificially increased prevalence rates—a concern raised by Croen, Grether, Hoogstrate, and Selvin (2002). However, the study did not rule out possible changes in case-finding methods over time, which may have resulted in fewer children with autistic disorder being referred to the regional centers in earlier years or, conversely, more children being referred in recent years; either or both of these phenomena could have contributed to the increased prevalence of autistic disorder in later years (Fombonne, 2003).

On the other hand, many investigators attribute the increased rates to the broadening of the definition of autism; the increased availability of and demand for services; and the increased awareness of ASDs on the part of physicians, teachers, and parents. A significant broadening of the criteria for autistic disorder occurred in the change from DSM-III (APA, 1980) to DSM-III-R (APA, 1987). What had been one- or two-sentence criteria for social, language, and stereotyped behavior in DSM-III became sets of criteria that covered a broad developmental range. For example, the single DSM-III social criterion of "pervasive lack of responsiveness to other people" became "qualitative impairment in reciprocal social interaction," as manifested by any two of a list of five characteristics ranging from "lack of awareness of others" to "gross impairment in ability to make friendships." Similar changes occurred in the criteria for language and restricted behavior patterns. As a result, many more high-functioning children were likely to receive a diagnosis of autistic disorder under DSM-III-R than had occurred with DSM-III (Hertzig, Snow, New, & Shapiro, 1990), or in the 1960s and 1970s with the earlier, even stricter criteria of Kanner. DSM-III-R also led to more diagnoses of children at the other end of the developmental continuum: Field trials showed that the DSM-III-R criteria resulted in an especially high rate of false positives among individuals with severe mental retardation (Volkmar, Bregman, Cohen, & Cicchetti, 1988). Then DSM-IV (APA, 1994) further enlarged the ASD/PDD category by adding Asperger's disorder, Rett's disorder, and CDD to the existing autistic disorder and PDD NOS categories of DSM-III-R. These changes in diagnostic criteria meant that prevalence studies conducted from about 1990 onward picked up many children whose severe symptoms would in the past have resulted in a primary diagnosis of mental retardation, as well as many children whose mild symptoms would not have qualified them for an autistic disorder diagnosis. Some evidence for this contention appears in the M.I.N.D Institute (2002) study. A comparison of children with autistic disorder born in 1983–1985 (16–18 years old at the time of the study) with those born in 1993–1995 (6–8 years old) showed that 50% of the older children had coexisting mental retardation, but only 20% of the younger children did. Even if allowance is made for delayed identification of mental retardation in some younger children with autistic disorder (and barring large reporting errors), it is likely that more children of average intelligence are being diagnosed with autistic disorder in recent years.

To turn to societal factors, expanded special education services under the Individuals with Disabilities Education Act and eligibility for federal Supplemental Security Insurance benefits are dependent on diagnosis, creating an incentive for diagnosing more children. Research documenting the value of intensive early intervention in ASDs was published in the late 1980s and became accessible to the general public by the early 1990s in books, magazine articles, and broadcast media, increasing the demand for diagnostic and treatment services for children as young as 2 years of age. Three trends in medicine during the 1990s increased the likelihood that ASD diagnoses would be made more frequently than in the past: (1) Residencies in pediatrics and family medicine began to include more training on developmental disabilities; (2) many children's hospitals established specialized clinics for developmental disabilities, and often for ASDs in particular; and (3) two of the most widely used screening and diagnostic instruments were published—the Checklist for Autism in Toddlers (Baron-Cohen et al., 1992) and the ADI-R (Lord et al., 1994)—greatly facilitating diagnosis by physicians and psychologists. As referrals for assessment continue to increase, more children are being diagnosed at earlier ages and with milder symptomatology (Prior, 2003). All of these trends—more inclusive diagnostic criteria, increased public awareness and funding, and increased availability of specialized services and trained professionals with new diagnostic tools—coincided with the increasing prevalence rates of the late 1980s and 1990s. They are believed by many experts to account for most if not all of the increase in ASDs (Barbaresi, Katusic, Colligan, Weaver, & Jacobsen, 2005; Caronna & Halfon, 2003; Fombonne, 2003; Gurney et al., 2003; Wing & Potter, 2002).

ETIOLOGY

The complexity of the central nervous system and the subtlety of its processes, combined with the wide range of expressions of ASDs, have made the task of charting the causes of ASDs profoundly difficult. When relatively large numbers of children are surveyed, a medical condition that is likely to be causally relevant can be identified in only 3–5% of cases (Challman, Barbaresi, Katusic, & Weaver, 2003), with a greater likelihood of finding genetic and prenatal conditions in the severe and profound ranges of mental retardation (Gillberg & Coleman, 1996). Virtually no modern investigator proposes that there is "a" cause of "autism"; instead, most expect to conquer it piecemeal as the causes of characteristic traits or particular subtypes within the ASDs are found (Eigisti & Shapiro, 2003). Because ASDs are present from birth or become apparent within the first 2–3 years, intensive effort has been directed toward possible genetic aberrations and early environmental events, including the possible role of routine childhood vaccinations.

Genetics

Most investigators now believe that ASDs result from multiple genes that interact in various combinations to increase liability for the different symptom profiles and degrees of severity that are seen clinically (Folstein & Rosen-Sheidley, 2001). Current research supports the possibility that 10–15 or more genes may interact to cause ASDs (Risch et al., 1999). The strongest evidence for the heritability of autism comes from twin and family studies. In twin studies, concordance for autistic disorder is found in at least 60% and for all ASDs in 90% of monozygotic (identical) twins, while low rates (0–10%) are found in dizygotic (fraternal) twins (Bailey et al., 1995; Stodgell, Ingram, & Hyman, 2000). Studies of families have indicated that 3–7% of the siblings of children with autistic disorder also have autism (a rate 50–100 times higher than the risk in unaffected families), and that 8% of the extended families include another member with autism (Smalley & Collins, 1996). Family studies reveal an increased prevalence of a constellation of characteristics referred to as the "broader autism phenotype," which includes social reticence, pragmatic communication difficulties, preference for routines, and difficulty with change (Lainhart et al., 2002; Spiker, Lotspeich, Dimiceli, Myers, & Risch, 2002). The working assumption is that these family members have some subthreshold number or combination of genes related to ASDs, and thus may show a range of effects from no impairment to one or more circumscribed impairments. Some are even high achievers in certain fields (Pickles et al., 2000; Piven, Palmer, Jacobi, Childress, & Arndt, 1997).

Identifying the specific genes contributing to ASDs has proved a formidable task. In genome-wide scans, chromosomes 2, 5, 7, 15, 16, 17, and 19 have been identified as likely sites for genes predisposing individuals to ASDs (Barnby & Manaco, 2003; Bass et al., 2000; Philippe et al., 1999; Turner, Barnby, & Bailey, 2000; Yonan et al., 2003). Linkage studies in families with more than one affected member have identified likely genetic loci on chromosomes 7 and 15 (Filipek et al., 1999; Philippe et al., 1999; Stodgell et al., 2000).

Considerable research effort has focused on chromosome 15, because it has an unstable region of genes involved in brain development and function, and it is known to be strongly associated with Angelman syndrome and Prader–Willi syndrome (Wassink & Piven, 2000). Abnormalities in a critical region known as 15q11–15q13 results in phenotypes ranging from developmental and language delays to autism (Herzing, Cook, & Ledbetter, 2002). A number of studies have found evidence that genes creating susceptibility to ASDs are located in this area (e.g., Bass et al., 2000; Maddox et al., 1999; Nurmi et al., 2003). The significance of 15q11–15q13 remains contro-

versial, however, due to some negative findings (Maestrini et al., 1999).

A region of chromosome 7 appears to be associated with ASDs involving significant language delays (Alarcon et al., 2002; Wassink et al., 2001). It is also associated with specific language disabilities, leading to the suggestion that it may be linked to all or most conditions that involve language disorders (O'Brien, Zhang, Nishimura, Tomblin, & Murray, 2003).

The high ratio of males to females with ASDs has led to investigations of the sex chromosomes. Two X-linked genes involved in synaptogenesis have been found to be associated with autistic disorder (Jamain et al., 2003). Skuse (2000) has proposed that there may be a protective factor controlled by a gene on the X chromosome transmitted from fathers to daughters that raises the threshold for the expression of the autism phenotype in girls. As a result, fewer girls meet the threshold and develop autistic disorder, even if they have other genes rendering them susceptible. Since boys inherit only maternally transmitted X chromosomes, where this protective gene is presumably silenced, they are more likely to develop autism if they have other genes making them susceptible.

The genetic picture is clearer for Rett's disorder, due to the recent discovery of the gene that is most clearly implicated in its etiology. Any of dozens of mutations of the MECP2 gene on the maternally derived X chromosome, which regulates other genes guiding early brain development, are found in 70–80% of cases of Rett's disorder (Van den Veyver & Zoghbi, 2002). These mutations are usually lethal to the male fetus, which explains why most individuals with Rett's disorder are girls (Bienvenu et al., 2000).

Still uncertain is the possibility that ASDs may be due to the interaction between genetics and an early environmental insult. For example, ASDs may result from an inherited susceptibility combined with a "second hit" from another factor during gestation or infancy (Folstein & Rosen-Sheidley, 2001). Factors such as prenatal infection, aberrant immune response, exposure to teratogens at critical periods of brain development (Rodier & Hyman, 1998), and vaccines or their components (Geier & Geier, 2003a; Wakefield et al., 1998) have all been proposed as possibilities.

Immunology

Increased autoantibody production in children with ASDs, and increased rates of family members with autoimmune diseases, suggest the possibility that ASDs may be the results of an autoimmune process that affects brain development (Comi, Zimmerman, Frye, Law, & Peeden, 1999; Connolly et al., 1999). However, differences in mean values of immunological variables for children with ASDs have been small when compared with those of nondisordered controls and usually have been within typical limits. Thus the etiological relevance of these findings is unknown; they could reflect genetic differences or an altered immune response to infectious agents yet to be identified (Halsey & Hyman, 2001).

Pregnancy and Perinatal Complications

Several known risks for ASDs can occur during pregnancy, but each of these has been reported in relatively few cases. Untreated maternal hypothyroidism, maternal use of thalidomide during a brief period in the first month of gestation, maternal use of valproic acid (an anticonvulsant medication), and maternal excessive use of alcohol have all been linked with ASDs (Folstein & Rosen-Sheidley, 2001). Prenatal infections with a number of viruses, including cytomegalovirus (Yamashita, Fujimoto, Nakajima, Isagai, & Matsuishi, 2003), toxoplasmosis (Todd, 1986), herpes simplex (Ghaziuddin, Tsai, Eilers, & Ghaziuddin, 1992), and especially rubella (Chess, 1977), increase the risk for ASDs. When strictly diagnosed cases were studied in the context of actual medical records and compared with population norms, the following pregnancy and perinatal factors were significantly higher in cases of ASDs: uterine bleeding in the second or third trimester, Rhesus factor incompatibility, induced or prolonged labor, precipitous labor, oxygen requirement at birth, and hyperbilirubinemia in the infant (Juul-Dam, Townsend, & Courchesne, 2001). Some progress is being made in using pregnancy and perinatal factors as predictors of autism. Wilkerson, Volpe, Dean, and Titus (2002) performed a discriminant analysis of several factors and found that 65% of subsequent diagnoses of autistic disorder could be predicted by prescription drugs taken during pregnancy; length of labor; viral infection; atypical presentation at delivery; low birthweight; and maternal urinary tract infection, fever, or depression.

The Brain

Neuropsychological, neuroimaging, and autopsy studies reveal a variety of brain abnormalities in ASDs. Evidence of deficits in executive function, joint attention, emotion perception, and theory of mind point to frontal lobe and midbrain impairment (Dawson, Osterling, Rinaldi, Carver, & McPartland, 2001; McEvoy, Rogers, & Pennington, 1993; Russell, 1998). A large number of studies have shown that executive functioning is deficient in individuals of various ages and intellectual levels with ASDs (Ozonoff, 1997). Executive functions include forming abstract concepts, flexible action planning, self-monitoring, and inhibiting impulsive responses. Flexibility in planning and verbal working memory are believed to be particularly impaired (Pennington & Ozonoff, 1996; Ozonoff, 1997). Mundy (2003) has summarized a body of evidence indicating that dysfunction in the frontal cortex and anterior cingulate may underlie deficits in social cognition in children with ASDs. However, executive function deficits are found in other disorders besides ASDs and have not always been found in high-functioning individuals with ASDs (Baron-Cohen, Wheelwright, Stone, & Rutherford, 1999) or young children with ASDs (Griffith, Pennington, Wehner, & Rogers, 1999); these results suggest that they are common but not necessary features of ASDs.

Other neuropsychological investigators have proposed that difficulties in perception of the human face and emotional expression are crucial (Marcus & Nelson, 2001). The most consistent abnormalities in perceptual processing of the face are focusing on parts of the face rather than the whole face, and making discriminations based on the mouth instead of the eyes (Hauck, Fein, Waterhouse, Feinstein, & Maltby, 1998; Joseph & Tanaka, 2003). Even when performance on face perception tasks is adequate, individuals with ASDs use a portion of the brain that typically processes objects to accomplish the task (Schultz et al., 2000), suggesting an equivalence between objects and people that contributes to the social deficits of ASDs.

Replicated findings from autopsy and structural magnetic resonance imaging (MRI) studies include increased total brain size, abnormal sizes of amygdala, hippocampus, and corpus callosum, delayed maturation of the frontal cortex, truncated development of neurons in the limbic system, and decreased number of Purkinje cells in the cerebellum (Brambilla et al., 2003; Zilbovicius et al., 1995). Functional MRI studies find patterns of relatively low activity in some regions of the brain, but both patterns and regions differ across studies (Muller, Kleinhans, Kemmotsu, Pierce, & Courchesne, 2003; Ring et al., 1999). The most consistent findings so far are abnormal localization of activity during various cognitive tasks and reduced activation of the frontal lobes and limbic system, particularly the amygdala (Baron-Cohen, Ring, et al., 1999; Howard et al., 2000). A dysfunctional amygdala in children with ASDs may account for their impairments in the recognition of facial expressions of fear, perception of eye gaze direction, and recognition memory for faces (Baron-Cohen et al., 2000; Howard et al., 2000). Although Baron-Cohen and colleagues (2000) also believe that the amygdala dysfunction accounts for theory-of-mind deficits, other recent work strongly implicates a region in the temporo-parietal junction (Saxe & Kanwisher, 2003).

Neurochemistry studies have generally been inconsistent, with the exception of a common finding of increased serotonin levels in platelets in about a third of children with ASDs. There appears to be no association between serotonin levels and overt behavior in ASDs (Medical Research Council, 2001), and trials of a serotonin antagonist, fenfluramine, were disappointing (Leventhal et al., 1993).

Recently, Courchesne, Carper, and Akshoomoff (2003) found that infants later diagnosed with autistic disorder tended to have much smaller than average head size at birth, but then showed a rapid and excessive increase in head size from 1–2 months to 6–14 months, compared to typical infants and to infants later diagnosed with PDD NOS. What determines such rapid growth remains to be discovered, but Courchesne and colleagues noted that repeated measurements of head circumference in infancy might serve as an early warning sign of autistic disorder and offered the following intriguing speculation about its implications. The developing brain is designed to benefit from an extended period of experience-guided growth, which provides the opportunity for a multitude

of experiences to direct neuron growth and to create, reinforce, or eliminate synapses as needed. In the abbreviated growth period seen in autistic disorder, the child's brain reaches its lifetime maximum by 4–5 years of age, 8 years before typical children. This shortened period of plasticity results in growth without guidance; the brain produces too many connections in too short a time that may not be adaptive. Faced with the neural noise that would result from such rapidly changing aberrant connections, the infant may be unable to make sense of the world and may withdraw. Some independent support for this account comes from a functional MRI study by Belmonte and Yurgelun-Todd (2003), implicating overconnected neural systems prone to noise and cross-talk during attention tasks.

Cognition

Baron-Cohen, Leslie, and Frith (1985) proposed that a fundamental deficit in children with ASD is their lack of a "theory of mind"—the ability to attribute mental states (knowledge, intentions, beliefs, feelings) to themselves and others. Baron-Cohen and his colleagues have shown that most children with ASDs fail at tasks requiring them to infer what someone else knows or expects, to distinguish between mental and physical events, and to distinguish between appearances and reality (Baron-Cohen, 2001). However, the centrality of theory-of-mind deficits to the etiology of ASDs is weakened by studies showing that theory of mind is highly related to verbal ability, age, and IQ (Bauminger & Kasari, 1999; Happe, 1995; Steele, Joseph, & Tager-Flusberg, 2003) and is intact or easily trained in many high-functioning children with ASDs. Explicit teaching of theory-of-mind principles improves performance on laboratory theory-of-mind tasks, but apparently not in communication or social competence in natural contexts (Hadwin, Baron-Cohen, Howlin, & Hill, 1997; Ozonoff & Miller, 1995).

The use of eye-tracking technology while individuals with ASDs and nondisabled controls watch selected movie scenes indicates that the former show a pronounced focus on mouths instead of eyes, and on physical features of the environment instead of social cues (Klin, Jones, Schultz, Volkmar, & Cohen, 2002b). In the first year of life, most infants establish a strong preference for looking at eyes instead of mouths and at people rather than inanimate objects (Haith, Bergman, & Moore, 1979; Spelke, Phillips, & Woodward, 1995). Failure to acquire this typical pattern of attention deployment means that profound limitations in opportunities to learn about the social world occur from early in life onward (Klin, Jones, Schultz, & Volkmar, 2003).

Klin and colleagues (2003) argue that to understand the social impairment of ASDs, it may be necessary to give up a traditional computational or modular model of cognition, which assumes that cognitive processes are rule-based manipulations of symbols representing the external environment. These authors' "enactive mind" model starts from the premise that social cognition results from social action. In a child with an ASD, the weak salience of social stimuli compared to that of inanimate objects results in a cascade of developmental events in which the child fails to act upon relevant social events. Instead, he or she acts repeatedly on the physical world, thus failing to accrue a personal history of interactive social experiences. As a result of missing the thousands of social experiences that most children have, children with ASDs have great difficulty with ever-changing social interactions and the moment-by-moment adaptations they require. Although most are able to acquire language and concepts, and some learn considerable information about people, their social repertoire remains truncated, slow, and inefficient.

Vaccination

When regression occurs in an ASD, correlated events such as immunization, illness/injury, or a change in the family are often suspected by the parents to be the cause. Serious concern about vaccination as a possible cause of regressive autism arose when a British gastroenterologist reported persistent measles virus infection in the ileum (the last part of the small intestine) in 8 of 12 children with ASDs and gastrointestinal problems, who reportedly had regressed within 2 weeks after receiving the measles–mumps–rubella (MMR) vaccine (Wakefield et al., 1998). In subsequent studies, Wakefield's group has identified a new variant of inflammatory bowel disease termed "autistic enterocolitis" in 80–90% of children with regressive autism and other developmental disorders (Uhlmann et al., 2002; Wakefield et al., 2000). Wakefield has hypothesized that the measles

virus in the MMR vaccine acts as an immunological trigger to cause inflammatory bowel disease, which in turn alters the permeability of the intestinal wall and allows certain neurotoxic proteins in food to reach the brain and cause damage. He has argued that widespread use of the MMR vaccine is a major determinant of the apparent increase in the rate of ASDs (Wakefield & Montgomery, 1999; Wakefield et al., 2000). Another mechanism by which the MMR vaccine may cause ASDs has been proposed by Singh, Lin, Newell, and Nelson (2002), who suggest that the measles component of the vaccine stimulates an unusual autoimmunity reaction in which antibodies attack the myelin basic protein in neurons.

Understandably, the Wakefield hypothesis generated widespread concern among parents and physicians. One unfortunate result of the publicity surrounding it was a decrease in MMR immunization rates in some areas below the rate considered adequate for population immunity, increasing the risk of measles outbreaks (Jefferson, Price, Demicheli, & Bianco, 2003; Taylor, 2000). The publicity surrounding the hypothesis has created "recall bias" in some parents whose children with ASDs showed developmental regression. That is, some parents are now more likely to recall the onset of symptoms as occurring shortly after their children received the MMR vaccination than were parents of similar children who were diagnosed before the publicity (Andrews et al., 2002).

The possible relationship between the MMR vaccine and ASDs has been subjected to intense scientific scrutiny. In reviewing the literature, it is helpful first to be aware of the known adverse effects of MMR vaccination. The main risks are temporary thrombocytopenia (decreased platelet count) at a rate of 1 in 25,000 children (Black, Kaye, & Jick, 2003), and febrile seizures at a rate of 25–34 per 100,000 children. These types of febrile seizures do not appear to increase the risk for subsequent seizures or for neurodevelopmental disabilities (Barlow et al., 2001). More serious complications can occur, but these are far less common. Postinfectious encephalomyelitis (inflammation of brain and spinal cord) is reported at a rate of about 1 per 1,000,000 after vaccination but 1 per 1,000 after natural measles infection. Anaphylaxis (systemic allergic reaction) occurs at a rate of 1 per 100,000–1,000,000 after vaccination and zero after natural infection

(Duclos & Ward, 1998). Clearly, if MMR vaccination is involved in the etiology of ASDs, it can affect at most only a small fraction of cases. On the other hand, other serious risks of natural measles infection but not vaccination include pneumonia (1–6% of cases), subacute sclerosing panencephalitis (dementia, seizures, and paralysis) (1 per 100,000), and death (0.1–1 per 1,000) (Duclos & Ward, 1998).

Regarding the possible link between measles vaccine and inflammatory bowel disease, Davis and Bohlke (2001) conducted a comprehensive review of epidemiological, case series, case–control, ecological, and laboratory studies of measles virus and inflammatory bowel disease. They concluded that the bulk of the available evidence does not support an association between either measles-containing vaccines or natural measles exposure and inflammatory bowel disease.

Disconfirming evidence directly bearing on a possible MMR-ASDs connection comes mostly from epidemiological studies addressing the logical implications of the hypothesized connection. Dales, Hammer, and Smith (2001) found no correlation between rates of MMR immunization and prevalence of ASDs in California children between 1980 and 1994, and similar findings were made in the United Kingdom by Kaye and colleagues (2001). Taylor and colleagues (1999) found no temporal association between the MMR vaccination and an ASD diagnosis over a 6-month interval; no clustering of cases of regression in development in the 2- to 4-month period after MMR immunization; and no increase in the rate of ASDs associated with the introduction of the MMR vaccine in the United Kingdom in 1988. Taylor and colleagues (2002) found no change in the proportion of children with ASDs and developmental regression or bowel symptoms across the 20-year period from 1979 to 1998, spanning the introduction of the MMR vaccine in the United Kingdom in 1988. Fombonne and Chakrabarti (2001) found that there was no difference in the percentage of children showing regression in a group first seen before the MMR vaccine was introduced in the United Kingdom and in a group first seen after its introduction. Among vaccinated children, the mean intervals from vaccination to parental recognition of autistic symptoms were similar in groups with and without regression. Finally, there was no association between developmental regression and gastrointestinal symptoms.

Madsen and colleagues (2002) conducted a population-based study in Denmark, where each infant or immigrant is given a unique number, and interlinked national databases allow tracking and analysis of significant medical information. There was no difference in the relative risk of autistic disorder or other ASDs between 441,000 vaccinated and 97,000 unvaccinated children.

In their recent review of 12 controlled epidemiological studies, Wilson, Mills, Ross, McGowan, and Jadad (2003) found no support for an association between ASDs and the MMR vaccine, although they noted that there is insufficient evidence to rule out a possible link between the vaccine and some rare variant form of ASD. Major reviews of available evidence have been conducted in the United States by the American Medical Association (Tan, 2003), the American Academy of Pediatrics (Halsey & Hyman, 2001), and the Institute of Medicine (Institute of Medicine, 2001); in Canada by the Population and Public Health Branch (Strauss & Bigham, 2001); and in the United Kingdom by the Medical Research Council (Medical Research Council, 2001). Each of these bodies concluded that the studies conducted so far do not support a link between MMR and ASDs, but noted that the studies have been too imprecise to rule out the prospect of the vaccine being involved in a small number of cases that would not affect prevalence rates.

Some parents ask about the value of administering measles, mumps, and rubella vaccines separately instead of in the MMR combination, based on Wakefield and Montgomery's (2000) speculation that combined vaccines could result in delayed clearance of the viruses and an increased risk of adverse outcomes. Reviews of multiple large studies have revealed no increased rate of adverse events with the combined vaccine compared with separate administration (Parkman, 1995; Redd, Markowitz, & Katz, 1999).

As evidence against an MMR-ASDs association accumulated, an alternative hypothesis emerged: that the mercury-containing preservative in vaccines, thimerosal, is what causes ASDs in certain children who are genetically susceptible (Bernard, Enayati, Redwood, Roger, & Binstock, 2001). Thimerosal is an antibiotic and stabilizer used in many vaccines since the 1930s. The current concern is that as the schedule of recommended immunizations has expanded over the years, increasing amounts of mercury are being injected along with the vaccines and damaging children's brains. A possible explanation for why so few children among the many who are vaccinated actually develop neurological problems comes from a recent study by Hornig, Chian, and Lipkin (2004). These investigators found that mice of a certain genetic strain were susceptible to the neurotoxic effects of thimerosal, while those of other strains were not.

Possible support for a role of mercury in ASDs came from a study by Holmes, Blaxill, and Haley (2003), who analyzed the mercury levels in hair clippings taken from children about 18 months old. The mean level of mercury in the hair of children later diagnosed as having autistic disorder was 0.47 parts per million, and that in typically developing children was 3.63 parts per million. Furthermore, mean mercury levels declined as the severity levels of ASDs increased. Holmes and colleagues suggested that their results might mean that children with ASDs have less mercury in their blood to be picked up by hair follicles because it is not being metabolized properly and is accumulating in their brains. Geier and Geier (2003a) found that more incidents of autism, mental retardation, and speech disorders were reported to occur shortly after the use of thimerosal-containing vaccines than occurred after vaccinations with thimerosal-free vaccines. However, the numbers involved are extremely small: Among millions of doses of vaccines, there were 18 reports of autism in the thimerosal group and 1 in the thimerosal-free group. Still, the 18:1 ratio is substantial and warrants further study to determine its meaning.

Comprehensive epidemiological studies of possible connections between thimerosal and ASDs are just beginning. Madsen and colleagues (2003) looked at annual counts of all cases with an autism diagnosis in Denmark from 1971 to 2000. There was no trend toward an increase in the incidence of autism during the period when thimerosal was used (1971–1990). From 1991 until 2000 the incidence increased, and it continued to rise after the removal of thimerosal from vaccines in 1992, including increases among children born after the discontinuation of thimerosal. Hviid, Stellfeld, Wohlfart, and Melbye (2003) extended these findings by studying the records of all children with ASDs born in Denmark between 1990

and 1996, and comparing children who had received thimerosal-containing pertussis vaccines with those receiving thimerosal-free pertussis vaccines. They found no difference in the relative risk of ASDs in each group, and no dose–response effect of the total amount of thimerosal received. Stehr-Green, Tull, Stellfeld, Mortenson, and Simpson (2003) compared rates of ASDs in the 1980s and 1990s in California, Sweden, and Denmark with levels of exposure to thimerosal-containing vaccines. In all three geographic regions, rates of ASDs began a steady increase in 1985–1989. However, during the 1990s the average childhood thimerosal dose increased in California, but it decreased in Sweden and Denmark after its discontinuation there in the early 1990s; these findings indicate no correlation between thimerosal-containing vaccines and the rising rates of ASDs.

The only established hazard of thimerosal at the doses found in vaccines is delayed-type hypersensitivity reaction (temporary redness and irritability) at the site of the injection in some individuals (Ball, Ball, & Pratt, 2001). In case studies of accidental overdoses, neurotoxicity occurred at levels of thimerosal greater than 100 times the amounts found in vaccines. Moreover, the symptom profile of mercury poisoning—including ataxia, dysarthria, visual field constriction, and peripheral neuropathy—is completely different from the profile of ASDs (Nelson & Bauman, 2003). Ball and colleagues (2001) calculated the maximum possible dose of mercury an infant could receive by 6 months of age under standard immunization schedules. They found that, depending on particular vaccine formulations, an infant could receive a cumulative amount of mercury exceeding the safe exposure limit published by the U.S. Environmental Protection Agency (EPA), but still below those of two other federal agencies and the World Health Organization. The clinical significance of this finding is unclear, since the EPA limits contain a 10-fold safety factor. Actual levels of mercury in the blood of 2- and 6-month-old babies receiving thimerosal-containing vaccines were measured by Pichichero, Cernichiari, Lopreiato, and Treanor (2002). They found that levels of mercury did not exceed safe limits and had a half-life of 7 days, suggesting that it cannot accumulate to toxic levels across multiple vaccinations. Nevertheless, given the paucity of knowledge about the possible long-term risks of thimerosal and as part of its effort to reduce mercury exposure from all sources, the American Academy of Pediatrics and the U.S. Public Health Service issued a joint statement in 1999 formally requesting that manufacturers eliminate or reduce the amount of thimerosal in vaccines (American Academy of Pediatrics, 1999).

At the current time, strong arguments and alternative interpretations of the data exist on both sides of the thimerosal debate, which must be regarded as unsettled. Parents who raise the question of whether or not to vaccinate their child should be referred to their physician for up-to-date information. Simple logic dictates that one cannot say that a vaccination could never cause an ASD, but current research does show that there are greater risks from natural measles infections than from vaccinations. The ethical issues involved for all who are advising parents—governments, scientists, physicians, journalists, and antivaccine advocates—are discussed by Clements and Ratzan (2003).

PROGNOSIS AND TREATMENT STRATEGIES

Predictions of outcome are hazardous at best with such a heterogeneous population, especially when children are very young. Severity of ASD symptomatology by itself is a poor predictor of outcome (Szatmari, Bartolucci, Bremner, Bond, & Rich, 1989). Verbal imitation ability, progress in initial learning tasks, IQ, and age at start of treatment are related to outcome in early intensive behavioral intervention programs (Harris & Handleman, 2000; Sallows & Graupner, 1999; Weiss, 1999). By middle and late childhood, standard measures of intelligence and language, and neuropsychological tests of flexibility and cognitive shift, are positively correlated with outcome (Korkmaz, 2000). Sigman and colleagues (1999) followed children with ASD from 2–6 years of age to 10–13 years. Joint attention skills were associated with language abilities and predicted long-term gains in expressive language, while early nonverbal communication and play skills were predictors of the extent of peer engagement.

In the absence of early intensive behavioral intervention, only 1–2% of individuals with autistic disorder become "normal" in the sense that there is little or no difference between them and children who have never been diagnosed with an ASD (Rutter, 1985). Ballaban-Gil, Rapin, Tuchman, and Shinnar (1996) reevaluated 45 clients with ASDs who had been

seen as children in adulthood. Over 90% had persisting social deficits of varying severity. Language improved with age, although only about a third showed relatively typical speech and comprehension. Slightly over half were living out of the home in residential placements. Only 11% held competitive jobs, and 16% worked in sheltered workshops. Similar findings are reported by Howlin, Goode, Hutton, and Rutter (2004), who found that about 60% of adults had "poor" or "very poor" adjustments in terms of living arrangement, friendships, and employment. Outcomes are equally poor whether the diagnosis is high-functioning autism or Asperger's disorder, even for those with IQs in the average range (Howlin, 2003).

Studies of adolescents and adults have shown that there are exacerbations of symptoms (hyperactivity, self-injury, stereotypy) during puberty or early adolescence (Gillberg & Steffenburg, 1987; Volkmar & Nelson, 1990). High-functioning children with ASDs tend to perform as well in school as typical peers do on mechanical reading, spelling, and computation, but less well on comprehension tasks. In later adolescence and adulthood, stereotypies, flat affect, anxiety, depression, and thought disorders are frequently observed (Dykens et al., 1991; Korkmaz, 2000). Loneliness, social ineptitude with poor insight, and employment are acute problems. Adaptive behavior skills and independent functioning tend to be significantly impaired even in adolescents with high intelligence (Green et al., 2000; Venter, Lord, & Schopler, 1992).

The practical usefulness of the foregoing outcome findings for making individual predictions is unknown. On the one hand, the emergence and gradual dissemination of effective early intervention programs, community-referenced educational curricula, supported employment opportunities, and varied community living options invite more optimism than was previously possible (Dawson & Osterling, 1997; Handleman & Harris, 2000; Koegel & Koegel, 1995; Kozloff, 1994; McEachin, Smith, & Lovaas, 1993; Rogers, 1998). On the other hand, these developments are still not widely available, and there may be little or no improvement in the measured intelligence or adaptive behavior levels of children and adolescents in conventional special education programs (Eaves & Ho, 1996; Freeman, Ritvo, Needleman, & Yokota, 1985; Lord & Schopler, 1989; Venter et al., 1992); however, some improvement in autistic symptomatology does occur, particularly in social relatedness (Fecteau, Mottron, Berthiaume, & Burack, 2003).

The most general conclusion that emerges both from the outcome studies mentioned above and from the early intervention studies to be described later is that outcome differs for the two large groups defined by general developmental level and language level (Lovaas & Smith, 1988; Stevens et al., 2000; Waterhouse et al., 1996). The prognosis for most children in the lower-functioning group—those with severe or profound mental retardation, and with minimal or no language—remains limited: Most such individuals require supervised living and work arrangements throughout life. The appropriate treatment strategy for children in this group emphasizes the acquisition of self-care skills, a reasonable degree of compliance with instructions and simple rules, basic social and affective behaviors, basic communication skills, appropriate play, and the reduction of harmful behaviors. In later childhood and adolescence, a steadily increasing emphasis on domestic living skills and work-related skills is crucial in preparation for supervised living and work environments. In working with the parents of such a child, the clinician must walk the narrow path between undue pessimism and unwarranted optimism. Communications that focus excessive attention on the child's deficiencies, or that conversely raise expectations for dramatic improvement, are not helpful. The main jobs are to teach the parents how to teach their child basic skills, how to control inappropriate behaviors, and how to solve the inevitable problems that arise within the family and between the family and service providers. Equally important are the celebration of progress, however slow and incremental at times, and the simple enjoyment of the child's unique and attractive characteristics.

For the second group of children—those with moderate to mild mental retardation or average intelligence, and with at least some useful language—outcome is dependent not only on intelligence, but also on when treatment begins and how intensive it is. As might be expected, when this group receives intensive behavioral treatment relatively early, it accounts for most of those who achieve the best outcomes (Harris & Handleman, 2000; Smith, 1999). The general treatment strategy for young children in this group should therefore assume the nature of a "total push," in which time is of the essence in order to take maximum advantage of the plasticity of neurological and behavioral processes early in life. There are major emphases on verbal language, age-appropriate social interactions with typical peers, and behaviors and skills expected in typical preschool and elementary classrooms (Green, 1996; Leaf & McEachin, 1999; Lovaas, 2003).

SOCIAL INTERACTION

The social domain is large, complex, and extensively interwoven with the domains of language and affect. The attainment of a significant level of social competence seems to require treatment strategies that include both direct training in key skills and the extensive involvement of typical peers. A brief review of procedures used to teach basic play and social interaction skills shows that a variety of approaches have been utilized effectively for children and adolescents with ASDs.

Toy Play

Prerequisite skills for learning social behaviors include responding to requests, imitation, and appropriate toy play (Taylor, 2001). Several studies have shown that basic play behaviors can be taught through observational learning procedures (Tryon & Keane, 1986), self-monitoring procedures (Stahmer & Schreibman, 1992), video modeling (D'Ateno, Mangiapanello, & Taylor, 2003), and prompting and reinforcement with edibles or the intrinsic sensory reinforcers available in some toys (Eason, White, & Newsom, 1982; Rincover, Cook, Peoples, & Packard, 1979; Santarcangelo, Dyer, & Luce, 1987). Although such procedures are effective in teaching independent play behaviors, and are therefore helpful early in treatment and for those times when children need to occupy themselves independently, the acquisition of such behaviors is not automatically followed by spontaneous social play among children with ASDs or between children with ASDs and typical peers. Thus mere physical proximity to other children in educational settings cannot be expected to improve socialization unless special training is carried out.

Teaching Typical Peers to Initiate Interactions

The most common strategy for remediating the social deficits of children with ASDs is teaching typical peers to engage in appropriate social interactions with them (Strain & Odom, 1986). The peer initiation paradigm that has received the most study is the one introduced by Strain and colleagues (Strain, 1977; Strain, Shores, & Timm, 1977). Several preliminary sessions are devoted to training a peer confederate to initiate toy play interactions. The teacher plays the role of a child with an ASD and uses instructions, modeling, and praise to teach the peer. On half the trials, the teacher complies with the peer's toy play initiations; on the other half, the teacher ignores the initiations, in order to prepare the peer for the other child's failures to respond (Jackson et al., 2003). The peer is taught to persist until the teacher finally complies (Odom, Hoyson, Jamieson, & Strain, 1985). In some studies, practice with a child who has an ASD while the teacher provides instructions and feedback to the typical peer is also a component of training (e.g., Odom & Strain, 1986; Shafer, Egel, & Neef, 1984). Rates of initiation by the peer can be facilitated with the use of a self-monitoring procedure that covers the elements of play interactions (Sainato, Goldstein, & Strain, 1992).

The content of the training for peers has varied across studies. In an empirical approach to content selection, Goldstein, Kaczmarek, Pennington, and Shafer (1992) based the content of peer training on previous research by Ferrel (1990), which identified specific types of interactions that were most likely to evoke a response in children with disabilities as well as typical children. They taught 3- to 5-year-old typical peers to engage in the following strategies: establishing mutual attention, commenting about ongoing activities, and acknowledging the partner's responses.

Although the peer initiation model is rapidly effective in bringing about increases in social interactions, it has long been known that little generalization occurs in settings where the peers do not initiate interactions (Ragland, Kerr, & Strain, 1978). Therefore, subsequent research has addressed procedural variables that might enhance generalization.

Several investigators have promoted generalization by including multiple peers who have all had social initiation training (Belchic & Harris, 1994; Mundschenk & Sasso, 1995), and by rewarding participants for social interactions on an individual or group basis (Gonzales-Lopez & Kamps, 1997; Kohler et al., 1995; Zanolli & Daggett, 1998). Gonzales-Lopez and Kamps (1997) found that social interaction between children with ASDs and typical peers was minimal until the peers were taught to give simple instructions, to prompt responses, to ignore disruptive behaviors, and to praise appropriate behavior. Another factor improving generalization is more realistic training. Instead of having a peer work with an adult in a role-play format during training, Shafer and colleagues (1984) and Brady, Shores, McEvoy, Ellis, and Fox (1987) taught the peer to interact directly with a child who had an ASD through modeling and coaching. Some investigators have found it possible to minimize the role of adults in natural settings by using pictures, scripts, or audiotaped prompts for either peers or children with ASDs (Goldstein & Cisar, 1992; Jolly, Test, & Spooner, 1993; Krantz & McClannahan, 1993; Odom, Chandler, Ostrosky, McConnell, & Reaney, 1992; Stevenson, Krantz, & McClannahan, 2000). For example, Goldstein and Cisar (1992) used scripts to teach social pretend play to preschoolers with autism and their classmates. The children were organized in triads consisting of one child with autism and two typical peers. Each triad was taught to act out each of three different scripts describing typical interactions in a pet shop, magic show, and carnival. After training, the children with autism showed increased use of the verbal and social behaviors of the scripts during pretend play, as well as increased social behaviors unrelated to the scripts.

A comprehensive approach to promoting generalization with adolescents is the social support network model developed by Haring and Breen (1992). These investigators enlisted groups of four or five nondisabled peers in a junior high school to prompt and reinforce social interactions in two socially withdrawn boys, one of whom had autistic disorder. The peers participated in weekly meetings to assess each week's interactions during breaks between classes and lunch periods, and to develop strategies for improving the target children's interactions in the coming week. Both boys showed increased frequencies of appropriate social interactions across the school day, as well as increased unprompted interactions outside school and improved attitudes and ratings of friendship toward the boys by their typical peers.

Teaching Children with ASDs to Initiate Interactions

Some investigators have addressed the possibility of teaching children with ASDs to initiate appropriate interactions, and thus not to be dependent on peers' initiations (Haring & Lovinger, 1989). Krantz and McClannahan (1993) taught teenagers with ASDs to read simple scripts, prompting them to engage in conversational exchanges with peers with ASDs, and then faded the scripts. Other investigators have successfully employed photographic prompts (Krantz, MacDuff, & McClannahan, 1993; McClannahan & Krantz, 1999) and prompts from a vibrating pager worn by a child (Taylor & Levin, 1998) to prompt social initiations and play. Oke and Schreibman (1990) compared the effects of peer initiation training with those of training a boy with autism to initiate play interactions with the same peers. A unique feature of this study was the use of videotaped examples of successful versus unsuccessful initiation strategies in teaching the peers and the boy with autism to initiate play interactions.

Because many individuals with autistic disorder have limited language for elaborating interactions, Brady and colleagues (1984) and Gaylord-Ross, Haring, Breen, and Pitts-Conway (1984) adopted the strategy of structuring social interactions around leisure objects that could be shared with typical peers in a context of brief verbal exchanges. This strategy of letting the objects carry the burden of the interaction was enhanced by selecting items that would be interesting to the typical peers, such as hand-held video games, an earphone radio, and a pack of gum. In the Gaylord-Ross and colleagues study, a training script was devised for each item; each script included phrases and sentences for each component (initiation, elaboration, and termination) of the interaction. Training sessions continued until each of two boys with autistic disorder had been exposed sequentially to six different peers as multiple exemplars of the typical students at the school. Both participants showed large increases in measures of generalized social interaction with naïve peers over baseline condi-

tions. Training scripts and sequentially introduced typical peers were also employed by Breen, Haring, Pitts-Conway, and Gaylord-Ross (1985) to teach four adolescents with ASDs to engage in appropriate social interactions during breaks at job sites.

Another approach to increasing the self-initiations of children with ASDs is to teach peers to respond appropriately to their initiations (Odom & Strain, 1986). Zanolli, Daggett, and Adams (1996) initially taught peers to respond positively to initiations by two preschool peers with ASDs, and then conducted "priming" sessions for children with ASDs just prior to play sessions. In priming sessions, the children were prompted to look at a peer, smile, touch the peer's hand, and make a verbal request. Both participants showed high levels of both trained and untrained spontaneous initiations in the play sessions. Social interaction opportunities in school can be supplemented at home by arranging "play dates" between a child with an ASD and typical peers of a similar age (Leaf & McEachin, 1999).

Social Skills Interventions for High-Functioning Individuals with ASDs

As part of their programmatic research on procedures to improve classroom instructional methods for children with ASDs and other disabilities, Kamps and her colleagues have studied procedures that improve social interaction (Dugan et al., 1995; Kamps, Barbetta, Leonard, & Delquadri, 1994; Kamps et al., 1992). Kamps and colleagues (1992) investigated the use of social skills training in groups to facilitate social interactions between high-functioning 7-year-olds with ASDs and their typical peers in an integrated first-grade classroom. Specific skills were selected from published social skills curricula and included initiating and maintaining interactions, giving and accepting compliments, taking turns and sharing, helping others and asking for help, and including others in activities. In other studies in integrated classrooms, classwide peer tutoring (Kamps et al., 1994) and cooperative learning groups (Dugan et al., 1995) resulted in increased social interaction between children with ASDs and their typical peers.

For higher-functioning children with ASDs, work on social interactions involves improving their conversational skills. Problems such as perseverating on particular topics, dominating the conversation, and not listening to the conversation partner lead easily to avoidance by peers. Frea (1995) described self-management procedures for teaching an adolescent boy to reduce the amount of time he spent speaking, to ask questions to invite the peer to take a turn speaking, and to comment on what the peer had just said. Koegel and Frea (1993) taught adolescents to discriminate their own appropriate and inappropriate social behaviors, to track their appropriate behaviors, and to obtain a reward when meeting a criterion.

The most common approach to teaching social behaviors to adolescents and adults with high-functioning autism and Asperger's disorder is to offer social skills groups (Ozonoff, Dawson, & McPartland, 2002). Ozonoff and colleagues (2002) recommend including the following topics in such groups:

1. *Friendship skills:* Greeting others, joining a group, taking turns, sharing, negotiating and compromising, following group rules, understanding the qualities of a good friend.
2. *Conversational skills:* Starting, maintaining, and ending a conversation; taking turns talking; commenting; asking questions; expressing interest; choosing appropriate topics; social body language (appropriate eye contact, personal space, voice volume, facial expression).
3. *Understanding thoughts and feelings:* Showing empathy, taking others' perspectives, handling difficult emotions.
4. *Social problem solving and conflict management:* Coping with being told "no," being teased or bullied, being left out.
5. *Self-awareness:* Learning about ASDs, personal strengths, unique differences, and self-acceptance.

To overcome generalization difficulties, Ozonoff et al. (2002) describe an *in vivo* modeling approach they call "implicit didacticism." The therapist demonstrates appropriate social behaviors in natural environments (e.g., a cafeteria or store), combining modeling, personal accounts of social dilemmas and their resolution, and feedback to the client about observed social behavior. A main goal is to teach the client how to learn social norms through observation. A number of additional procedures for social skills development can be found in Antonello (1996), Attwood (1998), Howlin

(1999), and Howlin, Baron-Cohen, and Hadwin (1999).

Some individuals with ASDs may benefit from individual or group cognitive-behavioral therapy (Attwood, 2003; Bauminger, 2002; Reaven & Hepburn, 2003). Bauminger (2002), working with 15 high-functioning children and adolescents with autism, found posttreatment improvements in initiations of positive social interactions with peers, social problem solving, and emotional knowledge. The children also received higher ratings from their teachers on assertiveness and cooperation. Ozonoff and colleagues (2002) suggest that the adolescents and adults most likely to benefit from such therapy will be those who have already shown some ability to understand their own and others' emotional states and behaviors. Treatment should be highly directive and should focus on concrete problems and coping methods.

Sibling-Mediated Procedures

In some families of children with ASDs, there are siblings who are willing to become peer trainers if given the opportunity (Celiberti & Harris, 1993; James & Egel, 1986; Schreibman, O'Neill, & Koegel, 1983; Taylor, Levin, & Jasper, 1999). Schreibman and colleagues (1983) noted that siblings can play an important role as facilitation agents for such children's social interactions with other children in the neighborhood, and can also provide continuity between school and home for educational programs. The training methods are like those used in peer initiation studies and have also included video modeling to teach children with ASDs to make appropriate play-related comments to their siblings (Taylor et al., 1999).

A note of caution should be sounded about working with the siblings of children who have ASDs. Although our experience has been that siblings usually respond very positively to the opportunity to learn better ways of interacting with these children, some siblings perceive themselves as having greater caretaking and supervision responsibilities than children whose siblings do not have disabilities (Harris, 1994). Therefore, sibling training programs should be designed with attention to the need to avoid adding to that burden (James & Egel, 1986). Helpful in this regard are negotiating schedules with a sibling to avoid conflicts with other activities, and letting the sibling establish some of the treatment priorities based on his or her own problems in living with the sibling who has an ASD.

Taylor (2001) and Taylor and Jasper (2001) have provided a comprehensive discussion of social skills training procedures and objectives designed for children with ASDs. Chandler, Lubek, and Fowler (1992) have analyzed generalization problems in social skills studies and have indicated that multiple procedures and extended training are essential. McConnell (2002) has provided recommendations for educational settings.

COMMUNICATION

The major strategies for establishing a basic repertoire of functional language are discrete-trials teaching (DTT; Leaf & McEachin, 1999; Lovaas, 2003) and several "natural environment" procedures: incidental teaching (Fenske, Krantz, & McClannahan, 2001), the Natural Language Paradigm (Koegel, O'Dell, & Koegel, 1987), and the Verbal Behavior approach (Sundberg & Partington, 1998). For children who show little or no progress in acquiring spoken language, the Picture Exchange Communication System (PECS; Frost & Bondy, 1994) and sign language training (Carr, 1981; Schaeffer, 1980) are commonly used. Basic overviews of these approaches are presented here, with the caveat that each approach in actual use is far more complex and technically sophisticated than can be indicated here. A comprehensive review of language interventions in ASDs has recently been presented by Goldstein (2002).

Discrete-Trials Teaching

DTT procedures have long been used in many different ways in teaching children with ASDs (as well as other disabilities) a variety of language and other skills, and their proper use is an essential skill for all intervention agents. The basic DTT instructional cycle is derived from operant discrimination-learning procedures and is designed to help lower-functioning children learn by reducing teaching interactions to their simplest components. DTT consists of repeated trials in which the teacher presents a cue, the child makes a response, and the teacher reinforces correct responses and ignores or corrects incorrect responses. Compre-

hensive presentations of DTT methodology appear in Leaf and McEachin (1999) and Lovaas (2003). In language training with nonverbal and minimally verbal children, DTT procedures are commonly used to teach an initial repertoire of attending, verbal and motor imitation, and receptive and expressive vocabularies. Once a child has learned to identify five or six objects receptively, generalization among exemplars of each object are used to teach the child to generalize within classes of objects while maintaining discriminations between classes of objects to create simple concepts. Next, the child is taught to identify the objects in different settings and with different individuals to ensure generalization.

When the child has learned to identify about 10 objects receptively, expressive training with the same objects begins in a successive discrimination-training format. The teacher places the first object on the table and, when the child looks at it, says its name as a verbal prompt for the child to name it. Over trials the verbal prompt is faded (MacDuff, Krantz, & McClannahan, 2001), in order to shift stimulus control from the teacher's verbal model to the sight of the object. The name of a second object is taught in the same way. Then the two objects are presented in random order across trials, until the child is able to name each object correctly without prompting on several consecutive trials. In subsequent training, the name of each new object is first taught in isolation; then trials with the new object are intermixed with trials on the previously trained objects. As is the case with receptive labeling, acquisition of each new expressive label after the first three or four is positively accelerated, but the rate of acquisition is highly variable across children. Once the child has learned to name several items, basic requests and answers to simple questions are taught, so as to make the newly acquired labels functional for the child in getting things. Special efforts to promote generalization across environments are usually necessary, because the tight control over attention and responding that is often required to teach beginning speech seems to combine with overselective attention to result in the frequent failure to generalize speech across settings and people. Therefore, from fairly early in training, DTT instruction is supplemented with procedures such as incidental teaching to promote communication in everyday environments.

Incidental Teaching

The main strategy for promoting generalized speech usage is to conduct brief teaching interactions requiring the child to use words to obtain natural reinforcers and to complete daily routines. The result has been the development of a group of procedures known collectively as "milieu teaching" or "incidental teaching" (Fenske et al., 2001; McGee, Morrier, & Daly, 1999). Incidental-teaching procedures vary in detail and specific purpose, but they share four features that distinguish them from the DTT procedures just described (Carr, 1985; Hwang & Hughes, 2000; McGee, Krantz, & McClannahan, 1985):

1. DTT is a massed-trials approach controlled and paced by the teacher; incidental-teaching episodes consist of only one trial or a few trials at a time, usually initiated by the child.
2. DTT occurs in time-limited, one-to-one sessions away from distractions; incidental teaching occurs intermittently throughout the day in everyday environments.
3. In DTT, the training stimuli are often teacher-selected objects, and the reinforcers may be arbitrary events such as food and praise; in incidental teaching, the training stimuli are child-selected items, and a reinforcer is access to such an item.
4. DTT is typically employed to teach new language *forms;* incidental-teaching procedures are employed to teach new language *functions*—that is, to help the child use existing language forms to influence others or to elaborate on existing forms in order to communicate better.

One of the most frequently used incidental teaching techniques is the time delay procedure (Charlop, Schreibman, & Thibodeau, 1985; Charlop & Trasowech, 1991; Ingenmey & Van Houten, 1991; Leung, 1994; Matson, Sevin, Box, Francis, & Sevin, 1993; Taylor & Harris, 1995), designed to shift stimulus control from the teacher's prompts to environmental cues. The time delay procedure can be used whenever the child wants an item or needs assistance. Instead of instructing or modeling an appropriate response, the teacher looks at the child and waits expectantly, either for gradually increasing durations across trials (e.g., 2, 4,

6, etc., seconds) or for a fixed duration on each trial (e.g., 10 seconds). If the child makes an appropriate response during the delay, the response is reinforced with assistance or the desired item. If an incorrect response or no response occurs, the teacher models the word or phrase and reinforces the child's correct imitation. With a more advanced child, a general request for the appropriate response can be made ("You need to tell me what you want"). The delay procedure teaches the child to respond to nonverbal cues; eventually, the objects and events are themselves sufficient to cue appropriate speech. To increase the frequency of opportunities, environmental prearrangement is usually necessary. For example, the teacher puts desired materials out of reach on a shelf or in a plastic container but in sight of the child, and keeps the incidental teaching interactions brief (Fenske et al., 2001).

Natural Language Paradigm

Koegel and colleagues (1987) used a modification of incidental teaching techniques in order to incorporate some correlates of typical speech acquisition that seem to be "pivotal" behaviors: turn taking, shared control, shared attention, and natural consequences. Pivotal behaviors are those expected to produce improvements in multiple behaviors simultaneously and thus make teaching more efficient (R. L. Koegel, Carter, & Koegel, 1998; Schreibman, Stahmer, & Pierce, 1996). The Natural Language Paradigm includes the following techniques:

1. Instructing the child to label the object is replaced by the teacher's playing with the object and modeling its name; if the child fails to imitate, the teacher simply plays with the object and models its name again.
2. Any spoken response, not just a correct response or an approximation, is reinforced.
3. Reinforcement consists of praise and the opportunity to play with the object for a few seconds.

Both of the children in the original study by Koegel and colleagues (1987) showed substantial increases in imitation, spontaneous vocalizations, and generalized imitation. Laski, Charlop, and Schreibman (1988) showed that parents could be successfully taught to use Natural Language Paradigm procedures, with corresponding increases in their children's imitations and answers to questions. The main value of the procedure seemed to be its ability to increase the frequency of existing speech, although it was noted anecdotally that novel words and phrases also occurred. Koegel, Koegel, and Surratt (1992) found that the use of Natural Language Paradigm procedures resulted in not only increased speech, but also reductions in problem behaviors such as aggression and tantrums. Koegel (1995) developed procedures to teach children with ASDs to ask for information about items in the environment, thus making them able to expand their vocabularies on their own. These and related studies (L. K. Koegel, Camarata, Valdez-Menchaca, & Koegel, 1998; R. L. Koegel, Camarata, Koegel, Ben-Tall, & Smith, 1998; Koegel, O'Dell, & Dunlap, 1988) show that developmental findings on typical language acquisition can serve a heuristic role in suggesting some novel teaching procedures. However, expertise in DTT techniques such as prompting and reinforcement is required, and careful attention must be paid to maintaining the subtle structure of the Natural Language Paradigm's approach, to avoid the risk of recreating the everyday situations in which autistic children fail to learn (Smith, 1993).

Verbal Learning

Sundberg and Partington (1998) have created a language training program based on Skinner's (1957) analysis of verbal behavior. Their Verbal Learning approach combines elements of DTT, incidental teaching, and the Natural Language Paradigm. Unlike traditional DTT approaches (but like the PECS, described below), the Verbal Learning approach begins by teaching "mands," or requests for reinforcers. Mands are typically the first type of communication acquired in typical development; they directly benefit the child because they let parents know exactly what is wanted at a particular moment (Sundberg & Partington, 1998). In the Verbal Learning approach, mand training is conducted with a variety of strong reinforcers many times a day. The child is shown the first reinforcer, is asked, "What do you want?", and is prompted to name (or sign) the reinforcer. Any prompts used to evoke the correct response are rapidly faded over trials. The second word taught is a reinforcer from a different

motivational category (e.g., a toy if the first word was a food). Once the child is reliably asking for two or three items, the object used as the reinforcer is faded out, then the question "What do you want?" is then faded out, so that the child is responding to his or her own motivation and not the sight of the object or the question. As in incidental teaching, opportunities are created to evoke requests throughout the day, and additional words are added to the child's repertoire. As mand training progresses, techniques for increasing vocal play and imitation are introduced. Then receptive commands, object identification, and matching to sample are introduced. Next, "tacts," or words controlled by nonverbal stimuli (e.g., names of objects), are taught by showing the child an object or picture and asking, "What is that?" A correct response is followed with an unrelated reinforcer in order to establish the sight of the object and not the child's current motivational state as the controlling stimulus for the word. Receptive discrimination training in a discrete-trials format occurs while expressive mand and tact training continue (i.e., there is no assumption that either receptive or expressive language must be mastered first).

After the child has acquired about 50 words for objects and actions, he or she is taught to respond to others' words in "receptive by function, feature, and class" training. For example, instead of learning only to "Touch the car," as in traditional receptive language training, the child is also taught to "Touch the one that's blue" (feature), "Show me the one you ride in" (function), and "Point to the one that has wheels" (class). Further programs expand responding to "intraverbals" (words spoken in response to other words) into beginning conversations by starting with simple word association games and verbal fill-in-the-blank exercises. More nouns, as well as verbs, adjectives, adverbs, prepositions, and pronouns—along with their combinations in simple sentences—are added as training progresses.

Sundberg and Partington (1998) noted that both DTT and natural environment approaches (the Natural Language Paradigm and incidental teaching) have been successful with children with ASDs, but that both have disadvantages when used alone and are not clearly based on the behavior analysis of language. They recommend blending the two approaches, emphasizing training in one or the other format at different points in training. For a nonverbal 3-year-old who rarely sits down, for example, Phase 1 training would emphasize natural environment training to shape initial mands, with some DTT (also focusing on mands) at a table or on the floor. In Phase 2, other verbal operants are introduced, and the child learns to work for extended periods of time at a table or desk. More academic tasks such as numbers and letters are introduced in Phase 3, along with more complex language relations such as prepositions and adjectives. Natural environment training continues to be used to help generalize these skills. Phases 4 and 5 move the child closer to a more typical educational setting and help the child learn from peers. These are general guidelines only; these phases are blended and overlapped, depending on each child's needs (Sundberg & Partington, 1998).

Considerable experimental research supports the efficacy of DTT, incidental teaching, and the Natural Language Paradigm as approaches to teaching language (e.g., Delprato, 2001; Elliott, Hall, & Soper, 1991; Howlin, 1981; R. L. Koegel, Carter, & Koegel, 1998; Spradlin & Siegel, 1982; Warren & Kaiser, 1986). The Verbal Learning approach is newer and less thoroughly researched, but has some support from studies of its components (e.g., Finkel & Williams, 2001; Hall & Sundberg, 1987; Miguel, Carr, & Michael, 2002; Partington, Sundberg, Newhouse, & Spengler, 1994; Sundberg, Loeb, Hale, & Eigenheer, 2002). Although we have highlighted the differences among these approaches for clarity, the differences are less marked in actual practice. Perhaps the main difference is that DTT procedures appear to be more effective in teaching language structures, whereas incidental teaching, the Natural Language Paradigm, and Verbal Learning procedures seem to excel at teaching and generalizing language functions (Carr & Kologinsky, 1983).

Picture Exchange Communication System

The PECS (Frost & Bondy, 1994), in which the child hands the teacher a picture of a desired item to request it, is especially useful with lower-functioning children because it does not require the imitation of complex hand movements or verbalizations. It is becoming a popular alternative to sign language training, both for this reason and because it does not require others in the child's environment to know a new form of language. The PECS includes training protocols for expanding communication from single words to phrases and for increasing communicative functions from requesting to labeling and commenting. By focusing on the use of symbols to teach requests from the beginning of training, the PECS seems to facilitate the acquisition of spoken language. Bondy and Frost (1994) provided a program review indicating that about 60% of 66 children who used the PECS for 2 years acquired independent speech, 30% used both speech and the PECS, and 10% used the PECS only. Similar results with smaller groups have been reported independently (Magiati & Howlin, 2003; Schwartz, Garfinkle, & Bauer, 1998). In an experimental study, Charlop-Christy, Carpenter, Le, LeBlanc, and Kellet (2002) found that PECS use could be mastered in a relatively short time by minimally verbal children with autism, who then showed increased spontaneous and imitative vocal speech, increased social behaviors, and a reduction in problem behaviors.

An alternative visual system teaches young children with autism to read and write to communicate (Watthen-Lovaas & Lovaas, 1999). It uses a carefully sequenced series of match-to-sample tasks to teach reading and writing, with programs for writing in longhand or using a computer keyboard, electronic communication devices, or PECS cards.

Sign Language Training

The basic techniques for teaching signing are similar to the DTT procedures used to teach initial speech (Carr & Dores, 1981). The teacher starts with two objects on the table and signs the name of one of the objects while simultaneously saying its name. Correct responses (touching the named object) are reinforced with praise and edibles. The positions of the objects on the table, and the names signed and spoken by the teacher, vary randomly across trials. Training continues until the child is able to respond correctly to both of the teacher's stimuli (sign + word) during randomly intermixed trials. One new object is added each time the child masters the current words. Prompting and fading procedures like those described earlier in connection with DTT for receptive speech are used if needed.

Expressive signing is also taught through procedures like those used in operant speech training (Carr, Binkoff, Kologinsky, & Eddy, 1978). The efficiency of learning will be enhanced if the child has already acquired generalized motor imitation, as modeling is the primary teaching technique. The size of the vocabulary the child acquires and the accuracy of sign formation are related to the child's fine motor abilities and motor planning skills (Seal & Bonvillian, 1997). An alternative to the procedures developed by Carr and his colleagues for teaching initial expressive signs has been described by Schaeffer (1980). Schaeffer's procedure is similar to the incidental teaching procedures described above for verbal language. The teacher begins by holding out a desired edible and waiting. When the child reaches for the food, the teacher catches the hand and moves it into position to make the sign for the edible, molds the hand and moves it through the sign, and only then gives the child the edible. The teacher's manual prompts are gradually faded over many trials, until the child makes the sign independently. Subsequent signs can be taught similarly by interrupting reaching for other reinforcers.

Adequate comparison studies providing clear guidance for the initial selection of a language teaching method are lacking. Generally speaking, the choice is made empirically on an individual basis, depending on the child's initial abilities and early progress. As is the case with social interaction skills, the attainment of a significant level of language competence and fluency seems to require both direct training in language skills and, when the child has acquired enough language to benefit from it, extensive exposure to typical peers.

ANALYSIS AND MANAGEMENT OF PROBLEM BEHAVIORS

Problem behaviors commonly observed in children with ASDs include tantrums, noncompliance, aggression, self-injury, property destruction, and repetitive, stereotyped behaviors, as well as dangerous behaviors such as running away, climbing on shelves or doors, and pica. Several characteristics that are inherent in the disorder seem to create difficulties in adapting to increasingly complex demands as a child grows older. Pragmatic language deficits make it difficult or impossible to assert oneself appropriately; to report anxiety, discomfort, or pain; or to make easily understood requests (Carr, Reeve, & Magito-McLaughlin, 1996). Social impairments result in insensitivity to social reinforcers, ignoring of others, and obliviousness to social cues (Dawson, Meltzoff, Osterling, Rinaldi, & Brown, 1998; Klin, 1991). High levels of stereotypy interfere with attention and learning; obsessions and perseverative interests and activities exclude social contacts and lead to rejection by peers (Lovaas, Litrownik, & Mann, 1971; Ozonoff et al., 2002). Cognitive disabilities impede learning; cognitive deviations, such as inability to read others' intentions, attention to parts rather than wholes, and preoccupation with the physical aspects of the environment, render many everyday situations and demands incomprehensible and frustrating (Frith, 1989; Klin et al., 2002a).

Problem behaviors can be characterized in several ways. At a basic descriptive level, they are behavioral excesses whose high rates and/or high intensities produce disruptive and harmful effects on a child's immediate social or physical environment and often on the child him- or herself. Even behaviors that are not physically harmful to the child or others, such as stereotyped behaviors, may be psychologically harmful to the child because they can interfere with learning and stigmatize the child in the community. Developmental considerations add the concept that many problem behaviors are continuations and elaborations of infantile behaviors that persist because the learning of more adaptive behaviors fails to occur in children with ASDs due to their social, language, and cognitive limitations (Carr et al., 1994; Lovaas et al., 1987). Problem behaviors can sometimes be viewed metaphorically as primitive communicative acts serving social functions, such as contacting adult attention or coercing escape from demands (Durand, 1990).

The emphasis in analyzing and understanding problem behaviors is on function over form: The relationship of a problem behavior to its context is more informative to treatment efforts than the topography of the behavior is. Functional analysis is the diagnostic process of behavior management efforts (O'Neill et al., 1997; Sturmey, 1996). Functional analysis engenders hypotheses about the causes of problem behaviors through interviews with caretakers, observation of the child and the contexts in which problem behaviors both occur and do not occur, and trial manipulations of antecedents and consequences believed to influence the behaviors. The applied behavior analysis (ABA) approach has led to a large literature of skill- and communication-building interventions for a wide variety of problem behaviors (e.g., Carr et al., 1994; Lucyshyn, Dunlap, & Albin, 2002; Luiselli & Cameron, 1998; Scotti & Meyer, 1999).

Initial decisions for limiting the scope of the variables to be assessed in a functional analysis can be informed by the body of research on problem behaviors in children with ASDs. Some of the classes of variables implicated by research are the following:

1. *Ecological and program variables.* These are characteristics of the general setting in which problem behaviors occur. How well organized versus chaotic is the home or classroom environment? Is the child's schedule and curriculum related to his or her developmental level, and does it seem to be meeting the child's identified needs? In the home, are there everyday household routines that regularly occasion problem behaviors? Does the parent or teacher have the material and human resources needed both to teach the child and to deal with problem behaviors? Do those who work with the child show skill in the use of empirically validated, effective teaching techniques (Leaf & McEachin, 1999; Lovaas, 2003; Maurice, Green, & Foxx, 2001; Maurice, Green, & Luce, 1996)? Is there adequate professional support on site or through consultation for ongoing analysis and treatment of learning difficulties and problem behaviors? Is the general emotional "climate" conducive to appropriate behavior, including a balance between nurturance- and control-oriented interactions with the child? Does the child have opportunities to indicate preferences and make choices consistent with his or her developmental level (Sigafoos, 1998)?

2. *Establishing operations or setting events.* These are prior events or conditions in the internal or external environments that interact with subsequent events to alter their impact on behavior (Iwata, Smith, & Michael, 2000; Kennedy & Meyer, 1998). More technically, establishing operations are prior events that alter the reinforcing effectiveness of some stimulus, object, or event and also alter the frequency of all behavior that has been reinforced by that stimulus, object, or event (Michael, 2000). Physiological setting events include painful or uncomfortable internal states (e.g., fatigue, hunger, illness, ear infections, toothaches, seizures, menses, allergies, constipation, the effects of drugs). Such states can make a child uninterested in typical reinforcers, less tolerant of everyday demands or frustrations, and more likely to engage in problem behaviors that have been reinforced in the past by escape or attention (Carr & Smith, 1995; Carr, Smith, Giacin, Whelan, & Pancari, 2003; Gunsett, Mulick, Fernald, & Martin, 1989; Kennedy & Meyer, 1996). Psychological setting events include mood, stress, and (in more able children and adolescents) distorted thinking and obsessions (Carr, Magito-McLaughlin, Giacobbe-Grieco, & Smith, 2003; Ozonoff et al., 2002). Social setting events include unpleasant interactions earlier in the day, the presence of certain other people in the environment, and extinction of appropriate behaviors when they go unnoticed by others (Taylor & Carr, 1992; Taylor, Ekdahl, Romanczyk, & Miller, 1994; Touchette, McDonald, & Langer, 1985). Environmental setting events include crowded or chaotic settings; settings lacking appropriate play and educational materials; a daily routine that lacks predictability and opportunities to make choices; and novel, difficult, or long-duration tasks (Brown, 1991; Flannery & Horner, 1994; Lalli, Casey, Goh, & Merlino, 1994; Mace, Browder, & Lin, 1987; R. G. Smith, Iwata, Goh, & Shore, 1995).

3. *Antecedents or stimuli.* These are discrete events that occur immediately before problem behaviors begin and can be shown to exert stimulus control over them. They include demands (requests, instructions, prompts, and interruptions), frustrating events (denial of access to reinforcing objects and activities), and loss of tangible reinforcers (Carr & Durand, 1985; Carr & Newsom, 1985; Durand & Crimmins, 1988; Iwata, Pace, Cowdery, Kalsher, & Cataldo, 1990; Zarcone, Iwata, Smith, Mazaleski, & Lerman, 1994).

4. *Consequences.* These are the relatively immediate effects of problem behaviors that function as positive or negative reinforcers. Positive reinforcers of problem behaviors for children with ASDs include attention; tangibles (food and preferred objects); preferred activities; and the automatic sensory feedback that is intrinsic to the performance of stereotypy, noise making, property destruction, and self-injury (Carr & McDowell, 1980; Durand & Crimmins, 1988; Lovaas et al., 1987; Rincover

& Devany, 1982). Examples of negative reinforcers include avoidance of, delay of, and escape from aversive tasks, events, or people, as well as automatic pain reduction or distraction (Carr & Smith, 1995; Durand & Crimmins, 1987, 1988; Iwata, Vollmer, & Zarcone, 1990; Lalli, Casey, & Kates, 1995).

The variables listed above are only a representative sample of those studied to date. The problem behaviors of individual children will usually prove to be influenced by idiosyncratic factors not listed here, but often discoverable through appropriate functional analysis procedures (Carr, Yarbrough, & Langdon, 1997; McAtee, Carr, & Schulte, 2004).

The treatment model most commonly used in home and school settings is the positive behavior support (PBS) model (Carr et al., 2002; Horner, Carr, Strain, Todd, & Reed, 2002; Koegel, Koegel, & Dunlap, 1996; Lucyshyn, Dunlap, et al., 2002). The PBS approach is a synthesis of nonaversive treatment procedures from ABA (Luiselli & Cameron, 1998; Scotti & Meyer, 1999), behavioral family intervention (Patterson, Reid, & Dishion, 1992), the family support movement (Dunst, Trivette, & Deal, 1994), and systems change strategies (Sailor, Gee, & Karasoff, 2000). In PBS interventions, "behavior support" plans emphasize the use of multiple interventions addressing environmental redesign, instruction in replacement behaviors, and consequences that eliminate rewards for problem behaviors and enhance rewards for appropriate behaviors. Aversive consequences such as restraint are avoided or used only as containment strategies in an emergency. Ideally, reductions in problem behaviors are accompanied by improvements in living, school/work, and leisure outcomes. Lifestyle goals for a child include successful participation in valued daily and weekly routines and activities in the home and community, the development of friendships with typical peers, and successful inclusion in the child's neighborhood school. Family-centered goals empower parents and other family members to implement behavior supports effectively and to use PBS to solve new or recurring problems. To its advocates, PBS represents an evolution of ABA into a new applied science that (1) views consumers of research as collaborative partners, (2) values ecological and social validity as much as internal validity, (3) seeks to effect lifestyle changes, and (4) views social systems as

units of analysis and intervention (Carr et al., 2002; Horner, Albin, Sprague, & Todd, 2000; Koegel et al., 1996). Reviews of PBS studies indicate that this approach can often be effective in achieving clinically significant, durable improvements in problem behaviors (Carr et al., 1999; Lucyshyn, Horner, Dunlap, Albin, & Ben, 2002).

The basic steps involved in conducting a PBS intervention in the home are summarized in Table 7.1 (Lucyshyn, Kayser, Irvin, & Blumberg,

---

TABLE 7.1. Steps in Collaborating with Families to Develop Positive Behavior Support Plans

1. Conduct a functional assessment:
   a. Conduct functional assessment interview.
   b. Conduct functional assessment observations.
2. Conduct an assessment of family routines and ecology:
   a. Conduct an interview about family activity settings (routines/activities) in the home and community.
   b. Select and prioritize valued but problematic activity settings for intervention, and define vision of realistic and successful activity settings.
   c. Conduct a supplemental interview to ascertain child positive contributions, family strengths, resources, and social supports, stressors, and goals.
3. Develop a summary hypothesis statement and a competing behavior pathways diagram for problem behavior in the targeted activity setting.
4. Design a technically sound and contextually appropriate behavior support plan:
   a. Identify strategies that are logically linked to features of the problem in the activity setting and that are likely to make problem behaviors irrelevant, ineffective, and inefficient at achieving their purposes. Brainstorm about:
      1. Setting event strategies
      2. Preventive strategies
      3. Teaching strategies
      4. Consequence strategies
   b. Finalize strategies that are likely to be effective and contextually appropriate:
      1. Select necessary and sufficient strategies.
      2. Select strategies that are acceptable, feasible, and a good fit with elements of the targeted activity setting.
5. As needed, select family-centered supports that may enhance implementation fidelity and long-term sustainability of the plan, as well as the overall quality of family life.

Note. From Lucyshyn, Kayser, Irvin, and Blumberg (2002, p. 110). Copyright 2002 by Paul H. Brookes. Reprinted by permission.

2002). After conducting functional assessment interviews and observations (Step 1), the clinician gathers information about family routines and family strengths and weaknesses (Step 2). In Step 3, a hypothesis about the likely function of the behavior is developed, and a diagram showing the connections among setting events, antecedents, problem behaviors, and consequences is created. In Step 4, the parents and the clinician jointly arrive at interventions designed to make problem behaviors irrelevant, ineffective, and inefficient by changing the setting events, introducing preventive strategies, teaching alternative behaviors, and eliminating the previous reinforcing consequences of the problem behavior. In Step 5, any equipment, financial, and personnel supports needed by the family are identified and accessed through the assistance of social service and educational agencies. Comprehensive descriptions and examples of the implementation of this model with families of children with ASDs can be found in Lucyshyn, Kayser, and colleagues (2002) and Fox, Benito, and Dunlap (2002).

The PBS approach expands the range of behavioral interventions to address multiple factors simultaneously in natural environments. Pursued rigorously in a setting open to significant change, it encourages not only better understanding of the individuals served, but also desirable organizational and system changes. However, the extent to which it is broadly applicable across settings, individuals with ASDs, and problem behaviors remains to be seen. In spite of its popularity, some cautions have been raised. Mulick and Butter (2005) point out that the individual behavioral procedures used in PBS interventions are not new, and that their combined use hardly constitutes a new science. Most importantly, the emphasis in PBS on such values as "normalization," person-centered planning, and universal inclusion in mainstream classrooms inappropriately mixes ideology and science. The danger is that when treatment decisions are based on ideological considerations first and scientific findings second, inappropriate and ineffective treatment can result. Newsom and Kroeger (2005) note that a policy of complete avoidance of aversive consequences (as recommended by some PBS proponents) ignores findings on optimal child development, which requires a balancing of nurturance and discipline (Baumrind, 1996). Moreover, an approach based solely on positive support may very well fail when applied to

problem behaviors more severe and complex than those typically addressed in the PBS literature. The right course to take in a particular clinical situation can be difficult to know. It is always necessary to keep the child's best long-term interests in mind, and to be prepared to weigh both scientific knowledge and worthy philosophical ideals in light of the circumstances of the case at hand.

PHARMACOTHERAPY

In the absence of definitive knowledge of the neurochemistry of ASDs, there is no medication specific to it that might be curative (Kwok, 2003). Psychotropic medications can sometimes serve a useful role as an adjunctive treatment with children showing unusually severe problem behaviors that are difficult to manage with behavioral procedures alone. They seem to be most helpful with symptoms such as hyperactivity, attention deficits, rituals, and obsessions. For problems usually responsive to behavioral interventions, such as aggression, anxiety, depression, impulsivity, and sleep disorders, the adjunctive use of medications may facilitate treatment. Medication is least likely to be helpful for problems requiring skill training, such as deficits in social, communication, and academic domains (Santosh & Baird, 2001). It is essential to collaborate with a physician who is familiar with pharmacotherapy in children with developmental disabilities, for the experience he or she can bring; the available research provides only rough guidance. Most reports are open-label case reports; relatively few double-blind, placebo-controlled studies exist (Volkmar, 2001), and almost no studies include direct observation of relevant behaviors (Crosland et al., 2003).

The most well-studied agents are the dopamine antagonists, especially haloperidol (Haldol). Several controlled studies have shown haloperidol to be superior to placebo for withdrawal, stereotypies, and hyperactivity (Anderson et al., 1984; Campbell, Schopler, Cueva, & Hallin, 1996). However, drug-induced dyskinesias tend to be relatively common with long-term administration (Campbell et al., 1997). As a result, most physicians today prefer to try the newer "atypical" antipsychotics (Hollander, Phillips, & Yeh, 2003), which have less risk of serious side effects; however, obesity is a common side effect of some of them, especially olanzapine (Zyprexa) (Kemner, Willemsen-Swinkels, de Jonge, Tuynman-Qua, & van Engeland, 2002). The most commonly prescribed atypical antipsychotic for ASDs is risperidone (Risperdal). In a double-blind, placebo-controlled study of adults with ASDs (McDougle et al., 1998), it was found to be superior to placebo on several measures and was well tolerated. In children, risperidone improves problem behaviors and affect dysregulation in about 50% of cases. Its main side effects are weight gain and elevated prolactin levels (Masi, Cosenza, Mucci, & Brovedani, 2003).

Several studies have been conducted with selective serotonin reuptake inhibitors (SSRIs), including fluoxetine (Prozac) (DeLong, Teague, & Kamran, 1998; Fatemi, Realmuto, Khan, & Thuras, 1998), fluvoxamine (Luvox) (McDougle et al., 1996), and clomipramine (Anafranil) (Gordon, Rapoport, Hamburger, State, & Mannheim, 1992; Gordon, State, Nelson, Hamburger, & Rapoport, 1993). Fluoxetine was found to be helpful in a subgroup of children who had hyperlexia, as well as a family history of bipolar disorder and unusual intellectual achievement (DeLong, Ritch, & Burch, 2002). However, some studies have indicated that children with ASDs respond less well to SSRIs than adolescents and adults do (Brasic et al., 1994; McDougle, Kresch, & Posey, 2000; Sanchez et al., 1996). SSRIs have shown significant rates of adverse effects, including seizures, constipation, weight gain, and excessive sedation (e.g., Brodkin, McDougle, Naylor, Cohen, & Price, 1997).

Panksepp (1979) proposed that autistic disorder results from an excess of opioid substances (beta-endorphins) in the central nervous system, which impairs social attachment. In addition to their euphoric effects, endorphins have analgesic properties, suggesting the possibility that their presence in excess might contribute to the maintenance of self-injurious behaviors. These considerations have led to numerous trials of naltrexone (ReVia), a potent opiate antagonist. Some studies have reported improved social behaviors; normalized pain sensitivity; and reductions in hyperactivity, self-injury, irritability and stereotypic behaviors (Barrett, Feinstein, & Hole, 1989; Bouvard et al., 1995; Campbell et al., 1993; Kolmen, Feldman, Handen, & Janosky, 1995; Willemsen-Swinkels, Buitelaar, & van Engeland, 1996). However, the effects are highly variable across children, and some reports show minimal or no

effects (Symons, Thompson, & Rodriguez, 2004). The best responders appear to be children in whom the drug reduces excessively high beta-endorphin and serotonin levels (Bouvard et al., 1995).

Currently under investigation are drugs typically used with Alzheimer disease, such as donezepil (Aricept) (Hardan & Handen, 2002). Recently, atomoxetine (Strattera) has been approved for the management of ADHD in children, teens, and adults (Christman, Fermo, & Markowitz, 2004). Studies are currently underway to determine whether this potent and specific noradrenergic reuptake inhibitor may be of benefit in the management of ASDs, particularly if ADHD is a comorbid condition (R. A. Barkley, personal communication, August 31, 2004; Jou, Handen, & Hardan, 2005). One other medical intervention, involving not a drug but the hormone secretin, has been extensively studied and found ineffective in numerous well-controlled trials (Esch & Carr, 2004). Dietary interventions derived from the excess opioid hypothesis and based on a gluten-free, casein-free diet have some anecdotal and single-case support (e.g., Whiteley, Rogers, Savery, & Shattock, 1999), but remain to be adequately investigated.

WORKING WITH FAMILIES

Behavioral Parent Training

Behavioral parent training for families that include children with challenging behaviors are the focus of some 30 years of research (Baker, 1996; Singer, Goldberg-Hamblin, Peckham-Hardin, Barry, & Santarelli, 2002). Nearly all this research is meaningfully applied to families that include children diagnosed with ASDs. The intense level of intervention required to create meaningful and lasting progress for children with ASDs necessitates the utilization of those closest and most frequently in contact with the children. Family involvement is also required by the simple need to manage challenging behaviors in the context of home and community environments. Parents are either in the leading role of the therapeutic endeavor or deeply embedded in a collaborative relationship that involves individualized as well as systemwide support (Becker-Cottrill, McFarland, & Anderson, 2003; Sperry, Whaley, Shaw, & Brame, 1999). In the absence of effective help, high levels of child behavior problems increase parents' levels of stress, which in turn contribute to a worsening of problem behaviors (Baker et al., 2003).

Common Problems in Using Behavioral Procedures

Although parent training is an integral component of treatment for children with challenging behaviors, 30% of parents cannot benefit from training unless other supportive interventions are included (Lutzker & Campbell, 1994; Sanders, 1996; Singer et al., 2002; Singer & Powers, 1993; Webster-Stratton, 1997). First, there are the ubiquitous problems of recruitment and attrition. Three other major problems are commonly encountered in parents' application of behavioral techniques.

Inconsistency in the application of behavioral procedures is a major problem that looms largest at the earliest stages of intervention, but remains problematic throughout intervention. Harris, Peterson, Filliben, Glassberg, and Favell (1998) targeted parents' interactions with each other in an attempt to improve consistency in application of behavior therapy. Behavioral techniques were initially taught to both parents. After this phase, researchers taught both parents specific and positive feedback skills to apply to one another. Harris and colleagues found that both parents showed increased skill levels long after the introduction of feedback techniques.

Application of behavioral techniques during "the heat of the moment" is a quite different skill from those that may be well learned in the clinic. There are subtle but pervasive difficulties in the application of an intervention in a specific context. Specific contexts that involve person variables—in both the parent and the child with ASD—include variability in energy, emotional availability, and mood throughout the day. There are also temporal and situational changes in the natural course of a day, and demands change with events. Occasions such as the morning rush out of the house or dinner at a restaurant require multiple tasks and perhaps are less forgiving of problem behavior than an afternoon spent at home during the weekend. Singer and Powers (1993) had parents keep diaries of their days for a week to identify stress levels during various routines. Predictable patterns of stress were identified. Many parents found that the times when their children displayed the most problem behavior

were during the stressful daily events that required split attention and completion of multiple tasks at once. To intervene, Singer and Powers taught parents stress management skills as well as behavioral procedures. For those children whose problem behaviors occurred at stressful times, attention seeking seemed to be a motivating factor. Awareness of these relationships allowed parents to create a plan for the times their attention would be compromised, allowing the parents to circumvent the disruptive attention-seeking behavior that was otherwise probable.

From the inception of behavioral parent training, concern about generalization and maintenance of the skills learned was present. In an older study of training for parents with young children with developmental disabilities, Baker, Heifetz, and Murphy (1980) found that 24% of the parents were unable to teach a new skill to their children 14 months after training. In a 4- to 7-year follow-up with 30 families who had received parent training, Harris (1986) found that parents whose children were not in behaviorally oriented educational programs were less likely to continue to use behavioral techniques than parents whose children attended schools with a behavioral orientation. Since then, some progress has been made toward improving the durability of parent training. Some of the techniques that have proved helpful for parents of children with ASDs include teaching general skills rather than task-specific training, teaching parents to self-monitor their parenting skills by means of checklists, and conducting training activities in natural family contexts at home and in the community instead of in a clinic (Horner, Dunlap, & Koegel, 1988). Most recently, Koegel, Koegel, and Brookman (2003) have emphasized teaching pivotal responses, behaviors that influence a number of others. For example, training parents to teach their children self-management skills for play and self-help routines can relieve the parents of some of the need for constant supervision.

Addressing Contextual Barriers

Identification of problems that limit the effectiveness of training has led to improvements in emphasis and focus. Overcoming contextual barriers to parent training involves the addition of strategies to improve both the content and delivery of training. The PBS model attempts to improve upon behavioral parent training by including a substantial emphasis on the family context (Koegel et al., 1996; Lucyshyn, Dunlap, et al., 2002; Singer et al., 2002). There is explicit attention to the quality of life of the child and the family as a whole. PBS emphasizes using a range of supportive contextual interventions to identify and alter barriers to family functioning. Challenges to successful behavioral parent training include a long list of interrelated problems, such as poverty and social isolation, marital/couple conflict, and depression (Baker, 1996; Lutzker & Campbell, 1994; Sanders, 1996; Singer & Powers, 1993; Webster-Stratton, 1998). These issues have in common the effect of interfering with the parents' ability to learn parenting skills or, having learned them, to implement them consistently.

A very significant percentage of the population lives below the poverty level. When families struggle for basic needs, they are less likely to seek parent training; even if parent training is begun, they are less likely to complete the full course of training (Webster-Stratton, 1997). Single mothers with few financial resources appear to have more difficulty applying behavioral techniques than do middle-class parents (Dumas, 1984; Wahler, 1980, 1988; Webster-Stratton, 1997). Some success has been demonstrated when supportive interventions are added (Lutzker, 1984; Lutzker & Campbell, 1994). In a study of single mothers who were socially isolated and had lower socioeconomic status, all were unable to utilize behavioral parent training successfully for their children with oppositional behavior (Wahler, Cartor, Fleischman, & Lambert, 1993). When supportive counseling focused on resolving conflicts with other adults was added to parent training, however, mothers were able to change their children's behavior and to maintain the improvement over a 6-month follow-up.

The presence of marital/couple problems has a detrimental effect on the effectiveness of parent training with parents of typically developing children (Sanders & Dadds, 1993). Surprisingly, little or no research has been conducted in this area on families that include children with ASDs (Singer et al., 2002), but it is likely that research on such families would show similarities. In a highly detailed study of families that include children with conduct disorder, Dadds, Sanders, Behrens, and James (1987) evaluated the relationship between marital discord and child problem behaviors. Positive par-

enting skills were taught to the parents. In three of the four couples, a decrease in challenging behavior from the children was found, but there was little concomitant change in the fighting between the parents. Partner support training was then added, which involved teaching the parents to be more positive toward one another as well less reactive. The addition of the latter component resulted in a reduction of child problem behavior as well as reduced marital conflict.

Approximately 25–30% of mothers of children with disabilities show evidence of mild depression, compared to about 20% of mothers with typically developing children (Singer & Yovanoff, 1993). These figures are clearly a source of concern. In families with typical children, parents with depression interact less with their children, are more random in their responses to their children, and are more likely to be inconsistent in their use of discipline techniques. There is some research suggesting that depressed parents of children with disabilities may not show these impairments (Singer et al., 2002), but the issue is far from closed. Robbins, Dunlap, and Plienis (1991) found that preintervention parental stress level may be one of the strongest predictors of a child's success in early intervention.

Families that include children with ASDs have multiple needs. Several different providers are often required to provide assistance and create the supportive context through which behavioral parent training may prove successful. A variety of family-focused treatments can be added to behavioral parent training such as supportive counseling, parent self-management, stress management, and interpersonal problem solving.

Although it is important to acknowledge the multiple and serious problems confronting family members, it is also important to avoid an exclusive emphasis on the negative aspects of having a child with an ASD. Most parents note that even a very difficult child can make positive contributions. These include helping the parents to learn love, patience, acceptance, and distinctions between the important and trivial aspects of life (Turnbull, Blue-Banning, Behr, & Kerns, 1986). Bristol (1984) identified successful coping strategies used by parents of children with ASDs that should be encouraged. The strategies ranked as most important by the parents fell into the following categories: (1) helping the child by learning effective teaching and behavior management skills; (2) controlling the meaning of the child's disability by endowing it with a higher significance, either through religious faith or through positive comparisons with the "worse" past and the "better" present; (3) seeking and receiving the spouse's or partner's support; (4) focusing on the relationships and needs within the family; and (5) self-development through the cultivation of interests and activities not directly related to the child with an ASD.

As a child with an ASD grows through adolescence and enters adulthood, the focus needs to shift from training and counseling to creating a social network of support that extends beyond the family. One promising model for doing so is the group action planning model of Turnbull and Turnbull (1996). An "action group" or "circle of support" consists of the individual with the ASD, family members, friends, teachers or job coaches, community citizens, and professionals having a strong commitment to helping the individual succeed in living as full and typical a life as possible. Regular meetings are held in which the desires of the individual set the agenda, and creative problem solving is used to address goals in each major life domain: family, friendships, supported living, education and work, and community participation. More able adolescents and adults with ASDs also find support in Internet forums and chat rooms focused on their needs and interests. Lists of active sites can be found on the websites of most state and national autism and Asperger's disorder organizations.

EARLY INTENSIVE BEHAVIORAL INTERVENTION

Brain development in the young child is strongly influenced by the timing and quality of early experience (Huttenlocher, 1988). As early as 1973, Lovaas's group at the University of California at Los Angeles had noticed that younger children in their intensive behavioral treatment program tended to make greater progress than older children (Lovaas, Koegel, Simmons, & Long, 1973; Lovaas & Newsom, 1976). Occasional reports of recovery to typical functioning in individual cases of children who clearly had autism when very young had also appeared by the early 1970s (DeMyer et al., 1973; Gajzago & Prior, 1974; Kanner, 1973; Lovaas et al., 1973; Rimland, 1964).

These developments challenged the "historical absolutism" of a bleak diagnosis (Maurice, 2001), and they encouraged the idea that more children might attain a good long-term outcome if appropriate treatment were provided early enough and intensively enough.

Preschool Programs

Most early intervention currently occurs in preschool classroom programs based in universities, private educational organizations, and public schools (Dawson & Osterling, 1997; Handleman & Harris, 2000; Schwartz, Sandall, Garfinkle, & Bauer, 1998). Dawson and Osterling (1997) reviewed the reports of the better-known model preschool programs for children with autism and found six common elements among them:

1. The curriculum emphasizes attention, imitation, language, play, and social skills. A behavioral or developmental–behavioral approach is the most common orientation to curriculum implementation.
2. Intensive one-to-one and small-group instruction are provided initially; these are then faded to more natural classroom conditions to enhance generalization. Most model programs also feature integrated classrooms, in order to promote social development through planned interactions with typical peers.
3. A high degree of structure exists in the organization of the environment and the daily routine.
4. Behavior management is addressed through functional analysis and the teaching of appropriate alternative behaviors.
5. Substantial effort is devoted to preparing each child and the receiving teachers for the transition to a kindergarten or first-grade classroom.
6. Parent training is offered, along with in-home consultations and treatment.

Overall, most children with ASDs in model preschool programs show substantial gains on standardized tests, and about 50% achieve placements in regular classrooms with varying levels of support ranging from none at all to a dedicated full-time aide (Dawson & Osterling, 1997; Rogers, 1998; Smith, 1999). Harris and Handleman (2000) found that age and IQ at intake were predictive of progress in their intensive behavioral preschool program. Nearly all children who were age 4 or younger at admission, and/or had IQs of 59 or higher, showed an average 26-point gain in IQ by the time they were discharged and were in regular public school classrooms 4–6 years later. The data on the progress of children in behaviorally oriented preschool programs show that most make clinically as well as statistically significant gains in intelligence, language, overall developmental rate, and reduction of autistic symptomatology (Anderson, Campbell, & Cannon, 1994; Eikeseth, Smith, Jahr, & Eldevik, 2002; Fenske, Zalenski, Krantz, & McClannahan, 1985; Harris & Handleman, 2000; Harris, Handleman, Gordon, Kristoff, & Fuentes, 1991; Howard, Sparkman, Cohen, Green, & Stanislaw, 2005; McClannahan & Krantz, 1994; Strain & Hoyson, 2000). Eikeseth and colleagues (2002) found that children older than those usually studied so far can make substantial progress in intensive classroom programs. Children between 4 and 7 years of age who received 30 hours a week of behavioral treatment in a school setting showed much greater gains in intelligence, language, and adaptive behavior in 1 year than a control group receiving 30 hours a week of eclectic special education. Children have also shown statistically significant gains in developmental rate in preschool programs with strong developmental orientations (Jocelyn, Casiro, Beattie, Bow, & Kneisz, 1998; Rogers, Hall, Osaki, Reaven, & Herbison, 2000; Salt et al., 2002). Direct comparisons of behavioral and clearly defined developmental programs have not yet been done, however.

Early Intensive Behavioral Intervention in the Home

In the early 1970s, Lovaas began treating very young children (under 4 years of age) with autistic disorder by teaching the parents to be the primary therapists, with the direction and help of graduate and undergraduate students who worked along with them in the home (Lovaas, 1987, 1996; Lovaas & Smith, 1988). The theoretical basis of the treatment was ABA, which relies heavily on principles of operant conditioning, especially reinforcement, shaping, discrimination learning, and chaining. Lovaas compared outcomes for an intensive treatment group of 19 children who received at least 40 hours a week of one-to-one instruction (Exper-

imental Group) with two control groups: a minimal-contact group receiving 10 or fewer hours a week of individual instruction (Control Group 1), and a no-contact control group (Control Group 2).

The first outcome data were obtained when the children were 7 years old (Lovaas, 1987). Of the 19 Experimental Group subjects, 9 (47%) were found to be educationally and intellectually "normal": They had successfully completed the regular first-grade class without support, had been recommended for promotion by their teachers to a regular second-grade class, and scored at or above average on standardized IQ tests. The mean IQs of these best-outcome children increased 37 points, from 70 to 107. Overall, the 19 Experimental Group children showed a 30-point increase in mean IQ, from 53 to 83. In contrast, only 1 of the 40 children in the two control groups obtained a regular class placement, and the two groups' mean IQs increased only 5 points.

McEachin and colleagues (1993) conducted a long-term follow-up of the Experimental Group children when their average age was 13, and compared them with the Control Group 1 children on measures of intelligence, adaptive behavior, and personality. The mean IQ of the entire Experimental Group was 85, and it was 111 for the best-outcome subgroup. When compared with typical children without a history of behavior disorder, eight of the nine best-outcome children showed no significant differences from the typical controls on independently administered intelligence, adaptive behavior, and personality scales. Residual deficits in language use or social behavior in some of the children were minor and not noticeable to school personnel. In Control Group 1, none of the 19 children was in a regular class, as had been true at the age 7 follow-up, and the mean IQ was 55.

Other investigators have reported impressive, if not as dramatic, results for young children with ASDs receiving less intensive behavioral treatment. A prospective study at Murdoch University in Western Australia (Birnbrauer & Leach, 1993) and a retrospective study at the University of California at San Francisco (Sheinkopf & Siegel, 1998) showed gains in IQ into the average range and improvements in language and adaptive behavior skills, along with decreases in problem behaviors, in about 45% of the young children involved in intensive behavioral home programs.

Weiss (1999) found improvements into the typical range in scores on the Vineland Adaptive Behavior Scales and the Childhood Autism Rating Scale, along with placement in regular classes for half the children receiving intensive behavioral treatment for 2 years. Similar results were reported by Sallows and Graupner (1999) for their home-based program. Several uncontrolled case studies have reported progress to typical or near-typical functioning in very young children with ASDs (Groden, Domingue, Chesnick, Groden, & Baron, 1983; Koegel, Koegel, Shoshan, & McNerney, 1999; Perry, Cohen, & DeCarlo, 1995), including one child who began treatment at 1 year of age (Green, Brennan, & Fein, 2002).

These findings are tempered by large individual differences across children and various methodological shortcomings, primarily the absence of truly random assignment to experimental and control groups (e.g., Gresham & MacMillan, 1998; Rogers, 1998; Smith, 1999). Consequently, reviewers (Chorpita et al., 2002; Rogers, 1998) have judged that no comprehensive interventions, including ABA programs, meet the standards of efficacy and effectiveness set by the Task Force on Promotion and Dissemination of Psychological Procedures, Division of Clinical Psychology, American Psychological Association (1995). (See also Lonigan, Elbert, & Johnson, 1998, regarding studies of child disorders generally.) More recent work is beginning to address such concerns. Using truly random assignment, Smith, Groen, and Wynn (2000) compared outcomes between a group of 3-year-olds who received intensive treatment like that given to the experimental group in Lovaas's (1987) study but for fewer hours a week (25 instead of 40), and a well-matched control group who received parent-directed behavioral treatment 5 hours a week and attended special education programs 10–15 hours a week. At follow-up at 7–8 years of age, the intensive treatment group had gained an average of 16 IQ points, compared to a loss of 1 point for the control group. Four (27%) of the 15 children in the intensive group were in regular education classes without support; none of the control children were. Smith and colleagues speculated that their results differed from those of Lovaas for several possible reasons, including lower levels of intelligence and language in their children at intake and fewer hours of treatment. The massive problems involved in conducting well-controlled outcome

research with different treatments for ASDs over a period of years have been thoroughly described by Rogers (1998) and Smith (1999).

For the most favorable outcomes to occur, the following four conditions appear to be necessary:

1. The child has average intelligence or mild to moderate mental retardation, and does not have a regressive neurological condition, such as CDD or Rett's disorder (Butter, 2003; Smith, Buch, & Gamby, 2000; Smith, Eikeseth, Klevstrand, & Lovaas, 1997; T. Smith, Klevstrand, & Lovaas, 1995).

2. Treatment begins at an early age—ideally by 2–3 years of age, or even younger when possible (Bryson, Rogers, & Fombonne, 2003; Harris & Handleman, 2000).

3. The treatment is behaviorally oriented and intensive, including 30–40 hours per week of high-quality one-to-one instruction and a high level of involvement by well-trained and supported parents (Johnson & Hastings, 2002; Sallows & Graupner, 1999).

4. The treatment is supervised by a professional with considerable experience in the application of behavioral methods with children with ASDs (Metz & Pinnock, 2003; Mudford, Martin, Eikeseth, & Bibby, 2001).

Since the publication of Maurice's (1993) popular account of the recovery of her two autistic children through early intensive behavioral intervention, there has been a continuing demand for this approach by parents of young children. There is consequently a high demand for professionals with expertise in ABA and curriculum design for young children with ASDs. Clinicians not thoroughly trained in these specialized skills should refer parents to the Behavior Analysis Certification Board (www.bacb.com) for the names of certified behavior analysts in their area, and to a nearby Families for Effective Autism Treatment support group for their consumer recommendations of qualified local service providers. The importance of qualified professional supervision even in parent-directed home programs is shown by studies indicating that such programs often fail to achieve the results of professionally directed programs based in a university clinic or a model school, although parents are generally satisfied with the gains their children do make (Bibby, Eikeseth, Martin, Mudford, & Reeves, 2001; Smith et al., 2000).

We are living in an unfortunate time in at least one respect: A beneficial technology has outpaced society's typical mechanisms for allocating the resources needed to provide it on a large scale. The four criteria listed above are difficult to meet, particularly at the level of the local school district—the default treatment setting for most children with ASDs. Society has not solved the problem of how to pay for early intensive behavioral treatment (which can cost from $30,000 to $60,000 a year in U.S. dollars) for every child who could benefit from it. School districts, burdened with many other mandated services, pay for it reluctantly if at all, and most do not (Mulick & Butter, 2002). Private health insurance carriers virtually never cover it (Freudenheim, 2004). The result has been a decade of contentious due process hearings and court battles, including a class action case appealed to the Supreme Court of Canada (*Auton v. British Columbia*, 2004). The Canadian case presented the compelling dilemma of a government committed to universal health care, faced with an expensive treatment while already squeezed by rapidly rising medical costs. Often lost in such disputes are careful cost–benefit estimates that demonstrate a savings to society of $1.6–2.8 million (U.S. dollars) over the lifetime of each child with an ASD who receives early intensive behavioral intervention in the United States (Jacobson, Mulick, & Green, 1998), and savings of $0.76–1.2 million per child (Canadian dollars) in Canada (Hildebrand, 1999).

CONCLUSIONS

A few general observations emerge from this review of some aspects of current approaches to the treatment of children with ASDs.

1. Procedures developed within the ABA framework remain the standard of treatment for children with ASDs (New York State Department of Health, 1999; U.S. Department of Health and Human Services, 1999). Even when recovery is not a realistic aim, as in the majority of cases, children show greater skill acquisition and less restrictive educational placements than with other approaches. Progress in helping more children to a greater degree might be

accelerated by improved functional analyses of important domains (e.g., language; Bondy, Tincani, & Frost, 2004) and by greater attention to the contributions of other fields, particularly basic research in developmental psychology. Regarding the latter, there are already signs of some convergence. For example, pivotal response training (Koegel, Koegel, & McNerney, 2001) relates to developmentalists' concern with what may be foundational skills for social interaction and communication, such as joint attention, turn taking, and social initiation. Whalen and Schreibman (2003) have used ABA procedures to teach joint attention and found improvement and generalization of social behaviors. Klin and colleagues' (2003) "enactive mind" theory of social development, with its emphasis on the importance of social learning, evokes concepts familiar to behavior analysts. In spite of considerable differences in philosophy of science, methodology, and language, cross-fertilization is beginning to occur and should become increasingly frequent. The difficulty lies in identifying true developmental *prerequisites* among the many developmental *correlates* revealed in basic research. As diagnosis and treatment within the first year of life become increasingly possible (Bryson et al., 2001; Cecil, 2004; Teitelbaum, Teitelbaum, Nye, Fryman, & Maurer, 1998), critical developmental targets for the very earliest intervention will need to be identified; these should then be taught through ABA methods tailored to infants and toddlers (Green et al., 2002). The problems presented by ASDs remain complex and require a broad-based assault with the best that science can offer.

2. Although progress on etiology is being made, the causes of ASDs remain frustratingly elusive. With our newfound capabilities to study the human genome and observe the working brain, it seems that finally the instrumentation is adequate to the task, but the right questions remain to be asked. At a minimum, it is clear that more discrimination in selecting samples for genetic and functional MRI studies is needed; existing diagnostic categories have proven to be overly broad and etiologically barren. Progress on the multiple etiologies of ASDs will require finer descriptions of important behavioral and cognitive features of subgroups, as well as better understanding of gene–brain–behavior–environment relationships.

3. The increase in the number of children with ASDs is real, but it reflects more of an epidemic of diagnoses than of any vaccine's adverse effects. A severe problem for the "true increase in affected cases" hypothesis is the failure so far to identify an environmental cause for such an increase. The magnitude of the contribution of vaccines or their components remains unknown, but seems likely to prove to be vanishingly small. No other chemicals, pollutants, or viruses have yet been implicated as serious candidates. However, science constantly surprises us, and this conclusion may change with further research.

4. Until appropriate genetic or neurochemical targets are identified and remediated very early in life, a medical cure for ASDs will remain out of reach. The progress of today's children will continue to depend critically on the timing, intensity, and quality of the teaching they receive. Simply stated, it will continue to be hard work, with no easy paths and no guarantees for the difficult job undertaken by committed, supported parents and teachers in building useful behaviors every day.

REFERENCES

Alarcon, M., Cantor, R. M., Liu, J., Gilliam, T. C., Geschwind, D. H., & Autism Genetic Research Exchange Consortium. (2002). Evidence for a language quantitative trait locus on chromosome 7q in multiplex autism families. *American Journal of Human Genetics, 70,* 60–71.

American Academy of Pediatrics. (1999). Joint statement of the American Academy of Pediatrics (AAP) and the United States Public Health Service (USPHS)(RE9937). *Pediatrics, 104,* 568–569.

American Psychiatric Association (APA). (1980). *Diagnostic and statistical manual of mental disorders* (3rd ed.). Washington, DC: Author.

American Psychiatric Association (APA). (1987). *Diagnostic and statistical manual of mental disorders* (3rd ed., revised). Washington, DC: Author.

American Psychiatric Association (APA). (1994). *Diagnostic and statistical manual of mental disorders* (4th ed.). Washington, DC: Author.

American Psychiatric Association (APA). (2000). *Diagnostic and statistical manual of mental disorders* (4th ed., text rev.). Washington, DC: Author.

Amir, R. E., Van den Veyver, I. B., Wan, M., Tran, C. Q., Francke, U., & Zoghbi, H. Y. (1999). Rett syndrome is caused by mutations in X-linked MECP2, encoding methyl-CpG-binding protein 2. *Nature Genetics, 23,* 127–128.

Anderson, L. T., Campbell, M., Grega, D. M., Perry, R., Small, A. M., & Green, W. H. (1984). Haloperidol in the treatment of infantile autism: Effects on learning and behavioral symptoms. *American Journal of Psychiatry, 141,* 1195–1202.

Anderson, S. R., Campbell, S., & Cannon, B. O. (1994). The May Center for Early Childhood Education. In S. L. Harris & J. S. Handleman (Eds.), *Preschool education programs for children with autism* (pp. 15–36). Austin, TX: Pro-Ed.

Andrews, N., Miller, E., Taylor, B., Lingam, R., Simmons, A., Stowe, J., et al. (2002). Recall bias, MMR, and autism. *Archives of Disease in Childhood, 87,* 493–494.

Antonello, S. (1996). *Social skills development: Practical strategies for adolescents and adults with developmental disabilities.* Boston: Allyn & Bacon.

Arvidsson, T., Danielsson, B., Forsberg, P., Gillberg, C., Goteborg, M. J., & Kjellgren, G. (1997). Autism in 3–6-year-old children in a suburb of Göteborg, Sweden. *Autism, 1,* 163–173.

Asarnow, J. R. (1994). Childhood-onset schizophrenia. *Journal of Child Psychology and Psychiatry, 35,* 1345–1371.

Asarnow, J. R., Tompson, M., & McGrath, E. P. (2004). Childhood-onset schizophrenia: Clinical and treatment issues. *Journal of Child Psychology and Psychiatry, 45,* 180–194.

Asperger, H. (1991). 'Autistic psychopathy' in childhood (U. Frith, Trans.). In U. Frith (Ed.), *Autism and Asperger syndrome* (pp. 37–92). Cambridge, UK: Cambridge University Press. (Original work published 1944)

Attwood, T. (1998). *Asperger's syndrome: A guide for parents and professionals.* London: Kingsley.

Attwood, T. (2003). Frameworks for behavioral interventions. *Child and Adolescent Psychiatric Clinics of North America, 12,* 65–86.

Auton v. British Columbia, S.C.C. 78. (2004). Retrieved from www.lexum.umontreal.ca/csc-scc/en/rec/html/2004scc078.wpd.html

Baieli, S., Pavone, L., Meli, C., Fiumara, A., & Coleman, M. (2003). Autism and phenylketonuria. *Journal of Autism and Developmental Disorders, 33,* 201–204.

Bailey, A., LeCouteur, A., Gottesman, L., Bolton, P., Simonoff, E., Yuzda, E., et al. (1995). Autism as a strongly genetic disorder: Evidence from a British twin study. *Psychological Medicine, 25,* 63–77.

Bailey, A., Phillips, W., & Rutter, M. (1996). Autism: Towards an integration of clinical, genetic, neuropsychological, and neurobiological perspectives. *Journal of Child Psychology and Psychiatry, 37,* 89–126.

Baird, G., Charman, T., Baron-Cohen, S., Cox, A., Swettenham, J., Wheelwright, S., et al. (2000). A screening instrument for autism at 18 months of age: A 6-year follow-up study. *Journal of the American Academy of Child and Adolescent Psychiatry, 39,* 694–702.

Baker, B. L. (1996). Parent training. In J. W. Jacobson & J. A. Mulick (Eds.), *Manual of diagnosis and professional practice in mental retardation* (pp. 289–299). Washington, DC: American Psychological Association.

Baker, B. L., Heifetz, L. J., & Murphy, D. M. (1980). Behavioral training for parents of mentally retarded children: One-year follow-up. *American Journal of Mental Deficiency, 85,* 31–38.

Baker, B. L., McIntyre, L. L., Blacher, J., Crnic, K., Edelbrock, C., & Low, C. (2003). Preschool children with and without developmental delay: Behaviour problems and parenting stress over time. *Journal of Intellectual Disability Research, 47,* 217–230.

Ball, L. K., Ball, R., & Pratt, R. D. (2001). An assessment of thimerosal use in childhood vaccines. *Pediatrics, 107,* 1147–1154.

Ballaban-Gil, K., Rapin, I., Tuchman, R., & Shinnar, S. (1996). Longitudinal examination of the behavioral, language, and social changes in a population of adolescents and young adults with autistic disorder. *Pediatric Neurology, 15,* 217–223.

Baranek, G. T. (1999). Autism during infancy: A retrospective video analysis of sensory–motor and social behaviours at 9–12 months of age. *Journal of Autism and Developmental Disorders, 29,* 213–224.

Barbaresi, W. J., Katusic, S. K., Colligan, R. C., Weaver, A. L., & Jacobsen, S. J. (2005). The incidence of autism in Olmsted County, Minnesota, 1976–1997. *Archives of Pediatrics and Adolescent Medicine, 159,* 37–44.

Barlow, W. E., Davis, R. L., Glasser, J. W., Rhodes, P. H., Thompson, R. S., Mullool, J. P., et al. (2001). The risk of seizures after receipt of whole-cell pertussis or measles, mumps, and rubella vaccine. *New England Journal of Medicine, 345,* 656–651.

Barnby, G., & Monaco, A. P. (2003). Strategies for autism candidate gene analysis. *Novartis Foundation Symposium, 251,* 48–63.

Baron-Cohen, S. (2001). Theory of mind and autism: A review. *International Review of Research in Mental Retardation, 23,* 170–184.

Baron-Cohen, S., Allen, J., & Gillberg, C. (1992). Can autism be detected at 18 months?: The needle, the haystack, and the CHAT. *British Journal of Psychiatry, 161,* 839–843.

Baron-Cohen, S., Leslie, A. M., & Frith, U. (1985). Does the autistic child have a "theory of mind"? *Cognition, 21,* 37–46.

Baron-Cohen, S., Ring, H. A., Bullmore, E. T., Wheelwright, S., Ashwin, C., & Williams, S. C. (2000). The amygdala theory of autism. *Neuroscience and Biobehavioral Reviews, 24,* 355–364.

Baron-Cohen, S., Ring, H. A., Wheelwright, S., Bullmore, E. T., Brammer, M. J., Simmons, A., et al. (1999). Social intelligence in the normal and autistic brain: An fMRI study. *European Journal of Neuroscience, 11,* 1891–1898.

Baron-Cohen, S., Wheelwright, S., Stone, V., & Rutherford, M. (1999). A mathematician, a physicist and a computer scientist with Asperger syndrome: Performance on psychology and folk physics tests. *Neurocase, 5,* 475–483.

Barrett, R. P., Feinstein, C., & Hole, W. T. (1989). Effects of naloxone and naltrexone on self injury: A double-blind, placebo-controlled analysis. *American Journal on Mental Retardation, 93,* 644–651.

Bass, M. P., Menold, M. M., Wolpert, C. M., Donnelly, S. L., Ravan, S. A., Hauser, E, R., et al. (2000). Genetic studies in autistic disorder and chromosome 15. *Neurogenetics, 2,* 219–226.

Bauman, M. L., Kemper, T. L., & Arin, D. M. (1995). Pervasive neuroanatomic abnormalities of the brain in three cases of Rett's syndrome. *Neurology, 45,* 1581–1586.

Bauminger, N. (2002). The facilitation of social-emotional understanding and social interaction in high-functioning children with autism: Intervention outcomes. *Journal of Autism and Developmental Disorders, 32,* 283–298.

Bauminger, N., & Kasari, C. (1999). Theory of mind in high-functioning children with autism. *Journal of Autism and Developmental Disorders, 29,* 81–86.

Baumrind, D. (1996). The discipline controversy revisited. *Family Relations: Journal of Applied Family and Child Studies, 45,* 405–414.

Becker-Cottrill, B., McFarland, J., & Anderson, V. (2003). A model of positive behavioral support for individuals with autism and their families: The family focus process. *Focus on Autism and Other Developmental Disabilities, 18,* 110–121.

Belchic, J. K., & Harris, S. L. (1994). The use of multiple peer exemplars to enhance the generalization of play skills to siblings of children with autism. *Child and Family Behavior Therapy, 16,* 1–25.

Belmonte, M. K., & Yurgelun-Todd, D. A. (2003). Functional anatomy of impaired selective attention and compensatory processing in autism. *Cognitive Brain Research, 17,* 651–664.

Bernard, S., Enayati, A., Redwood, L., Roger, H., & Binstock, T. (2001). Autism: A novel form of mercury poisoning. *Medical Hypotheses, 56,* 462–471.

Bertrand, J., Mars, A., Boyle, C., Bove, F., Yeargin-Allsopp, M., & Decoufle, P. (2001). Prevalence of autism in a United States population: The Brick Township, New Jersey, investigation. *Pediatrics, 108,* 1155–1161.

Bibby, P., Eikeseth, S., Martin, N. T., Mudford, O. C., & Reeves, D. (2001). Progress and outcomes for children with autism receiving parent-managed intensive interventions. *Research in Developmental Disabilities, 23,* 81–104.

Bienvenu, T., Carrie, A., de Roux, N., Vinet, M. C., Jonveaux, P., Couvert, P., et al. (2000). MECP2 mutations account for most cases of typical forms of Rett syndrome. *Human Molecular Genetics, 9,* 1377–1384.

Birnbrauer, J. S., & Leach, D. J. (1993). The Murdoch early intervention program after two years. *Behaviour Change, 10,* 63–74.

Black, C., Kaye, J. A., & Jick, H. (2003). MMR vaccine and idiopathic thrombocytopaenic purpura. *British Journal of Clinical Pharmacology, 55,* 107–111.

Bondy, A. S., & Frost, L. A. (1994). The Picture Exchange Communication System. *Focus on Autistic Behavior, 9,* 1–19.

Bondy, A., Tincani, M., & Frost, L. (2004). Multiply controlled verbal operants: An analysis and extension to the Picture Exchange Communication System. *The Behavior Analyst, 27,* 247–261.

Bouvard, M., Leboyer, M., Launay, J., Recasens, C., Plunet, M. I I., Waller-Perotte, D., et al. (1995). Low-dose naltrexone effects on plasma chemistries and clinical symptoms in autism: A double-blind, placebo-controlled study. *Psychiatry Research, 58,* 191–201.

Brady, M. P., Shores, R. E., Gunter, P., McEvoy, M. A., Fox, J. J., & White, C. (1984). Generalization of an adolescent's social interaction behavior via multiple peers in a classroom setting. *Journal of the Association for Persons with Severe Handicaps, 9,* 278–286.

Brady, M. P., Shores, R. E., McEvoy, M. A., Ellis, D., & Fox, J. J. (1987). Increasing social interactions of severely handicapped autistic children. *Journal of Autism and Developmental Disorders, 17,* 375–390.

Brambilla, P., Hardan, A., Ucelli di Nemi, S., Perez, J., Soares, J. C., & Barale, F. (2003). Brain anatomy and development in autism: Review of structural MRI studies. *Brain Research Bulletin, 61,* 557–569.

Brasic, J. R., Barnett, J. Y., Kaplan, D., Sheitman, B. B., Aisemberg, P., Lafargue, R. T., et al. (1994). Clomipramine ameliorates adventitious movements and compulsions in prepubertal boys with autistic disorder and severe mental retardation. *Neurology, 44,* 1309–1312.

Breen, C., Haring, T., Pitts-Conway, V., & Gaylord-Ross, R. (1985). The training and generalization of social interaction during breaktime at two job sites in the natural environment. *Journal of the Association for Persons with Severe Handicaps, 10,* 41–50.

Bristol, M. M. (1984). Family resources and successful adaptation to autistic children. In E. Schopler & G. B. Mesibov (Eds.), *The effects of autism on the family* (pp. 289–310). New York: Plenum Press.

Brodkin, E. S., McDougle, C. J., Naylor, S. T., Cohen, D. J., & Price, L. H. (1997). Clomipramine in adults with pervasive developmental disorders: A prospective open-label investigation. *Journal of Child and Adolescent Psychopharmacology, 7,* 109–121.

Brown, F. (1991). Creative daily scheduling: A nonintrusive approach to challenging behaviors in community residences. *Journal of the Association for Persons with Severe Handicaps, 16,* 75–84.

Bryson, S. E., Clark, B. S., & Smith, I. M. (1988). First report of a Canadian epidemiological study of autistic syndromes. *Journal of Child Psychology and Psychiatry, 29,* 433–446.

Bryson, S. E., Rogers, S. J., & Fombonne, E. (2003). Autism spectrum disorders: Early detection, intervention, education, and psychopharmacological man-agement. *Canadian Journal of Psychiatry, 48,* 506–516.

Bryson, S. E., Rombough, V., McDermott, C., Wainwright, A., Szatmari, P., & Zwaigenbaum, L. (2001, November). *Autism Observation Scale for Infants: Scale development and preliminary reliability data.* Poster presented at the International Meeting for Autism Research, San Diego, CA.

Butter, E. M. (2003, August). What parents have learned about autism intervention. In J. A. Mulick (Chair), *Preliminary reports from the Ohio Autism Recovery Project.* Symposium conducted at the convention of the American Psychological Association, Toronto.

California Department of Developmental Services. (1999, March 1). *Changes in the population of persons with autism and pervasive developmental disorders in California's developmental services system: 1987 through 1998. Report to the Legislature.* Retrieved from www.dds.ca.gov/Autism/pdf/Autism_Report_1999.pdf

California Department of Developmental Services. (2003, April). *Autistic spectrum disorders: Changes in the California caseload. An update: 1999 through 2002.* Retrieved from www.dds.ca.gov/Autism/pdf/AutismReport2003.pdf

Campbell, M., Anderson, L., Small, A., Adams, P., Gonzalez, N., & Ernst, M. (1993). Naltrexone in autistic children: Behavioral symptoms and attentional learning. *Journal of the American Academy of Child and Adolescent Psychiatry, 32,* 1283–1291.

Campbell, M., Armenteros, J. L., Malone, R. P., Adams, P. B., Eisenberg, Z. W., & Overall, J. E. (1997). Neuroleptic-related dyskinesias in autistic children: A prospective, longitudinal study. *Journal of the American Academy of Child and Adolescent Psychiatry, 35,* 134–143.

Campbell, M., Schopler, E., Cueva, J. E., & Hallin, A. (1996). Treatment of autistic disorder. *Journal of the American Academy of Child and Adolescent Psychiatry, 35,* 134–143.

Caronna, E. B., & Halfon, N. (2003). Dipping deeper into the reservoir of autistic spectrum disorder. *Archives of Pediatrics and Adolescent Medicine, 157,* 619–621.

Carpentieri, S. C., & Morgan, S. B. (1994). A comparison of patterns of cognitive functioning of autistic and nonautistic retarded children on the Stanford–Binet—Fourth Edition. *Journal of Autism and Developmental Disorders, 24,* 215–223.

Carr, E. G. (1977). The motivation of self-injurious behavior: A review of some hypotheses. *Psychological Bulletin, 84,* 800–816.

Carr, E. G. (1981). Sign language. In O. I. Lovaas (Ed.), *Teaching developmentally disabled children* (pp. 153–161). Austin, TX: Pro-Ed.

Carr, E. G. (1985). Behavioral approaches to language and communication. In E. Schopler & G. B. Mesibov (Eds.), *Communication problems in autism* (pp. 37–57). New York: Plenum Press.

Carr, E. G., Binkoff, J. A., Kologinsky, E., & Eddy, M. (1978). Acquisition of sign language by autistic children: I. Expressive labelling. *Journal of Applied Behavior Analysis, 11,* 489–501.

Carr, E. G., & Dores, P. A. (1981). Patterns of language acquisition following simultaneous communication with autistic children. *Analysis and Intervention in Developmental Disabilities, 1,* 347–361.

Carr, E. G., Dunlap, G., Horner, R. H., Koegel, R. L., Turnbull, A. P., Sailor, W., et al. (2002). Positive behavior support: Evolution of an applied science. *Journal of Positive Behavior Interventions, 4,* 4–16.

Carr, E. G., & Durand, V. M. (1985). Reducing behavior problems through functional communication training. *Journal of Applied Behavior Analysis, 18,* 111–126.

Carr, E. G., Horner, R. H., Turnbull, A. P., Marquis, J. G., Magito-McLaughlin, D., McAtee, M. L., et al. (1999). *Positive behavior support for people with developmental disabilities: A research synthesis.* Washington, DC: American Association on Mental Retardation.

Carr, E. G., & Kologinsky, E. (1983). Acquisition of sign language by autistic children: II. Spontaneity and generalization effects. *Journal of Applied Behavior Analysis, 16,* 297–314.

Carr, E. G., Levin, L., McConnachie, G., Carlson, J. I., Kemp, D. C., & Smith, C. E. (1994). *Communication-based intervention for problem behavior.* Baltimore: Brookes.

Carr, E. G., Magito-McLaughlin, D., Giacobbe-Grieco, T., & Smith, C. E. (2003). Using mood ratings and mood induction in assessment and intervention for severe problem behavior. *American Journal on Mental Retardation, 108,* 32–55.

Carr, E. G., & McDowell, J. J. (1980). Social control of self-injurious behavior of organic etiology. *Behavior Therapy, 11,* 402–409.

Carr, E. G., & Newsom, C. (1985). Demand-related tantrums: Conceptualization and treatment. *Behavior Modification, 9,* 403–426.

Carr, E. G., Reeve, C. E., & Magito-McLaughlin, D. (1996). Contextual influences on problem behavior in people with developmental disabilities. In L. K. Koegel, R. L. Koegel, & G. Dunlap (Eds.), *Positive behavioral support: Including people with difficult behavior in the community* (pp. 403–423). Baltimore: Brookes.

Carr, E. G., & Smith, C. E. (1995). Biological setting events for self-injury. *Mental Retardation and Developmental Disabilities Research Reviews, 1,* 94–98.

Carr, E. G., Smith, C. E., Giacin, T. A., Whelan, B. M., & Pancari, J. (2003). Menstrual discomfort as a biological setting event for severe problem behavior: Assessment and intervention. *American Journal on Mental Retardation, 108,* 117–133.

Carr, E. G., Yarbrough, S. C., & Langdon, N. A. (1997). Effects of idiosyncratic stimulus variables on functional analysis outcomes. *Journal of Applied Behavior Analysis, 30,* 673–686.

Cecil, S. (2004). Autism interrupted?: Baby sibs study holds hope for reversing behaviors before they become embedded. *CAIRN Review of Evidence-Based Diagnosis and Treatment in Autism, 1,* 2.

Celiberti, D. A., & Harris, S. L. (1993). Behavioral intervention for siblings of children with autism: A focus on skills to enhance play. *Behavior Therapy, 24,* 573–599.

Ceponiene, R., Lepisto, T., Shestakova, A., Vanhala, R., Alku, P., Naatanen, R., et al. (2003). Speech–sound–selective auditory impairment in children with autism: They can perceive but do not attend. *Proceedings of the National Academy of Sciences USA, 100,* 5567–5572.

Chakrabarti, S., & Fombonne, E. (2001). Pervasive developmental disorders in preschool children. *Journal of the American Medical Association, 285,* 3093–3099.

Chakrabarti, S., & Fombonne, E. (2005). Pervasive developmental disorders in preschool children: Confirmation of high prevalence. *American Journal of Psychiatry, 162,* 1133–1141.

Challman, T. D., Barbaresi, W. J., Katusic, S. K., & Weaver, A. (2003). The yield of the medical evaluation of children with pervasive developmental disorders. *Journal of Autism and Developmental Disorders, 33,* 187–192.

Chandler, L. K., Lubek, R. C., & Fowler, S. A. (1992). Generalization and maintenance of preschool children's social skills: A critical review and analysis. *Journal of Applied Behavior Analysis, 25,* 415–428.

Charlop, M. H., Schreibman, L., & Thibodeau, M. G. (1985). Increasing spontaneous verbal responding in autistic children using a time delay procedure. *Journal of Applied Behavior Analysis, 18,* 155–166.

Charlop, M. H., & Trasowech, J. E. (1991). Increasing autistic children's daily spontaneous speech. *Journal of Applied Behavior Analysis, 24,* 747–761.

Charlop-Christy, M. H., Carpenter, M., Le, L., LeBlanc, L. A., & Kellet, K. (2002). Using the Picture Exchange Communication System (PECS) with children with autism: Assessment of PECS acquisition, speech, social-communicative behavior, and problem behavior. *Journal of Applied Behavior Analysis, 35,* 213–231.

Charman, T., & Baird, G. (2002). Practitioner review: Diagnosis of autism spectrum disorder in 2- and 3-year-old children. *Journal of Child Psychology and Psychiatry, 43,* 289–305.

Chess, S. (1977). Follow-up report on autism in congenital rubella. *Journal of Autism and Childhood Schizophrenia, 7,* 79–81.

Chorpita, B. F., Yim, L. M., Donkervoet, J. C., Arensdorf, A., Amundsen, M. J., McGee, C., et al. (2002). Toward large-scale implementation of empirically supported treatments for children: A review and observations by the Hawaii Empirical Basis to Services Task Force. *Clinical Psychology: Science and Practice, 9,* 165–189.

Christman, A. K., Fermo, J. D., & Markowitz, J. S.

(2004). Atomoxetine, a novel treatment for attention-deficit-hyperactivity disorder. *Pharmacotherapy, 24,* 1020–1036.

Clements, C. J., & Ratzan, S. (2003). Misled and confused?: Telling the public about MMR vaccine safety. *Journal of Medical Ethics, 29,* 22–26.

Cohen, D. J., Paul, R., & Volkmar, F. R. (1986). Issues in the classification of pervasive and other developmental disorders: Toward DSM-IV. *Journal of the American Academy of Child Psychiatry, 25,* 213–220.

Comi, A. M., Zimmerman, A. W., Frye, V. H., Law, P. A., & Peeden, J. N. (1999). Familial clustering of autoimmune disorders and evaluation of medical risk factors in autism. *Journal of Child Neurology, 14,* 388–394.

Connolly, A. M., Chez, M. G., Pestronk, A., Arnold, S. T., Mehta, S., & Deuel, R. K. (1999). Serum autoantibodies to brain in Landau–Kleffner variant, autism, and other neurologic disorders. *Journal of Pediatrics, 134,* 607–613.

Courchesne, E., Carper, R., & Akshoomoff, N. (2003). Evidence of brain overgrowth in the first year of life in autism. *Journal of the American Medical Association, 290,* 337–344.

Courchesne, E., Townsend, J., Akshoomoff, N. A., Saitoh, O., Yeung-Courchesne, R., Lincoln, A. J., et al. (1994). Impairment in shifting attention in autistic and cerebellar patients. *Behavioral Neuroscience, 108,* 848–865.

Croen, L. A., Grether, J. K., Hoogstrate, J., & Selvin, S. (2002). The changing prevalence of autism in California. *Journal of Autism and Developmental Disorders, 32,* 207–215.

Crosland, K. A., Zarcone, J. R., Lindauer, S. E., Valdovinos, M. G., Zarcone, T. J., Hellings, J. A., et al. (2003). Use of functional analysis methodology in the evaluation of medication effects. *Journal of Autism and Developmental Disorders, 33,* 271–279.

Dadds, M. R., Sanders, M. R., Behrens, B. C., & James, J. E. (1987). Marital discord and child behavior problems: A description of family interactions during treatment. *Journal of Clinical Child Psychology, 16,* 192–203.

Dales, L., Hammer, S. J., & Smith, N. J. (2001). Time trends in autism and in MMR immunization coverage in California. *Journal of the American Medical Association, 285,* 1183–1185.

D'Ateno, P., Mangiapanello, K., & Taylor, B. A. (2003). Teaching complex play sequences to a preschooler with autism using video modeling. *Journal of Positive Behavioral Interventions, 5,* 5–11.

Davidovitch, M., Glick, L., Holtzman, G., Tirosh, E., & Safir, M. P. (2000). Developmental regression in autism: Maternal perception. *Journal of Autism and Developmental Disorders, 30,* 113–119.

Davis, R. L., & Bohlke, K. (2001). Measles vaccination and inflammatory bowel disease: Controversy laid to rest? *Drug Safety, 24,* 939–946.

Dawson, G., Meltzoff, A. N., Osterling, J., Rinaldi, J., & Brown, E. (1998). Children with autism fail to orient to naturally occurring social stimuli. *Journal of Autism and Developmental Disorders, 28,* 479–485.

Dawson, G., & Osterling, J. (1997). Early intervention in autism: Effectiveness and common elements of current approaches. In M. J. Guralnick (Ed.), *The effectiveness of early intervention* (pp. 307–326). Baltimore: Brookes.

Dawson, G., Osterling, J., Rinaldi, J., Carver, L., & McPartland, J. (2001). Recognition memory and stimulus–reward associations: Indirect support for the role of ventromedial prefrontal dysfunction in autism. *Journal of Autism and Developmental Disorders, 31,* 337–341.

De Bona, C., Zappella, M., Hayek, G., Meloni, I., Vitelli, F., Bruttini, M., et al. (2000). Preserved speech variant is allelic of classic Rett syndrome. *European Journal of Human Genetics, 8,* 325–330.

DeLong, G. R., Ritch, C. R., & Burch, S. (2002). Fluoxetine response in children with autistic spectrum disorders: Correlation with familial major affective disorder and intellectual achievement. *Developmental Medicine and Child Neurology, 44,* 652–659.

DeLong, G. R., Teague, L. A., & Kamran, M. M. (1998). Effects of fluoxetine treatment in young children with idiopathic autism. *Developmental Medicine and Child Neurology, 40,* 551–562.

Delprato, D. J. (2001). Comparisons of discrete-trial and normalized behavioral language interventions for young children with autism. *Journal of Autism and Developmental Disorders, 31,* 315–325.

DeMyer, M. K., Barton, S., DeMyer, W. E., Norton, J. A., Allen, J., & Steele, R. (1973). Prognosis in autism: A follow-up study. *Journal of Autism and Childhood Schizophrenia, 3,* 199–246.

Dennis, M., Lazenby, A. L., & Lockyer, L. (2001). Inferential language in high-function children with autism. *Journal of Autism and Developmental Disorders, 31,* 47–54.

Duclos, P., & Ward, B. J. (1998). Measles vaccines: A review of adverse events. *Drug Safety, 19,* 435–454.

Dugan, E., Kamps, D., Leonard, B., Watkins, N., Rheinberger, A., & Stackhaus, J. (1995). Effects of cooperative learning groups during social studies for students with autism and fourth-grade peers. *Journal of Applied Behavior Analysis, 28,* 175–188.

Dumas, J. E. (1984). Indiscriminate mothering: Empirical findings and theoretical speculations. *Advances in Behaviour Research and Therapy, 6,* 13–27.

Dunst, C. J., Trivette, C. M., & Deal, A. G. (1994). *Supporting and strengthening families: Methods, strategies, and practices.* Cambridge, MA: Brookline Books.

Durand, V. M. (1990). *Severe behavior problems: A functional communication training approach.* New York: Guilford Press.

Durand, V. M., & Carr, E. G. (1987). Social influences on "self-stimulatory" behavior: Analysis and treatment application. *Journal of Applied Behavior Analysis, 20,* 119–132.

Durand, V. M., & Crimmins, D. B. (1987). Assessment and treatment of psychotic speech in an autistic child. *Journal of Autism and Developmental Disorders, 17,* 17–28.

Durand, V. M., & Crimmins, D. B. (1988). Identifying the variables maintaining self-injurious behavior. *Journal of Autism and Developmental Disorders, 18,* 99–117.

Dykens, E., Volkmar, F., & Glick, M. (1991). Thought disorder in high-functioning autistic adults. *Journal of Autism and Developmental Disorders, 21,* 291–301.

Eason, L. J., White, M. J., & Newsom, C. (1982). Generalized reduction of self-stimulatory behavior: An effect of teaching appropriate play to autistic children. *Analysis and Intervention in Developmental Disabilities, 2,* 157–169.

Eaves, L. C., & Ho, H. H. (1996). Brief report: Stability and change in cognitive and behavioral characteristics of autism through childhood. *Journal of Autism and Developmental Disorders, 26,* 557–569.

Eigisti, I. M., & Shapiro, T. (2003). A systems neuroscience approach to autism: Biological, cognitive and clinical perspectives. *Mental Retardation and Developmental Disabilities Research Reviews, 9,* 205–215.

Eikeseth, S., Smith, T., Jahr, E., & Eldevik, S. (2002). Intensive behavioral treatment at school for 4- to 7-year-old children with autism: A 1-year comparison controlled study. *Behavior Modification, 26,* 49–68.

Elliott, R. O., Hall, K., & Soper, H. V. (1991). Analog language teaching versus natural language teaching: Generalization and retention of language learning for adults with autism and mental retardation. *Journal of Autism and Developmental Disorders, 21,* 433–447.

Epstein, L. J., Taubman, M. T., & Lovaas, O. I. (1985). Changes in self-stimulatory behaviors with treatment. *Journal of Abnormal Child Psychology, 13,* 281–294.

Esch, B. E., & Carr, J. E. (2004). Secretin as a treatment for autism: A review of the evidence. *Journal of Autism and Developmental Disorders, 34,* 543–556.

Fatemi, S. H., Realmuto, G. M., Khan, L., & Thuras, P. (1998). Fluoxetine in treatment of adolescent patients with autism: A longitudinal open trial. *Journal of Autism and Developmental Disorders, 28,* 303–307.

Fecteau, S., Mottron, L., Berthiaume, C., & Burack, J. A. (2003). Developmental changes of autistic symptoms. *Autism, 7,* 255–268.

Fein, D., Lucci, D., Braverman, M., & Waterhouse, L. (1992). Comprehension of affect in context in children with pervasive developmental disorders. *Journal of Child Psychology and Psychiatry, 33,* 1157–1167.

Fenske, E. C., Krantz, P. J., & McClannahan, L. E. (2001). Incidental teaching: A not-discrete-trial teaching procedure. In C. Maurice, G. Green, & R.

M. Foxx (Eds.), *Making a difference: Behavioral intervention for autism* (pp. 75–82). Austin, TX: Pro-Ed.

Fenske, E. C., Zalenski, S., Krantz, P. J., & McClannahan, L. E. (1985). Age at intervention and treatment outcome for autistic children in a comprehensive intervention program. *Analysis and Intervention in Developmental Disabilities, 5,* 49–58.

Ferrel, D. R. (1990). *Communicative interaction between handicapped and nonhandicapped preschool children: Identifying facilitative strategies.* Unpublished doctoral dissertation, University of Pittsburgh.

Filipek, P. A., Accardo, P. J., Baranek, G. T., Cook, E. H., Dawson, G., Gordon, B., et al. (1999). The screening and diagnosis of autistic spectrum disorders. *Journal of Autism and Developmental Disorders, 29,* 439–484.

Finkel, A. S., & Williams, R. L. (2001). A comparison of textual and echoic prompts on the acquisition of intraverbal behavior in a six-year-old boy with autism. *Analysis of Verbal Behavior, 18,* 61–70.

Flannery, K. B., & Horner, R. H. (1994). The relationship between predictability and problem behavior for students with severe disabilities. *Journal of Behavioral Education, 4,* 157–176.

Folstein, S. E., & Rosen-Sheidley, B. (2001). Genetics of autism: Complex aetiology for a heterogeneous disorder. *Nature Reviews, 2,* 943–954.

Fombonne, E. (2003). Epidemiological surveys of autism and other pervasive developmental disorders: An update. *Journal of Autism and Developmental Disorders, 33,* 365–382.

Fombonne, E., & Chakrabarti, S. (2001). No evidence for a new variant of measles–mumps–rubella-induced autism. *Pediatrics, 108,* E58.

Fombonne, E., du Mazaubrun, C., Cans, C., & Grandjean, H. (1997). Autism and associated medical disorders in a French epidemiological survey. *Journal of the American Academy of Child and Adolescent Psychiatry, 36,* 1561–1569.

Fombonne, E., Simmons, H., Ford, T., Meltzer, H., & Goodman, R. (2003). Prevalence of pervasive developmental disorders in the British nationwide survey of child mental health. *International Review of Psychiatry, 15,* 158–165.

Fox, L., Benito, N., & Dunlap, G. (2002). Early intervention with families of young children with autism and behavior problems. In J. M. Lucyshyn, G. Dunlap, & R. W. Albin (Eds.), *Families and positive behavior support* (pp. 251–266). Baltimore: Brookes.

Frances, A., First, M. B., & Pincus, H. A. (1995). *DSM-IV guidebook.* Washington, DC: American Psychiatric Press.

Frea, W. D. (1995). Social-communicative skills in higher-functioning children with autism. In R. L. Koegel & L. K. Koegel (Eds.), *Teaching children with autism* (pp. 53–66). Baltimore: Brookes.

Freeman, B. J., Ritvo, E. R., Needleman, R., & Yokota, A. (1985). The stability of cognitive and linguistic parameters in autism: A five-year prospective study. *Journal of the American Academy of Child Psychiatry, 24*, 459–464.

Freudenheim, M. (2004, December 21). Battling insurers over autism treatment. *The New York Times*, p. C1. Retrieved from http://query.nytimes.com/gst/abstract.html?res=F30711FA38540C728EDDAB0994DC404482

Frith, U. (1989). *Autism: Explaining the enigma*. Cambridge, MA: Blackwell.

Frith, U. (1991). Asperger and his syndrome. In U. Frith (Ed.), *Autism and Asperger syndrome* (pp. 1–36). Cambridge, UK.: Cambridge University Press.

Frost, L. A., & Bondy, A. S. (1994). *The picture exchange communication system training manual*. Cherry Hill, NJ: Pyramid Educational Consultants.

Gajzago, C., & Prior, M. (1974). Two cases of "recovery" in Kanner syndrome. *Archives of General Psychiatry, 31*, 264–268.

Gaylord-Ross, R. J., Haring, T. G., Breen, C., & Pitts-Conway, V. (1984). The training and generalization of social interaction skills with autistic youth. *Journal of Applied Behavior Analysis, 17*, 229–247.

Geier, M. R., & Geier, D. A. (2003a). Neurodevelopmental disorders after thimerosal-containing vaccines: A brief communication. *Experimental Biology and Medicine, 228*, 660–664.

Geier, M. R., & Geier, D. A. (2003b). Thimerosal in childhood vaccines, neurodevelopment disorders, and heart disease in the United States. *Journal of American Physicians and Surgeons, 8*, 6–11.

Ghaziuddin, M., & Butler, E. (1998). Clumsiness in autism and Asperger syndrome: A further report. *Journal of Intellectual Disability Research, 42*, 43–48.

Ghaziuddin, M., Ghaziuddin, N., & Greden, J. (2002). Depression in persons with autism: Implications for research and clinical care. *Journal of Autism and Developmental Disorders, 32*, 299–306.

Ghaziuddin, M., Tsai, L. Y., Eilers, L., & Ghaziuddin, N. (1992). Autism and herpes simplex encephalitis. *Journal of Autism and Developmental Disorders, 22*, 107–113.

Gilchrist, A., Green, J., Cox, A., Burton, D., Rutter, M., & Le Couteur, A. (2001). Development and current functioning in adolescents with Asperger syndrome: A comparative study. *Journal of Child Psychology and Psychiatry, 42*, 227–240.

Gillberg, C. (1992). The Emanuel Miller Memorial Lecture 1991. Autism and autistic-like conditions: Subclasses among disorders of empathy. *Journal of Child Psychology and Psychiatry, 33*, 813–842.

Gillberg, C. (2001). Asperger syndrome and high functioning autism: Shared deficits or different disorders? *Journal of Developmental and Learning Disorders, 5*, 79–94.

Gillberg, C., & Billstedt, E. (2000). Autism and Asperger syndrome: Coexistence with other clinical disorders. *Acta Psychiatrica Scandinavica, 102*, 321–330.

Gillberg, C., & Coleman, M. (1996). Autism and medical disorders: A review of the literature. *Developmental Medicine and Child Neurology, 38*, 191–202.

Gillberg, C., & Forsell, C. (1984). Childhood psychosis and neurofibromatosis: More than a coincidence? *Journal of Autism and Developmental Disorders, 14*, 1–8.

Gillberg, C., Gillberg, C., Rastam, M., & Wentz, E. (2001). The Asperger Syndrome (and high-functioning autism) Diagnostic Interview (ASDI): A preliminary study of a new structured clinical interview. *Autism, 5*, 57–66.

Gillberg, C., & Steffenburg, S. (1987). Outcome and prognostic factors in infantile autism and similar conditions: A population-based study of 46 cases followed through puberty. *Journal of Autism and Developmental Disorders, 17*, 273–287.

Gillberg, C., Steffenburg, S., & Schaumann, H. (1991). Is autism more common now than 10 years ago? *British Journal of Psychiatry, 158*, 403–409.

Gillberg, I. C., & Gillberg, C. (1989). Asperger's syndrome—some epidemiological considerations: A research note. *Journal of Child Psychology and Psychiatry, 30*, 631–638.

Gilliam, J. E. (2003). *Gilliam Asperger's Disorder Scale*. Lutz, FL: Psychological Assessment Resources.

Gillham, J. E., Carter, A. S., Volkmar, F. R., & Sparrow, S. S. (2000). Toward a developmental operational definition of autism. *Journal of Autism and Developmental Disorders, 30*, 269–278.

Goldstein, H. (2002). Communication intervention for children with autism: A review of treatment efficacy. *Journal of Autism and Developmental Disorders, 32*, 373–396.

Goldstein, H., & Cisar, C. L. (1992). Promoting interaction during sociodramatic play: Teaching scripts to typical preschoolers and classmates with disabilities. *Journal of Applied Behavior Analysis, 25*, 265–280.

Goldstein, H., Kaczmarek, L., Pennington, R., & Shafer, K. (1992). Peer-mediated intervention: Attending to, commenting on, and acknowledging the behavior of preschoolers with autism. *Journal of Applied Behavior Analysis, 25*, 289–305.

Gonzales-Lopez, A., & Kamps, D. M. (1997). Social skills training to increase social interactions between children with autism and their typical peers. *Focus on Autism and Other Developmental Disabilities, 12*, 2–14.

Gordon, C. T., Rapoport, J. L., Hamburger, S. D., State, R. C., & Mannheim, G. B. (1992). Differential response of seven subjects with autistic disorder to clomipramine and desipramine. *American Journal of Psychiatry, 149*, 363–366.

Gordon, C. T., State, R. C., Nelson, J. E., Hamburger, S. D., & Rapoport, J. L. (1993). A double-blind comparison of clomipramine, desipramine, and placebo in the treatment of autistic disorder. *Archives of General Psychiatry, 50*, 441–447.

Green, G. (1996). Early behavioral intervention for autism: What does research tell us? In C. Maurice, G. Green, & S. C. Luce (Eds.), Behavioral intervention for young children with autism (pp. 2–44). Austin, TX: Pro-Ed.

Green, G., Brennan, L. C., & Fein, D. (2002). Intensive behavioral treatment for a toddler at high risk for autism. Behavior Modification, 26, 69–102.

Green, J., Gilchrist, A., Burton, D., & Cox, A. (2000). Social and psychiatric functioning in adolescents with Asperger syndrome compared with conduct disorder. Journal of Autism and Developmental Disorders, 30, 279–293.

Gresham, F. M., & MacMillan, D. L. (1998). Early Intervention Project: Can its claims be substantiated and its effects replicated? Journal of Autism and Developmental Disorders, 28, 5–13.

Griffith, E. M., Pennington, B. F., Wehner, E. A., & Rogers, S. J. (1999). Executive functions in young children with autism. Child Development, 70, 817–832.

Groden, G., Domingue, D., Chesnick, M., Groden, J., & Baron, G. (1983). Early intervention with autistic children: A case presentation with pre-program, program and follow-up data. Psychological Reports, 53, 715–722.

Guess, D., & Carr, E. (1991). Emergence and maintenance of stereotypy and self-injury. American Journal on Mental Retardation, 96, 299–319.

Gunsett, R. P., Mulick, J. A., Fernald, W. B., & Martin, J. L. (1989). Briefreport: Indications for medical screening prior to behavioral programming for severely and profoundly mentally retarded clients. Journal of Autism and Developmental Disorders, 19, 167–172.

Gunter, H. L., Ghaziuddin, M., & Ellis, H. D. (2002). Asperger syndrome: Tests of right hemisphere functioning and interhemispheric communication. Journal of Autism and Developmental Disorders, 32, 263–281.

Gurney, J. G., Fritz, M. S., Ness, K. K., Sievers, P., Newschaffer, C. J., & Shapiro, E. G. (2003). Analysis of prevalence trends of autism spectrum disorder in Minnesota. Archives of Pediatrics and Adolescent Medicine, 157, 622–627.

Hagberg, B. (1995). Clinical delineation of Rett syndrome variants. Neuropediatrics, 26, 62.

Hadwin, J., Baron-Cohen, S., Howlin, P., & Hill, K. (1997). Does teaching theory of mind have an effect on the ability to develop conversation in children with autism? Journal of Autism and Developmental Disorders, 27, 519–537.

Haith, M. M., Bergman, T., & Moore, M. J. (1979). Eye contact and face scanning in early infancy. Science, 198, 853–855.

Hall, G. A., & Sundberg, M. L. (1987). Teaching mands by manipulating conditioned establishing operations. Analysis of Verbal Behavior, 5, 41–53.

Halsey, N. A., & Hyman, S. L. (2001). Measles–mumps–rubella vaccine and autistic spectrum disorder: Report from the New Challenges in Childhood Immunizations Conference convened in Oak Brook, Illinois, June 12–13, 2000. Pediatrics, 107, E84.

Handleman, J. S., & Harris, S. L. (Eds.). (2000). Preschool education programs for children with autism (2nd ed.). Austin, TX: Pro-Ed.

Happe, F. G. E. (1991). The autobiographical writings of three Asperger syndrome adults: Problems of interpretation and implications for theory. In U. Frith (Ed.), Autism and Asperger syndrome (pp. 207–242). Cambridge, UK: Cambridge University Press.

Happe, F. G. E. (1993). Communicative competence and theory of mind: A test of relevance theory. Cognition, 48, 101–119.

Happe, F. G. E. (1995). The role of age and verbal ability in the theory of mind task performance of subjects with autism. Child Development, 66, 843–855.

Happe, F. G. E. (1996). Studying weak central coherence at low levels: Children with autism do not succumb to visual illusions. A research note. Journal of Child Psychology and Psychiatry, 37, 873–877.

Happe, F. G. E. (1997). Central coherence and theory of mind in autism: Reading homographs in context. British Journal of Developmental Psychology, 15, 1–12.

Hardan, A. Y., & Handen, B. L. (2002). A retrospective open trial of adjunctive donepezil in children and adolescents with autistic disorder. Journal of Child and Adolescent Psychopharmacology, 12, 237–241.

Haring, T. G., & Breen, C. G. (1992). A peer-mediated social network intervention to enhance the social integration of persons with moderate and severe disabilities. Journal of Applied Behavior Analysis, 25, 319–131.

Haring, T. G., & Lovinger, L. (1989). Promoting social interaction through teaching generalized play initiation responses to preschool children with autism. Journal of the Association for Persons with Severe Handicaps, 14, 58–67.

Harris, S. L. (1986). A 4- to 7-year questionnaire follow-up of participants in a training program for parents of autistic children. Journal of Autism and Developmental Disorders, 16, 377–383.

Harris, S. L. (1994). Siblings of children with autism: Guide for families. Bethesda, MD: Woodbine House.

Harris, S. L., & Handleman, J. S. (2000). Age and IQ at intake as predictors of placement for young children with autism: A four- to six-year follow-up. Journal of Autism and Developmental Disorders, 30, 137–142.

Harris, S. L., Handelman, J. S., Gordon, R., Kristoff, B., & Fuentes, F. (1991). Changes in cognitive and language functioning of preschool children with autism. Journal of Autism and Developmental Disorders, 21, 281–290.

Harris, T. A., Peterson, S. L., Filliben, T. L., Glassberg, M., & Favell, J. E. (1998). Evaluating a more cost-efficient alternative to providing in-home feedback to parents: The use of spousal feedback. Journal of Applied Behavior Analysis, 31, 131–134.

Hauck, M., Fein, D., Waterhouse, L., Feinstein, C., &

Maltby, N. (1998). Memory for faces in autistic children. *Child Neuropsychology, 4,* 187–198.

Heller, T. (1954). About dementia infantilis (W. Hulse, Trans.). *Journal of Nervous and Mental Disease, 119,* 610–616. (Original work published 1908)

Hermelin, B., & O'Connor, N. (1964). Effects of sensory input and sensory dominance on severely disturbed children and on subnormal controls. *British Journal of Psychology, 55,* 201–206.

Hertzig, M. E., Snow, M. E., New, E., & Shapiro, T. (1990). DSM-III and DSM-III-R diagnosis of autism and pervasive developmental disorder in nursery school children. *Journal of the American Academy of Child and Adolescent Psychiatry, 29,* 123–126.

Herzing, L. B. K., Cook, E. H., & Ledbetter, D. H. (2002). Allele-specific expression analysis by RNA-FISH demonstrates preferential maternal expression of UBE3A and imprint maintenance within 15q11–q13 duplications. *Human Molecular Genetics, 11,* 1707–1718.

Hewett, F. M. (1965). Teaching speech to an autistic child through operant conditioning. *American Journal of Orthopsychiatry, 35,* 927–936.

Hildebrand, D. G. (1999). *Cost–benefit analysis of Lovaas treatment for autism and autism spectrum disorder (ASD).* Vancouver, BC: Columbia Pacific Consulting. Retrieved from http://featbc.org/downloads/Hildebrand_Lovaas_ABA.pdf

Hollander, E., Phillips, A. T., & Yeh, C. C. (2003). Targeted treatments for symptom domains in child and adolescent autism. *Lancet, 362,* 732–734.

Holmes, A. S., Blaxill, M. F., & Haley, B. E. (2003). Reduced levels of mercury in first baby haircuts of autistic children. *International Journal of Toxicology, 22,* 277–285.

Honda, H., Shimizu, Y., Misumi, K., Niimi, M., & Ohashi, Y. (1996). Cumulative incidence and prevalence of childhood autism in children in Japan. *British Journal of Psychiatry, 169,* 228–235.

Horner, R. H., Albin, R. W., Sprague, J. R., & Todd, A. W. (2000). Positive behavior support for students with severe disabilities. In M. E. Snell & F. Brown (Eds.), *Instruction of students with severe disabilities* (5th ed., pp. 207–243). Upper Saddle River, NJ: Prentice Hall.

Horner, R. H., Carr, E. G., Strain, P. S., Todd, A. W., & Reed, H. K. (2002). Problem behavior interventions for young children with autism: A research synthesis. *Journal of Autism and Developmental Disorders, 32,* 423–446.

Horner, R. H., Dunlap, G., & Koegel, R. L. (Eds.). (1988). *Generalization and maintenance: Lifestyle changes in applied settings.* Baltimore: Brookes.

Hornig, M., Chian, D., & Lipkin, W. I. (2004). Neurotoxic effects of postnatal thimerosal are mouse strain dependent. *Molecular Psychiatry, 9,* 833–845.

Howard, J. S., Sparkman, C. R., Cohen, H. G., Green, G., & Stanislaw, H. (2005). A comparison of intensive behavior analytic and eclectic treatments for young children with autism. *Research in Developmental Disabilities, 26,* 359–383.

Howard, M. A., Cowell, P. E., Boucher, J., Broks, P., Mayes, A., Farrant, A., et al. (2000). Convergent neuroanatomical and behavioural evidence of an amygdala hypothesis of autism. *Neuroreport, 11,* 2931–2935.

Howlin, P. (1981). The effectiveness of operant language training with autistic children. *Journal of Autism and Developmental Disorders, 11,* 89–105.

Howlin, P. (1999). *Children with autism and Asperger syndrome: A guide for practitioners and carers.* New York: Wiley.

Howlin, P. (2003). Outcome in high-functioning adults with autism with and without early language delays: Implications for the differentiation between autism and Asperger syndrome. *Journal of Autism and Developmental Disorders, 33,* 3–13.

Howlin, P., Baron-Cohen, S., & Hadwin, J. (1999). *Teaching children with autism to mind-read: A practical guide.* Chichester, UK: Wiley.

Howlin, P., Goode, S., Hutton, J., & Rutter, M. (2004). Adult outcome for children with autism. *Journal of Child Psychology and Psychiatry, 45,* 212–229.

Huttenlocher, P. R. (1988). Developmental neurobiology: Current and future challenges. In F. J. Menolascino & J. A. Stark (Eds.), *Preventive and curative intervention in mental retardation* (pp. 101–111). Baltimore: Brookes.

Hviid, A., Stellfeld, M., Wohlfart, J., & Melbye, M. (2003). Association between thimerosal-containing vaccine and autism. *Journal of the American Medical Association, 290,* 1763–1766.

Hwang, B., & Hughes, C. (2000). Increasing early social-communicative skills of preverbal children with autism through social interactive training. *Journal of the Association for Persons with Severe Handicaps, 25,* 18–28.

Ingenmey, R., & Van Houten, R. (1991). Using time delay to promote spontaneous speech in an autistic child. *Journal of Applied Behavior Analysis, 24,* 591–596.

Institute of Medicine. (2001, April 23). *Immunization safety review: Measles–mumps–rubella (MMR) vaccine and autism.* Washington, DC: National Academy Press. Retrieved from http://books.nap.edu/html/mmr

Itard, J. M. G. (1962). *The wild boy of Aveyron* (G. Humphrey & M. Humphrey, Trans.). New York: Appleton-Century-Crofts. (Original work published 1801)

Iwata, B. A., Pace, G. M., Kalsher, M. J., Cowdery, G. E., & Cataldo, M. F. (1990). Experimental analysis and extinction of self-injurious escape behavior. *Journal of Applied Behavior Analysis, 23,* 11–27.

Iwata, B. A., Smith, R. G., & Michael, J. (2000). Current research on the influence of establishing operations on behavior in applied settings. *Journal of Applied Behavior Analysis, 33,* 411–418.

Iwata, B. A., Vollmer, T. R., & Zarcone, J. R. (1990). The experimental (functional) analysis of behavior disorders: Methodology, applications, and limitations. In A. C. Repp & N. N. Singh (Eds.), *Perspectives on the use of nonaversive and aversive interventions for persons with developmental disabilities* (pp. 301–330). Sycamore, IL: Sycamore.

Jackson, C. T., Fein, D., Wolf, J., Jones, G., Hauck, M., Waterhouse, L., et al. (2003). Responses and sustained interactions in children with mental retardation and autism. *Journal of Autism and Developmental Disorders, 33,* 115–121.

Jacobson, J. W., Mulick, J. A., & Green, G. (1998). Cost–benefit estimates for early intensive behavioral intervention for young children with autism: General model and single state case. *Behavioral Interventions, 13,* 201–226.

Jamain, S., Quach, H., Betancur, C., Råstam, M., Colineaux, C., Gillberg, I. C., et al. (2003). Mutations of the X-linked genes encoding neuroligins NLGN3 and NLGN4 are associated with autism. *Nature Genetics, 34,* 27–29.

James, S. D., & Egel, A. L. (1986). A direct prompting strategy for increasing reciprocal interactions between handicapped and nonhandicapped siblings. *Journal of Applied Behavior Analysis, 19,* 173–186.

Jefferson, T., Price, D., Demicheli, V., & Bianco, E. (2003). Unintended events following immunization with MMR: A systematic review. *Vaccine, 21,* 3954–3960.

Jocelyn, L. J., Casiro, O. G., Beattie, D., Bow, J., & Kneisz, J. (1998). Treatment of children with autism: A randomized controlled trial to evaluate a caregiver-based intervention program in community day-care centers. *Journal of Developmental and Behavioral Pediatrics, 19,* 326–334.

Johnson, E., & Hastings, R. P. (2002). Facilitating factors and barriers to the implementation of intensive home-based behavioural intervention for young children with autism. *Child: Care, Health and Development, 28,* 123–129.

Jolly, A. C., Test, D. W., & Spooner, F. (1993). Using badges to increase initiations of children with severe disabilities in a play setting. *Journal of the Association for Persons with Severe Handicaps, 18,* 46–51.

Joseph, R. M., & Tanaka, J. (2003). Holistic and part-based face recognition in children with autism. *Journal of Child Psychology and Psychiatry, 44,* 529–542.

Jou, R. J., Handen, B. L., & Hardan, A. Y. (2005). Retrospective assessment of atomoxetine in children and adolescents with pervasive developmental disorders. *Journal of Child and Adolescent Psychopharmacology, 15,* 325–330.

Juul-Dam, N., Townsend, J., & Courchesne, E. (2001). Prenatal, perinatal, and neonatal factors in autism, pervasive developmental disorder-not otherwise specified, and the general population. *Pediatrics, 107,* E63.

Kamps, D. M., Barbetta, P. M., Leonard, B. R., & Delquadri, J. (1994). Classwide peer tutoring: An integration strategy to improve reading skills and promote peer interactions among students with autism and general education peers. *Journal of Applied Behavior Analysis, 27,* 49–61.

Kamps, D. M., Leonard, B. R., Vernon, S., Dugan, E. P., Delquadri, J. C., Gershon, B., et al. (1992). Teaching social skills to students with autism to increase peer interactions in an integrated first-grade classroom. *Journal of Applied Behavior Analysis, 25,* 281–288.

Kanner, L. (1973). Autistic disturbances of affective contact. In L. Kanner (Ed.), *Childhood psychosis: Initial studies and new insights* (pp. 1–50). Washington, DC: Winston. (Original work published 1943)

Kanner, L. (1973). How far can autistic children go in matters of social adaptation? In L. Kanner (Ed.), *Childhood psychosis: Initial studies and new insights* (pp. 189–213). Washington, DC: Winston.

Kaye, J. A., Melero-Montes, M. D. M., & Jick, H. (2001). Mumps, measles, and rubella vaccine and the incidence of autism recorded by general practitioners: A time trend analysis. *British Medical Journal, 322,* 460–463.

Kemner, C., Willemsen-Swinkels, S. H., de Jonge, M., Tuynman-Qua, H., & van Engeland, H. (2002). Open-label study of olanzapine in children with pervasive developmental disorder. *Journal of Clinical Psychopharmacology, 22,* 455–460.

Kennedy, C. H., & Meyer, K. A. (1996). Sleep deprivation, allergy symptoms, and negatively reinforced problem behavior. *Journal of Applied Behavior Analysis, 29,* 133–135.

Kennedy, C. H., & Meyer, K. A. (1998). Establishing operations and the motivation of challenging behavior. In J. K. Luiselli & M. J. Cameron (Eds.), *Antecedent control: Innovative approaches to behavioral support* (pp. 329–346). Baltimore: Brookes.

Klin, A. (1991). Young autistic children's listening preferences in regard to speech: A possible characterization of the symptom of social withdrawal. *Journal of Autism and Developmental Disabilities, 21,* 29–42.

Klin, A., Jones, W., Schultz, R., & Volkmar, F. (2003). The enactive mind, or from actions to cognition: Lessons from autism. *Philosophical Transactions of the Royal Society of London, Series B, 358,* 345–360.

Klin, A., Jones, W., Schultz, R., Volkmar, F., & Cohen, D. (2002a). Defining and quantifying the social phenotype in autism. *American Journal of Psychiatry, 159,* 895–908.

Klin, A., Jones, W., Schultz, R., Volkmar, F., & Cohen, D. (2002b). Visual fixation patterns during viewing of naturalistic social situations as predictors of social competence in individuals with autism. *Archives of General Psychiatry, 59,* 809–816.

Klin, A., & Volkmar, F. R. (1995). *Asperger's syndrome: Guidelines for assessment and diagnosis.* Retrieved from http://info.med.yale.edu/chldstdy/autism/asdiagnosis.html

Klin, A., Volkmar, F. R., & Sparrow, S. S. (1992). Autistic social dysfunction: Some limitations of the theory of mind hypothesis. *Journal of Child Psychology and Psychiatry, 33*, 861–876.

Klin, A., Volkmar, F. R., Sparrow, S. S., Cicchetti, D. V., & Rourke, B. P. (1995). Validity and neuropsychological characterization of Asperger syndrome: Convergence with nonverbal learning disabilities syndrome. *Journal of Child Psychology and Psychiatry, 36*, 1127–1140.

Koegel, L. K. (1995). Communication and language intervention. In R. L. Koegel & L. K. Koegel (Eds.), *Teaching children with autism* (pp. 17–32). Baltimore: Brookes.

Koegel, L. K., Camarata, S. M., Valdez-Menchaca, M. C., & Koegel, R. L. (1998). Setting generalization of question-asking by children with autism. *American Journal on Mental Retardation, 102*, 346–357.

Koegel, L. K., Koegel, R. L., & Dunlap, G. (Eds.). (1996). *Positive behavioral support: Including people with difficult behavior in the community.* Baltimore: Brookes.

Koegel, L. K., Koegel, R. L., Shoshan, Y., & McNerney, E. (1999). Pivotal response intervention: II. Preliminary long-term outcome data. *Journal of the Association for Persons with Severe Handicaps, 24*, 186–198.

Koegel, R. L., Camarata, S., Koegel, L. K., Ben-Tall, A., & Smith, A. E. (1998). Increasing speech intelligibility in children with autism. *Journal of Autism and Developmental Disorders, 28*, 241–251.

Koegel, R. L., Carter, C. M., & Koegel, L. K. (1998). Setting events to improve parent-teacher coordination and motivation for children with autism. In J. K. Luiselli & M. J. Cameron (Eds.), *Antecedent control: Innovative approaches to behavioral support* (pp. 167–186). Baltimore: Brookes.

Koegel, R. L., & Frea, W. D. (1993). Treatment of social behavior in autism through the modification of pivotal social skills. *Journal of Applied Behavior Analysis, 26*, 369–377.

Koegel, R. L., & Koegel, L. K. (Eds.). (1995). *Teaching children with autism.* Baltimore: Brookes.

Koegel, R. L., Koegel, L. K., & Brookman, L. I. (2003). Empirically supported pivotal response interventions for children with autism. In A. E. Kazdin & J. R. Weisz (Eds.), *Evidence-based psychotherapies for children and adolescents* (pp. 341–357). New York: Guilford Press.

Koegel, R. L., Koegel, L. K., & McNerney, E. (2001). Pivotal behaviors in the treatment of autism. *Journal of Clinical Child Psychology, 30*, 19–32.

Koegel, R. L., Koegel, L. K., & Surratt, A. (1992). Language intervention and disruptive behavior in preschool children with autism. *Journal of Autism and Developmental Disorders, 22*, 141–153.

Koegel, R. L., O'Dell, M. C., & Dunlap, G. (1988). Producing speech use in nonverbal autistic children by reinforcing attempts. *Journal of Autism and Developmental Disorders, 18*, 525–538.

Koegel, R. L., O'Dell, M. C., & Koegel, L. K. (1987). A natural language teaching paradigm for nonverbal autistic children. *Journal of Autism and Developmental Disorders, 17*, 187–200.

Kohler, F. W., Strain, P. S., Hoyson, M., Davis, L., Donina, W. M., & Rapp, N. (1995). Using a group-oriented contingency to increase social interactions between children with autism and their peers. *Behavior Modification, 19*, 10–32.

Kolmen, B., Feldman, H., Handen, B., & Janosky, J. (1995). Naltrexone in young autistic children: A double-blind, placebo-controlled crossover study. *Journal of the American Academy of Child and Adolescent Psychiatry, 34*, 223–231.

Konstantareas, M. M., & Hewitt, T. (2001). Autistic disorder and schizophrenia: Diagnostic overlaps. *Journal of Autism and Developmental Disorders, 31*, 19–28.

Korkmaz, B. (2000). Infantile autism: Adult outcome. *Seminars in Clinical Neuropsychiatry, 5*, 164–170.

Kozloff, M. A. (1994). *Improving educational outcomes for children with disabilities: Principles for assessment, program planning, and evaluation.* Baltimore: Brookes.

Krantz, P. J., MacDuff, M. T., & McClannahan, L. E. (1993). Programming participation in family activities for children with autism: Parents' use of photographic schedules. *Journal of Applied Behavior Analysis, 26*, 137–138.

Krantz, P. J., & McClannahan, L. E. (1993). Teaching children with autism to initiate to peers: Effects of a script-fading procedure. *Journal of Applied Behavior Analysis, 26*, 121–132.

Kwok, H. W. M. (2003). Psychopharmacology in autism spectrum disorders. *Current Opinion in Psychiatry, 16*, 529–534.

Lainhart, J. E., Ozonoff, S., Coon, H., Krasny, L., Dinh, E., Nice, J., & McMahon, W. (2002). Autism, regression, and the broader autism phenotype. *American Journal of Medical Genetics, 113*, 231–237.

Lalli, J. S., Casey, S., Goh, H., & Merlino, J. (1994). Treatment of escape-maintained aberrant behavior with escape extinction and predictable routines. *Journal of Applied Behavior Analysis, 27*, 705–714.

Lalli, J. S., Casey, S., & Kates, K. (1995). Reducing escape behavior and increasing task completion with functional communication training, extinction, and response chaining. *Journal of Applied Behavior Analysis, 28*, 261–268.

Laski, K. E., Charlop, M. H., & Schreibman, L. (1988). Training parents to use the natural language paradigm to increase their autistic children's speech. *Journal of Applied Behavior Analysis, 21*, 391–400.

Lauritsen, M., & Ewald, H. (2001). The genetics of autism. *Acta Psychiatrica Scandinavica, 103*, 411–427.

Leaf, R., & McEachin, J. (1999). *A work in progress.* New York: DRL Books.

Leonard, H., Silberstein, J., Falk, R., Houwink-Manville, I., Ellaway, C., Raffaele, L. S., et al. (2001). Occurrence of Rett syndrome in boys. *Journal of Child Neurology, 16*, 333–338.

Leung, J. (1994). Teaching spontaneous requests to children with autism using a time delay procedure with multi-component toys. *Journal of Behavioral Education, 4,* 21–31.

Leventhal, B. L., Cook, E. H., Morford, M., Ravitz, A. J., Heller, W., & Freedman, D. X. (1993). Clinical and neurochemical effects of fenfluramine in children with autism. *Journal of Neuropsychiatry and Clinical Neurosciences, 5,* 307–315.

Lewine, J. D., Andrews, R., Chez, M., Patil, A. A., Devinsky, O., Smith, M., et al. (1999). Magnetoencephalographic patterns of epileptiform activity in children with regressive autism spectrum disorders. *Pediatrics, 104,* 405–418.

Lewis, M. H., Bodfish, J. W., Powell, S. B., Wiest, K., Darling, M., & Golden, R. N. (1996). Plasma HVA in adults with mental retardation and stereotyped behavior: Biochemical evidence for a dopamine deficiency model. *American Journal on Mental Retardation, 100,* 413–427.

Lingam, R., Simmons, A., Andrews, N., Miller, E., Stowe, J., & Taylor, B. (2003). Prevalence of autism and parentally reported triggers in a northeast London population. *Archives of Disease in Childhood, 88,* 666–670.

Lonigan, C. J., Elbert, J. C., & Johnson, S. B. (1998). Empirically supported psychosocial interventions for children: An overview. *Journal of Clinical Child Psychology, 27,* 138–145.

Lord, C., Risi, S., Lambrecht, L., Cook, E. H., Leventhal, B. L., DiLavore, P. C., et al. (2000). The Autism Diagnostic Observation Schedule—Generic: A standard measure of social and communication deficits associated with the spectrum of autism. *Journal of Autism and Developmental Disorders, 30,* 205–223.

Lord, C., Rutter, M., & Le Couteur, A. (1994). Autism Diagnostic Interview—Revised: A revised version of a diagnostic interview for caregivers of individuals with possible pervasive developmental disorders. *Journal of Autism and Developmental Disorders, 24,* 659–685.

Lord, C., & Schopler, E. (1989). The role of age at assessment, developmental level, and test in the stability of intelligence scores in young autistic children. *Journal of Autism and Developmental Disorders, 19,* 483–499

Lovaas, O. I. (1987). Behavioral treatment and normal educational and intellectual functioning in young autistic children. *Journal of Consulting and Clinical Psychology, 55,* 3–9.

Lovaas, O. I. (1996). The UCLA Young Autism model of service delivery. In C. Maurice, G. Green, & S. C. Luce (Eds.), *Behavioral intervention for young children with autism* (pp. 241–248). Austin, TX: Pro-Ed.

Lovaas, O. I. (2003). *Teaching individuals with developmental delays.* Austin, TX: Pro-Ed.

Lovaas, O. I., Berberich, J. P., Perloff, B. F., & Schaeffer, B. (1966). Acquisition of imitative speech by schizophrenic children. *Science, 151,* 705–707.

Lovaas, O. I., Freitag, G., Gold, V. J., & Kassorla, I. C. (1965). Experimental studies in childhood schizophrenia: Analysis of self-destructive behavior. *Journal of Experimental Child Psychology, 2,* 67–84.

Lovaas, O. I., Koegel, R. L., & Schreibman, L. (1979). Stimulus overselectivity in autism: A review of research. *Psychological Bulletin, 86,* 1236–1254.

Lovaas, O. I., Koegel, R. L., Simmons, J. Q., & Long, J. S. (1973). Some generalization and follow-up measures on autistic children in behavior therapy. *Journal of Applied Behavior Analysis, 6,* 131–166.

Lovaas, O. I., Litrownik, A., & Mann, R. (1971). Response latencies to auditory stimuli in autistic children engaged in self-stimulatory behaviour. *Behaviour Research and Therapy, 9,* 39–49.

Lovaas, O. I., & Newsom, C. (1976). Behavior modification with psychotic children. In H. Leitenberg (Ed.), *Handbook of behavior modification and behavior therapy* (pp. 303–360). Englewood Cliffs, NJ: Prentice-Hall.

Lovaas, O. I., Newsom, C., & Hickman, C. (1987). Self-stimulatory behavior and perceptual reinforcement. *Journal of Applied Behavior Analysis, 20,* 45–68.

Lovaas, O. I., & Smith, T. (1988). Intensive behavioral treatment for young autistic children. In B. B. Lahey & A. E. Kazdin (Eds.), *Advances in clinical child psychology* (Vol. 11, pp. 285–324). New York: Plenum Press.

Lucyshyn, J. M., Dunlap, G., & Albin, R. W. (Eds.). (2002). *Families and positive behavior support.* Baltimore: Brookes.

Lucyshyn, J. M., Horner, R. H., Dunlap, G., Albin, R. W., & Ben, K. R. (2002). Positive behavior support with families. In J. M. Lucyshyn, G. Dunlap, & R. W. Albin (Eds.), *Families and positive behavior support* (pp. 3–43). Baltimore: Brookes.

Lucyshyn, J. M., Kayser, A. T., Irvin, L. K., & Blumberg, E. R. (2002). Functional assessment and positive behavior support at home with families. In J. M. Lucyshyn, G. Dunlap, & R. W. Albin (Eds.), *Families and positive behavior support* (pp. 97–132). Baltimore: Brookes.

Luiselli, J. K., & Cameron, M. J. (Eds.). (1998). *Antecedent control: Innovative approaches to behavioral support.* Baltimore: Brookes.

Luteijn, E., Luteijn, F., Jackson, S., Volkmar, F., & Minderaa, R. (2000). The Children's Social Behavior Questionnaire for milder variants of PDD problems: Evaluation of the psychometric characteristics. *Journal of Autism and Developmental Disorders, 30,* 317–330.

Lutzker, J. R. (1984). A review of Project 12–Ways: An ecobehavioral approach to the treatment and prevention of child abuse and neglect. *Advances in Behavior Research and Therapy, 6,* 63–73.

Lutzker, J. R., & Campbell, R. (1994). *Ecobehavioral family interventions in developmental disabilities.* Pacific Grove, CA: Brooks/Cole.

MacDuff, G. S., Krantz, P. J., & McClannahan, L. E.

(2001). Prompts and prompt-fading strategies for people with autism. In C. Maurice, G. Green, & R. M. Foxx (Eds.), *Making a difference: Behavioral intervention for autism* (pp. 37–50). Austin, TX: Pro-Ed.

Mace, F. C., Browder, D. M., & Lin, Y. (1987). Analysis of demand conditions associated with stereotypy. *Journal of Behavior Therapy and Experimental Psychiatry, 18,* 25–31.

Maddox, L. O., Menold, M. M., Bass, M. P., Rogala, A. R., Pericak-Vance, M. A., Vance, J. M., & Gilbert, J. R. (1999). Autistic disorder and chromosome 15q11–q13: Construction and analysis of a BAC/PAC contig. *Genomics, 62,* 325–331.

Madsen, K. M., Hviid, A., Vestergaard, M., Schendel, D., Wohlfahrt, J., Thorsen, P., et al. (2002). A population-based study of measles, mumps, and rubella vaccination and autism. *New England Journal of Medicine, 347,* 1477–1482.

Madsen, K. M., Lauritsen, M. B,, Pedersen, C. B., Thorsen, P., Plesner, A. M., Andersen, P. H., et al. (2003). Thimerosal and the occurrence of autism: Negative ecological evidence from Danish population-based data. *Pediatrics, 112,* 604–606.

Maestrini, E., Lai, C., Marlow, A., Matthews, N., Wallace, S., Bailey, A., et al. (1999). Serotonin transporter (5–HTT) and gamma-aminobutyric acid receptor subunit beta3 (GABRB3) gene polymorphisms are not associated with autism in the IMGSA families. *American Journal of Medical Genetics, 88,* 492–486.

Magiati, I., & Howlin, P. (2003). A pilot evaluation study of the Picture Exchange Communication System (PECS) for children with autistic spectrum disorders. *Autism, 7,* 297–320.

Malhotra, S., & Gupta, N. (2002). Childhood disintegrative disorder: Re-examination of the current concept. *European Child and Adolescent Psychiatry, 11,* 108–114.

Manjiviona, J., & Prior, M. (1995). Comparison of Asperger's syndrome and high-functioning autistic children on a test of motor impairment. *Journal of Autism and Developmental Disorders, 25,* 23–39.

Manjiviona, J., & Prior, M. (1999). Neuropsychological profiles of children with Asperger syndrome and autism. *Autism, 3,* 327–356.

Marcus, D. J., & Nelson, C. A. (2001). Neural bases and development of face recognition in autism. *CNS Spectrums, 6,* 36–59.

Masi, G., Cosenza, A., Mucci, M., & Brovedani, P. (2003). A 3-year naturalistic study of 53 preschool children with pervasive developmental disorders treated with risperidone. *Journal of Clinical Psychiatry, 64,* 1039–1047.

Matson, J. L., Sevin, J. A., Box, M. L., Francis, K. L., & Sevin, B. M. (1993). An evaluation of two methods for increasing self-initiated verbalizations in autistic children. *Journal of Applied Behavior Analysis, 26,* 389–398.

Matsuishi, T., Shiotsuki, Y., Yoshimura, K., Shoji, H.,

Imuta, F., & Yamashita, F. (1987). High prevalence of infantile autism in Kurume City, Japan. *Journal of Child Neurology, 2,* 268–271.

Maudsley, H. (1867). *The physiology and pathology of the mind.* New York: Appleton.

Maurice, C. (1993). *Let me hear your voice: A family's triumph over autism.* New York: Knopf.

Maurice, C. (2001). Autism advocacy or trench warfare? In C. Maurice, G. Green, & R. M. Foxx (Eds.), *Making a difference: Behavioral intervention for autism* (pp. 1–9). Austin, TX: Pro-Ed.

Maurice, C., Green, G., & Foxx, R. M. (Eds.). (2001). *Making a difference: Behavioral intervention for autism.* Austin, TX: Pro-Ed.

Maurice, C., Green, G., & Luce, S. C. (Eds.). (1996). *Behavioral intervention for young children with autism.* Austin, TX: Pro-Ed.

McAtee, M., Carr, E. G., & Schulte, C. (2004). A contextual assessment inventory for problem behavior: Initial development. *Journal of Positive Behavior Interventions, 6,* 148–165.

McClannahan, L. E., & Krantz, P. J. (1994). The Princeton Child Development Institute. In S. L. Harris & J. S. Handleman (Eds.), *Preschool education programs for children with autism* (pp. 107–126). Austin, TX: Pro-Ed.

McClannahan, L. E., & Krantz, P. J. (1999). *Activity schedules for children with autism: Teaching independent behavior.* Bethesda, MD: Woodbine House.

McConnell, S. R. (2002). Interventions to facilitate social interaction for young children with autism: Review of available research and recommendations for educational intervention and future research. *Journal of Autism and Developmental Disorders, 32,* 351–352.

McDougle, C. J., Holmes, J. P., Carlson, D. C., Pelton, G., Cohen, D. J., & Price, L. H. (1998). A double-blind, placebo-controlled study of risperidone in adults with autistic disorder and other pervasive developmental disorders. *Archives of General Psychiatry, 55,* 633–641.

McDougle, C. J., Kresch, L. E., & Posey, D. J. (2000). Repetitive thoughts and behavior in pervasive developmental disorders: Treatment with serotonin reuptake inhibitors. *Journal of Autism and Developmental Disorders, 30,* 427–435.

McDougle, C. J., Naylor, S. T., Cohen, D. J., Volkmar, F. R., Heninger, G. R., & Price, L. H. (1996). A double-blind, placebo-controlled study of fluvoxamine in adults with autistic disorder. *Archives of General Psychiatry, 53,* 1001–1008.

McEachin, J. J., Smith, T., & Lovaas, O. I. (1993). Long-term outcome for children with autism who received early intensive behavioral treatment. *American Journal on Mental Retardation, 97,* 359–372.

McEvoy, R., Rogers, S., & Pennington, R. (1993). Executive function and social communication deficits in young autistic children. *Journal of Child Psychology and Psychiatry, 34,* 563–578.

McGee, G. G., Krantz, P. J., & McClannahan, L. E.

(1985). The facilitative effects of incidental teaching on preposition use by autistic children. *Journal of Applied Behavior Analysis, 18,* 17–31.

McGee, G. G., Morrier, M. J., & Daly, T. (1999). An incidental approach to early intervention for toddlers with autism. *Journal of the Association for Persons with Severe Handicaps, 24,* 133–146.

Medical Research Council. (2001). *MRC review of autism research: Epidemiology and causes.* Retrieved from www.mrc.ac.uk/pdf-autism-report.pdf

Metz, B., & Pinnock, N. (2003, August). Maximizing the benefits: Implications for research and service delivery of early intensive behavioral intervention for children with autism. In J. A. Mulick (Chair), *Preliminary reports from the Ohio Autism Recovery Project.* Symposium conducted at the convention of the American Psychological Association, Toronto.

Michael, J. (2000). Implications and refinements of the establishing operation concept. *Journal of Applied Behavior Analysis, 33,* 401–410.

Miguel, C., Carr, J. E., & Michael, J. (2002). The effects of a stimulus–stimulus pairing procedure on the vocal behavior of children diagnosed with autism. *Analysis of Verbal Behavior, 18,* 3–13.

M.I.N.D. Institute. (2002). *Report to the legislature on the principal findings from the epidemiology of autism in California: A comprehensive pilot study.* Retrieved from www.dds.ca.gov/Autism/pdf/study_final.pdf

Molloy, C. A., & Manning-Courtney, P. (2003). Prevalence of chronic gastrointestinal symptoms in children with autism and autistic spectrum disorders. *Autism, 7,* 165–171.

Mouridsen, S. E., Rich, B., & Isager, T. (2000). A comparative study of genetic and neurobiological findings in disintegrative psychosis and infantile autism. *Psychiatry and Clinical Neurosciences, 54,* 441–446.

Mudford, O. C., Martin, N. T., Eikeseth, S., & Bibby, P. (2001). Parent-managed behavioral treatment for preschool children with autism: Some characteristics of UK programs. *Research in Developmental Disabilities, 22,* 173–182.

Mulick, J. A., & Butter, E. M. (2002). Educational advocacy for children with autism. *Behavioral Interventions, 17,* 57–74.

Mulick, J. A., & Butter, E. M. (2005). Positive behavior support: A paternalistic utopian delusion. In J. W. Jacobson, R. M. Foxx, & J. A. Mulick (Eds.), *Controversial therapies for developmental disabilities: Fad, fashion, and science in professional practice* (pp. 385–404). Mahwah, NJ: Erlbaum.

Muller, R., Kleinhans, N., Kemmotsu, N., Pierce, K., & Courchesne, E. (2003). Abnormal variability and distribution of functional maps in autism: An fMRI study of visuomotor learning. *American Journal of Psychiatry, 160,* 1847–1862.

Mundschenk, N. S., & Sasso, G. S. (1995). Assessing sufficient social exemplars for students with autism. *Behavior Disorders, 21,* 62–78.

Mundy, P. (2003). The neural basis of social impairments in autism: The role of the dorsal medial–frontal cortex and anterior cingulate system. *Journal of Child Psychology and Psychiatry, 44,* 793–809.

Nelson, K. B., & Bauman, M. L. (2003). Thimerosal and autism? *Pediatrics, 111,* 674–679.

New York State Department of Health. (1999). *Clinical practice guideline: Report of the recommendations. Autism/pervasive developmental disorders, assessment and intervention for young children (age 0–3 years)* (Publication No. 4215). Albany: Author. Retrieved from www.health.state.ny.us/nysdoh/eip/autism/index.htm

Newsom, C., & Kroeger, K. A. (2005). Nonaversive treatment. In J. W. Jacobson, R. M. Foxx, & J. A. Mulick (Eds.), *Controversial therapies for developmental disabilities: Fad, fashion, and science in professional practice* (pp. 405–422). Mahwah, NJ: Erlbaum.

Nurmi, E. L., Amin, T., Olson, L. M., Jacobs, M. M., McCauley, J. L., Lam, A. Y., et al. (2003). Dense linkage disequilibrium mapping in the 15q11–q13 maternal expression domain yields evidence for association in autism. *Molecular Psychiatry, 8,* 624–634.

O'Brien, E. K., Zhang, X., Nishimura, C., Tomblin, J. B., & Murray, J. C. (2003). Association of specific language impairments (SLI) to the region of 7q31. *American Journal of Human Genetics, 72,* 1536–1543.

Odom, S. L., Chandler, L. K., Ostrosky, M., McConnell, S. R., & Reaney, S. (1992). Fading teacher prompts from peer-initiation interventions for young children with disabilities. *Journal of Applied Behavior Analysis, 25,* 307–317.

Odom, S. L., Hoyson, M., Jamieson, B., & Strain, P. S. (1985). Increasing handicapped preschoolers' peer social interactions: Cross-setting and component analysis. *Journal of Applied Behavior Analysis, 18,* 3–16.

Odom, S. L., & Strain, P. S. (1986). A comparison of peer-initiation and teacher-antecedent interventions for promoting reciprocal social interaction of autistic preschoolers. *Journal of Applied Behavior Analysis, 19,* 59–71.

Oke, N. J., & Schreibman, L. (1990). Training social initiations to a high-functioning autistic child: Assessment of collateral behavior change and generalization in a case study. *Journal of Autism and Developmental Disorders, 20,* 479–497.

O'Neill, R. E., Horner, R. H., Albin, R. W., Sprague, J. R., Storey, K., & Newton, J. S. (1997). *Functional assessment and program development for problem behavior: A practical handbook.* Pacific Grove, CA: Brooks/Cole.

Osterling, J., & Dawson, G. (1994). Early recognition of children with autism: A study of first birthday home video tapes. *Journal of Autism and Developmental Disorders, 24,* 247–259.

Ozonoff, S. (1997). Components of executive function

deficits in autism and other disorders. In J. Russell (Ed.), *Autism as an executive disorder* (pp. 179–211). Oxford: Oxford University Press.

Ozonoff, S., Dawson, G., & McPartland, J. (2002). *A parent's guide to Asperger syndrome and high-functioning autism.* New York: Guilford Press.

Ozonoff, S., Goodlin-Jones, B. L., & Solomon, M. (2005). Evidence-based assessment of autism spectrum disorders in children and adolescents. *Journal of Clinical Child and Adolescent Psychology, 34,* 523–540.

Ozonoff, S., & Miller, J. N. (1995). Teaching theory of mind: A new approach to social skills training for individuals with autism. *Journal of Autism and Developmental Disorders, 25,* 415–433.

Ozonoff, S., Rogers, S. J., & Pennington, B. F. (1991). Asperger's syndrome: Evidence of an empirical distinction from high-functioning autism. *Journal of Child Psychology and Psychiatry, 32,* 1107–1122.

Panksepp, J. (1979). A neurochemical theory of autism. *Trends in Neurosciences, 2,* 174–177.

Parkman, P. D. (1995). Combined and simultaneously administered vaccines: A brief history. *Annals of the New York Academy of Sciences, 754,* 1–9.

Partington, J. W., Sundberg, M. L., Newhouse, L., & Spengler, S. M. (1994). Overcoming an autistic child's failure to acquire a tact repertoire. *Journal of Applied Behavior Analysis, 27,* 733–734.

Patterson, G. R., Reid, J. B., & Dishion, T. J. (1992). *Antisocial boys.* Eugene, OR: Castalia.

Pennington, B. F., & Ozonoff, S. (1996). Executive functions and developmental psychopathology. *Journal of Child Psychology and Psychiatry, 37,* 51–87.

Perry, R., Cohen, I., & DeCarlo, R. (1995). Case study: Deterioration, autism, and recovery in two siblings. *Journal of the American Academy of Child Psychiatry, 34,* 232–237.

Petty, L., Ornitz, E. M., Michelman, J. D., & Zimmerman, E. G. (1984). Autistic children who later become schizophrenic. *Archives of General Psychiatry, 41,* 129–135.

Philippe, A., Martinez, M., Guilloud-Bataille, M., Gillberg, C., Rastam, M., Sponheim, E., et al. (1999). Genome-wide scan for autism susceptibility genes: Paris Autism Research International Sibpair Study. *Human Molecular Genetics, 8,* 805–812.

Pichichero, M. E., Cernichiari, E., Lopreiato, J., & Treanor, J. (2002). Mercury concentrations and metabolism in infants receiving vaccines containing thimerosal: A descriptive study. *Lancet, 360,* 1737–1741.

Pickles, A., Starr, E., Kazak, S., Bolton, P., Papanikolaou, K., Bailey, A., et al. (2000). Variable expression of the autism broader phenotype: Findings from extended pedigrees. *Journal of Child Psychology and Psychiatry, 41,* 491–502.

Piven, J., Palmer, P., Jacobi, D., Childress, D., & Arndt, S. (1997). Broader autism phenotype: Evidence from a family history study of multiple-incidence families. *American Journal of Psychiatry, 154,* 185–190.

Potter, H. W. (1933). Schizophrenia in children. *American Journal of Psychiatry, 89,* 1253–1270.

Powell, J. E., Edwards, A., Edwards, M., Pandit, B. S., Sungum-Paliwal, S. R., & Whitehouse, W. (2000). Changes in the incidence of childhood autism and other autistic spectrum disorders in preschool children from two areas of the West Midlands, U.K. *Developmental Medicine and Child Neurology, 42,* 624–628.

Prior, M. (2003). Is there an increase in the prevalence of autism spectrum disorders? *Journal of Pediatrics and Child Health, 39,* 81–82.

Prior, M., Eisenmajer, R., Leekam, S., Wing, L., Gould, J., Ong, B., at el. (1998). Are there subgoups within the autistic spectrum?: A cluster analysis of a group of children with autistic spectrum disorders. *Journal of Child Psychology and Psychiatry, 39,* 893–902.

Pronovost, W., Wakstein, M. P., & Wakstein, D. J. (1966). A longitudinal study of speech behaviour and language comprehension of fourteen children diagnosed as atypical or autistic. *Exceptional Children, 33,* 19–26.

Ragland, E. U., Kerr, M. M., & Strain, P. S. (1978). Behavior of withdrawn autistic children: Effects of peer social initiations. *Behavior Modification, 2,* 565–578.

Rasmussen, P., Borjesson, O., Wentz, E., & Gillberg, C. (2001). Autistic disorders in Down syndrome: Background factors and clinical correlates. *Developmental Medicine and Child Neurology, 43,* 750–754.

Reaven, J., & Hepburn, S. (2003). Cognitive-behavioral treatment of obsessive–compulsive disorder in a child with Asperger syndrome: A case report. *Autism, 7,* 145–164.

Redd, S. C., Markowitz, L. E., & Katz, S. L. (1999). Measles vaccine. In S. A. Plotkin & W. A. Orenstein (Eds.), *Vaccines* (3rd ed., pp. 222–266). Philadelphia: Saunders.

Richdale, A. L. (1999). Sleep problems in autism: Prevalence, cause, and intervention. *Developmental Medicine and Child Neurology, 41,* 60–66.

Rimland, B. (1964). *Infantile autism.* New York: Appleton-Century-Crofts.

Rincover, A., Cook, R., Peoples, A., & Packard, D. (1979). Using sensory extinction and sensory reinforcement principles for programming multiple adaptive behavior change. *Journal of Applied Behavior Analysis, 12,* 221–233.

Rincover, A., & Devany, J. (1982). The application of sensory extinction procedures to self-injury. *Analysis and Intervention in Developmental Disabilities, 2,* 67–81.

Ring, H. A., Baron-Cohen, S., Wheelwright, S., Williams, S. C. R., Brammer, M., Andrew, C., et al. (1999). Cerebral correlates of preserved cognitive skills in autism: A functional MRI study of embedded figures task performance. *Brain, 122,* 1305–1315.

Risch, N., Spiker, D., Lotspeich, L., Nouri, N., Hinds, D., Hallmayer, J., et al. (1999). A genomic screen of autism: Evidence for a multilocus etiology. *American Journal of Human Genetics, 65,* 493–507.

Risley, T. R., & Wolf, M. (1967). Establishing functional speech in echolalic children. *Behaviour Research and Therapy, 5,* 73–88.

Robbins, F. R., Dunlap, G., & Plienis, A. J. (1991). Family characteristics, family training, and the progress of young autistic children with autism. *Journal of Early Intervention, 15,* 173–184.

Robinson, R. O., Baird, G., Robinson, G., & Simonoff, E. (2001). Landau–Kleffner syndrome: Course and correlates with outcome. *Developmental Medicine and Child Neurology, 43,* 243–247.

Rodier, P. M., & Hyman, S. L. (1998). Early environmental factors in autism. *Mental Retardation and Developmental Disabilities Research Reviews, 4,* 121–128.

Rogers, S. J. (1998). Empirically supported comprehensive treatments for young children with autism. *Journal of Clinical Child Psychology, 27,* 168–179.

Rogers, S. J., Hall, T., Osaki, D., Reaven, J., & Herbison, J. (2000). The Denver Model: A comprehensive, integrated educational approach to young children with autism and their families. In J. S. Handleman & S. L. Harris (Eds.), *Preschool education programs for children with autism* (2nd ed., pp. 95–113). Austin, TX: Pro-Ed.

Rosenhall, U., Nordin, V., Sandstrom, M., Ahlsen, G., & Gillberg, C. (1999). Autism and hearing loss. *Journal of Autism and Developmental Disorders, 29,* 349–357.

Russell, J. (Ed.). (1998). *Autism as an executive disorder.* Oxford: Oxford University Press.

Rutter, M. (1978). Diagnosis and definition. In M. Rutter & E. Schopler (Eds.), *Autism: A reappraisal of concepts and treatment* (pp. 1–25). New York: Plenum Press.

Rutter, M. (1985). Infantile autism and other pervasive developmental disorders. In M. Rutter & L. Hersov (Eds.), *Child and adolescent psychiatry* (2nd ed., pp. 545–566). Oxford: Blackwell.

Rutter, M. (1988). Biological basis of autism: Implications for intervention. In F. J. Menolascino & J. A. Stark (Eds.), *Preventive and curative intervention in mental retardation* (pp. 265–294). Baltimore: Brookes.

Rutter, M., & Lockyer, L. (1967). A five to fifteen year follow-up study of infantile psychosis: I. Description of sample. *British Journal of Psychiatry, 113,* 1169–1182.

Rutter, M., & Schopler, E. (1987). Autism and pervasive developmental disorders: Concepts and diagnostic issues. *Journal of Autism and Developmental Disorders, 17,* 159–186.

Sailor, W., Gee, K., & Karasoff, P. (2000). Inclusion and school restructuring. In M. E. Snell & F. Brown (Eds.), *Instruction of students with severe disabilities* (5th ed., pp. 1–30). Upper Saddle River, NJ: Prentice Hall.

Sainato, D. M., Goldstein, H., & Strain, P. S. (1992). Effects of self-evaluation on preschool children's use of social interaction strategies with their classmates with autism. *Journal of Applied Behavior Analysis, 25,* 127–141.

Sallows, G. O., & Graupner, T. D. (1999, July). *Replicating Lovaas' treatment and findings: Preliminary results.* Paper presented at the conference of the Autism Society of America, Kansas City, KS.

Salt, J., Shemilt, J., Sellars, V., Boyd, S., Coulson, T., & McCool, S. (2002). The Scottish Centre for autism preschool treatment programme: II. The results of a controlled treatment outcome study. *Autism, 6,* 33–46.

Sanchez, L. E., Campbell, M., Small, A. M., Cueva, J. E., Armenteros, J. L., & Adams, P. B. (1996). A pilot study of clomipramine in young autistic children. *Journal of the American Academy of Child and Adolescent Psychiatry, 35,* 537–544.

Sanders, M. R. (1996). New directions in behavioral family intervention with children. In T. H. Ollendick & R. J. Prinz (Eds.), *Advances in clinical child psychology* (Vol. 18, pp. 283–329). New York: Kluwer Academic/Plenum.

Sanders, M. R., & Dadds, M. R. (1993). *Behavioral family intervention.* Needham Heights, MA: Allyn & Bacon.

Santarcangelo, S., Dyer, K., & Luce, S. C. (1987). Generalized reduction of disruptive behavior in unsupervised settings through specific toy training. *Journal of the Association for Persons with Severe Handicaps, 12,* 38–44.

Santosh, P. J., & Baird, G. (2001). Pharmacotherapy of target symptoms in autistic spectrum disorders. *Indian Journal of Pediatrics, 68,* 427–431.

Saxe, R., & Kanwisher, N. (2003). People thinking about thinking people: The role of the temporo-parietal junction in "theory of mind." *NeuroImage, 19,* 1835–1842.

Scambler, D., Rogers, S. J., & Wehner, E. A. (2001). Can the Checklist for Autism in Toddlers differentiate young children with autism from those with developmental delays? *Journal of the American Academy of Child and Adolescent Psychiatry, 40,* 1457–1463.

Schaeffer, B. (1980). Spontaneous language through signed speech. In R. L. Schiefelbusch (Ed.), *Nonspeech language and communication* (pp. 421–446). Baltimore: University Park Press.

Schain, R. J., & Yannet, H. (1960). Infantile autism: An analysis of 50 cases and a consideration of certain neurophysiologic concepts. *Journal of Pediatrics, 57,* 560–567.

Schopler, E., Reichler, R. J., & Renner, B. R. (1988). *Childhood Autism Rating Scale.* Los Angeles: Western Psychological Services.

Schover, L. R., & Newsom, C. (1976). Overselectivity, developmental level, and overtraining in autistic and normal children. *Journal of Abnormal Child Psychology, 4,* 289–298.

Schreck, K. A., & Mulick, J. A. (2000). Parental report of sleep problems in children with autism. *Journal of Autism and Developmental Disorders, 30,* 127–135.

Schreibman, L., O'Neill, R. E., & Koegel, R. L. (1983). Behavioral training for siblings of autistic children. *Journal of Applied Behavior Analysis, 16,* 129–138.

Schreibman, L., Stahmer, A. C., & Pierce, K. L. (1996). Alternative applications of pivotal response training: Teaching symbolic play and social interaction skills. In L. K. Koegel, R. L. Koegel, & G. Dunlap (Eds.), *Positive behavior support: Including people with difficult behavior in the community* (pp. 353–371). Baltimore: Brookes.

Schultz, R. T., Gauthier, I., Klin, A., Fulbright, R., Anderson, A., Volkmar, F. R., et al. (2000). Abnormal ventral temporal cortical activity among individuals with autism and Asperger syndrome during face discrimination. *Archives of General Psychiatry, 57,* 331–340.

Schwartz, I. S., Garfinkle, A. N., & Bauer, J. (1998). The Picture Exchange Communication System: Communicative outcomes for young children with disabilities. *Topics in Early Childhood Special Education, 18,* 144–159.

Schwartz, I. S., Sandall, S. R., Garfinkle, A. N., & Bauer, J. (1998). Outcomes for children with autism: Three case studies. *Topics in Early Childhood Special Education, 18,* 132–143.

Scotti, J. R., & Meyer, L. H. (1999). *Behavioral intervention: Principles, models, and practices.* Baltimore: Brookes.

Seal, B., & Bonvillian, J. (1997). Sign language and motor functioning in students with autistic disorder. *Journal of Autism and Developmental Disorders, 27,* 437–466.

Shafer, M. S., Egel, A. L., & Neef, N. A. (1984). Training mildly handicapped peers to facilitate changes in the social interaction skills of autistic children. *Journal of Applied Behavior Analysis, 17,* 461–476.

Shattuck, R. (1994). *The forbidden experiment: The story of the wild boy of Aveyron.* Tokyo: Kodansha International.

Sheinkopf, S. J., & Siegel, B. (1998). Home based behavioral treatment of young children with autism. *Journal of Autism and Developmental Disorders, 28,* 15–23.

Sigafoos, J. (1998). Choice making and personal selection strategies. In J. K. Luiselli & M. J. Cameron (Eds.), *Antecedent control: Innovative approaches to behavioral support* (pp. 187–221). Baltimore: Brookes.

Sigman, M., Ruskin, E., Arbeile, S., Corona, R., Dissanayake, C., Espinosa, M., et al. (1999). Continuity and change in the social competence of children with autism, Down syndrome, and developmental delays. *Monographs of the Society for Research in Child Development, 64*(1), 115–130.

Singer, G. H. S., Goldberg-Hamblin, S. E., Peckham-Hardin, K. D., Barry, L., & Santarelli, G. E. (2002). Toward a synthesis of family support practices and positive behavior support. In J. M. Lucyshyn, G. Dunlap, & R. W. Albin (Eds.), *Families and positive behavior support* (pp. 155–183). Baltimore: Brookes.

Singer, G. H. S., & Powers, L. E. (Eds.). (1993). *Families, disability, and empowerment: Active coping skills and strategies for family interventions.* Baltimore: Brookes.

Singer, G. H. S., & Yovanoff, P. (1993). *A meta-analysis of depression in parents of children with developmental disabilities and parents of typically developing children.* Unpublished manuscript, Graduate School of Education, University of California at Santa Barbara.

Singh, V. K., Lin, S. X., Newell, E., & Nelson, C. (2002). Abnormal measles–mumps–rubella antibodies and CNS autoimmunity in children with autism. *Journal of Biomedical Science, 9,* 359–364.

Skinner, B. F. (1957). *Verbal behavior.* New York: Appleton-Century-Crofts.

Skuse, D. H. (2000). Imprinting, the X-chromosome, and the male brain: Explaining sex differences in the liability to autism. *Pediatric Research, 47,* 9–16.

Smalley, S. L., & Collins, F. (1996). Genetic, prenatal, and immunologic factors. *Journal of Autism and Developmental Disorders, 26,* 195–198.

Smith, R. G., Iwata, B. A., Goh, H. L., & Shore, B. A. (1995). Analysis of establishing operations for self-injury maintained by escape. *Journal of Applied Behavior Analysis, 28,* 515–535.

Smith, T. (1993). Autism. In T. R. Giles (Ed.), *Effective psychotherapies* (pp. 107–133). New York: Plenum Press.

Smith, T. (1999). Outcome of early intervention for children with autism. *Clinical Psychology: Science and Practice, 6,* 33–49.

Smith, T., Buch, G. A., & Gamby, T. E. (2000). Parent-directed, intensive early intervention for children with pervasive developmental disorder. *Research in Developmental Disabilities, 21,* 297–309.

Smith, T., Eikeseth, S., Klevstrand, M., & Lovaas, O. I. (1997). Intensive behavioral treatment for preschoolers with severe mental retardation and pervasive developmental disorder. *American Journal on Mental Retardation, 102,* 238–249.

Smith, T., Groen, A. D., & Wynn, J. W. (2000). A randomized trial of intensive early intervention for children with pervasive developmental disorder. *American Journal on Mental Retardation, 105,* 269–285.

Smith, T., Klevstrand, M., & Lovaas, O. I. (1995). Behavioral treatment of Rett's disorder: Ineffectiveness in three cases. *American Journal on Mental Retardation, 100,* 317–322.

Soderstrom, H., Rastam, M., & Gillberg, C. (2002). Temperament and character in adults with Asperger syndrome. *Autism, 6,* 287–297.

Sparrow, S. S., Balla, D., & Cicchetti, D. (1984).

Vineland Adaptive Behavior Scales. Circle Pines, MN: American Guidance Service.

Sparrow, S. S., Rescorla, L. A., Provence, S., Condon, S. O., Goudreau, D., & Cicchetti, D. V. (1986). Follow-up of "atypical" children: A brief report. *Journal of the American Academy of Child Psychiatry, 25,* 181–185.

Spelke, E. S., Phillips, A., & Woodward, A. L. (1995). Infants' knowledge of object motion and human action. In D. Sperber, D. Premack, & A. J. Premack (Eds.), *Causal cognition: A multidisciplinary debate* (pp. 44–78). Oxford: Oxford University Press.

Sperry, L. A., Whaley, K. T., Shaw, E., & Brame, K. (1999). Services for young children with autism spectrum disorder: Voices of parents and providers. *Infants and Young Children, 11,* 17–33.

Spiker, D., Lotspeich, L. J., Dimiceli, S., Myers, R. M., & Risch, N. (2002). Behavioral phenotypic variation in autism multiplex families: Evidence for a continuous severity gradient. *American Journal of Medical Genetics, 114,* 129–136.

Spradlin, J. E., & Siegel, G. (1982). Language training in natural and clinical environments. *Journal of Speech and Hearing Disorders, 47,* 2–6.

Stahmer, A. C., & Schreibman, L. (1992). Teaching children with autism appropriate play in unsupervised environments using a self-management treatment package. *Journal of Applied Behavior Analysis, 25,* 447–459.

Steele, S., Joseph, R. M., & Tager-Flusberg, H. (2003). Developmental change in theory of mind abilities in children with autism. *Journal of Autism and Developmental Disorders, 33,* 461–467.

Stefanatos, G. A., Kinsbourne, M., & Wasserstein, J. (2002). Acquired epileptiform aphasia: A dimensional view of Landau–Kleffner syndrome and the relation to regressive autistic spectrum disorders. *Child Neuropsychology, 8,* 195–228.

Steffenburg, S., Gillberg, C., Steffenburg, U., & Kyllerman, M. (1996). Autism in Angelman syndrome: A population-based study. *Pediatric Neurology, 14,* 131–136.

Stehr-Green, P., Tull, P., Stellfeld, M., Mortenson, P. B., & Simpson, D. (2003). Autism and thimerosal-containing vaccines: Lack of consistent evidence for an association. *American Journal of Preventive Medicine, 25,* 101–106.

Stevens, M. C., Fein, D. A., Dunn, M., Allen, D., Waterhouse, L. H., Feinstein, C., et al. (2000). Subgroups of children with autism by cluster analysis: A longitudinal examination. *Journal of the American Academy of Child and Adolescent Psychiatry, 39,* 346–352.

Stevenson, C. L., Krantz, J. P., & McClannahan, L. E. (2000). Social interaction skills for children with autism: A script-fading procedure for nonreaders. *Behavioral Interventions, 15,* 1–20.

Stodgell, C. J., Ingram, J. L., & Hyman, S. L. (2000). The roll of candidate genes in unraveling the genetics of autism. *International Review on Research in Mental Retardation, 20,* 57–81.

Strain, P. S. (1977). Effects of peer social initiations on withdrawn preschool children: Some training and generalization effects. *Journal of Abnormal Child Psychology, 5,* 445–455.

Strain, P. S., & Hoyson, M. H. (2000). On the need for longitudinal, intensive social skill intervention: LEAP follow-up outcomes for children with autism as a case-in-point. *Topics in Early Childhood Special Education, 20,* 116–122.

Strain, P. S., & Odom, S. L. (1986). Peer-social initiations: Effective intervention for social skills development of exceptional children. *Exceptional Children, 52,* 543–552.

Strain, P. S., Shores, R. E., & Timm, M. A. (1977). Effects of peer initiations on the social behavior of withdrawn preschool children. *Journal of Applied Behavior Analysis, 10,* 289–298.

Strauss, B., & Bigham, M. (2001). Does measles–mumps–rubella (MMR) vaccination cause inflammatory bowel disease and autism? *Canada Communicable Disease Report, 27,* 65–72.

Sturmey, P. (1996). *Functional analysis in clinical psychology.* New York: Wiley.

Sundberg, M. L., Loeb, M., Hale, L., & Eigenheer, P. (2002). Contriving establishing operations to teach mands for information. *Analysis of Verbal Behavior, 18,* 15–29.

Sundberg, M. L., & Partington, J. W. (1998). *Teaching language to children with autism or other developmental disabilities.* Pleasant Hill, CA: Behavior Analysts.

Symons, F. J., Thompson, A., & Rodriguez, M. C. (2004). Self-injurious behavior and the efficacy of naltrexone treatment: A quantitative synthesis. *Mental Retardation and Developmental Disabilities Research Reviews, 10,* 193–200.

Szatmari, P., Bartolucci, G., Bremner, R., Bond, S., & Rich, S. (1989). A follow-up study of high-functioning autistic children. *Journal of Autism and Developmental Disorders, 19,* 213–225.

Szatmari, P., Tuff, L., Finlayson, A. J., & Bartolucci, G. (1990). Asperger's syndrome and autism: Neurocognitive aspects. *Journal of the American Academy of Child and Adolescent Psychiatry, 29,* 130–136.

Tager-Flusberg, H. (1992). Autistic children's talk about psychological states: Deficits in the early acquisition of a theory of mind. *Child Development, 63,* 161–172.

Tan, L. J. (2003, June 6). *The relationship between the MMR vaccine and autism.* Retrieved from www.ama-assn.org/ama/pub/article/1824–6108.html

Tani, P., Lindberg, N., Nieminen-von Wendt, T., von Wendt, L., Alanko, L., Appelberg, B., et al. (2003, October 16). Insomnia is a frequent finding in adults with Asperger syndrome. *BMC Psychiatry, 3,* 1–23. Retrieved from www.biomedcentral.com/content/pdf/1471-244x-3-12.pdf

Task Force on Promotion and Dissemination of Psychological Procedures, Division of Clinical Psychology,

American Psychological Association. (1995). Training in and dissemination of empirically-validated psychological treatments: Report and recommendations. *The Clinical Psychologist, 48,* 3–23.

Taylor, B. (2000, April 6). *Testimony to the Congress of the United States House of Representatives Committee on Government Reform. Hearing on "The challenges of autism: Why the increased rates?"* Retrieved from www.hpa.org.uk/infections/topics_az/vaccination/Taylor_paper.pdf

Taylor, B., Miller, E., Farrington, C. P., Petropoulos, M. C., Favot-Mayaud, I., Li, J., et al. (1999). Autism and measles, mumps, and rubella vaccine: No epidemiological evidence for a causal association. *Lancet, 353,* 2026–2029.

Taylor, B., Miller, E., Lingam, R., Andrews, N., Simmons, A., & Stowe, J. (2002). Measles, mumps, and rubella vaccination and bowel problems or developmental regression in children with autism: Population study. *British Medical Journal, 324,* 393–396.

Taylor, B. A. (2001). Teaching peer social skills to children with autism. In C. Maurice, G. Green, & R. M. Foxx (Eds.), *Making a difference: Behavioral intervention for autism* (pp. 83–96). Austin, TX: Pro-Ed.

Taylor, B. A., & Harris, S. L. (1995). Teaching children with autism to seek information: Acquisition of novel information and generalization of responding. *Journal of Applied Behavior Analysis, 28,* 3–14.

Taylor, B. A., & Jasper, S. (2001). Teaching programs to increase peer interaction. In C. Maurice, G. Green, & R. M. Foxx (Eds.), *Making a difference: Behavioral intervention for autism* (pp. 97–162). Austin, TX: Pro-Ed.

Taylor, B. A., & Levin, L. (1998). Teaching a student with autism to make verbal initiations: Effects of a "tactile prompt." *Journal of Applied Behavior Analysis, 31,* 651–654.

Taylor, B. A., Levin, L., & Jasper, S. (1999). Increasing play-related statements in children with autism toward their siblings: Effects of video modeling. *Journal of Developmental and Physical Disabilities, 11,* 253–264.

Taylor, J., & Carr, E. G. (1992). Severe problem behaviors related to social interaction: I. Attention seeking and social avoidance. *Behavior Modification, 16,* 305–335.

Taylor, J., Ekdahl, M., Romanczyk, R. G., & Miller, M. (1994). Escape behavior in task situations: Task versus social antecedents. *Journal of Autism and Developmental Disorders, 24,* 331–344.

Teitelbaum, P., Teitelbaum, O., Nye, J., Fryman, J., & Maurer, R. G. (1998). Movement analysis in infancy may be useful for early diagnosis of autism. *Proceedings of the National Academy of Sciences USA, 95,* 13982–13987.

Thelen, E. (1979). Rhythmical stereotypies in normal human infants. *Animal Behavior, 27,* 699–715.

Todd, R. D. (1986). Pervasive developmental disorders and immunological tolerance. *Psychiatric Developments, 4,* 147–165.

Touchette, P. E., MacDonald, R. F., & Langer, S. N. (1985). A scatter plot for identifying stimulus control of problem behavior. *Journal of Applied Behavior Analysis, 18,* 343–351.

Tryon, A. S., & Keane, S. P. (1986). Promoting imitative play through generalized observational learning in autisticlike children. *Journal of Abnormal Child Psychology, 14,* 537–549.

Tubbs, V. K. (1966). Types of linguistic disability in psychotic children. *Journal of Mental Deficiency Research, 10,* 230–240.

Tuchman, R. F., & Rapin, I. (1997). Regression in pervasive developmental disorders: Seizures and epileptiform electroencephalogram correlates. *Pediatrics, 99,* 560–566.

Tuchman, R. F., & Rapin, I. (2002). Epilepsy in autism. *Lancet Neurology, 6,* 352–358.

Turnbull, A. P., Blue-Banning, M., Behr, S., & Kerns, G. (1986). Family research and intervention: A value and ethical examination. In P. R. Dokecki & R. M. Zaner (Eds.), *Ethics of dealing with persons with severe handicaps* (pp. 119–140). Baltimore: Brookes.

Turnbull, A. P., & Turnbull, H. R. (1996). Group action planning as a strategy for providing comprehensive family support. In L. K. Koegel, R. L. Koegel, & G. Dunlap (Eds.), *Positive behavioral support: Including people with difficult behavior in the community* (pp. 99–114). Baltimore: Brookes.

Turner, M. (1999). Repetitive behavior in autism: A review of psychological research. *Journal of Child Psychology and Psychiatry, 40,* 839–849.

Turner, M., Barnby, G., & Bailey, A. (2000). Genetic clues to the biological basis of autism. *Molecular Medicine Today, 6,* 238–244.

Uhlmann, V., Martin, C. M., Sheils, O., Pilkington, L., Silva, I., Killalea, A., et al. (2002). Potential viral pathogenic mechanism for new variant inflammatory bowel disease. *Molecular Pathology, 55,* 84–90.

U.S. Department of Health and Human Services. (1999). *Mental health: A report of the Surgeon General.* Rockville, MD: Author. Retrieved from www.surgeongeneral.gov/library/mentalhealth/chapter3/sec6.html#autism

Van den Veyver, I. B., & Zoghbi, H. Y. (2002). Genetic basis of Rett syndrome. *Mental Retardation and Developmental Disabilities Research Reviews, 8,* 82–86.

Venter, A., Lord, C., & Schopler, E. (1992). A follow-up study of high-functioning autistic children. *Journal of Child Psychology and Psychiatry, 33,* 489–507.

Volkmar, F. R. (2001). Pharmacological interventions in autism: Theoretical and practical issues. *Journal of Clinical Child Psychology, 30,* 80–87.

Volkmar, F. R., Bregman, J., Cohen, D. J., & Cicchetti, D. V. (1988). DSM-III and DSM-III-R diagnosis of autism. *American Journal of Psychiatry, 145,* 1404–1408.

Volkmar, F. R., & Nelson, D. S. (1990). Seizure disorders in autism. *Journal of the American Academy of Child and Adolescent Psychiatry, 29,* 127–129.

Volkmar, F. R., & Rutter, M. (1995). Childhood disintegrative disorder: Results of the DSM-IV autism field trial. *Journal of the American Academy of Child and Adolescent Psychiatry, 34,* 1092–1095.

Volkmar, F. R., Sparrow, S. S., Goudreau, D., Cicchetti, D. V., Paul, R., & Cohen, D. J. (1987). Social deficits in autism: An operational approach using the Vineland Adaptive Behavior Scales. *Journal of the American Academy of Child and Adolescent Psychiatry, 26,* 156–161.

Wahler, R. G. (1980). The insular mother: Her problems in parent–child treatment. *Journal of Applied Behavior Analysis, 13,* 207–208.

Wahler, R. G. (1988). Skill deficits and uncertainty: An interbehavioral view on the parenting problems of multi-stressed mothers. In R. D. Peters & R. McMahon (Eds.), *Social learning and systems approaches to marriage and the family* (pp. 45–71). New York: Brunner/Mazel.

Wahler, R. G., Cartor, P. G., Fleischman, J., & Lambert, W. (1993). The impact of synthesis teaching and parent training with mothers of conduct-disordered children. *Journal of Abnormal Child Psychology, 21,* 425–440.

Wainwright-Sharp, J. A., & Bryson, S. E. (1993). Visual orienting deficits in high-functioning people with autism. *Journal of Autism and Developmental Disorders, 23,* 1–13.

Wakefield, A. J., Anthony, A., Murch, S. H., Thomson, M., Montgomery, S. M., Davies, S., et al. (2000). Enterocolitis in children with developmental disorders. *American Journal of Gastroenterology, 95,* 2285–2295.

Wakefield, A. J., & Montgomery, S. M. (1999). Autism, viral infection and measles–mumps–rubella vaccination. *Israel Medical Association Journal, 1,* 183–187.

Wakefield, A. J., Murch, S. H., Anthony, A., Linnell, J., Casson, D. M., Malik, M., et al. (1998). Ileal-lymphoid-nodular hyperplasia, non-specific colitis, and pervasive developmental disorder in children. *Lancet, 351,* 637–641.

Walker, D. R., Thompson, A., Zwaigenbaum, L., Goldberg, J., Bryson, S. E., Mahoney, W. J., et al. (2004). Specifying PDD NOS: A comparison of PDD NOS, Asperger syndrome, and autism. *Journal of the American Academy of Child and Adolescent Psychiatry, 43,* 172–180.

Warren, S. F., & Kaiser, A. P. (1986). Incidental language teaching: A critical review. *Journal of Speech and Hearing Disorders, 51,* 291–299.

Wassink, T. H., & Piven, J. (2000). The molecular genetics of autism. *Current Psychiatry Reports, 2,* 170–175.

Wassink, T. H., Piven, J., Vieland, V. J., Huang, J., Swiderski, R. E., Pietila, J., et al. (2001). Evidence supporting WNT2 as an autism susceptibility gene. *American Journal of Medical Genetics, 105,* 406–413.

Waterhouse, L. (1988). Speculations on the neuroanatomical substrate of special talents. In L. Obler & D. Fein (Eds.), *The exceptional brain* (pp. 493–512). New York: Guilford Press.

Waterhouse, L., Morris, R., Allen, D., Dunn, M., Fein, D., Rapin, I., & Wing, L. (1996). Diagnosis and classification in autism. *Journal of Autism and Developmental Disorders, 26,* 59–86.

Watthen-Lovaas, N., & Lovaas, E. E. (1999). *The reading-writing program: An alternative form of communication.* Austin, TX: Pro-Ed.

Webb, E., Morey, J., Thompsen, W., Butler, C., Barber, M., & Fraser, W. I. (2003). Prevalence of autistic spectrum disorder in children attending mainstream schools in a Welsh education authority. *Developmental Medicine and Child Neurology, 45,* 377–384.

Webster-Stratton, C. (1997). From parent training to community building. *Families in Society, 78,* 156–171.

Webster-Stratton, C. (1998). Parent training with low-income families: Promoting parental engagement through a collaborative approach. In J. R. Lutzker (Ed.), *Handbook of child abuse research and treatment* (pp. 183–210). New York: Kluwer Academic/Plenum Press.

Weiss, M. J. (1999). Differential rates of skill acquisition and outcomes of early intensive behavioral intervention for autism. *Behavioral Interventions, 14,* 3–22.

Werner, E., Dawson, G., Osterling, J., & Dinno, H. (2000). Recognition of autism spectrum disorder before one year of age: A retrospective study based on home videotapes. *Journal of Autism and Developmental Disorders, 30,* 157–162.

Whalen, C., & Schreibman, L. (2003). Joint attention training for children with autism using behavior modification procedures. *Journal of Child Psychology and Psychiatry, 44,* 456–468.

Whiteley, P., Rogers, J., Savery, D., & Shattock, P. (1999). A gluten free diet as an intervention for autism and associated spectrum disorders. *Autism, 3,* 45–65.

Wilkerson, D. S., Volpe, A. G., Dean, R. S., & Titus, J. B. (2002). Perinatal complications as predictors of infantile autism. *International Journal of Neuroscience, 112,* 1085–1098.

Willemsen-Swinkels, S. H. N., Buitelaar, J., & van Engeland, H. (1996). The effects of chronic naltrexone treatment in young children: A double-blind, placebo-controlled crossover study. *Biological Psychiatry, 39,* 1023–1031.

Wilson, K., Mills, E., Ross, C., McGowan, J., & Jadad, A. (2003). Association of autistic spectrum disorder and the measles, mumps, and rubella vaccine: A systematic review of current epidemiological evidence. *Archives of Pediatrics and Adolescent Medicine, 157,* 628–634.

Wing, L. (1981a). Asperger's syndrome: A clinical account. *Psychological Medicine, 11,* 115–129.

Wing, L. (1981b). Language, social, and cognitive impairments in autism and severe mental retardation.

Journal of Autism and Developmental Disorders, 11, 31–44.

Wing, L. (1991). The relationship between Asperger's syndrome and Kanner's autism. In U. Frith (Ed.), *Autism and Asperger syndrome* (pp. 93–121). Cambridge, UK: Cambridge University Press.

Wing, L. (1993). The definition and prevalence of autism: A review. *European Child and Adolescent Psychiatry, 2,* 61–74.

Wing, L., & Attwood, A. (1987). Syndromes of autism and atypical development. In D. J. Cohen & A. M. Donnellan (Eds.), *Handbook of autism and pervasive developmental disorders* (pp. 3–19). New York: Wiley.

Wing, L., & Gould, J. (1979). Severe impairments of social interaction and associated abnormalities in children: Epidemiology and classification. *Journal of Autism and Developmental Disorders, 9,* 11–29.

Wing, L., & Potter, D. (2002). The epidemiology of autistic spectrum disorders: Is the prevalence rising? *Mental Retardation and Developmental Disabilities Research Reviews, 8,* 151–161

Wolff, S. (1995). *Loners: The life path of unusual children.* London: Routledge.

World Health Organization. (1992). *The ICD-10 classification of mental and behavioral disorders: Clinical descriptions and diagnostic guidelines.* Geneva: Author.

Yamashita, Y., Fujimoto, C., Nakajima, E., Isagai, T., & Matsuishi, T. (2003). Possible association between congenital cytomegalovirus infection and autistic disorder. *Journal of Autism and Developmental Disorders, 33,* 455–459.

Yeargin-Allsopp, M. (2003, September). *Past and future perspectives on the epidemiology of autism.* Paper presented at the Fourth Annual Collaborative Conference on Autism Spectrum Disorders, Cincinnati, OH.

Yeargin-Allsopp, M., Rice, C., Karapurkar, T., Doernberg, N., Boyle, C., & Murphy, C. (2003). Prevalence of autism in a US metropolitan area. *Journal of the American Medical Association, 289,* 49–55.

Yonan, A. L., Alarcon, M., Cheng, R., Magnusson, P. K., Spence, S. J., Palmer, A. A., et al. (2003). A genomewide screen of 345 families for autism-susceptibility loci. *American Journal of Human Genetics, 73,* 886–897.

Zanolli, K., & Daggett, J. (1998). The effects of reinforcement rate on the spontaneous social initiations of socially withdrawn preschoolers. *Journal of Applied Behavior Analysis, 31,* 117–125.

Zanolli, K., Daggett, J., & Adams, T. (1996). Teaching preschool age autistic children to make spontaneous initiations to peers using priming. *Journal of Autism and Developmental Disorders, 26,* 407–422.

Zarcone, J. R., Iwata, B. A., Smith, R. G., Mazaleski, J. L., & Lerman, D. C. (1994). Reemergence and extinction of self-injurious escape behavior during stimulus (instructional) fading. *Journal of Applied Behavior Analysis, 27,* 307–316.

Zilbovicius, M., Garreau, B., Samson, Y., Remy, P., Barthelemy, C., Syrota, A., et al. (1995). Delayed maturation of frontal cortex in childhood autism. *American Journal of Psychiatry, 152,* 248–252.

8

Learning Disabilities

G. Reid Lyon, Jack M. Fletcher, Lynn S. Fuchs, and Vinita Chhabra

An extraordinarily complex task confronting researchers, clinicians, and educators is to identify and understand the instructional factors and decisions that should be considered in teaching children with learning disabilities (LDs). Frequently, students with LDs do not process information in a manner that allows them to profit from typical classroom instruction, even though the children are seemingly as capable as their classmates and have (at least initially) similar opportunities to learn. As such, the importance of instruction and treatment is central to the concept of LDs as disabling conditions. From clinical and educational standpoints, the validity of the construct of LDs is linked directly to its ability to inform intervention decisions. If identifying students with LDs does not facilitate intervention, the concept would be virtually meaningless except as a legal definition of a group of people with disabilities requiring civil rights protection.

In the past decade, substantial converging scientific research indicates that those conditions eventuating as LDs can, for many students, be prevented through early intervention (Donovan & Cross, 2002; Jenkins & O'Connor, 2002; Snow, Burns, & Griffin, 1998). In the context of this research, the proposal that the magnitude of a student's response to instruction could serve as a critical diagnostic marker for the identification of an LD has gained momentum (Bradley, Danielson, & Hallahan, 2002; Donovan & Cross, 2002; Fuchs & Fuchs, 1998; President's Commission on Excellence in Special Education, 2002; Vaughn & Fuchs, 2003). This proposal is not really new, given that identification of LDs has always required assurances of adequate instructional opportunities. *The emphasis now is on measuring response to high-quality instruction as documented through assessments of progress and through assessments of the quality and integrity of the intervention.* For older students with LDs who have not had the opportunity to benefit from early intervention, there is increasing evidence that high-quality, intense remedial interventions can successfully improve their reading, math, and writing skills (Swanson, Harris, & Graham, 2003; Swanson with Hoskyn & Lee, 1999).

Such research raises the question of why legislation supporting services for students with LDs—legislation that permeates all sectors involved with LDs (clinics, public schools, private schools, and vocational settings)—persists with the traditional analysis on extensive diagnostic testing. The alternative is to prioritize intervention—in a sense reserving LD identification for students who do not respond adequately to high-quality instruction—and then to pursue diagnostic evaluations and labeling. Even in an approach based on instructional response, it is likely that there is a continuum of response to instruction. The goal will be to identify the lower part of the continuum, with identification predicated on falling below some criterion. Then it will be a question of how much additional instruction is needed to reach that criterion, which may be most strongly predicted by progress to date. The focus of testing revolves around instruction, and the continuum is not a univariate achievement or IQ–

achievement distribution, but one derived from assessments of response to instruction. In the absence of systematic, high-quality instruction, all students are at risk for LDs, with variation in the amount and intensity required to teach academic skills. This "treat and test" notion of LDs is a marked departure from the historical emphasis on "test and treat," but it is an approach that does not depart from historical conceptualizations of LDs (Fletcher, Morris, & Lyon, 2003), and that may lead to improved outcomes for these students (Donovan & Cross, 2002).

The primary goal of this chapter is to identify and discuss what we believe are critical issues in the treatment of LDs. Before we embark upon this examination, several themes that guide the organization of this chapter should be summarized. First, the construct of LDs and the many definitions that serve as conceptual frameworks for the identification and treatment of LDs continue to be frequently misunderstood. Even a cursory review of the literature relevant to the history and current status of LDs reveals that the field is beset by pervasive disagreements about the definition of LDs, diagnostic criteria, assessment practices, treatment procedures, and educational policies (Lyon, 1996a; Lyon et al., 2001). During the past decade, and particularly within the past 5 years, substantial progress has been made in developing a reliable and valid classification system for at least some specific types of LDs (Fletcher et al., 2002, 2003; Lyon, 1995a, 1996a, 1996b; Lyon, Fletcher, & Barnes, 2003; Torgesen, 1993). To understand advances in the treatment of LDs, one must understand the field's struggle for a scientific foundation. Accordingly, the first major section of this chapter addresses the field's ongoing transition from clinical intuition to clinical science.

Second, in order to fully understand the diversity of treatment concepts and methods for each type of LD, one must appreciate that they emanate from a wide range of frameworks, models, and theories. Issues relevant to the purposes of treatment, to the ways in which assessments should be conducted and related to treatment, and to the validity of different treatment protocols can be best addressed by identifying the historical and contemporary models and theories that guide instructional decision making for individuals with LDs (Fletcher et al., 2003; Lyon & Moats, 1988). Thus, in a subsequent section of the chapter, we focus on selected schools of thought that serve as a basis for contemporary intervention methods.

Third, the conduct of intervention research with individuals with LDs is complex and can be labor-intensive. Within the context of this complexity, several factors have consistently impeded attempts to study the effectiveness and the efficacy of different interventions in a well-controlled manner. For future research and treatment efforts to be as productive and informative as possible, these factors need to be specifically identified and discussed. Thus a section of this chapter is devoted to methodological issues that affect intervention research.

Fourth, LDs are not a single disorder; rather, they constitute a general category of disabilities in a number of specific domains. Thus, for clarity, we have elected to examine research relevant to the prevention and/or remediation of disabilities in three domains—reading (including deficiencies in word recognition, fluency, and comprehension), written language, and mathematics—and have organized most of the remaining chapter text for this purpose. These domains have been selected both because of their prominence in current definitions of LDs, and because many children and adults are identified as having LDs due to unexpected underachievement or atypical development in these areas.

Finally, some caveats are in order. Given the enormous volume and complexity of literature on topics associated with treatment and instruction, our review of relevant research is necessarily selective rather than exhaustive. For example, given space limitations, it was not possible to address research related to intervention for disorders of attention or for social and emotional difficulties—areas of development that are clearly problematic for many students with LDs. These types of problems are discussed in other chapters of this book. Moreover, although various theoretical and conceptual models related to treatment are reviewed, as are specific intervention methods, we do not view the work emanating from these different sources and perspectives as necessarily contradictory. Rather, thoughtful integration of these models is resulting in more efficacious interventions for individuals with different types of LDs. Lastly, the literature is replete with claims for instructional and treatment methods that are based on subjective, nonreplicated clinical reports, testimonial information, and anecdotal statements. For purposes of brevity and clarity, we have limited our discussion to methods and approaches with some empirical basis that extend beyond testimony or evidence of efficacy in the absence of appropriate comparison groups or clearly defined groups of students with specific academic types of LDs. We do not review intervention research on students broadly defined as having LDs when the form of academic impairment is not indicated. In the absence of this type of specification, the groups are too heterogeneous to determine the real impact of the intervention. However, the reader should note that wide variation exists among studies of the different intervention and teaching methods we have selected for discussion.

THE FIELD'S PASSAGE FROM CLINICAL INTUITION TO CLINICAL SCIENCE

Since their recognition as federally designated disabling conditions in 1968, LDs now represent approximately one-half of all students receiving special education nationally (Donovan & Cross, 2002; President's Commission on Excellence in Special Education, 2002). Yet LDs have traditionally been among the least understood and most debated disabling conditions that affect students (Bradley et al., 2002; Fuchs & Fuchs, 1998; Lyon, 1996a; Lyon et al., 2001; Moats & Lyon, 1993). To reiterate, LDs are not a single disorder, but a general category composed of disabilities in specific academic domains. In U.S. federal regulations governing special education, these are usually organized into seven areas: (1) listening comprehension (receptive language), (2) oral expression (expressive language), (3) basic reading skills (decoding and word recognition), (4) reading comprehension, (5) written expression, (6) mathematics calculation, and (7) mathematics reasoning. These separate types of LDs frequently co-occur with one another, and also with deficits in social skills, emotional disorders, and disorders of attention that usually represent comorbid problems; that is, a child may well have a problem in more than one area (Fletcher, Shaywitz, & Shaywitz, 1999). The reader should note that LDs are not synonymous with reading disability or dyslexia, although they are frequently misinterpreted as such (Lyon, 1995b; Lyon, Shaywitz, & Shaywitz, 2003). However, much of the available information concerning LDs relates to reading disabilities (Lyon, 1996a, 1996b; Lyon

et al., 2001), and the majority of students with LDs have their primary deficits in reading. For students identified for special education in the LD area, reading disabilities represent 80–90% of all LDs (Kavale & Reese, 1992; Lerner, 1989; Lyon et al., 2001). Indeed, two of every five students served in special education in the United States were identified because of difficulties learning to read (President's Commission on Excellence in Special Education, 2002).

Historical Background

Given these numbers, it is not surprising that LDs have been a concern of scientists and educators for over 100 years. The field of LDs in the United States was not born primarily of scientific inquiry, but was developed over time to assist students with clinical and educational needs that were not being addressed by existing policies and programs (Doris, 1993; Hallahan & Mock, 2003; Kavale & Forness, 2003; Lyon, 1996a, 1996b; Lyon et al., 2001; Moats & Lyon, 1993). Research involving LDs was initiated because of the practical need (1) to understand individual differences among children and adults who displayed *specific* deficits in spoken and written language, while maintaining integrity in general intellectual functioning; and (2) to provide services to students who were not being adequately served by the general educational system (Lyon et al., 2001; Torgesen, 1991; Zigmond, 1993).

In the early 1960s, special services were not provided to children who manifested learning difficulties but who were average or above in general intellectual abilities. These children did not manifest behaviors or characteristics typically associated with individuals identified as having mental retardation, emotional disturbances, or physical impairments (visual, hearing-related, or orthopedic/motor). Thus their intervention needs were often overlooked or not addressed. Because of this void, parents and educators, under the leadership of Samuel Kirk, established the Association for Children with Learning Disabilities and convened its first meeting in Chicago in 1963. At this meeting, a rigorous advocacy agenda was developed to promote recognition of LDs as significant disabilities. At the same time, a scientific focus was identified that reflected the views of several disciplines with a tradition of interest in learning problems—neurology, psychology, remedial education, neurology, and speech–

language pathology. Pioneers within each of these disciplines promoted theories of disability, designed tests presumed to measure information-processing dysfunctions, and developed remedial techniques that were appealing because they were logically designed to address deficits in learning. The field progressed rapidly through many developmental stages after the initial formal recognition of LDs as disabling conditions in 1968 (Doris, 1993; Hallahan & Mock, 2003; Kavale & Forness, 1985, 2003; Myers & Hammill, 1990).

In brief, the diagnostic concept of LDs gained significant momentum during the 1970s and 1980s. The proliferation of students diagnosed as having LDs during these two decades was related to multiple factors. First, it was clear that many students had difficulties in learning to read, to write, and to understand and apply mathematics concepts in a manner commensurate with age and grade expectations. Thus the newly developed category provided such youngsters with a clinical "home" and eligibility for special education services. Second, it became clear that identification of an LD on the basis of deficits in a specific area of academic achievement did not necessarily imply mental retardation, behavioral difficulties, or sensory disabilities. On the contrary, many students with LDs manifest difficulties in learning *despite* having adequate intelligence, and they typically also have intact vision, hearing, and emotional status. Within this context, the fact that many students with LDs displayed average or above-average intelligence gave parents and teachers hope that difficulties in learning to read, write, or calculate could be surmounted if only the right arrangement of instructional conditions and settings could be identified. Third, it emerged that the LD label is not a stigmatizing one. Parents and teachers were (and are) more comfortable with the term than with etiologically based labels such as "minimal brain dysfunction" or "perceptual handicap" (Lyon, 1996a; Lyon et al., 2001).

The fact that LDs were initially identified as disabling conditions on the basis of advocacy rather than systematic scientific inquiry is certainly not uncommon in the domains of psychology, medicine, education, or public policy. In fact, many scientific advances are stimulated by vocal critics of the educational or medical status quo. Rarely is a psychological condition, disease, or educational problem afforded attention until political forces are mobilized by parents, patients, or other advocates expressing their concerns about the quality of life to their elected officials. Clearly this was the case in the field of LDs, where parents and child advocates successfully lobbied Congress to enact legislation in 1970 via the Education of the Handicapped Act (P.L. 91-230), which authorized funds for research and intervention programs to address the needs of students with specific LDs (Doris, 1993; Lyon et al., 2001).

Definitional Issues

A fundamental historical assumption underlying the construct of LDs is that the academic difficulties manifested by individuals with LDs are *unexpected*, given the often recognized disparity between such difficulties and other factors (such as intellectual capabilities, opportunities to learn, and freedom from extreme social disadvantage or emotional disturbance). In addition, traditional definitions of LDs provide statements that emphasize what the condition is not, rather than what it is. For example, the statutory definition of LDs contained in the Individuals with Disabilities Education Act (IDEA) Amendments of 1997 and 2004, as well as the U.S. federal formulation of LDs in 1968, is as follows:

> The term "specific learning disability" means a disorder in one or more of the basic psychological processes involved in understanding or in using language, spoken or written, which may manifest itself in an imperfect ability to listen, speak, read, write, spell, or to do mathematical calculations. The term includes such conditions as perceptual handicaps, brain injury, minimal brain dysfunction, dyslexia, and developmental aphasia. The term does not include students who have learning disabilities which are primarily the result of visual, hearing, or motor handicaps, or mental retardation, or emotional disturbance, or of environmental, cultural, or economic disadvantage. (34 C.F.R. 300)

As can be seen, an important part of the definition of LDs under the IDEA is its use of exclusionary language. Specifically, LDs cannot be attributed primarily to mental retardation, emotional disturbance, cultural differences, or environmental or economic disadvantage. This aspect of the definition clearly reflects the historical underpinnings of the category that were discussed earlier, as well as initial concerns by the U.S. Congress concerning (1) commingling of funds for special education and compensatory education, and (2) confusion of LDs with other categories in the special education legislation. However, another important component involves heterogeneity—the idea that there are multiple types of LDs. Despite the evidence supporting heterogeneity, most definitions of LDs are the same, regardless of the type of LDs (Fletcher et al., 2002). Finally, given this heterogeneity and the exclusions, what is the marker for key concepts of LDs: Is it a discrepancy between aptitude and achievement, indicating a disorder of psychological processing? In 1977, largely in response to concerns about states concerning the need for *inclusionary* criteria, the U.S. Department of Education proposed that an LD be identified as a discrepancy between scores on IQ and achievement tests. This regulatory emphasis is maintained by most states as the cornerstone for LD eligibility, now for over 27 years (Reschly, Hosp, & Schmied, 2003).

The result is that the concept of LDs embedded in U.S. federal regulations focuses on the notion of a discrepancy between a child's academic achievement and his or her capacity and opportunity to learn. More succinctly, Zigmond (1993) notes that typical definitions of "learning disabilities reflect unexpected learning problems in a seemingly capable child" (p. 254). Despite the significant role that a definition should play in the scientific and clinical understanding of LDs, the federal definitions currently encased in law are far too vague and ambiguous to provide clear guidance for educational and research practices (Fletcher & Morris, 1986; Fletcher et al., 2002, 2003; Lyon, 1996a; Lyon et al., 2001). The federal definition fails to provide specific and valid *inclusionary* criteria for distinguishing individuals with LDs from those with other disabilities or generalized learning difficulties (Fletcher et al., 2002; Lyon, 1996a, 1996b; Lyon et al., 2001). Attempts to tighten the definition have not fared appreciably better, as can be seen in the revised definition produced by the National Joint Committee on Learning Disabilities (NJCLD, 1988):

> Learning disabilities is a general term that refers to a heterogeneous group of disorders manifested by significant difficulties in the acquisition and use of listening, speaking, reading, writing, reasoning, or mathematical abilities. These disorders are intrinsic to the individual, presumed to be due to central nervous system dysfunction, and may occur across the life span. Problems in self-regulatory behaviors, social perception, and social interaction may exist with learning disabilities but do not by themselves constitute a learning disability. Although learning disabilities may occur concomitantly with other handicapping conditions (for example, sensory impairment, mental retardation, serious emotional disturbance) or with extrinsic influences (such as cultural differences, insufficient or inappropriate instruction), they are not the result of those conditions or influences. (p. 1)

On the positive side, the NJCLD definition reflects consensus on the concept of LDs in clinical, educational, and political arenas; it eliminates the word "children"; and it adopts a life span perspective, which is more consistent with the wide age range of individuals in need of identification and services in adulthood and in occupational/vocational settings (Hammill, 1990). Unfortunately, this revised definition does not provide specific guidance on identification criteria that would indicate how people should be defined as having LDs.

Clinically, the criteria for assigning support services for individuals with LDs are typically not clear or justified by research findings; this situation leads to numerous inequities in who does and who does not receive specialized services and programs. Similarly, vague descriptions of the nature of LDs provided in current definitions fail to provide guidance about which specific academic and adaptive functioning skills are impaired and require remedial attention. Unfortunately, the lack of emphasis in current definitions on the salience of specific academic, cognitive, and information-processing skills necessary for learning contributes to inadequate training for professionals concerned with children's school performance (Lyon et al., 2001; Moats, 1994b; Moats & Lyon, 1996). Concerns about the limitations of these types of omnibus exclusionary definitions have prompted many scholars to call for a moratorium on the development of broad definitions, at least for research purposes. As Stanovich (1993) has stated,

> Scientific investigations of some generically defined entity called "learning disability" simply make little sense given what we already know about heterogeneity across various learning domains. Research investigations must define groups

specifically in terms of the domain of deficit (reading disability, arithmetic disability). (p. 273)

Stanovich (1993) makes it clear that the problems with the federal statutory definition of LDs, as well as the NJCLD definition, begin with the failure to specify marker variables that can be used to indicate the presence of LDs. These variables are most likely to exist in the achievement domain, as these difficulties are the most overt manifestations of LD. Attempts to define LDs by a focus on exclusionary criteria, cognitive processing skills, or "biological" markers have not met with much success unless anchored with a focus on academic skills (Fletcher, Francis, Morris, & Lyon, 2005). In line with this suggestion, recent attempts to develop definitions for specific types of LDs have been made. For example, a working group composed of clinicians, educators, and scientists from universities within the United States; representatives from the International Dyslexia Association (IDA); and representatives from the National Institute of Child Health and Human Development (NICHD) recently revised an inclusionary definition of dyslexia (reading disability) (see Lyon et al., 2003) that was initially developed by the IDA in 1994 (see Lyon, 1995b). This most current definition elaborates on the inclusionary definition published in 1995 by including relationships between and among word-level reading skills, fluency, reading comprehension, and vocabulary development:

> Dyslexia is a specific learning disability that is neurobiological in origin. It is characterized by difficulties with accurate and/or fluent word recognition and by poor spelling and decoding abilities. These difficulties typically result from a deficit in the phonological component of language that is often unexpected in relation to other cognitive abilities and the provision of effective classroom instruction. Secondary consequences may include problems in reading comprehension and reduced reading experience that can impede growth of vocabulary and background knowledge. (Lyon et al., 2003, p. 2)

The construction of this revised definition provides an example of how current research continues to inform policy and practice, and shows how the field of LDs continues to progress from a context of clinical intuition toward one of clinical science. Note that in contrast to the general definitions of LDs, the revised IDA

research-based definition is composed of specific, evidence-based *inclusionary* statements that can be operationalized.

In addition, the revised IDA definition does not emphasize the need for a discrepancy between IQ and achievement scores in the identification of dyslexia, although it maintains the concept of unexpected unevenness in development. This is because in the last 15 years, a number of studies addressing the validity of IQ–achievement discrepancy as a diagnostic marker have provided little evidence that such a discrepancy demarcates a specific type of LD that differs from other forms of underachievement (Fletcher et al., 2002, 2003; Francis et al., 1996, 2005; Hoskyn & Swanson, 2000; Stuebing et al., 2002). Although the case against the use of IQ–achievement discrepancy is strongest for word-level reading disabilities, enough research has been completed on the underlying *psychometric* model to cast doubt on applications to others forms of LDs in reading, math, and written expression (Francis et al., 2005; Stuebing et al., 2002).

Heterogeneity of LDs

The field of LDs is a long way from constructing inclusionary definitions for the different types of LDs that are included in typical general exclusionary definitions, such as the first two definitions given above. The domain-specific definition developed for dyslexia (reading disability)—the most prevalent type of the different LDs—represents a continued attempt at constructing a classification system that identifies different types of LDs, as well as the distinctions and interrelationships among these types and other developmental disorders (Fletcher et al., 2002, 2003; Lyon, 1995b, 1996a; Lyon et al., 2001; Torgesen, 1993).

These types of inclusionary definitions are becoming increasingly important. Fletcher and colleagues (2002) reviewed the evidence for the seven forms of LDs in the federal regulatory definition, observing that disorders of oral expression and listening comprehension do not represent academic skill deficiencies and are more properly described as disorders of spoken language, which are typically covered in classifications of speech and language disorders. Listening comprehension and reading comprehension are highly correlated, especially beyond grade 3, so why identify these areas of difficulty separately? They also found little evidence to support a separate disorder of math reasoning, asking what aspect of math does not involve reasoning. In addition to LDs in reading involving word recognition and comprehension, there are specific reading difficulties that involve fluency, and these may represent a form of reading LD. Noting the evidence suggesting differences in math disorders with and without a word recognition/fluency component, Fletcher and colleagues suggested that co-occurring reading and math disability be separately identified. Thus there is evidence for the six forms of LDs summarized in Table 8.1: reading disorders involving word recognition, fluency, and comprehension; math disability; both reading and math disability; and disorders of written expression. The evidence base is weakest for disorders of written expression, partly because of the high co-occurrence of reading and writing difficulties, and the presence of writing problems in students with difficulties involving math and attention-deficit/hyperactivity disorder (ADHD).

Note that this proposed classification specifically identifies academic skills as one marker for LDs. Most of the evidence for the construct of LDs is based on achievement typologies (Fletcher et al., 2005). In the absence of this type of marker, it is difficult to support the validity of LDs as entities (Stanovich, 1993). Some may argue for the primacy of cognitive processing deficits as implied by the federal definition, but other than phonological awareness and its link with word recognition, no cognitive process stands out as a specific marker for other LDs. There is little evidence that intervening in cognitive processes generalizes to academic gains (Reschly, Tilly, & Grimes, 1999). In older students, processing assessments do not appear to provide information that is significantly independent of the data provided by a thorough assessment of academic skills, and the tools are not adequately

developed to reliably indicate LDs (Torgesen, 2002). In kindergarten and grade 1, processing assessments may help identify students at risk for LDs, but even here interventions need to be conceptualized in terms of the links with academic outcomes. In reading, measures associated with print knowledge (e.g., letter names and sounds) are better predictors of outcomes than phonological awareness is (Schatschneider, Fletcher, Francis, Carlson, & Foorman, 2004). This does not mean that processing deficits do not "cause" academic deficits, or that such deficits are not mediated by the brain. Rather, from a classification and identification perspective, these assessments are not necessary except to establish risk in younger students, and are redundant in older students because of the evidence base showing links of processing deficits to academic skills and neurological processes. Thus the construct of LDs has no validity independent of classification and identification procedures anchored in academic skills. Finally, contrary to some arguments (Kavale & Forness, 2000, 2003), the notion that LDs must be defined as a unitary construct does not seem feasible, and certainly are not reliably demarcated by discrepancies between IQ and achievement.

Despite the time that it has taken the scientific community to generate more parsimonious research-based definitions and coherent classifications for specific types of LDs, various conceptual approaches for treatment, intervention, and remediation have emerged from the clinical community over the past three decades. The major issue has been the types of LDs with which these models are most effectively applied. These models are reviewed in the next section.

CONCEPTUAL APPROACHES TO TREATMENT

The types of instructional treatment methods that are applied to individuals with LDs are influenced significantly by the conceptual approaches or models that are used to formulate the rationale, purposes, and expected outcomes of these interventions. Researchers and clinicians differ in their views with respect to such approaches. For example, if one believes that specific academic deficits are a function of aberrant neural processing of information, the treatment method might target the hypothesized underlying neurological substrate respon-

TABLE 8.1. Evidence-Based Classification of Learning Disabilities

1. Reading disability—word recognition
2. Reading disability—comprehension
3. Reading disability—fluency
4. Math disability—computations/problem solving
5. Reading disability and math disability
6. Written expression disability—spelling, text, handwriting

sible for the deficits, in the hope that improvements in underlying processes will result in improvements in the academic behavior. On the other hand, if one minimizes the role of the nervous system in understanding learning deficits, then the processing dimensions or academic behaviors become the target for treatment. Obviously, these are overly simplistic examples of complex approaches, but they indicate how approaches to treatment are influenced by conceptual and/or theoretical points of view. In point of fact, different conceptual approaches to the treatment of individuals with LDs are more easily discussed at a general level, but lose their explanatory power when one attempts to employ them to generate specific instructional methods (see Lyon & Moats, 1988).

Historical Perspectives on Treatment

When LDs were first recognized in the early 1960s as disabling conditions, even before the field of LDs became a category of special education, the treatment approaches prominent at that time were reflected in three conceptual models (Bateman, 1967; Hallahan, Kauffman, & Lloyd, 1996; Hallahan & Mock, 2003): (1) the medical or etiological model; (2) the psychoeducational or diagnostic–remedial model; and (3) the behavioral or task-analytic model (Figure 8.1).

Medical or Etiological Model

Medically oriented approaches viewed LDs as overt symptoms of underlying biological pa-

thology. For example, a number of theorists hypothesized that deficits in underlying neurological processes could impede development of language abilities, visual and auditory perception, perceptual–motor organization, and ocular–motor functioning (see Mann, 1979, and Vellutino, 1979; see Vellutino, Fletcher, Scanlon, & Snowling, 2004, for a review). More specifically, deficits in oral language could be described as a primary language disorder due to organic impairment resulting from putative anoxia. Recommended treatment might involve patterning exercises in which a child repeated the sequence of oral language acquisition to "stimulate" brain regions thought to subserve the language process in question.

It is difficult to find evidence (beyond testimonials and anecdotal reports) to support the assumptions, treatment methods, and stated outcomes associated with these early medical or etiological approaches (Lyon & Moats, 1988). Given the noticeable lack of validity for such methods, the use of medical or etiological approaches to guide treatment declined substantially over the years, but has seen some recent reemergence. Intervention involving auditory processing, eye movements, the use of special lenses to correct visual processing deficits, "brain-based" learning, and perceptual skills are again becoming more prominent, despite lack of efficacy and generalization to actual development of academic skills (e.g., reading). For instance, the Fast ForWord (FFW) family of programs claims to "train the brain" to process information more effectively through a set of computer games that slow and

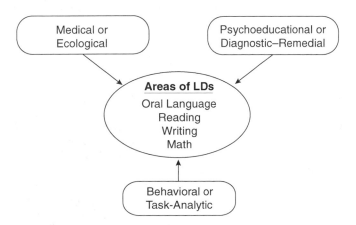

FIGURE 8.1. Historical approaches to the treatment of learning disabilities.

magnify the acoustic changes within typical speech (Scientific Learning Corporation, 1999). A recent randomized study of the effectiveness of FFW programs involving language purported to improve reading indicated that although some aspects of students' language skills improved, actual reading skills were not significantly enhanced (Rouse & Krueger, 2004). Similar results were obtained by Pokorni, Worthington, and Jamison (2004) and by Hook, Macaruso, and Jones (2001). As we see in the next section, if there is one cardinal intervention principle for students with LDs, it is that training only in motor, visual, neural, or cognitive processes does not generalize to the academic area. Because this version of FFW does not have a print component, no generalization to reading would be expected.

Psychoeducational or Diagnostic–Remedial Model

Proponents of psychoeducational models of LDs interpreted academic deficits as reflecting aberrations in the ability to perceive, integrate, and remember auditory and visual information, associated with the development of listening, speaking, reading, and writing behaviors (Frostig, 1967; Kirk & Kirk, 1971). Assessment procedures were developed to identify specific strengths and weaknesses in, for example, auditory and visual processes hypothesized to be related to academic functioning, and this information was considered in the process known as "clinical teaching." In contrast to the medical model, the psychoeducational approach advocated teaching academic skills as well as information-processing abilities (not underlying biological processes), by taking into account the student's modality preferences or areas of information-processing strength (visual, auditory, and/or kinesthetic), the nature of the content to be learned (verbal or nonverbal), and the response required (oral or written).

Psychoeducational or diagnostic–remedial approaches have not received a great deal of support in the scientific literature (Lyon & Moats, 1988). There is little evidence that such approaches have incorporated the essential elements of learning, and the notions of modality preferences and learning styles have been reported to be conceptually and empirically weak (Liberman & Shankweiler, 1985; Reschly et al., 1999). In addition, many of the assessment measures designed to evaluate auditory and vi-

sual processing characteristics and other learning styles were flawed with respect to reliability and validity, and were related only minimally to academic content (Vellutino, 1979).

As we see below, even more contemporary approaches have not fared much better. In the neuropsychological area, there is little evidence for subtype × treatment interactions (Lyon, Fletcher, et al., 2003). Despite extravagant claims, newer aptitude tests based on, for example, variations in sequential and simultaneous processing have not been shown to interact with intervention outcomes in math, much less reading (Reschly et al., 1999). Even models with strong theoretical foundations, such as teaching phonological awareness skills, do not generalize to reading without a component that involves letters and their sounds (National Reading Panel [NRP], 2000). These findings are not unlike those apparent for the medical model in showing lack of generalization of process training to the academic area.

Behavioral or Task-Analytic Model

In contrast to medical and psychoeducational models and approaches, behavioral approaches have conceptualized LDs as resulting from a mismatch between enabling behaviors and the characteristics of the academic task (Lyon & Moats, 1988). There is no assumption of underlying pathology or information-processing deficiency. Instead, assessment and instructional activities are directed toward evaluating academic skill deficits and modifying them with techniques derived from learning theory. The major assumption guiding this approach is that academic content consists of skill hierarchies, and that complex academic behaviors such as reading, writing, and mathematics can be task-analyzed into component subskills. Explicit instruction is then applied to ensure that all prerequisite subskills are mastered and the target behaviors taught.

Reviews of the effectiveness of behavioral interventions with individuals with LDs have generally indicated favorable results with respect to increasing academic skills (see Gadow, Torgesen, & Dahlem, 1985). However, there has been some concern that academic skills acquired through the application of behavioral procedures do not generalize to contexts not incorporated in the teaching paradigm, and that some behavioral interventions are neither practical nor cost-effective (Myers & Hammill,

1990). As Torgesen (1986) pointed out, early behavioral models provided no conceptual framework for the ultimate understanding of individual differences in cognitive processing or neurological functioning, and this could have limited understanding of why certain teaching procedures succeed or fail with particular learners.

The strengths of these models, however, is the focus on explicit intervention on academic skills, or other behaviors sometimes associated with LDs. As we discuss next, these three historical approaches to the assessment and treatment of students with LDs have, despite their stated shortcomings, contributed substantially to the intervention models that are in use today. This is particularly true of behavioral approaches to intervention, which continue to demonstrate efficacy with specific types of academic deficits.

Contemporary Perspectives

A review of the current literature relevant to the treatment of LDs indicates that a number of approaches have evolved in recent years to guide instruction. Prominent among them are cognitive, cognitive-behavioral, task-analytic, neuropsychological, and constructivist models (Figure 8.2). Even more recently, intraindividual-differences models and models based on response to instruction (e.g., problem-solving models) have emerged. These models have been shaped by some of the approaches depicted in Figure 8.2 and are also discussed below. It should be noted that the theoretical roots and emphases of all these models often overlap, and

they are distinguished largely by their relative degree of attention to various factors.

Cognitive Models

The cognitive models that serve as frameworks for treatment and intervention today are descendants of the psychoeducational models discussed earlier. Cognitive models typically emphasize the processes involved in human thinking and are frequently referred to as "information-processing models" (Hallahan et al., 1996). Whereas the earlier psychoeducational models focused on the reception, perception, integration, and expression of information, contemporary cognitive models address specific information-processing abilities related to such domains as memory (e.g., rehearsal), thinking (e.g., metacognition), and more specific cognitive skills (e.g., the role of phonological awareness in the development of basic reading skills). Cognitive models are typically derived from cognitive and developmental psychology, and their views of LDs suggest that instruction should be directed toward enabling students to exercise self-conscious, deliberate, and strategically applied efforts when learning academic content (Brown & Campione, 1986). With respect to teaching an individual with an LD problem-solving behaviors, assessment procedures are designed to determine whether the student can analyze the nature of the problem, relate the nature of the problem to previous experience, devise a strategic plan for operating on the information, and monitor and adjust performance (Flavell, 1979; Hallahan et al., 1996). Instructional emphasis is then

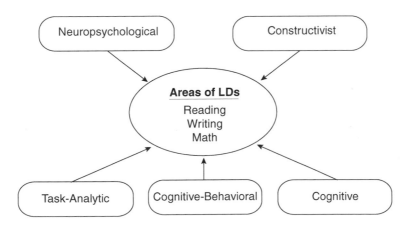

FIGURE 8.2. Contemporary approaches to the treatment of learning disabilities.

directed toward (1) increasing the learner's awareness of task demands, (2) teaching the student to employ appropriate strategies to facilitate task completion, and (3) teaching the student to monitor the success of the strategy (Lyon & Moats, 1988).

Support for the application of cognitive (e.g., metacognitive) principles to the assessment and instruction of problem-solving behaviors has accrued from studies that have characterized individuals with LDs as failing to enlist efficient, task-appropriate strategies and to orchestrate their use (Palinscar & Brown, 1987). For example, Torgesen (1987) found that poor readers were less likely than good readers to use organization and memory strategies spontaneously to aid in the grouping and subsequent recall of pictorial stimuli. However, following explicit instruction in the use of categorization as a mnemonic aid, differences in recall between the groups were reduced. Similar procedures teach students with LDs how to use existing academic skills in a strategically optimal manner, so that content information can be acquired, manipulated, stored, retrieved, and expressed. Such procedures have been applied to instructional situations involving thinking and organizational skills (Borkowski & Burke, 1996; Graham & Harris, 1996), reading comprehension (Palinscar & Brown, 1987; Vaughn & Klingner, 2004), arithmetic problem solving (Cawley & Miller, 1986; L. S. Fuchs, Fuchs, Hamlett, & Appleton, 2002), written language skills (Englert, Hiebert, & Stewart, 1986; Graham & Harris, 2003), memory skills (Swanson & Saez, 2003), and study skills (Hughes, Ruhl, Schumaker, & Deshler, 2002; Wong, 1986). These approaches, often provided at a classroom level, appear effective in enhancing the performance of students with LDs if they involve a link to an academic domain (Swanson et al., 1999).

A narrower conceptualization and application of a cognitive model can be seen in studies of cognitive/linguistic factors in skill acquisition. In the main, these studies have employed (1) language-based models, which are used primarily to conceptualize the nature of linguistic deficits associated with reading, writing, and spelling disorders (Siegel, 2003; Vellutino et al., 2004); and (2) various forms of cognitive strategy instruction (Lovett, Barron, & Benson, 2003; Swanson et al., 1999). More specifically, deficiencies in phonological coding and short-term memory for linguistic material have been causally linked to poor reading decoding, poor spelling, word retrieval problems, and reading comprehension difficulties (Adams, 1990; Shankweiler & Liberman, 1989; Share & Stanovich, 1995; Siegel, 2003; Vellutino et al., 2004). The major deficiency associated with poor reading, according to this conceptual model, is neither auditory, visual, nor kinesthetic; it is a linguistic deficit that interferes with the reader's ability to grasp the concept that words have parts (phonemes, syllables, and morphemes), and that these are parts represented by the abstract alphabetical code. In turn, this point of view has provided a rationale for language-based interventions that teach word recognition and comprehension in a logical, sequential, and explicit manner, regardless of the learner's general cognitive profile. In word recognition interventions, students are taught to analyze the sound structure of words, sound–symbol relations, inflectional and derivational forms of words, syntactic transformations, and text structure (Lyon & Moats, 1988; Moats & Lyon, 1996). Intervention approaches based on this type of cognitive/linguistic conceptualization have received a good deal of support in the research literature, particularly with respect to beginning reading development, but only when the intervention is tied specifically to academic content (Snow et al., 1998). Similarly, intervention in different cognitive strategies improves word recognition and comprehension (Lovett et al., 2003; Swanson et al., 1999).

Cognitive-Behavioral Models

As the name suggests, cognitive-behavioral models integrate the empirical principles of behavioral approaches with the notion that affective and cognitive states influence behavior. In contrast to traditional behavioral approaches, this view includes mental activities in the active determination of behavior. In addition, unlike the strictly cognitive approaches, cognitive-behavioral models recognize the considerable influence of contingencies of reinforcement on learning (Hallahan et al., 1996). A critical concept in the development of cognitive-behavioral approaches to intervention is "reciprocal determinism"—that is, the idea that behavior, environmental events, and internal variables such as thoughts and feeling interact with and influence one another. Within this context, the application of behavioral principles to modify external behavior is a legitimate intervention method, as is the application of strategies to alter cognitive processing and metacognitive behavior (see Meichenbaum, 1977). In contrast to strict cognitive approaches to intervention, cognitive-behavioral interventions emphasize actively involving students in learning, particularly with respect to monitoring and directing their thinking and then measuring the outcomes of the intervention in an objective manner (Borkowski & Burke, 1996; Hallahan et al., 1996). Thus, in teaching a student word attack and word recognition skills, the student not only is exposed to the specific subskills involved, but also is taught a strategy for applying these skills to the reading process (Lovett et al., 2003).

A strong argument for utilizing cognitive-behavioral approaches with individuals with LDs is that multicomponent, integrative interventions are necessary to address interrelated problems of an affective, behavioral, and cognitive nature. An excellent example of such an integrated model is "self-regulated strategy development" (SRSD; Graham & Harris, 1996, 2003), which was designed to help students (1) master higher-level cognitive processes and strategies underlying effective performance on academic tasks; (2) develop autonomous, self-regulated use of these processes and strategies; and (3) form positive attitudes about themselves and their academic capabilities. According to Graham and Harris (1996), students learn specific strategies for successfully engaging in academic tasks, in conjunction with procedures for applying and regulating the use of these strategies in the tasks, and for modifying undesirable behaviors such as impulsivity that may interfere with performance. This approach has been employed effectively to teach strategies and self-regulation procedures in reading and mathematics (Case, Harris, & Graham, 1992), as well as writing (Graham & Harris, 2003). The Learning Strategies Curriculum is an example of a comprehensive set of teaching routines addressing multiple domains of academic and behavior functioning in students with LDs (Schumaker, Deshler, & McKnight, 2002).

Task-Analytic Models

Interventions that are guided by a task-analytic perspective have a rich theoretical and experimental history. In essence, task-analytic models place the student's actions and the environment foremost, and deemphasize underlying causal mechanisms or thought processes. Functionally, task-analytic models require that an operational learning objective first be specified, followed by a detailed description and sequencing of the specific steps necessary to achieve the objective (Hallahan et al., 1996; Reschly et al., 1999). A number of different theories of learning have contributed to the design and implementation of task-analytic models, with stimulus control factors being emphasized by researchers studying concept learning (Carnine, Silbert, & Kame'enui, 1997; Engelmann & Carnine, 1982), and reinforcement contingencies being emphasized by radical behaviorists (Bijou, 1970; Lovitt, 1967; Skinner, 1968). Many of the intervention concepts inherent within task-analytic models are exemplified within the context of "direct instruction" (Rosenshine & Stevens, 1986). In the main, direct instruction consists of nine teaching functions: (1) a review of prerequisite learning; (2) a short statement of goals at the beginning of the lesson; (3) a presentation of new concepts and material in small steps, with student practice after each step; (4) the provision of clear and detailed instructions and explanations; (5) the provision of a high level of practice for all students; (6) a continual checking of student understanding of concepts through responses to teacher questions; (7) the explicit guidance of students during initial practice; (8) the provision of systematic feedback and corrections; and (9) the provision of explicit instruction and practice for seatwork exercises. Where necessary, it also includes (10) the monitoring of students during seatwork.

Direct Instruction methods have been expanded and elaborated by Englemann and his colleagues at the University of Oregon (Adams & Carnine, 2003; Carnine, 1980; Englemann & Carnine, 1982; Gersten, White, Falco, & Carnine, 1982). Specifically, although the Oregon group's approach is similar to that of Rosenshine and Stevens (1986) with respect to placing a strong emphasis on the teacher's behavior in the form of explicit correction, reinforcement, and provision of practice opportunities for students, Englemann and his colleagues also stress the logical analysis of the instructional communication between the teacher and the student. A central feature of this logical analysis is that instruction should provide the opportunity for only one interpretation of the concept that has been presented ("faultless instruction"). As Adams and Carnine (2003) have noted, if the instructional presentation fosters more than one interpretation, some students will learn the wrong interpretation and thus prolong or inhibit learning of the correct concept. Within the teaching lesson itself, the interaction between teachers and students is structured by having lessons presented according to field-tested scripts. In the typical lesson, a teacher works with a small group of students. The teacher asks questions of the students at a rate as high as 10–12 per minute, and the students answer chorally, with the teacher then providing reinforcement or corrective feedback (depending on the accuracy of the students' answers).

Although the instructional principles associated with Direct Instruction and other task-analytic methods have been criticized because of the extensive structure provided by the teacher, the effectiveness of such methods has clearly been demonstrated with both typically achieving students (Carnine, 1980) and students with LDs (Adams & Carnine, 2003; Gersten et al., 1982). When compared to students receiving instruction via standard classroom practices, students in groups provided with direct instruction typically outperform controls by at least three-fourths of a standard deviation (Adams & Carnine, 2003; White, 1988).

Neuropsychological and Intraindividual-Difference Models

Neuropsychological approaches to the instruction of individuals with LDs incorporate assessment and remediation concepts from both traditional medical and psychoeducational theories and models; they thus share some shortcomings of these models, particularly with respect to the reliability and construct validity of assessment procedures (Brown & Campione, 1986; Lyon & Moats, 1988; Reschly et al., 1999; Torgesen, 2002) and to ecological validity (Lyon & Moats, 1988). We consider neuropsychological models to be variants of medical models, in that they stress the role of neurobiology in learning.

We are addressing neuropsychological models separately in this chapter, because they are chronologically more current than traditional medical models and because they emphasize remediation of the academic learning defi-

ciencies. Neuropsychological approaches proliferated in the last decade, commensurate with advances in the basic neurosciences, but their importance has begun to fade because implementation has not been linked to improved intervention outcomes (Lyon, Fletcher, et al., 2003). Interestingly, many of the individuals conducting successful intervention research are trained as neuropsychologists and have considerable experience with this model.

In general, neuropsychological models and theories of LDs conceptualize learning strengths and weaknesses as manifestations of efficient and inefficient brain regions or systems (Fisk & Rourke, 1983; Obrzut & Hynd, 1983; Rourke, 1995). Within this context, instruction is designed so that intact neural systems will be exploited in bypassing the areas of dysfunction. For example, several researchers (see Kirby & Robinson, 1987) have extended theoretical concepts relevant to cerebral asymmetry and hemispheric specialization to explain both the information-processing and response characteristics of students with LDs. Others (see Lovett, Steinbach, & Frijters, 2000; Wolf & Bowers, 1999) have hypothesized that LDs can result from a number of independent neurobehavioral deficiencies in information processing, thus underscoring the need to identify LD subtypes and subtype-specific interventions. In implementations of these approaches, neuropsychological aptitudes such as simultaneous and sequential processing, linguistic (phonological, semantic, syntactic) processing, and visual–spatial capacities are considered when instruction of academic skills is undertaken.

Evidence to support the clinical efficacy and scientific validity of these neuropsychological approaches remains sparse. Lyon and his colleagues (see Lyon, 1985; Lyon, Moats, & Flynn, 1988) adduced preliminary data suggesting that LD subtypes, identified on the basis of subtype members' performance on neuropsychological tasks, differ significantly with respect to response to reading instruction. However, Lyon (1996a) and Newby and Lyon (1991) have cautioned against the overinterpretation of these data.

Bakker and his associates (Bakker, 1984; Bakker & Vinke, 1985) reported experiments wherein hemisphere-specific stimulation increased the reading capabilities of two subtypes of children with dyslexia. Although Bakker's data provide some support for the practice of classifying LDs by processing subtype, the results of these experiments should likewise be interpreted with caution. The subjects in the Bakker and Vinke (1985) study were inadequately described with respect to marker variables, were drawn from a low-IQ school-identified population, and were not well differentiated with regard to subtypes of dyslexia. Furthermore, procedures with known reliability constraints (dichotic listening paradigms and patterns of oral reading errors) were used to form the subtypes, which places in question the internal validity of this type of classification (Lyon & Risucci, 1988). There were no controls. Recent attempts to replicate these findings have not met with success (Berends & Reitsma, 2005).

Despite some strides in the use of neuropsychological theories and models to guide instruction for students with LDs, it appears premature to accept without qualification the validity of such practices. For example, the Cognitive Assessment System (CAS; Naglieri & Das, 1997) has been aggressively promoted as a vehicle for planning instruction. The CAS involves assessments of four constructs (Planning, Attention, Simultaneous, Sequential), which have been hypothesized to produce profiles of strengths and weaknesses that interact with response to intervention. Naglieri and Johnson (2000) subdivided a group of 19 students into those with significantly lower scores in Planning ($n = 3$) and compared them with the other 16 students, 6 of whom had lower scores on one of the other CAS scales and 10 of whom had no weaknesses. The students had been identified for special education under several eligibility categories, including LDs. An intervention was provided that emphasized planning in math problem solving. Naglieri and Johnson found that students with Planning difficulties benefited more from the intervention than students who did not have low Planning scores. Note, however, that the samples were small and that the study could not even test for differential response to different types of interventions (i.e., subtype × intervention interactions).

In a recent large-scale study, Kroesbergen, Van Luit, and Naglieri (2003) identified 267 students with LDs in math. Administration of the CAS to these students showed lower scores on all scales in the group with LDs in math than in a normative reference group. Comparing students with different kinds of math

problems showed variations in different CAS scales. In an evaluation of the effects of intervention, no relationships between type of cognitive deficit and outcome were found in this large sample. Thus evidence supporting subtype × treatment interactions based on the CAS does not appear to be robust.

More recent variations involve rate–accuracy classifications, which are actually based on an assessment of *reading* skills (Lovett, Steinbach, et al., 2000), and models based on the double-deficit model, which focus on *processing* skills (Wolf & Bowers, 1999). Lovett (1984; Lovett, Steinbach, et al., 2000) proposed subtypes of reading disability based on impairments in the accuracy and fluency of word and text reading. Children are identified as "accuracy-disabled" if they struggle with reading words in isolation. Those who are stronger at word recognition but weaker in the fluency of word and text reading are identified as "rate-disabled." In intervention studies, Lovett, Lacerenza, and colleagues (2000) found some differences in intervention outcomes between the accuracy- and rate-disabled groups on contextual reading, whereas word recognition improved for both groups.

In the double-deficit model, Wolf and Bowers (1999) propose three subtypes of impaired reading. The first subtype involves problems with phoneme awareness processes, accuracy and fluency in decoding, and comprehension. The second subtype involves no problems in phoneme awareness and accuracy in decoding, but consists of deficits in rapid automatized naming, fluency in decoding, and comprehension. The most severe subtype involves difficulties in both phonological processing and rapid naming, as well as all other reading processes. Despite the focus on cognitive processes, interventions focus on reading, combining explicit instruction in word decoding and strategies designed to enhance fluency and comprehension, with additional emphases on vocabulary, syntax, orthography, morphology, and processing speed. Evidence that phonological processing and rapid naming predict how different subtypes respond to intervention has not yet been demonstrated, but is under active investigation (see Bowers, 2001; Levy, 2001). Certainly, interventions can be tailored to address different components of the reading process. If word recognition is strong and fluency weak, why teach word recognition? If the problem is only at the level of comprehension, why teach word recognition and fluency? We return to specific interventions from these approaches in the section on remedial interventions.

More recent applications of this type of model focus on intraindividual differences in cognitive processes. As stated in a recent consensus document (Learning Disabilities Roundtable, 2002),

> while IQ tests do not measure or predict a student's response to instruction, measures of neuropsychological functioning and information processing could be included in evaluation protocols in ways that document the areas of strength and vulnerabilities needed to make informed decisions about eligibility for services, and more importantly, what services are needed. An essential characteristic of [specific LDs] is failure to achieve at a level of expected performance based upon the student's other abilities. (p. 18)

Building on reading research, proponents of this model call for better classifications that more clearly delineate the different cognitive profiles associated with LDs. A major assumption is that better classifications lead to enhanced treatment of LDs. The weakness of the model is the focus on assessments of processing skills to describe a child's performance in isolation from the child's actual classroom performance (Reschly et al., 1999). Moreover, this model, like medical and earlier neuropsychological models, focuses on behaviors that are not directly related to intervention, such as processing skills (Torgesen, 2002). Little empirical evidence supports the validity of this model (Fletcher et al., 2003), particularly the notion of focusing on processing strengths and weaknesses as a specific marker for LDs, or as a guide for intervention.

Constructivist Models

Constructivist models rely heavily on the work of Piaget (see, e.g., Piaget & Inhelder, 1969). These models stress, with respect to intervention and treatment, the "holistic" presentation of material to the student. Constructivist models have often rejected behavioral and task-analytic principles (Hallahan et al., 1996). Some constructivists argue that academic material that is analyzed into constituent objectives is meaningless to students. The holistic perspective espoused in constructivist models is captured in this statement by Poplin (1988):

> Structuralist philosophy, constructivist theory, and holistic beliefs define the learning enterprise in opposition to reductionist behavioral learning theory and suggest that the task of schools is to help students develop new meanings in response to new experiences rather than to learn the meanings others have created. This change in the very definition of learning reveals principles of learning that beg consideration in designing classroom instruction. (p. 401)

In a more specific vein, Poplin (1988) outlined 14 holistic/constructivist principles that should guide instruction. Some of these principles are as follows: New experiences are integrated into the whole spiral of knowledge, so that new pieces of knowledge, the new meanings, are much larger than the sum of their parts; the learner is always learning, and the process of self-regulation, not reinforcement theory, determines best when, what, and how things are learned; instruction is best derived from student interest and talent, not from deficits or curriculum materials; the assessment of student development, interests, and involvement is more important to teachers than is student performance on reductionist subskills and subprocesses; problems in learning are the result of interactions of personalities, interests, development expectations, and previous experiences; and passion, trust, and interest are paramount—subjectivity surrounding learning, and cognitive processes, are only part of the picture.

Several themes can be observed with respect to the application of such models to teaching. These themes include (1) teacher empowerment; (2) child-centered instruction; (3) the integration of listening, speaking, reading, and writing with the student's interests and background; (4) a disavowal of the value of teaching subskills; and (5) a view that children are naturally predisposed to learning, and that instruction provides activities (in the broadest sense) to facilitate the learner's ability to construct meaning from experience (see Reid & Hresko, 1981).

More recent applications of constructivist approaches to LDs emphasize the social context of learning and are often described as "sociocultural" models (Englert & Mariage, 2003). These models focus on the situated nature of the learning process. Students do not learn abilities in isolation from their relationships with teachers, other students, and the community in which they learn. The learning context is described as an "apprenticeship" through which teachers provide opportunities for students to think and analyze by guiding and mentoring them in complex cognitive tasks. This form of scaffolding is believed to support more independence in learning, which is a key to the development of critical reasoning, analysis, and higher-order thinking.

Contemporary applications of this model in LDs have moved away from the radical holism of "whole language," which is demonstrably ineffective for students with or at risk for LDs, and toward cognitive models that emphasize strategy instruction. Thus Englert and Mariage (2003) identify forms of strategy instruction in reading comprehension and writing (discussed below) as evidence-based examples of a sociocultural model. This linking reflects the increasing integration of different models of instruction, as well as the importance of establishing an evidence base supporting different instructional activities (Vaughn, Gersten, & Chard, 2000).

The Problem-Solving Model

The problem-solving model is informed by concepts inherent in earlier cognitive-behavioral and task-analytic models. It is based on the view that what is paramount for LDs is how to treat it. According to proponents of this model, classifications, intraindividual differences, and subtypes are all notions that have not proved beneficial for intervention and are therefore not useful (Reschly et al., 1999). It reflects an empirical approach to "what works."

In implementation, the model is often non-categorical, similar to task-analytic models, and relies on the functional analysis of learning and behavior in an ipsative model. The referent population is typically locally defined. The model implicitly retains the concepts of unexpectedness and discrepancy, but bases them on assessments of learning and progress over time. For example, the initial decision regarding whether a child is discrepant from school and/or parent expectations, essential to this model, is a discrepancy classification (Ysseldyke & Marston, 1999). The decision is fraught with the same difficult issues that the more normative classification systems possess. If children are from a low-performing school, does this mean that they are not poor readers if their performance is in line with school expecta-

tions? Similarly, if children are from a high-performing school, should parental expectations that their children should be superior readers represent the basis for such decisions? Even if one uses curriculum-based measurement (CBM) as an alternative to more traditional norm-referenced psychometric measures, there is always the decision to be made as to whether the child has met, or not met, the specified academic skill or ability level of their group.

In the problem-solving model, the progress of students (e.g., their response to instruction) is constantly monitored, and those who do not show adequate progress in reading, math, and other subjects receive targeted interventions on a phased in basis (to be discussed in detail in a later section). In contrast to all models discussed previously, which involve the use of a single assessment, the identification of LDs is potentially based on a failure to respond to well-defined intervention protocols, which requires an assessment of change over time. Thus the classification of LDs involves explicit criteria for assigning students according to criteria based on instructional response. Any determination of change requires a postintervention attribute comparison, which is another type of discrepancy model. These are decisions that reflect implicit classifications of students, interventions, intervention/treatment effectiveness, and how they should be matched. Otherwise all students would receive the same interventions. Although problem-solving approaches have great conceptual appeals, few data are available to support many of the implementations (D. Fuchs, Mock, Morgan, & Young, 2003).

Conceptual Models: Conclusions

Although there are clear differences among the cognitive, cognitive-behavioral, task-analytic, neuropsychological, intraindividual-difference, constructivist, and problem-solving models, they have evolved to a point where they implicitly reflect common themes and assumptions about LDs. Integration of these models into identification, assessment, and intervention practices will involve incorporation of the concept of response to instruction, as well as normative and CBM approaches to assessment (Fuchs & Fuchs, 1998; Vaughn & Fuchs, 2003). The key to LD identification is to measure students over time, and to observe the strengths and weaknesses of both normative and ipsative assessments and their contributions to guiding and measuring response to instruction. Otherwise, identification models based on single assessments are underidentified and not linked to intervention (Fletcher et al., 2005). Although progress monitoring of individual students via CBM is emerging as vital for both the identification of LDs and for guiding instruction (Fuchs & Fuchs, 1998), the snapshots of behavior provided by norm-referenced achievement tests can complement this approach. Both types of measures complement identification for special education services and help remove the inherently relative orientation of CBM in documenting response to instruction. At the end of an intervention, the student should approximate average levels of proficiency on a norm-referenced assessment, even when the amount of change demonstrated by CBM indicates a positive response. This expectation may not be possible for some students, especially if the effort required reaching that goal is unreasonable. These are students who may well need the protections afforded by different forms of disability legislation. But the best way to identify these students is by assessing instructional response.

The primary goal is to identify intervention needs by systematically evaluating academic achievement and to monitor a child's progress in responding to instruction, which can be complemented by methods derived from both models. Because students do learn in social contexts, specifications of the learning environment are essential to establishing positive responses to instruction, which extends to the school and community levels of analysis. As an example, consider that an instructional reading program that has been found effective in research has been selected for application in a particular school district. No matter how effective that program has been in research contexts, it is only as good as the teacher's knowledge of academic development and instruction, and as the district's and school's ability to implement programs with robust fidelity. Extra time on task is required, so that remedial instruction must increase the amount of time the child spends in reading instruction and in independent reading outside of school.

In looking at all the conceptual models reviewed in this chapter, we acknowledge that the limited nature of the discussion has prevented us from including all of the fine points that characterize the different perspectives. However, this discussion has made it clear that the models differ with respect to whether instruction should proceed from specific subskills to the academic area or vice versa; whether a highly structured or an unstructured type of instruction is advocated; whether the teaching strategies recommended are specific or more general in nature; and whether the effects of particular methods should be directly and explicitly evaluated or inferred from general student performance. In practice, a combination of these models is frequently employed, with the finer distinctions blurred by the dynamic nature of the intervention/treatment process. As our review of interventions with LDs will show, tying a particular intervention to one or more of these models is difficult, because efficacious methods involve aspects of many different models.

IMPROVING THE METHODOLOGICAL QUALITY OF TREATMENT RESEARCH

The previous edition of this chapter (Lyon & Cutting, 1998) reported on only a limited number of treatment/intervention studies that yielded reliable and valid information on the effectiveness of different instructional programs, approaches, and strategies for students with LDs. In 1998, the reason why effectiveness data were scarce was not that interventions were unavailable, but that the data on effectiveness were difficult to interpret because of various methodological problems. Since 1998, improvements in the methodological rigor of intervention research has led to high-quality converging evidence on a number of specific instructional factors that significantly improve the academic capabilities of students with LDs, particularly in the area of reading. Although the quality of research has improved, the current treatment/intervention literature still includes studies that are difficult to interpret because of methodological issues. It is the responsibility of consumers of the intervention literature, as well as of intervention products and programs, to have a basic understanding of the types of methodological shortcomings that make interpretation of intervention studies difficult and implementation of the results problematic. Not only is an understanding of these shortcomings critical to an accurate analysis of existing treatment studies and approaches, but it should be taken into account in the design of future intervention studies. We reiterate these issues in this section of the chapter.

Random Assignment

As in much of education research, there continues to be a shortage of high-quality randomized controlled experiments (RCEs) to determine the effectiveness of interventions for well-defined LDs (Towne & Hilton, 2004). In an RCE, individuals are randomly assigned to one of more intervention and comparison groups, in order to objectively assess the effects of the intervention. The value of RCEs lies in their ability to provide consumers of the research with a high degree of confidence that there are no systematic differences between groups in any observed or unobserved characteristics, except that the intervention group receives the treatment and the control group does not (Coalition for Evidence-Based Policy, 2002; Lyon & Chhabra, 2004; Morris, 2004; Stanovich & Stanovich, 2003; Towne & Hilton, 2004). In contrast, pre–post intervention designs without control groups or appropriate statistical controls do not permit determination of whether improvements would have occurred over time without the benefit of the intervention. In addition, these designs do not permit assignment of a causal role to the intervention. Although a variety of designs may support inferences about the causal effects of interventions, RCEs make the fewest assumptions about causality and are therefore strongest in supporting inferences about causality (Shavelson & Towne, 2002; Vaughn & Dammann, 2001).

Heterogeneity of LDs

It is still the case that many studies addressing the efficacy of different treatment intervention methods continue to enroll heterogeneous groups of students with LDs who are identified by vague and inconsistent criteria and who demonstrate unaccounted-for differences in demographic features (e.g., socioeconomic status, race, ethnicity, number of parents, etc.), in number and severity of behavioral and academic disabilities, and in the comorbidity of these disabilities (Morris et al., 1994). As such, not only have replication efforts been impeded, but the influence of uncontrolled variables has made it difficult to determine specific treatment effects and outcomes (especially in the absence

of an RCE). Moreover, this lack of clarity about students' demographic, academic, behavioral, and information-processing characteristics has made it difficult to identify which intervention methods are most efficacious for which particular students and under what specific ecological (contextual) conditions (Lyon & Moats, 1997).

Descriptions of Interventions

Although there have been substantial improvements, some studies of how students with LDs respond to teaching methods and approaches have employed instructional procedures that are poorly described and defined. For instance, some intervention studies do not critically describe how and why intervention/task stimuli are represented to the students. In addition, the type of response that the procedure requires of a child may not be defined in detail. For example, in intervention studies involving reading disorders, many studies do not provide sufficiently detailed answers to the following questions (Johnson, 1994): What is the nature of the structure of the spoken and written language used in the teaching methodology? What is the nature of the vocabulary? Is the vocabulary controlled? Is the sequence of phonological representations controlled? On what basis were the words to be read in the intervention phase selected? Do the word stimuli possess a consistent phoneme–grapheme relationship? How many meaningful nouns and verbs are used? Is the sentence structure similar to the child's oral language? What is the nature of the content of the reading material used in the intervention?

Unpacking Effective Interventions

Intervention studies using methods that consist of several treatment components or procedures often do not have the capability of addressing which component or procedure, or which combination or sequence of procedures, is most critical to promoting gains in learning (Zigmond, 1993). Likewise, intervention studies employing multimodal methods frequently fail to identify how and why different interventions are selected, or what roles different interventions play in achieving treatment gains. This information is critical, because some students with LDs may require a more intensive emphasis, a different sequence, or a longer duration of exposure to and teaching on particular components of the intervention program (Lyon & Moats, 1997).

Durations of Interventions

Many intervention studies conducted with students with LDs continue to be of relatively brief duration (Berninger, 1994; Lyon & Moats, 1997). Thus, when limited effects of a method or intervention are reported, it is not clear whether the limited efficacy is due to the intervention itself or to the fact that it was employed for a duration that was too short to promote long-term change, no matter how robust the intervention. Moreover, it is likely that even the most powerful interventions may not result in measurable effects if traditional pretest–posttest designs are employed and only two measurement points are sampled. Difference scores in this type of design can be confounded by regression toward the mean, although randomization will help with this problem. Measurement methods must be able to assess both the rate *and* degree of change over time, and must be able to predict the slope and intercept of individual growth curves with multiple measures, including type of intervention, individual-difference variables, ecological variables, and other factors that explain why some students respond and others do not (Francis, Shaywitz, Stuebing, Shaywitz, & Fletcher, 1994; Fuchs & Fuchs, 1998; Lyon & Moats, 1997).

Effects of Prior Interventions

Some studies assessing the efficacy of different interventions may have been confounded by the effects of previous and concurrent interventions (Lyon & Flynn, 1991). It is unclear whether a history of a particular type of intervention significantly influences response to an ongoing intervention. Likewise, it is not well understood whether concurrent interventions or methods being used in either regular or special class settings influence response to ongoing experimental interventions. These issues must be addressed, in order to separate specific treatment effects from additive practice or inhibitory effects produced by previous or concurrent interventions. Again, the use of randomization in assigning students to interventions would help in accounting for this type of concurrent and/or historical bias.

Teacher and Contextual Variables

Many intervention studies involving students with LDs have not separated specific treatment effects from clinician or teacher effects. That is, limited attention has been paid to delineating those teacher and contextual variables (e.g., teacher experience and preparation, teacher–student relationship, etc.) that influence change within any treatment program (Lyon & Moats, 1997). This may include attention to the fidelity of implementation essential to employing the intervention in other contexts. Many intervention studies do not analyze the degree of fidelity with respect to the administration of the intervention (Berninger, 1994). This is unfortunate, given that even teachers who are prepared in similar ways have been found to deviate significantly from their application of a method outside the research setting (Lovett, 1991).

Generalization

It still remains unclear in many intervention studies whether gains in academic skills developed under highly controlled intervention conditions generalize to less controlled naturalistic settings (Lyon, 1996a). For example, follow-up studies of intervention benefits have typically shown a decrease in intervention gains, particularly when measurements are taken in settings that differ from those employed in the original intervention study (Lyon & Moats, 1997).

Methodological Issues: Summary

Taken individually or in combination, the methodological issues and limitations described here can limit the interpretability of an intervention study or can undermine confidence in a particular intervention method. To assist in the evaluation of the scientific quality of intervention studies, three recently published papers provide an overview of principles and criteria that can be applied to research reports to ensure that the evidence provided is reliable, valid, and ready for implementation in the classroom (Coalition for Evidence-Based Policy, 2002; Lyon & Chhabra, 2004; Stanovich & Stanovich, 2003). Given the complexity inherent in this type of evaluation process, readers are referred to these sources for specific information relevant to (1) the use of appropriate research methodologies, (2) peer review and publication in appropriate archival journals,

(3) the principle of converging evidence, and (4) the generalizability of the treatment protocol(s).

DOMAIN-SPECIFIC INTERVENTION METHODS: A SELECTIVE REVIEW

Space does not permit a comprehensive review of all treatment and teaching methods employed with students with or at risk for LDs— that is, those who manifest difficulties in learning to read, write, and carry out mathematical operations. Thus the following sections are devoted to reviewing research that is programmatic (as opposed to relatively isolated studies) and that attempts to identify principles supporting effective intervention. We have focused on RCEs and quasi-experimental intervention studies that (1) were conducted in naturalistic settings (e.g. school and classroom environments), or in clinical settings commonly used for students with LDs; (2) addressed and quantified the fidelity with which the treatment was implemented; and (3) involved students with specific reading, math, and written language disabilities, alone or in combination. In addition, due to the importance of early intervention, this review is largely limited to work conducted at the kindergarten through grade 5 levels, although some of the methods have been extended to secondary levels.

Paralleling previous literature reviews (e.g., Lyon & Cutting, 1998), we selected studies to highlight three principles about effective instruction for students with LDs. The first principle is that these students do not learn easily or incidentally. Explicit instruction that increases intensity and/or time on task, guided by a task-analytic perspective with cumulative review of previously mastered content, is a cornerstone of effective teaching practice for these students. The second principle is that higher-order processing, which is the long-term goal of most instructional programs, involves fluent foundational skills: Word reading is required for text comprehension; math fact retrieval and algorithmic computation provide the foundation for mathematics problem solving; and letter formation and word spelling are necessary to express thoughts in writing. For students with LDs, attention to these foundational skills must precede or occur concurrently with instruction on higher-order processes. The third principle is that teachers must carefully plan for transfer

to render new skills, strategies, and knowledge usable for students with LDs. In particular, teaching processes in the absence of an emphasis on the application of the skill in the targeted academic domain may not generalize to academic improvement.

We organize this review in terms of major academic domains (reading, written expression, and mathematics). Within each domain, we first review studies targeting foundational skills and then highlight research on higher-order processes. After summarizing these studies to illustrate the critical components of instruction for students with LDs, we consider why, despite the existence of highly effective practices, so many students with LDs continue to experience serious academic deficiencies. In response, we propose a framework for helping the field enhance practice.

Intervention programs have been developed to enhance the memory skills (e.g., Swanson & Saez, 2003), metacognitive abilities (Borkowski, 1992; Borkowski & Burke, 1996; Case et al., 1992; Flavell, 1979; Graham & Harris, 1996), attentional skills (Barkley, 2006; see also Smith, Barkley, & Shapiro, Chapter 2, this volume), and social behavior (Dunlap et al., 1994) of students with LDs. These references should be perused for specific examples of intervention programs in these domains. In addition, Lyon, Fletcher, and colleagues (2003) provide a recent review of literature related to etiologies, epidemiology, developmental course, and common comorbidities for reading, written language, and mathematics disorders.

Reading

Of all the LDs, reading disabilities are the most common, significantly impeding the development of many academic skills and the acquisition of content knowledge. Vocabulary development, writing ability, the development of mathematical reasoning skills, and knowledge about science, social studies, and English—all are critically dependent upon accurate and fluent decoding and comprehension of written language. Moreover, students with specific LDs in reading are at substantial risk for poor adolescent and adult outcomes. Approximately 70% of students with disabilities in reading that are not identified until the third grade continue to have reading problems through high school and into adulthood (Shaywitz et al., 1999).

The issue of reading and LDs occurs in the context of national concerns about the number of children who suffer from reading problems in the United States. A recent National Assessment of Educational Progress (NAEP) found that 37% of fourth graders read below the "basic" level of proficiency (National Center for Education Statistics [NCES], 2003). The basic achievement level is defined as partial mastery of the skills that are necessary for proficient grade-level work (NCES, 2003). Even more alarming is the finding that when the NAEP fourth-grade data are disaggregated by subgroups, 63% of black students and 58% of Hispanic students score below the basic level on the reading assessment, as compared to 27% of white non-Hispanic fourth-grade students. To be sure, it is not race or ethnicity that is responsible for these extreme rates of reading failure, but economic disadvantage, which cuts across ethnicities. For example, when the NAEP data are disaggregated according to socioeconomic status, 60% of poor children score below basic levels in reading (NCES, 2003).

LDs are not responsible for all forms of educational difficulty. We know that youngsters from disadvantaged environments begin school significantly behind their more affluent agemates in literacy-related skills and experiences (Snow et al., 1998). For example, Hart and Risley (1999) reported that the average child from a family on public assistance has half as much experience listening and speaking to parents during the period from birth to 3 years of age (616 words per hour) as the average working-class child (1,251 words per hour), and less than one-third as much as the average child in a professional family (2,153 words per hour). These types of oral language interactions play a significant role in building the foundational vocabulary abilities essential for later reading growth (Tumner, Chapman, & Prochnow, 2003). Moreover, because of financial stress and low levels of adult literacy, parents of disadvantaged preschoolers are less likely to engage in reading interactions with their children, are less likely to have a positive regard for literacy, and may feel less comfortable communicating with teachers about literacy development (Tumner et al., 2003). The end result is that critical reading-related skills such as phonological awareness and vocabulary, which contribute significantly to the later acquisition of reading skills, are typically un-

derdeveloped (Share & Stanovich, 1995). Similar factors are also present in families where parents have reading difficulties. Such families do not have books and magazines in the home, read to children less frequently than families with better-reading parents, and generally place less emphasis on the development of literacy. These represent shared environmental factors that interact with genetic factors to produce LDs in reading (Wadsworth, Olson, Pennington, & DeFries, 2000).

Regardless of their putative causes, reading disabilities have a deleterious effect on educational, social, and occupational well-being. As such, a substantial amount of research in the development of reading-related skills during the preschool period, the early identification and prevention of reading failure in kindergarten and the early grades, and the remediation of reading problems in later elementary and middle school grades has taken place in the last decade. We begin with research on children who struggle because of word recognition difficulties. This research, and the specific teaching methods and approaches that have been studied, are described here within the categories of (1) early identification and intervention methods and procedures to prevent reading failure at classroom and tutorial levels; and (2) reading remediation methods and procedures for older students. Whenever possible, we begin with a well-known commercial program and then discuss specific methods derived from research.

Prevention of Reading Disabilities

Prevention programs typically include assessments to identify students with difficulties acquiring foundational skills in word recognition and fluency, and targeted interventions to address specific deficits. Some of these programs also address academic needs in the area of vocabulary and comprehension. Studies designed to assess the capability of specific approaches to prevent reading disabilities have accumulated in recent years, because of the increased ability to predict which students will develop such difficulties as they enter and proceed through school (see Torgesen, Wagner, & Rashotte, 1994). In the main, this enhanced predictive ability has emerged from research demonstrating (1) that most reading difficulties are the result of deficits in word recognition (Bruck, 1990; Stanovich, 1991; Vellutino et al.,

2004); (2) that problems in word recognition are related to deficits in phonological awareness, or the ability to notice, think about, or manipulate sounds in words (Adams, 1990; Brady & Shankweiler, 1991; Liberman & Shankweiler, 1991); and (3) that poor reading can be predicted during kindergarten and first grade by analyzing children's performance on measures assessing letter knowledge, phonological awareness skills, and initial sight word reading. Thus these studies largely target students who are at risk for reading difficulties because of early phonological processing and/or word recognition difficulties. The research has largely been supported by the NICHD as part of a large intervention initiative for reading disabilities, as well as research programs from the Office of Special Education. In this section, we distinguish studies that attempt to intervene at a classroom level from those that attempt to identify students who are at risk and pull them out for intervention. We only review studies that begin in kindergarten or grade 1, but we note that preschool interventions are also demonstrably effective (Lonigan, 2003).

There is considerable evidence supporting the use of specific instructional procedures addressing word recognition difficulties in poor readers. This research parallels studies demonstrating at a classroom level the importance of explicit instruction in the alphabetic principle as a component of any reading program. A national panel convened by the NICHD (NRP, 2000) conducted meta-analyses on the efficacy of phonemic awareness instruction as well as phonics instruction. Although the report has been both misinterpreted and misrepresented (see Shanahan, 2004), the results show that these components in reading instructional programs are effective for most students, and are especially effective for students who are struggling with the development of these skills.

The NRP conducted a meta-analysis of 96 studies designed to improve phonemic awareness skills. The analysis yielded effect sizes that were in the large range immediately after intervention (0.86) and remained strong over the long term (0.73). There was evidence of generalization to reading and spelling in the moderate range (0.53–0.59). The NRP found that phonemic awareness instruction was most effective when it included a letter component, when instruction focused on one or two types of phonemic manipulations as opposed to multiple types, and when students were taught in

small groups. Programs lasting less than 20 hours were typically more effective than longer programs, with single sessions lasting about 25 minutes on average. There was little difference in the effectiveness of classroom teachers and computers.

Similar findings were apparent in the NRP's meta-analysis of data derived from studies of the effectiveness of phonics instruction on a variety of reading outcomes, most often word recognition. Seventy-five studies were screened, and 38 were retained for meta-analysis. The overall effect size of phonics instruction was in the moderate range (0.44). Programs that included phonics instruction were more effective than comparisons that provided either implicit or no phonics instruction. Programs in which phonics was taught "systematically" were more effective than programs that taught phonics less systematically. Phonics instruction was effective in individual tutorial programs (0.57), small-group programs (0.42), and whole-class programs (0.39). It was much more effective when introduced in kindergarten (0.56) or grade 1 (0.54) than in grades 2–6 (0.27). Phonics instruction was more effective in kindergarten (0.58) and grade 1 (0.74) for students at risk for reading problems. It tended to be less effective for students who were defined with LDs in reading (0.32) and had a negligible effect size for low-achieving readers in grades 2–6. As suspected, word recognition skills were most significantly affected (0.60–0.67), with smaller effects on spelling (0.40), and reading comprehension (0.51). Again, gains were smaller in poor readers after first grade (0.32).

In contrast to misrepresentations of the NRP (2000) report (Garan, 2001), it was never suggested that the studies that were identified only involved phonics instruction or attempted to isolate the effects of phonics instruction (Shanahan, 2004). In a subsequent meta-analysis that is best described as a replication because it essentially produced the same results as the NRP report, Camilli, Vargas, and Yuecko (2003) proposed that effect sizes were larger when phonics instruction was accompanied with instruction that involved other aspects of reading or oral language development. In the studies reviewed below, it is clear that programs incorporating explicit instruction in the alphabetic principle are more effective than programs that do not make this instruction explicit. How this instruction is delivered varies considerably, with some studies (e.g., Mathes et al., 2005; Torgesen et al., 1999; Vellutino et al., 1996) finding that explicit phonics instruction, taught in the context of reading and writing, was as effective as more decontextualized approaches. In all three studies, the reading interventions were comprehensive, addressing word recognition, fluency, and comprehension. The important finding, however, is the focus on explicitness, which is a guiding principle of instruction for all readers at risk of or with LDs.

At this point in the development of reading interventions, the issue is not whether or not to provide phonics instruction; rather, the question is how to integrate phonics instruction with instruction in other components central for learning to read. Individuals who argue that the solution to reading difficulties is simply to introduce more phonics instruction in the classroom, without incorporating instruction in other critical reading skills (e.g., fluency, vocabulary, comprehension), are not attending to the converging scientific evidence. This is true for programs that attempt to enhance the reading abilities of all students in the classroom, as well as programs that attempt to enhance reading in students with LDs.

CLASSROOM STUDIES

Classroom studies either attempt to introduce new comprehensive reading programs into the classroom with an accompanying emphasis on professional development, or provide a classroom-level intervention that the teacher provides or directs. It is well known that introducing reading curricula into the classroom with professional development linked explicitly to the curriculum typically results in improved reading scores for the classroom as a whole, as well as accelerated reading development in students at risk for reading difficulties (Snow et al., 1998). We present three examples, involving (1) Direct Instruction; (2) the University of Texas–Houston classroom intervention study; and (3) Peer-Assisted Learning Strategies (PALS).

Direct Instruction. We use the term Direct Instruction to refer to the method of intervention developed by Engelmann and colleagues. Adams and Engelmann (1996) provided a review of research based on this particular reading methodology. The review was updated recently by Adams and Carnine (2003). At a classroom level, there are different versions of

Direct Instruction programs, which vary depending on the instructional goals in the target population. In the Adams and Englemann (1996) analysis, effect sizes comparing direct instruction programs versus contrast groups receiving standard practice yielded large effect sizes that generally exceeded 0.75. In more recent studies, similar effect sizes are apparent for students at a variety of achievement levels, including students with LDs (Adams & Carnine, 2003).

Direct Instruction programs include an extensive professional development component that helps teachers understand the rationale for this approach to reading instruction, lesson plans, methods for error correction, grouping strategies, and related issues. Although it is common to characterize Direct Instruction programs (usually in a derogatory manner) as "scripted," "teacher-proof" methods for teaching phonics, scripts for teachers do not make them immune to error in implementation or eliminate the need for judgment and decision making. The curriculum extends beyond phonics into fluency and comprehension. Direct Instruction lessons are typically fast-paced and follow a prescribed lesson plan. The lessons usually last 35–45 minutes and contain 12–20 tasks. These methods are based on task-analytic and behavior management systems, including opportunities for practice using individualized workbooks that match the content in the group lesson. The program that is typically used with students who have specific reading difficulties is Corrective Reading, which includes both decoding and comprehension components (Engelmann, Becker, Hanner, & Johnson, 1978). Although we focus on reading, these are also programs for spelling, math, and writing.

Adams and Carnine (2003) summarized research studies that support different aspects of the Direct Instruction model, including a meta-analysis that updated the Adams and Engelmann (1996) analysis. In a comprehensive review of approximately 300 studies involving reading that utilized Direct Instruction methods, 17 were research studies that met very specific inclusion and exclusion criteria, including presence of a comparison group, pretest scores, and the ability to isolate Direct Instruction as the primary reading methodology. The average effect size for those studies that specifically included students with LDs was 0.93, which is in the large range. This is comparable to the effect sizes reported by Adams and Engelmann for students in general education classrooms (0.82) and in all special education categories (0.84). Disaggregating the results showed that the effect sizes tended to be larger for secondary/adult groups (1.37) relative to elementary groups (0.73). Gains were apparent on criterion-referenced measures (1.14) as well as norm-referenced tests (0.77). Quasi-experimental studies yielded an average effect size of 0.90, while experimental studies that included an RCE yielded an average effect size of 0.95, supporting findings reported by the NRP (2000). For studies that lasted up to 1 year, the average effect size was 1.08, relative to studies that persisted over 1 year (0.77).

One limitation of the Adams and Carnine (2003) analysis is that it does not compare effect sizes within domains of reading. Often the outcome measures are reading composites, and it would be useful to know more about differences in the impact of Direct Instruction programs on word recognition, reading fluency, and comprehension. More recent studies do break apart these components. Carlson and Francis (2002) carried out an RCE of a program (Rodeo Institute for Teacher Excellence, or RITE) that involved schoolwide implementation of a Direct Instruction model. The evaluation involved 20 schools that implemented the RITE program and 20 comparison schools that were not significantly different in the number of students who received free lunch, belonged to an ethnic minority group, were characterized by limited English proficiency, and met minimum expectations on state assessments of reading. The RITE program included implementation of a Direct Instruction curriculum and extensive professional development through an institute providing teachers with professional development in the model as well as ongoing coaching. In the target schools, all teachers in kindergarten, grade 1, and grade 2 were provided with professional development and a Direct Instruction curriculum including instructional materials and generic professional development, largely over the summer. Each school was assigned a master reading teacher to provide on-site support with monthly meetings for the teachers. Another focus of the RITE program was on classroom management methods, including student-directed models as well as teachers' ability to manage the classroom environment.

The evaluation was conducted over a 4-year period. Outcome measures were largely based on the state-mandated tests in grade 3 and the Stanford Achievement Test in grades 1 and 2, with some individualized kindergarten assessments. Results revealed that the overall program was successful in increasing the reading abilities of students in the targeted schools relative to comparison schools. The effect sizes in both word recognition and reading comprehension were in the large range. Those students who were exposed to the program early and spent more years in the program outperformed all other students, including those within the target schools. Thus students who began in kindergarten and were assessed for the final time in grade 3 had the best outcomes. There were direct links of intervention and professional development with teachers to improvements in teaching skills, fidelity of implementation, and student performance. The number of students reading at levels in word recognition and reading comprehension that would be considered potential evidence of LDs was reduced over time in both domains. This study adds to the research base on Direct Instruction, showing that it is effective for many students and a model for other programs that propose evaluations of efficacy.

Direct Instruction programs have been widely criticized, despite the significant evidence base. The criticisms include the possibility that the results of Direct Instruction programs do not extend to comprehension skills and begin to fade in upper elementary grades. Others suggest that the scripting of programs "deprofessionalizes" teachers. Another concern is the behavioral component of Direct Instruction programs, which some have suggested impairs critical thinking. Although there is evidence in some early studies that the effects begin to fade, this is a characteristic of many of the types of schools in which programs like Direct Instruction are implemented. It also reflects the use of norm-referenced achievement tests, which represent comparisons against age-based cohorts that are cross-sectional samples. As such, the drop in scores is not really a decline, but a reduction in the rate of acceleration. Some of the same concerns have been expressed about Reading Recovery (RR), a widely used early intervention program that we discuss later (Shanahan & Barr, 1995). The concerns about scripting, deprofessionalization of teachers, and the negative impact on critical thinking do not appear to be supported by objective evidence. Using a scope and sequence does not eliminate the need for teacher judgment and skill, content expertise, and the ability to assess and monitor student progress. More research is needed to evaluate the apparent decline in effect sizes—a problem apparent in many intervention studies.

The University of Texas–Houston Intervention Study. Foorman, Francis, Fletcher, Schatschneider, and Mehta (1998) contrasted the effects of reading curricula that varied in the explicitness of instruction in word recognition for at-risk students receiving Title 1 services in eight schools in grades 1–2. The students were taught by one of three approaches:

1. A basal curriculum (Open Court Reading, 1995), which provided explicit instruction in word recognition in text.
2. An embedded-phonics program (Hiebert, Colt, Catto, & Gury, 1992), which emphasized the learning of phonics concepts within the context of whole words.
3. A curriculum that stressed contextual reading; responses to literature; writing, spelling, and phonics in context; integration of reading, writing, listening, and speaking; and no decontextualized instruction in phonemic awareness or phonics.

All students received the same amount of time in the respective programs, with comparable student–teacher ratios. The teachers received professional development and support for implementing each of the approaches.

Growth curve analyses were conducted on measures of phonological awareness, word reading, and spelling administered at four time points between September and April. The results showed that students in the explicit-code group improved at a faster rate than students who received the implicit-code condition, and had significantly higher April scores in word reading, phonological processing, and spelling. The means for students in the embedded-phonics condition were between those of the other two groups. A significantly higher percentage of students in the implicit-code and embedded-phonics groups than in the explicit instruction group showed little improvement in word reading over the year. In addition, Foorman and colleagues (1998) found that the relationship between phonological analysis and

word reading was stronger for the explicit-code group than for the implicit-code group, suggesting that the effects of explicit instruction on word reading stemmed from its effects on phonological awareness. Altogether, Foorman and colleagues indicate that for students whose reading is markedly below age and grade expectations, a classroom-based early intervention program that integrates the explicit teaching of phonological awareness, phonics, and textual reading skills is superior to methods based on less explicit teaching of the alphabetic principle. It also shows the value of introducing comprehensive reading curricula with professional development as an early intervention model.

Peer-Assisted Learning Strategies. An alternative and cost-effective classroom-level intervention based on cooperative learning has been developed (Jenkins & O'Connor, 2003). "Cooperative learning" refers to a set of practices involving small-group instruction and students' working together in learning activities. Such activities emerge from a number of the models reviewed above, often integrating cognitive, behavioral, and constructivist principles. As a set of practices, cooperative learning has a large empirical base that provides strong support for its use at a classroom level (Jenkins & O'Connor, 2003). This is partly because such practices facilitate classroom management and differentiated instruction by their focus on smaller groups with the classroom.

In the reading area, the best-developed form of cooperative learning intervention is PALS, most fully elaborated in a systematic research program involving over 30 studies over the past 20 years by a research group at Vanderbilt University led by Doug and Lynn Fuchs (D. Fuchs & Fuchs, 2005; L. S. Fuchs & Fuchs, 2000). These studies are described in the classroom intervention section, because PALS is a classroom-level intervention in which students who are stronger and weaker in academic skills are typically paired for about 30 minutes of instruction three to five times per week. Often the instruction efforts are divided into strategies that involve word recognition and decoding skills and other strategies involving comprehension. There is an extensive literature on the efficacy of PALS, which has been developed for reading and math, and used in research from kindergarten into secondary school (D. Fuchs & Fuchs, 2005; L. S. Fuchs & Fuchs,

2000). We provide examples of studies in which PALS was implemented in different formats in kindergarten and grade 1, although we note that the research base extends beyond grade 1.

In a kindergarten study, D. Fuchs, Fuchs, Thompson, and colleagues (2001) compared three groups of students who received phonemic awareness instruction based on the Ladders to Literacy program (O'Connor, Notar-Syverson, & Vadasy, 1998). O'Connor, Notar-Syverson, and Vadasy (1996) found that this program enhanced phonological awareness skills in kindergarteners who varied in levels of such skills. A second group received instruction in both phonemic awareness and beginning word recognition skills, and a classroom comparison group received neither of these interventions. The decoding instruction was based on PALS. The results indicated that the two treatment groups did not differ in phonological awareness skills at the end of kindergarten, but exceeded levels apparent in the comparison group that received standard instruction. On decoding and spelling tests, students who also received the decoding component of PALS exceeded the group that only received phonological awareness instruction, whose performance was comparable to that of the comparison group.

A second study utilized the same comparison groups with different students, but focused on non-Title 1 schools. Thus D. Fuchs and Fuchs (2005) compared kindergarten groups that received (1) PALS with and without phonological awareness training; (2) only phonological awareness training; and (3) neither intervention. The two intervention groups were generally comparable on a variety of phonological awareness, reading, and spelling measures, but performed at higher levels than the comparison group. There was little evidence that the phonological awareness training added to the value of PALS, which emphasized decoding skills. These studies demonstrate that classroom-level interventions involving the teaching of word recognition skills are not enhanced when phonological awareness instruction is added. They also attest to the power of classroom-level interventions that result in more differentiated instruction in the classroom.

Other researchers have developed versions of peer-mediated instruction for older students. For example, Mathes, Torgesen, and Allor (2001) utilized PALS with first graders. The PALS intervention in first grade provided 15 minutes of instruction in word recognition and 15 minutes in story reading, which represent a standard PALS implementation. However, the researchers also evaluated a phonological awareness component using a computer-assisted methodology. At-risk students who received both PALS and the computer-assisted phonological awareness training did not perform better than students who received only PALS. Additional training in phonological awareness did not add to the impact of the intervention.

In other intervention studies involving first-grade PALS, D. Fuchs and Fuchs (2005) report evidence that PALS improved not only word recognition skills, but also reading fluency and comprehension. Mathes, Howard, Allen, and Fuchs (1998) found that first-grade PALS improved reading skills in both low- and average-performing first graders, documenting that PALS is not detrimental to higher achievers. In summarizing the results of several studies involving PALS in first grade, Denton and Mathes (2003) found that 69–82% of the poorest readers in the classroom had progressed to the average range by the end of the PALS intervention, based on an admittedly arbitrary criterion of word reading above the 25th percentile. Nonetheless, extrapolating this reduction to the total school population indicates that PALS potentially reduces the population base rate for reading difficulties from 25% to 5–6%. These results are similar to those reported by Foorman and colleagues (1998).

Classroom Studies: Summary. We have reviewed three examples of classroom-level intervention. All three examples showed efficacy in preventing reading difficulties in at-risk students. Enhancing classroom instruction is clearly a front-line strategy for reducing the number of students who might eventually develop LDs in reading. An advantage of this approach is that it also affects students who are at risk because of poverty and other causes of academic difficulties.

TUTORIAL STUDIES

In this section, we review studies that are largely independent of classroom-level interventions. These studies typically utilize a tutoring model in which at-risk students are pulled out of the classroom for additional instruction.

Although initial studies focused on individualized tutoring, more recent implementations utilize small groups of three to five students. We begin with a widely available program and then examine specific studies of tutoring.

Reading Recovery. A popular early intervention program for first-grade students reading in the lower 20% of their classes is RR (Clay, 1985, 1993). This intervention provides daily, individual 30-minute lessons to students in grade 1 who are identified as at risk on the basis of a survey of reading skills. A complete RR program includes 20 weeks of lessons, although the actual duration of the program varies from student to student. The RR program stresses that basic decoding and phonics skills should be taught in the context of authentic reading and writing activities; it also emphasizes teaching students to employ multiple strategies (use of context clues, word attack, etc.) to identify words, rather than focusing on only one strategy, such as "sounding out" words. The RR teacher is responsible for selecting text for each individual student, so that the student will be challenged but not frustrated and can be successful with teacher support. In essence, RR stresses the need to screen students for reading difficulties early in the first grade, and to provide intensive one-to-one tutorial instruction that emphasizes reading new and familiar text, writing words in a manner that encourages the induction of phonemic awareness and sound–symbol relationships, and integrating reading and writing activities. A major emphasis is placed on the teacher's observational skills and judgment in planning instruction.

Shanahan and Barr (1995) provided a comprehensive review of the effectiveness studies conducted to date with RR, reporting that the program does result in substantial gains in reading for approximately 70% of participating students. However, they noted that many of the studies reviewed were methodologically deficient. A recent meta-analysis also found that RR was effective for many grade 1 students (D'Agostino & Murphy, 2004). This study disaggregated RR outcomes by whether the outcomes involved standardized achievement tests or the Observation Survey (Clay, 2002), which parallels the RR curriculum. It also separated results for students who successfully completed RR (i.e., met program criteria and were discontinued) versus those who were unsuccessful or left the program before receiving

20 lessons (i.e., were not discontinued). Finally, it divided results according to the methodological rigor of the studies. When the comparison group consisted of low-achieving students, average effect sizes on standardized achievement tests for all discontinued and not-discontinued students were in the small range (0.32), and higher for discontinued (0.48) than for not-discontinued (–0.34) students. This finding was consistent with Elbaum, Vaughn, Hughes, and Moody's (2000) report that RR was less effective for students with more severe reading problems. D'Agostino and Murphy (2004) found that analyses based on just the more rigorous studies included in their meta-analysis, in which evaluation groups were more comparable on pretests, showed smaller but significant effect sizes on standardized measures. Disaggregation according to whether the students were discontinued or not was not possible. Effect sizes were much larger for the Observation Survey measures, but these assessments are tailored to the curriculum and also have severely skewed distributions at beginning and end of grade 1, which suggest the Observation Survey should not be analyzed as a continuous variable in program evaluation studies (Denton, Ciancio, & Fletcher, in press). D'Agostino and Murphy found evidence for persistence of effects through grade 2, with less evidence of diminished efficacy than reported by Shanahan and Barr.

Recent concerns about the efficacy of RR revolve around two issues: (1) Is RR successful with the lowest-performing students? (2) Is RR cost-effective? In regard to the first concern, RR has typically targeted students who perform in the lowest 20% of their classes. The actual performance levels of participants varies from school to school. Although the research from the developers of RR continues to indicate efficacy for about 70% of the students in the program, its reported effects are much weaker when students who do not meet the program's exit criteria are included in the analyses of outcomes. It should also be noted that most of the research reported by the developers of RR has not been scrutinized by rigorous peer review prior to publication. In their review, Elbaum and colleagues (2000) found that gains for the poorest readers were often minimal, which they suggested might be related to the need for more explicit instruction in decoding. Several studies support this observation. Iverson and Tunmer (1993) compared the reading growth of students enrolled in the standard RR program with students enrolled in a modified RR program supplemented with explicit instruction in the alphabetic principle. Although both RR groups significantly outperformed control students on a variety of reading measures, students in the modified RR program progressed significantly faster than those in the standard program. Tumner and colleagues (2003) noted that in New Zealand (which, as RR's country of origin, has implemented it widely), there remains a large gap in the reading skills of economically advantaged and economically disadvantaged students. In one study, Chapman, Tumner, and Prochnow (2001) followed students who were placed in RR programs, observing that many experienced severe difficulties in phonological awareness and decoding skills before entering the program. Participation in RR did not reduce these difficulties, which they attributed to the absence of attention to explicit instruction in the alphabetic principle. More recently, Tumner and colleagues modified an RR program in New Zealand to include phonological awareness and explicit phonics instruction, implementing it with economically disadvantaged minority students. Comparing the modified program in seven schools with a historical control cohort from the same schools revealed that students who received the modified program scored more highly than the historical controls on all phonological awareness and reading measures, including standardized measures of reading achievement and measures like those employed in RR. These gains persisted through grade 2. There was evidence that the modified program reduced the achievement gap characteristic of economically disadvantaged students in New Zealand.

A second issue with RR involves its cost-effectiveness. The professional development component is expensive, and because RR requires one-on-one tutoring, many schools find it difficult to implement on a long-term basis. Hiebert (1994) reported that RR cost over $8,000 per student, a contention disputed by RR's developers. The issue, however, concerns whether any reading intervention in elementary schools needs to be provided on a one-to-one basis. In their meta-analysis, Elbaum and colleagues (2000) found that larger groupings of three students to one teacher were just as effective as one-to-one groupings across a range of interventions. In a series of studies summarized by Vaughn and Linan-Thompson (2003), group size was systematically manipulated in order to compare interventions delivered at three student–teacher ratios: 1:1, 3:1, and 10:1. Across a variety of reading assessments involving word recognition, fluency, and comprehension, outcomes were comparable for the 3:1 and 1:1 interventions, and both group sizes were significantly better than interventions in group sizes of 10:1. These findings support conclusions reached by the NRP (2000).

Perhaps the most significant question is why RR has not been modified in the face of the current research base in early reading. There is no doubt that RR is effective with many students, particularly those with less severe reading difficulties. With modifications involving a more explicit phonics component, a focus on the use of letter–sound relationships rather than context in the identification of words, and larger group sizes, RR would probably be more beneficial to many students and more cost-effective. The resistance of RR's developers to participation in well-designed studies contrasting such elements to the traditional RR approach is puzzling, and appears to be based on philosophical and ideological factors.

Other Tutorial Studies. Torgesen and colleagues (1999) evaluated the long-term effects of a prevention study that began in kindergarten and followed students through grade 4, with intervention through grade 2. Students were identified for the study in the first semester of kindergarten, based on scores on tests of letter name knowledge and phonological awareness (Torgesen et al., 1994). The 180 students in the final sample were randomly assigned to four treatment conditions: (1) phonological awareness plus synthetic phonics (PASP) instruction embedded within real-word reading and spelling activities (embedded phonics); (2) phonics instruction embedded with real-word reading and spelling activities; (3) a regular kindergarten classroom support group receiving individual instruction to support the goals of the regular classroom program; and (4) a best-practice control group. Students in each treatment condition were provided with 80 minutes of one-on-one instruction each week during kindergarten and the first grade. Results revealed that the PASP program was related to significantly higher gains in alphabetic reading skills (decoding) and spelling than were the embedded-phonics and the regular-classroom-based treatments. Students in the embedded-phonics and regular-classroom-based intervention groups outperformed the best-practices group. Students in all three treatment groups performed equally well on measures of single-word reading, indicating that enhanced preventive instruction is beneficial, no matter what the training format.

At the end of the second grade, students who received the most explicit instruction in the alphabetic principle had much stronger word-reading skills than students in all the other groups. In addition, students who received the most explicit instruction showed the lowest retention rate (9%), with retention rates in the other three conditions ranging from 25% (implicit phonics), 30% (classroom support condition), and 41% (no-treatment comparison group). As a group, students in the most explicit condition demonstrated word-level reading skills that were in the middle of the average range. However, in this same group, 24% of the students were still well below average levels in these skills (a criterion of word reading above the 25th percentile was used). Extrapolated to the entire population, this would lead to an overall failure rate in the population from which these students were selected of 2.4%. This figure, of course, is far below the approximate 20% figure reported for students commonly assumed to be at risk for reading disabilities, and the 37% of fourth-grade students performing below the basic level in reading on the NAEP. Other analyses showed that growth in reading skills was mediated by improvements in phonological processing skills.

Torgesen (2004) presented preliminary data from a new generation of studies introducing preventive instruction to first graders at risk for reading difficulties. The provision of PASP in groups of three to five students for 45 minutes a day (about 30 weeks) led to significant improvement, with only 8% of the at-risk individuals performing below the average range (as defined by word recognition skills below the 26th percentile at the end of first grade). This suggests a population failure rate of 1.6%. These results persisted through second grade, although outcomes were slightly poorer for comprehension than for word recognition, with a comprehension test suggesting that 4.1% were reading below average levels.

In a series of studies, Blachman (1997; Blachman, Ball, Black, & Tangel, 1994; Tangel & Blachman, 1995) exposed 84 low-income,

inner-city kindergarten students to 11 weeks of instruction, with one teacher instructing a small group of four to five students in several aspects of phonological awareness and letter–sound knowledge for 15–20 minutes per day, 4 days a week. The students completed 41 of these lessons, for a total of 10–13 hours of instruction. At the end of the 11 weeks, students receiving the phonological treatment significantly outperformed control students on tasks assessing the reading of phonetically regular words and related tasks. A follow-up study conducted in February and May of first grade showed that these gains were maintained if the curriculum contained the same emphasis on phonological skill development and on the relation of these skills to decoding, word recognition, and textual reading.

Vellutino and colleagues (1996) identified students who had scores below the 15th percentile in reading real words and pseudowords at the beginning of the second semester of first grade. These students were in schools that were selected because of the high probability of the students' having strong literacy backgrounds. The schools were largely middle-class or above, and the sample was predominantly white. These students received 30 minutes of daily individualized tutoring. Approximately half of this tutorial was devoted to explicit-code-based activities, as well as word recognition and writing activities; the other half was devoted to activities involving the use of decoding and other strategies for word recognition and comprehension in text reading (see Vellutino & Scanlon, 2002). At the end of only one semester of remediation, approximately 70% of the students were reading within the average or above-average range, based on national norms. These results translated to a reading failure rate (based on those reading below the 26th percentile in word recognition skills) of approximately 1.5–3% of the overall population, depending on whether severely impaired and moderately impaired readers were both included in the tally (3%), or only severely impaired readers (1.5%). Furthermore, students who responded well to remediation and "caught up" to their typically reading peers generally maintained these performance levels once the intervention was discontinued.

In a follow-up evaluation, Vellutino, Scanlon, and Jaccard (2003) reported on outcomes through fourth grade, exploring differences in students according to the amount of progress made in the intervention. Poor readers who were most difficult to remediate performed well below the typical readers, as well as below the poor readers who were readily remediated, on kindergarten, first-, and third-grade tests evaluating phonological abilities. They did not differ on semantic, syntactic, and visual measures, although all tutored groups tended to perform below the typical readers on these measures as well as on most of the phonological measures. Vellutino and colleagues found that although most students maintained their gains, a significant number did not maintain their progress, especially those who were the most difficult to remediate. The investigators suggested that these students may not have received the type of individualized, comprehensive, and integrated approach to reading instruction they needed to consolidate their initial gains and become functionally independent readers after tutoring was discontinued.

MULTITIERED INTERVENTION STUDIES

The examples of prevention research reviewed to this point have involved *either* classroom intervention or tutorial intervention. As both approaches demonstrate efficacy, why not evaluate the effects of layering classroom and tutorial interventions (O'Connor, 2000; Vaughn, Linan-Thompson, & Hickman, 2003)? Such implementations must involve a determination of who needs tutoring—that is, which students do not respond to the classroom level intervention. In this section, six recent studies involving multitiered classroom (tier 1) and tutorial (tier 2) interventions are reviewed.

O'Connor, Fulmer, Harty, and Bell (2001) evaluated a multitiered intervention program for students in grade 1 who were identified as at risk. In tier 1, classroom teachers were provided with professional development addressing differentiated reading instruction geared toward low-achieving students. In tier 2, supplemental small-group reading instruction was provided for about 30 minutes per day, three times per week. The content varied depending on needs for word recognition and fluency instruction. At the end of grade 2, comparisons with a group that did not receive the tiered interventions showed higher levels of performance on word recognition, fluency, and comprehension in the tutored students.

In an earlier study, O'Connor (2000) evaluated the effects of multitiered intervention in kindergarten. Fifty-nine students representing the lowest-scoring 40% of kindergarteners were identified as at risk on an assessment battery involving vocabulary, memory, letter identification, rapid naming, and phonological awareness measures. The intervention focused on the provision of professional development to kindergarten teachers, with an emphasis on differentiated instruction in the classroom. In addition, students who seemed to struggle received one-on-one tutoring. The study found that 28% of students who received both levels of intervention continued to struggle. The provision of additional intervention involving small-group or one-on-one intensive interventions substantially reduced the number of students who continued to struggle at the end of grade 1. Following these students into grade 2 revealed, however, that the tutored students tended to lose ground in comparison with students who were not at risk.

Simmons, Kame'enui, Stoolmiller, Coyne, and Harn (2003) summarized a kindergarten through grade 1 intervention program that also layered classroom and supplemental interventions. This study began in kindergarten, identifying 113 students who performed in the bottom 25% of all students in seven schools. Identification was based on CBM of letter naming and initial sound fluency. The at-risk kindergarteners were assigned to one of three interventions. All interventions provided 30-minute, small-group, pull-out supplements to typical kindergarten instruction. One intervention (code emphasis) provided 30 minutes of strategic and systematic instruction in the alphabetic principle, phonological awareness, and decoding, as well as practice and application through handwriting, spelling, and related tasks. The second program (code/comprehension emphasis) provided two 15-minute segments involving (1) phonological and alphabetic skills and (2) vocabulary and comprehension activities. The third intervention represented a comparison group that received 30 minutes of instruction emphasizing phonological awareness and decoding skills derived from a commercial program. Results revealed that the code emphasis group obtained higher scores in word recognition than either the coding/comprehension emphasis group or the commercial program group did.

In grade 1, students who scored at or above a specified benchmark of 20 letter sounds per minute on a nonsense word fluency measure received either the monitoring condition or a maintenance intervention. The maintenance intervention involved 30 minutes of instruction focused on decoding, word recognition, and connected text reading. Findings revealed an interaction of entry-level skills and benefit from the maintenance program. Students who entered with higher scores on nonsense word fluency performed comparably whether they received the maintenance or the monitoring condition. Students whose scores met the fall benchmark but were at the low end of the score continuum revealed lower rates of growth on an oral reading fluency measure. A third group of students who received kindergarten intervention but did not respond strongly to it continued small-group instruction in first grade. Three conclusions were drawn from these findings: (1) Students who responded strongly to kindergarten intervention and scored well above fall benchmarks did not require further intervention to reach end-of-first-grade benchmarks; (2) students who received kindergarten intervention and barely reached fall benchmarks required additional intervention to maintain adequate growth; and (3) students who did not respond strongly to kindergarten and fell far below fall first-grade benchmarks required extensive intervention in first grade. These latter results support the adjustment of instruction according to student needs and show that certain forms of kindergarten instruction led to improved reading in at-risk students in first grade (Coyne, Kame'emui, Simmons, & Harn, 2004).

Vaughn and colleagues (2003) provided a multitiered intervention that began with kindergarten students in six schools. In this study, kindergarten teachers were provided with professional development and in-class support. Students identified as at risk were randomly assigned to supplemental small-group intervention (i.e., the multitiered intervention) or to only to the enhanced classroom intervention. Interestingly, in addition to generic professional development, the classroom implementations included support through kindergarten PALS. The interventions included an emphasis on phonological awareness and beginning decoding, as well as elements of the Direct Instruction model (including error correction, explicit instruction, and purposeful examples). The lesson plan was sequenced, and progress was monitored in all at-risk students. The intervention involved approximately 50 daily

sessions over 13 weeks and supplemented the tier 1 instruction. Results revealed that at-risk students who received multitiered intervention performed at significantly higher levels than historical control students on measures involving word recognition, fluency, and comprehension. In addition, students who received multitiered intervention outperformed students who were at risk and received enhanced classroom instruction, although the effect sizes were smaller than in the comparison with the historical controls.

Mathes and colleagues (2005) evaluated the effectiveness of two small-group pull-out interventions in grade 1, relative to enhanced classroom instruction alone, in a sample of students who were identified as at risk for reading difficulties. These students represented the lowest-performing 20% of students in terms of early reading development in about 30 classrooms in six non-Title 1 schools. All identified students received enhanced classroom reading instruction; the researchers provided classroom teachers with professional development in the use of assessment to inform instruction and in a peer tutoring reading strategy, along with ongoing graphs of participating students' progress in oral reading fluency. The two pull-out interventions, provided to subgroups of the at-risk students in addition to this classroom instruction, were constructed to reflect different philosophies in early reading intervention. One intervention (Proactive Reading) was modeled on Direct Instruction principles. It consisted of 120 fully articulated lessons designed in five strands targeting phonological awareness, alphabetic decoding, orthographic knowledge, fluency development in decodable text, and comprehension strategies. The other intervention (Responsive Reading) also involved explicit instruction in the alphabetic principle, as well as fluency and comprehension strategy instruction. Teachers provided phonemic awareness and phonics instruction both in isolation and in the context of reading and writing. There was no predetermined scope or sequence. Rather, teachers were provided with guidelines consisting of a sequence of useful phonic elements, a list of high-frequency words, and designed lessons to respond to student needs reflected in daily assessments and observations. In contrast to Proactive Reading, Responsive Reading had students read text that was leveled for difficulty but not explicitly phonetically decodable. A typical lesson would involve fluency work (repeated reading with modeling) and assessment of one student in the group for the first 8–10 minutes, 10–12 minutes of explicit instruction in phonemic awareness and phonics, and supported reading and writing for the remaining 20 minutes. Both interventions were provided in small groups of three students to one teacher for about 40 minutes each day for about 8 months. A third group of students received the typical instruction provided in their schools, which in most cases consisted only of enhanced classroom instruction.

The results revealed that although these students were in the bottom-scoring 20% at the beginning of the year, all three groups obtained scores that were in the average range at the end of the year on measures of word recognition, fluency, comprehension, and spelling. The two groups that received pull-out intervention generally did not differ from one another, but had higher outcomes involving phonological awareness, word reading, and oral reading fluency than the group that received only enhanced classroom instruction. Based on a criterion of the 30th percentile in word recognition skills, about 16% of the group that stayed in the classroom did not achieve in the average range at the end of the year, which translates to 3% of the schools' first-grade populations. Fewer than 8% of students who received the two pull-out interventions failed to achieve in the average range, representing population rates that were under 1.5%. These results demonstrate that pull-out intervention has a value-added impact relative to classroom instruction alone, even instruction of generally high quality. It is important to recognize that the participating classroom teachers had been provided by their school district with an aggressive professional development program targeting reading instruction, and that these students received the beneficial effects of the professional development, screening, and progress monitoring provided by the researchers.

In what is emerging as an interesting integration of reading intervention and neuroimaging studies, Simos and colleagues (in press) used a functional neuroimaging technique that measures changes in the biomagnetic energy generated by the brain to assess changes in brain function in a subset of the students followed by Mathes and colleagues (2005). For the purpose of this imaging study, students in the three intervention conditions were combined into one

group to increase the size of the sample of students at risk for reading difficulty, to enable comparison with students who are not at risk. Students were imaged at the end of kindergarten and again at the end of first grade. Comparisons of spatial–temporal profiles of brain activation obtained during performance on letter–sound and pseudoword-naming tasks showed clear differences at the end of kindergarten between low-risk and high-risk students. In general, the high-risk students showed early development of neurophysiological processes like those seen in older students with severe reading difficulties—namely, much greater activity in the right hemisphere, and little activation in the areas of the left hemisphere that have been identified as key to successful reading acquisition. At the end of first grade, the high-risk group was subdivided into those who responded and those who did not respond adequately to first-grade reading instruction (which, for some students, included the pull-out interventions described above). At this point, the high-risk students who responded well to instruction showed significant increases in activation in areas of the left hemisphere associated with phonological processing, particularly the superior temporal gyrus in the left hemisphere. Students who did not respond adequately to intervention showed patterns like those described above, which, again, are typically seen in older students with severe reading difficulties. It is noteworthy that the changes were seen not only in students who responded well to the pull-out interventions, but also in at-risk students who responded adequately to classroom instruction with no additional intervention. Even students who were not at risk for reading difficulties at the beginning of first grade showed significant activation increases in the same areas in the left hemisphere associated with the development of reading proficiency after first-grade reading instruction. Such results imply that the neural systems mediating the development of reading skills are malleable and dependent on experience in order to develop. As we show below, remedial studies have revealed similar, and often more dramatic, changes in activation patterns.

The last study we describe examining the effects of multitiered interventions incorporated RCEs at the classroom level as well as at the tutoring level. McMaster, Fuchs, Fuchs, and Compton (2005) randomly assigned 33 first-grade teachers, half in high-poverty schools and half in middle-class schools, to validated classroom treatment with PALS (22 teachers) or to their standard practice (11 control classrooms). The researchers monitored students' response to whole-class instruction each week over 7 weeks. On the basis of (1) the students' level of performance at the end of 7 weeks, combined with (2) the amount of improvement they showed over the 7-week period, results showed that the use of PALS reduced the proportion of nonresponders from 28% to 15%. The students who failed to demonstrate adequate response to PALS were then randomly assigned to three secondary service conditions: none (i.e., continuing in classroom PALS without modification), classroom adaptations to PALS (i.e., receiving a modified form of classroom PALS), or one-to-one adult tutoring. The amount of reading instructional time across these three secondary service conditions was held constant. Adult tutoring involved three weekly sessions that combined a strong focus on word-level instruction and story-reading practice with self-regulation. Results showed that adult tutoring was more effective than the other two secondary conditions, further reducing unresponsiveness to 2–5%, depending on how unresponsiveness was calculated (D. Fuchs, Fuchs, & Compton, 2004).

PREVENTION STUDIES: CONCLUSIONS

The classroom and tutorial studies reviewed in this section show that early intervention may reduce the number of students who are at risk for reading difficulties—including those who might eventually be characterized with LDs in reading, as well as those who are economically disadvantaged and might be served in compensatory education programs. The limitation to this statement is the need for long-term follow-up of these students to assess the persistence of the effects. Nonetheless, as several reviews attest, intervention studies that address the lowest-performing 10–25% of the student population may reduce the number of at-risk students to rates that approximate 2–10% (Denton & Mathes, 2003; Torgesen, 2000). From the studies of these programs, it is clear that both classroom and tutorial programs are effective, and that small groups can be involved in the intervention (i.e., successful intervention programs do not require one-on-one tutoring). In addition, the most effective programs were comprehensive, integrated programs that em-

phasized instruction in the alphabetic principle, teaching for meaning, and opportunities for practice. As these components differentially affect word recognition, comprehension, and fluency, respectively, such findings are not surprising. Moreover, although tutorial programs often vary in emphasis, these instructional features were apparent in both classroom and tutorial programs.

Of particular interests were the results of studies that attempted to layer classroom and tutorial interventions. When this layering occurs—as in the provision of tutorial instruction for at-risk students from classrooms with an intervention emphasizing PALS, or in schools where the core reading program is apparently strong—the number of students who are at risk appears to go below 2%. Moreover, outcome studies show that these changes are effective through grade 5, and that domains involving word recognition, fluency, and comprehension are affected.

In the next section, we will see that the principles underlying successful remediation of reading difficulties in older students are similar in many respects, but also somewhat different because the students are typically further behind in their reading skills. As such, fluency skills, which depend greatly on practice and experience, typically lag behind gains in word recognition and comprehension. Moreover, there is typically more differentiation of specific instructional components, usually beginning with significant, explicit emphasis on the alphabetic principle; this reflects the fact that most students with reading difficulties lag behind in the development of word recognition principles. However, if word recognition is the only component that is emphasized, gains in other areas are less apparent. Some of these studies also involve neuroimaging components, which highlight the increased integration of the neuroscience and education fields in studies of LDs in reading.

Reading Remediation Programs

Unfortunately, not all students with reading disabilities have the benefit of appropriate prevention and intervention programs. In fact, the majority of such youngsters are not identified for special education services before the late second-grade or third-grade year, and often even later. Even more unfortunate is the finding that severe reading disabilities diagnosed after age 8 may be more refractory to treatment, especially in the area of fluency (Torgesen, Rashotte, & Alexander, 2001). Shaywitz (1996) reported that approximately 70% of students identified as having a reading disability in the third grade continue to manifest reading difficulties through the end of high school, despite the fact that many have received special education. The problem may reflect the format of instructional service delivery and the content of reading interventions, as many of the remedial studies cited below show stronger intervention effects.

Although remediation programs applied at later elementary grades do not yield the same degree of improvement as early intervention programs do, gains in reading skills are possible if the remediation is directly related to the academic deficiencies, if the teacher is well prepared, and if both the intensity and duration of the remediation are sufficient. In a comprehensive meta-analysis of intervention studies for students defined broadly as having LDs, Swanson and colleagues (1999) grouped intervention studies into four instructional models: those providing only direct instruction, those providing only strategy instruction, those providing both direct instruction and strategy instruction, and those providing interventions that could not be categorized as either direct instruction or strategy instruction. Various interventions were placed under each of those domains. "Direct instruction" as defined here included interventions that involved breaking tasks into smaller steps, administering probes, use of feedback and diagrams, modeling of skills and behaviors, and related interventions. In contrast, "strategy instruction" included attempts at student collaboration, teacher modeling, reminders to use strategies, multiprocessing instructions, dialogue, and other interventions related to the attempt to teach students strategies. Overall, the results indicated that interventions providing both direct instruction and strategy instruction were more effective than those only involving either direct instruction or strategy instruction. The studies that included strategy instruction resulted in larger effect sizes than those that did not (0.84 vs. 0.67); methods that included direct instruction had larger effect sizes than those that did not (0.82 vs. 0.66). Combining direct instruction and strategy instruction yielded larger effect sizes (0.84) vs. either direct instruction alone (0.68) or strategy instruction alone

(0.72). Note that these effect sizes are in the moderate to large range, showing that remedial reading interventions across a variety of different methods improve reading outcomes. These effects were observed in word recognition, comprehension, and fluency.

There are many examples of remedial reading programs. In the next section, we begin with a commonly utilized overarching approach and then move to highlight some of the more recent studies.

MULTISENSORY METHODS

Historically, reading remediation approaches were characterized as "multisensory" in nature, were provided in an individualized fashion, and were used to develop spelling and writing skills as well as reading skills. An early example of this type of method was the Fernald approach (Fernald, 1943), which incorporated principles of language experience and whole-word (not whole-language) instruction in the teaching format. In essence, the reading material to be learned was provided by the students through the dictation of their own stories. Fernald (1943) argued that this type of approach could help to overcome the negative feelings that many students have because of their prolonged difficulties in learning to read. From these stories, the students selected words that they wished to learn and worked directly on them, repeatedly saying and tracing the words until they could be written from memory. Words that were mastered were kept in a file, and the words were used to generate additional reading material. The Fernald approach emphasized learning words as wholes and discouraged teaching students how to "sound out" new words. Given what is now known about the importance of decoding skills in the learning-to-read process, it is not surprising that the Fernald method has not been substantiated by research evidence (Lyon & Moats, 1988; Myers, 1978).

Other programs considered "multisensory" were derived from the early work of Samuel and June Orton under the general rubric of "Orton–Gillingham" approaches. Early versions of these programs emphasized the need for instruction in all sensory modalities. These approaches required the student to learn associations between letters and sounds that are required in reading, spelling, and writing tasks. Students were taught to see a letter (visual), hear its sound (auditory), say its sound (auditory), trace the letter (tactile), and write the letter (kinesthetic). Words mastered were eventually inserted into sentences and passages to promote textual reading and reading comprehension. There was an emphasis on understanding the structure of language and sounding out words.

These early efforts were reformulated by Anna Gillingham and Betsy Stillman in the 1960s and have continued to evolve. Many of the remedial approaches reviewed in this chapter—including approaches used in research by Blachman, Berninger, Wolf, and others, which emphasize the importance of explicitly and systematically teaching students about the structure of language—reflect this influence of these earlier remedial approaches (Moats & Farrell, 1999). Similarly, commercial programs such as the Lindamood Phoneme Sequencing Program for Reading, Spelling, and Speech (Lindamood & Lindamood, 1998) and Phono-Grafix (McGuiness, McGuiness, & McGuiness, 1996) reflect the influence of Orton–Gillingham instruction. Reflecting the type of student of interest, these programs also initially focused primarily on word recognition, but have expanded to incorporate activities related to reading fluency and comprehension, writing, and oral language development under the rubric of "multisensory structured language education." As outlined in Birsh (1999), the content of multisensory structure language instruction involves six components: (1) phonology and phonological awareness, (2) sound–symbol association, (3) syllable instruction, (4) morphology, (5) syntax, and (6) semantics. This content is embedded in five principles of instruction: (1) simultaneous, multisensory teaching to all learning modalities (visual, auditory, kinesthetic), to enhance memory and learning; (2) systematic and cumulative organization of material; (3) direct teaching through continued teacher–student interaction; (4) diagnostic teaching involving continued assessment of individual needs; and (5) both synthetic (putting parts of language together to form a whole) and analytic (presenting the whole and breaking it down into constituent parts) instruction. With the exception of the multisensory component, which remains controversial, principles 2–5 characterize many effective approaches to reading remediation for students with word recognition and fluency

difficulties, along with the focus on explicit teaching of the structure of language.

Older versions represented as Orton–Gillingham approaches have received little research support (Hallahan et al., 1996), and more recent versions are just beginning to be rigorously evaluated. The NRP (2000) found only four studies with adequate methodological quality that involved variations of older multisensory Orton–Gillingham programs. Two of these programs yielded positive effect sizes, and two did not. For example, Oakland, Black, Stanford, Nussbaum, and Balise (1998) implemented the Dyslexia Training Program (an adaptation of the widely employed Alphabetic Phonics program developed at the Texas Scottish Rite Hospital) for 2 years of daily instruction in small groups. In relation to a comparison group of students who were served in "regular-practice" classrooms, effect sizes associated with the Dyslexia Training Program were not regarded as significant (NRP, 2000). Although the students in the intervention had severe reading skill deficits, 2 years of instruction resulted in changes from about the 3rd percentile of word recognition ability to the 10th percentile.

In another study, students with identified reading disabilities in grades 2 and 3 who were provided services in public school special education resource rooms received one of two programs in which phonics was taught explicitly. One of these was an alphabetic (synthetic) phonics program based on an Orton–Gillingham model, and the other an analytic phonics method (Recipe for Reading). Students in these two groups were compared with a group that received an intervention involving the teaching of sight word recognition skills (Foorman et al., 1997). Although there was a clear tendency for students who received the alphabetic phonics program to show better gains in phonological analysis and word-reading skills at the end of 1 year of intervention, these differences were not apparent when verbal intelligence scores (higher in this group) were controlled for in the analysis. Unfortunately, Foorman and colleagues (1997) also noted that the instructional groups were too large to promote adequate implementation of any of the programs.

There are efficacy data from less rigorous evaluation studies that support these types of programs, and more rigorous studies are emerging. There is concern about the necessity of the traditional multisensory components, because studies that compare instruction with and without these components do not indicate differences in outcomes (Bryant, 1979; Clark, 1988; Moats & Farrell, 1999; Moats & Lyon, 1993). Wise, Ring, and Olson (1999) also did not find that a multisensory articulatory component (such as the one in the Lindamood program) was a necessary component of their own intervention.

The strengths of these programs probably include the intense, systematic approach to instruction, the link with specific types of struggling readers, and possibly the explicit attention to the structure of language. Although there is limited evidence for the efficacy of programs under the multisensory rubric, other programs reviewed below that are similar in content and structure do show positive effects. It is important for practitioners to attend to the findings of research and to alter traditional practices as necessary. Any remedial approach to reading for students with problems at the level of word recognition and fluency needs to teach phonics explicitly, provide sufficient practice to promote fluency, include comprehension lessons that integrate instruction in word recognition, and identify and instruct struggling readers as early as possible.

HOSPITAL FOR SICK CHILDREN STUDIES

The longest continual program on reading remediation research is directed by Maureen Lovett at the Hospital for Sick Children in Toronto. In the initial phase of this research, children with severe reading disabilities were randomly assigned to (1) an intervention that is a modification of Reading Mastery, a Direct Instruction program called Phonological Analysis and Blending/Direct Instruction (PHAB/DI); or (2) a program with a metacognitive focus that teaches word recognition through the application of different strategies, called Word Identification Strategy Training (WIST). Both programs recognized the importance of decoding instruction that helps children break apart words, as well as the importance of instruction that maximizes transfer of learning. The PHAB/DI program emphasizes letter–sound units, while the WIST program focuses on larger subsyllable units. In the initial evaluations, both programs were more effective than an active comparison group (classroom sur-

vival skills) on standardized and experimental measures (Lovett, Warren-Chaplin, Ransby, & Borden, 1990). These programs resulted in different patterns of transfer of learning, thus showing treatment-specific effects. For example, PHAB/DI was specifically associated with stronger results in phonological decoding, such as psuedowords; the WIST program, resulted in generalization to regular *and* exception words in English. As Lovett and colleagues (2003) observed, these programs did not fully remediate reading skills, and 35 hours of instruction did not seem to be adequate. Note, however, that the students in these interventions were largely at upper elementary and middle school levels when they began the intervention, and that they entered with very severe reading difficulties (often around the 2nd–5th percentiles, and more than half consistently below the 1st percentile in word recognition ability).

Lovett, Lacerenza, and colleagues (2000) conducted an RCE in which PHAB/DI and WIST were combined and compared to longer-term intervention with PHAB/DI or WIST alone and to an active control condition. The study provided about 70 hours of instruction in different sequences that involved going from PHAB/DI to WIST, going from WIST to PHAB/DI, or receiving either intervention alone for the same amount of overall instructional time. Generalized treatment effects on standardized measures of word identification, passage comprehension, and phonological decoding were demonstrated for all four reading instruction sequences. Results showed that the combination of PHAB/DI and WIST, in either order, was more effective than either intervention alone on measures of nonword reading, letter–sound knowledge, and different word identification measures. Thus 35 hours of instruction in PHAB/DI combined with 35 hours of instruction in either WIST or Wolf's RAVE-O program (see below) was more effective than 70 hours of PHAB/DI or WIST, and the latter interventions alone were more effective than teaching math and study skills.

These studies occurred in special research classrooms where children were referred for reading difficulties. Subsequent research has employed these programs in school settings. A combined program (PHAB/DI and WIST) is now called the PHAST (Phonological and Strategy Training) Track Reading Program

(Lovett, Lacerenza, et al., 2000). In an ongoing study in which the PHAST Track Reading Program is implemented in community schools in Toronto, initial data showed that the students who received these interventions made substantial gains on standardized and experimental measures, achieving on average about two-thirds of the program gains achieved in the laboratory-based interventions. There was considerable variability in the response to the community-based interventions, which may reflect differences in the fidelity and the vitality of implementation. Many children who were served in the community schools obtained remedial gains similar to those observed in a laboratory setting. The PHAST Track Reading Program has been extended to include systematic teaching of text comprehension strategies, and a special program called PHAST PACES has been developed for implementation with struggling readers in high school. Both the expanded PHAST Comprehension Program and PHAST PACES are being evaluated in ongoing studies conducted in community school settings in Toronto.

MORRIS, LOVETT, AND WOLF STUDIES

The PHAST Track Reading Program has also been employed in recent multisite intervention studies involving collaboration by Lovett's group, Wolf's group in Boston, and Morris and colleagues at Georgia State University (Lovett et al., 2005; Wolf et al., 2003). In the initial 5 years, a group of students received different combinations of the interventions in schools in Toronto, Atlanta, and Boston. The samples were carefully constructed to control for variations in socioeconomic status, ethnicity, and intellectual levels, all involving students in second and third grade. About half the children in each site and group were from lower socioeconomic backgrounds, and within the lower and not-lower socioeconomic levels, half were white and half were black. Four treatment groups were compared. One group received the original PHAST Track Reading Program (decoding and word identification focus). The second group received a combination of PHAB/DI and Wolf's RAVE-O program (for Retrieval, Automaticity, Vocabulary Elaboration, and Orthography; Wolf, Miller, & Donnelly, 2002), which is described more fully in the section on fluency. These two programs, which combine direct instruction methods emphasizing the al-

phabetic principle with different forms of language focus and strategy instruction, were contrasted with two comparison groups—one that was taught Direct Instruction math and study skills, and one that received PHAB/DI along with study skills training. Results showed that students who received either combined condition achieved higher levels of word recognition and comprehension ability than students who received only PHAB/DI; all three groups performed at higher levels than the math comparison group did. This intervention, which involved approximately 70 hours of instruction, resulted in changes of about 0.5 standard deviation. Approximately 50% of students who received the two combined interventions showed word recognition ability that approximated the average range. This study revealed that these multidimensional programs yielded equivalent gains for children with lower versus higher IQs at entry, and equal benefit for children from disadvantaged versus more advantaged environments.

UNIVERSITY OF COLORADO STUDIES

Olson and Wise (in press) summarized a series of computer-based remedial studies for students with significant reading problems defined on the basis of difficulties with decoding skills. These students were generally identified with disabilities in grades 2–5 and had word recognition scores that were in the lowest 10% of their classes. In their initial studies, Olson and Wise (1992) pulled students from regular reading or language arts classes to read interesting instruction-level stories on a computer during approximately 28 half-hour sessions over a semester. Decoding support for targeted words in the stories was available in various forms through the use of synthetic speech. The group that received computer-based instruction showed significantly better gains in phonological decoding skills and word recognition than a randomly assigned control group of poor readers who remained in their regular remedial reading or language arts classes. However, the gains in the computer-trained group were much less dramatic in poor readers with the lowest scores on measures of phoneme awareness.

Therefore, Wise, Ring, and Olson (2000) developed a longer computer-based Phonological intervention, which instructed students in groups of three with a main focus on phonological awareness and decoding in 50–60 half-hour sessions over a semester. One-third of the intervention time was devoted to computer-based and small-group interactive instruction in phonological and articulatory awareness, based in part on the program developed by Lindamood and Lindamood (1998). Another third of the intervention time was spent on practice in the phonological decoding of nonwords and in building nonwords and words spoken by the computer. The final third of the intervention included reading instruction-level stories on the computer (with decoding assistance when requested for difficult words), answering occasional multiple-choice comprehension questions, and reviewing targeted words at the end of the session.

The Phonological intervention was compared with an Accurate Reading in Context intervention, which also devoted a third of its time to small-group interaction and discussions regarding use of comprehension strategies (Palinscar & Brown, 1987), to balance with the highly motivating small-group phonological awareness activities in the Phonological condition. The remaining two-thirds of the Accurate Reading intervention involved reading stories independently on the computer as described for the Phonological condition. The main purpose of this second intervention was to compare the benefits of the Phonological condition with benefits from Accurate Reading practice with stories without explicit phonological instruction.

Two hundred students were randomly assigned to the two intervention conditions. There was no regular-reading-class control group as in earlier studies, since these studies had already shown significantly greater gains from less intensive intervention, and a main objective of the Wise and colleagues (2000) study was to maximize statistical power for detecting differential treatment main effects and potential treatment interactions with subject characteristics and specific reading skills. A separate large study of the Phonological condition focused on the specific contribution of intervention involving articulatory awareness (there was none) and included a regular-reading-class control group; those who received the intervention showed substantially greater gains in phoneme awareness (effect size = 0.92–1.73), phonological decoding (effect size = 1.46), and word reading (effect size = 0.73–0.98) (Wise et al., 1999).

When compared to the Accurate Reading in Context group at the end of the study period, the Phonological group in Wise and colleagues (2000) made three times more improvement in phonological awareness and two times more improvement in the phonological decoding of nonwords. However, the results for standard score gains in word reading varied depended on the poor readers' grade/reading levels, and on whether the measure of word reading was time-limited or unlimited. Combined across grades 2–5, those in the Phonological condition showed significantly greater standard score gains on two untimed measures of word reading, but this main effect was qualified by a significant interaction with their grade/reading level: Phonologically trained poor readers in grades 2–3 showed substantially greater gains in untimed word reading, but there was no significant advantage for phonologically trained students in grades 4–5, in spite of their superior phonological skills. An *opposite* treatment main effect was found for an experimental measure of time-limited word reading: The Phonological group actually had significantly smaller gains, and this treatment difference tended to be larger for the poor readers in grades 4–5, where growth in rapid and accurate word reading was clearly better in the group that spent most of the time accurately reading stories on the computer. This result is consistent with those of other studies reviewed later in the chapter's section on fluency training, which showed significant fluency gains from text-reading practice (e.g., Stahl, 2004). One additional treatment × grade level interaction was found for spelling, where the Phonological group had the advantage in grades 2–3, but the Accurate Reading group had the advantage in grades 4–5.

The Wise and colleagues (2000) study included follow-up tests 1 and 2 years after the end of intervention. The authors reasoned that if the Phonological group continued to maintain its advantage in phoneme awareness and phonological decoding in follow-up tests, these skills might eventually support more rapid postintervention growth in reading and spelling across all grade levels, when compared to the Accurate Reading in Context group. However, although the Phonological group's advantages in phonological skills did remain significant 1 and 2 years after intervention, there were no significant differential main effects of training group or interactions for any of the reading or spelling measures at follow-up tests. Wise and colleagues were encouraged by the substantial short- and long-term gains in word-reading standard scores for *both* conditions, and by the support these gains provided for computer-based reading intervention, but the absence of an additional long-term reading advantage resulting from the Phonological group's superior phonological skills was not expected.

Wise and colleagues (2000) hypothesized that better long-term transfer to reading from improved phonological skills might be attained through longer and more intensive intervention to "automatize" phonological skills, and through continued support for the application of those skills in reading. However, after reviewing the results from other more recent and intensive intervention studies that included comparisons of intervention conditions varying in their emphasis on phonological skills, Olson and Wise (in press) concluded that there is still little evidence for older poor readers experiencing specific long-term benefits that can be specifically attributed to a heavy emphasis on sublexical phonological intervention as provided in many interventions (e.g., (Lindamood & Lindamood, 1998). They cited the intensive individualized-tutoring intervention study by Torgesen, Alexander, and colleagues (2001; see below) with 67 hours of instruction for five poor readers in grades 3–5, which resulted in similar and strong reading gains at the end of intervention and at 1- and 2-year follow-up tests for two conditions that, like those in Wise and colleagues, were quite different in their emphasis on explicit phonological intervention (although Torgesen and colleagues' Embedded Phonics intervention did include a sublexical component). These results parallel others from the prevention section, showing that the addition of phonological awareness training to the decoding component of PALS (which also has a sublexical component) has no value-added impact on reading outcomes. Mathes and colleagues (2005) also found comparable gains for two reading interventions that varied the amount of phonological awareness and sublexical phonics intervention. The Colorado interventions provide the most extreme distinctions, but keep in mind that the computer reading condition provided pronunciations as targeted words were highlighted, so implicit learning of their print–speech relations was supported (Foorman, 1994).

SYRACUSE UNIVERSITY STUDIES

The emphasis on interventions that combine different components including explicit instruction in the alphabetic principle with different aspects of strategy instruction can be found in other interventions, both older and more recent ones. Blachman and colleagues (2004) reported the results of a reading intervention compared with standard-practice intervention in a sample of second and third graders with poor word recognition ability. The intervention involved 8 months of individualized tutoring (average of 105 hours) in a program that emphasized explicit instruction in phonological and orthographic connections in words as well as text-based reading. Each lesson was built around a five-step core: (1) review of sound–symbol associations; (2) practice in word building to develop new decoding skills; (3) review of previously learned regular words and high-frequency sight words; (4) oral reading of stories; and (5) writing words and sentences from earlier components of the lesson. Each lesson also included activities that involved additional reading of narrative and expository text to enhance fluency, comprehension, and engagement, along with other writing activities and games.

Results revealed significantly greater gains in the students who received the intervention than students who received their interventions through the schools in word recognition, fluency, comprehension, and spelling. These gains were maintained at a 1-year follow-up. These students generally began the intervention with word recognition scores that approximated the 10th–12th percentiles; at the end of the intervention their scores approximated the 23rd percentile in word recognition, with higher scores in spelling, slightly lower scores on measures of reading fluency, and comparable scores on comprehension. The effect sizes were generally in the moderate to large range across reading domains, ranging on standardized tests from 0.55 for reading comprehension to 1.69 for word recognition.

Shaywitz and colleagues (2004) performed functional MRI on the students who received the Blachman and colleagues (2004) intervention in Syracuse and on comparison groups of students in New Haven, Connecticut, who were either typical achievers or students with reading problems who received standard interventions from the school. This study required the Syracuse students to fly to New Haven, because logistical factors precluded imaging community controls from Syracuse. The results showed that prior to the intervention, students with reading difficulties exhibited much less activation of brain areas in the left hemisphere commonly associated with reading difficulties. After the intervention, students who received the experimental intervention showed greater activation of bilateral inferior frontal gyri, the left superior temporal sulcus, the occipital temporal region of the brain involving the middle and inferior temporal gyri, and the interior aspect of the middle occipital gyrus, as well as other regions. Shaywitz and colleagues interpreted these results as showing "normalization" of left occipital temporal regions associated with efficiency in reading.

FLORIDA STATE UNIVERSITY STUDY

Other intervention studies parallel these results, generally showing that the nature of the program is less important than its comprehensiveness and intensity. For example, Torgesen, Alexander, and colleagues (2001) enrolled students reading below the 3rd percentile in word recognition ability in grades 3–5 in an intense 8-week program in which the student received 2 hours of instruction per day, 5 days per week (about 67 hours over the 8-week period). The interventions involved either the well-known Lindamood–Bell Auditory Discrimination in Depth program or a program called Embedded Phonics, which was developed by the authors. Both interventions incorporated intervention principles that have been found to be effective for students with significant reading difficulties. These included ample opportunities for structured practice of new skills, the cuing of appropriate strategies in context, and explicit instruction in the alphabetic principle. A comparison of time × activity analyses showed that the Lindamood–Bell program involved about 85% time in instruction in phonological decoding, about 10% in sight word instruction, and 5% time in reading and writing connected text. The Embedded Phonics program, in contrast, involved about 20% instructional time in phonological decoding, 30% in sight word instruction, and 50% in reading or writing connected text. There was little difference in the relative efficacy of the two interventions. The results showed that there was significant improvement of about 1 standard deviation in word recogni-

tion, about 0.66 standard deviation in comprehension, and little change in fluency. The gains in word recognition and comprehension persisted for 2 years past the intervention. About 70% of the students who received one of these interventions were able to read in the average range, defined as word recognition scores above the 25th percentile, after the intervention; most remarkably, 40% exited special education. Disappointing, however, was the absence of changes in fluency.

In explaining the absence of improvement in fluency, Torgesen, Alexander, and colleagues (2001) suggested that reading rate was limited because the number of words in grade-level passages that the students could read "on sight" was much smaller than for average readers. Thus, when fluency rates on stories that were at the students' instructional level were compared, there were no rate differences. However, grade-level passages reduced the fluency differences, because there were too many words the students did not have as part of their sight word vocabulary. There is a strong relationship between reading fluency and practice, so that if students are not able to access print for 3–5 years, it may be very difficult to close this gap. Torgesen (2002) estimated that students in the interventions would have to read for 8 hours per day for a year in order to close the gap induced by the students' access to print.

Torgesen (2004) reported on preliminary data that represented another attempt to evaluate a cohort similar in age and decoding impairment. In this study, students with severe reading difficulties in grades 3–5 received either an intense phonologically based intervention, or an intervention that included a fluency-oriented component addressing repeated reading of words and passages. Initial results did not show differences between the two interventions. Although both interventions led to significant improvement in word-reading accuracy and in comprehension, little change in norm-referenced fluency scores was apparent, paralleling the findings of Torgesen, Alexander, and colleagues (2001).

UNIVERSITY OF TEXAS–HOUSTON STUDY

At the University of Texas–Houston, Simos and colleagues (2002) performed MSI on eight students with severe dyslexia (ranging from 7 to 17 years of age) before and after an 8-week, 2-hour-per-day intervention paralleling that of

Torgesen and colleagues (2001) in its format and intensity. Students received one of two programs designed to teach phonological skills and word recognition. After 8 weeks, all eight students had word recognition skills in the average range, with scores ranging from the 38th to the 60th percentile. Before intervention, imaging responses to a pseudoword-decoding task paralleled those seen in other studies of dyslexia (Simos et al., 2000), showing little activation of a neural network in the left hemisphere associated with proficient word recognition, as well as a predominance of activation in the homologous right-hemisphere region. In all 8 cases, intervention resulted in a significant increase in activation of the left-hemisphere network, particularly involving the left superior temporal gyrus, an area associated with phonological processing. This pattern paralleled that seen in typical readers, leading Simos and colleagues to suggest that the pattern reflected "normalization" of brain function as opposed to a compensatory pattern.

UNIVERSITY OF WASHINGTON STUDIES

Berninger and colleagues (2003) identified 20 students in grades 4–6 who were participating in a family genetics study. These students read 1 standard deviation below their Verbal IQ on one of several different measures. The selection criteria resulted in a sample that tended to be much higher in Verbal IQ than other samples, with the students also tending to have higher reading scores at baseline. These students were randomly assigned to an intervention involving about 28 hours of either extensive phonological awareness intervention or intervention in morphological awareness. The phonological intervention emphasized word building through phonological analysis and synthesis, while the morphological treatment emphasized word building and generation with larger units of words. Each student received intervention in groups of 10 over a 3-week period. Results showed gains of about 0.5 standard deviation in word recognition for both conditions compared to pretreatment scores. It should be noted that the students in this sample had much higher language development scores and fewer attentional problems than those in the other remedial studies reviewed in this chapter.

Aylward and colleagues (2003) evaluated functional neuroimaging changes in these students before and after the intervention, using a letter–sound task and a task involving morphological judgments. At baseline, comparisons of students with reading problems with controls showed different patterns of brain activation for two tasks. These did not change in controls. In contrast, students with reading difficulties showed significant changes in neuroimaging responses after the intervention, again largely suggesting "normalization" of brain function. As in Simos and colleagues (2002), changes were especially apparent in the superior temporal gyrus of the left hemisphere, a region strongly associated with phonological processing.

REMEDIAL STUDIES: SUMMARY

Remedial studies show that foundational skills can be improved in students with LDs in reading, which are typically characterized by word recognition difficulties. The effects are most apparent in word recognition, but also show transfer to comprehension. Fluency gains are often smaller, but vary across studies and may reflect the age and severity of reading difficulties of the students addressed by the study. For example, Blachman and colleagues (2004) obtained stronger gains in fluency than Torgesen, Alexander, and colleagues (2001), but many of the Blachman and colleagues' students were younger and less severely impaired than Torgesen and colleagues' were. Wise and colleagues (2000) also found age-related changes in fluency gains. Various approaches are associated with improvement, including commercial programs that were reviewed (Lindamood-Bell, Phono-Graphix), research-based approaches (PHAB/DI, RAVE-O, PHAST Track, PASP), and programs that were not reviewed (e.g., Spell-Read PAT; Rashotte, MacPhee, & Torgesen, 2001). It is clear that the program is less important than how it is delivered, with the most impressive gains associated with more intensity and an explicit and systematic delivery (Torgesen, Alexander, et al., 2001). There are also associations with the length of instruction; many hours are required to accelerate reading development in older students (grade 2 and beyond). To reiterate a critical finding, programs that are explicit, teach to mastery, provide scaffolding and emotional support, and monitor progress are particularly effective. Outcomes are specific to the content of instruction, so that more comprehensive programs are emerging. It is clear that the future development of remedial programs must involve instructional interactions to improve reading fluency, which seems least responsive to intervention. We address this topic in detail in the next section.

Fluency Interventions

In contrast to studies that target either the prevention or remediation of word recognition difficulties, there are few examples of specific interventions for problems primarily in reading fluency. It is likely that interventions addressing fluency deficits could be applied to these students if they were identified as a separate subgroup. But most attempts to intervene in the fluency area usually involve students who began with problems with word recognition, and typically attempt to include both word recognition and fluency components in the intervention. The NRP (2000) reviewed classroom and tutorial studies addressing intervention studies involving fluency. The panel identified 16 studies that included 398 students who were poor readers and 281 students who were good readers. The NRP found comparable, moderate effect sizes (about 0.50) for both poor readers and average readers. Although a variety of intervention programs were examined, the only domains that could be characterized as effective interventions involved repeated reading and other guided reading oral interventions. In general, these types of interventions involve repeated oral readings with a model or with a peer or parent. They did not necessarily focus on students who were poor readers.

In a subsequent analysis, Kuhn and Stahl (2003) followed the NRP report on fluency with a review of a broader range of studies. These authors expanded the NRP report by including studies of repeated reading, assisted reading in clinical settings, and approaches to fluency development that involved the entire classroom. In evaluating this literature, Kuhn and Stahl confirmed the NRP finding that interventions involving fluency were efficacious, with virtually all of the studies examined showing gains in response to instruction. However, gains were generally lower in students with reading difficulties. Approaches that involved some form of assistance, such as reading with a model or listening during reading, appeared more effective than approaches that did not involve assistance, such as silent sustained reading. These findings suggest that teacher guidance and monitoring are critical components of

fluency instruction. Kuhn and Stahl noted that little evidence supported simple repeated reading of passages and stories; they suggested that time spent in oral reading of connected text, as opposed to repetition, may be responsible for the effect of repeated reading on fluency and comprehension.

In a more recent empirical synthesis of interventions for reading fluency specifically addressing students with LDs, Chard, Vaughn, and Tyler (2002) found 24 published and unpublished studies that reported specific findings involving fluency. These studies included repeated reading both with and without a model, as well as sustained silent reading; they also evaluated issues involving the number of repetitions, text difficulty, and the extent of improvement. Chard and colleagues found 21 studies that addressed whether repeatedly reading text resulted in improved reading fluency in students defined with LDs. These studies yielded an average effect size in the moderate range (0.68). In 14 studies, almost all single cases involving modeling by an adult, all studies were associated with positive effect sizes in the small to large range. Peer modeling was also associated with small to moderate effect sizes. Modeling with an audiotape or computer in four small studies showed small to moderate effects. A variety of factors influenced effect size estimates, including the amount of text, text difficulty, number of repetitions, types of feedback, and criteria for repeated reading. Like the NRP (2000), Chard and colleagues concluded that more research is needed to redress the lack of attention to fluency development. At the same time, it is apparent that an emphasis on fluency building as part of either classroom or tutorial interventions is essential to improving performance in this domain.

As the study by Torgesen, Alexander, and colleagues (2001) graphically demonstrates, a common finding in reading remedial approaches for students with word recognition deficiencies is improvement in word reading and comprehension, but little change in fluency. Although early intervention will help address some of these difficulties for many students, the reduced efficacy of many remedial studies may be due to persistent word recognition difficulties that could have been reduced through earlier intervention. For example, early intervention programs do seem to have an impact on fluency as well as word recognition (Torgesen, 2002). Nonetheless, remedial studies may continue to produce a population of students who respond to instruction in the alphabetic principle, but continue to have fluency difficulties. In turn, many of these students may not be able to comprehend what is read, primarily because their slow reading rate places too many demands on their ability to remember what they have read. In addition, students who are not fluent do not enjoy reading, so they are less likely to read, which contributes to the failure to build sight word vocabulary—a key to the development of accurate and fluent of reading skills.

One commercial program specifically targeting fluency is Read Naturally (Ihnot, 2000). In Read Naturally, students read nonfiction passages designed for students in grades 1–8. Students practice oral reading of short, interesting passages (i.e., repeated reading); read with a videotape at a challenging pace; and time and graph their reading rates (e.g., words correct per minute) so that they are constantly aware of their progress. A comprehension component involves discussing passages with the teacher and answering questions about what they have read. There is little research on Read Naturally. Hasbrouck, Ihnot, and Rogers (1999) reported cases that had benefited from Read Naturally, but these were not controlled evaluations. More research on the effectiveness of this approach to reading fluency would be useful.

Stahl, Heubach, and Cramond (1997) developed a "fluency-oriented reading instruction" approach to facilitate automatic word recognition and fluency in second graders. This approach had three components: (1) a redesign of the basal reading lesson to include specific components involving fluency; (2) a period involving free reading in school; and (3) a component involving reading at home. The redesign of the basal reader largely involved an attempt to introduce differentiated instruction by dividing students into two groups based on their reading levels, with modifications of fluency instruction based on the amount of assistance needed. The school and home components were designed to increase the amount of time spent reading connected text. An initial evaluation of the program (4 teachers and 2 schools, eventually expanded to 10 teachers and 3 schools) showed positive results. On average, students gained about 2 years in overall reading growth on an informal inventory. Of particular importance was the finding that over the 2-year period, even struggling readers improved in fluency, with only 2 of about 105 students reading below second-grade level by the end of the year. Reading practice clearly improved fluency in this study.

Stahl (2004) summarized the initial findings from a larger-scale attempt to evaluate fluency-oriented reading instruction that included control groups. The first year of the study involved 9 schools and 28 classrooms across three sites and compared fluency-oriented reading instruction with a program that emphasized repeated reading of a wide range of materials. A third group served as a classroom curriculum control and was simply followed over time. Historical controls were also included and evaluated. Stahl reported that both interventions involving fluency instruction resulted in better outcomes than those for the historical controls, and there were no systematic differences between the two treatments. Results were especially dramatic for the students who were struggling readers when the fluency program was supplemented with Direct Instruction principles to address decoding weaknesses (following Lovett et al., 1990). When the performance of these students was compared to that of students who had been in the same school programs in the past (historical controls), improvements in word recognition, oral reading rate and accuracy, and comprehension were apparent. The effects on these struggling readers, many of whom would have had LDs, were especially interesting. A second wave of the initial study is underway to replicate and extend these initial findings, suggesting that more time spent reading leads to growth in fluency.

Not surprising, fluency is emerging as a major emphasis in the remedial area, with newer efforts perhaps best characterized by the RAVE-O program developed by Wolf and colleagues (2002). RAVE-O is designed to facilitate the development of automaticity in reading subskills, to facilitate fluency in decoding and comprehension processes, and to enhance interest and engagement in reading and language use in students with LDs in this area. It is based on a developmental model of fluency (Wolf & Katzir-Cohen, 2001), which emphasizes the multiple contributions to proficient comprehension made by a student's familiarity with common orthographic patterns, as well as a student's knowledge of a word's meaning(s), morpheme parts, and grammatical uses. A major premise is that the more a student knows about a word, the faster the student will retrieve and read it. The game-like format includes intensive work on rapid orthographic pattern recognition; building word webs; learning word retrieval and comprehension strategies; playing games with language through computer games enhanced with animation; and rapid, repeated reading of short (1-minute) mystery stories that incorporate the multiple meanings and syntactic uses of core words. This program is typically used in conjunction with a word recognition program and is being evaluated along with the PHAST Track Reading Program by the Morris, Wolf, and Lovett research group, described above (Lovett et al., 2005; Wolf et al., 2003). Preliminary results indicate that RAVE-O enhances word recognition, fluency, and comprehension better than instruction based only on decoding skills does. To date, there is no strong evidence from these studies that RAVE-O produces larger gains in fluency at the word level than a program like PHAST Track, which teaches strategies for generalizing from the alphabetic principle to higher-level reading skills; however, this evaluation is not complete. One question is whether a program like RAVE-O leads to more improvement in reading connected text, as well as comprehension. This possibility would reflect the focus of programs like RAVE-O on fluency not only at the sublexical and word levels, but at the connected text level. Previous theories of fluency's emergence have focused on accurate and fluent word recognition, which is supported by the comparable word-level fluency results for programs like WIST. If RAVE-O leads to stronger gains in fluency at the connected text level and in comprehension, such findings would support a more comprehensive approach to intervention at the text level of proficiency and comprehension.

In a series of remedial studies specifically addressing fluency deficits (Levy, 2001), students identified with fluency difficulties received a variety of interventions. Most of these students also had word recognition problems. These studies were specifically designed to evaluate whether transfer in fluency is mediated at the level of word recognition or at the level of text. In general, the studies summarized by Levy (2001) showed that the reading fluency of poor readers was limited by their slow rate of processing at the level of the individual word. She found that simple practice in a "repetition of names" game led to significant gains in word recognition skills, particularly for poor readers.

Words were learned best through word-training study, in which the students were taught to read a list of words as fast as possible. The alternative involved having students read a story four times in succession that contained the same word. For the poor readers, transfer to improved reading speed occurred, regardless of whether a similar or a different story context was used. However, Levy reported that context was not an essential component of the experience, and that teaching automaticity of word reading was less difficult for poor readers and also made them more successful. There was clear evidence for transfer across linguistic levels in context. In other studies, there appeared to be little additional benefit of highlighting shared orthographic units. However, blocking according to the orthographic unit, which has the effect of making the orthographic relation more explicit, resulted in more automaticity. These results are consistent with the premises of RAVE-O, showing that grouping words into similar orthographic patterns accelerates fluency.

FLUENCY STUDIES: SUMMARY

Fluency is an emerging area of research. The key is practice in reading and exposure to sight words in an effort to develop automatic word recognition skills. Unfortunately, few studies have isolated students whose primary problem is with fluency. The Levy (2001) studies, like many others, largely involved students who were poor in both word recognition and fluency. In the future, it will be interesting to observe the development of new alternatives to repeated reading techniques and practice, as well as interventions that specifically target students with fluency difficulties. As students with reading difficulties enter the middle and high school grades, where proficient reading of context texts is critical, evidence-based interventions that specifically address fluency will be of significant importance.

Reading Comprehension

As summarized in Lyon, Fletcher, and colleagues (2003), comprehension difficulties in reading tend to affect older students (grades 3 and above). There is an extensive research base showing that specific comprehension disorders in reading commonly parallel comprehension problems in spoken language (Lyon, Fletcher, et al., 2003). Impairments involving vocabulary development and comprehension of spoken language are most frequently described in the literature, but limitations in higher-order metacognitive processes that involve application of comprehension strategies are also involved in reading comprehension difficulties, regardless of whether a child's reading is accurate and/or fluent at the word and text levels.

Problems with accuracy and fluency are major causes of reading comprehension difficulties in students with LDs. Leach, Scarborough, and Rescorla (2003) compared students in grades 4–5 with LDs in reading identified before and after grade 3, and evaluated relations of word recognition, listening comprehension, and both word recognition and listening comprehension problems in students with LDs. Very few students (6%) in the "early identified" group had specific comprehension problems. This group was comparable in the number of students with specific word recognition (49%) or with both word recognition and listening comprehension (46%) problems. In the "late identified" group, approximately one-third showed specific comprehension problems, and another third showed both problems. In other words, a third had only word recognition problems that were not identified until after grade 3, and two-thirds had problems that involved word recognition. In a study of comprehension in adults with a history of dyslexia, Ransby and Swanson (2003) found that scores on assessments of phonological processing and naming speed continued to contribute to reading comprehension scores. Scores on assessments of vocabulary, listening comprehension, and working memory also independently contributed to reading comprehension scores in this sample. Comprehension problems may not be identified until later in development, but are persistent and sometimes occur in isolation from word-level difficulties. The latter situation is much less frequent, accounting for LDs in less than 20% of the Leach and colleagues (2003) sample.

Although difficulties with decoding inevitably have an impact on reading comprehension, there are other causes for comprehension deficiencies. Garner, Alexander, and Hare (1991) cited five possible causes for comprehension failure, aside from difficulty with decoding: confusion about task demands, meager domain knowledge, weak comprehension monitoring, low self-esteem, and low interest. Many of the intervention methods described below are efforts to remediate these causes of reading failure. These methods are often classified into two general types of instruction: "specific skills instruction" and "strategy instruction" (Clark & Uhry, 1995; Swanson et al., 1999). As the name suggests, specific skills instruction focuses on teaching specific skills that can be applied to texts, such as vocabulary skills, finding the main idea, making inferences, and finding facts. Vocabulary skills can be taught through either direct instruction approaches or contextual approaches to learning vocabulary (Carlisle, 1993). Skills such as finding the main idea and making inferences can be taught by reading short passages and answering questions. However, for these to be effective, the teacher must provide the instruction in an explicit and systematic manner.

In contrast to specific skills instruction, strategy instruction is "viewed as [training in] cognitive processes requiring decision making and critical thinking" (Clark & Uhry, 1995, p. 107). Strategy instruction in reading comprehension is an outgrowth of several cognitive psychology theories and concepts, notably schemas, metacognition, and mediated learning. For example, a reader is viewed as bringing certain psychological frameworks, or "mental schemas," to a text. During reading, in order for the reader to comprehend, facts must be added or adjusted to the reader's mental schemas. The study of metacognition has also had considerable influence on reading comprehension research. It has been found that "good readers who possess metacognitive skills in reading are aware of the purpose of reading and differentiate between task demands. They actively seek to clarify the purposes or task demands through self-questioning prior to reading the given materials . . . [and] evaluate their own comprehension of materials read" (Wong, 1991, pp. 239–240). Research has shown that readers who have deficits in comprehension lack these metacognitive skills (Baker & Brown, 1984a, 1984b; Wong, 1985). As is true for other skill domains (e.g., memory), the teaching of metacognitive strategies is beneficial to poor comprehenders, even though metacognition is not causally related to comprehension skill.

Finally, the concept of mediated learning, which involves the effects of student–teacher interactions on students' later ability to solve problems independently, has also influenced reading comprehension theory and instruction. For example, Maria (1990) has conceptualized reading instruction as an interaction among reader, text, and teacher. The reader brings decoding ability, oral vocabulary, and background knowledge to the text. The text is no longer perceived as having a single meaning for all students; rather, meaning is constructed through this interaction. The teacher is viewed as a manager and facilitator who provides direct instruction in strategies, but who also encourages independence (Clark & Uhry, 1995).

Several intervention methods based on these types of cognitive strategies have been developed to teach reading comprehension. For example, as discussed earlier, Palinscar and Brown (1983, 1985) have developed a method called "reciprocal teaching" that has been found to enhance reading comprehension skills. In addition, Pressley and his colleagues have developed interventions known as "transactional strategies," which are based in part on Vygotskian concepts, to increase reading comprehension skills (Pressley, 2006; Pressley et al., 1991). In this method of instruction, students are "provided with direct instruction in a number of comprehension strategies and are encouraged to talk about and choose a strategy for understanding what they read ... students are provided with positive instruction when a strategy is successful" (Clark & Uhry, 1995, p. 111). Transactional instruction also involves teacher modeling of different comprehension strategies.

Bos and Anders (1990) have developed an interactive teaching model similar to Pressley and colleagues' (1991) transactional teaching method. This model, which is also based on Vygotskian principles, incorporates six teaching–learning characteristics: (1) activating prior knowledge; (2) integrating new knowledge with old knowledge; (3) cooperative knowledge sharing and learning; (4) predicting, justifying, and confirming concepts and text meaning; (5) predicting, justifying, and confirming relationships among concepts; and (6) purposeful learning. Initially, a teacher models these strategies for the students, but gradually moves away from being an instructor to being more of a facilitator.

The characteristics of any effective instruction for students with reading comprehension disabilities include explicit instruction, multiple opportunities for instruction, and carefully sequenced lessons (Clark & Uhry, 1995). Although specific skills instruction and strategy instruction have some similarities, strategies based on cognitive concepts (i.e., strategy instruction) appear to be the most effective *methods* of intervention for reading comprehension, and have provided the best results to date for improving comprehension in readers with LDs.

Several interventions, especially strategy-based ones, are specifically effective in the reading comprehension area with students who vary in the extent of impairment in word recognition, fluency, and listening comprehension. In Swanson and colleagues' (1999) meta-analysis, strategy instruction was specifically effective with students with LDs who had comprehension difficulties. The NRP (2000) report identified 47 studies involving vocabulary instruction and 203 studies involving text comprehension. However, because many of the studies had limitations in their research designs, the final database was not adequate for empirical synthesis. It was difficult to separate and classify the many different variables and methodologies involved in experimental research involving vocabulary instruction. The 203 studies on text comprehension instruction identified 16 different types of instruction, with 8 providing a firm scientific basis indicating that they improved comprehension. These included comprehension monitoring, cooperative learning, graphic and semantic organizers, instruction in story structure, question answering, question generating, summarization, and multiple-strategy teaching.

For students with LDs, recent meta-analyses of cooperative learning (Jenkins & O'Connor, 2003) and the role of graphic organizers (Kim, Vaughn, Wanzek, & Wei, 2004) suggest moderate to large aggregated effect sizes for these kinds of interventions. In another review, Vaughn and Klingner (2004) found that several practices show some evidence for facilitating reading comprehension in students with LDs. These include (1) assistance in activating background knowledge; (2) various aspects of comprehension monitoring during and after reading; (3) procedures using questioning; (4) various methods focusing on the main idea in summarization of text; (5) explicit teaching of vocabulary development that facilitate students' understanding of concepts, as opposed to surface-level memorization; and (6) graphic organizers, including semantic maps, word maps, and semantic feature analysis. In addition, strategies that facilitate the understanding of unknown words, including the use of context cues, morphonemic analysis, and external references, can be helpful. Explicit instruction in understanding the organization of text structure, particularly expository effects, has been effective. Finally, paralleling findings in the NRP, the teaching of multiple strategies appears to be effective.

Among the strategy-based methods used for students with LDs in reading, reciprocal teaching, transactional strategies instruction, collaborative strategic reading, and PALS have all been found to be effective. Consistent with Mastropieri and Scruggs (1997), Vaughn and Klingner (2004) concluded that students with LDs can improve reading comprehension (1) when teachers provide instruction in strategies that have been documented as effective for reading comprehension; (2) design instruction that is explicit and not dependent on contextual or incidental learning; (3) model, support, and guide instruction; (4) provide opportunities to promote generalization across different kinds of text; and (5) systematically monitor student progress and make indicated adjustments in the instructional plan.

A review of collaborative strategic reading is an interesting example of approaches that are used at the classroom level (Vaughn, Klingner, & Bryant, 2001). In collaborative strategic reading, the teacher presents strategies to the class as a whole, using modeling, role playing, and think-alouds. Students are explicitly taught to apply strategies involving why, when, and how events occur in the text they are reading. After they develop some proficiency with the strategies, they are divided into groups on the basis of their proficiency in applying the strategies. In the groups, students perform in defined roles as they collaboratively implement the strategies in expository text. In collaborative strategic reading, four strategies are taught to students: (1) a preview component, in which students essentially attempt to activate background knowledge; (2) monitoring comprehension during reading by identifying difficult words and concepts in the passage, and using strategies that address what to do when text does not make sense; (3) restudying the most important idea in the paragraph; and (4) summarizing/asking questions. The results of several studies showed that many students made significant gains in reading comprehension and academic content. However, some students showed little response, highlighting the importance of carefully monitoring the progress of students receiving a classroom-based intervention. In a similar way, the line of work on PALS at grades 2–6, where the instructional focus is on comprehension strategies, has documented impressive effects for students with LDs, as well as for their low-, average-, and high-performing classmates, in settings where English is the dominant language (D. Fuchs, Fuchs, Mathes, & Simmons, 1997; Saenz, Fuchs, & Fuchs, 2005). However, as in Vaughn's line of work, an unacceptable proportion of students with LDs demonstrate insufficient response to PALS.

As an illustration of research involving remediation of comprehension difficulties in primary school students with LDs, Williams and colleagues have completed studies that focused on middle school students with LDs (e.g., Wilder & Williams, 2001; Williams, Brown, Silverman, & deCani, 1994) as well as second- and third-grade students (Williams, 2003).

This research is based on the Theme Identification Program, which consists of 14 lessons (Williams, 2002). The goal of the program is to help students derive themes (the overall meaning of stories abstracted from the specific plot components). In the Theme Identification Program, 2 introductory sessions focus on plot components; the remaining 12 lessons address the identification of a story's theme. Each lesson is organized around a single story and includes prereading discussion of the theme concept; reading the story aloud; discussing the important story information, using organizing questions as a guide (i.e., the "theme scheme"); transfer and application of the theme to other story examples and real-life situations; review; and an activity. The heart of this program is the theme scheme, which is a set of questions organizing the important story components to help students follow the plot and derive the theme. The teacher models how to answer the eight questions leading to a theme, and students gradually assume increasing responsibility for asking the questions and identifying the theme. In addition, the students rehearse these questions and commit them to memory, so they can apply the theme scheme to untaught stories. Toward that end of instruction, transfer instruction is provided in an explicit manner, with two additional questions employed to help students generalize the theme to other relevant situations.

Williams and colleagues (2002) applied this program in five second-grade and five third-grade inclusion classes in Harlem in New York City, representing students who were performing at high, average, and low levels in relation to their classmates. Of these 120 students, 12 of the low-performing children had been identified with LDs. The 10 classrooms were assigned randomly to the Theme Identification Program or to a more traditional comprehension program that emphasized vocabulary and plot. Students were assessed on a variety of acquisition and transfer measures. Results showed that as a function of the Theme Identification Program, students acquired the concept of a theme (effect size = 2.17) and learned the theme scheme questions (effect size = 2.11). More importantly, on novel passages, students in the experimental condition were more skilled at identifying themes (effect size = 0.68). Effects pertained to high-, average-, and low-achieving classmates, including the students with LDs, in second and third grades. The methods illustrate how teachers can address a high-level comprehension skill (i.e., identification of a story's theme) even among students with word-reading difficulties.

To extend this line of research, Williams, Hall, and Lauer (2004) focused on the compare/contrast expository text structure. Again relying on an explicit and structured instructional model, with systematic guided and then independent practice, these researchers developed the Text Structure Program to address three strategies: (1) using clue words to identify a passage as a compare/contrast text; (2) using a graphic organizer to lay out the relevant information in the text; and (3) using a series of questions to focus on the important information in the text.

In a study conducted in second grade, the researchers incorporated the Text Structure Program into a unit on animal classification (i.e., the five classes of vertebrates)—content included in the elementary-level science standards in New York State. The program comprised nine lessons, taught in 15 sessions. Each lesson focused on two of the five animal classes and incorporated the following segments: clue words (where the teacher previewed the lesson's purpose and introduced the eight clue words); trade book reading and discussion; vocabulary development; reading and analysis of a target paragraph; graphic organizer (where students used a matrix representing the com-

pare/contrast structure to compare each animal feature explained in the paragraph); compare/contrast questions; summary (where students wrote summaries of the paragraph); and review. Williams and colleagues (2004) tested the effectiveness of this program by contrasting it to a more traditional program on animal classification and to a no-treatment control group. Teachers of 10 second-grade classes in three New York City public schools volunteered to participate and were randomly assigned to treatments (text structure, $n = 4$; content, $n = 4$; no instruction, $n = 2$). Participants were 128 students among whom approximately 6% had been identified as having LDs. The researchers first looked at students' ability to summarize a compare/contrast paragraph that had been explicitly taught in the program. The text structure group outperformed the other two groups on the number of summary statements that were accurate and that included an appropriate clue word. The researchers also examined students' ability to transfer, with three novel compare/contrast texts that were structured analogously to those used for instruction but that incorporated novel content (the content of the three texts was increasingly different from the materials included in class). Across the near- and far-transfer measures, students in the text structure group scored significantly higher than both contrast groups. At the same time, the researchers also explored whether the instruction on compare/contrast would transfer to a new text structure; it did not, suggesting the need for explicit instruction on a variety of text structures.

Across these studies—one addressing story themes and the other focusing on compare/contrast text structure—this work illustrates how systematic, explicit instruction, with gradual fading of teacher support and with cumulative review, can enhance young students' reading comprehension. This is the case for second- and third-grade students with and without LDs. It indicates that an explicit focus on high-level comprehension can yield positive results. It is possible that this type of instruction can help poor readers navigate the transition from "learning to read" to "reading to learn" more successfully. Longitudinal studies exploring how this kind of instruction affects long-term outcomes are required before we can understand the potential for this kind of comprehension treatment to enhance long-term schooling experiences for students with LDs. Presently we do not have much information on whether such programs produce lasting effects on growth in reading comprehension, several years following intervention. Do the students continue to apply the strategies long after training? With any reading instruction, do students develop sufficient interest in reading to spend time doing it? As with fluency, long-term growth in reading comprehension is achieved partly through the growth in vocabulary and word knowledge that comes from reading.

COMPREHENSION RESEARCH: SUMMARY

The comprehension studies highlight the role of strategy instruction for students with LDs. In the studies cited that involved students with accuracy and fluency difficulties, research programs that incorporated both skills instruction and strategy instruction involving word recognition and fluency were found to be more effective than programs that simply taught the skills involved in word recognition and fluency (e.g., Lovett, Lacerenza, et al., 2000). The Swanson and colleagues (1999) meta-analysis also found that teaching both skills and strategies seemed to be more effective than teaching either alone.

Strategy instruction can be extended beyond the area of reading comprehension. For example, a long-term program of research from the Center for Research on Learning at the University of Kansas (Schumaker & Deshler, 1992; Schumaker et al., 2002) has identified a series of strategies or "teaching routines" that improve the learning not just of students with LDs, but of all students in the classroom. These teaching routines involve several academic domains, including reading comprehension and writing, as well as a variety of organizational skills both in and out of school (e.g., homework). Largely implemented in secondary school environments and at a classroom level, these routines have been organized into the Learning Strategies Curriculum, which focuses on three major demands presented by a standard curriculum: acquisition, storage, and expression of information. For acquisition, the teaching routines involve strategies that facilitate word recognition and reading comprehension (paraphrasing, visual imagery, recall of narrative text, self-questioning, and related strategic activities). A series of research studies, many of them involving probe assessments in single-case designs, have shown that adolescents with LDs can be taught complex learning

strategies and that implementation of these strategies results in improved academic performance (Schumaker & Deshler, 1992; Schumaker et al., 2002). Effect sizes are consistently in the large range for different strategies. Studies of explicit, strategic classroom-level instruction in organizational skills show that such instruction improves organizational skills and overall performance not only in students with LDs, but in students without LDs (Hughes et al., 2002).

In the next section, the importance of strategic instruction for students with LDs is expanded to the written language domain. Although there is a role for skills instruction, particularly in handwriting and spelling, it will be apparent that the overall impact of instruction involving written language for students with LDs focuses largely on the development of strategies. It is well known that students with LDs in a variety of domains do not spontaneously identify strategies. If they are taught strategies, they do not implement them in the absence of specific instruction that promotes generalization. Strategic instruction promotes self-regulation and increases the student's level of independence. Such instruction addresses the executive function deficiencies commonly observed in students with various types of LDs.

Written Language

Lyon and Cutting (1998) reported that interventions for LDs affecting handwriting, spelling, and written composition have been developed, but studied less extensively than those for reading disabilities. At the time, the relative paucity of intervention research in the area of written language was seen as due in part to the complexity of the multiple linguistic tasks that must be negotiated in the writing process. In expressing oneself in writing, one has to formulate the ideas to be expressed, organize and sequence them in a coherent fashion, produce the ideas in a syntactically correct format, spell the words correctly, and produce the content legibly via motor response. Furthermore, once one gains competence in these foundation skills, they must be integrated within a broader cognitive system that superimposes organizational strategies on issues of genre structure, text coherence and cohesion, and sense of audience. Given the number of variables that could be studied in research on written language intervention, it is not surprising that many investigations have focused on only parts of the process. Since Lyon and Cutting's report, however, a substantial research base on written language interventions has emerged.

Handwriting

Handwriting is composed of a set of complex behaviors that are developed over a period of time. Difficulties in both printing and cursive writing stem from a number of factors, including motor deficits, visual–motor coordination problems, visual memory deficits, and reading disabilities. The term "dysgraphia" has been used historically to refer to a difficulty in transducing visual information to the motor system (Johnson & Myklebust, 1967) that manifests itself in an inability to copy. Bain (1991) observed that students with handwriting difficulties have four characteristics that appear in contiguity: (1) unconventional grip, (2) fingers very near the pencil point, (3) difficulty in erasing, and (4) trouble with letter alignment. Intervention methods for handwriting difficulties have traditionally been based on clinical observation and clinical models. Johnson and Myklebust (1967) conducted a substantial amount of clinical research involving written language disorders, including handwriting deficits. From their research, they developed a comprehensive task-analytic model for the treatment of handwriting difficulties.

An older method for the remediation of handwriting deficits is the Gillingham and Stillman (1965) approach. This is a method used by many teachers working with students with LDs and is characterized by the following: (1) The teacher models a large letter on the blackboard, writing and saying the name; (2) the student traces the letter while saying the name (this tracing stage continues until the student is secure with both the letter formation and the name); (3) the student copies the letter while saying the name; and (4) the student writes the letter from memory while saying the name. In addition to these types of multisensory intervention methods, some studies have assessed the utility of improving handwriting by teaching students to guide themselves verbally through the process (Hayes & Flower, 1980).

Mechanically, letter formation and word spelling are necessary to express thoughts in written fashion. In addition, however, handwriting and spelling difficulties can have se-

rious deleterious consequences for written expression. They can (1) result in misinterpretations of the author's meaning (cf. Graham, Harris, & Chorzempa, 2002; Graham, Harris, & Fink, 2000); (2) create negative perceptions about the writer, which taint overall impressions about the quality of an essay (Chase, 1986; Hughes, Keeling, & Tuck, 1983); (3) interfere with the execution of composing processes, because cognitive resources are unduly allocated to the mechanical aspects of the process (Berninger & Graham, 1998); or (4) lead students to avoid writing, which constrains writing development (Berninger, Mizokawa, & Bragg, 1991; Graham, 1999). For these reasons, an explicit focus on the development of handwriting and spelling skills is important, especially for students with LDs, who are most likely to experience these deficits. In this section, we describe a series of studies from two primary settings (University of Washington and University of Maryland) that illustrate critical instructional features for enhancing handwriting and spelling outcomes for students with LDs. (Interventions specifically for spelling are described separately below.)

Berninger and Amtmann (2003) reviewed a series of studies involving early intervention for handwriting difficulties. For example, Berninger and colleagues (1997) randomly assigned first graders with poor legibility and automaticity in handwriting to one of five interventions: conventional repeated copying of letters; conventionally imitating the motor components of letter formations; providing visual cues for letter formations; writing letters from memory with increasing delays; and combinations of the visual cues/memory component. After 24 lessons over a 4-month period, the combined treatment was more effective than control or other conditions in improving handwriting. These findings were replicated by Graham and colleagues (2000) and Jones and Christensen (1999).

Graham and colleagues (2000) conducted an experimental intervention study with first-grade students who were experiencing handwriting and writing difficulties. Thirty-eight students were assigned randomly to two groups: handwriting or phonological awareness instruction. Handwriting instruction comprised 27 lessons lasting 15 minutes each and divided into nine units. In each unit, three lowercase letters that shared common formational characteristics were introduced and practiced.

Each lesson incorporated four activities. The first activity, Alphabet Warm-Up, focused on learning to name each letter, matching the name with its letter, and knowing the sequence of the letters in the alphabet. The second activity, Alphabet Practice, provided tracing and writing individual letters. The third activity was Alphabet Rockets, designed to increase students' handwriting fluency; and the fourth activity, Alphabet Fun, allowed students to play with the letter in a creative manner. Across these four components, the instruction was explicit, relying on a task analysis of the letters to focus each child's attention on the critical features and demands of the task and to provide adequate support for the child to enjoy success until independent mastery was demonstrated. Results showed that students in the handwriting condition made greater handwriting gains by posttest (effect size = 1.39), which were maintained 6 months later (effect size = 0.87). Effects were also demonstrated on posttest compositional fluency (effect size = 1.46), which dropped to a nonsignificant effect size of 0.45 at the 6-month maintenance assessment. This pattern held for low-performing students with and without identified LDs. At the same time, at posttest, students in the handwriting condition did not produce qualitatively better stories than their peers in the phonological awareness condition. This suggests that additional work on strengthening handwriting, perhaps in conjunction with composition tasks, may be needed.

Spelling

The English spelling system, or orthography, is an alphabetical system in which phonemic units (speech sounds) are represented by graphemes (letters or letter combinations) (Bailet, 1991). For both students and primary-grade teachers, this fundamental relationship between spoken and written language is the most important aspect underlying literacy development. Spelling disabilities are ubiquitous among individuals with LDs and frequently co-occur with disorders of oral language, reading, motor skills, and attention (Moats, 1994a). Spelling is never mastered by most individuals with reading disabilities, who after appropriate intervention can usually improve their decoding skills, but typically continue to be poor spellers (Bruck, 1987). This finding, as well as the number of people who read well but spell poorly (Frith, 1980), suggests that reading and spelling are to some extent dissociated and that theoretical models of one skill will not necessarily explain the other (Moats, 1994a). However, as in reading, phonemic awareness training procedures that provide concrete visual materials for students to manipulate, in parallel with auditory input, appear to be effective in improving spelling abilities (Bradley & Bryant, 1985). These types of methods are probably successful for at least two reasons (Bailet, 1991). First, they provide a concrete, visual means of representing abstract spoken phonemes. Second, they provide students with an opportunity for physically manipulating chips or plastic letters to match their spoken counterparts, rather than requiring mental manipulation.

In addition to the Orton–Gillingham and Fernald multisensory methods to improve reading and spelling (also described earlier), a number of behavioral/task-analytic interventions have been applied to improve spelling behavior in students with LDs. For example, Lovitt, Guppy, and Blattner (1969) found that providing free time contingent upon improved spelling accuracy had positive effects on spelling performance. In addition, Gerber (1986) and Kauffman, Hallahan, Haas, Brame, and Boren (1978) reported that imitating students' spelling errors and then requiring the students to write the words correctly boosted performance significantly.

In a more contemporary approach that involved rigorous evaluation, Graham and colleagues (2002) addressed spelling interventions for poor spellers in grade 2, who were randomly assigned to receive spelling or math supplementary instruction. Forty-eight sessions, each 20 minutes in duration, were conducted. The lessons were divided into eight units, each focusing on two or more related spelling patterns. The first lesson was a word-sorting activity, in which students categorized words by the spelling pattern featured in that unit. The teacher, modeling the thinking process by which words might be sorted into their appropriate category, engaged the students in thinking about similarities and differences among the words. Gradually, students assumed responsibility for sorting while articulating the features by which they categorized. Once all the words were sorted, the teacher provided the rule for the patterns emphasized in the word sort. After that, students generated words of their own. Then the pack of words was shuffled, and students completed the sorting while trying to beat previous times. During lesson 2, the teacher gave each student eight study words that (1) occurred in the student's writing frequently and (2) the child had missed on the pretest. In lessons 2–5, students employed two study procedures to learn these eight words: self-study using a set of steps, and dyadic practice using games. Also as part of lessons 2–5, teachers provided students explicit instruction and practice in identifying the sound patterns associated with each unit's content and worked in pairs to build words that corresponded to the spelling pattern emphasized in that unit. In lesson 6, students took a test to determine their mastery of the eight words. They scored their test performance and graphed the score; then they set a goal for how many words they would spell correctly on the next unit test. Also, students completed a test assessing their spelling of nine words that contained the rimes emphasized during word sorting. Cumulative review was conducted systematically, beginning with the second unit. Results demonstrated the value of this systematic and explicit approach to spelling instruction. Compared to peers in the math control condition, students who received the spelling intervention made greater improvements on norm-referenced spelling tests (effect sizes = 0.64–1.05), a writing fluency test (effect size = 0.78), and a reading word attack measure (effect size = 0.82). Six months later, students in the spelling treatment maintained their advantage in spelling (effect sizes = 0.70–1.07), but not on the writing fluency (effect size = 0.57) or reading word attack (effect size = 0.47) measures. Spelling instruction did, however, have a positive effect at maintenance on the reading word recognition skills of students whose pretest scores on the latter measure were lowest.

Berninger and colleagues (2002) assigned third graders to interventions that involved training only in spelling, training in essay composition, and combined training in spelling and essay composition, along with a control condition involving keyboard training. The spelling component emphasized orthographic patterns in words, particularly at the morphological level. Both interventions that included spelling instruction produced more gains in spelling than the essay condition that did not involve explicit intervention in spelling. Together, these latter studies highlight that many students with LDs do improve in spelling when it is taught, and that gains are maximized with explicit focus on letter patterns (orthography) and opportunities to practice in writing.

Compensatory Devices

Berninger and Amtmann (2003) reviewed evidence for the efficacy of various compensatory tools to support handwriting and spelling, including keyboarding, voice recognition systems that allow students to dictate, and word prediction programs. Keyboarding did not seem to improve the mechanical components of writing if typing was slow. Students who had difficulty with automatic production of letters in paper-and-pencil format also had difficulty with keyboard production. Ultimately, keyboarding may well be an effective bypass tool for students who write poorly, but a research base on its effective implementation has not emerged. In regard to the use of voice recognition methodologies for dictation, all students, including those with LDs, produced more material if they could dictate instead of write. Presently, however, there is little evidence indicating that such programs enhance written language performance, which may reflect the need to develop voice recognition technologies more fully. Finally, word prediction software for students with written language difficulties has yet to show significant effects for students with LDs. This may reflect such students' comorbid difficulties with working memory or attention.

Altogether, there is a need to evaluate all forms of compensatory tools for individuals who have mechanical difficulties with the transcriptional component of written language. The weak results for compensatory tools probably reflect what has been learned in the reading area, which is the importance of integrating any type of compensatory tool into the actual process of writing (and reading).

Written Expression

The ability to produce one's thoughts in writing is a complex form of communication requiring a number of cognitive abilities. In producing a written composition, the student must simultaneously attend to the subject, the text, and the reader. Deficits in oral language and reading are often precursors to difficulties in the writing process, and attention and memory play critical roles as well (Gregg, 1991). As simple as it sounds, some researchers (e.g., Higgins & Raskind, 2000; Kraetsch, 1981) have found that increased writing practice can be a significant force in improving not only written composition, but also reading ability. In more detailed interventions, methods that require students to take two related sentences and write them as one ("sentence combining") have produced significant gains in written composition (O'Hare, 1973). More recently, "story grammar" techniques have been studied in relation to written composition and expression (Hallahan et al., 1996). Story grammar involves teaching students to employ a strategic outline to ensure that the necessary components are present in their compositions (Montague & Graves, 1993). A number of cognitive-behavioral intervention techniques have been employed to increase composition skills.

Graham and Harris (1996) developed self-regulated strategy development (SRSD; mentioned earlier in the discussion of cognitive-behavioral models) to assist students in mastering the higher-level cognitive processes involved in written composition, and in developing the self-regulated use of these processes. Using SRSD, Graham and Harris stimulated significant gains in the length and quality of story writing in students with LDs (Graham & Harris, 1993), and found that such gains were maintained over time and generalized across settings and persons (Graham, Harris, MacArthur, & Schwartz, 1991). Although this body of work was conducted primarily with students in intermediate and middle schools (see Graham & Harris, 2003), recently Graham, Harris, and colleagues have moved their work on SRSD to second and third grades, targeting low-performing students with and without LDs for intervention. Effects with these younger struggling students are encouraging.

First targeting third graders, Graham, Harris, and Mason (2005) taught struggling writers two genre-specific strategies. These genre-specific strategies were embedded in a more general strategy for planning and writing a paper, which reminded students to pick a topic, organize ideas into a writing plan, and use/upgrade this plan while writing. Within the second step of this general strategy (i.e., organizing ideas into a writing plan), students were taught the two genre-specific strategies for generating ideas: the first for writing a story, and the second for writing a persuasive essay. Furthermore, students learned about the basic parts of a story and a persuasive essay, the importance of using words that make a paper more interesting, and self-talk to facilitate performance. Finally, a self-regulation component was overlaid onto the instruction, whereby students set goals to write complete papers, monitored and graphed their success in achieving this goal, compared their preinstructional performance with their performance during instruction, and credited their success to the use of the target strategies. At the same time, the study examined the effect of peer mediation in enhancing the effects of the strategy instruction, especially for the purposes of maintenance and generalization. In the peer-mediated condition, peers worked together to promote strategy use, identifying other places or instances where they could apply the strategies and brainstorming about how they might need to modify the strategies for the new application. They were then encouraged to remind each other to apply what they were learning to those transfer situations, and in the next session, they identified when, where, and how they had applied the strategies. Thus this study incorporated three conditions: Writers' Workshop (control condition), explicit and systematic SRSD, and SRSD with peer mediation. The control condition represents a popular approach to expressive writing in many public schools. Seventy-two students, screened into the study because of difficulty with writing, were assigned to pairs to ensure compatibility. Then pairs (which were the unit of analysis for the study) were assigned randomly to the three conditions. Instructors worked with students three times weekly for 20 minutes each time, with approximately 11 hours' total instruction across the two genres.

Results showed the advantage of both SRSD conditions over Writers' Workshop for planning and composing stories and persuasive essays. Students in the SRSD conditions wrote longer, more complete, and qualitatively better papers for both genres, with effect sizes ranging between 0.82 and 3.23. These effects were maintained over time for story writing and generalized to a third uninstructed genre, informative writing. The peer mediation component augmented SRSD by increasing students' knowledge of planning and enhancing generalization to informative and narrative writing.

With encouraging effects at third grade, Harris, Graham, and Mason (in press) moved down to second grade with a parallel study that incorporated the same three conditions. Results were again strong. Among the struggling writers, SRSD produced greater knowledge about writing and stronger performance in the two instructed genres (story and persuasive writing), as well as two uninstructed genres (personal narrative and informative writing). Effect sizes were similarly strong. Peer support augmented SRSD by enhancing specific aspects of students' performance in the instructed and uninstructed genres. Across the two studies, findings revealed (1) the capacity to enhance relatively young students' writing performance, even within the high-poverty communities where this series of studies was conducted; (2) the added value of a peer support component to effect generalization of the targeted genres to untaught genres; and (3) the superiority of a structured, explicit, systematic approach to writing instruction over the more popular Writers' Workshop.

The latter finding illustrates the continued predominance of relatively unstructured approaches to writing instruction, despite persuasive evidence for more explicit, strategy-based approaches. Research on SRSD in writing represents a comprehensive, long-term program of research. Graham and Harris (2003; see also Graham, 2005) conducted a meta-analysis of 26 studies addressing strategy-based instruction in writing. Many of the studies included students identified with LDs, but actually involved students with a range of achievement levels as well as different comorbidities. Overall, strategic approaches to writing instruction yielded effect sizes in the large range for a variety of different components of writing (quality, elements, length, story grammar) across different groups, including students with LDs. For students with LDs, effect sizes ranged from 1.14 for quality to effect sizes above 2.0 for elements in story grammar. Similar effect sizes were found for average writers. There was evidence for maintenance and generalization of the effects, as well as large effect sizes with younger and older students and across a variety of instructional environments.

Evaluating the components of strategic instruction in writing showed that those involved in self-regulation are most significant in improving writing performance for those students with LDs (Graham, 2005). These findings were noteworthy, because SRSD is typically provided at a classroom level, and the provision of written language instruction is difficult for many teachers. It is not surprising that explicit teaching of writing strategies—as is the case with explicit teaching of comprehension strategies—is beneficial for all students in the classroom.

Written Language Studies: Summary

Together, the studies in handwriting, spelling, and written expression demonstrate how systematic, explicit instruction can result in better outcomes for students with LDs on skills that are foundational to the use of written language. Results also suggest how work targeting these foundational skills may simultaneously enhance related skills, such as word attack and word recognition, as well as higher-order processes.

There are many emerging intervention methods for the remediation of deficits in handwriting, spelling, and written composition. As in other content areas, clinicians and teachers, must be aware that written language is a complex domain, requiring the integration of oral language, written language, cognitive, and motor skills. Within this context, a combination of the different intervention methods discussed in this section is likely to net the greatest improvements in the writing skills of students with LDs. The key is to identify the basis for a student's impairment(s) in this domain (handwriting, spelling, and/or written expression) and to provide explicit instruction, using one or more of the evidence-based approaches outlined in this section.

Mathematics

In general, students who manifest LDs in mathematics typically display deficits in arithmetic calculation and/or mathematics reasoning skills (Lyon, 1996a). Rourke and Finlayson (1978) and Fleishner (1994) have reported that mathematics LDs often co-occur with deficits in reading, writing, and/or oral language. However, when comorbidity occurs to this degree, an LD in mathematics should not be construed as a selective impairment, but rather as a feature of a generalized problem (Feagans & McKinney, 1981; Fleishner & Frank, 1979). As is the case for interventions in written language, solid research in the treatment of mathematics disorders is beginning to emerge. A major difficulty in diagnosing LDs in this domain is that in mathematics, more than in any other content area, learning is tied closely to the teacher's knowledge and preparation in the teaching of math skills.

Difficulties in developing arithmetic calculation skills are frequently linked to difficulties in writing numerals and mathematical symbols correctly, recalling the meanings of symbols and answers to basic facts, counting, and following the steps in a multistep algorithm (Glennon & Cruickshank, 1981). In turn, the ability to reason mathematically in the context of word problems is negatively influenced by the presence of extraneous information, complex syntactic structures, change in numbers and types of nouns used, and the use of certain verbs (Blankenship & Lovitt, 1976; Hallahan et al., 1996).

As with instruction in other content areas, the teaching of arithmetic and mathematics skills has the following characteristics: (1) The instruction takes place in groups; (2) it is teacher-directed; (3) it is academically focused; and (4) it is individualized for each student in the group (Stevens & Rosenshine, 1981). Some basal or developmental programs used for students with LDs have many of these characteristics. For example, Connecting Math Concepts (Englemann, Carnine, Englemann, & Kelly, 1991) is a basal program based on a behavioral/task-analytic model that is frequently used for primary- and elementary-age students with LDs. This program grew out of the DISTAR Arithmetic program (Engelmann & Carnine, 1975). Both programs contain highly structured lessons involving frequent teacher questions and student answers. A number of studies have demonstrated the efficacy of Connecting Math Concepts and DISTAR Arithmetic with students identified with LDs (Carnine, 1991). In a similar way, controlled research on math PALS documents the importance of explicit instruction targeting procedural skill as well as conceptual knowledge, with carefully guided peer-mediated practice; it also shows how such an approach can be used in general classrooms to improve outcomes for students with LDs, as well as their low-, average-, and high-performing classmates at kindergarten through grade 6 (e.g., L. S. Fuchs et al., 1997; L. S. Fuchs, Fuchs, & Karns, 2001; L. S. Fuchs, Fuchs, Yazdian, & Powell, 2002).

A number of early intervention programs were developed specifically for students with LDs in mathematics (Hallahan et al., 1996). One such program is Structural Arithmetic, developed by Stern and Stern (1971). This program is designed to help students in kindergarten through the third grade better understand numeration and relationships between numbers. Different-colored blocks and sticks represent numbers from 1 to 10. Numerical relationships are represented to the students through combinations of these manipulatives. Little evaluative research is available. Similarly, Project MATH (Cawley et al., 1976) was designed to help students with LDs in kindergarten through sixth grade discover meaningful principles underlying mathematics. Specifically, six highly structured "strands" are used to teach patterns, sets, numbers, fractions, geometry, and measurement concepts. These concepts are made more meaningful to the students by integrating them with the students' daily experiences and by individualizing the instruction. Field tests of Project MATH demonstrated positive results (see Cawley, Fitzmaurice, Shaw, Kahn, & Bates, 1978).

In addition to basal programs and specialized instructional programs, a number of teaching techniques have been shown to be useful in helping students with LDs develop arithmetic and mathematics concepts. For example, Rivera and Smith (1987), summarizing research on the value of modeling in teaching computational skills, found teacher demonstrations of calculation algorithms and higher-level procedural steps to be effective in increasing both computational and problem-solving behaviors in students. In addition, Lloyd and his colleagues (Cullinan, Lloyd, & Epstein, 1981; Lloyd, 1980) have tested the value of strategy training with students who are deficient in math skills. In this type of intervention, a task analysis of the relevant cognitive operation is demonstrated and explained to the students. When students have mastered the component skills, strategies are provided that help the students integrate the steps and apply them in different problem-solving contexts. Finally, cognitive-behavioral models of intervention have given rise to the development of self-instructional strategy techniques to help guide students with LDs through a variety of problem-solving contexts (Hallahan et al., 1996). A key component in this type of technique is to teach a student first to verbalize the steps that should be used in solving a particular mathematics problem. Once the student has mastered the application of the problem-solving algorithm, the student is taught to use subvocal self-instruction. This type of technique has been shown to be useful with both elementary-age students (Lovitt & Curtiss, 1968) and adolescents (Seabaugh & Schumaker, 1993).

In summary, although deficits in arithmetic and mathematics reasoning abilities are common among individuals with LDs, research-based interventions are just beginning to emerge. In the main, the most useful treatment methods and techniques have evolved from cognitive and behavioral models of intervention. It should also be pointed out that students with mathematics-based LDs are extremely vulnerable to the negative effects of limited teacher experience and the improper application of pedagogical principles. Consistent with this finding, twin studies show stronger shared environment effects on math deficits than on reading deficits (Knopik & DeFries, 1999). The next two sections examine more recent intervention studies.

Fact Retrieval and Procedural Math

The majority of prior intervention work for students with LDs in mathematics has focused on lower-order skills, including fact retrieval and procedural math (i.e., multidigit computation). This research provides guidance on how to structure effective remediation, which includes explicit explanations, pictorial or concrete representations, verbal rehearsal with fading, intensive timed practice on mixed problem sets, cumulative review of previously mastered skills, and self-regulation strategies.

With respect to all these remediation components except the last one (self-regulation strategies), research substantiates beneficial effects on student outcomes. For example, Fuchs and colleagues cumulatively designed and tested a set of instructional components for enhancing students' math competence. Three studies conducted at grades 2–6 in general education classrooms addressed procedural math (L. S. Fuchs, Fuchs, Hamlett, Phillips, & Bentz, 1994; L. S. Fuchs et al., 1997; L. S. Fuchs, Fuchs, Phillips, Hamlett, & Karns, 1995). Two additional studies assessed fact retrieval along with procedural math (i.e., multidigit computation and estimation) at kindergarten (L. S. Fuchs et al.,

2001) and first grade (L. S. Fuchs, Fuchs, Yazdian, et al., 2002). Effects were assessed separately for students with LDs and for students not identified with LDs who had low, average, and high initial achievement status. For students throughout the primary and intermediate grades, a combination of (1) explicit, procedurally clear, conceptually based explanations; (2) pictorial representations of the math; (3) verbal rehearsal with gradual fading; (4) timed practice on mixed problem sets; and (5) systematically provided cumulative review of previously mastered problem types resulted in statistically significant effects across all four types of learners (those with LDs and with low, average, and high achievement). Effect sizes ranged from 0.35 to 1.27.

This set of instructional principles was incorporated into an expert system, which was tested experimentally among 33 teachers who provided math instruction to students with LDs in grades 2–8 (L. S. Fuchs, Fuchs, Hamlett, & Stecker, 1991). The focus of the study was procedural math, which represented a deficient area for all participating students with LDs. Teachers were assigned to three conditions: (1) ongoing, systematic assessment of student growth with descriptive profiles of students' strengths/weaknesses; (2) ongoing, systematic assessment of student growth with descriptive profiles of students' strengths/weaknesses, plus use of an expert system incorporating task analyses for supplying clear explanations, pictorial representations, verbal rehearsal with fading recommendations for instruction, and intensive timed practice that featured cumulative review with mixed problem sets; and (3) best-practice controls. Teachers implemented treatments for 20 weeks. Analyses indicated that only the expert system resulted in superior learning. This provides additional evidence for the effectiveness of this combination of instructional principles.

With respect to self-regulation strategies, studies demonstrate the contribution of ongoing monitoring of performance, as well as of student goal setting and feedback, to improvement in fact retrieval and procedural math. For example, L. S. Fuchs, Bahr, and Rieth (1989) randomly assigned 20 students with LDs who had math fact retrieval deficits to self-selected versus assigned goals and to contingent versus noncontingent game play—all within the context of computer-mediated fact retrieval drill and practice. Performance was assessed prior to and following a 3-week treatment. Results indicated stronger learning for students who selected their own goals than for those who were assigned goals, with an effect size of 0.68. No differences were found between the contingency conditions.

Using similar methods, L. S. Fuchs, Fuchs, Hamlett, and Whinnery (1991) examined the effects of student feedback. Twice weekly for 20 weeks, students completed math procedure tests on computer and immediately received feedback. Each special educator ($n = 20$) identified two students with LDs who experienced chronic procedural math difficulties. One student in each pair was assigned to see a graph of performance over time, with a goal line superimposed over the graph; the other student saw the graph without the goal line. Goal line feedback was associated with greater performance stability, with an effect size of 0.70. As these studies illustrate, engaging students in the monitoring of their own performance as they work via computer on math fact retrieval and procedural math provides substantial benefit.

Problem Solving

As noted above, most treatment research for students with LDs has focused on math fact retrieval and algorithmic computation (e.g., Cawley, Parmar, Yan, & Miller, 1998; Harris, Miller, & Mercer, 1995; Howell, Sidorenko, & Jurica, 1987; Woodward, Howard, & Battle, 1997). At the same time, as students acquire competence with foundational math skills, an additional challenge is to improve their application of those skills to problem-solving situations. Toward that end, some attention has been allocated to arithmetic word problems, which exclude irrelevant information, keep syntactic structure straightforward, and require one-step solutions.

To promote competence with arithmetic word problems, Case and colleagues (1992) assessed the effects of SRSD among four students with LDs. They found that overall performance improved, with less probability of applying the wrong operation, but that only two of the four students maintained effects. Montague, Applegate, and Marquard (1993) and Hutchinson (1993) corroborated the short-term effects of this sort of cognitive strategy instruction.

Another line of work substantiates the value of concrete materials and diagrams in helping elementary-age students with LDs master arith-

metic word problems (e.g., Jitendra & Hoff, 1996; Mercer & Miller, 1992; Miller & Mercer, 1993). Jitendra and colleagues (1998) also tested and showed the value of combining diagrams with methods designed to induce schemas. Little attention, however, has been focused on mathematics problem solving (MPS) as it appears in school curricula, where problems are more varied and complex than arithmetic word problems. This more complex form of MPS incorporates irrelevant information and more varied syntactic structures, with many problems requiring two or more computational steps and other related mathematics skills (e.g., computing fractions or reading graphs) for solution.

This lack of attention to MPS, which is especially acute at the primary grades, is unfortunate on three counts. First, for students with LDs in mathematics, the critical outcome of schooling is MPS as it occurs in the real world. Second, research with typical students reveals the challenges associated with improving MPS. Researchers cannot assume that interventions designed to promote success with arithmetic word problems will translate into improved MPS. Finally, even when students have severe challenges with foundational mathematical skills (Jordan & Hanich, 2000), waiting for mastery of those foundational skills before beginning to develop MPS competence may create MPS deficits that are impossible to address later in school.

To address this gap in the literature, Fuchs and their colleagues have focused on MPS at grade 3. This work falls into two categories. One strand of research has been conducted classwide in general education settings, exploring the effects of innovative MPS treatments on students who enter third grade with varying achievement histories (LDs, as well as low, average, and high initial math achievement). The second category of research examines the effects of tutoring treatments to enhance MPS among students with LDs. In both lines of work, the instruction has been explicit and systematic. That is, the teacher begins with worked examples illustrating the problem-solving rules targeted for a particular problem type. The teacher explains the solutions in the worked examples and displays a poster listing the steps of the solution strategy. Moving to partially worked examples, with one step of the solution missing, the teacher asks students to complete the solution and then debriefs the activity, with students explaining their work and the teacher providing corrective feedback. Gradually, the teacher provides increasing opportunities for students to contribute more and more of the solutions to sample problems. Next, the teacher pairs higher- and lower-achieving students, so they can help each other to complete entire problems; as problems are completed, the teacher reviews solutions with correct feedback. Before the completion of each lesson, students complete problems independently (with teacher-led debriefing) and receive homework assignments. Instruction is clear and concise, with lots of opportunities for students to participate via choral and individual responding in the whole-class portions of the lessons and via peer mediation. Moreover, as mastery of the problem types is accomplished, cumulative review is routinely provided.

This form of explicit, systematic, scaffolded instruction is applied not only to instruction on problem-solving rules, but also to instruction designed to enhance transfer. Theoretically, the instructional approach is based on schema theory. Within schema theory, MPS is deemed a form of transfer, because students are solving problems they have never seen before. To achieve this transfer, three kinds of development are required (Cooper & Sweller, 1987). First, for any given problem type, students must master the problem-solving rules. Second, students must develop schemas—in this context, generalized descriptions of two or more problems, which individuals use to sort problems into groups requiring similar solutions (Gick & Holyoak, 1980). The broader the schema, the greater the probability individuals will recognize connections between familiar and novel problems (Cooper & Sweller, 1987). Third, students must be vigilant for the connections between teaching and transfer tasks (e.g., Asch, 1969; Bransford, Sherwood, Vye, & Rieser, 1986; Catrambone & Holyoak, 1989; Gick & Holyoak, 1980; Keane, 1988; Ross, 1989).

Salomon and Perkins (1989) provided a framework for broadening schemas and evoking independent searches for connections between novel and familiar tasks. Within this framework, schemas provide the bridge from one context to the other, and metacognition is the conscious recognition and effortful application of that schema. Salomon and Perkins asserted that this framework represents an un-

tapped instructional opportunity for explicitly teaching students to transfer.

In addressing MPS at the third grade, L. S. Fuchs and colleagues (2003a, 2003b) operationalized Cooper and Sweller's (1987) and Salomon and Perkins's (1989) frameworks: teaching problem-solving rules; familiarizing students with the notion of transfer; teaching them to build schemas by showing how superficial problem features change without altering the problem-solving rules; and cautioning students to search novel-looking problems to recognize superficial problem features and thereby identify familiar problem types for which solutions are known. In a series of studies conducted classwide, L. S. Fuchs and colleagues (2003a) used this framework to teach students explicitly to transfer for MPS. Classrooms were assigned randomly to four study conditions: (1) teacher-designed instruction; (2) instruction in word problem solution rules (20 sessions); (3) instruction in word problem solution rules + explicit transfer instruction (20 sessions, with half as much problem solution rule instruction to control for time); and (4) instruction in word problem solution rules + explicit transfer instruction (30 sessions, with full doses of both components). Instruction was delivered in a whole-class arrangement over 16 weeks with strong fidelity. Effects were assessed on immediate, near, and far transfer to complex MPS, with condition as a between-classroom variable and student achievement type (high, average, low) as a within-classroom variable. Effects were also explored for students with LDs ($n = 30$).

Results showed that problem solution rule instruction was sufficient to improve performance on problems very similar to those used in intervention; that transfer instruction was necessary to enhance performance on less similar problems; and that for students with LDs and other low-performing students, the full dose of both components was most effective. For students without disability, effect sizes for the best condition (4 above) were 1.82 for immediate transfer, 2.25 for near transfer, and 1.16 for far transfer. For students with LDs, effect sizes for the best condition (also 4) were 1.78 for immediate transfer, 1.18 for near transfer, and 0.45 for far transfer.

Owen and Fuchs (2002) obtained similar findings for a 3-week instructional unit focusing on word problems requiring students to calculate halves. To strengthen this prevention treatment, the contribution of self-regulation strategies was assessed in a subsequent study (L. S. Fuchs et al., 2003b). Classrooms were assigned randomly to three 16-week conditions: (1) teacher-designed instruction; (2) explicit transfer instruction (which included teaching rules for problem solutions); and (3) explicit transfer instruction (including teaching rules for problem solutions) + self-regulated learning strategies (graphing and monitoring performance and goal setting). Treatment fidelity was strong. Effects were assessed on immediate, near, and far transfer to complex word problems, with condition as a between-classroom variable and student achievement type (high, average, low) as a within-classroom variable. Effects were also explored for students with LDs (n = 40). Results supported the effectiveness of the combined treatment (3 above). Across all student types, effect sizes for the combined treatment were 2.81 on immediate transfer, 2.43 on near transfer, and 1.81 on far transfer. For students with LDs, effects on the three respective measures were 1.43, 0.95, and 0.58.

A second line of MPS intervention research involving complex problems concerns tutoring. The Fuchs and Fuchs group has examined the effects of the schema-based explicit transfer approach to classroom-level MPS intervention when the treatment is delivered in small-group tutoring. The goal is to remediate existing deficits among fourth-grade students with LDs in math, while exploring the potential for computer-assisted instruction to enhance effects (L. S. Fuchs, Fuchs, Hamlett, et al., 2002).

Stratified by resource teacher/class, students were assigned randomly to: (1) checking/labeling work (control); (2) checking/labeling work + computer-assisted practice on a far-transfer task; (3) checking/labeling work + small-group explicit tutoring on problem solution rules and transfer; (4) checking/labeling work + computer-assisted practice on a far-transfer task + small-group explicit tutoring on problem solution rules and transfer. Instruction was delivered for 16 weeks with strong fidelity. Effects were assessed on immediate, near, and far transfer to complex word-problems. Results documented the effectiveness of small-group tutoring on immediate and near transfer. On far transfer, moderate effects were revealed, but without statistical significance. Interestingly, findings revealed that computer work added little when small-group tutoring was in place.

Effect sizes for tutoring versus control ranged from 0.64 to 2.10; for computer versus control, 0.51 to 0.64; for tutoring versus computer, –1.60 to 0.05; and for tutoring versus tutoring + computer, –0.03 to 0.14.

To extend this work, L. S. Fuchs, Fuchs, and Prentice (2004) described responsiveness to the classroom-level schema-based treatment as a function of LD subtype: math disability (abbreviated here as MD), reading disability (abbreviated here as RD), or both math and reading disability (MD-RD). Classrooms were assigned randomly to validated prevention or control (i.e., teacher-designed instruction) conditions. Students were assigned to disability status based on the preceding spring's TerraNova achievement test scores. Instruction was delivered in a whole-class arrangement over 16 weeks with strong fidelity. Effects were assessed on immediate and near transfer to complex MPS, with performance dimension (problem solving, computation, communication) as a within-subjects variable and treatment condition as a between-subjects variable. Students with all LD subtypes improved less than nondisabled students on computation and communication. However, only students with MD-RD improved less than nondisabled students on problem-solving accuracy.

To gain some insight into the relative role that reading versus math deficits play in the differentially poor MPS capacity of students with MD-RD, L. S. Fuchs and colleagues (2004) also conducted exploratory regression analyses. Results suggested that these students' multidigit computational deficits explained a greater proportion of the variance in responsiveness to MPS treatment than did their reading comprehension deficits.

Mathematics Interventions: Summary

This review of interventions for students with LDs in mathematics shows that effective interventions are emerging both for foundational skills and for higher-order skills involving MPS. As is the case for reading and writing, interventions often include not only skills instruction, but also explicit instruction in strategies that include a focus on self-regulation. In addition, many research studies specifically address the importance of transfer to the classroom environment, as well as to broader environments that involve application of academic skills. Given the evidence reviewed throughout this chapter for the efficacy of research-based interventions, the next set of questions concerns translating these kinds of interventions into practice.

PROBLEMS IN PUTTING EDUCATIONAL INTERVENTIONS INTO PRACTICE

As this selective literature review illustrates, considerable progress has been made in designing instructional components that boost learning in impressive ways for students with LDs. In light of the strong effects associated with these best practices, it is perplexing and disturbing that so many students with LDs continue to suffer dramatic deficits in reading, writing, and math. We offer eight possible reasons to explain this apparent contradiction: (1) inadequate implementation; (2) difficulties in matching instructional components to students' needs; (3) students' multifaceted problems; (4) diluted intervention fidelity; (5) need for systematic progress monitoring; (6) prevention versus remediation; (7) lack of sufficient engagement and practice; and (8) clinical intuition versus scientific evidence.

Inadequate Implementation

The first reason why best-practice instructional components fail to meet the needs of so many students with LDs in schools today is inadequate implementation. Many classroom settings are not configured in ways that support the requirements of research-validated innovations (L. S. Fuchs et al., 1996). Policymakers, administrators, and teachers require tools to help them achieve classroom contexts required to support sound instructional practices, even as researchers need to disseminate their methods in a manner that facilitates implementation (Denton, Vaughn, & Fletcher, 2003). There are effective interventions with adequate research bases, but the research base is often not a factor in decision making for students with LDs.

Implementation is of particular concern, given the move toward full inclusion of students with LDs in general education classrooms in many schools. Although the goals of inclusion are laudatory, there exists little evidence that students with LDs show significant growth in reading in many standard general education settings (Vaughn, Moody, & Schumm, 1998; Zigmond, 2003). These findings are in stark contrast to the results of many of the classroom-based interventions reviewed in this chapter, which are often designed for inclusive environments. Moreover, no single approach works with every student, and even these successful classroom interventions do not appear to work adequately with up to 30% or more of students with LDs. Because a range of intervention strategies is needed (Zigmond, 2003), multitiered intervention strategies are of great potential value. However, all research-based strategies must be implemented with fidelity, and no approach can prevent or remediate all forms of academic difficulties.

Difficulties in Matching Instructional Components to Students' Needs

Of course, even with adequate levels of implementation, validated instructional components fail to meet the needs of some students with LDs. As demonstrated in research where high levels of treatment fidelity are achieved, an unacceptably high proportion of students with LDs fail to profit. For example, with strong implementation of PALS, D. Fuchs and colleagues (1997) demonstrated statistically significant effects for PALS with students with LDs on a variety of reading measures. Nevertheless, 20% of students with LDs failed to make adequate progress, in terms of performance levels in the average range at the end of intervention. In the Foorman and colleagues (1998) study, about 30% of students in the bottom 20% of readers who received the most effective reading curriculum continued to struggle, with word reading scores below the 25th percentile after classroom-based instruction.

It should not, however, be surprising to find that generally effective programs do not meet the needs of all students with LDs. As noted in more detail below, students with LDs have multifaceted problems, reflecting processing deficiencies that make fluent, generalized performances difficult to achieve; deficits in domain-relevant background knowledge; and poor self-regulation, metacognition, task persistence, and motivation (Gersten et al., 1982). Although each promising instructional component is designed to address some of these difficulties, none is sufficiently comprehensive to address the particular constellation of deficits and the range of severity that any given child may manifest. Moreover, there are domains for which instructional components do not appear to be adequate, particularly in areas involving reading comprehension, writing, and math. Finally, although many different instructional components have been developed, their integration into comprehensive instructional packages remains to be addressed. There are some emerging examples, such as collaborative reading comprehension instruction (Vaughn & Klingner, 2004), the strategy instruction research by Graham and Harris (2003), and the Learning Strategies Curriculum from the University of Kansas (Schumaker & Deshler, 1992). More integration of instruction that involves both skills and strategies needs to be provided. In addition, research that begins to unpack the contribution of different instructional components across different academic domains needs to be emphasized, although it could be argued that LDs typically involve multiple cognitive skills and academic components, so that the issue is less one of unpacking than of simply finding effective combinations of integrated methods.

Students' Multifaceted Problems

Students with LDs are heterogeneous, even if their LDs are defined in specific academic domains. Most students with LDs have problems that involve more than one domain. Even within a domain, students with LDs present with a variety of cognitive difficulties and comorbidities. In many instances, explaining the academic problem does not provide a full explanation of an LD, particularly if comorbidities are not addressed. Although variation at the level of major disorders (e.g., intellectual, academic, behavioral) accounts for much of the heterogeneity in people with LDs, variability remains substantial, largely because many students with LDs have more than one problem.

Research on interventions has not done an adequate job in identifying the contribution of these different sources of heterogeneity to intervention outcomes. For example, one reason why strategy instruction emphasizing self-regulation may be effective is that many students with LDs have difficulties in areas involving executive functions. However, executive function deficits in students whose problems are restricted to word recognition are not dramatic. Similarly, cognitive morbidity in students with ADHD but with no impairment of academic domains is much less significant than the cognitive morbidity associated with both

academic impairment and ADHD (Fletcher et al., 1999). It may be that the self-regulation component is especially critical for students who have comorbid LDs and ADHD, reflecting the executive function component derived from ADHD. Understanding intervention outcomes in terms of these major sources of heterogeneity may emerge as the next step in intervention for a variety of childhood conditions. It seems shortsighted, for example, not to systematically evaluate students with ADHD for academic difficulties, given the greater cognitive difficulties associated with comorbid associations that involve LDs, as well as the differential treatment implications associated with academic versus behavioral problems. Similarly, intervening for students with LDs without considering comorbid ADHD may dilute the academic intervention. Not only do instructional components need better integration, but the tailoring of interventions for students at the level of major sources of heterogeneity is an urgent problem.

Diluted Intervention Fidelity

It goes without saying that interventions will only be as effective as the fidelity for which they are implemented. Many interventions demonstrate efficacy when they are controlled by researchers. But when the interventions are translated into everyday practice, there is often less fidelity, and contextual variables dilute the efficacy apparent in a more controlled condition. Given the evidence for effective interventions at a variety of levels—classroom, preventive, and remedial—it is becoming increasingly apparent that a range of interventions could be used in conjunction with "response to instruction" models (Vaughn & Fuchs, 2003). Many recent consensus documents have suggested that students with LDs should not be identified in the absence of adequate instructional opportunities for them, or the inability to ensure such opportunities (Bradley et al., 2002). Thus, as part of the identification process for providing special education services to students with LDs, students would pass through a sequence of instructional opportunities, often in a multitiered process that begins at the level of the classroom. Students might be identified as at risk for either academic problems or LDs. They would be placed in increasingly intense interventions with curriculum-based assessments of progress. Those students who do not show adequate response to high-quality instruction would be candidates for highly specialized interventions in special education.

The key to this process is not just progress monitoring, which is a well-developed technology (Fuchs & Fuchs, 1999; Shinn, 1998; Stecker, Fuchs, & Fuchs, in press). Faithful implementation of the interventions and the monitoring of fidelity are also key aspects of this process. Thus future research on interventions should carefully evaluate the conditions under which interventions can be implemented in everyday educational environments. Strategies that facilitate acceptance by schools and teachers of evidence-based interventions should be delineated. Barriers to implementations of interventions that work should be identified and eliminated. In the current climate—which involves significant accountability under acts like No Child Left Behind, and the fact that students with LDs have to be included in the state-based accountability systems—such intervention research that addresses scaling and implementation is absolutely critical.

Need for Systematic Progress Monitoring

As illustrated in this chapter, research supports the efficacy of a variety of instructional methods for promoting academic achievement among students with LDs. At the same time, the heterogeneity of this population, combined with the severe and multifaceted nature of their needs, results in a high rate of unresponsiveness to validated interventions—ranging between 10% and 50%, depending on intervention and criteria for "inadequate response." For this reason, academic outcomes for students with LDs can be enhanced substantially when teachers systematically monitor student progress while validated interventions are being implemented.

With careful progress monitoring, teachers can gauge the extent to which an individual student with a LD is responding to an instructional intervention. When response is inadequate, teachers can quickly revise the program and then monitor the impact of those revisions. Progress can be monitored in various ways. For example, it is possible to use widely adopted tests, such as the Test of Word Reading Efficiency (Torgesen & Wagner, 1999) or the Woodcock–Johnson III Tests of Achievement (Woodcock, McGrew, & Mather, 2001). With such tests, alternate forms can be used repeatedly to model student improvement as a function of intervention, but only over relatively long periods of time. Other tools, which have been developed specifically for the purpose of progress monitoring, provide many alternate forms for frequent data collection. One well-established approach to progress monitoring is curriculum-based measurement (CBM), of which the Test of Reading Fluency (Deno & Marston, 2001), AIMSweb (Germann, 2002), the Dynamic Indicators of Basic Early Reading Skills (Good, Simmons, & Kame'enui, 2001), Monitoring Basic Skills Progress (L. S. Fuchs, Hamlett, & Fuchs, 1990), and Yearly Progress Pro (McGraw-Hill Digital Learning, 2002) are examples. Although these tests vary considerably in the extent of their reliability data, research substantiates that CBM provides teachers with reliable and valid information about how well students are progressing. Controlled studies also document that teachers who use CBM to determine when revisions to student programs are needed obtain substantially better end-of-year academic outcomes than teachers who do not use CBM. CBM efficacy studies have examined the effects of alternative data utilization strategies; they have also assessed CBM's overall contribution to instructional planning and student learning.

With respect to the effects of alternative data utilization strategies, CBM has been shown to enhance teacher planning and student learning by helping teachers set ambitious student goals, by assisting teachers in determining when instructional adaptations are necessary to prompt better student growth, and by providing ideas for potentially effective teaching adjustments. With respect to goal setting, L. S. Fuchs, Fuchs, and Hamlett (1989a) explored the contribution of goal-raising guidelines within CBM decision-making rules. Teachers were assigned randomly to, and participated in, one of three treatments for 15 weeks in mathematics: no CBM, CBM without a goal-raising rule, and CBM with a goal-raising rule. The goal-raising rule required teachers to increase goals whenever a student's actual rate of growth exceeded the growth rate anticipated by a teacher. Teachers in the CBM goal-raising condition raised goals more frequently (for 15 of 30 students) than teachers in the non-goal-raising conditions (for 1 of 30 students). Moreover, differential student achievement on pre–post standardized achievement tests was concurrent with teachers' goal-raising behavior: The effect size comparing the pre–post change of the two CBM conditions (i.e., with and without the goal-raising rule) was 0.52. Consequently, using CBM to monitor the appropriateness of instructional goals and to adjust goals upward whenever possible is one way in which teachers can use CBM in their instructional planning.

A second key way in which teachers can use CBM to enhance instructional decision making is to assess the adequacy of student progress and to determine whether (and, if so, when) instructional adaptation is necessary. When the actual growth rate is less than the expected growth rate (slope of the goal line), a teacher can modify an instructional program to promote stronger learning. L. S. Fuchs, Fuchs, and Hamlett (1989b) estimated the contribution of this CBM decision-making strategy with 29 special educators who implemented CBM for 15 school weeks with 53 students who had mild to moderate disabilities. Teachers in a CBM "measurement only" group measured students' reading growth as required, but did not use the assessment information to structure students' reading programs. Teachers in a CBM "change the program" decision rule group measured students' performance and used the assessment information to determine when to introduce programmatic adaptations to enhance growth rates. Results indicated that although teachers in both groups measured students' performance, important differences were associated with the use of the "change the program" decision rule. On the Reading Comprehension subtest of the Stanford Achievement Test, students in the "change the program" group scored higher than a no-CBM control group (effect size = 0.72), whereas students in the "measurement only" group did not (effect size = 0.36). Moreover, the slopes of the two CBM treatment groups were significantly different, favoring the achievement of the "change the program" group (effect size = 0.86). As suggested by these findings and the results of other researchers (e.g., Stecker & Fuchs, 1990; Wesson, Skiba, Sevcik, King, & Deno, 1984), collecting CBM data in and of itself exerts only a small effect on student learning. To enhance student outcomes in important ways, teachers need to use the CBM data experimentally to build effective programs for students with LDs.

For helping teachers determine when adjustments are required in students' programs and for identifying when goal increases are war-

ranted, the CBM total scores are used. In addition, by inspecting the graph of performance indicators over time, the teachers may formulate ideas for potentially effective instructional adaptations. For example, a flat or decelerating slope might generate hypotheses about lack of maintenance of previously learned material or about motivational problems. Nevertheless, to obtain rich descriptions of student performance, alternative ways of summarizing and describing student performance are necessary. Because CBM assesses performance on the year's curriculum at each testing, rich descriptions of strengths and weaknesses in the curriculum can be generated. The effects of CBM diagnostic profiles were investigated in three studies: one in math (L. S. Fuchs, Fuchs, Hamlett, & Stecker, 1991), one in reading (L. S. Fuchs, Fuchs, & Hamlett, 1989c), and one in spelling (L. S. Fuchs, Fuchs, Hamlett, & Allinder, 1991). In each investigation, teachers were assigned randomly to one of three conditions: no CBM, CBM with goal-raising and "change the program" decision rules, and CBM with goal-raising and "change the program" decision rules along with CBM diagnostic profiles. In all three studies, teachers in the diagnostic profile treatment group generated instructional plans that were more varied and more responsive to individuals' learning needs. Moreover, they effected better student learning, as indicated by change between pre- and posttest performance on global measures of achievement. Effect sizes associated with the CBM diagnostic profile groups ranged from 0.65 to 1.23. This series of studies demonstrated how structured, well-organized CBM information about students' strengths and difficulties in the curriculum can help teachers build better programs and effect greater learning.

Research has also provided evidence of CBM's overall utility in helping teachers plan more effective programs (e.g., L. S. Fuchs, Deno, & Mirkin, 1984; L. S. Fuchs, Fuchs, Hamlett, & Allinder, 1991; L. S. Fuchs, Fuchs, Hamlett, & Ferguson, 1992; Jones & Krouse, 1988; Wesson, 1991; Wesson et al., 1984). To illustrate this database, we describe one study in reading. L. S. Fuchs and colleagues (1984) conducted a study in the New York City Public Schools. Teachers participated for 18 weeks in a contrast group or a CBM treatment group, where teachers measured students' reading performance at least twice weekly, scored and graphed those performances, and used pre-scriptive CBM decision rules for planning the students' reading programs. Students whose teachers employed CBM to develop reading programs achieved better than students whose teachers used conventional monitoring methods on the Passage Reading Test and on the Decoding and Comprehension subtests of the Stanford Diagnostic Reading Test, with respective effect sizes of 1.18, 0.94, and 0.99. This suggests that, despite the exclusive focus on passage-reading fluency for progress monitoring, teachers planned better reading programs comprehensively to include foci on fluency, decoding, and comprehension.

In sum, many controlled investigations provide corroborating evidence of dramatic effects on student outcomes in reading, spelling, and math when teachers rely on CBM to inform instructional planning. When this form of progress monitoring is used to assess the effects of validated interventions on individual students with LDs and to revise programs responsively to those data, academic outcomes for students with LDs improve.

Prevention versus Remediation

Given the evidence cited in this chapter for the greater efficacy of early identification and preventive interventions than of remedial interventions, the widespread failure to implement early intervention programs in general education and in special education is frustrating. Students vary in their instructional needs. Those who do not receive instruction addressing their developmental needs in grades K–2 develop academic difficulties that parallel those typically observed in students with LDs. Yet many are instructional "casualties" who are not identified until grade 3 and beyond. The "wait and fail" model in itself makes the process orientation of special education cumbersome, simply because there are more students than the system can handle. More importantly, the key to remediation is intensity, especially for students who do not respond to high-quality classroom intervention. Unless early instruction programs are enhanced, it seems that special education will continue to be a process for protecting civil rights, but will not be successful in helping students develop academic and adaptive behavior skills. Widespread implementation of early intervention programs could potentially reduce the number of students who emerge as possibly

eligible for special education. This could be done through universal screening for reading and behavior problems, progress monitoring of those who show risk characteristics, and specialized intervention for those who do not make adequate progress (Donovan & Cross, 2002; Vaughn & Fuchs, 2003). Special education would reflect the opportunity to provide highly specialized and intense interventions like those reviewed in the section on reading remediation, in cases where implementation requires the power and flexibility of IDEA. How else could a struggling student receive 2 hours of reading instruction per day over an 8-week period, which seems to accelerate development in many struggling students (Torgesen, Alexander, et al., 2001)? Similarly, special education could support early intervention as part of the prereferral process, or even as part of its mission. Until general education and special education work together in a seamless system toward the same goal—enhancing academic outcomes for all students—many will struggle. The key is to embrace prevention whenever possible, and to be prepared to respond with intense specialized remediation when preventive efforts are not adequate. Remediation can be effective, and this chapter has identified effect sizes for many remedial interventions that were just as large as those for prevention studies. But interventions of the type implemented in research are generally more intense than those used in schools. In the LD area, the size of the instructional group in many settings is just not adequate to promote the level of intensity need to accelerate growth in academic skills.

Insufficient Engagement and Practice

We can make our prevention and intervention efforts more efficient in the schools and elsewhere by applying some of the instructional methods and interventions reviewed in this chapter. However, for many students, much more time on task may be required to reach a given criterion in any area. Remedial interventions are commonly substituted for time in the general education curriculum, and it is commonly observed that students who attend remedial reading classes read less than they would have if they had simply remained in the general education classroom (Allington, Stuetzel, Shake, & Lamarch, 1987). Thus the first thing that should happen in considering how to accelerate academic development in either a preventive or a remedial mode is to increase the time devoted to instruction in the area in which a student is struggling. In order to further accelerate development, it may be necessary to ensure that the student spends time reading and engaging in other academic tasks outside of school. Extra time outside of school means that the student must become engaged in the task to such an extent that he or she is independently motivated to spend time on it (as opposed to all the other priorities competing for the student's nonschool time). More reading instruction and practice time in school can be added, as many schools in the United States have done to respond to the No Child Left Behind legislation—but that additional time comes out of other important educational activities, especially in middle school and secondary school. In elementary school, learning to read, write, and do math are clearly priorities, and some students need lots of time in these domains. However, as the studies of reading practice in the fluency section demonstrate, time spent on reading outside of school promotes practice, which in turn promotes the opportunity to develop vocabulary and other capabilities that support comprehension. In addition, extra engagement affords the opportunity to practice what is being taught and to consolidate the skills; such practice and consolidation promote transfer from the remedial environment. Intervention programs must look more systematically at the practice and engagement issues.

Clinical Intuition versus Scientific Evidence

The field of LDs, like other areas of education, is in the process of transforming itself from a discipline based largely on clinical intuition and experience to one that utilizes information from scientific research. Although intuition and experience must temper judgment, especially with individual students, instruction needs to be informed by research on effectiveness and on the mechanisms that underlie this effectiveness. The field of LDs, in particular, continues to be hampered by reliance on faddish interventions that persist despite absence of any evidence for their effectiveness or for their underlying mechanisms: learning styles, perceptual and motor training, auditory or visual training, multisensory integration, and even less reasonable interventions (involving special lenses, metronomes, neural patterning, etc.). For all these interventions, wise instructors, parents, and students, will testify that these interventions were effective. However, in the absence of scientific investigation, it is not possible to sort through competing claims about effectiveness and mechanisms, much less to prescribe specific interventions for individual students. Consumers must have the information they need to make informed choices. Clinicians must be prepared to modify and update their practice on the basis of research, or at least to identify the shortcomings of research that contradicts traditional beliefs. Without this concerted effort, the field of LDs will remain a mysterious, belief-based, and murky domain, and will not mature into an area with a basis in scientific research.

CONCLUSIONS

The road to establishing the efficacy of treatment approaches and methods designed for students with LDs is a long one. Until the past decade, little progress had been made in developing an understanding of the core clinical and diagnostic features of each of the major LD types (Table 8.1), and even this understanding is not equally robust for all types of LDs. The best-developed domain of our current knowledge about students' difficulties in learning academic concepts is the area of reading development in general and word-level skills in particular.

A substantial number of converging studies strongly support the hypothesis that difficulties in learning to read are highly related to linguistic deficits in the phonological processing area. These findings have provided a foundation for the development and experimental test of treatment modalities that target the linguistic deficiencies as well as the basic reading skill deficits. From this work, the data are clear that in order for an individual with or at risk for an LD in reading to gain access to print, the individual must receive a comprehensive, integrated intervention program composed of explicit instruction in the alphabetic principle; the opportunity to learn comprehension strategies; and many opportunities to practice these competencies within the context of reading meaningful, interesting, and controlled texts. The sooner in a child's school career that this can take place, the better.

Our current knowledge of what works best for students with deficits in written language and mathematics is less well developed. This is due in part to the fact that we simply know less about the etiological factors that presage these difficulties, the core cognitive deficits that define the disorders, and the developmental courses associated with these types of LDs. It goes without saying that a substantial increase in intervention research for different types of well-defined LDs will have to occur if students are to receive the best treatment that we can offer. To provide a full understanding of the many factors that will influence a youngster's response to treatment, such research must be primarily longitudinal in design. Although this type of research is time-consuming and expensive, it is probably the only way to identify clearly which teaching approaches or combinations of teaching approaches have the highest probability of success with which students, at which age, in which setting, and with which types of teachers.

Across reading, written expression, and mathematics—and within each domain, across foundational skills and higher-order processes—these studies (along with other corroborating studies in the literature) provide the basis for drawing a smaller set of 10 conclusions about how to design instruction to enhance academic outcomes for students with LDs.

1. Students with LDs require an instructional approach that is explicit, that is well organized, and that routinely provides opportunity for cumulative review of previously mastered content. This appears to represent the cornerstone of effective practice. It is important to highlight that this conclusion applies whether teachers are addressing foundational skills and higher-order processes, for which transfer and generalization are critical challenges.

2. Self-regulation strategies, whereby students monitor their academic progress and set goals for their academic performance, provide an added value beyond systematic, explicit instruction.

3. Peer mediation provides a potentially feasible and effective method for extending scaffolded instruction. It creates structured opportunities for supported practice in ways that enhance acquisition of knowledge and extend transfer of learned content.

4. It is possible to produce impressive growth in higher-order processes even when students' foundational skills are weak. This argues that educators should provide systematic instruction on both dimensions of academic performance, so that as foundational skills are strengthened, teachers are simultaneously working explicitly to improve students' text comprehension, written expression, and MPS.

5. Gains are specific to what is taught. If interventions do not teach academic content, little transfer occurs. Similarly, if academic content in one domain is learned, it does not lead to improvement in another domain if that domain is not explicitly taught.

6. Instructional programs needed to be integrated. It is not enough simply to provide instruction in specific skills. The focus needs to be on the ultimate sets of competencies that are desirable for students with LDs. In reading, for example, intervention programs ultimately need to account for word recognition, fluency, and comprehension, as the goal of any instructional program in reading is the development of proficient comprehension. Engagement and practice must be incorporated into the intervention.

7. Research must increasingly take into account the heterogeneity of students with LDs. The strongest formulation of this issue is to focus on heterogeneity at the level of major comorbidities, especially those that involve combinations of academic difficulties and those behaviors subsumed under ADHD. In addition, the multifaceted nature of LDs in many students needs to be taken into account.

8. Progress must be frequently monitored and used to inform instruction intervention at all levels of intervention.

9. Practice must be grounded in and modified on the basis of scientific evidence, which in turn must be tempered by experience and judgment.

10. Interventions designed for students with LDs must be better integrated with general education practices.

The last conclusion recognizes the recent explosion of systematic, empirical research on interventions that work both for students who have LDs in reading, written language, and mathematics and for typically developing students. This explosion is likely to continue over the next decade. In addition, research will probably focus increasingly on policy-based issues that are highly relevant for students with

LDs and that require more integration with general education. Major changes in identification procedures for LDs can be expected that will require a close working relationship between special education and general education. It is likely that the current practice of waiting for students to fail, identifying them with LDs, and placing them in educational environments that do not result in closing the gap will begin to change, and that more emphasis on preventing LDs through effective general education practices will emerge.

In order for this change to occur, general education and special education must take responsibility for preventing academic difficulties whenever possible (President's Commission on Excellence in Special Education, 2002). Students must be identified and instructed earlier in their development than is presently the case, which will require better teacher preparation programs in both general education and special education. Teachers need exposure to research-based interventions in the classroom and to remedial interventions, regardless of their area of specialization, with the focus on evidence for effectiveness. The ultimate goal of identifying students with LD should be to provide instructional experiences that will allow them to overcome the adaptive difficulties associated with LDs. Special education should be an environment that involves relatively few students, and the power of the legislation underlying special education should be used to provide alternative interventions that cannot be provided in the classroom or through small-group instruction in general education.

To accomplish this goal, the numbers of students in special education have to be reduced, or funding needs to be significantly increased. The purpose of reducing the numbers is not to cut funding for special education, but to put the funding that is available to better use. Our hope is that through a focus on prevention, effective early instruction, and progress monitoring, the number of students who require unusually intense interventions can be reduced. Special education can then become an environment where instructional "casualties" have been eliminated and the development of students with LDs can be accelerated, so that they return and function effectively in general education environments and elsewhere.

Presently, as many consensus reports have noted, the focus of special education is on process and legal rights, which often has the effect of making special education a separate system. Although ensuring the rights of students with disabilities is very important and should continue to be a priority, special education should also be an environment where results are achieved and where the goal is maximal involvement in general education. The research studies reviewed in this chapter show that the evidence base is increasing, and that there are interventions that would work with many students identified with LDs if they were effectively implemented. It can only be hoped that over the next decade, more of these interventions will be implemented and will have some systematic impact on students with LDs. In the meantime, the research base will continue to flourish, which gives us great hope for the future.

ACKNOWLEDGMENTS

Grants from the National Institute of Child Health and Human Development (No. P50 21888, Center for Learning and Attention Disorders, and No. P01 HD46261, Cognitive, Instructional, and Neuroimaging Factors in Math); the National Science Foundation (No. 9979968, Early Reading Development: A Cognitive Neuroscience Approach); and the U.S. Department of Education, Office of Special Education Programs (No. H324V980001, Center for Accelerated Student Learning) supported this chapter. We gratefully acknowledge the contribution of Rita Taylor to manuscript preparation.

REFERENCES

Adams, G., & Carnine, D. (2003). Direct instruction. In H. L. Swanson, K. R. Harris, & S. Graham (Eds.), *Handbook of learning disabilities* (pp. 403–416). New York: Guilford Press.

Adams, G. L., & Engelmann, S. (1996). *Research on Direct Instruction: 25 years beyond DISTAR*. Portland, OR: Educational Achievement Systems.

Adams, M. J. (1990). *Beginning to read: Thinking and learning about print*. Cambridge, MA: MIT Press.

Allington, R. L., Stuetzel, H., Shake, M. C., & Lamarch, L. (1987). What is remedial reading?: A descriptive study. *Reading Research and Instruction, 26*, 15–30.

Asch, S. E. (1969). A reformulation of the problem of associations. *American Psychologist, 24*, 92–102.

Aylward, E. H., Richards, T. L., Berninger, V. W., Nagy, W. E., Field, K. M., Grimme, A. C., et al. (2003). Instructional treatment associated with changes in brain activation in children with dyslexia. *Neurology, 22*, 212–219.

Bailet, L. L. (1991). Development and disorders of spelling in the beginning school years. In A. M. Bain, L. L. Bailet, & L. C. Moats (Eds.), *Written language disorders: Theory into practice* (pp. 1–22). Austin, TX: Pro-Ed.

Bain, A. M. (1991). Handwriting disorders. In A. M. Bain, L. L. Bailet, & L. C. Moats (Eds.), *Written language disorders: Theory into practice* (pp. 43–64). Austin, TX: Pro-Ed.

Baker, L., & Brown, A. L. (1984a). Cognitive monitoring in reading. In P. D. Pearson (Ed.), *Understanding reading comprehension* (pp. 21–44). Newark, DE: International Reading Association.

Baker, L., & Brown, A. L. (1984b). Metacognitive skills in reading. In P. D. Pearson (Ed.), *Handbook of reading research* (pp. 126–140). New York: Longman.

Bakker, D. J. (1984). The brain as a dependent variable. *Journal of Clinical Neuropsychology, 6,* 1–16.

Bakker, D. J., & Vinke, J. (1985). Effects of hemispheric-specific stimulation on brain activity and reading in dyslexics. *Journal of Clinical Neuropsychology, 7,* 505–525.

Barkley, R. A. (2006). *Attention-deficit hyperactivity disorder: A handbook for diagnosis and treatment* (3rd ed.). New York: Guilford Press.

Bateman, B. (1967). An educator's view of a diagnostic approach to learning disorders. In J. Hellmuth (Ed.), *Learning disorders* (Vol. 1, pp. 219–239). Seattle, WA: Special Child.

Berends, I. E., & Reitsma, P. (2005). Lateral and central presentation of words with limited exposure duration as remedial training for reading disabled children. *Journal of Clinical and Experimental Psychology, 27,* 886–896.

Berninger, V. W. (1994). Future directions for research on writing disabilities: Integrating endogenous and exogenous variables. In G. R. Lyon (Ed.), *Frames of reference for the assessment of learning disabilities: New views on measurement issues* (pp. 419–440). Baltimore: Brookes.

Berninger, V. W., & Amtmann, D. (2003). Preventing written expression disabilities through early and continuing assessment and intervention for handwriting and/or spelling problems: Research into practice. In H. L. Swanson, K. R. Harris, & S. Graham (Eds.), *Handbook of learning disabilities* (pp. 345–363). New York: Guilford Press.

Berninger, V. W., & Graham, S. (1998). Language by hand: A synthesis of a decade of research in handwriting. *Handwriting Review, 12,* 11–25.

Berninger, V. W., Mizokowa, D. T., & Bragg, R. (1991). Theory-based diagnosis and remediation of writing disabilities. *Journal of School Psychology, 29,* 57–79.

Berninger, V. W., Nagy, W. E., Carlisle, J., Thomson, J., Hoffer, D., Abbott, S., et al. (2003). Effective treatment for children with dyslexia in grades 4–6: Behavioral and brain evidence. In B. R. Foorman (Ed.), *Preventing and remediating reading difficulties,* (pp. 381–418). Baltimore: York Press.

Berninger, V. W., Vaughan, K., Abbott, R., Abbott, S., Brooks, A., Rogan, L., et al. (1997). Treatment of handwriting fluency problems in beginning writing: Transfer from handwriting to composition. *Journal of Educational Psychology, 89,* 652–666.

Berninger, V. W., Vaughan, K., Abbott, R., Begay, K., Cyrd, K., Curtin, G., et al. (2002). Teaching spelling and composition alone and together: Implications for the simple view of writing. *Journal of Educational Psychology, 94,* 291–304.

Bijou, S. (1970). What psychology has to offer education—now. *Journal of Applied Behavior Analysis, 3,* 65–71.

Birsh, J. (Ed.). (1999). *Multisensory teaching of basic language skills.* Baltimore: Brookes.

Blachman, B. A. (1997). Early intervention and phonological awareness: A cautionary tale. In B. Blachman (Ed.), *Foundations of reading acquisition and dyslexia* (pp. 408–430). Mahwah, NJ: Erlbaum.

Blachman, B. A., Ball, E. W., Black, R. S., & Tangel, D. M. (1994). Kindergarten teachers develop phoneme awareness in low-income, inner-city classrooms: Does it make a difference? *Reading and Writing: An Interdisciplinary Journal, 6,* 1–18.

Blachman, B. A., Schatschneider, C., Fletcher, J. M., Francis, D. J., Clonan, S., Shaywitz, B., et al. (2004). Effects of intensive reading remediation for second and third graders. *Journal of Educational Psychology, 96,* 444–461.

Blankenship, C., & Lovitt, T. C. (1976). Story problems: Merely confusing or downright befuddling? *Journal for Research in Mathematics Education, 7,* 290–298.

Borkowski, J. G. (1992). Metacognitive theory: A framework for teaching literacy, writing, and math skills. *Journal of Learning Disabilities, 25,* 253–257.

Borkowski, J. G., & Burke, J. E. (1996). Theories, models, and measurements of executive functioning: An information processing perspective. In G. R. Lyon & N. A. Krasnegor (Eds.), *Attention, memory and executive functioning* (pp. 235–278). Baltimore: Brookes.

Bos, C. S., & Anders, P. L. (1990). Interactive teaching and learning: Instructional practices for teaching content and strategic knowledge. In T. E. Scruggs & B. Y. L. Wong (Eds.), *Intervention research in learning disabilities* (pp. 161–185). New York: Springer-Verlag.

Bowers, P. G. (2001). Exploration of the basis for rapid naming's relationship to reading. In M. Wolf (Ed.), *Dyslexia, fluency, and the brain* (pp. 41–64). Timonium, MD: York Press.

Bradley, L., & Bryant, R. (1985). *Rhyme and reason in reading and spelling* (International Academy for Research in Learning Disabilities, Monograph Series No. 1). Ann Arbor: University of Michigan Press.

Bradley, R., Danielson, L., & Hallahan, D. P. (Eds.). (2002). *Identification of learning disabilities: Research to practice.* Mahwah, NJ: Erlbaum.

Brady, S. A., & Shankweiler, D. P. (Eds.). (1991). *Phonological processes in literacy.* Hillsdale, NJ: Erlbaum.

Bransford, J. D., Sherwood, R., Vye, N., & Rieser, J. (1986). Teaching thinking and problem solving. *American Psychologist, 41*, 1078–1089.

Brown, A. L., & Campione, J. (1986). Psychological theory and the study of learning disabilities. *American Psychologist, 41*, 14–21.

Bruck, M. (1987). The adult outcomes of children with learning disabilities. *Annals of Dyslexia, 37*, 252–263.

Bruck, M. (1990). Word-recognition skills of adults with childhood diagnoses of dyslexia. *Developmental Psychology, 26*, 439–454.

Bryant, S. (1979). *Relative effectiveness of visual–auditory vs. visual–auditory–kinesthetic–tactile procedures for teaching sight words and letter sounds to young disabled readers.* Unpublished doctoral dissertation, Teachers College, Columbia University.

Camilli, G., Vargas, S., & Yreka, M. (2003). Teaching children to read: The fragile link between science and federal policy. *Education Policy Analysis Archives, 11*, 1–52.

Carlisle, J. F. (1993). Selecting approaches to vocabulary instruction for the reading disabled. *Learning Disabilities Research and Practice, 8*, 97–105.

Carlson, C. D., & Francis, D. J. (2002). Increasing the reading achievement of at-risk children through Direct Instruction: Evaluation of the Rodeo Institute for Teacher Excellence (RITE). *Journal of Education for Students Placed at Risk, 7*, 141–166.

Carnine, D. W. (1980). Preteaching versus concurrent teaching on the component skills of a multiplication problem-solving strategy. *Journal for Research in Mathematics Education, 11*, 370–379.

Carnine, D. W. (1991). Increasing the amount and quality of learning through direct instruction: Implications for mathematics. In J. W. Lloyd, N. N. Singh, & A. C. Repp (Eds.), *The regular education initiative: Alternative perspectives on concepts, issues, and models* (pp. 163–175). Sycamore, IL: Sycamore.

Carnine, D. W., Silbert, J., & Kame'enui, E. J. (1997). *Direct Instruction reading.* Upper Saddle River, NJ: Prentice Hall.

Case, L. P., Harris, K. R., & Graham, S. (1992). Improving the mathematical problem-solving skills of students with learning disabilities: Self-regulated strategy development. *Journal of Special Education, 26*, 1–19.

Catrambone, R., & Holyoak, K. J. (1989). Overcoming contextual limitations on problem-solving transfer. *Journal of Experimental Psychology: Learning, Memory, and Cognition, 15*, 1127–1156.

Cawley, J. F., Fitzmaurice, A. M., Goodstein, H. A., Lepore, A. V., Sedlak, R., & Althause, V. (1976). *Project MATH.* Tulsa, OK: Educational Development.

Cawley, J. F., Fitzmaurice, A. M., Shaw, R., Kahn, H., & Bates, H., III. (1978). Mathematics and learning disabled youth: The upper grade levels. *Learning Disability Quarterly, 1*, 37–52.

Cawley, J. F., & Miller, J. H. (1986). Selected views on metacognition, arithmetic problem-solving, and learning disabilities. *Learning Disabilities Focus, 2*, 36–48.

Cawley, J. F., Parmar, R. S., Yan, W., & Miller, J. H. (1998). Arithmetic computation performance of students with learning disabilities: Implications for curriculum. *Learning Disabilities Research and Practice, 13*, 68–74.

Chapman, J. W., Tunmer, W. E., & Prochnow, J. E. (2001). Does success in the Reading Recovery program depend on developing proficiency in phonological processing skills?: A longitudinal study in a whole language instruction context. *Scientific Studies of Reading, 5*, 141–176.

Chard, D. J., Vaughn, S., & Tyler, B. (2002). A synthesis of research on effective interventions for building reading fluency with elementary students with learning disabilities. *Journal of Learning Disabilities, 35*, 386–406.

Chase, C. (1986). Essay test scoring: Interaction of relevant variables. *Journal of Educational Measurement, 23*, 33–41.

Clark, D. B. (1988). *Dyslexia: Theory and practice of remedial instruction.* Timonium, MD: York Press.

Clark, D. B., & Uhry, J. K. (1995). *Dyslexia: Theory and practice of remedial instruction* (2nd ed.). Baltimore: York Press.

Clay, M. M. (1985). *The early detection of reading difficulties* (3rd ed.). Portsmouth, NH: Heinemann.

Clay, M. M. (1993). *Reading Recovery: A guidebook for teachers in training.* Portsmouth, NH: Heinemann.

Clay, M. M. (2002). *An Observation Survey of Early Literacy Achievement* (2nd ed.). Portsmouth, NH: Heinemann.

Coalition for Evidence-Based Policy. (2002). *Bringing evidence-driven progress to education: A recommended strategy for the U.S. Department of Education.* Washington, DC: William T. Grant Foundation.

Cooper, G., & Sweller, J. (1987). Effects of schema acquisition and rule automation on mathematical problem solving transfer. *Journal of Educational Psychology, 79*, 347–362.

Coyne, M. D., Kame'enui, E. J., Simmons, D. C., & Harn, B. A. (2004). Beginning reading intervention as inoculation or insulin: First-grade reading performance of strong responders to kindergarten intervention. *Journal of Learning Disabilities, 37*, 90–104.

Cullinan, D., Lloyd, J., & Epstein, M. H. (1981). Strategy training: A structured approach to arithmetic instruction. *Exceptional Education Quarterly, 2*, 41–49.

D'Agostino, J. V., & Murphy, J. A. (2004). A meta-analysis of Reading Recovery in the United States schools. *Educational Evaluation and Policy Analysis, 26*, 23–38.

Deno, S. L., & Marston, D. (2001). *Test of Oral Reading Fluency.* Minneapolis, MN: Educators Testing Service.

Denton, C. A., Ciancio, D. J., & Fletcher, J. M. (in press). Validity, reliability, and utility of the Observation Survey of Early Literacy Achievement. *Reading Research Quarterly.*

Denton, C. A., & Mathes, P. G. (2003). Intervention for struggling readers: Possibilities and challenges. In B. R. Foorman (Ed.), *Preventing and remediating reading difficulties* (pp. 229–252). Baltimore: York Press.

Denton, C. A., Vaughn, S., & Fletcher, J. M. (2003). Bringing research-based practice in reading intervention to scale. *Learning Disabilities Research and Practice, 18,* 201–211.

Donovan, M. S., & Cross, C. T. (2002). *Minority students in special and gifted education.* Washington, DC: National Academy Press.

Doris, J. L. (1993). Defining learning disabilities: A history of the search for consensus. In G. R. Lyon, D. B. Gray, J. F. Kavanagh, & N. A. Krasnegor (Eds.), *Better understanding learning disabilities: New views from research and their implications for education and public policies* (pp. 97–116). Baltimore: Brookes.

Dunlap, G., dePerczel, M., Clarke, S., Wilson, D., Wright, S., White, R., et al. (1994). Choice making to promote adaptive behavior for students with emotional and behavioral challenges. *Journal of Applied Behavior Analysis, 27,* 505–518.

Elbaum, B., Vaughn, S., Hughes, M. T., & Moody, S. W. (2000). How effective are one-to-one tutoring programs in reading for elementary students at risk for reading failure?: A meta-analysis of the intervention research. *Journal of Educational Psychology 92,* 605–619.

Engelmann, S., Becker, W. C., Hanner, S., & Johnson, G. (1978). *Corrective Reading Program: Series guide.* Chicago: Science Research Associates.

Engelmann, S., & Carnine, D. W. (1975). *DISTAR Arithmetic I* (2nd ed.). Chicago: Science Research Associates.

Engelmann, S., & Carnine, D. W. (1982). *Theory of instruction: Principles and applications.* New York: Irvington.

Engelmann, S., Carnine, D. W., Engelmann, O., & Kelly, B. (1991). *Connecting math concepts.* Chicago: Science Research Associates.

Englert, C. S., Hiebert, E. H., & Stewart, S. R. (1986). Spelling unfamiliar words by an analogy strategy. *Journal of Special Education, 19,* 291–306.

Englert, C. S., & Mariage, T. (2003). The sociocultural model in special education interventions: Apprenticing students in higher-order thinking. In H. L. Swanson, K. R. Harris, & S. Graham (Eds.), *Handbook of learning disabilities* (pp. 450–470). New York: Guilford Press.

Feagans, L., & McKinney, J. D. (1981). The pattern of exceptionality across domains of learning disabled children. *Journal of Applied Developmental Psychology, 1,* 313–328.

Fernald, G. (1943). *Remedial techniques in basic school subjects.* New York: McGraw-Hill.

Fisk, J. L., & Rourke, B. P. (1983). Neuropsychological subtyping of learning disabled children: History,

methods, implications. *Journal of Learning Disabilities, 16,* 529–531.

Flavell, J. H. (1979). Metacognition and cognitive monitoring: A new area of cognitive developmental inquiry. *American Psychologist, 34,* 906–911.

Fleishner, J. E. (1994). Diagnosis and assessment of mathematics learning disabilities. In G. R. Lyon (Ed.), *Frames of reference for the assessment of learning disabilities: New views on measurement issues* (pp. 441–458). Baltimore: Brookes.

Fleishner, J. E., & Frank, B. (1979). Visual–spatial ability and mathematics achievement in learning disabled and normal boys. *Focus on Learning Problems in Mathematics, 1,* 7–22.

Fletcher, J. M., Francis, D. J., Morris, R. D., & Lyon, G. R. (2005). Evidence-based assessment of learning disabilities in children and adolescents. *Journal of Clinical Child and Adolescent Psychology, 34,* 506–522.

Fletcher, J. M., Lyon, G. R., Barnes, M. Stuebing, K. K., Francis, D. J., Olson, R., et al. (2002). Classification of learning disabilities: An evidence-based evaluation. In R. Bradley, L. Danielson, & D. P. Hallahan (Eds.), *Identification of learning disabilities: Research to practice* (pp. 185–250). Mahwah, NJ: Erlbaum.

Fletcher, J. M., & Morris, R. (1986). Classification of disabled learners: Beyond exclusionary definitions. In S. J. Cici (Ed.), *Handbook of cognitive, social, and neuropsychological aspects of learning disabilities* (Vol. 1, pp. 55–80). Hillsdale, NJ: Erlbaum.

Fletcher, J. M., Morris, R. D., & Lyon, G. R. (2003). Classification and definition of learning disabilities: An integrative perspective. In H. L. Swanson, K. R. Harris, & S. Graham (Eds.), *Handbook of learning disabilities* (pp. 30–56). New York: Guilford Press.

Fletcher, J. M., Shaywitz, S. E., & Shaywitz, B. A. (1999). Comorbidity of learning and attention disorders: Separate but equal. *Pediatric Clinics of North America, 46,* 885–897.

Foorman, B. R. (1994). The relevance of a connectionist model of reading for "the great debate." *Educational Psychology Review, 16*(1), 25–47.

Foorman, B. R., Francis, D. J., Fletcher, J. M., Schatschneider, C., & Mehta, P. (1998). The role of instruction in learning to read: Preventing reading failure in at-risk-children. *Journal of Educational Psychology, 90,* 37–55.

Foorman, B. R., Francis, D. J., Winikates, D., Mehta, P., Schatschneider, C., & Fletcher, J. (1997). Early interventions for children with reading disabilities. *Scientific Studies of Reading, 1,* 255–276.

Francis, D. J., Fletcher, J. M., Stuebing, K. K., Lyon, G. R., Shaywitz, B. A., & Shaywitz, S. E. (2005). Psychometric approaches to the identification of learning disabilities: IQ and achievement scores are not sufficient. *Journal of Learning Disabilities, 38,* 98–110.

Francis, D. J., Shaywitz, S. E., Stuebing, K. K., Shaywitz, B. A., & Fletcher, J. M. (1994). Measurement of change: Assessing behavior over time and within a developmental framework. In G. R. Lyon (Ed.), *Frames of reference for the assessment of learning disabilities: New views on measurement issues* (pp. 29–68). Baltimore: Brookes.

Frith, U. (Ed.). (1980). *Cognitive processes in spelling.* New York: Academic Press.

Frostig, M. (1967). Education of children with learning disabilities. In E. C. Frierson & W. B. Barbe (Eds.), *Educating children with learning disabilities* (pp. 387–398). New York: Appleton-Century-Crofts.

Fuchs, D., & Fuchs, L. S. (2005). Peer-Assisted Learning Strategies: Promoting word recognition, fluency, and reading comprehension in young children. *Journal of Special Education, 39,* 34–44.

Fuchs, D., Fuchs, L. S., & Compton, D. L. (2004). Identifying reading disability as inadequate response to treatment: Methodological challenges. *Learning Disability Quarterly, 27,* 216–228.

Fuchs, D., Fuchs, L. S., Mathes, P., & Simmons, D. (1997). Peer-Assisted Learning Strategies: Making classrooms more responsive to student diversity. *American Educational Research Journal, 34,* 174–206.

Fuchs, D., Fuchs, L. S., Thompson, A., Al Otaiba, S., Yen, L., Yang, N. J., et al. (2001). Is reading important in reading readiness program?: A randomized field trial with teachers as program implementers. *Journal of Educational Psychology, 93,* 251–267.

Fuchs, D., Mock, D., Morgan, P., & Young, C. (2003). Responsiveness-to-intervention: Definitions, evidence, and implications for the learning disabilities construct. *Learning Disabilities Research and Practice, 18,* 157–171.

Fuchs, L. S., Bahr, C. M., & Rieth, H. J. (1989). Effects of goal structures and performance contingencies on the math performance of adolescents with learning disabilities. *Journal of Learning Disabilities, 22,* 554–560.

Fuchs, L. S., Deno, S. L., & Mirkin, P. K. (1984). The effects of frequent curriculum-based measurement and evaluation on student achievement, pedagogy, and student awareness of learning. *American Educational Research Journal, 21,* 449–460.

Fuchs, L. S., & Fuchs, D. (1998). Treatment validity: A simplifying concept for reconceptualizing the identification of learning disabilities. *Learning Disabilities Research and Practice, 4,* 204–219.

Fuchs, L. S., & Fuchs, D. (1999). Monitoring student progress toward the development of reading competence: A review of three forms of classroom-based assessment. *School Psychology Review, 28,* 659–671.

Fuchs, L. S., & Fuchs, D. (2000). Building student capacity to work productively during peer-assisted reading activities. In B. Taylor, M. Graves, & P. van den Broek (Eds.), *Reading for meaning: Fostering comprehension in the middle grades* (pp. 95–115). New York: Teachers College Press.

Fuchs, L. S., Fuchs, D., & Hamlett, C. L. (1989a). Effects of alternative goal structures within curriculum-based measurement. *Exceptional Children, 55,* 429–438.

Fuchs, L. S., Fuchs, D., & Hamlett, C. L. (1989b). Effects of instrumental use of curriculum-based measurement to enhance instructional programs. *Remedial and Special Education, 102,* 43–52.

Fuchs, L. S., Fuchs, D., & Hamlett, C. L. (1989c). Monitoring reading growth using student recalls: Effects of two teacher feedback systems. *Journal of Educational Research, 83,* 103–111.

Fuchs, L. S., Fuchs, D., Hamlett, C. L., & Allinder, R. M. (1991). Effects of expert system advice within curriculum-based measurement on teacher planning and student achievement in spelling. *School Psychology Review, 20,* 49–66.

Fuchs, L. S., Fuchs, D., Hamlett, C. L., & Appleton, A. C. (2002). Explicitly teaching for transfer: Effects on the mathematical problem solving performance of students with disabilities. *Learning Disabilities Research and Practice, 17,* 90–106.

Fuchs, L. S., Fuchs, D., Hamlett, C. L., & Ferguson, C. (1992). Effects of expert system consultation within curriculum-based measurement using a reading maze task. *Exceptional Children, 58,* 436–450.

Fuchs, L. S., Fuchs, D., Hamlett, C. L., Phillips, N. B., & Bentz, J. (1994). Class wide curriculum-based measurement: Helping general educators meet the challenge of student diversity. *Exceptional Children, 60,* 518–537.

Fuchs, L. S., Fuchs, D., Hamlett, C. L., Phillips, N. B., Karns, K., & Dutka, S. (1997). Enhancing students' helping behavior during peer-mediated instruction with conceptual mathematical explanations. *Elementary School Journal, 97,* 223–250.

Fuchs, L. S., Fuchs, D., Hamlett, C. L., & Stecker, P. M. (1991). Effects of curriculum-based measurement and consultation on teacher planning and student achievement in mathematics operations. *American Educational Research Journal, 28,* 617–641.

Fuchs, L. S., Fuchs, D., Hamlett, C. L., & Whinnery, K. (1991). Effects of goal line feedback on level, slope, and stability of performance within curriculum-based measurement. *Learning Disabilities Research and Practice, 6,* 65–73.

Fuchs, L. S., Fuchs, D., & Karns, K. (2001). Enhancing kindergartners' mathematical development: Effects of Peer-Assisted Learning Strategies. *Elementary School Journal, 101,* 495–510.

Fuchs, L. S., Fuchs, D., Karns, K., Hamlett, C. L., Dutka, S., & Katzaroff, M. (1996). The relation between student ability and the quality and effectiveness of explanations. *American Educational Research Journal, 33,* 631–664.

Fuchs, L. S., Fuchs, D., Phillips, N. B., Hamlett, C. L., & Karns, K. (1995). Acquisition and transfer effects of class wide Peer-Assisted Learning Strategies in mathematics for students with varying learning histories. *School Psychology Review, 24,* 604–620.

Fuchs, L. S., Fuchs, D., & Prentice, K. (2004). Responsiveness to mathematical problem-solving treatment among students with risk for mathematics disability, with and without risk for reading disability. *Journal of Learning Disabilities, 27,* 273–306.

Fuchs, L. S., Fuchs, D., Prentice, K., Burch, M., Hamlett, C. L., Owen, R., et al. (2003). Explicitly teaching for transfer: Effects on third-grade students' mathematical problem solving. *Journal of Educational Psychology.*

Fuchs, L. S., Fuchs, D., Prentice, K., Burch, M., Hamlett, C. L., Owen, R., et al. (2003). Enhancing third-grade students' mathematical problem solving with self-regulated learning strategies. *Journal of Educational Psychology.*

Fuchs, L. S., Fuchs, D., Yazdian, L., & Powell, S. R. (2002). Enhancing first-grade children's mathematical development with peer-assisted learning strategies. *School Psychology Review, 31,* 569–584.

Fuchs, L. S., Hamlett, C. L., & Fuchs, D. (1990). *Monitoring Basic Skills Progress.* Austin, TX: Pro-Ed.

Gadow, K., Torgesen, J. K., & Dahlem, W. E. (1985). Learning disabilities. In M. Herson, V. B. Hanslet, & J. L. Matson (Eds.), *Behavior therapy for the developmentally and physically disabled: A handbook* (pp. 310–351). New York: Academic Press.

Garan, E. (2001). Beyond the smoke and mirrors: A critique of the National Reading Panel report on phonics. *Phi Delta Kappan, 82,* 500–506.

Garner, R., Alexander, P. A., & Hare, V. C. (1991). Reading comprehension failure in children. In B. Y. L. Wong (Ed.), *Learning about learning disabilities* (pp. 283–307). San Diego, CA: Academic Press.

Gerber, M. M. (1986). Generalization of spelling strategies by LD students as a result of contingent imitation/modeling and mastery criteria. *Journal of Learning Disabilities, 19,* 530–537.

Germann, G. (2002). *AIMSweb General Outcome Measure of Curriculum-Based Measurement.* Retrieved from www.aimsweb.com

Gersten, R. M., White, W. A., Falco, R., & Carnine, D. (1982). Teaching basic discriminations to handicapped and non-handicapped individuals through a dynamic presentation of instructional stimuli. *Analysis and Intervention in Developmental Disabilities, 2,* 305–317.

Gick, M. L., & Holyoak, K. J. (1980). Analogical problem solving. *Cognitive Psychologist, 12,* 306–355.

Gillingham, A., & Stillman, B. (1965). *Remedial training for children with specific disability in reading, spelling and penmanship* (7th ed.). Cambridge, MA: Educators.

Glennon, V. J., & Cruickshank, W. M. (1981). Teaching mathematics to children and youth with perceptual and cognitive deficits. In V. J. Glennon (Ed.), *The mathematical education of exceptional children and youth: An interdisciplinary approach* (pp. 50–94). Reston, VA: National Council of Teachers of Mathematics.

Good, R. H., III, Simmons, D. C., & Kame'enui, E. J. (2001). The importance and decision-making utility of a continuum of fluency-based indicators of foundational reading skills for third-grade high-stakes outcomes. *Scientific Studies of Reading, 5,* 257–288.

Graham, S. (1999). Handwriting and spelling instruction for students with learning disabilities: A review. *Learning Disability Quarterly, 22,* 78–79.

Graham, S. (2005). Strategy instruction and the teaching of writing: A meta-analysis. In C. MacArthur, S. Graham, & J. Fitzgerald (Eds.), *Handbook of writing research.* New York: Guilford Press.

Graham, S., & Harris, K. R. (1993). Self-regulated strategy development: Helping students with learning problems develop as writers. *Elementary School Journal, 94,* 169–181.

Graham, S., & Harris, K. R. (1996). Addressing problems in attention, memory, and executive function. In G. R. Lyon & N. A. Krasnegor (Eds.), *Attention, memory, and executive function* (pp. 349–366). Baltimore: Brookes.

Graham, S., & Harris, K. R. (2003). Students with learning disabilities and the process of writing: A meta-analysis of SRSD studies. In H. L. Swanson, K. R. Harris, & S. Graham (Eds.), *Handbook of learning disabilities* (pp. 323–344). New York: Guilford Press.

Graham, S., Harris, K. R., & Chorzempa, B. F. (2002). Contribution of spelling instruction to the spelling, writing, and reading of poor spellers. *Journal of Educational Psychology, 94,* 669–686.

Graham, S., Harris, K. R., & Fink, B. (2000). Is handwriting causally related to learning to write?: Treatment of handwriting problems in beginning writers. *Journal of Educational Psychology, 92,* 620–633.

Graham, S., Harris, K. R., MacArthur, C., & Schwartz, S. (1991). Writing and writing instruction with students with learning disabilities: A review of a program of research. *Learning Disability Quarterly, 14,* 89–114.

Graham, S., Harris, K. R., & Mason, L. (2005). Improving the writing performance, knowledge, and motivation of struggling young writers: The effects of self-regulated strategy development. *Contemporary Educational Psychology, 30,* 207–241.

Gregg, N. (1991). Disorders of written expression. In A. Bain, L. Bailet, & L. Moats (Eds.), *Written language disorders: Theory into practice* (pp. 65–97). Austin, TX: Pro-Ed.

Hallahan, D. P., Kauffman, J., & Lloyd, J. (1996). *Introduction to learning disabilities.* Needham Heights, MA: Allyn & Bacon.

Hallahan, D. P., & Mock, D. R. (2003). A brief history of the field of learning disabilities. In H. L. Swanson, K. R. Harris, & S. Graham (Eds.), *Handbook of learning disabilities* (pp. 16–29). New York: Guilford Press.

Hammill, D. D. (1990). On defining learning disabilities: An emerging consensus. *Journal of Learning Disabilities, 23,* 74–84.

Harris, C. A., Miller, S. P., & Mercer, C. D. (1995). Teaching initial multiplication skills to students with disabilities in general education classrooms. *Learning Disabilities Research and Practice, 10,* 190–195.

Harris, K. R., Graham, S., & Mason, L. (in press). Improving the writing performance, knowledge, and self-efficacy of struggling writers in second grade: The effects of self-regulated strategy development. *American Educational Research Journal.*

Hart, B., & Risley, T. R. (1999). *Meaningful differences in the everyday experience of young American children.* Baltimore: Brookes.

Hasbrouck, J. E., Ihnot, C., & Rogers, G. (1999). Read Naturally: A strategy to increase oral reading fluency. *Reading Research and Instruction, 39,* 27–37.

Hayes, J. R., & Flower, L. S. (1980). Identifying the organization of the writing process. In L. W. Gregg & E. R. Steinbery (Eds.), *Cognitive processes in writing* (pp. 3–30). Hillsdale, NJ: Erlbaum.

Hiebert, E. H. (1994). Reading Recovery in the United States: What difference does it make to an age cohort? *Educational Researcher, 23,* 15–25.

Hiebert, E. H., Colt, J. M., Catto, S. L., & Gury, E. C. (1992). Reading and writing of first grade students in a restructured Chapter I program. *American Educational Research Journal, 29,* 545–572.

Higgins, E., & Raskind, M. (2000). Speaking to read: A comparison of continuous vs. discrete speech recognition in the remediation of learning disabilities. *Journal of Special Education Technology, 15,* 19–30.

Hook, P. E., Macaruso, P., & Jones, S. (2001). Efficacy of Fast ForWord training on facilitating acquisition of reading skills by children with reading difficulties: A longitudinal study. *Annals of Dyslexia, 51,* 75–96.

Hoskyn, M., & Swanson, H. L (2000). Cognitive processing of low achievers and children with reading disabilities: A selective meta-analytic review of the published literature. *School Psychology Review, 29,* 102–119.

Howell, R., Sidorenko, E., & Jurica, J. (1987). The effects of computer use on the acquisition of multiplication facts by students with learning disabilities. *Journal of Learning Disabilities, 20,* 336–341.

Hughes, C. A., Ruhl, K. L., Schumaker, J. B., & Deshler, D. D. (2002). Effects of instruction in an assignment completion strategy on the homework performance of students with learning disabilities in general education classes. *Learning Disabilities Research, 17,* 1–18.

Hughes, D. C., Keeling, B., & Tuck, B. F. (1983). Effects of achievement expectations and handwriting quality on scoring essays. *Journal of Educational Measurement, 20,* 65–70.

Hutchinson, N. L. (1993). Effects of cognitive strategy instruction on algebra problem solving of adolescents with learning disabilities. *Learning Disability Quarterly, 16,* 34–63.

Ihnot, C. (2000). *Read naturally.* St. Paul, MN: Read Naturally.

Individuals with Disabilities Education Act (IDEA) Amendments of 1997, P.L. 105-17, 20 U.S.C. 1400 et seq. [statute], 34 C.F.R. 300 [regulations] (1997).

Iverson, S., & Tumner, W. (1993). Phonological processing skills and the Reading Recovery program. *Journal of Educational Psychology, 85,* 112–120.

Jenkins, J. R., & O'Connor, R. E. (2002). Early identification and intervention for young children with reading/learning disabilities. In R. Bradley, L. Danielson, & D. P. Hallahan (Eds.), *Identification of learning disabilities: Research to practice* (pp. 99–149). Mahwah, NJ: Erlbaum.

Jenkins, J. R., & O'Connor, R. E. (2003). Cooperative learning for students with learning disabilities: Evidence from experiments, observations, and interviews. In H. L. Swanson, K. R. Harris, & S. Graham (Eds.), *Handbook of learning disabilities* (pp. 417–430). New York: Guilford Press.

Jitendra, A. K., Griffin, C. C., McGoey, K., Gardill, M. C., Bhat, P., & Riley, T. (1998). Effects of mathematical word problem solving by students at risk or with mild disabilities. *Journal of Educational Research, 91,* 345–355.

Jitendra, A. K., & Hoff, K. (1996). The effects of schema-based instruction on the mathematical problem-solving performance of students with learning disabilities. *Journal of Learning Disabilities, 29,* 422–431.

Johnson, D. J. (1994). Measurement of listening and speaking. In G. R. Lyon (Ed.), *Frames of reference for the assessment of learning disabilities: New views on measurement issues* (pp. 201–227). Baltimore: Brookes.

Johnson, D. J., & Myklebust, H. (1967). *Learning disabilities.* New York: Grune & Stratton.

Jones, D., & Christensen, C. (1999). The relationship between automaticity in handwriting and students' ability to generate written text. *Journal of Educational Psychology, 91,* 44–49.

Jones, E. D., & Krouse, J. P. (1988). The effectiveness of data-based instruction by student teachers in classrooms for pupils with mild learning handicaps. *Teacher Education and Special Education, 11,* 9–19.

Jordan, N. C., & Hanich, L. B. (2000). Mathematical thinking in second-grade children with different forms of LD. *Journal of Learning Disabilities, 33,* 567–578.

Kauffman, J. M., Hallahan, D. P., Haas, K., Brame, T., & Boren, R. (1978). Imitating children's errors to improve their spelling performance. *Journal of Learning Disabilities, 11,* 217–222.

Kavale, K., & Forness, S. R. (1985). *The science of learning disabilities.* San Diego, CA: College-Hill Press.

Kavale, K. A., & Forness, S. R. (2000). What definitions of learning disability say and don't say: A critical analysis. *Journal of Learning Disabilities, 33,* 239–256.

Kavale, K. A., & Forness, S. R. (2003). Learning disability as a discipline. In H. L. Swanson, K. R. Harris, & S. Graham (Eds.), *Handbook of learning disabilities* (pp. 76–93). New York: Guilford Press.

Kavale, K. A., & Reese, L. (1992). The character of learning disabilities: An Iowa profile. *Learning Disability Quarterly, 15,* 74–94.

Keane, M. (1988). *Analogical problem solving.* Chichester, UK: Ellis Horwood.

Kim, A., Vaughn, S., Wanzek, J., & Wei, S. (2004). Graphic organizers and their effects on the reading comprehension of students with LD: A synthesis of research. *Journal of Learning Disabilities, 37,* 105–118.

Kirby, J. R., & Robinson, G. L. (1987). Simultaneous and successive processing in reading disabled children. *Journal of Learning Disabilities, 20,* 243–252.

Kirk, S. A., & Kirk, W. D. (1971). *Psycholinguistic learning disabilities: Diagnosis and remediation.* Chicago: University of Chicago Press.

Knopik, V. S., & DeFries, J. C. (1999). Etiology of covariation between reading and mathematics performance: A twin study. *Twin Research, 2,* 226–234.

Kraetsch, G. A. (1981). The effects of oral instructions and training on the expansion of written language. *Learning Disability Quarterly, 4,* 82–90.

Kroesbergen, E. H., Van Luit, J. E. H., & Naglieri, J. A. (2003). Mathematical learning difficulties and PASS cognitive processes. *Journal of Learning Disabilities, 36,* 574–562.

Kuhn, M. R., & Stahl, S. A. (2003). Fluency: A review of developmental and remedial practices. *Journal of Educational Psychology, 95,* 3–21.

Leach, J. M., Scarborough, H. S., & Rescorla, L. (2003). Late-emerging reading disabilities. *Journal of Educational Psychology, 95,* 211–224.

Learning Disabilities Roundtable. (2002). *Specific learning disabilities: Finding common ground.* Washington, DC: U.S. Department of Education, Office of Special Education Programs, Office of Innovation and Development.

Lerner, J. (1989). Educational intervention in learning disabilities. *Journal of the American Academy of Child and Adolescent Psychiatry, 28,* 326–331.

Levy, B. A. (2001). Moving the bottom: Improving reading fluency. In M. Wolf (Ed.), *Dyslexia, fluency, and the brain* (pp. 357–382). Timonium, MD: York Press.

Liberman, I. Y., & Shankweiler, D. (1985). Phonology and the problems of learning to read and write. *Remedial and Special Education, 6,* 8–17.

Liberman, I. Y., & Shankweiler, D. (1991). Phonology and beginning reading: A tutorial. In L. Rieben & C. A. Perfetti (Eds.), *Learning to read: Basic research and its implications* (pp. 3–17). Hillsdale, NJ: Erlbaum.

Lindamood, P., & Lindamood, P. (1998). *The Lindamood Phoneme Sequencing Program for Reading, Spelling, and Speech.* Austin, TX: Pro-Ed.

Lloyd, J. W. (1980). Academic instruction and cognitive-behavior modification. *Exceptional Education Quarterly, 1,* 53–63.

Lonigan, C. J. (2003). Development and promotion of emergent literacy skills in children at-risk of reading difficulties. In B. R. Foorman (Ed.), *Preventing and remediating reading difficulties* (pp. 23–50). Baltimore: York Press.

Lovett, M. W. (1984). A developmental perspective on reading dysfunction: Accuracy and rate criteria in the subtyping of dyslexic children. *Brain and Language, 22,* 67–91.

Lovett, M. W. (1991). Reading, writing, and remediation: Perspectives on the dyslexic learning disability from remedial outcome data. *Learning and Individual Differences, 3,* 295–305.

Lovett, M. W., Barron, R. W., & Benson, N. J. (2003). Effective remediation of word identification and decoding difficulties in school-age children with reading disabilities. In H. L. Swanson, K. Harris, & S. Graham (Eds.), *Handbook of learning disabilities* (pp. 273–292). New York: Guilford Press.

Lovett, M. W., Lacerenza, L., Borden, S. L., Frijters, J. C., Steinbach, K. A., & DePalma, M. (2000). Components of effective remediation for developmental reading disabilities: Combining phonological and strategy-based instruction to improve outcomes. *Journal of Educational Psychology, 92,* 263–283.

Lovett, M. W., Lacerenza, L., Murphy, D., Steinbach, K. A., De Palma, M., & Frijters, J. C. (2005). The importance of multiple-component interventions for children and adolescents who are struggling readers. In S. O. Richardson & J. W. Gilger (Eds.), *Research-based education and intervention: What we need to know* (pp. 67–102). Baltimore: International Dyslexia Association.

Lovett, M. W., Steinbach, K. A., & Frijters, J. C. (2000). Remediating the core deficits of reading disability: A double-deficit perspective. *Journal of Learning Disabilities, 33,* 334–358.

Lovett, M. W., Warren-Chaplin, P., Ransby, M., & Borden, S. L. (1990). Training the word recognition skills of reading disabled children: Treatment and transfer effects. *Journal of Educational Psychology, 82,* 769–780.

Lovitt, T. C. (1967). Assessment of children with learning disabilities. *Exceptional Children, 34,* 233–239.

Lovitt, T. C., & Curtiss, K. A. (1968). Effects of manipulating an antecedent event on mathematics response rate. *Journal of Applied Behavior Analysis, 1,* 329–333.

Lovitt, T. C., Guppy, T. E., & Blattner, J. E. (1969). The use of a free time contingency with fourth graders to increase spelling accuracy. *Behaviour Research and Therapy, 7,* 151–156.

Lyon, G. R. (1985). Identification and remediation of learning disability subtypes. *Learning Disability Focus, 1,* 21–35.

Lyon, G. R. (1995). Toward a definition of dyslexia. *Annals of Dyslexia, 45,* 3–30.

Lyon, G. R. (1996a). Learning disabilities. In E. Mash & R. A. Barkley (Eds.), *Child psychopathology* (pp. 390–435). New York: Guilford Press.

Lyon, G. R. (1996b). Learning disabilities: Past, present, and future perspectives. *The Future of Children, 6,* 24–46.

Lyon, G. R., & Chhabra, V. (2004). The science of reading research. *Educational Leadership, 61,* 12–17.

Lyon, G. R., & Cutting, L. E. (1998). Treatment of learning disabilities. In E. J. Mash & R. A. Barkley (Eds.), *Treatment of childhood disorders* (pp. 468–500). New York: Guilford Press.

Lyon, G. R., Fletcher, J. M., & Barnes, M. C. (2003). Learning disabilities. In E. J. Mash & R. A. Barkley (Eds.), *Child psychopathology* (2nd ed., pp. 520–588). New York: Guilford Press.

Lyon, G. R., Fletcher, J. M., Shaywitz, S. E., Shaywitz, B. A., Torgesen, J. K., Wood, F. B., et al. (2001). Rethinking learning disabilities. In C. E. Finn, Jr., R. A. J. Rotherham, & C. R. Hokanson, Jr. (Eds.), *Rethinking special education for a new century* (pp. 259–287). Washington, DC: Thomas B. Fordham Foundation and Progressive Policy Institute.

Lyon, G. R., & Flynn, J. M. (1991). Assessing subtypes of learning disabilities. In H. L. Swanson (Ed.), *Handbook on the assessment of learning disabilities: Theory, research, and practice* (pp. 59–74). Austin, TX: Pro-Ed.

Lyon, G. R., & Moats, L. C. (1988). Critical issues in the instruction of the leaning disabled. *Journal of Consulting and Clinical Psychology, 56,* 830–835.

Lyon, G. R., & Moats, L. C. (1997). Critical conceptual and methodological considerations in reading intervention research. *Journal of Learning Disabilities, 30,* 578–588.

Lyon, G. R., Moats, L. C., & Flynn, J. M. (1988). From assessment to treatment: Linkages to interventions with children. In M. Tramontana & S. Hooper (Eds.), *Assessment issues in child neuropsychology* (pp. 182–210). New York: Plenum Press.

Lyon, G. R., & Risucci, D. (1988). Issues in the classification of learning disabilities. In K. Kavale (Ed.), *Learning disabilities: State of the art and practice* (pp. 48–61). San Diego, CA: College-Hill Press.

Lyon, G. R., Shaywitz, S. E., & Shaywitz, B. A. (2003). A definition of dyslexia. *Annals of Dyslexia, 53,* 1–14.

Mann, L. (1979). *On the trail of process.* New York: Grune & Stratton.

Maria, K. (1990). *Reading comprehension instruction: Issues and strategies.* Parkton, MD: York Press.

Mastropieri, M. A., & Scruggs, T. E. (1997). Best practices in promoting reading comprehension in students with learning disabilities: 1976 to 1996. *Remedial and Special Education, 18,* 197–214.

Mathes, P. G., Denton, C. A., Fletcher, J. M., Anthony, J. L., Francis, D. J., & Schatschneider, C. (2005). An evaluation of two reading interventions derived from diverse models. *Reading Research Quarterly, 40,* 148–183.

Mathes, P. G., Howard, J. K., Allen, S. H., & Fuchs, D. (1998). Peer-assisted learning strategies for first-grade readers: Responding to the needs of diverse learners. *Reading Research Quarterly, 33,* 62–94.

Mathes, P. G., Torgesen, J. K., & Allor, J. H. (2001). The effects of peer-assisted literacy strategies for first-grade readers with and without additional computer assisted instruction in phonological awareness. *American Educational Research Journal, 38,* 371–410.

McGraw-Hill Digital Learning. (2003). *Yearly Progress Pro.* Available from www.mhdigitallearning.com

McGuiness, C., McGuiness, D., & McGuiness, G. (1996). Phono-Graphix: A new method for remediating reading difficulties. *Annals of Dyslexia, 46,* 73–96.

McMaster, K. L., Fuchs, D., Fuchs, L. S., & Compton, D. L. (2005). Responding to nonresponders: An experimental field trial of identification and intervention methods. *Exceptional Children, 71,* 445–463.

Meichenbaum, D. (1977). *Cognitive behavior modification.* New York: Plenum Press.

Mercer, C. D., & Miller, S. P. (1992). Teaching students with learning problems in math to acquire, understand, and apply basic math facts. *Remedial and Special Education, 13,* 19–35, 61.

Miller, S. P., & Mercer, C. D. (1993). Using a graduated word problem sequence to promote problem solving skills. *Learning Disabilities Research and Practice, 8,* 169–174.

Moats, L. C. (1994a). Honing the concepts of listening and speaking: A prerequisite to the valid measurement of language behavior in children. In G. R. Lyon (Ed.), *Frames of reference for the assessment of learning disabilities: New views on measurement issues* (pp. 229–241). Baltimore: Brookes.

Moats, L. C. (1994b). The missing foundation in teacher education: Knowledge of the structure of spoken and written language. *Annals of Dyslexia, 44,* 81–102.

Moats, L. C., & Farrell, M. L. (1999). Multisensory instruction. In J. Birsh (Ed.), *Multisensory teaching of basic language skills* (pp. 1–18). Baltimore: Brookes.

Moats, L. C., & Lyon, G. R. (1993). Learning disabilities in the United States: Advocacy, science, and the future of the field. *Journal of Learning Disabilities, 26,* 282–294.

Moats, L. C., & Lyon, G. R. (1996). Wanted: Teachers with knowledge of language. *Topics in Language Disorders, 16,* 73–86.

Montague, M., Applegate, B., & Marquard, K. (1993). Cognitive strategy instruction and mathematical problem-solving performance of students with learning disabilities. *Learning Disabilities Research and Practice, 8,* 223–232.

Montague, M., & Graves, A. (1993). Improving students' story writing. *Teaching Exceptional Children, 25,* 36–37.

Morris, R. D. (2004). Clinical trials as a model for intervention research studies in education. In P. McCardle

& V. Chhabra (Eds.), *The voice of evidence in reading research* (pp. 127–149). Baltimore: Brookes.

Morris, R. D., Lyon, G. R., Alexander, D., Gray, D., Kavanagh, J., Rourke, B., et al. (1994). Proposed guidelines and criteria for describing samples of persons with learning disabilities. *Learning Disability Quarterly, 17,* 106–109.

Myers, C. A. (1978). Reviewing the literature on Fernald's technique of remedial reading. *Reading Teacher, 31,* 614–619.

Myers, P., & Hammill, D. D. (1990). *Learning disabilities: Basic concepts, assessment practices, and instructional strategies.* Austin, TX: Pro-Ed.

Naglieri, J. A., & Das, J. P. (1997). *Cognitive Assessment System interpretive handbook.* Itasca, IL: Riverside.

Naglieri, J. A., & Johnson, D. (2000). Effectiveness of a cognitive strategy intervention in improving arithmetic computation based on the PASS theory. *Journal of Learning Disabilities, 33,* 591–597.

National Center for Educational Statistics (NCES). (2003). *National Assessment of Educational Progress: The nation's report card.* Washington, DC: U.S. Department of Education.

National Joint Committee on Learning Disabilities (NJCLD). (1988). *Letter to NJCLD member organizations.* Author.

National Reading Panel (NRP). (2000). *Report of the National Reading Panel. Teaching children to read: An evidence-based assessment of the scientific research literature on reading and its implications for reading instruction: Reports of the subgroups (NIH Publication No. 00-4754).* Washington, DC: U.S. Government Printing Office.

Newby, R. F., & Lyon, G. R. (1991). Neuropsychological subtypes of learning disabilities. In J. E. Obrzut & G. W. Hynd (Eds.), *Neuropsychological foundations of learning disabilities: A handbook of issues, methods, and practice* (pp. 355–385). San Diego, CA: Academic Press.

Oakland, T., Black, J., Stanford, G., Nussbaum, N., & Balise, R. (1998). An evaluation of the dyslexia training program: A multisensory method for promoting reading in students with reading disabilities. *Journal of Learning Disabilities, 31,* 140–147.

Obrzut, J. E., & Hynd, G. W. (1983). The neurobiological and neurophysiological foundations of learning disabilities. *Journal of Learning Disabilities, 16,* 515–520.

O'Hare, F. (1973). *Sentence-combining: Improving student writing without formal grammar instruction.* Urbana, IL: National Council of Teachers of English.

O'Connor, R. E. (2000). Increasing the intensity of intervention in kindergarten and first grade. *Learning Disabilities Research and Practice, 15,* 43–54.

O'Connor, R. E., Fulmer, D., Harty, K., & Bell, K. (2001). *Total awareness: Reducing the severity of reading disability.* Paper presented at the American Educational Research Conference, Seattle, WA.

O'Connor, R. E., Notari-Syverson, N., & Vadasy, P. (1996). Ladders to Literacy: The effects of teacher-led phonological activities for kindergarten children with and without disabilities. *Exceptional Children, 63,* 117–130.

O'Connor, R. E., Notari-Syverson, N., & Vadasy, P. (1998). *Ladders to Literacy: A kindergarten activity book.* Baltimore: Brookes.

Olson, R. K., & Wise, B. W. (1992). Reading on the computer with orthographic and speech feedback: An overview of the Colorado Remedial Reading Project. *Reading and Writing: An Interdisciplinary Journal, 4,* 107–144.

Olson, R. K., & Wise, B. (in press). Computer-based remediation for reading and related phonological disabilities. In M. McKenna, L. Labbo, R. Kieffer, & D. Reinking (Eds.), *Handbook of literacy and technology* (Vol. 2). Mahwah, NJ: Erlbaum.

Open Court Reading. (1995). *Collections for young scholars.* Peru, IL: Science Research Associates/McGraw-Hill.

Owens, R. L., & Fuchs, L. S. (2002). Mathematical problem-solving strategy instruction for third-grade students with learning disabilities. *Remedial and Special Education, 23,* 268–278.

Palinscar, A., & Brown, A. (1983). *Reciprocal teaching of comprehension-monitoring activities* (Technical Report No. 269). Urbana: University of Illinois, Center for the Study of Reading.

Palinscar, A., & Brown, A. (1985). Reciprocal teaching: A means to a meaningful end. In J. Osborn, P. T. Wilson, & R. C. Anderson (Eds.), *Reading education: Foundations for a literate America* (pp. 66–87). Lexington, MA: Heath.

Palinscar, A., & Brown, A. (1987). Enhancing instructional time through attention to metacognition. *Journal of Learning Disabilities, 20,* 66–75.

Piaget, J., & Inhelder, B. (1969). *Memory and intelligence.* New York: Basic Books.

Pokorni, J. I., Worthington, C. K., & Jamison, P. J. (2004). Phonological awareness intervention: Comparison of Fast ForWord, Earobics, and LiPS. *Journal of Educational Research, 97,* 147–157.

Poplin, M. S. (1988). Holistic/constructivist principles of the teaching/learning process: Implications for the field of learning disabilities. *Journal of Learning Disabilities, 21,* 401–416.

President's Commission on Excellence in Special Education. (2002). *A new era: Revitalizing special education for children and their families.* Washington, DC: U.S. Department of Education.

Pressley, M. (2006). *Reading instruction that works* (3rd ed.). New York: Guilford Press.

Pressley, M., Gaskins, I. W., Cunicelli, E. A., Burdick, N. J., Schaub-Matt, M., Lee, D. S., et al. (1991). Strategy instruction at Benchmark School: A faculty interview study. *Learning Disability Quarterly, 14,* 19–48.

Ransby, M. J., & Swanson, H. L. (2003). Reading comprehension skills of young adults with childhood diagnosis of dyslexia. *Journal of Learning Disabilities, 36,* 538–555.

Rashotte, C. A., MacPhee, K., & Torgesen, J. K. (2001). The effectiveness of a group reading instruction program with poor readers in multiple grades. *Learning Disability Quarterly, 24,* 119–134.

Reid, D. K., & Hresko, W. P. (1981). *A cognitive approach to learning disabilities.* New York: McGraw-Hill.

Reschly, D. J., Hosp, J. L., & Smied, C. M. (2003). *And miles to go . . . : State SLD requirements and professional association recommendations.* Retrieved from www.nrcld.org

Reschly, D. J., Tilly, W. D., & Grimes, J. P. (1999). *Special education in transition: Functional assessment and noncategorical programming.* Longmont, CO: Sopris West.

Rivera, D., & Smith, D. D. (1987). Influence of modeling on acquisition and maintenance of computational skills: A summary of research findings from three sites. *Learning Disability Quarterly, 10,* 69–80.

Rosenshine, B., & Stevens, R. (1986). Teaching functions. In M. C. Wittrock (Ed.), *Handbook of research on teaching* (3rd ed., pp. 376–391). New York: Macmillan.

Ross, B. H. (1989). Distinguishing types of superficial similarities: Different effects on the access and use of earlier problems. *Journal of Experimental Psychology: Learning, Memory, and Cognition, 15,* 456–468.

Rourke, B. P., & Finlayson, M. A. J. (1978). Neuropsychological significance of variations in patterns of academic performance: Verbal and visual–spatial abilities. *Journal of Abnormal Child Psychology, 6,* 121–133.

Rouse, C. E., & Krueger, A. B. (2004). Putting computerized instruction to the test: A randomized evaluation of a "scientifically based" reading program. *Economics of Education Review, 23,* 323–338.

Saenz, L., Fuchs, L. S., & Fuchs, D. (2005). Effects of peer-assisted learning strategies on English language learners: A randomized controlled study. *Exceptional Children, 71,* 231–247.

Salomon, G., & Perkins, D. N. (1989). Rocky roads to transfer: Rethinking mechanisms of a neglected phenomenon. *Educational Psychologist, 24,* 113–142.

Schatschneider, C., Fletcher, J. M., Francis, D. J., Carlson, C. D., & Foorman, B. R. (2004). Kindergarten prediction of reading skills: A longitudinal comparative analysis. *Journal of Educational Psychology, 96,* 265–282.

Schumaker, J. B., & Deshler, D. D. (1992). Validation of learning strategy interventions for students with learning disabilities: Results of a programmatic research effort. In B. Y. L. Wong (Ed.), *Contemporary intervention research in learning disabilities: An international perspective* (pp. 22–46). New York: Springer-Verlag.

Schumaker, J. B., Deshler, D. D., & McKnight, P. (2002). Ensuring success in the secondary general education curriculum through the use of teaching routines. In M. A. Shinn, H. M. Walker, & G. Stoner (Eds.), *Interventions for academic and behavior problems II: Preventive and remedial approaches* (pp. 791–823). Bethesda, MD: National Association of School Psychologists.

Scientific Learning Corporation. (1999). *Fast ForWord companion: A comprehensive guide to the training exercises.* Berkeley, CA: Author.

Seabaugh, G. O., & Schumaker, J. B. (1993). The effects of self-regulation training on the academic productivity of secondary students with learning problems. *Journal of Behavioral Education, 4,* 109–133.

Shanahan, T. (2004). Critiques of the National Reading Panel Report: Their implications for research, policy, and practice. In P. McCardle & V. Chhabra (Eds.), *The voice of evidence in reading research* (pp. 235–265). Baltimore: Brookes.

Shanahan, T., & Barr, R. (1995). Reading Recovery: An independent evaluation of the effects of an early instructional intervention for at-risk learners. *Reading Research Quarterly, 30,* 958–996.

Shankweiler, D., & Liberman, I. Y. (1989). *Phonology and reading disability.* Ann Arbor: University of Michigan Press.

Share, D., & Stanovich, K. (1995). Cognitive processes in early reading development: Accommodating individual differences into a model of acquisition. *Issues in Education: Contributions to Educational Psychology, 1,* 1–57.

Shavelson, R., & Towne, L. (2002). *Science and education.* Washington, DC: National Academy of Sciences.

Shaywitz, B. A., Shaywitz, S. E., Blachman, B., Pugh, K. R., Fulbright, R. K., Skudlarski, P., et al. (2004). Development of left occipitotemporal systems for skilled reading children after a phonologically-based intervention. *Biological Psychiatry, 55,* 926–933.

Shaywitz, S. E. (1996). Dyslexia. *Scientific American, 275,* 98–104.

Shaywitz, S. E., Fletcher, J. M., Holahan, J. M., Schneider, A. E., Marchione, K. E., Stuebing, K. K., et al. (1999). Persistence of dyslexia: The Connecticut longitudinal study at adolescence. *Pediatrics, 104,* 1351–1359.

Shinn, M. R. (1998). *Advanced applications of curriculum-based measurement.* New York: Guilford Press.

Siegel, L. S. (2003). Basic cognitive processes and reading disabilities. In H. L. Swanson, K. R. Harris, & S. Graham (Eds.), *Handbook of learning disabilities* (pp. 158–181). New York: Guilford Press.

Simmons, D. C., Kame'enui, E. J., Stoolmiller, M., Coyne, M. D., & Harn, B. (2003). Accelerating growth and maintaining proficiency: A two-year intervention study of kindergarten and first-grade children at-risk for reading difficulties. In B. R. Foorman (Ed.), *Preventing and remediating reading difficulties* (pp. 197–228). Baltimore: York Press.

Simos, P. G., Breier, J. I., Fletcher, J. M., Foorman, B. R., Bergman, E., Fishbeck, K., et al. (2000). Brain activation profiles in dyslexic children during nonword reading: A magnetic source imaging study. *Neuroscience Reports, 290,* 61–65.

Simos, P. G., Fletcher, J. M., Bergman, E., Breier, J. I., Foorman, B. R., Castillo, E. M., et al. (2002). Dyslexia-specific brain activation profile becomes normal following successful remedial training. *Neurology, 58,* 1203–1213.

Simos, P. G., Fletcher, J. M., Sarkari, S., Billingsley, R. L., Francis, D. J., Castillo, E. M., et al. (in press). Early development of neurophysiological processes involved in normal reading and reading disability. *Neuropsychology.*

Skinner, B. F. (1968). *The technology of teaching.* New York: Appleton-Century-Crofts.

Snow, C., Burns, M. S., & Griffin, P. (Eds.). (1998). *Preventing reading difficulties in young children.* Washington, DC: National Academy Press.

Stahl, S. A. (2004). What do we know about fluency?: Findings of the National Reading Panel. In P. McCardle & V. Chhabra (Eds.), *The voice of evidence in reading research* (pp. 187–212). Baltimore: Brookes.

Stahl, S. A., Heubach, K., & Cramond, B. (1997). *Fluency-oriented reading instruction.* Athens, GA/ Washington, DC: National Reading Research Center/U.S. Department of Education, Office of Educational Research and Improvement, Educational Resources Information Center.

Stanovich, K. E. (1991). Discrepancy definitions of reading disability: Has intelligence led us astray? *Reading Research Quarterly, 26,* 7–29.

Stanovich, K. E. (1993). The construct validity of discrepancy definition of reading disabilities. In G. R. Lyon, D. B. Gray, J. F. Kavanagh, & N. A. Krasnegor (Eds.), *Better understanding learning disabilities: New views from research and their implications for education and public policies* (pp. 273–307). Baltimore: Brookes.

Stanovich, P., & Stanovich, K. (2003). *Using research and reason in education.* Washington, DC: Partnership for Reading (U.S. Department of Education/U.S. Department of Health and Human Services).

Stecker, P. M., & Fuchs, L. S. (2000). Effecting superior achievement using curriculum-based measurement: The importance of individual progress monitoring. *Learning Disabilities Research and Practice, 15,* 128–134.

Stecker, P. M., Fuchs, L. S., & Fuchs, D. (in press). Using curriculum-based measurement to improve student achievement: Review of research. *Psychology in the Schools.*

Stern, C. A., & Stern, M. B. (1971). *Children discover arithmetic: An introduction to structural arithmetic* (rev. ed.). New York: Harper & Row.

Stevens, R., & Rosenshine, B. (1981). Advances in research on teaching. *Exceptional Education Quarterly, 2,* 1–9.

Stuebing, K. K., Fletcher, J. M., LeDoux, J. M., Lyon, G. R., Shaywitz, S. E., & Shaywitz, B. A. (2002). Validity of IQ-discrepancy classifications of reading dis-

abilities: A meta-analysis. *American Educational Research Journal, 39,* 469–518.

Swanson, H. L., Harris, K., & Graham, S. (Eds.). *Handbook of learning disabilities.* New York: Guilford Press.

Swanson, H. L., with Hoskyn, M., & Lee, C. (1999). *Interventions for students with learning disabilities: A meta-analysis of treatment outcome.* New York: Guilford Press.

Swanson, H. L., & Sachse-Lee, C. (2001). Mathematical problem solving and working memory in children with learning disabilities: Both executive and phonological processes are important. *Journal of Experimental Child Psychology, 79,* 294–321.

Swanson, H. L., & Saez, L. (2003). Memory difficulties in children and adults with learning disabilities. In H. L. Swanson, K. R. Harris, & S. Graham (Eds.), *Handbook of learning disabilities* (pp. 182–198). New York: Guilford Press.

Tangel, D. M., & Blachman, B. A. (1995). Effect of phoneme awareness instruction on the invented spelling of first-grade children: A one-year follow-up. *Journal of Reading Behavior, 27,* 153–185.

Torgesen, J. K. (1986). Learning disabilities theory: Its current state and future prospects. *Journal of Learning Disabilities, 19,* 399–407.

Torgesen, J. K. (1987). Thinking about the future by distinguishing between issues that have answers and those that do not. In S. T. Vaughn & C. S. Bos (Eds.), *Issues and future directions for research in learning disabilities* (pp. 55–64). San Diego, CA: College-Hill Press.

Torgesen, J. K. (1991). Learning disabilities: Historical and conceptual issues. In B. Wong (Ed.), *Learning about learning disabilities* (pp. 3–39). San Diego, CA: Academic Press.

Torgesen, J. K. (1993). Variations on theory in learning disabilities. In G. R. Lyon, D. B. Gray, J. F. Kavanagh, & N. A. Krasnegor (Eds.), *Better understanding learning disabilities: New views from research and their implications for education and public policies* (pp. 27–56). Baltimore: Brookes.

Torgesen, J. K. (2000). Individual responses in response to early interventions in reading: The lingering problem of treatment resisters. *Learning Disabilities Research and Practice, 15,* 55–64.

Torgesen, J. K. (2002). Empirical and theoretical support for direct diagnosis of learning disabilities by assessment of intrinsic processing weaknesses. In R. Bradley, L. Danielson, & D. Hallahan (Eds.), *Identification of learning disabilities: Research to practice* (pp. 565–650). Mahwah, NJ: Erlbaum.

Torgesen, J. K. (2004). Lessons learned from research on interventions for students who have difficulty learning to read. In P. McCardle & V. Chhabra (Eds.), *The voice of evidence in reading research* (pp. 355–382). Baltimore: Brookes.

Torgesen, J. K., Alexander, A. W., Wagner, R. K., Rashotte, C. A., Voeller, K. K. S., & Conway, T. (2001). Intensive remedial instruction for children with severe reading disabilities: Immediate and long-term outcomes from two instructional approaches. *Journal of Learning Disabilities, 34,* 33–58.

Torgesen, J. K., Rashotte, C. A., & Alexander, A. W. (2001). Principles of fluency instruction in reading: Relationships with established empirical outcomes. In M. Wolf (Ed.), *Dyslexia, fluency, and the brain* (pp. 333–356). Timonium, MD: York Press.

Torgesen, J. K., & Wagner, R. (1999). *Test of Word Reading Efficiency.* Austin, TX: Pro-Ed.

Torgesen, J. K., Wagner, R. K., & Rashotte, C. A. (1994). Longitudinal studies of phonological processing and reading. *Journal of Learning Disabilities, 27,* 276–286.

Torgesen, J. K., Wagner, R. K., Rashotte, C. A., Rose, E., Lindamood, P., Conway, J., et al. (1999). Preventing reading failure in young children with phonological processing disabilities: Group and individual responses to instruction. *Journal of Educational Psychology, 91,* 579–594.

Towne, L., & Hilton, M. (Eds.). (2004). *Implementing randomized trials: Report of a workshop.* Washington, DC: National Academy Press.

Tunmer, W. E., Chapman, J. W., & Prochnow, J. E. (2003). Preventing negative Matthew effects in at-risk readers: A retrospective study. In B. R. Foorman (Ed.), *Preventing and remediating reading difficulties* (pp. 121–164). Baltimore: York Press.

Vaughn, S., & Dammann, J. E. (2001). Science and sanity in special education. *Behavior Disorders, 27,* 21–29.

Vaughn, S., & Fuchs, L. S. (2003). Redefining learning disabilities as inadequate response to instruction: The promise and potential problems. *Learning Disabilities Research and Practice, 18,* 137–146.

Vaughn, S., Gersten, R., & Chard, D. J. (2000). The underlying message in LD intervention research: Findings from research syntheses. *Exceptional Children, 67,* 99–114.

Vaughn, S., & Klingner, J. K. (2004). Reading comprehension: Instructional/intervention frameworks. In C. A. Stone, E. R. Silliman, B. Ehren, & K. Apel (Eds.), *Handbook of language and literacy: Development and disorders.* New York: Guilford Press.

Vaughn, S., Klingner, J. K., & Bryant, D. P. (2001). Collaborative strategic reading as a means to enhance peer-mediated instruction for reading comprehension and content-area learning. *Remedial and Special Education, 22,* 66–74.

Vaughn, S., & Linan-Thompson, S. (2003). Group size and time allotted to intervention: Effects for students with reading difficulties. In B. R. Foorman (Ed.), *Preventing and remediating reading difficulties* (pp. 299–324). Baltimore: York Press.

Vaughn, S., Linan-Thompson, S., & Hickman, P. (2003). Response to treatment as a means of identifying students with reading/learning disabilities. *Exceptional Children, 69,* 391–409.

Vaughn, S., Moody, S. W., & Schumm, J. S. (1998). Broken promises: Reading instruction in the resource room. *Exceptional Children, 64,* 211–225.

Vellutino, F. R. (1979). *Dyslexia: Theory and research.* Cambridge, MA: MIT Press.

Vellutino, F. R., Fletcher, J. M., Scanlon, D. M., & Snowling, M. J. (2004). Specific reading disability (dyslexia): What have we learned in the past four decades? *Journal of Child Psychiatry and Psychology, 45,* 2–40.

Vellutino, F. R., Scanlon, D. M., & Jaccard, J. (2003). Toward distinguishing between cognitive and experiential deficits as primary sources of difficulty in learning to read: A two-year follow-up to difficult to remediate and readily remediated poor readers. In B. R. Foorman (Ed.), *Preventing and remediating reading difficulties* (pp. 73–120). Baltimore: York Press.

Vellutino, F. R., Scanlon, D. M., Sipay, E. R., Small, S. G., Pratt, A., Chen, R., et al. (1996). Cognitive profiles of difficult-to-remediate and readily remediated poor readers: Early intervention as a vehicle for distinguishing between cognitive and experimental deficits as basic causes of specific reading disability. *Journal of Educational Psychology, 88,* 601–638.

Wadsworth, S. J., Olson, R. K., Pennington, B. F., & DeFries, J. C. (2000). Differential genetic etiology of reading disability as a function of IQ. *Journal of Learning Disabilities, 33,* 192–199.

Wesson, C. L. (1991). Curriculum-based measurement and two models of follow-up consultation. *Exceptional Children, 57,* 246–257.

Wesson, C. L., Skiba, R., Sevcik, B., King, R., & Deno, S. (1984). The effects of technically adequate instructional data on achievement. *Remedial and Special Education, 5,* 17–22.

White, W. A. T. (1988). A meta-analysis of the effects of direct instruction in special education. *Education and Treatment of Children, 11,* 364–374.

Wilder, A. A., & Williams, J. P. (2001). Students with severe learning disabilities can learn higher-order comprehension skills. *Journal of Educational Psychology, 93,* 268–278.

Williams, J. P. (2002). Using the Theme Scheme to improve story comprehension. In C. C. Block & M. Pressley (Eds.), *Comprehension instruction: Research-based best practices* (pp. 126–139). New York: Guilford Press.

Williams, J. P. (2003). Teaching text structure to improve reading comprehension. In H. L. Swanson, K. R. Harris, & S. Graham (Eds.), *Handbook of learning disabilities* (pp. 293–305). New York: Guilford Press.

Williams, J. P., Brown, L. G., Silverman, A. K., & deCani, J. S. (1994). An instructional program for adolescents with learning disabilities in the comprehension of narrative themes. *Learning Disability Quarterly, 17,* 205–221.

Williams, J. P., Hall, K. M., & Lauer, K. D. (2004). Teaching expository text structure to young at-risk learners: Building the basics of comprehension instruction. *Exceptionality, 12,* 129–144.

Williams, J. P., Lauer, K. D., Hall, K. M., Lord, K. M., Gugga, S. S., Bak, S. J., et al. (2002). Teaching elementary students to identify story themes. *Journal of Educational Psychology, 94*, 235–248.

Wise, B., Ring, J., & Olson, R. K. (1999). Training phonological awareness with and without attention to articulation. *Journal of Experimental Child Psychology, 72*, 271–304.

Wise, B., Ring, J., & Olson, R. K. (2000). Individual differences in gains from computer-assisted remedial reading with more emphasis on phonological analysis or accurate reading in context. *Journal of Experimental Child Psychology, 77*, 197–235.

Wolf, M., & Bowers, P. G. (1999). The double deficit hypothesis for the developmental dyslexias. *Journal of Educational Psychology, 91*, 415–438.

Wolf, M., & Katzir-Cohen, T. (2001). Reading fluency and its intervention. *Scientific Studies of Reading, 5*, 211–239.

Wolf, M., Miller, L., & Donnelly, K. (2002). Retrieval, Automaticity, Vocabulary Elaboration, Orthography (RAVE-O): A comprehensive, fluency-based reading intervention program. *Journal of Learning Disabilities, 33*, 375–386.

Wolf, M., O'Brien, B., Adams, K. D., Joffe, T., Jeffrey, J., Lovett, M., et al. (2003). Working for time: Reflections on naming speed, reading fluency, and intervention. In B. R. Foorman (Ed.), *Preventing and remediating reading difficulties* (pp. 355–380). Baltimore: York Press.

Wong, B. Y. L. (1985). Issues in cognitive-behavior interventions in academic skill areas. *Journal of Abnormal Child Psychology, 13*, 425–442.

Wong, B. Y. L. (1986). Metacognition and special education: A review of a view. *Journal of Special Education, 20*, 9–29.

Wong, B. Y. L. (1991). The relevance of metacognition to learning disabilities. In B. Y. L. Wong (Ed.), *Learning about learning disabilities* (pp. 231–258). San Diego, CA: Academic Press.

Woodcock, R., McGrew, K., & Mather, N. (2001). *Woodcock–Johnson III Tests of Achievement*. Itasca, IL: Riverside.

Woodward, J., Howard, J., & Battle, R. (1997). *Learning subtraction in the third and fourth grade: What develops over time* (Tech. Rep. No. 97-21). Tacoma, WA: University of Puget Sound.

Ysseldyke, J. E., & Marston, D. (1999). Origins of categorical special education services in schools and a rationale for changing them. In D. Reschly, W. Tilly, & J. Grimes (Eds.), *Special education in transition* (pp. 1–18). Longmont, CO: Sopris West.

Zigmond, N. (1993). Learning disabilities from an educational perspective. In G. R. Lyon, D. B. Gray, J. F. Kavanagh, & N. A. Krasnegor (Eds.), *Better understanding learning disabilities: New views from research and their implications for education and public policies* (pp. 251–272). Baltimore: Brookes.

Zigmond, N. (2003). Searching for the most effective service delivery model for students with learning disabilities. In H. L. Swanson, K. R. Harris, & S. Graham (Eds.), *Handbook of learning disabilities* (pp. 110–124). New York: Guilford Press.

V

CHILDREN AT RISK

9

Child Physical Abuse and Neglect

Sandra T. Azar and David A. Wolfe

Although the number of children reported as abused and neglected in the United States continues to remain high (almost 3 million cases are reported to authorities each year; Administration on Children, Youth and Families [ACYF], 2004), systems put in place to combat this problem have not kept pace with children's needs or those of their families (Burns et al., 2004; Cicchetti & Toth, 2003; Swenson, Brown, & Sheidow, 2003). As many as one-half of maltreated children have clinically significant emotional and behavioral problems; yet only one-third to one-fourth receive mental health services (Burns et al., 2004; National Research Council, 1993), even if they are placed under state care (Garland, Landsverk, Hough, & Ellis-McLeod, 1996). More importantly, a significant proportion cannot return home once placed in foster care, because the services needed by their families are not available to make their homes safe enough for their return. Another group return home only to be maltreated again and return to foster care.

Research evidence has grown documenting the many negative sequelae of maltreatment for children and the many other inadequacies that have been found in their lives—such as the lack of a stable home environment, of positive interactions with adults and siblings, and of opportunities for learning prosocial behavior—that often coexist with maltreatment and potentiate its impact (Azar & Bober, 1999; Wolfe, 1999). Despite the fact that a federal panel dubbed the situation a national emergency over a decade ago (U.S. Advisory Board on Child Abuse and Neglect [USABCAN], 1990, 1993), empirically

validated treatment efforts have not been carefully implemented in any widespread manner. Approaches that have been implemented (e.g., family preservation efforts) have been inconsistent in terms of their effectiveness (Fraser, Nelson, & Rivard, 1997; Fraser, Pecora, & Haapala, 1997; Staudt & Drake, 2002).

In the wake of children languishing in foster care and the unclear effectiveness of such approaches, society has become restless. Instead of calling for the implementation of better interventions, legal efforts have stepped up that allow children to be more easily removed from their parents once abuse and neglect has occurred (e.g., the Adoption and Safe Families Act of 1997; laws allowing for long-term guardianship by kin). As well, limited funding has been directed at efforts to prevent abuse and neglect from occurring in the first place. Whether the emphasis on the latter two approaches will mean better lives for children, as opposed to more concerted efforts at treating identified parents using the approaches outlined in this chapter, remains to be seen. According to some observers, the biggest obstacle for preventing harm to children has been the lack of persistence in carrying out any one policy in the field (Daro & Donnelly, 2002).

This chapter describes available promising behavioral and cognitive behavioral approaches to the treatment of child physical abuse and neglect (see also Saunders, Berliner, & Hanson, 2003). (Child sexual abuse, another form of maltreatment that can occur with physical abuse and neglect, is covered by V. V. Wolfe in Chapter 10 of this volume.) We outline many of the critical issues that have arisen in the child abuse and neglect treatment field over the past decade (e.g., legal changes that have occurred affecting families), and offer suggestions for advancing clinical practice and research. Reasons for the lack of progress in the treatment arena are many and are discussed at the end of this chapter.

We first provide an overview of the child, parent, and family factors that contribute to or result from child maltreatment (the term "maltreatment" is used to refer to physical abuse and to physical and emotional neglect; the more specific terms are used in referring to each specific type). A conceptual framework is presented to offer a theoretical basis for understanding the development of abusive and neglectful behavior over time, and to assist treatment planners in the recognition of major family "symptoms" that foretell greater risk of maltreatment. This framework is accompanied by an assessment overview that focuses on the general needs of the family and the specific needs of the parent and child. Treatment methods that have shown promise or have received empirical support with maltreating families are then discussed in detail. Although our understanding of the impact of maltreatment on children has progressed considerably (Cicchetti & Toth, 2003; Wekerle & Wolfe, 2003), strategies for treatment and prevention remain inadequate (Becker et al., 1995). In particular, studies of treatment outcomes with children continue to be few and far between (Azar, 2005; Azar & Bober, 1999; Fantuzzo, 1990).

In our overview of treatments, we emphasize the use of behavioral and cognitive-behavioral approaches, since these methods have received the most empirical support. The data on family preservation efforts that mix an intensive case management approach with other treatment modalities are also highlighted, as well as newer approaches that have arisen from attachment theory and are directed at parents of infants and toddlers. In some respects, these latter efforts overlap with many techniques based on social learning theory (e.g., attachment interventions that work with parental narratives and involve strategies that are similar to cognitive restructuring; Azar, Nix, & Makin-Byrd, 2005). We also outline special issues and precautions required with this population (e.g., difficulties regarding engagement and trust). New directions in prevention are given special consideration, with the hope that these promising approaches will receive further expansion and research.

DEFINITION AND SCOPE

Conceptual Definition

Parents who abuse their children are often seen as being categorically distinct from nonabusive parents. That is, abusive behavior is so difficult to comprehend that a false dichotomy can surface inadvertently to separate and define "abusive" parents in relation to "normal" parents (Wolfe, 1999). However, such a clear distinction does not exist. All parents' behavior toward their offspring changes dramatically at any given moment in response to child- or situation-related demands, and at times this behavior includes negative interactions. What most often distinguishes parents who have been reported for abuse from socioeconomically matched parents who have not is the chronic and escalating pattern of parent–child conflict, culminating in more and more serious harm over time (Knutson & Bower, 1994). Similarly, neglectful parents are usually distinguished by the chronicity and severity of their behavior over time, rather than by single exceptional events (Hildyard & Wolfe, 2002). Moreover, what may make this pattern most detrimental to children is that it occurs in the absence of compensatory factors (e.g., positive interactions, a strong social support network), which are crucial in facilitating their social, cognitive, and emotional development. Thus, rather than being distinct from other parental actions, child abuse and neglect must be conceived along a continuum with other parenting behavior (Azar, Barnes, & Twentyman, 1988; Wolfe, 1991). At one extreme of the continuum are those practices considered to be most harmful and inappropriate (such as striking a child with a dangerous object, burns, physical and emotional rejection, etc.); at the other extreme are methods that promote the child's social, emotional, and intellectual development. From this perspective, child abuse and neglect can be defined, for treatment purposes, in terms of the degree to which a parent (1) uses aversive or inappropriate control strategies with his or her child, and/or (2) fails to provide minimal standards of caregiving and nurturance (Wolfe, 1999), and/or (3) adopts a negative and rejecting stance toward the child that fails to promote the child's positive development (Azar, 1989a). Accordingly, child abuse is not necessarily viewed as a symptom of an undefined personality disorder, but rather is conceptualized as a breakdown in a parent's emotional and behavioral self-regulation and control during interactions with his or her child. The psychological mechanisms associated with such lack of control (e.g., thought processes, emotional responses, behavioral skills deficits) have received greater attention in recent studies (Azar, Robinson, Hekimian, & Twentyman, 1984; Bugental et al., 1993; Caselles & Milner, 2000), clarifying the extent to which abusive behavior is a function of characteristics of the individual (e.g., personality disturbance, cognitive styles, executive functioning problems) and of situational factors that foster such behavior (e.g., aversive child behavior, marital/couple conflict, unmanageable stress, violent neighborhoods).

The previous definition of child abuse and neglect for treatment-planning purposes does not imply that the consequences of maltreatment are not serious for children. Maltreatment was responsible for over 1,400 child deaths in 2000 alone, with 30% of these from physical abuse, 38% from neglect alone, and another 29% from multiple maltreatment types combined (ACYF, 2004). Rather, this viewpoint focuses our attention on those aspects of abuse that resemble "typical" parenting methods except in terms of their severity. Furthermore, it broadens our view of parental capacities that are inadequate to meet the child's needs, such as the absence of physical attention or praise, failures in supervision, or the delivery of unclear directives from the parent (Azar, 1986, 1989a).

This view of child maltreatment as a part of a breakdown in the caretaking system suggests that such caretakers possess maladaptive schemas regarding the socialization process (i.e., cultural values; overly rigid, inappropriate, and inflexible parent–child role schemas and norms). These schemas permit the use of violence as a means of interpersonal control and problem solving, and justify failures in care (Azar & Weinzierl, 2005). Essentially, in maltreating families the usual balances between reward and punishment and between discipline and affection have broken down, and failures exist in the contingencies between parent

and child behavior (e.g., maternal negative responses to prosocial child behavior; Cerezo, D'Ocon, & Dolz, 1996). As a result, these children's developmental accomplishments and progress often fall behind. Families have ceased to promote healthy socialization.

Incidence and Profile of Child Abuse and Neglect

In 2002, over 3 million reports of suspected child abuse and neglect occurred—a figure that has changed very little over the last decade (ACYF, 2004). Numbers identified officially by child protection services (CPS) are often smaller than those found in community surveys (Sedlak & Broadhurst, 1996). A national survey, for example, estimated that only 28% of the cases found through sampling in the community (e.g., hospitals, schools) that met criteria for abuse were known to CPS, which was a sharp decline from previous figures (Sedlak & Broadhurst, 1996). Since national incidence data do not show a change in identified cases, this discrepancy suggests that agencies have reached their capacities in terms of resources to investigate cases, or that underreporting is occurring. More importantly, not all reported cases are substantiated, due to lack of evidence or subthreshold forms of abuse or neglect; even if a case is substantiated, limited resources may mean that the family receives little in terms of services needed. Thus many children may remain unprotected despite the fact that someone sees them as at risk, and their families may not be provided with needed resources.

Maltreatment situations are classified into four major types: physical abuse, neglect, sexual abuse, and emotional abuse. (As noted earlier, we concentrate in this chapter on physical abuse and on neglect. See V. V. Wolfe, Chapter 10, this volume, for a discussion of sexual abuse.) The legally identified categories of neglect and physical abuse are umbrella terms for heterogeneous sets of events. For example, Zuravin (1991) defined the following types of behaviors included in neglect: supervisory neglect; refusal to provide, or delay in providing, health or mental health care; custody refusal or related neglect; abandonment/desertion; failure to provide a home; personal hygiene; housing hazards or poor sanitation; nutritional neglect; and educational neglect. Some definitions of neglect also include emotional neglect (a marked indifference to children's need for affection, attention and emotional support), as well as exposure to chronic or extreme spousal abuse. Emotional abuse has been seen as both central to all maltreatment and as a distinct entity. It includes acts that are psychologically damaging to children (e.g., rejecting, terrorizing, degrading; Brassard, Germain, & Hart, 1987; Hart, Brassard, Binggeli, & Davidson, 2002). Although somewhat less heterogeneous, physical abuse can include everything from restraining a child inappropriately (e.g., locking him or her in closets for long periods) to beating with an electric cord, breaking bones, or threatening with a gun or knife. Clearly, such heterogeneity has been difficult to capture in a single theory of etiology and makes understanding the impact difficult. The reader is referred to a report by the World Health Organization (1999) for further clarification of these definitions and distinctions.

The rate of maltreatment reports has remained constant in recent years (35.9 per 1,000 children in the U.S. population). Based on official cases substantiated by CPS, child neglect continues to be the most common form of maltreatment: 60.5% of cases in 2002 (or almost 7.22 children out of every 1,000 children in the United States). Physical abuse accounted for 18.6% of child protection cases, or 2.2 children per 1,000 children in the United States. These figures have remained relatively stable over the last few years, after many decades of dramatic increases (ACYF, 2004). However, these figures may underestimate the actual number of children exposed to these forms of maltreatment by more than 300%, based on community surveys. Types of maltreatment often co-occur, and over multiple reports, many cases appear to move from one type to another (English, Marshall, & Orme, 1999). The sequelae of maltreatment may vary with the forms experienced, as well as their severity, their frequency, and the points at which they occurred in children's lives. Although maltreatment occurs at all ages, younger children are more likely to be reported for physical neglect, latency-age children for emotional neglect (such as witnessing spousal abuse), and teens for physical abuse (Sedlak & Broadhurst, 1996). Gender differences in rates of child victims in physical abuse and neglect are generally insignificant.

A sociodemographic profile of families reported for child abuse and neglect illuminates many of the cultural and social forces that determine child-rearing methods, and that at the same time may contribute to family discord and violence. Although maltreatment occurs in all socioeconomic groups, clinical reports, surveys, and official statistics consistently find that it is most likely to happen among the poor or disadvantaged (Sedlak & Broadhurst, 1996; Freissthler, 2004). Although the association with poverty has been found consistently (Pelton, 1994), more fine-grained studies have found that situational factors may determine rates of maltreatment within families that are faced with economic deprivation. Garbarino and Sherman (1980) found, for example, that the available resources within poor neighborhoods may determine the rates of maltreatment that occur. Similarly, the relationship of family structure to maltreatment deserves consideration. Children living in single-parent homes are at significantly greater risk of both physical abuse and neglect, and those living in father-only homes are almost twice as likely to be physically abused as those living with mothers alone (Sedlak & Broadhurst, 1996). Furthermore, qualitative work suggests that biases may exist in where CPS directs its efforts. Farmer and Owen (1998) found that work is often directed at mothers as opposed to fathers, even if the fathers are the perpetrators. They suggest that this shift in focus may in part be due to fears of violent males on the part of largely female caseworkers.

Perpetrator characteristics are also relevant to treatment approaches. Children's birth parents or parent figures (stepparents, adoptive parents) are the predominant perpetrators of all forms of child maltreatment (81.0% of cases in 2002; ACYF, 2004). Figures vary by gender and type of maltreatment, however. Consistent with the fact that mothers and mother substitutes tend to be the primary caretakers, mothers are labeled as the perpetrators in 87% of all neglect cases and 93% of cases of child physical neglect. This is true despite the fact that fathers or male parental figures may be equally culpable (e.g., neglect may be in part due to their lack of child support payments or to the fact that available funds are used for their substance abuse). In contrast, community survey data indicate that abuse in all categories was more often perpetrated by males: 67% of all abused, 89% of sexual abuse, 63% of emotional abuse, and 58% of physical abuse was committed by males (Sedlak & Broadhurst, 1996).

THEORETICAL–CONCEPTUAL FORMULATIONS

Distinctions between different theoretical formulations of child abuse and neglect have become less clear, which may reflect the fact that they share important commonalities and do not necessarily represent radically opposed viewpoints of maltreating parents (Wolfe, 1985). Much of the theoretical work in the area has focused on physical abuse, although there has been some attempts to address both abuse and neglect together (see Wekerle & Wolfe, 2003, and Azar, Povilaitis, Lauretti, & Pouquette, 1997, for further details on available theories). Attempts have also been made at models that view maltreatment as sharing causal antecedents with other forms of harm to children (e.g., unintentional childhood injury; Azar & Weinzierl, 2005; Peterson & Brown, 1994). Available models vary in emphasis placed on the cause of maltreatment as nested within the parent/family versus the situation or the broader sociocultural milieu (Azar, 1991b; Belsky, 1980).

The major theories of child abuse focus primarily on explanations as to *why* a parent might abuse a child, and *how* family process can develop into violent interactions (see Azar, 1991b; Azar et al., 1997; Wekerle & Wolfe, 2003). Three major tenets are at the core of these discussions. The first of these tenets relates to the importance of recognizing and studying the *context* of maltreatment, such as the nature of family life, environmental stressors, and sociodemographic factors. Maltreatment most often occurs in a context of social, family, and community deprivation. Such deprivation may be the force that transforms predisposed, high-risk parents into abusive or neglectful ones (see Freissthler, 2004, and Garbarino & Stocking, 1980).

Level of stress in the environment of an abusive parent increases the probability that family violence will surface as an attempt to gain control or cope with irritating, stressful events. In the case of neglect, stress may be so great as to cause parents to withdraw entirely from their responsibilities as an avoidant coping strategy. Thus maltreatment is not seen as an isolated social phenomenon or a personality defect of the parents per se; rather, this view maintains that "normal" parents may be socialized into harmful child care practices through the interaction of cultural, community, and familial influences (Belsky, 1980; Parke, 1977).

Supporting this tenet are studies indicating that, for example, socioeconomic factors (e.g., unemployment, restricted opportunities, poor housing) account for a large proportion of the variance in rates of child abuse and neglect reports (Freissthler, 2004; Garbarino, 1976; Steinberg, Catalano, & Dooley, 1981), and that even within these overt indicators of deprivation, important qualities of the social fabric of communities and social networks can further increase risk (e.g., neighborhood social and environmental resources; Freissthler, 2004; Garbarino & Sherman, 1980). Context is a critical factor in determining treatment goals and obstacles to treatment gains, as discussed later in this chapter.

The second major tenet of child abuse theories relates to the social-interactional *process* that is ongoing between parent and child. This process resembles similar ones that occur in "normal" and in clinically distressed parent–child relationships, such as the reciprocation of aversive/coercive behavior, reinforcement of inappropriate behavior, ineffective use of punishment, avoidance, and conditioned emotional arousal. This transactional process approaches the etiology and maintenance of abuse in terms of the dynamic interplay among individual, family, and social factors in relation to both past events (e.g., parents' attachment relationships with their own caregivers; Lieberman & Zeanah, 1999) and present conditions (e.g., a demanding child, domestic violence, parental depression) that shape the parent–child relationship. Although parental characteristics are considered important determinants of an abusive episode, the emphasis is mostly upon the *processes* that define the relationship between the parent and child; these are not limited only to observable behaviors, such as parental criticisms, child behavior problems, yelling, or displays of anger and aggression. The relevance of cognitive and affective processes—such as intelligence, relational schema or expectancies of relationships, executive functioning capacities (e.g., problem-solving capacities, appraisal or attributional style), depression, and anger—also emerge in studies as potentially relevant to how abusive parents process the stressful aspects of their environment (Azar & Weinzierl, 2005; Balge & Milner, 2000; Caselles & Milner, 2003; Mammen, Kolko, & Pikonis, 2002, 2003; Milner, 2003).

The third tenet involves the learning-based explanations for aggressive behavior that are implicit in the two previous explanations. Particularly relevant to an understanding of the escalation from punishment to abuse are the psychological processes linking mood states and emotional arousal to the disinhibition of aggression. It comes as no surprise that an individual's behavior can be greatly influenced by his or her mood and/or relative state of quiescence versus arousal. Negative experiences with intimate others have affective "tags" when stored in memory (Bower, 1981). When memories of these negative experiences are primed by current situations, the recollection of the event may bias or overshadow the person's mood at the time. Thus a parent's previous mood of distress and anger toward others or the child may be recalled by the child's current expression or behavior, even though it is not necessarily provocative. In turn, an overgeneralized (i.e., more angry, more aggressive) response by the parent may occur. Presumably, the adult's behavior toward the child may be potentiated by these conditioning experiences (Berkowitz, 1983; Todorov & Bargh, 2002; Vasta, 1982). Cognitive formulations have also emphasized the role that stable, maladaptive, preexisting relational schemas and scripts play in triggering an abusive episode, as well as misjudgments in providing care (Azar, 1986, 1989a, 1997; Azar et al., 2005). That is, the abusive parent's schemas for the parent's and child's roles are overly rigid and inappropriate, such that the realities of parenting constantly violate them and produce distress.

The person's level of arousal and his or her beliefs about the *source* of this arousal play a critical role in determining the actual expression of aggression. An abusive parent, for example, may have been angered and aroused (i.e., hyperalert, tense, anxious, in a state of emotional reactivity) by a previous encounter with someone (an employer, neighbor, motorist, etc.), which lowers his or her threshold for anger and aggression with others (e.g., family members). These feelings of anger create a need for justification, such as blaming others for feeling angry, upset, and bothered, which in return encourages further anger and aggression. Because of the child's availability and lower-status position, he or she becomes a likely target for this blaming process. The resulting anger and arousal interfere with rational problem solving, such that the parent's awareness of the outcome of his or her actions is diminished, and the disciplinary behaviors come under control of emotional and reflexive factors (Vasta, 1982). In this state, the physical punishment may be prolonged, and the act itself can become invigorating or cathartic (see Zillman, 1979). Short of losing emotional control, the parent may avoid the child altogether and, as a result, be unavailable to monitor her or his behavior or to provide needed caregiving; this unavailability can lead in the extreme to neglectful behavior (Azar & Weinzierl, 2005).

Cognitive formulations have also argued for preexisting parental executive functioning deficits (e.g., maladaptive expectancies, generally poor problem-solving capacities), which increase the probability of heightened frustration and of narrowed information-processing capacities under conditions of situational and child-rearing stress (Azar, 1989a, 1997; Milner, 1993). In addition, over time, the blaming of a child may solidify into an attributional bias, so that even unintentional aversive child behavior becomes cause for an excessive negative retaliation. How parents gradually acquire the preconditions that lead to the rather sudden onset of an abusive episode or to chronic rejection and neglect remains a critical concern for treatment planning. Different approaches to intervention may be more relevant at different stages in the development of the preconditions of maltreatment.

The role of information-processing disturbances has been highlighted (see Azar, 1989a, 1997; Azar & Twentyman, 1986; Azar et al., 2005; Crittenden, 1993; Milner, 2003). This perspective attempts to explain the full breadth of disturbed transactions in abusive and neglectful families beyond those involving child noncompliance. Parents may misperceive or mislabel typical child behavior in ways that lead to developmentally maladaptive responses (e.g., neglectful behavior), and disturbances in executive functioning capacities (e.g., problem solving) may lead as well as to greater frustration and aggression. One possibility is that parents at risk for abusive and neglectful behavior have disturbed assumptions regarding the role of parents in children's lives (e.g., "A good parent has absolute control over his or her children"), as well as appropriate behaviors to expect from children (Azar et al., 2005). For example, some abusive and neglectful parents view children as having the perspective-taking capacities of adults—that is, as being capable of understanding from a young age what their parents are thinking and feeling—and adjust their behavior accordingly. Children inevitably violate these unrealistic standards, and this can result in tension in the family system. Such schemas also lead parents to fail to respond in appropriate ways regarding the developmental needs of children. Parents may make less use of explanation, because they believe that children "know" what they are doing or what is expected of them. Even when a child is behaving appropriately, a parent may believe that he or she is being noncompliant. Because such parents misperceive the meaning of child behavior, their children's needs for information, stimulation, and basic care and monitoring are less likely to be met, resulting in potential neglect situations (e.g., leaving young children alone in an apartment, with the belief that they can handle such situations).

Over time, because children continually fail to behave as parents believe children "should," children may be seen as intentionally withholding appropriate responses and resisting the parents' efforts. Parents may attribute such behavior to children's "disposition," which strengthens their expectations for further misbehavior. Negative self-attributions may result (e.g., "I'm a lousy mother; other mothers can get their kids to do these things"), leaving parents with a lowered sense of self-efficacy in their role as parents and making the tasks involved less rewarding (Christensen, Brayden, Dietrich, & McLaughlin, 1994). Parents may consequently avoid attempts to address their children's needs. At other times they may take actions to discipline what they see as their children's blatant provocative behavior, but because their responses are coercive, they do not facilitate the children's emotional, social, and behavioral development. Indeed, through processes of reciprocity, children may actually become more coercive in response, validating parental biases.

Research has begun to document the existence of such cognitive disturbances and to link them to parental responses. Abusive and at-risk parents, for example, have been shown to have higher levels of unrealistic expectations regarding both the social-cognitive and physical care capacities of children (e.g., beliefs that a 3-year-old can comfort them when they are upset, that a 4-year-old can pick out the right clothing for the weather, or that a teenager can help patch up their marital/couple problems) (Azar et al., 1984; Azar & Rohrbeck, 1986; Haskett, Scott, Grant, Ward, & Robinson, 2003). Child-

abusing parents have also shown a negative attributional bias in interpreting child behavior (Azar, 1989a; Caselles & Milner, 2000; Haskett et al., 2003; Larrance & Twentyman, 1983). Unrealistic expectations and attributions of negative intent to children have both been linked to higher levels of punishment assigned to aversive child behavior and to lower use of explanation (a more adaptive parenting strategy; Azar, 1991a, 1991b; Barnes & Azar, 1990). Indeed, maltreating parents are more likely to define punishment as a central feature of what they should do in rearing their children, and are less likely to see inductive reasoning strategies as effective (Caselles & Milner, 2000). These cognitive factors have also been linked to social workers' ratings of family dysfunction and child jeopardy, as well as to lower parental empathy (Azar, 1989b).

Finally, Miller and Azar (1996) showed that mothers at risk for child abuse displayed a more generalized attributional bias, making more internal attributions for negative outcomes for others as well as themselves. The finding that child-abusing parents appear to assign more responsibility to their children for negative outcomes (e.g., the children are intentionally misbehaving or "out to get" the parents; Haskett et al., 2003; Larrance & Twentyman, 1983) is particularly important, in light of evidence suggesting that the extent to which children are held responsible for negative behavior influences the severity of punishment deemed appropriate by parents (Dix, Ruble, & Zambarano, 1989). Such an attributional bias may also explain why abusive parents see themselves as having less control as parents, which has likewise been associated with parents' physiological arousal and negative affect when interacting with behaviorally challenging children (Bugental et al., 1993; Bugental, Brown, & Reiss, 1996). Such appraisals would heighten the probability that children will be harshly treated.

Similar processes may play a role in neglect. Peterson and Brown (1994) argue that unrealistic expectations may lead to a lack of supervision, which can result in childhood injuries. Parents may underestimate their infants' motor abilities and curiosity (Roberts & Wright, 1982) and overestimate their children's ability to maintain their own physical safety. The same types of self-appraisals and child appraisals discussed above have been linked to neglectful parental behavior. Perceptions of low parental control have been shown to predict parental neglect and failure to provide a physically safe environment (Bugental & Happaney, 2004). Parents who believe that children's injuries are due to fate and beyond their control (misattributions) are less likely to take the remedial actions necessary for children to learn safety rules (Peterson, Bartelstone, Kern, & Gillis, 1995).

The task of professionals dealing with such distressed families is to interrupt these processes and to intervene in such a way as to restore the families' ability to cope with external demands and provide for the developmental and socialization needs of their children. Cognitive and behavioral assessment and intervention approaches show much promise in assisting in this task.

TREATMENT ISSUES WITH MALTREATING FAMILIES

Early treatments for physical abuse (e.g., lay counseling, psychotherapy, and provisions of support services) were too narrow in scope to produce changes in the disturbed family interaction patterns that are central to maltreatment. By the late 1970s, national evaluation studies indicated high recidivism rates both during and after treatment (Cohn, 1979; Herrenkohl, Herrenkohl, Egolf, & Seech, 1979). Family preservation efforts followed, in which short-term intensive case management was instituted for families where parents were in danger of losing custody of their children due to safety concerns (Staudt & Drake, 2002). However, such efforts were found to produce inconsistent results. Better results were found for families of older children with behavioral problems than for families of younger children (Fraser, Nelson, et al., 1997), and for more motivated families than for families with lower levels of motivation (Bitoni, 2002).

Approaches based on social learning theory have targeted child-rearing attitudes, skill deficiencies (e.g., ability to identify safety hazards, child management skills), and anger control. These efforts adapted well-developed behavioral methods such as child management skills training, stress and anger management training, and cognitive restructuring approaches (e.g., Barkley, 2000; Dangel & Polster, 1984; McMahon & Forehand, 1984; Novaco, 1975) for use with this population, to improve parents' abilities to address all areas driving maltreating behavior (e.g., managing context, improving individual skill deficits, and facilitating more positive social-interactional processes).

Approaches based on social learning theory also address characteristics of abusive and neglectful parents that often impede treatment efforts (e.g., lower cognitive functioning; Feldman, 1998; Schilling & Schinke, 1984; Tymchuk, 1992, 1998). Such approaches are often more effective than insight-oriented ones with less sophisticated clients and those of lower socioeconomic status, because they are concrete and problem-focused (Kazdin & Polster, 1973), and they match such clients' expectations that psychological treatments should be prescriptive like medical treatments (Lorion, 1978; Wood & Baker, 1999).

Along with these benefits, there are some limitations in the use of behavioral approaches. First, some parents suffer from long-standing personality disorders or severe disturbances (e.g., psychosis, substance abuse), which may require long-term psychiatric and pharmacological treatment. Such approaches may precede or replace behavioral treatment when necessary. For example, material from parents' own childhood may require specific attention. This can be done within cognitive work through a focus on attachment history. Clearly, child psychopathology and disabilities must be attended to as well. For example, a child with a pervasive developmental disability may tax even a well-functioning parent, and efforts to provide respite may be required. The intervention needs of the child need to be addressed as well. Some of the treatments discussed later have built-in strategies to address children's issues (e.g., multisystemic approaches with adolescents involved with the juvenile court system). Second, legal involvement may interfere with clients' motivation (e.g., fear that the observations required in such work may be used against them). More is said about this problem later in the chapter.

A third limitation in behavioral methods is related to the requirement that parents practice new strategies with children, which may not be possible if children are in foster care and parents have limited visitation. Role playing and special supervised visitation arrangements may be viable interim solutions to this problem in cases where reunification is a goal. Fourth, behavioral approaches alone may not be enough for families with many other pressing needs, such as unemployment and homelessness. Supplemental efforts may be required. For example, the requirements of Temporary Assistance to Needy Families (TANF; i.e., welfare funding) that parents work may compete with attendance at parenting programs.

Finally, a more general and less easily resolved limitation to the application of behavioral treatment strategies has to do with our understanding of child maltreatment as a "behavioral" problem. When behavioral treatments were initially developed, rigorously devised research on the causal factors for child abuse was limited (Azar, Fantuzzo, & Twentyman, 1984). Some progress (although slow) has been made since then, but a complete understanding of the antecedents and consequences that elicit and maintain maltreating behavior is still limited. Some of the most relevant dimensions to be assessed and then targeted in treatment may still be unknown. Finally, some of the antecedents of maltreatment require social changes that are beyond the reach of individual clinicians (e.g., poverty, violent neighborhoods). These issues are addressed throughout the remainder of this chapter. A discussion of the need for advocacy efforts is provided briefly at the end.

ASSESSMENT ISSUES

The causes and outcomes of child maltreatment are entwined with parents' childhood and early adult histories, child-rearing skills, stressful events, and social relationships, and the features of children, among other factors. In view of this complexity, the assessment and treatment of abusive and neglectful families must be approached as a multistage process. Assessment typically begins with impressionistic data from reporting and referral sources, and then narrows toward the evaluation of more specific intervention needs. Unique elements of assessment and treatment most relevant to abusive and neglectful families must also be included, and these will be highlighted (Wolfe & McEachran, 1997). A clinician typically begins the assessment of a family by consulting with the family's social worker to review the allegations, evidence, proceedings, and decisions that affect the evaluation, leading to the formulation of appropriate assessment questions. Typically, a service plan has already been drawn up by the social worker involved in the case. The goals for parents outlined by this

plan may be especially crucial if the child has been placed in foster care. Returning the child home may hinge on the parents' meeting these goals. If these are not met in a timely fashion, then proceedings for the termination of parental rights may occur. As will be discussed later, recent legislation has shortened this time frame significantly; therefore, throughout treatment, the therapist cannot lose sight of these goals, as they may play the most significant role in determining the family's future legal viability. As a result of the clinician's evaluations, modifications of the original service plan may be undertaken. The views of the social worker also should be solicited, as he or she may have valuable information that can affect treatment. Establishing this relationship with the family's caseworker may be crucial as treatment progresses, because the caseworker may be aware of changes in the family's situation that the therapist may not be.

Following this initial consultation, several intermediate goals must be met prior to making case management decisions and starting intervention with a maltreating family. These goals include two general concerns requiring initial screening and attention: (1) determining danger and risk to the child, and (2) identifying general strengths and problem areas of the family system. These are followed by more specific goals: (3) identifying parental needs vis-à-vis child-rearing demands, and (4) identifying the child's needs.

This assessment strategy has been summarized in Table 9.1, which highlights decisions to be made and precautions that must be heeded. In light of the first two general concerns (see above), the examiner often must first address the degree of dangerousness or risk to the child that currently exists, in order to assist the CPS agency and/or courts in deciding on whether the child needs alternative placement or can remain in his or her own home. Although violence prediction is controversial, evaluating level of risk may have some utility (see "Determining Treatment Priorities," below, for suggestions here) both at the outset of treatment and when return of a child in foster care is being considered. Risk assessment protocols are now being used at the reporting stage (Pecora, 1991) and may ultimately have utility for ongoing risk assessment by clinicians. This overriding concern of CPS is typically approached in conjunction with other community professionals involved with the family (e.g., physicians, social workers, public health nurses), although the psychologist's role is critical in identifying the major strengths and problem areas of the family system that guide the decision for child placement. An interview with the parent or parents can begin to establish the significance of different etiological factors, such as parental background, the couple relationship, perceived areas of stress and support, and psychiatric or physical symptomatology that may have a bearing on a parent's behavior toward the child. Assessment findings that have more specific relevance to behavioral treatment emerge during the detailed identification of parental and child needs (see Table 9.1). At this point, the examiner is concerned with identification or development of possible treatment alternatives; this requires more specialized assessment instruments and skills, as discussed below. Materials collected may ultimately serve legal purposes (e.g., in hearings concerning the termination of parental rights, establishing parental lack of progress in treatment), and therefore evaluators must have specific knowledge of legal criteria and measurement issues and be very attentive to the specifics of a parent's CPS service plan (Azar, Benjet, Furmann, & Cavallaro, 1995).

It needs to be kept in mind that the process of assessment is the beginning of the engagement process with families. Parents' motivation for change may hinge in part on the relationships developed during this process. For some parents, poor histories of relationships and their own histories of trauma may interfere with this initial relationship building. See Azar and Soysa (2000) for methods of maximizing relationship building during assessments.

Assessing Parental Responses to Child-Rearing Demands

Child maltreatment is strongly linked to events that involve the child in some manner, despite the formidable influence of parental background, psychological functioning, and situational stressors (Wolfe, 1985). Therefore, data should be collected on the parent's typical daily behavior with his or her child, using self-report and observational procedures of situations that may lead to parent–child conflict and maladaptive caretaking responses. This work should include an analysis of idiosyncratic cognitions, executive functioning, arousal patterns, fluctuations in mood and affect, and characteristic response styles during everyday child-rearing situations. Executive functioning, for example, pertains to parents' ability to perceive information from the environment accurately; to plan, implement, and evaluate their efforts to prevent harm to children (e.g., anticipate risks, self-regulate); and to adapt their responses to changing situations and children's developmental needs.

Parenting involves considerable cognitive activity. Parents must balance long- and short-term socialization goals, and must make continual judgments regarding the meaning of child behavior, its causes, and whether intervention is required. This is especially true before the child has language. Cognitive disturbances can occur at the pre-cue level (e.g., preexisting expectancies regarding child behavior), in the assignment of causality after a child cue has been labeled as noncompliant (e.g., negative dispositional attributions), or in the active selection of responses (e.g., problem-solving capacities). Initial assessment (as well as ongoing work), therefore, should include examining what a parent thinks is "normal" child and parenting behavior and the "typical" meaning the parent assigns to his or her own behavior and a child's responses (i.e., the parent's expectations). (See Wolfe & McEachran, 1997, for comprehensive discussion of assessment and specific instruments.) Parents should also be questioned regarding their assignment of causality for aversive child behavior, which may provide evidence of attributional biases that may need to be addressed in anger management work and that may interfere with parents' engaging in child management strategies. For example, it will be difficult for parents to remain calm if they believe that their child is "out to get" them. Parents keeping diaries have also been used to solicit parental thought patterns, antecedents to emotion-producing events, and behavioral responses in child rearing (Peterson, Tremblay, Ewigman, & Popkey, 2002). Attributions of children's behavior can be obtained through parental self-report, and in response to hypothetical vignettes describing children's ambiguous behavior (Bugental, Johnston, New, & Silvester, 1998). When hypothetical scenarios are used, rather than events more directly tied to the respondent's experience, respondents rely on their stable ways of interpreting the stimulus.

In addition to parental cognitions, a parent's emotional reactivity or displeasure in response

TABLE 9.1. Child Abuse and Neglect Assessment Strategy: An Overview

1. Determining dangerousness and risk to the child in cases of detected or undetected maltreatment

   Decisions

   - Apprehension of child risk
   - Alternative placement of child

   Precautions

   - Removing and returning child to family is highly stressful
   - Initial impression of family may be distorted

2. Identifying general strengths and problem areas of the family system

   Decisions

   - Family background
   - Marital/couple relationship
   - Perceived areas of stress and supports
   - Symptom pattern
   - Major factors (antecedents, consequences, and individual characteristics) suspected to be operative within the family
   - Directions for protective services, supports, additional community services

   Precautions

   - Involvement of too many professionals may overwhelm family
   - "Crises" that family members report may change dramatically
   - Parent–child problems may be embedded in chronic family problems (e.g., financial, marital/couple) that resist change

3. Identification of parental needs vis-à-vis child-rearing demands

   Decisions

   - Child-rearing methods and skills
   - Anger and arousal toward child
   - Perceptions and expectations of children
   - Behavioral intervention planning and establishing priority of needs

   Precautions

   - Parental behavior toward child may be a function of both proximal (e.g., child behavior) and distal (e.g., job stress) events
   - Numerous factors that may interfere with treatment must be identified (e.g., resistance, socioeconomic status, marital/couple problems)

4. Identification of the child's needs

   Decisions

   - Child behavior problems with family members
   - Child adaptive abilities and cognitive and emotional development
   - Referral to school-based intervention
   - Behavioral interventions (e.g., parent training)
   - Returning child to family
   - Unclear or delayed expression of symptoms/impairments

   Precautions

   - Child's behavior may be partially a function of recent family separation and change

Note. From Wolfe and McEachran (1997, p. 543). Copyright 1997 by The Guilford Press. Adapted by permission.

to aversive environmental demands merits careful attention, because of the role it is believed to play as a mediator of anger and aggression (Berkowitz, 1983; Wolfe, 1985). Although maltreating parents may be unwilling to acknowledge the full extent of their culpability, they are often willing to describe their feelings of anger and irritation that they believe are "provoked" by their children or by family events. They are also more willing to describe their feelings of anger and "loss of control" if provided with distinctive cues or examples, such as interacting with their children in high-conflict situations (e.g., Koverola, Elliot-Faust, & Wolfe, 1984). Alternatively, self-monitoring of annoyance, anger, or similar feelings that lead to conflict with a child can be achieved by using an "anger diary" (Wolfe, Kaufman, Aragona, & Sandler, 1981), in which the parent records his or her feelings of anger or frustration in response to incidents of child misbehavior, or by having the parent review videotapes from previous parent–child interactions in the clinic and identify changes in affect and/or irritation during an ongoing, realistic interchange with the child. In reviewing such videotapes, parents are put in the role of observers and problem solvers in reference to their own situation. This is typically well received by parents and is useful for assessing their unique pattern of emotional arousal and cognitive attributions.

Assessment of child-rearing methods that a parent uses on a daily basis is critical for developing behavioral treatment objectives, as maltreating parents have been observed to differ from nonmaltreating ones in the quality of their interactions with their children. In particular, maltreating parents are less interactive and less positive toward their children (Bousha & Twentyman, 1984; Burgess & Conger, 1978); they fail to modify their behavior in response to the children's needs; they are more inclined to make inappropriate demands of young children (Crittenden, 1982; Trickett & Kuczynski, 1986); and they are less likely to take into consideration mitigating information in response to their children's misbehavior (Milner & Froody, 1994).

Maltreating parents also show less ability to change set (e.g., shift to another solution when the first one fails; Nayak & Milner, 1998), and less cognitive flexibility (Robyn & Fremouw, 1996). Problems in "tracking" their children's behavior have also been found by Wahler and Dumas (1989), and these may indicate problems in sustaining attention. Failures in the contingencies between parent and child behaviors have also been suggested as distinguishing aspects of abusive families' transactions (Cerezo et al., 1996). All of this evidence suggests executive functioning problems. Such difficulties with reading child cues, shifting set when a problem is encountered, sustained attention, insensitive caregiving can have a far-reaching negative impact on children's development and the organization of the home (e.g., consistent basic care—maintaining regular mealtimes/bedtimes, following through with medical appointments), and may account for many of the disturbances found in maltreated children (Azar et al., 1988; Azar & Bober, 1999).

Neglect-related issues deserve special consideration (Lutzker & Bigelow, 2002). Family resource scales exist (Dunst, 1986; Magura & Moses, 1986), as well as scales for rating home cleanliness (Rosenfield-Schlicter, Sarber, Bueno, Greene, & Lutzker, 1983; Watson-Perczel, Lutzker, Green, & McGimpsey, 1988), safety (e.g., Tertinger, Greene, & Lutzker, 1984), and provision of health care (Magura & Moses, 1986). Skills-oriented assessment in areas relevant to neglect may also be useful, such as ability to recognize and act on medical problems (Delgado & Lutzker, 1985), ability to identify safety risks (Tymchuk, Lang, Sewards, Lieberman, & Koo, 2003) and emergency response skills (e.g., ability to respond effectively to a grease fire; Tymchuk, 1990). Because of cognitive limitations that often occur in maltreating populations, consideration should be given to pictorial presentations of assessment materials, as literacy is often an issue (see Tymchuk, 1998, for a discussion of such assessment). Importantly, careful consideration should also be given to cultural differences and child-rearing practices in interpreting assessment findings (Azar & Benjet, 1994; Azar & Cote, 2002). For example, high levels of parental control may be seen negatively by children in one culture, but may be seen as signs of caring and stability by children in another (Thompson, 1994). Knowledge of the culture may also influence an evaluator's interpretation of social cues. For example, a child's turning his or her eyes downward when speaking to an adult family member may be mistakenly seen as fear, when it may in fact represent a sign of respect.

Assessing the Needs of the Child

Although abused children are often not found to display problem behaviors indicative of one specific clinical disorder (Azar & Bober, 1999; Wolfe & Mosk, 1983), maltreated children show a wide range of developmental changes and deviations, and their parents describe them as being extremely difficult and annoying. Assessment must be sensitive to ongoing circumstances (e.g., exposure to other forms of family violence, foster placement) that work in combination either to attenuate the effects of powerful traumatic events or to turn a minor developmental crisis into a major impairment (Azar & Bober, 1999). The physical consequences of maltreatment (e.g., neurological damage due to head injuries, anemia due to poor nutrition) also need to be considered therapeutically. They may produce psychological outcomes (e.g., embarrassment due to disfiguring scars, which may increase children's social distance from peers) and/or interfere with children's ability to deal with therapeutic intervention itself (e.g., attentional problems) (Azar, Breton, & Miller, 1998).

In each era of development, disturbances in social, intellectual, and socioemotional realms are seen in maltreated children and may need to be targeted in treatment, but also may act to interfere with the formation of a therapeutic relationship. Early disruptions in the parent–infant relationship appear to result in anxious and disorganized attachment patterns (e.g., clinging, rigidity, withdrawal) and problems in later development (e.g., speech and language, social interaction; Aber & Allen, 1987; Egeland & Farber, 1984; Egeland & Sroufe, 1981).

Abused preschool children show delays in their ability to discriminate emotions in others (Frodi & Smetana, 1984; Smetana et al., 1999; Smetana, Kelly, & Twentyman, 1984), and show lower expectations of support from their mothers in response to their displays of emotion (Rogosch, Cicchetti, & Aber, 1995; Shipman & Zeaman, 1999). They have been shown to have more marked delays in self-control and peer interactions than nonclinic children. Heightened aggressiveness and hostility toward others (especially authority figures), as well as angry outbursts with little or no provocation, are also prominent (Howes & Eldredge, 1985; Kolko, 1992; Wekerle & Wolfe, 2003). These very basic emotion deficits

(e.g., identification of emotional states) and affective and behavioral dysregulation may be targets of intervention during this stage of development.

In contrast, neglected preschoolers appear more socially avoidant (Hoffman-Plotkin & Twentyman, 1984), show more evidence of lacking empathy (George & Main, 1979), and seem to have more difficulty dealing with challenging tasks or interpersonal situations than either abused or typical children do (Egeland, Sroufe, & Erickson, 1983). Parent, teacher, and child report measures of behavior problems (e.g., destructiveness, fighting with siblings) have consistently indicated that abused school-age children are perceived as more difficult to manage, less socially mature, and less capable of developing trust with others (Wekerle & Wolfe, 2003). Crittenden (1992), on the other hand, found that neglected preschool and school-age children tended to remain isolated during opportunities for free play with other children. Neglected school-age children, compared to nonmaltreated children, have been found to be more passive, to display fewer overtures of affection, and to produce less frequent initiations of play behavior in interactions with their mothers (Bousha & Twentyman, 1984; Crittenden, 1992). These findings suggest targeting social skills capacities with greater emphasis on very basic skills (e.g., peer initiation skills).

Studies of physically abused school-age children concur with those of younger children, showing similar learning and motivational problems at school, as well as higher rates of aggressive and destructive behavior and social impairment as they enter unfamiliar peer and school situations (Feldman et al., 1995). A study of the social relationships of physically abused 8- to 12-year-old children (Salzinger, Feldman, Hammer, & Rosario, 1993) found them to be at increased risk for lower social status in the classroom (especially peer rejection), which is the strongest predictor of school dropout and delinquency in adolescence. These negative interactional patterns have also been observed in the home setting (e.g., yelling, hitting, and destructiveness) during this period (Lorber, Felton, & Reid, 1984; Reid, Taplin, & Lorber, 1981).

Abused and neglected children appear to suffer from many academic, cognitive, and language delays during both the preschool and school-age years (Eckenrode, Laird, & Doris,

1993; Fox, Long, & Langlois, 1988; Wodarski, Kurtz, Gaudin, & Howing, 1990). Neglected children are at particularly increased risk (Crouch & Milner, 1993). Salzinger, Kaplan, Pelcovitz, Samit, and Krieger (1984) found that both abused children ($n = 30$) and neglected children ($n = 26$) performed at 2 years below grade level in verbal and math abilities compared to nonmaltreated children ($n = 480$), with approximately one-third of the maltreated children failing one or more subjects and/or being placed in a special classroom. Intervention in academic skill areas has been less studied.

Socioemotional problems (e.g., lower self-esteem, depression) have also been observed (Allen & Tarnowski, 1989; Kaufman, 1991; Kaufman & Cicchetti, 1989; Toth, Manly, & Cicchetti, 1992). There is some evidence of posttraumatic stress disorder (PTSD) symptoms in physically abused children, although these seem less prominent than in sexually abused children (Naar-King, Silvern, Ryan, & Sebring, 2002; Pelcovitz et al., 1994).

Although maltreated adolescents have been seldom studied, some evidence for problems in this period has emerged as well. Abuse and neglect have been linked to delinquent behavior, including fighting, stealing, skipping school, and traffic violations (Brown, 1984; Mak, 1994), and to heightened risk-taking behaviors such as early sexual activity and teenage parenthood (Kaplan, Pelcovitz, & LaBruna, 1999). In adulthood, an increased risk of alcohol abuse has been seen (Widom, 1998), as well as arrests for violent crimes and diagnoses of antisocial personality disorder (Cahill, Kaminer, & Johnson, 1999; Widom, 1998). Moreover, youths from violent and neglectful families begin social dating with inappropriate expectations about relationships and report more violence—especially verbal abuse and threats—toward their dating partners (Wolfe, Wekerle, Scott, Straatman, & Grasley, 2004). Dating violence and a past history of family violence are strong prerelationship predictors of intimate violence in early adulthood and marriage (Murphy, Meyer, & O'Leary, 1994; O'Leary, Malone, & Tyree, 1994).

Importantly, not all abused and neglected children show clinical symptoms or problem behaviors. Salzinger and colleagues (1993), for example, found that 13 of the 87 abused children they studied were seen as popular by peers. A 20-year follow-up of a group of abused and neglected children found females who had experienced abuse to be more resilient than males across several domains of functioning. "Resilience" was defined by meeting criteria for success across six of eight domains of functioning, including employment, homelessness, education, social activity, psychiatric disorder, substance abuse, and criminal behavior (both self-reported and official arrests) (McGloin & Widom, 2001). Indeed, 22% of abused and neglected children followed into young adulthood met the criteria for resilience; this finding should caution clinicians against an automatic assumption of psychopathology.

Clinical assessment of the child must take into consideration the parent's subjective perceptions of the child, as well as other sources (e.g., self-report, reports of significant others such as teachers and social workers, and observations in the home or school). Since the needs of abused and neglected children are extensive, a broad-spectrum screening that includes clinical interviews and traditional global screening devices can be used to begin the process, followed by a more targeted assessment to follow up on specific problems related to the child's unique history. Parents are usually quite willing to provide behavior problem information, since they feel that their behavior stems directly from their children's difficulties. Because of parents' potential to distort the level of a child's aversive behavior, however, ancillary reports from other adults who know the child (e.g., foster parents, teachers) are crucial. These reports also provide data regarding the child's adjustment in other settings.

Child self-report can also assist the examiner in understanding the child's overall functioning and can provide insight into current fears, anxieties, or unhappiness, which may be quite disruptive. A semistructured child interview provides a good beginning point for eliciting a child's feelings and perceptions about the family. In one study involving 160 maltreated youths, McGee, Wolfe, and Olson (1995) found that the majority viewed the offenders as the major causes of their maltreatment; however, for physical and emotional abuse, one-third of the sample identified their own misbehavior as the major cause for what happened. This finding suggests that targeting self-blame statements, as well as children's underlying beliefs that they could have prevented such acts and are somewhat to blame, may be needed.

As with parent protocols, see Wolfe and McEachran (1997) for more details regarding specific child-based assessment protocols. Observations (during interviews) can also be useful. The interviewer should be sensitive to verbal and somatic indices of anxiety or negative affect (e.g., poor eye contact, twitching movements, long silences, sadness) and should explore the origins or reference for such emotions, which are often linked to foster care placement, uncertainty over family reunion, and/or fear of further maltreatment. All may become the focus of treatment. For adolescents, assessing the types of issues that give rise to family conflict may also be useful and may provide situations for use in discussing negotiation skills and communication. Because maltreated children's and adolescent's problems are often manifested with peers, observations with peers and/or dating partners are useful, as well as using self-report instruments (Wolfe et al., 2001).

Determining Treatment Priorities

Once a child's abilities and needs are assessed, findings can be integrated with those of the parent's report and observations of current behavior to establish treatment priorities. First and foremost, the feasibility of the parent's and child's remaining together must be decided, and then treatment recommendations to support the family unit must be formulated. The most specific question is clearly the potential for future violence or continued neglect.

Research has attempted to provide better decision-making tools and risk prediction protocols. Until recently, such prediction was thought to have limited scientific foundation (Monahan, 1981). More recent data with psychiatric populations, however, have shown some predictive validity for actuarial methods in narrowly defined groups (e.g., psychiatric patients with specific diagnoses), in specific settings (e.g., hospitals) and within certain limited time frames (e.g., immediately after discharge) (e.g., Gardner, Lidz, Mulvey, & Shaw, 1996). Even then, risk statements are only possible when a certain level and quality of scientific data are available regarding recidivism (Grisso & Appelbaum, 1992). Scientific data in abuse in many ways fail to meet these criteria, especially given the type of risk involved (within a specific relationship) and the period over which prediction is needed (e.g., for a 2-year-old, it would be 16 years until adulthood) (Azar & Soysa, 1999; Melton & Limber, 1989). Also,

general violence risk models have been less studied for females (Lidz, Mulvey, & Gardner, 1993).

A literature has begun to emerge on predicting risk in abuse. Predictors of recidivism and treatment variables include case level and perpetrator dimensions (Fuller & Wells, 2003; Hamilton & Browne, 1998). Child resilience factors also have risk prediction value (e.g., rapid responses to danger, information seeking, formation and utilization of relationships for survival; Hamilton & Browne, 1998). Although controversial, along with situational and perpetrator factors, these risk factors may provide a more comprehensive picture of a child's vulnerability.

Based on such research, some CPS agencies are now employing risk assessment "systems" that use a variety of parent, child, family, and environmental factors as predictors, as well as the nature of the abuse identified to date (Camasso & Jagannathan, 2000; DePanfilis & Zuravin, 2001; Milner, Murphy, Valle, & Tolliver, 1998; Pecora, 1991). Although these systems are still in their early stages, some do show evidence of ability to predict length of time cases remain open, response to services, substantiation rates, and (to a limited extent) further abuse. False-positive rates are too high for making more permanent legal decisions, but such systems may improve screening and service planning. These methods have not been used in clinical settings to date, but may have potential to be helpful here as well. Along with risk models, specific child abuse risk prediction instruments are available (e.g., the Child Abuse Potential Inventory; Milner, 1986, 1994). Sensitivity and specificity for both physical and sexual abuse are too poor as yet to justify use in clinical and court decision making (i.e., high false-positive and false-negative classifications, Caldwell, Bogat, & Davidson, 1988; Milner et al., 1998).

Given that risk prediction can only occur over short time frames, risk assessment must be an ongoing task in treatment. Kolko (1996a) describes the use of weekly self-reports of behavioral risk indicators in treatment, which may be useful in such ongoing monitoring.

The second step in the treatment plan is typically to establish a timetable and hierarchy of priorities for addressing the major parental and child needs revealed by assessment. The order in which targets are addressed must be carefully considered with maltreating families. For example, teaching a parent to ignore a child's tantrums may place the child at higher risk if the parent does not yet have well-established ways for dealing with the child's increased attempts to gain attention. The following is a point summary of empirical and clinical findings concerning individual and family characteristics of child maltreatment that warrant assessment and treatment consideration (Wolfe & McEachran, 2003; Wekerle & Wolfe, 2003):

Child intervention needs

1. Deficits in social sensitivity and relationship development (these include problems with attachment formation, the development of empathy, interpersonal trust, and affective expression).
2. Deficits in cognitive, language, and moral development (these refer to poor social judgment, communication skills, and school performance in particular).
3. Problems with self-control and aggression.
4. Concerns about health, safety, and protection from harm.

Parent intervention needs

1. Symptoms of emotional distress, learning impairments, parental psychopathology, and personality deficits that limit adult adjustment and coping.
2. Emotional arousal and reactivity to child provocation, and poor control of anger and hostility.
3. Inadequate and inappropriate methods of teaching, discipline, and child stimulation.
4. Inappropriate perceptions and expectations of children, reflected in rigid and limited beliefs about child rearing and in negative biases.
5. Negative lifestyle and habits related to the use of alcohol and drugs, prostitution, and/or subcultural peer groups, which interfere with the parent–child relationship and parental problem-solving capacities.

Family/situational intervention needs

1. Couple discord and/or coercive family interactions, and/or (for mothers) a history of violent male partners.
2. Chronic economic problems and associated socioeconomic stressors.
3. Social isolation and the inability to establish meaningful social supports.

SPECIAL TREATMENT CONSIDERATIONS

Before we discuss applications of behavioral techniques to the treatment of child abuse and neglect, a number of more general cautions regarding maltreating families need to be discussed. These concerns fall under three general headings: the characteristics of maltreating parents, the characteristics of their children, and contextual factors that influence the development of therapeutic relationships.

Characteristics of Maltreating Parents

Abusive parents typically do not identify themselves as having a problem and are not self-referred for treatment (Azar & Twentyman, 1986). Because many families commonly use corporal punishment as a means of controlling child behavior, some parents may believe (falsely) that society places no bounds or restraints on such techniques. Because of ambiguity or subcultural differences in where such limits may exist despite legal sanctions, parents may not accept their designation as having violated community standards (Conger, 1982). The therapist also may experience feelings about what the parent has done (e.g., disgust, vicarious trauma responses) or have reactions if parents become belligerent. Biases may result that interfere with engagement and that must be guarded against (Azar, 1996; Azar & Makin-Byrd, in press; Farber & Azar, 1999).

This fundamental disagreement between society's judgment and that of a maltreating parent is important to keep in mind. Resistance to treatment is usually high, and motivation for change is often an issue. This fact is reflected in the high treatment dropout rates found among abusive parents, ranging from 32% to 87% (Reid, 1985; Wolfe, Aragona, Kaufman, & Sandler, 1980). This issue often needs to be resolved before treatment can effectively begin, as ruptures in the therapeutic alliance may occur that will decrease the success of treatment (Azar & Makin-Byrd, 2004). It is important to note that although clinicians may want to see treatment failure or dropout as the parents' "fault," therapists have also been shown to display nonfacilitating behaviors in parent training more generally (e.g., a tendency to withdraw, disengage, and dislike their clients; Patterson & Chamberlain, 1988, 1994), and this may occur with maltreating families in particular.

One solution to parent-based motivation problems in the initial phases of work is to help the family reframe the problem in terms of day-to-day difficulties that a parent can identify. "Child noncompliance," "poor ability to deal with stress," "vocational difficulties," and "lack of supports" may all be more easily accepted problem definitions than "abuse" or "neglect" for such parents. A therapist's openness to such redefinitions and acceptance of the parent's way of seeing the problem is crucial to reducing resistance, for two reasons. First, it may reduce the parent's fear of being evaluated and labeled as a "bad" parent by the therapist. Being labeled as a person who "has trouble handling children" or as someone who is "very lonely" (e.g., without social supports) or "stressed" may be easier for the parent to accept. Second, such redefinitions may serve to differentiate the therapist from the referral source (e.g., CPS or the court), which the parent may see as the "cause" of the family's trouble.

In developing this reformulation, the therapist must take care not to collude with the client's assertion that no problem exists or that the child is the only source of the problem. A delicate balance must be achieved. For some clients, the only problem definition that they are initially willing to accept is that they are "in trouble," and that the therapist may help them to learn ways to interact with their children that will assist them in getting "out of trouble." Lack of compliance with treatment may still occur despite such reformulations.

Many maltreating families have competing life crises that may interfere with participation in treatment (e.g., evictions, domestic violence). The requirements of treatment may be one of the few stresses that they can put aside. The use of lay therapists as adjunct treatment agents may assist treatment compliance by helping family members deal with life problems and reduce some of their ambient stress levels.

Behaviorally oriented clinicians have cited incentives to improve attendance as being important with these families (Azar & Twentyman, 1986; Conger, 1982; Wolfe, Kaufman, et al., 1981), but typical behavioral methods for increasing participation may not work with this population. The fact that many of these parents do not have telephones, for example, precludes the widespread use of telephone prompts, shown to improve attendance in parent training and other mental health ser-vices with other clients (Ayllon & Roberts, 1975; MacDonald, Brown, & Ellis, 2000). Initial monetary deposits, another commonly used technique (Hagen, Foreyt, & Durham, 1976), may represent a hardship for such families. More appropriate strategies include use of tangible incentives for attendance (e.g., movie tickets) (Ambrose, Hazzard, & Haworth, 1980), provision of transportation and babysitting (Azar & Twentyman, 1986), and behavioral contracting (Gambrill, 1983; Wolfe, Kaufman, et al., 1981). One aspect of contracts might be contingencies for the therapist to act as an advocate for the parent with CPS or the court if certain objectives are met (Conger, 1982). (See Katz et al., 2001, for a discussion of the use of incentives with low-socioeconomic-status parents.) Court ordering of treatment attendance has produced gains in completion of treatment by the parents (Wolfe et al., 1980); however, few child maltreatment cases become involved in the criminal justice system (as opposed to child welfare), and court-ordered treatment can have undesirable side effects. Hansen and Warner (1994), in a self-report survey of professionals working with maltreating parents, indicated that the most common "incentive" used to improve attendance and compliance with homework assignments was verbal praise. This survey, however, did not find the high levels of attrition found in other studies. Overall, despite the discussion of the use of such strategies, the effectiveness of these methods (except for court orders) has not been examined in controlled studies.

Although such incentives may produce better attendance at sessions, they do not ensure that clients will make the investment required to make lasting behavioral changes. For example, a mother who had been court-ordered to complete a parenting group run by one of us conscientiously *attended* every session, but spent her time looking out the window each session, not participating.

The social isolation and poor relationship histories of the maltreating parent are final factors that need to be addressed as the therapeutic relationship begins. Wahler and his colleagues have shown that a combination of social isolation and socioeconomic disadvantage reduces the probability that changes in parent–child interactions will occur, and also limits the generalization of such changes over time (Wahler, 1980). Because of poor relationship skills, a parent may also act inappropriately toward the therapist (e.g., testing limits, making excessive demands). Early in treatment, the therapist may need to define clearly the parameters of the relationship, and along the way inform the parent of what is expected in such relationships. Studies of therapy preparation techniques with disadvantaged clients indicate that such efforts improve success (Heitler, 1976). This process can also be an important source of role modeling for relationship-building skills.

Treatment Needs of Abused and Neglected Children

Specific treatment considerations involving maltreated children have received little attention in the behavioral literature. Also, treatment efforts to date have primarily focused on families of preschool-age or elementary-school-age children; there has been little mention of work with families of toddlers or adolescents. This is noteworthy, given that the most dangerous period for maltreatment occurs in the first year of life (ACYF, 2004), with the majority of deaths occurring before age 6 (85.1%). Moreover, community surveys show a second peak in maltreatment incidence rates occurs in adolescence, although abuse during this period may go unreported (Burgdorf, 1988).

The characteristics of these two age groups may explain their absence in the treatment literature. The participation of young abused infants or toddlers in treatment may be limited because of developmental considerations, and priority may be given to parental behavior changes. When an abuse report involves a child in this age group, treatment commonly focuses on changing a parent's negative responses to typical developmental behavior, such as crying (e.g., Lieberman & Zeanah, 1999; Sandford & Tustin, 1974). In addition, given the greater vulnerability of this younger age group, intervention is more likely to include placement outside of the home; if abuse or neglect is severe, parental rights to the child may be terminated.

The lack of treatment studies regarding abused and neglected adolescents may be explained by different concerns. For this older age group, the consequences of maltreatment most often surface as disruptive behaviors, such as running away (Farber, McCord, Kinast, & Baum-Faulkner, 1984) and delinquency (Lewis, Shanok, Pincus, & Glaser, 1979), and

such behaviors have probably overshadowed parental abuse or neglect as a focus of treatment. There also may be a bias toward seeing adolescents as participants in family violence (i.e., they may hit back) and not as victims (Azar, 1991a). Clearly, additional investigations need to be conducted to address the behavioral treatment needs of younger and older groups of maltreated children. Some recent efforts have begun to appear (see Stovall & Dozier, 2000; Swenson, Saldana, Joyner, & Henggeler, in press; Toth, Maughan, Manly, Spagnola, & Cicchetti, 2002), and these are discussed later.

Behavioral treatment efforts can involve preschool-age or elementary-school-age children in two ways: The children may participate in parent–child interaction training, or may be treated in other settings, such as the day care center or school. With some exceptions (Azar et al., 1998; Haskett & Myers, 1994; Kolko, 1996b; Urquiza & McNeil, 1996), only the former approach has been discussed in detail. Child maltreatment cases have unique features that need to be addressed. The majority of these issues have to do with the unusual experiences of these children in their relationships with caretakers. Psychological maltreatment (e.g., exploitation, humiliation), which often accompanies abuse or neglect, gives rise to a number of common themes in therapy to which therapists need to be sensitive. These include issues of trust, anticipation of rejection, feelings of loss, and fear.

First, hypervigilance and fearfulness has been commonly noted in abused children when they encounter a new adult (Crittenden, 1992; Mann & McDermott, 1983), especially if the abuse was very recent. Therefore, developing trust may be crucial for intervention work. Such children, for example, may require greater control over what happens in treatment sessions. Keeping the door open or allowing children to leave sessions when they choose may be important in building a therapeutic relationship.

As previously noted, an abused child may exhibit aggressive behavior, either during work with the child alone or in the presence of the parent. In such circumstances, the therapist's calm handling of the behavior may provide the child with a different experience (e.g., a desensitizing experience); if the parent is present, it may also model appropriate responses for the parent. Given that parents may feel inadequate or be dogmatic about their parenting, care must be taken not to undermine a parent's role with a child during work with the dyad.

A third area of concern in undertaking treatment involving a maltreated child is how much faith to put in the child's reports of home interactions. Maltreated children have learned not to report difficulties. Previous disclosures, for example, may have resulted in foster care placement—an event that a child may have perceived as punishment for "telling." The child may have also encountered further abuse from the parent, if no actions were taken. The child's readiness and comfort for sharing information regarding home interactions should determine how much is asked of him or her in this regard. If disclosures of abuse or neglect are made, the child needs to be prepared for the actions that may be taken. This should be done at a level that is developmentally appropriate.

Observations of parent–child interactions also need to be approached with caution. In our work, abusive parents sometimes threaten or bribe their children to perform in a particular way during observational sessions, prior to arriving at the clinic for a session. A therapist must be alert to the stress that such observations place on a family and, ultimately, on the child. For example, the therapist's presence in the home may intensify parental responses to child noncompliance (e.g., parents may feel that the child is purposefully trying to make them "look bad"). The negative consequences may not be evident while the therapist is present, but may only erupt once he or she has left. A "cooling-down" period before the therapist's departure, in which any residual parental anger can be discussed and resolved, is helpful. Such protections are essential to ensure the safety of the child. Therapy will be of little use if the child must continue to devote energy to concerns about harm.

If the child remains in parental custody, concurrent work with parents should be required if the child is in individual treatment. Concurrent work with foster or adoptive parents may also be useful during the course of individual work with maltreated children, to help foster parents cope with the children's response to their past maltreatment (Azar & Bober, 1999). The number of children in kin care as a foster/adoptive placement has risen, and there is some evidence that the mental health needs of children in kin care may not be monitored as carefully by CPS. There may be special issues specific to these children and their caregivers that have not been explored by the mental health field. (See Azar & Hill, in press, and Geen, 2004, for discussions of the issues involved in kin care.) In addition, sometimes children who have sustained physical abuse or been subjected to chronic neglect will have developmental impairments, such as attention or language disorders and difficulties in emotional understanding. In such instances, therapists may need to make adaptations, such as simplifying their language in presenting new skills, breaking down complex tasks into smaller pieces, providing written as well as oral instructions, and providing controlled outlets for activity (e.g., greater use of role plays and other activities).

Contextual Factors Affecting the Therapeutic Relationship

The last area of concern in approaching treatment relates to the development of a therapeutic relationship. The nature of child maltreatment and the referral source introduce a number of factors not present in most therapy situations. First and foremost, therapists may have personal reactions to the serious injury and neglect of children, which, depending on their intensity, may impair the therapists' ability to work effectively with offenders. Steele (1975) noted two reactions of therapists: (1) denial, or (2) a surge of anger and an urge to scold the parents. Both reactions can be destructive to establishing a therapeutic relationship. The assumptions underlying the behavioral approach may inhibit such reactions, since abusive and neglectful behaviors are viewed as environmentally determined (e.g., learned) and are not viewed as something "intrinsically bad" about the parents. Referral of an abusive family by a social service agency or the court system often can result in a different kind of role strain for the behavior therapist. Two conflicting goals present themselves in treatment—therapeutic intervention with the family versus physical protection of the child. Training for accomplishing the latter is often lacking in a therapist's preparation and experience. Moreover, actions here may negatively affect the family's chance of success in treatment. There is no easy solution to this conflict; rather, it requires cooperative efforts with the social service agencies responsible for child protection (see Wolfe, Kaufman, et al., 1981).

Another area where role strain occurs is in the area of client confidentiality. Given the figures cited earlier indicating a high rate of recidivism *during* treatment, the probability of the need to report maltreatment is high. As in all family treatment work, this legal requirement should be discussed at the outset with parents (Azar & Twentyman, 1986), and this discussion can be referred to and resumed if it becomes necessary to report. Clearly, though this precaution does not entirely alleviate the obstacles to maintaining a therapeutic relationship once reporting has occurred, at the very least it defines overtly for the clients the limitations of confidentiality.

If reporting becomes necessary, following certain steps may be helpful to minimize the effects on the relationship. If possible, a report should not be made without first informing the client. An offer should be made to the client to make the report him- or herself or with the therapist's assistance, rather than the therapist's making it alone. These steps may reduce some of the client's anger at being "betrayed" and may act as a positive element in therapy. In making a self-referral, the client is also taking the first step toward acknowledging a problem, which may motivate change (Prochaska, DiClemente, & Norcross, 1992). Follow-up with the client in dealing with the authorities can also act to enhance the therapeutic relationship; that is, the first time such a report was made the client had to go through the process alone, and now he or she has the therapist to help. In addition, such self-referral is often viewed as a hopeful sign by authorities, and in less serious cases it may actually lessen the repercussions of having reoffended.

Court involvement can hamper work, because full disclosure of assessment findings and treatment progress is required. Clients need to be made aware that this will take place at the beginning of treatment, and the content of any written report should be discussed with them whenever feasible. Such behavior on the therapist's part will help to differentiate the therapist's role from that of the "authorities" and may facilitate cooperation. The fact that a maltreating parent is often "pushed" into treatment can also result in conflicting agendas. The parent and the therapist may differ in their goals for treatment. The parent's position may be "I want to get the social service agency off my back, so I'll come to sessions, but don't expect me to do anything." Here, the therapist needs to make his or her own position and the goals of intervention clear, and to work out a

compromise with the client that is within the bounds of treatment. Written contracts with the family, discussed earlier, may be useful in this regard to spell out clearly expectations. The social service agency's and the therapist's agendas may also conflict. The agency's goal in seeking treatment for the family may be to demonstrate that the agency has tried every possible alternative for reuniting the family before starting proceedings for permanent removal of the child, whereas the therapist's assumption may be that he or she is working to reunite the family (of course, the reverse situation can also occur). Again, goals must be clearly specified before treatment proceeds and revisited periodically during the course of treatment.

Working with children may result in agenda conflict as well. Children may want to return to their maltreating parents, and the therapist's task may be to help them deal with their reactions to permanent removal. Conversely, children may wish to remain with their foster families, and the therapist may be asked to help them adjust to being returned home. These conflicting agendas can produce role strain for everyone involved. At the outset of therapy, therefore, the goals of the referral source, the family, the child, and the therapist need to be expressed and agreed upon.

Two final areas have to do with the value system of the therapist. First, the maltreating parent and the therapist may come from different racial/ethnic backgrounds or socioeconomic strata. Since "good parenting" can be thought of as a relativistic goal, therapists must be careful not to generalize their own personal views on parenting to the families they are asked to treat (Azar, 1996). A culturally relativistic point of view, which attempts to define treatment goals in relation to cultural, community, and personal expectations and capabilities, has been advocated in the literature (Azar & Benjet, 1994; Azar & Makin-Byrd, in press). Second, unrealistic expectations by the therapist and the family of what progress will be made should be anticipated. Highly stressed and disadvantaged families are slow to make detectable changes and require much patience. Such families may also expect all their problems to be handled by the therapist. Even with the elimination of maltreatment, parents in such families may still not be "ideal" parents or even "ideal" clients. A goal that may be the most realistic is to help them to become *ade-*

quate parents. Each of these areas must be considered as the therapist begins treating an abusive or neglectful parent and his or her family, as well as during the course of treatment. Failure to address these issues carefully may limit the progress that might be achieved.

TREATMENT FOCUS, FORMAT, AND SUPPORT PERSONNEL

Parent versus Child Focus

Treatments of child abuse and neglect via behavioral strategies have included a number of different cognitive and behavioral targets. Treatment outcome studies have been carried out with individual parents, children, parent–child dyads, families, and parent groups, both in clinic and in home settings. Most studies have treated maternal caregivers. The bulk of this work has focused on changing parent–child interaction patterns through the use of training in child management skills, role playing, and feedback. In addition to attempts to change parent–child interactions directly, other efforts have been aimed at broad-spectrum skill deficits associated with the occurrence of maltreatment. These have included systematic desensitization to increase tolerance for aversive child behavior, stress management and anger control training, and cognitive restructuring of distorted interpretations of child behavior. Neglect has also been targeted (e.g., home safety, hygiene, budgeting), and combinations of these approaches have been utilized. A few studies have tailored programs, selecting as targets unique antecedent conditions specific to the parents involved (e.g., marital/couple discord, migraines, alcohol use, etc.). Other potential targets have been discussed in descriptive reports of behavioral programs, such as vocational assistance (Lutzker & Rice, 1984), but empirical work has not yet documented the success of such targets.

As noted earlier, parental treatment has clearly been predominant in efforts to date, despite the occurrence of child behavioral and developmental problems resulting from parental inadequacies. The most commonly addressed child behavior is noncompliance, but even this behavior has been approached through parent training. A number of reasons exist for this emphasis on parental treatment as the method of choice for intervention work, even where child needs are evident. Child behavior therapy in general has turned to parent training as the method of choice for intervention work, based on the assumption that parents constitute a "continuous treatment resource" who are the most powerful agents in a child's environment. Furthermore, in the general clinical child population, the use of such training has been shown to be highly effective in producing favorable changes in child behavior across a number of problem areas (Barkley, 2000), and similar findings have been reported with abusive populations (Azar & Cote, 2005; Skowron & Reinemann, 2005).

Furthermore, behavioral parent training has been shown to have differential treatment effectiveness in changing child behavior with parents of lower socioeconomic status (Knapp & Deluty, 1989; Rieppi et al., 2002), and in at least one study it showed better child outcomes than individual child therapy (Love, Kaswan, & Bugental, 1972). Despite the emphasis on parent treatment in the literature, some recent work has suggested (after global training of parenting strategies in groups) the use of dyadic therapy, in which children and parents are coached through interactions to promote a more positive relationship (e.g., Chaffin et al., 2004; Urquiza & McNeil, 1996). Parallel treatment, in which parents and elementary-school-age children have received comparable interventions, has also been attempted (Kolko, 1996b).

Treatment focusing on the child and his or her difficulties should also be carefully considered. As discussed earlier, maltreated children have been shown to exhibit a wide range of behavioral and emotional problems. This maladaptive behavior has also been shown to extend beyond the home setting to include interactions with others (e.g., foster care parents, teachers, and peers; George & Main, 1979; Hoffman-Plotkin & Twentyman, 1984), and it may continue to be maintained in these settings despite changes in the family. Training efforts may need to be conducted in each of these settings to enhance home changes. Because of the heterogeneity of behavioral problems exhibited by maltreated children, one standard approach cannot be outlined.

Content, Format, and Setting

The decision as to whether the abusing or neglectful parent, the couple (if one exists), the parent–child dyad, or the child should be treated, as well as decisions about the structure and content of that treatment, should be made according to the specific needs of the family. Although parent training is the most commonly used strategy, this approach may not be the treatment of choice if parental or child characteristics or aspects of the family's situation indicate that child-rearing problems are not the biggest source of difficulty. An issue that arises during assessment is whether the child or children are actually exhibiting deviant behavior that warrants change, or whether the problem is primarily due to inappropriate expectations on the part of the parent(s). In the latter case, a cognitive-behavioral strategy to deal with such inappropriate perceptions may be the starting point of treatment (see the later discussion).

Other significant parent-related problems may also need to be handled before changes in parent–child interactions are attempted. For example, a parent who has a significant alcohol problem may require treatment prior to working on parent–child interactional problems, since attempts to produce parenting changes may be doomed to failure due to the effects of alcoholism. Extreme marital/couple conflict is another factor associated with maltreatment that may have its own effects on child outcome (Wolfe, Crooks, Lee, McIntyre-Smith, & Jaffe, 2003). Such relationship problems may preclude the parents' working together in a collaborative manner, and may therefore mean that a lower priority must be placed at first on parent training. Similarly, if parents' stress level is high and resources are so low that they are incapable of altering their social environment, then the effectiveness of parent training strategies will also be severely limited unless support services can be provided (Azar, Ferguson, & Twentyman, 1992). And, as noted by Smith, Barkley, and Shapiro (Chapter 2, this volume), parental attention-deficit/hyperactivity disorder (ADHD) may be a major hindrance to successful parent training, warranting the treatment of the parent with ADHD prior to or coincident with the treatment program for the child. It is conceivable that other parental disorders may likewise interfere with efforts to work with parents of maltreated children.

In each of the scenarios above, other problem areas may require treatment either before or simultaneously with behavioral interventions for parent–child problems. Despite these other treatment needs, however, it is important

to reaffirm that in the majority of cases, treatment of abusive or neglectful families must focus on the parent–child relationship and its context (e.g., the family, financial limits, alcohol usage, etc.). If parent training is to be utilized, a decision needs to be made as to whether a parent will be seen individually or with other parents in a group. If parental deficit areas are highly specific, or a parent is too low-functioning or socially avoidant to benefit from material presented in a group session, individual treatment may be preferred. Both individual and group parent training have been used with maltreating parents, and some researchers have used a combination of both methods. For example, Wolfe, Sandler, and Kaufman (1981) and Azar and Twentyman (1984; Azar, 1989a, 1997) combined group parenting sessions with weekly individual home visits. The role of the home visitor was to promote generalization of the gains made during group sessions and to provide extra practice in the trained techniques with the child present. Both studies provide sound arguments, and supportive results, for combining individual and group training. Urquiza and McNeil (1996) adapted parent–child interaction therapy (PCIT), an empirically validated treatment developed by Eyberg (1988) for use with maltreating parents (and discussed in more detail later). In a randomized trial of this approach, Chaffin and colleagues (2004) combined separate parent and child group work with individualized parent–child dyadic work. The coaching was done through a one-way mirror. Motivational enhancements have also been discussed in these studies (e.g., behavioral contracting; Wolfe, Kaufman, et al., 1981) as useful.

In addition to decisions regarding the structure of treatment, the choice of setting must also be made. Three different settings have been used with abusive families in research efforts to date: (1) the standard clinic office or educational group, (2) a controlled learning environment in the clinic, and (3) the home. As before, a combination of these settings has often been utilized (e.g., group didactic training and home practice sessions, or individual office discussions followed by practice with the child in a structured laboratory analogue situation). As mentioned above, the controlled learning environment can be equipped with a one-way mirror and bug-in-the-ear transmitter device to guide parents through interactions with their children. This approach is well suited for parents who need concrete demonstrations and feedback, but it requires extensive therapist time and effort.

Support Services as an Adjunct to Treatment

High levels of stress and low levels of resources for some families may be obstacles to treatment effectiveness and/or long-term maintenance of effects. New learning requires freedom from distraction and gentle scaffolding by more experienced others. We know that stress interferes with cognition. Distractibility, narrowing of perceptual capacities, and problem solving in crises may lead to misjudgments or oversights. For example, negative child attributions are especially common when parents are in a negative mood state (Dix, Rheinhold, & Zambarano, 1990). Some evidence has begun to emerge that chronic levels of stress may influence brain functioning, thus producing more chronic cognitive problems in executive functioning (McEwen, 2001; Stein, Hanna, Koverola, Torchia, & McClarty, 1997). Providing instrumental supports (e.g., help with housing, marital/couple problems, or money difficulties) can reduce stress and free up the attentional capacities needed for new learning in behavioral and cognitive-behavioral approaches. These supports might also include homemaker services, day care, respite care, and crisis hotlines. One study with neglectful parents (Gaudin, Wodarksi, Arkinson, & Avery, 1990) attempted to decrease neglect through strengthening informal support networks, using personal networking, linking volunteers with families, employing neighborhood helpers, and providing social skills training. One study, however, did not show that offering enhanced adjunct services added to the positive outcomes obtained when behavioral approaches were employed (Chaffin et al., 2004).The approach used, however, has been demonstrated to have effects on marital/couple functioning and maternal depression, and this may account for the lack of added effects of enhanced services.

SPECIFIC TREATMENT METHODS

Once the decisions about treatment target areas, structure, and format have been made, the choice of specific intervention methods remains. A limited number of standard cognitive

and behavioral methods have been employed with maltreating parents to date, such as behavioral rehearsal, cognitive restructuring, feedback, skills training (e.g., parent training, anger and self-control training, and stress management training), and treatment of antecedent conditions. In addition to programs that focus on just one of these skill areas, several treatment programs have utilized a package approach that works on a number of target areas simultaneously. In many cases, however, the techniques being employed have been modified to meet the special needs of maltreating families. Therefore, each of these commonly used methods is discussed with specific consideration to their application with maltreating families (Wolfe & Werkele, 1993). Several single-case and group studies involving behavioral efforts with maltreating parents have appeared in the literature. In addition, there have been four comparative treatment studies (Azar & Twentyman, 1984; Brunk, Henggeler, & Whelan, 1987; Egan, 1983; Kolko, 1996b). Methods that hold promise but have not been fully evaluated are also mentioned, in anticipation that future efforts will be directed toward these areas (e.g., specific child treatments, behavioral consultation).

Parent-Focused Treatment

Modeling and Behavioral Rehearsal

Modeling and role playing of newly acquired behaviors are probably the most common components in behavioral treatments of child abuse or neglect, and in parent training in particular (see Denicola & Sandler, 1980; Wolfe, Kaufman, et al., 1981). Maltreating parents' feelings of inadequacy regarding their parenting behavior or general interpersonal skills may make them more reluctant than most clients to undertake role playing. Presenting a clear rationale and therapist modeling of "role-playing" behavior may initially be useful in reducing parents' anxiety. An early program developed by Barth, Blythe, Schinke, Stevens, and Schilling (1983) demonstrated how parents might gradually be worked into role playing (shaping). Examples of desirable child management approaches were first presented via videotape, followed by therapist modeling of the behaviors. Finally, parents were provided with scripts to follow in their initial role-play attempts, and they were praised for their efforts. In group interventions, asking other parents to act out particular parents' situations or to act as coaches in a role play may also reduce the pressure in using such a technique. A danger of using role plays with this population, however, is that on occasion inappropriate parental responses (e.g., coercive responses) may be volunteered by group members during "coaching." Therapists must be careful to deal with such responses immediately; otherwise, parents are likely to incorporate such negative responses into their repertoire.

Feedback

An important component of role playing is the provision of feedback. Care needs to be taken here, however: Negative feedback (both given and received) is common in such families, and there is danger that the therapist will be perceived as negative or harsh. Parents will not benefit from their experience and/or will become overly sensitive to any comments about their child-rearing methods and leave treatment if sessions are perceived as too critical. Feedback during role plays help refine parents' response toward the desired goal behavior; more importantly, it models for them a different way of responding when faced with needing to correct the behavior of another. It is especially important, therefore, that feedback be presented in a positive manner (e.g., what a parent is doing right, not wrong). Initially, the frequency of praise for attempting or acquiring new behaviors must be higher than with other populations, and/or commensurate with each parent's preferences (e.g., some prefer quiet recognition, and others prefer a lot of attention and fanfare). The therapist can also model acceptance of negative feedback by describing instances of self-criticism.

Cognitive Restructuring

Cognitive restructuring is a method of addressing irrational or dysfunctional beliefs that may lead to inappropriate responses (e.g., misattributions, distorted beliefs, unrealistic expectancies) (Azar, 1984, 1986, 1997; Azar et al., 2005; Azar & Twentyman, 1986). Evidence has supported the idea that maltreating parents possess cognitive styles and belief systems (maladaptive schemas, negative appraisal styles) that could play such a mediational role. For example, abusive parents have been shown to as-

cribe greater negative intentionality to their children's behavior than do other parents, even when that behavior is within developmental norms (Haskett et al., 2003; Larrance & Twentyman, 1983; Plotkin, 1983); to view themselves as having less control in relation to their children (Bugental et al., 1993, 1996); and to have more unrealistic ideas of what is appropriate to expect in children's behavior (Azar, Robinson, et al., 1984; Azar & Rohrbeck, 1986). Such appraisals can increase the risk of aggression, and can also lead to a decrease in or lack of responses that facilitate child development (e.g., less use of explanation; Barnes & Azar, 1990).

Along with child-based cognitions, disturbances in more general models of relationships have been posited (e.g., by attachment theorists). When maltreating parents are interacting with their children, these child-specific or more generally disturbed schemas regarding relationships are activated. Once activated, these schemas bring with them affective and cognitive material that may interfere with responding to the actual cues children are presenting (i.e., they may disturb information processing) and lead to overly harsh reactions or withdrawal, or at the very least mismatches between parental responses and child needs. The low perceptions of parental control found among abusive parents (see above) have been associated with parents' physiological arousal and negative affect when interacting with behaviorally challenging children (Bugental et al., 1993, 1996), as well as with neglectful behavior (e.g., failing to provide physically safe environments and taking remediative actions following an injury; Bugental & Happaney, 2004; Peterson et al., 1995).

Cognitive restructuring involves, first of all, clients' recognition that their thoughts/assumptions about situations and others affect their behavior. Once this relationship is acknowledged, clients are required to generate their own "personalized cognitions" about situations that are problematic. An example is a father's interpretation of his 2-year-old's unwillingness to go take a nap as an active attempt to devalue him as a parent (e.g., "He must think I'm really stupid"), rather than typical 2-year-old behavior. The therapist then challenges those cognitions, and an attempt is made to replace them with ones that are more appropriate (e.g., "Here we go again—I've just got to be patient"). Generating such "personalized" cognitions may be very difficult for maltreating parents. Role plays of problematic situations are useful to activate maladaptive schemas, and parents can then be assisted in identifying their dysfunctional thoughts *in vivo*. Imagery techniques have also been used (Azar, 1984). Extremely stressful situations, for example, can be described in which a potentially triggering child event is introduced. An example is the following:

> Your landlord just came by and said that he is evicting you. Your welfare check that was due yesterday still hasn't arrived, and you and your boyfriend had a bad fight last night. You have on your new white dress that you saved for weeks to buy and your child comes up to you and despite telling him to be careful, he spills his Kool-Aid all over it. (Azar, 1984, p. 166)

Once the client has successfully imagined this situation (or a self-generated problem situation), questioning can take place regarding what the parent would be saying to him- or herself at that moment, and how these statements would affect his or her actions. Dramatizations of examples clients spontaneously provide can be particularly useful. Questioning can start with what a parent is feeling. Once a feeling is stated, the parent can then be asked what the parent expected of the child in this situation or what he or she was thinking. It is also helpful to ask the parent whether other people besides the child make him or her feel the same way. One mother, for example, found conflict with her 3-year-old son very difficult to take and perceived him as intentionally trying to make her feel "stupid." When she was asked about others in her life, it became clear that the child's father, her ex-boyfriend, used to belittle her in conflict situations, and that the boy looked very much like his father. Such priming of critical others has been shown to make individuals more self-critical and to generate negative affect in experimental work (Baldwin, 1997).

Attachment theorists have recently argued for a heavy emphasis on the historical roots of such schemas (i.e., they contend that early representational models are at the root of parenting difficulties; Lieberman & Zeanah, 1999; Marvin, Cooper, Hoffman, & Powell, 2002; van IJzendoorn, Juffer, & Duyvesteyn, 1994), although even these writers suggest that identifying historical roots for the parent may not be necessary. The contribution of this approach is

its more explicit emphasis on emotion in the work—something that has been more implicit in strict cognitive approaches. In any case, it has been shown experimentally that when individuals are made aware a schema has been primed, it has less impact on their responses (Baldwin, 1997).

In building a rationale for going through this exercise, it is important for therapists to model the process by sharing examples of their own where cognitions resulted in responses that were inappropriate. The exact process of rational reevaluation can then be modeled, with alternative cognitive statements generated as solutions. If clients still have difficulty generating cognitions, therapists may need to provide examples (e.g., scripts that include such cognitive statements; Barth et al., 1983). In group treatment, exercises designed to generate parents' ideas regarding their definitions of "good" parenting or a "good" child can also elicit what may be considered overly idealized parental expectations regarding themselves and those around them (Azar, 1984). Once such statements and belief systems are identified, challenging them can be undertaken. Parents can be questioned as to whether such self-statements help or hinder their job as parents (e.g., whether they allow them to act as good teachers to their children). Beliefs regarding the similarity of children's understanding and ability to those of adults can also be disputed by using concrete demonstrations. For example, with parents of preschoolers, Piagetian conservation tasks can be shown in a group situation as concrete evidence that children do not think in the same way that adults do.

Clinicians also can help parents articulate the benefits and consequences of particular socialization goals they may have. For example, clinicians can recast children's demands for attention as an indication of their respect for parents and desire for closeness. They can help parents articulate how it would be nice to have a child who is always compliant, but not so desirable to have a nation of adults who never question authority. Similarly, they can gently challenge parents' previously unexamined beliefs with statements such as "Where did you learn that parents must always maintain absolute control over their children? That sounds like a lot of pressure to bear."

At times, work requires helping parents understand potential conflicts that may exist between cultural and religious beliefs and functioning in society at large (Peterson, Gable, Doyle, & Ewigman, 1997). For example, many parents who live in dangerous neighborhoods believe their children need to fight to avoid being picked on, but those same behaviors can cause problems at school. Of course, therapists must be careful to be respectful when they do this. For example, parental belief in the maxim "Spare the rod, spoil the child" might be challenged by offering alternative Biblical interpretations: "The saying actually referred to the rod of a shepherd who used it to 'guide' his sheep, not physically punish them" (Peterson et al., 1997, p. 61).

The use of metaphors may be particularly effective in helping parents understand and differentiate core beliefs in their schemas. Metaphors function to overlay new meaning on a set of beliefs in a salient and easily accessible form. For example, clinicians can discuss—and even demonstrate—how punishing a child is like driving a nail into a piece of wood: Although a sledgehammer can accomplish that one goal, it is likely to do much damage in the process; a small finishing hammer is much more likely to get the job done without undesirable consequences (Peterson et al., 1997). Developmental immaturity can be illustrated by using phrases such as "Asking your child to do that is like my asking you to fix a carburetor. No matter how much you might want to do it, it is simply beyond your capacity. It would be unfair of me to punish you for not listening" (Azar, Nix, & Makin-Byrd, 2005, p. 53). Metaphors enhance persuasion by helping to facilitate, organize, and process a large amount of information (Sopory & Dillard, 2002). They appear to be most effective when presented at the beginning of a message.

Clinicians can then carefully provide alternative assumptions or self-talk. The faulty belief systems and inappropriate self-statements can then be replaced with ones like these: "He's only 2," "He doesn't know any better," "It may feel like I can't take any more, but I can handle it. She's only a child. She doesn't know what I've been through today," or "It was an accident. Kids do these things." These alternative narratives give parents more "space" within which to do their job.

The Use of Resources and Technology

Each of the methods described above may be augmented by the use of other resources and technology. For instance, coaching can be carried out through the use of a bug-in-the-ear transmitter and a one-way mirror. Such training allows for prompting, shaping, and reinforcement of new responses as they happen, which may be more powerful training methods than demonstration alone. Videotaped observations of staged parenting situations (Barth et al., 1983) and of the clients and their children (Wolfe & Manion, 1984) may make therapist suggestions more salient to maltreating parents. Videotaped modeling has been used successfully as part of parent training with other populations (Connolly, Sharry, & Fitzpatrick, 2001; Webster-Stratton, 1984, 1994). Over the course of treatment, previous parent–child tapes can be replayed to illustrate the progress clients have made, and also to note how a relapse might appear. Board games to train social skills among adults with mental retardation (Foxx, McMorrow, & Schloss, 1983) have been adapted for use with low-functioning maltreating parents (Fantuzzo, Wray, Hall, Goins, & Azar, 1986). Using a common board game, Sorry, parents make moves on the board dependent upon their responses to various parenting and social problem situations. More elaborate responses to situations are gradually shaped and socially reinforced. In group programs, films may also be useful adjuncts to provide material for discussion. Films and audiotapes are available illustrating behavioral techniques, as well as the handling of general parenting and child development issues.

Skills Training

Skills training has been done with maltreating parents in three general areas: parent training, anger control, and stress management. Work in each area may be broad, going beyond parent–child relationships to include general social skills training. In each case, standardized training packages developed for other groups have been employed, with modifications carried out to meet the specific needs of this population.

PARENT TRAINING

Child management skills training has been described in detail in the literature. Standard parent training packages typically include (1) teaching parents to track child problem behaviors that they have selected; (2) education in techniques based on social learning theory, such as the identification of antecedents and the use of reinforcement, extinction, time out, and punishment to change behavior (usually presented didactically); and (3) home application of techniques. Record keeping (e.g., charting of child behavior) is often required, and reading often supplements didactic presentations. Care must be taken in assigning reading to make sure that literacy is not a problem.

The most basic of issues in undertaking parent training with maltreating parents (especially abusive ones) is their willingness to give up physical forms of punishment and to utilize more positive means of control. Even if a parent is willing to attempt a different approach, attending to the child's good behavior takes time to produce results, and the parent may become frustrated. Rather than completely removing the parent's only means of control, the therapist can establish a contractual agreement with the parent at the outset of treatment to practice a nonphysical form of punishment for a specified period of time, thus allowing for a gradual shift in behavior (Wolfe, Kaufman, et al., 1981). As described later, DuCharme, Atkinson, and Poulton (2000) focus entirely on positive strategies in their approach to work with maltreating parents, to avoid the stress that might be produced by emphasizing compliance.

The requirements of standard training packages may also be difficult for the typical maltreating parent. A parent's chaotic lifestyle, for example, may interfere with the consistent collection of data usually required in such programs, making simplification of data collection procedures necessary. Collecting data for a single day or afternoon, rather than a week, may be more practical with such families. With some parents, reviewing over the phone what occurred in a given day may be the only way to collect such information consistently. Training parents in the use of reinforcement and punishment techniques may also present problems. Parents' own state of economic and emotional deprivation, for example, may interfere with their use of reinforcement with their children. A clinical example of this occurred in a case where a child's bedwetting was the target of intervention. This behavior resulted in the mother's becoming angry and at times aggressive. When a reinforcement procedure was worked out with the family, it quickly became clear that despite the initial success of the program, the maltreating mother was sabotaging it

by failing to maintain consistent use. It was only after a parental reward (i.e., special attention from her spouse) was introduced contingent on her carrying out the program that progress could be made.

High levels of therapist encouragement are also needed initially to motivate such a parent to try the new techniques. Even if a parent reports active use of the new techniques and desired improvement in a child's behavior, observation of the parent's application of the methods is needed. Parents may engage in manipulative behavior because of their legal status or because of a sincere desire to "please" the therapist. Particular dangers exist in training abusive parents in behavioral punishment strategies. Because of the inappropriate judgment of such parents, there is a greater potential for misuse of techniques. Time-out procedures, such as placing a child in his or her own room for misbehavior, need to be carefully reviewed and rehearsed with parents; otherwise, they may proceed to lock children in closets or other closed spaces. "Grandma's rule" (e.g., "If you do X, then Y will happen"; Becker, 1971) can easily be twisted into a new form of parental tyranny unless extreme caution is used in training. The types of behavior most appropriate for targeting with this technique should be carefully specified with each client. Extinction (e.g., ignoring of negative child behavior), another common behavioral method, can also have negative side effects, because it usually results in an increase in a child's aversive behavior before a reduction occurs. Clients should be warned that this may take place, and should be provided with coping strategies to get them through this stressful period (e.g., they can be told to *interpret* this increase as a sign of success).

Overall, parent training efforts have shown success in changing interaction patterns in the abusing and neglectful parents studied (Wolfe & Wekerle, 1993). In addition, reductions in abuse and neglect rates have been found (Azar & Twentyman, 1984; Chaffin et al., 2004; DuCharme et al., 2000; Kolko, 1996b; Lutzker & Rice, 1984, Wolfe, Sandler, et al., 1981). A recent use of PCIT with maltreating parents in a randomized controlled trial showed reductions in maltreatment re-reports, compared to typical community-based parenting programs; it also showed that behavioral parent–child interaction changes mediated the effects (Chaffin et al., 2004). This study supports strongly the effectiveness of behavioral approaches with this population of parents. These studies, however, have used more highly trained professionals (e.g., psychologists) than is typical with CPS clients, which must be considered in generalization of their effects.

ANGER CONTROL STRATEGIES

Along with parenting skills training, instruction in self-control and anger control strategies is useful with abusive parents, given their heightened arousal and poor ability to cope with stress. Cognitive and behavioral techniques have been used with other populations to reduce anger and to increase coping ability (Novaco, 1975). Such techniques have obvious applicability to this population (Acton & During, 1992; Azar & Twentyman, 1984; Barth et al., 1983; Nomellini & Katz, 1983; Sanders et al., 2004; Wolfe, Sandler, et al., 1981). The most common strategies include the following components: (1) early detection of physiological and cognitive cues associated with anger arousal; (2) replacing anger-producing thoughts with more appropriate cognitions; and (3) developing self-control skills to modulate the expression of anger in anger eliciting situations. Systematic desensitization has also been employed when discrete aversive child behaviors that trigger extreme anger incidents can be identified (e.g., babies' crying). There is evidence to suggest that training in anger control may not be sufficient to change an abusive parent's behavior toward a child (Egan, 1983). It may reduce aggressive responses, but it does not change parental use of appropriate ones. Over time, the lack of child management capacities may lead situations to deteriorate to such an extent that anger control alone will not be sufficient to prevent abuse from occurring.

STRESS REDUCTION STRATEGIES

Stress reduction techniques are a third skills training approach employed with abusive parents. This type of training, like anger control, is usually included as part of a larger package of treatment. Training typically includes instruction in relaxation techniques and cognitive-behavioral methods of reducing stress. Parents are trained to recognize how the negative ways they interpret situations lead them to become stressed, and to substitute stress-reducing self-statements for negative ones. They are also trained to perform actions to reduce their stress level (e.g., leave the situation, seek outside advice, increase resources). Parents may be required to read written material on stress reduction techniques between treatment sessions, and to keep notebooks on class material and do homework assignments (Egan, 1983). Parents have also been provided with relaxation tapes to practice this strategy between sessions (Wolfe, Kaufman, et al., 1981). Since general coping abilities in this population may be low, a broad range of situations—parenting as well as nonparenting—need to be included for maximum benefit.

Stress reduction techniques and anger control training are subject to many of the same problems as parenting skills training (e.g., lack of client sophistication, manipulation, etc.), and modifications of presentations may be needed, depending on the characteristics of the individuals being served. Given the highly stressed nature of this parent population, consideration should be given to parenting skills training that emphasizes positive approaches exclusively. DuCharme and colleagues (2000), for example, have described "errorless compliance training." This strategy involves hierarchical introduction of more demanding parental requests at a gradual pace that greatly reduces noncompliance and obviates the need for constraining consequences (e.g., time out). They showed it to be effective with a group of parents whose children exhibited oppositional defiant behavior and whose families had long histories of family violence. Barkley (2000) cites this approach as a solution to the concerns raised when working with parents who are prone to violence and who may use punishment contingencies inappropriately, although he points out that comparisons with the more routine and manual-based parent training approaches used in clinical settings have yet to be done.

Treatment of Antecedents of Abuse and Strategies for Addressing Neglect-Related Issues

Along with addressing parental skills and cognitive processes related to maltreatment, some work has been directed to stressful antecedent conditions that might set up situations where maltreatment is more likely. Outcome studies have tailored their treatment to specific and most relevant needs of the families. Multiple targets, including depression, marital/couple discord, migraine headaches, and vocational goals, are typically chosen (Campbell, O'Brien, Bickett, & Lutzker, 1983; Conger, Lahey, & Smith, 1981). Neglect-related issues have been successfully addressed by behavioral interventions. Strategies include teaching parents home safety skills to "childproof" their homes; meal planning and budgeting to improve the nutrition provided to children; symptom recognition skills to improve parents' ability to identify illness in their children and to make appropriate responses; emergency skills; and home cleanliness (Lutzker, Bigelow, Doctor, Gershater, & Greene, 1998; Tymchuk, 1992). Because neglect affects more children and may have more far-reaching consequences than other forms of maltreatment (Dubowitz, 1991), expansion of methods for this population is sorely needed. Large-scale efforts to employ these approaches are discussed below (Lutzker et al., 1998; Lutzker & Bigelow, 2002).

Multicomponent Treatment Approaches

Behavioral efforts have evaluated the impact of multicomponent (package) approaches to treatment, given the complexity of factors leading to maltreatment. Packages can also be delivered in group formats by agencies that serve families, thereby meeting the differing needs of a larger number of families at one time. Social service agencies usually have limited resources available, and the development of effective packages may have utility. Furthermore, the urgency of the problem often requires immediate changes in a family, and lengthy assessment periods to determine specific target areas are not always possible. Several treatment studies have shown how a multicomponent approach may be successfully applied. Wolfe, Sandler, and colleagues (1981) used a group treatment format that emphasized several behavioral methods in their competency-based program for abusive parents. Individual home-based sessions served as adjuncts to group training sessions. Eight abusive families referred by CPS were provided with eight sessions of group training, while another eight abusive families received the usual level of monitoring provided by the referring agency. Training focused on child management skills and anger control, as taught via didactic instruction, problem solving, role modeling, rehearsal, self-control training, and in-home implementation with each parent and child together. During observations of parent–child interactions in the home, treated subjects were found to use appropriate child management procedures (e.g., positive reinforcement, effective punishment and commands) significantly more than waiting-list controls did. This difference was maintained at a 1-year follow-up, and the treated group showed no recidivism, whereas one abuse report occurred in the control group.

Another multicomponent approach that has been applied to child maltreatment is a commonly used evidence-based treatment, PCIT (Eyberg, 1988; Hembree-Kigin & McNeil, 1995), which has been adapted for use with maltreating parents (Urquiza & McNeil, 1996). This approach has two key components: parent–child relational enhancement through teaching parents better and more positive communication skills (using training in reflective listening skills, narrating of child behavior, and high levels of praise), and training parents in strategies to improve compliance. Parents are provided with information, practice skills to the point of mastery with therapist coaching, and work to generalize adaptation of skills to other settings. The original approach was developed for children ages 2–8 years, but has been used with maltreating parents of 4- to 12-year-olds, where the most common contexts for physical abuse are disciplinary situations. In a randomized controlled trial, Chaffin and colleagues (2004) examined the effectiveness of this two-component approach in preventing re-reports of physical abuse. Physically abusive parents (n = 110) were randomly assigned to one of three intervention conditions: (1) PCIT; (2) PCIT plus individualized enhanced services (e.g., marital/couple and family psychotherapy, services targeting parental depression); and (3) a standard community-based parenting group. Participants had multiple past child welfare reports; severe parent-to-child violence; low household income; and significant levels of depression, substance abuse, and antisocial behavior. At a median follow-up of 850 days, 19% of parents assigned to PCIT had a re-report for physical abuse, compared with 49% of the parents receiving a standard parenting group. Enhanced services did not improve the efficacy of PCIT. Greater reductions in negative parent–child interactions mediated the relative superiority of PCIT. This study provides strong support for a skills-based approach with maltreating parents. The lack of added effectiveness for the adjunct services is puzzling, but may be due to the fact that such services were offered to all parents who had problems, without consideration of whether the problems had a direct impact on the parent–child relationship. The problems addressed, however, may result in long-term reduction of risk to children beyond the risk of abuse. Furthermore, it has been shown that PCIT itself has a positive impact on marital/couple relationships and depression in parents, and thus greater effects may not have been possible.

Two large-scale programs that are based on social learning theory, and that operate in the community with large numbers of maltreating clients, have also been evaluated: Project 12-Ways and Project SafeCare. Both use a variety of behavioral techniques to deal with child maltreatment (Gershater, Ronit, Lutzker, & Wesch, 2003; Lutzker & Rice, 1984, Lutzker et al., 1998). In-home services (treatment and training) are provided to families referred to the projects by CPS. Areas of treatment include parent–child training, stress reduction, self-control training, social support, assertiveness training, use of leisure time, health maintenance and nutrition, home safety, job placement, marital/couple discord counseling, alcoholism referral, and money management. Selection of treatment provided is based on individual case needs. Evaluations of these programs have indicated that they are successful in reducing numbers of reports of maltreatment in participating families, relative to carefully matched control groups receiving typical CPS interventions (e.g., family preservation services). Because of the variations in the specific treatments offered to each individual family, solid conclusions regarding the effectiveness of any one type of treatment are difficult to draw from the results of these evaluations. However, smaller-scale evaluations of components suggest they are highly effective for the behaviors targeted (Lutzker et al., 1998; Lutzker & Bigelow, 2002).

In two other interesting community-based studies, Szykula and Fleischman (1985) demonstrated the impact that social-learning-theory-based intervention programs might have on out-of-home placement of abused and neglected children. The families treated in the two studies were referred by state CPS agencies and were selected because they were considered at risk for placement of their children outside the home due to abuse. In the first study, families all had children between the ages of 3 and 12 years of age; they were described as primar-

ily white and of lower socioeconomic status, and about 50% of the parents were single. The treatment package included methods based on social learning theory: training parents in the tracking of problem behavior; the use of reinforcement and time-out procedures to modify behavior; problem solving; and cognitive self-control training to deal with anger, guilt, depression, and anxiety. Phone supervision of assignments was also employed. Each family received 15–25 hours of treatment-oriented contact time. The investigators found that there was an 85% drop in out-of-home placements during the program's operation, but that placements rebounded to previous levels during a 9-month break in the program. Out-of-home placements for reasons other than abuse showed no change over the entire period of study. There was also no recidivism for abuse among treated families during treatment and at a 1-year follow-up (unfortunately, the number of families involved was not reported). A noteworthy aspect of this program was that it used bachelor's- and master's-level caseworkers as treatment agents, providing a better demonstration of the utility of such techniques in typical treatment settings.

Szykula and Fleischman's (1985) second study used an experimental design with 48 abusive families and the same treatment package described above, with out-of-home placement again used as the outcome measure. Families were first divided into two levels of severity, "less difficult" and "more difficult," based on review of each family's social history and case file. Less difficult cases ($n = 26$) had fewer than three reports of abuse, had no serious difficulty with housing or transportation, and had a child's conduct identified as a major problem. More difficult cases ($n = 22$) had three or more reports of abuse, had serious problems with unemployment, had consistent transportation and housing difficulties, and had been identified as having major problems outside of a parent's relationship with a child (e.g., frequent fights with boyfriends or extended family, extreme feelings of anger and/or depression, and frequent difficulties with others in their community). Families within each severity level were randomly assigned to either the treatment package or a control condition of standard social services (ranging from limited supervision to other forms of therapy available in the community). Outcome data indicated that the treatment package was most successful in reducing out-of-home placement for the less difficult group (1 of 13 of the treated families vs. 5 of 13 of the controls), but not for the more difficult group (7 of 11 of the treated families vs. 5 of 11 of the controls). In their conclusions, the researchers point out that the success rates for the first study may have been due to differential referrals of less difficult cases. Their findings also show a need for refining methods to discriminate between those families that will or will not benefit from social-learning-theory-based treatments.

These community-based projects suggest the viability of programmatic application of social-learning-theory-based interventions for child maltreatment. Findings suggest that they may be effective in reducing maltreatment incidence and out-of-home placement of children for a broader range of maltreating families. Packages also may allow the widespread dissemination of such methods. However, because of the use of multiple components, the specific methods responsible for their effectiveness await further determination.

Other innovative large-scale multicomponent approaches have been implemented and are also worthy of mention. Fantuzzo, Weiss, and Coolahan (1998) describe an attempt to intervene with maltreating parents within already existing community structures—in this case, already existing Head Start services for at-risk preschoolers. The project involved a partnering of researchers and community groups (CPS, community-based agencies, schools, parents). Interesting components included the use of Head Start parents to recruit maltreating parents who were not currently involved in Head Start; focus groups to determine parents' needs; work aimed at empowering parents (e.g., showing parents how their stress might affect their parent–child interactions and how they could become change agents on stress-related issues, informing parents on how to transact with school systems on behalf of their children); and an intervention that involved peers to increase children's social competence (see a later section for description of this peer-to-peer intervention). This "mainstreaming" of maltreating parents with nonmaltreating ones within an intervention is a unique element of this project. To date, only evaluation of the social competence intervention is available and showed promising results (Fantuzzo et al., 1996); positive findings are described regarding the other elements (Fantuzzo et al., 1998).

An ecological model, multisystemic therapy (MST; see below for comparative findings), has also been recently applied to work with parent-to-adolescent abuse (Swenson et al., in press). MST has been employed successfully for juveniles with violent and chronic offenses, and has shown decreases in long-term rates of rearrest and rates of days in out-of-home placements. The approach is characterized by a "family-friendly" engagement process (e.g., family members are seen as needing to trust the system providing therapy, and the approach must reduce the fear that the therapist is collaborating with CPS to take the child away); a strong focus on family strengths; recruitment of the key individuals in the child's natural ecology (e.g., family members, teachers, caseworker, etc.) to achieve success; and the development of goals that involve and prioritize interactions within this ecology and the relationship changes that are needed. These goals may be narrow (e.g., parental behavioral change) or fairly broad (e.g., decreasing parental depression, promoting interaction between the school and the parent, and monitoring of the intervention success by all participants).

Evidence-based treatment techniques are integrated that address problematic behaviors by multiple members of the system, and the treatment is home-based to address barriers to service delivery. Adaptations to typical MST for use with maltreating families include safety planning (written contracting that draws on family, extended family, and friends or neighbors as resources); treatment for PTSD and anger management with parents and children; treatment of substance abuse; family communication training; and clarification of the abuse (which is a method for helping the parent [who typically blames the child for the abuse] to rethink the incidences of abuse, to accept responsibility for the abuse, and apologize to the child and the family). The clarification takes place through writing a letter that is drafted over multiple sessions, where the therapist can work on distortions the parent might have regarding the abuse, culminating in a family meeting where clarification work takes place. The CPS caseworker is involved in treatment, and the MST therapist works on facilitating a relationship between the family and the caseworker in a manner that is most beneficial to the family. Highly supportive supervision of the therapist is seen as key, given the depth of problems in the family and ecological system. A major evaluation is underway of PEACE (Project Empowering Adults, Children, and Their Ecology), a 5-year project utilizing this package approach that is targeting 10- to 17-year-olds in Charleston, South Carolina, who are involved with the CPS system; however, data are not yet available on outcomes.

Comparative Treatment Effectiveness

Six studies have evaluated differential treatment effectiveness in order to specify methods that are most beneficial with this population. Comparisons involved different types of behavioral treatments (Egan, 1983); different forms of cognitive-behavioral treatment (CBT) versus an insight- oriented intervention (Azar & Twentyman, 1984); systemic treatment versus social-learning- theory-based treatment (Brunk et al., 1987); CBT versus family therapy (Kolko, 1996b); and an attachment intervention versus a psychoeducational approach that was labeled a "CBT" intervention (Toth et al., 2002).

Across the studies, some differential treatment effects were found. For example, Egan (1983) found that stress management training led to changes in the feelings of parents, and that child management training produced changes in specific child management skills. Brunk and colleagues (1987) compared MST in the home (which included reframing, joining, and prescribed tasks, with content varying depending on family needs—e.g., marital/couple work, work with extended family, child management education, work on expectations of children) to a social-learning-based approach presented in group format. Results favored the MST for restructuring parent–child relationships, whereas the group parent training decreased parents' social problems. The latter finding may be due to the effect of group participation on social isolation, although the lack of a control condition and differences in formats and settings make firm conclusions difficult. Arguably, the MST approach may have been more effective because it worked on changing cognitive distortions and relationship skills across multiple relationships.

Others did not find many differential treatment effects at the end of treatment, but found differences in recidivism or child abuse risk. Kolko (1996b) compared individual child and parent CBT to family therapy, and had a comparison group that received routine community services. This study is interesting, in that both children and parents in the CBT condition received social-learning-theory-based work to address their cognitive, affective, and behavioral repertoires. For children, this involved reviewing their perspectives on family stressors and violence, and receiving training in coping and self-control skills (e.g., safety and support planning, relaxation). Parents also reviewed their perspectives on violence and physical punishment, attributional style and expectations, self-control (e.g., anger control, cognitive coping), and contingency management (e.g., attention, reinforcement, time out). The family therapy condition (functional family therapy) also had a base in social learning theory. The control condition received typical CPS programs (e.g., support groups, homemaking, home-based services). Although all treatment groups showed improvement over time, the CBT and family therapy groups were associated with improvements in parent-reported child-to-parent violence and child externalizing behaviors, parental distress and abuse risk, and family conflict and cohesion. No differences were found between CBT and family therapy on consumer satisfaction or maltreatment risk at termination. Only one family in both of these two groups showed another incident of maltreatment over a 1-year period, whereas in the community group there were three such cases. Both treatment conditions included cognitive elements (e.g., work on attributions in CBT and problem-solving training in family therapy), so it cannot be determined whether the treatments were sufficiently different to produce differential treatment results.

Azar and Twentyman (1984) compared two versions of a CBT group package approach (child management skills training, stress and anger management, and communication skills training) with insight-oriented group treatment and a waiting-list control comparison group. One of the CBT groups received additional home visits that involved further active training, whereas the other received only supportive home visiting. The insight-oriented group also received supportive home visiting. From caseworkers' perspectives, treated groups showed improvements compared to controls, but few differential treatment effects were found at the completion of a 10-week parenting program. At a 1-year follow-up, however, no recidivism was found for the CBT group with generalization training (0 of 13 cases), but recidivism rates for the other treatment conditions were typical of those found in CPS caseloads generally (25–37%).

One last comparative outcome study that has been published compared a psychoeducational/"CBT" intervention with another intervention labeled an "attachment" intervention (Toth et al., 2002). The former condition was a psychoeducational home visitation approach and differed from the CBT approach described elsewhere in this chapter, in that there was no description of efforts directed at altering parental appraisals or skills. The attachment approach used followed that of Lieberman, Silverman, and Pawl (2000). This approach focuses on the parent–infant dyad and works on changing parental internal models (similar to CBT described above, with a heavy emphasis on historical roots of present transactions between parent and child—"processing of maternal attachment histories," p. 882) and fewer attempts "to modify parenting behavior or verbalizations through direct instruction" (p. 891). As in CBT, work focuses on the parental narrative (see Azar et al., 2005, for a discussion of the common links between attachment models and CBT approaches. Although the psychoeducational/"CBT" condition did not fare as well in this comparison (e.g., there was less change in a child's "internal self-representational model"), the lack of distinction between the two approaches limited conclusions.

Overall, the effectiveness of behavioral approaches in the treatment of maltreating parents, especially physically abusive parents, is supported by these comparative studies. Although the question of differential effectiveness of behavioral versus other treatments is equivocal, the combination of behavioral group training with active home training seems effective at reducing recidivism. Recent work on relationship-enhancing approaches as an adjunct to cognitive and behavioral approaches seems promising. Future efforts need to use larger sample sizes to permit a test of what treatment works best for which type of client.

Child-Focused Treatments

Studies involving specific treatments for abused or neglected children are uncommon. Our discussion focuses primarily on the special issues and adaptations required to work with this population. Types of treatments that have been used with abused and neglected children include therapeutic day care and foster care to provide safety and fostering of developmental skills (Ayoub, 1991; Culp, Heide, & Richardson, 1987), behavioral skills training (e.g., social skills; Fantuzzo et al., 1988), and initial efforts to address PTSD symptoms (Deblinger, McLeer, & Henry, 1990). We discuss these methods in reference to four major categories of intervention: removal of a child from the home; developmental stimulation work; behavioral consultation; and studies aimed at treating trauma symptoms in children with other forms of maltreatment (which may be applicable to abused children as well).

Foster Care Placement and Day Care

Since its recognition as a major social problem, the most commonly used "intervention" for abused and neglected children has been to remove them from their homes. Two types of removal have occurred: foster care placement outside the home for a specified period of time, or day care placement for a limited number of hours each day. Foster care placement was originally advocated as a means of dealing with child maltreatment for two reasons. First, it was assumed to remove a child from harm and provide a stable and therapeutic environment. Second, it was also believed to provide a brief time for the family to undergo rehabilitation before the child was returned. Foster care placement has, however, recently come under criticism for economic and social reasons. The child welfare system was originally designed for short-term evaluation and placement, with the hope that children would soon be returned home or adopted. But for many, it has become a purgatory (B. Azar, 1995).

In any given year, more than 500,000 U.S. children reside in foster care (U.S. Department of Health and Human Services, 2001). Although foster care is intended to be short-term, fewer than 40% of children under 10 years of age who remain in care longer than 2 years will ever return home, and 60% of children born to parents with substance use problems and discharged from the hospital to foster care are still there 3 years later (B. Azar, 1995). Health and mental health care for children placed in foster care has been limited. One study found that 87% of children entering foster care over a 1-year period had at least one physical problem at the time of placement (Risley-Curtiss, Coombs-Orme, Chernoff, & Heisler, 1996). Despite this need, only about 61% of the children with urgent problems and fewer than half of children with important or routine care needs received services. The shortage of trained foster parents results in shifting children from one home to the next, and often in separating siblings (Shealy, 1995). Shifting care to kin has been one solution. Although this perhaps increases stability for children, care needs in kin care may go unmonitored by CPS or unattended to by caretakers, who are often unaware of the rights of their children to services and are not informed of them by caseworkers (Azar & Hill, in press).

Even though the child welfare system has been the main line of defense in assisting child victims of abuse and neglect (as well as related family crises) for almost a century, we know very little about the effectiveness of this system (Thompson & Wilcox, 1995). Accordingly, it is no secret that child welfare systems in North America are considered failures. The performance of the U.S. system was evaluated by the USABCAN (1990), which concluded that there were emergency needs in every part of the system. A further criticism involves the assumption that rehabilitation of a parent is occurring while a child is in placement. Only limited treatment services were typically provided to parents, and treatment deliverers still tend to be inadequately trained and to carry heavy caseloads, making intervention spotty. In addition, parental contact with a child in foster care may be quite limited. Lack of contact may make the child's return home and the family's reunification after foster placement difficult for both parent and child. In some cases, children who have spent most of their lives in foster placement, after much court litigation, are being returned to parents they hardly know.

Research on the impact of foster placement is limited, and much of it is flawed methodologically, making it difficult to reach definitive conclusions on its effects. Foster children show high levels of mental health problems both in childhood and in adulthood (Heflinger, Simpkins, & Coombs-Orme, 2000). More refined studies, however, suggest that perhaps those children showing the poorest outcomes as adults (e.g., incarceration) following foster care also had shown poor adjustment prior to foster placement (Widom, 1991). On the other hand, foster care itself has been blamed for long-term negative outcomes in adulthood,

such as higher levels of homelessness (Mangine, Royse, Wieche, & Nietzel, 1990). In one study that controlled for poverty, effects of foster placement were found over and above those associated with economic deprivation (e.g., an external attributional style, higher peer rejection; McIntyre, Launsbury, Bernton, & Steel, 1988). These diverse outcomes in relation to foster care may vary with the age of the child (Hurwitz, Simms, & Farrington, 1994; Rutter, 1989).

As an alternative to foster placement, day care is often used, especially for young children. Specially designed programs are rare, and more often than not such children are placed in day care settings with nonmaltreated children, without any modifications to programming. Nevertheless, a few therapeutic day care centers/preschools have arisen, aimed at more than providing children with a safe place during the day and relieving parental stress. These settings provide opportunities for maltreated children to develop and sustain basic trust in others, to have positive social interactions with peers, and to explore alternative affective and behavioral responses through activities (Ayoub, 1991). Key to such settings is the ongoing modeling of nonviolent conflict resolution by staff members. One such program is the Kempe Early Education Project, which incorporates a therapeutic preschool and home visitation for young abused children (see www.kempecenter. org/about/KempeTherapeuticPreschool.html). One evaluation found that children in the program showed improvements in general intellectual functioning and receptive language by discharge 1 year later (Oates, Gray, Schweitzer, Kempe, & Harmon, 1995). Intensive group-based treatment and developmental programming, with other family services, have been associated with improvements in children's functioning (e.g., perceived cognitive competence, peer acceptance, maternal acceptance, and developmental scores on standardized measures; Culp, Little, Letts, & Lawrence, 1991). For example, when exposed to caretakers who are more flexible and attentive than those found in their own homes, the maltreated children may behave differently at home. They may become more demanding of attention and less compliant, as well as showing a preference for the day care staff. These new behaviors may be perceived negatively by the parents and, paradoxically, may increase child abuse risk.

One solution may be to integrate parents into the day care program in some way; this can be accomplished by prearranged observation sessions of the program or by actual involvement of the parents in classroom activities. In such centers, parents can take part in classroom activities and attend supportive or educational groups with other parents (Ayoub, 1991; Crittenden, 1983). With their permission, they can also be videotaped while interacting with teachers and children. Later, these videotapes can be used as a source of group discussion with staff members or with outside consultants (Ayoub, 1991). Such informal instruction can be a valuable adjunct to treatment of such parents.

Developmental Stimulation Training

Because of the low levels of interaction in a maltreating family, developmental delays are often noted. These may further exacerbate risk for child maltreatment, in that the child may be more difficult to handle and require more effort on parents' part (e.g., more calls from school, day care, etc.). Use of interventions that increase parental stimulation and sensitivity may be helpful here. Wolfe and his colleagues describe a competency-based program that used modeling and feedback to increase positive parent–child interaction (e.g., physical contact, positive parent–child experiences, and use of nonaversive control) (Wolfe, Edwards, Manion, & Koverola, 1988; Wolfe & Manion, 1984). The attachment interventions described earlier also focus on parental sensitivity.

Behavioral Consultation with Day Care, School, and Foster Care Settings

While efforts are being directed at improving interactions in the home, inappropriate child behaviors that were acquired from an abusive or neglectful environment may be maintained by caretakers' reactions in other settings. Behavioral consultation with staff members in these other settings may help to support the changes made at home by parents, to assist reunification if children are in foster care, and to facilitate the overall adjustment of children. Unfortunately, such consultation has not been discussed in the literature.

Programs to reduce aggressive behavior in school settings (e.g., training day care staff in the use of reward with aggressive children for periods when they are behaving in a non-aggressive or prosocial way; use of time out) have been undertaken with other populations

by teachers and other staff members. Such programs may also be useful for aggressive abused children, promoting generalization of the children's responsiveness to these methods.

Socially withdrawn behavior has also been handled via behavioral techniques, such as peer prompting of social initiations (Strain, Shores, & Timm, 1977; Strain & Timm, 1974). In three intervention studies using such techniques with maltreated children who were either withdrawn or aggressive, Fantuzzo and his associates (Davis & Fantuzzo, 1989; Fantuzzo, Stovall, Schachtel, Goins, & Hall, 1987; Fantuzzo et al., 1988) found that positive, prosocial responses and initiations improved for the withdrawn children as a function of peer- and adult-mediated play sessions conducted in a playroom setting. It is noteworthy, however, that the maltreated children who tended to be aggressive showed an increase in negative behaviors in response to peer-initiated social interaction, and thus may have required more adult contact (Davis & Fantuzzo, 1989), whereas the withdrawn maltreated children were more responsive to peer-initiated strategies. Similarly, Fantuzzo and colleagues (1988) discovered that withdrawn neglected children actually responded more favorably to peer-initiated social interaction, but decreased their social behavior in response to adult initiations. A large-scale implementation of this program within Head Start programs targeting both maltreated and nonmaltreated preschoolers showed effectiveness in increasing peer-interactive play behavior and decreasing solitary play behavior (Fantuzzo et al., 1996). Teacher ratings of classroom social functioning indicated improvements 2 months following treatment. Children also demonstrated significantly higher self-control and interpersonal skills, and lower rates of internalizing and externalizing behavior problems.

Consultation with foster parents has also received some attention. Although there are not many data surrounding the effects on young children of placement outside the home, one study recently found that young children's adaptive behavior as reported by the current caregiver improved significantly during the 12 months following placement (Horwitz, Balestracci, & Simms, 2001).

Infant mental health approaches have been adapted for use with foster parents, and evaluations have been undertaken. Horwitz, Owens, and Simms (2000) studied the effects of a multidisciplinary clinic that provided health, mental health, and developmental outcomes for all children from 11 to 74 months of age who entered foster care in one county. Comparisons with children who received the usual services in a nearby county found that children in the intervention county had greater identification of developmental and mental health problems, a greater number of referrals, and were more likely to receive follow-up care at 6 and 12 months after placement. Although such systemic effects are important, no data were reported on the children's outcomes.

The attachment approaches discussed earlier have been adapted for work with foster parents of infants (Stovall & Dozier, 2000). The intent is to support infants' emotional development within the context of the new caretaking relationship. Because of these infants' idiosyncratic caretaking history and presumably insecure attachment, the foster caregivers are provided with assistance to read the infants' emotional cues; to increase their emotional sensitivity and responsiveness; to decrease harsh and inconsistent parenting; to foster a consistent, predictable environment; and to promote the development of secure caregiver–infant attachments. The general goal is to help caregivers to understand the infants' maltreatment experience, to see how it might have affected them, and to adapt their own parenting to meet these infants' unique needs (Clyman, Harden, & Little, 2002). Attachment approaches use observational work extensively and involve careful questioning of the meaning foster parents are making of the infants' interactive cues, as well as modeling of alternative appraisals. Suggestions of how to interact are modeled and prompted. The strategies employed, while drawing on ethological theory, appear to be very like those used by cognitive-behavioral and behavioral intervention agents (Azar et al., 2005). Indeed, traditional behavioral interventions to address children's specific problematic behaviors—such as depression; sleep and feeding problems; posttraumatic stress responses (e.g., sexualized behavior, heightened fear, and hypervigilance); and oppositional, aggressive, and impulse control difficulties—are also incorporated (Bonner, 2000; Webster-Stratton & Herbert, 1993).

Rigorous evaluations of the approaches described above have not yet been undertaken (e.g., random assignment to interventions, measures of intervention integrity, etc.). Better-controlled studies involving foster care have been undertaken with older children and involved social-learning-theory-based approaches, notably the work of Chamberlain and her colleagues (Chamberlain, Fisher, & Moore, 2002; Chamberlain & Smith, 2003; Fisher, Ellis, & Chamberlain, 1999; Fisher, Gunnar, Chamberlain, & Reid, 2000). This research has employed a modified version of the Oregon Social Learning Center Multidimensional Treatment Foster Care Model, used with juvenile offenders in foster care (Chamberlain et al., 2002).

The Early Interventions Foster Care model involves intensive training of foster parents to work with younger children (ages 3–7 years) who are in foster care due to child maltreatment. Community families are recruited, trained, and supported to provide placements, and no more than two youngsters are placed in a home. Both foster parents and biological parents receive intervention. The foster homes have a relatively high degree of ecological similarity to the children's former home environments in terms of day-to-day activities and systems of authority. Both sets of parents are trained in the use of behavioral management strategies (e.g., frequent reinforcement of appropriate child behavior, close supervision, and clear rules and limits), to ensure commonality when the children are returned to their homes. Mental health professionals with small caseloads oversee the work with parents and provide individual contact with each child. Group support meetings are held with foster parents. During daily phone contacts with the foster parents, data are collected on each child's progress/problems, and solutions are discussed where needed. Children receive skill-building interventions weekly and are slowly transitioned home when they are ready. Case managers are on call 24 hours a day to provide assistance throughout the program for both foster care and biological parents. Pilot work suggests that this model produces decreases in child symptoms, compared to more typical foster care. Foster parents showed greater use of positive reinforcement and lower stress than typical foster parents.

Interventions Aimed at Trauma Symptoms

The chronicity of the abuse and related stressors (e.g., number of out-of-home placements, need for hospitalization, etc.) have a bearing on how a child may adapt in both the short and the long term (Famularo, Kinscherff, & Fenton, 1990; Terr, 1991). Many abused children have been subjected to a series of traumas rather than a single traumatic event. Also, unlike children experiencing other kinds of trauma, abused children may not only lack the support of loved ones in coping with the trauma; the loved ones may in fact be the perpetrators. This fact may engender greater withdrawal and mistrust in abused children than in other traumatized youngsters. Lipovksy (1991) emphasizes four goals for the treatment of children and adolescents with PTSD: education, facilitation of emotional expression, anxiety control, and controlled exposure to memories of the event. Clinicians may find that pursuit of some of these goals may be enhanced by group treatment, whereas others may be best attempted in individual work.

In an individual setting, therapists must be sensitive to the possibility that an abused child may be too fearful to confide quickly in an adult (Aber & Allen, 1987; Steward, Farquhar, Dicharry, Glick, & Martin, 1986). Exposure to memories of the abusive event through play therapy techniques or imaginal exposure, however, may be best accomplished in an individual setting, because it is more difficult to monitor each child and control the emotional dynamics involved in a group setting. In contrast, education goals, which emphasize teaching children about typical reactions to stress and general coping strategies (Lipovsky, 1991), may be facilitated by a group. Seeing that other abused children share similar symptoms and concerns, for example, may help to "destigmatize" the experience. However, the clinician must be careful to monitor individual reactions, for what may be an innocuous topic of discussion for one child may bring back painful memories of abuse for another.

With some exceptions, outcome studies for treatment of PTSD-related symptoms have largely focused on adults, and they have been criticized for lack of adherence to experimental design (e.g., random assignment to treatment condition; McFarlane, 1989). Controlled exposure techniques have been used successfully to alleviate trauma due to other types of stressors in adults (McMillan, 1991; Richards & Rose, 1991) and children (Jones & Peterson, 1993). Anxiety management interventions such as biofeedback (Peniston, 1986) have also been used successfully with adults. Such approaches have been adapted successfully for use with sexually abused children and may have utility for physically abused youngsters as well. Deblinger and colleagues (1990) reduced PTSD-related symptoms among sexually abused children with a treatment package that included gradual exposure, modeling, education, coping, and prevention skills training. Nonoffending parents received cognitive-behavioral coping strategies concurrently, to help them respond appropriately to their children's behavioral difficulties and emotional symptoms. Treatment produced reductions in PTSD symptoms with this population, paving the way for its application with children from other backgrounds of maltreatment (Runyon, Deblinger, Ryan, & Thakkar-Kolar, 2004).

Summary of Treatment Methods

The limited child-focused treatment outcome research continues to be striking. Further work needs to be directed toward gathering information on how best to deal with a maltreated child's problems, as well as to enhance family functioning enough to ensure his or her safety and continued growth. In teaching new child-rearing skills to maltreating parents, a therapist must be aware of the contextual factors that interact with the family's acquisition of new parenting methods, as well as the potential misuse of the material presented. Consistent monitoring of information the parents have acquired during sessions is needed, and careful evaluations of parental use of techniques need to be carried out if failures occur. Regrettably, the modifications needed for work with these families have not received much attention in the literature. Finally, there is a pressing need to develop methods for assisting children with histories of physical and emotional abuse and neglect. Stimulation training, behavioral consultations, and stress management/coping are promising approaches.

PREVENTION AND EARLY INTERVENTION EFFORTS

Prevention and early intervention efforts using social-learning-theory-based methods constitute an important area for research at all levels of causation (Wekerle & Wolfe, 1993). At a societal level, mass media campaigns are emerging as a universal way of enhancing parenting skills, based on various behavioral and family systems strategies (Sanders, 1996). At the community and school levels, increased awareness of risk indicators allows for early identification of individuals at risk of child maltreatment, and services can be offered without coercion or labeling. Mothers and fathers can be offered assistance during pregnancy, or provided with education and skills training related to child development during high school. Adolescents who have experienced negative parental role models, or who have other special needs related to cognitive or behavioral abilities, can be offered preventive prepaTenting training programs (Azar, 1991b), as well as ones focused on general relationship skills (Wolfe, Wekerle, et al., 2003).

At the individual level, the need for support, instruction, and resource linkage among new parents is best met by a personalized outreach strategy, such as home visitation. This approach is illustrated by the Prenatal/Early Infancy Project of Olds and colleagues (Olds, Henderson, Chamberlin, & Tatelbaum, 1986; Olds, Henderson, & Kitzman, 1994; Olds et al., 1997), which began in the late 1970s. This team targets first-time parents with one or more child maltreatment risk factors, such as teen parents, single parents, and low-income families. Child care services and pre- and postnatal nurse home visits are offered to establish resource linkages and provide child development education. Notably, individuals receiving this intervention are viewed in terms of their strengths and abilities rather than their deficits, which translates into an empowerment strategy. Women are assisted in understanding and meeting their own needs and those of their newborn children, and are taught skills necessary to enhance this relationship as well as their own development.

The encouraging findings from this prospective prevention program support these methods of influencing major psychological determinants of healthy parent–child relationships. Relative to controls, mothers receiving the program have developed or changed their understanding of child health and development, their expectations for their own development, and their self-efficacy. Therapeutic alliances are also formed with each mother and other family members during pregnancy, so that when family stressors become significant, family members can be linked with needed health and human services (e.g., families are assisted in locating financial aid, subsidized housing, family counseling, nutritional supplementation, cloth-

ing and furniture, and proper medical care). This program is underway at three U.S. sites, and a variation of the program is underway in Canada. Encouragingly, a 15-year follow-up with 324 mothers and 315 of their firstborn adolescents has revealed that this program of prenatal and early childhood home visitation by nurses can reduce subsequent pregnancies, use of welfare, child maltreatment, and criminal behavior among low-income mothers and children (Olds et al., 1997). It has also shown long-term effects on health outcomes (e.g., child injuries and ingestions; Olds et al., 1998).

Many other universal prevention programs designed to influence children's lives for the better may also produce reductions in maltreatment risk for children (e.g., Head Start) when they include parenting components. In one study, Reynolds and Robertson (2003) explored the incidence of maltreatment in children who participated in an early education school-based prevention program, the Chicago Child–Parent Center. This program not only was designed to enhance children's outcomes, but placed a heavy emphasis on environmental supports to parents as children made the transition to school (e.g., program activities for parents in resource rooms and in community contexts; parenting skills, vocational skills; and social supports with the goal of increasing parents' involvement in their children's education). The parent centers were located in high-poverty areas. A large group of children ($n = 1,408$), with 93% being African American, were included in this study. After adjustments for preprogram maltreatment and background factors, those participating in the prevention program showed lower rates of court petitions for child maltreatment by age 17 than children who participated in alternative kindergarten interventions (5.0% vs. 10.5%, a 52% reduction). Longer participation was also associated with lower rates of maltreatment. Parent involvement in school and school mobility were significant mediators of intervention effects, suggesting that the parent and family changes reduced maltreatment.

Other efforts have utilized more specific cognitive strategies, along with either universal prevention approaches or child management training based on social learning theory. Such work has recently appeared and shows promising reductions in child maltreatment and childhood injury. The efforts involving child management training have been directed at parents with older children, while the universal prevention approaches target parents of infants and toddlers. Bugental and her colleagues (2002) targeted maternal appraisals and problem solving as an enhancement to an existing nationally disseminated program for preventing child maltreatment, Healthy Start (Daro, 1998). When the enhanced Healthy Start program was compared with the typical program and a control condition, it was found to significantly decrease levels of child abuse (4% vs. 23% and 26%) among high-risk mothers versus those receiving the standard Healthy Start package and the control condition. Similar results for spanking favored the intervention with the cognitive appraisal element (i.e., 18% for the enhanced group compared to 42% for the other conditions, a figure close to that found in college-educated parents; Holden, Buck, & Stickeis, 2000). Finally, when child health was examined, the enhanced program had the best outcomes, followed by the standard Healthy Start program, with both better than the control condition.

Peterson and colleagues (Peterson, Tremblay, Ewigman, & Saldana, 2003; Peterson et al., 1997) described another such program that addressed abuse prevention in a group of isolated young mothers. The program included 16 weeks of group treatment that included both behavioral and cognitive components. Decreases in use of harsh discipline were shown at a 1-year follow-up. Sanders and colleagues (2004) added an attributional and anger control component to the Triple P-Positive Parenting Program, a highly successful behaviorally based prevention program, and found similar improvements. At postintervention, both the standard and enhanced programs produced behavioral changes in parenting, increased parental efficacy, and decreased distress, but the enhanced program showed greater decreases in negative attributions for child misbehavior, risk of abuse, and unrealistic expectations of children. At a 6-month follow-up, the enhanced program maintained its advantage in decreasing negative attributions to children.

These findings offer convincing opportunities to prevent maltreatment and related social and family problems on the basis of early intervention services. Clearly, efforts to enhance positive experiences at an early stage in the development of the parent–child relationship hold considerable promise for the prevention of child maltreatment and its consequences.

LEGAL INTERVENTIONS AFFECTING MALTREATED CHILDREN

Many statutory efforts provide for children's safety and protection, and they deserve a place in this chapter on interventions for children who are abused and neglected. They provide safety nets for families and give society rights to intervene when families are not functioning well. We briefly discuss four types of these that are most relevant: (1) economic, health, and child care supports to families functioning below the poverty line; (2) statutes providing for reductions for health and safety hazards in children's environments; (3) statutes that assist families where domestic violence has occurred; and (4) statutes addressing timelines and supports for reunification or termination of parental rights once maltreatment has occurred.

As noted earlier, many of the families involved in CPS actions are ones who are operating at the bottom socioeconomic levels of our society. Thus changes in the welfare supports to families have a direct effect on those most at risk for maltreatment. Indeed, much overlap exists between CPS caseloads and cash assistance groups (Ovwigho, Leavitt, & Born, 2003). Concerns exist about recent U.S. welfare reform and effects on this population. This reform has shortened the time parents remain on welfare and its lifetime use. New legislation pushes parents toward acquiring work to receive supports, and provides provisions for child care to support work efforts.

Fears have arisen (1) that the changes in resources might increase children's risk of abuse, neglect, or out-of-home placement; and (2) that parents' work might affect stress and increase risk of abuse, and might decrease supervision or support at times of crisis. Recent research has examined patterns of entrances/exits (i.e., how consistently the families have economic support). Negative effects in some cognitive and behavioral areas were found for children with mothers who cycle on and off welfare, and for mothers with high levels of job training and work (Yoshikawa & Seidman, 2001). Stresses due to juggling work and shifting family organizational arrangements may be to blame. Work following short-term welfare use was associated with positive effects on child reading scores, whereas work in the context of cycling was linked with increased internalizing symptoms, suggesting that the effects may vary by family. Because of sampling issues, these data must be viewed cautiously, but they indicate that statutes affecting the income of the poor ultimately affect children.

Although the recent reform was intended to move mothers into work, an important underlying theme was the promotion of responsible parenting. Two-thirds of states have used funds to promote better parenting through programs such as home visits to new parents and parenting classes. These programs, unfortunately, have not been evaluated, so their preventive impact is unknown. Evidence appears to indicate that their impact on parenting has been minimal, except that some programs have significantly affected choice of child care and extracurricular child activities (Chase-Lansdale & Pittman, 2002). The better programs had more generous work supports and more flexible work requirements. Some family effects were also found (i.e., more stable marriages and less violence between partners, both of which lead to better parenting) (Chase-Lansdale & Pittman, 2002).

Of most interest are studies of the links between welfare reform and patterns of TANF use on abuse. Patterns of leaving TANF rolls (either returning to work or exceeding the time limits of participation) have in fact been linked to increases in maltreatment rates, with parents who are later leavers showing significantly higher rates (Ovwigho et al., 2003). This finding is a concern.

A second area of law that has attempted to fill gaps in protecting children consists of statutes ensuring environmental safety and reduction of health hazards. Something as simple as safety caps on dangerous medicines can decrease risk due to failures in parental supervision of children. Safety of playground equipment, licensing of amusement park rides, safety guards on escalators, requirements for swimming pools in residential settings (fences, locks), and the presence of state-funded guards at street crossings and lifeguards at public pool facilities are all legal efforts to ensure safe environments for children. All children benefit (not only those who are living in neglectful homes), but clearly such efforts act as buffers for parents whose vigilance regarding child safety is lower.

A third area where legislative actions have assisted in protecting children is the area of domestic violence (Jaffe, Crooks, & Wolfe, 2003). At the state level, provisions for restraining orders (compelling violent persons to stay a specified distance away from victims, their homes, and their places of work) protect children as well. Statutes have been aimed at increasing public awareness, funding shelters, and providing other assistance for victims of family violence and their children. Restraining orders vary in their duration and breadth (Matthews, 1999), and some have included provisions for support during their tenure, thus sparing victims the need for separate actions for financial support of children. Some states have fee waivers for low-income women, and/or the perpetrators pay the filing fees, thus removing one barrier.

The final area of legal efforts on behalf of children consists of laws governing maltreatment and procedures on removing children permanently from families unable to care for them. Legal changes have made identification of child maltreatment possible and allowed the state to intervene in family life. This clearly has meant positive things in terms of protecting children and providing families in trouble with needed services. As the depth of the problem of child maltreatment has become more apparent, society has become increasingly concerned about swifter intervention by the state, and this has resulted in various changes. The Adoption and Safe Families Act of 1997, and the revisions made since, have shortened timelines for reunification once children are placed in foster care and started the process for adoptive placement earlier. Recent statutes have allowed the use of long-term guardianship (often by kin) as another form of permanency. In Illinois, for example, adoption increased from 1,640 children to 7,315 over a 4-year period (Testa, 2001). Despite these positive benefits, concerns have arisen regarding whether adequate services are being provided to foster reunification for parents. For certain groups of parents in particular (e.g., substance-abusing parents, intellectually low-functioning parents, incarcerated parents), their difficulties may not be resolved quickly enough to meet these new timelines, or specialized services designed for their special needs are limited in most areas of the United States.

Clearly, legislation directly protects children from harm, and auxiliary laws have been enacted that are aimed at supporting their families and the safety of their general environments. This ensemble of statutes and policies forms a safety net for children and their families, although some continue to fall through the spaces. However, legislation in and of itself is not enough; additional resources must be provided to carry out the intent of the legislation, and drift in carrying out the original intent of laws must be carefully monitored. Moreover, everyday procedures developed by courts, social welfare agencies, and institutions can lead to inconsistent and inadequate coverage of the factors affecting children's outcomes. These issues may seem far afield from providing therapeutic services to abused and neglected children. As members of fields charged with intervening to produce better functioning in children, however, we must not only be aware of statutes, but play an active role in supporting their passage and monitoring their implementation through research and advocacy efforts. The profession of psychology has played an active role in related issues (e.g., American Psychological Association *amicus curiae* briefs regarding protections for children testifying in sexual abuse cases; Small & Melton, 1994).

CONCLUSIONS AND FUTURE DIRECTIONS

Treatment initiatives for child abuse and neglect saw a flurry of activity over two decades ago, followed by a long period of relative silence. Only recently have investigators brought new energy into this important field, resulting in a number of promising initiatives and broader clinical involvement with multiproblem families. Behavioral and cognitive-behavioral approaches continue to show real promise as effective means of changing interaction patterns within families. (To date, most of this work has focused on changing the parents' behavior, with less emphasis on the needs of the children.) Fortunately, large-scale efforts to validate the effectiveness of these approaches with larger samples are underway, as is work identifying the families for whom these strategies are most useful.

We hope that the next decade brings increased awareness of, and efforts toward encouraging, diversity and opportunities for the development of unique resources among high-risk parents and children. Societal influences that play a role in child abuse and neglect—especially in circumstances where families are exposed to major effects of poverty, health risks, and environmental conflict—require concerted efforts. The special risks and strengths of diverse cultural and ethnic groups need to be addressed, along with greater sensitivity to eth-

nic and cultural issues in the planning of services. Such a cross-cultural perspective on child abuse and neglect intervention and prevention would redirect the focus away from individuals and families, and explore societal and cultural conditions that worsen or improve these problems.

Despite the promising efforts described above for effectively intervening with maltreating parents, these approaches are seldom available in many communities. This failure to disseminate evidence-based approaches is puzzling, but may be understood from a number of viewpoints. First, child maltreatment has been primarily a problem associated with the poor, although this may be an anomaly of surveillance systems and biases in which parents are identified by formal systems. Although society has clearly indicated its interest in supporting the needs of poor children, it has been more ambivalent regarding providing support to the adults associated with them (Heclos, 1997). Providing costly assistance in parenting to maltreating parents, who tend to dwell on the lowest rungs of the socioeconomic ladder, may therefore be met with resistance. Furthermore, it has been a long-held societal belief that nurturant parenting is the foundation of maternal behavior toward offspring and is invariant (an instinct). Yet we know that maternal behavior toward offspring can vary strongly with environmental conditions, and that under certain conditions of social deprivation during early years (1ack of good models), nurturant behavior may be less likely to occur (Hrdy, 1999). Because of the strong and pervasive societal belief that parenting is entirely instinct-driven, there may be strong psychological forces operating against the idea of parenting as a "teachable" role, and society may instead believe that parents who maltreat their children are constitutionally "damaged" permanently. If such societal beliefs and reluctance are valid explanations for the lack of dissemination of social-learning-theory-based interventions, then more effort needs to be made to counter these beliefs before such interventions can be undertaken on a wide scale.

Other explanations may be the strength of the data supporting such dissemination. Most of the studies to date are small-scale efforts, and the number of treatment agents trained in these approaches is still quite limited. In practice, interventions for this population are the province of the social work profession, whose members are not traditionally trained in social learning theory or approaches based on it. Therefore, training efforts on a wide scale are needed. One possible approach would be to develop a network of treatment researchers who have accrued a foundation of experience in interventions, and to encourage this consortium to conduct more multisite examinations of treatment effectiveness, develop more manuals, and make more efforts to train a cadre of treatment agents/researchers.

REFERENCES

Aber, J. L., & Allen, J. P. (1987). The effects of maltreatment on young children's socio-emotional development. *Developmental Psychology, 23,* 406–414.

Acton, R. G., & During, S. M. (1992). Preliminary results of aggression management training for aggressive parents. *Journal of Interpersonal Violence, 7,* 410–417.

Administration for Children, Youth and Families (ACYF). (2004). *Child maltreatment 2002: Reports from the states to the National Center on Child Abuse and Neglect.* Washington, DC: U.S. Department of Health and Human Services.

Adoption and Safe Families Act of 1997, P.L. 105-89, 42 U.S.C. 1305 (1997).

Allen, D. M., & Tarnowski, K. J. (1989). Depressive characteristics of physically abused children. *Journal of Abnormal Child Psychology, 17,* 1–11.

Ambrose, S., Hazzard, A., & Haworth, J. (1980). Cognitive-behavioral parenting groups for abusive families. *Child Abuse and Neglect, 4,* 119–125.

Ayllon, T., & Roberts, M. D. (1975). Mothers as educators for their children. In T. Thompson & W. S. Dockens (Eds.), *Applications of behavior modification* (pp. 107–137). New York: Academic Press.

Ayoub, C. (1991). Physical violence and preschoolers: The use of therapeutic day care in the treatment of physically abused children and children from violent families. *The Advisor, 4,* 1–18.

Azar, B. (1995, September). Foster care has bleak history. *APA Monitor,* p. 8.

Azar, S. T. (1984). *An evaluation of the effectiveness of cognitive behavioral versus insight oriented mothers groups with child maltreaters.* Unpublished doctoral dissertation, University of Rochester.

Azar, S. T. (1986). A framework for understanding child maltreatment: An integration of cognitive behavioural and developmental perspectives. *Canadian Journal of Behavioural Science, 18,* 340–355.

Azar, S. T. (1989a). Training parents of abused children. In C. E. Schaefer & J. M. Briesmeister (Eds.), *Handbook of parent training* (pp. 414–441). New York: Wiley.

Azar, S. T. (1989b, November). *Unrealistic expectations and attributions of negative intent among teenage mothers at risk for child maltreatment: The validity of a cognitive view of parenting.* Poster presented at the annual meeting of the Association for Advancement of Behavior Therapy, Washington, DC.

Azar, S. T. (1991a, April). *Concern about the physical abuse of adolescents: A case of neglect.* Paper presented at the annual meeting of the Eastern Psychological Association, New York.

Azar, S. T. (1991b). Models of physical child abuse: A metatheoretical analysis. *Criminal Justice and Behavior, 18,* 30–46.

Azar, S. T. (1996). Cognitive restructuring of professionals' schema regarding women parenting in poverty. *Women and Therapy, 18,* 149–163.

Azar, S. T. (1997). A cognitive behavioral approach to understanding and treating parents who physically abuse their children. In D. Wolfe & R. McMahon (Eds.), *Child abuse: New directions in prevention and treatment across the life span* (pp. 78–100). Thousand Oaks, CA: Sage.

Azar, S. T. (2005). Physical abuse and neglect in girls. In D. J. Bell, S. L. Foster, & E. J. Mash (Eds.), *Handbook of behavioral and emotional problems in girls* (pp. 321–356). New York: Kluwer/Academic/Plenum.

Azar, S. T., Barnes, K. T., & Twentyman, C. T. (1988). Developmental outcomes in physically abused children: Consequences of parental abuse or the effects of a more general breakdown in caregiving behaviors? *The Behavior Therapist, 11,* 27–32.

Azar, S. T., & Benjet, C. L. (1994). A cognitive perspective on ethnicity, race and termination of parental rights. *Law and Human Behavior, 18,* 249–268.

Azar, S. T., Benjet, C., Fuhrmann, G., & Cavallaro, L. (1995). Termination of parental rights: Can behavioral research help Solomon? *Behavior Therapy, 26,* 599–623.

Azar, S. T., & Bober, S. L. (1999). Developmental outcomes in abused children: The result of a breakdown in socialization environment. In W. Silverman & T. Ollendick (Eds.), *Group intervention in the school and the community* (pp. 376–400). Needham Heights, MA: Allyn & Bacon.

Azar, S. T., Breton, S. J., & Miller, L. P. (1998). Cognitive behavioral group work and physical child abuse: Intervention and prevention. In K. C. Stoiber & T. Kratochwill (Eds.), *Group intervention in the school and the community* (pp. 376–400). Needham Heights, MA: Allyn & Bacon.

Azar, S. T., & Cote, L. (2002). Sociocultural issues in the evaluation of the needs of children in custody decision-making: What do our current frameworks for evaluating parenting practices have to offer? *International Journal of Law and Psychiatry, 25,* 193–217.

Azar, S. T., & Cote, L. (2005). Cognitive behavioral interventions with neglectful parents. In F. Talley (Ed.), *Handbook of interventions in child abuse and neglect* (pp. 145–182). Binghamton, NY: Haworth Press.

Azar, S. T., Fantuzzo, J., & Twentyman, C. T. (1984). An applied behavioural approach to child maltreatment: Back to basics. *Advances in Behaviour Research and Therapy, 6*, 6–11.

Azar, S. T., Ferguson, E., & Twentyman, C. T. (1992). Social competence. In P. H. Wilson (Ed.), *Principles and practice of relapse prevention* (pp. 329–348). New York: Guilford Press.

Azar, S. T., & Hill, L. K. (in press). Adoption, foster care, and guardianship in minority families. In K. Wegar (Ed.), *Adoptive families in a diverse society*. New Brunswick, NJ: Rutgers University Press.

Azar, S. T., & Makin-Byrd, K. N. (in press). Violent families; When family values clash with therapists' goals and treatment delivery. In T. A. Cavrell & K. Malcolm (Eds.), *Anger, aggression, and interventions for interpersonal violence*. Mahwah, NJ: Erlbaum.

Azar, S. T., Nix, R. L., & Makin-Byrd, K. N. (2005). Parenting schemas and the process of change. *Journal of Marriage and Family Therapy, 31*, 45–58.

Azar, S. T., Povilaitis, T., Lauretti, A., & Poquette, C. (1997). Theory in child abuse. In J. Lutzker (Ed.), *Child abuse: A handbook of theory, research and treatment* (pp. 3–30). New York: Plenum Press.

Azar, S. T., Robinson, D. R., Hekimian, E., & Twentyman, C. T. (1984). Unrealistic expectations and problem solving ability in maltreating and comparison mothers. *Journal of Consulting and Clinical Psychology, 52*, 687–691.

Azar, S. T., & Rohrbeck, C. A. (1986). Child abuse and unrealistic expectations: Further validation of the Parent Opinion Questionnaire. *Journal of Consulting and Clinical Psychology, 54*, 867–868.

Azar, S. T., & Soysa, K. (1999). Legal and system issues in the assessment of family violence involving children. In R. T. Ammerman & M. Hersen (Eds.), *Assessment of family violence: A clinical and legal sourcebook* (2nd ed., pp. 48–72), New York: Wiley.

Azar, S. T., & Soysa, K. (2000). How do I assess a caregiver's parenting attitudes, knowledge, and level of functioning? In H. Dubowitz & D. DePanfilis (Eds.), *Handbook for child protection practice* (pp. 308–313). Thousand Oaks, CA: Sage.

Azar, S. T., & Twentyman, C. T. (1984, November). *An evaluation of the effectiveness of behaviorally versus insight oriented group treatments with maltreating mothers*. Paper presented at the annual meeting of the Association for Advancement of Behavior Therapy, Philadelphia.

Azar, S. T., & Twentyman, C. T. (1986). Cognitive-behavioral perspectives on the assessment and treatment of child abuse. In P. C. Kendall (Ed.), *Advances in cognitive-behavioral research and therapy* (Vol. 5, pp. 237–267). New York: Academic Press.

Azar, S. T., & Weinzierl, K. M. (2005). Child maltreatment and childhood injury research: A cognitive behavioral approach. *Journal of Pediatric Psychology, 31*, 1–17.

Baldwin, M. W. (1997). Relational schema as a source of if-then self inference procedures. *Review of General Psychology, 1*, 326–335.

Balge, K. A., & Milner, J. S. (2000). Emotion recognition ability in mothers at high and low risk for child physical abuse. *Child Abuse and Neglect, 24*, 1289–1298.

Barkley, R. A. (2000). Issues in training parents to manage children with behavior problems. *Journal of the American Academy of Child and Adolescent Psychiatry, 39*, 1004–1006.

Barnes, K. T., & Azar, S. T. (1990, August). *Maternal expectations and attributions in discipline situations: A test of a cognitive model of parenting*. Poster presented at the annual meeting of the American Psychological Association, Boston.

Barth, R. P., Blythe, B. J., Schinke, S. P., Stevens, P., & Schilling, R. F. (1983). Self-control training with maltreating parents. *Child Welfare, 62*, 313–324.

Becker, J. V., Alpert, J. L., Bigfoot, D. S., Bonner, B. L., Geddie, L. F., Henggeler, S. W., et al. (1995). Empirical research on child abuse treatment: Report by the Child Abuse and Neglect Treatment Working Group, American Psychological Association. *Journal of Clinical Child Psychology, 24*, 23–46.

Becker, W. C. (1971). *Parents are teachers*. Champaign, IL: Research Press.

Belsky, J. (1980). Child maltreatment: An ecological integration. *American Psychologist, 35*, 320–335.

Berkowitz, L. (1983). Aversively stimulated aggression: Some parallels and differences in research with animals and humans. *American Psychologist, 38*, 1135–1144.

Bitoni, C. (2002). Formative evaluation in family preservation: Lessons from Nevada. *Children and Youth Services Review, 24*, 653–672.

Bonner, B. (2000). What are effective strategies to address common behavior problems? In H. Dubowitz & D. DePanfilis (Eds.), *Handbook for child protection practice* (pp. 414–419). Thousand Oaks, CA: Sage

Bousha, D., & Twentyman, C. T. (1984). Abusing, neglectful and comparison mother–child interactional style. *Journal of Abnormal Psychology, 93*, 106–114.

Bower, G. H. (1981). Mood and memory. *American Psychologist, 36*, 129–148.

Brassard, M. R., Germain, R., & Hart, S. N. (1987). *Psychological maltreatment of children and youth*. New York: Pergamon Press.

Brown, S. E. (1984). Social class, child maltreatment, and delinquent behavior. *Criminology, 22*, 259–278.

Brunk, M., Henggeler, S. W., & Whelan, J. P. (1987). Comparison of multisystemic therapy and parent training in the brief treatment of child abuse and neglect. *Journal of Consulting and Clinical Psychology, 55*, 171–178.

Bugental, D. B., Blue, J., Cortez, V., Fleck, Kopeikin, H., Lewis, J. C., et al. (1993). Social cognitions as organizers of autonomic and affective responses to social challenge. *Journal of Personality and Social Psychology, 64*, 94–103.

Bugental, D. B., Brown, M., & Reiss, C. (1996). Cognitive representations of power in caregiving relationships: Biasing effects on interpersonal interaction and information processing. *Journal of Family Psychology, 10,* 397–407.

Bugental, D. B., Ellerson, P. C., Lin, E. K., Rainey, B., Kokotovic, A., & O'Hara, N. (2002). A cognitive behavioral approach to child abuse prevention. *Journal of Family Psychology, 16,* 243–258.

Bugental, D. B., & Happaney, K. (2004). Predicting infant maltreatment in low-income families. *Developmental Psychology, 40,* 234–243.

Bugental, D. B., Johnston, C., New, M., & Silvester, J. (1998). Measuring parental attributions. Conceptual and methodological issues. *Journal of Family Psychology, 12,* 459–480.

Burgdorf, K. (1988). *Study of national incidence and prevalence of child abuse and neglect.* Washington, DC: National Center on Child Abuse and Neglect.

Burgess, R. L., & Conger, R. D. (1978). Family interaction in abusive, neglectful and normal families. *Child Development, 49,* 1163–1173.

Burns, B., Phillips, S. D., Wagner, H., Barth, R. P., Kolko, D. J., Campbell, Y., et al. (2004). Mental health needs and access to mental health services by youth involved with child welfare: A national survey. *Journal of the American Academy of Child and Adolescent Psychiatry, 43,* 960–970.

Cahill, L. T., Kaminer, R. K., & Johnson, P. G. (1999). Developmental, cognitive, and behavioral sequelae of child abuse. *Child and Adolescent Psychiatric Clinics of North America, 8,* 827–843.

Caldwell, R. A., Bogat, G. A., & Davidson, W. S. (1988). The assessment of child abuse potential and the prevention of child abuse and neglect: A policy analysis. *American Journal of Community Psychology, 16,* 609–624.

Camasso, J. J., & Jagannathan, R. (2000). Modeling the reliability and predictive validity of risk assessment in child protective services. *Children and Youth Services Review, 22,* 873–896.

Campbell, R. V., O'Brien, S., Bickett, A. D., & Lutzker, J. R. (1983). In-home parent training of migraine headaches and marital counselling as an ecobehavioral approach to prevent child abuse. *Journal of Behavior Therapy and Experimental Psychiatry, 14,* 147–154.

Caselles, C. E., & Milner, J. S. (2000). Evaluation of child transgressions, disciplinary choices, and expected child compliance and a crying infant condition in physically abused and comparison mothers. *Child Abuse and Neglect, 24,* 477–491.

Cerezo, M. A., D'Ocon, A., & Dolz, L. (1996). Mother–child interactive patterns in abusive families versus non-abusive families: An observational study. *Child Abuse and Neglect, 20,* 573–587.

Chaffin, M., Silovsky, J. F., Funderurk, B., Valle, L. A., Brestan, E. V., Balachova, T., et al. (2004). Parent–child interaction therapy with physically abusive parents: Efficacy for reducing future abuse reports. *Journal of Consulting and Clinical Psychology, 72,* 500–510.

Chamberlain, P., Fisher, P. A., & Moore, K. (2002). Multidimensional treatment foster care: Applications of the OSLC intervention model to high-risk youth and their families. In J. B. Reid, G. R. Patterson, & J. Snyder (Eds.), *Antisocial behavior in children and adolescents* (pp. 203–218). Washington, DC: American Psychological Association.

Chamberlain, P., & Smith, K. (2003). Antisocial behavior in children and adolescents: The Oregon Multidimensional Treatment Foster Care Model. In A. E. Kazdin & J. R. Weisz (Eds.), *Evidence-based psychotherapies for children and adolescents* (pp. 282–300). New York: Guilford Press.

Chase-Lansdale, P. L., & Pittman, L. D. (2002). Welfare reform and parenting: Reasonable expectations. *The Future of Children, 9,* 167–186.

Christensen, M. J., Brayden, R. M., Dietrich, M. S., & McLaughlin, F. J. (1994). The prospective assessment of self concept in neglectful and physically abusive low income mothers. *Child Abuse and Neglect, 18,* 225–232.

Cicchetti, D., & Toth, S. L. (2003). Child maltreatment: Past, present, and future perspectives. In R. P. Weissberg, H. J. Walberg, M. U. O'Brien, & C. B. Kuster (Eds.), *Long-term trends in the well-being of children and youth* (pp. 181–206). Washington, DC: Child Welfare League of America Press.

Clyman, R. B., Harden, B. J., & Little, C. (2002). Assessment, intervention, and research with infants in out-of-home placement. *Infant Mental Health Journal, 23,* 435–453.

Cohn, A. H. (1979). Essential elements of successful child abuse and neglect treatment. *Child Abuse and Neglect, 3,* 491–496.

Conger, R. D. (1982). Behavioral intervention for child abuse. *The Behavior Therapist, 5,* 49–53.

Conger, R. D., Lahey, B. B., & Smith, S. S. (1981, July). *An intervention program for child abuse: Modifying maternal depression and behavior.* Paper presented at the Family Violence Research Conference, University of New Hampshire, Durham.

Connolly, L., Sharry, J., & Fitzpatrick, C. (2001). Evaluation of a group treatment programme for parents of children with behavioural disorders. *Child and Adolescent Mental Health, 6,* 159–165.

Crittenden, P. M. (1982). Abusing, neglecting, problematic, and adequate dyads: Differentiating by patterns of interaction. *Merrill–Palmer Quarterly, 27,* 201–218.

Crittenden, P. M. (1983). The effects of mandatory protective daycare on mutual attachment in maltreating mother–infant dyads. *Child Abuse and Neglect, 3,* 297–300.

Crittenden, P. M. (1992). Treatment of anxious attachment in infancy and early childhood. *Development and Psychopathology, 4,* 575–602.

Crittenden, P. M. (1993). An information processing perspective on the behavior of neglectful parents. *Criminal Justice and Behavior, 20,* 27–48.

Crouch, J. L., & Milner, J. S. (1993). Effects of child neglect on children. *Criminal Justice and Behavior, 20,* 49–65.

Culp, R. E., Heide, J. S., & Richardson, M. T. (1987).

Maltreated children's developmental scores: Treatment versus nontreatment. *Child Abuse and Neglect, 11,* 2934.

Culp, R. E., Little, V., Letts, D., & Lawrence, H. (1991). Maltreated children's self concept: Effects of a comprehensive treatment program. *American Journal of Orthopsychiatry, 61,* 114–121.

Dangel, R. F., & Polster, R. A. (Eds.). (1984). *Parent training: Foundations of research and practice.* New York: Guilford Press.

Daro, D. A. (1998). Child abuse prevention: New directions and challenges. In D. J. Hansen (Ed.), *Nebraska Symposium on Motivation* (Vol. 46, pp. 160–219). Lincoln: University of Nebraska Press.

Daro, D. A., & Donnelly, A. C. (2002). Charting the waves of prevention: Two steps forward, one step back. *Child Abuse and Neglect, 26,* 731–742.

Davis, S., & Fantuzzo, J. W. (1989). The effects of adult and peer social initiations on social behavior of withdrawn and aggressive maltreated preschool children. *Journal of Family Violence, 4,* 227–248.

Deblinger, E., McLeer, S. V., & Henry, D. (1990). Cognitive behavioral treatment for sexually abused children suffering from post-traumatic stress: Preliminary findings. *Journal of the American Academy of Child and Adolescent Psychiatry, 29,* 747–752.

Delgado, A. E., & Lutzker, J. R. (1985, November). *Training parents to identify and report their children's illness.* Paper presented at the annual convention of the Association for Advancement of Behavior Therapy, Houston, TX.

Denicola, J., & Sandler, J. (1980). Training abusive parents in cognitive behavioral techniques. *Behavior Therapy, 11,* 263–270.

DePanfilis, D., & Zuravin, S. J. (2001). Assessing risk to determine the need for services. *Children and Youth Services, 23,* 3–20.

Dix, T. H., Rheinhold, D. P., & Zambarano, R. J. (1990). Mothers' judgments in moments of anger. *Merrill–Palmer Quarterly, 36,* 465–486.

Dix, T. H., Ruble, D. N., & Zambarano, R. J. (1989). Mothers' implicit theories of discipline: Child effects, parent effects, and the attribution process. *Child Development, 60,* 1373–1391.

Dubowitz, H. (1991). The impact of child maltreatment on health. In R. H. Starr & D. A. Wolfe (Eds.), *The effects of child abuse and neglect* (pp. 278–294). New York: Guilford Press.

DuCharme, J., Atkinson, L., & Poulton, L. (2000). Success based, noncoercive treatment of oppositional behavior in children from violent homes. *Journal of the American Academy of Child and Adolescent Psychiatry, 39,* 995–1004.

Dunst, C. H. (1986). *Family resources, personal well-being, and early intervention.* Unpublished manuscript, Family Infant and Preschool Program, Western Carolina Center, Morganton, NC.

Eckenrode, J., Laird, M., & Doris, J. (1993). School performance and disciplinary problems among abused and neglected children. *Developmental Psychology, 29,* 53–62.

Egan, K. (1983). Stress management and child management with abusive parents. *Journal of Clinical Child Psychology, 12,* 292–299.

Egeland, B., & Farber, E. A. (1984). Infant–mother attachment: Factors related to its development and changes over time. *Child Development, 55,* 753–771.

Egeland, B., & Sroufe, L. A. (1981). Attachment and early maltreatment. *Child Development, 52,* 44–52.

Egeland, B., Sroufe, L. A., & Erickson, M. (1983). The developmental consequence of different patterns of maltreatment. *Child Abuse and Neglect, 7,* 459–469.

English, D. J., Marshall, D. B., & Orme, M. (1999). Characteristics of repeated referrals to child protective services in Washington State, US. *Child Maltreatment, 4,* 297–307.

Eyberg, S. (1988). Parent–child interaction therapy: Integration of traditional and behavioral concerns. *Child and Family BehaviorTherapy, 10,* 33–46.

Famularo, R., Kinscherff, R., & Fenton, T. (1990). Symptom differences in acute and chronic presentation of childhood post-traumatic stress disorder. *Child Abuse and Neglect, 14,* 439–444.

Fantuzzo, J. W. (1990). Behavioral treatment of the victims of child abuse and neglect. *Behavior Modification, 14,* 316–339.

Fantuzzo, J. W., Jurecic, L., Stovall, A., Hightower, A. D., Goins, C., & Schachtel, D. (1988). Effects of adult and peer social initiations on the social behavior of withdrawn, maltreated preschool children. *Journal of Consulting and Clinical Psychology, 56,* 34–39.

Fantuzzo, J. W., Stovall, A., Schachtel, D., Goins, C., & Hall, R. (1987). The effects of peer social initiations on the social behavior of withdrawn maltreated preschool children. *Journal of Behavior Therapy and Experimental Psychiatry, 18,* 357–363.

Fantuzzo, J. W., Sutton-Smith, B., Atkins, M., Meyers, R., Stevenson, H., Coolahan, K., et al. (1996). Community-based resilient peer treatment of withdrawn maltreated preschool children. *Journal of Consulting and Clinical Psychology, 64,* 1377–1386.

Fantuzzo, J. W., Weiss, A. D., & Coolahan, K. C. (1998). Community-based partnership-directed research: Actualizing community strengths to treat child victims of physical abuse and neglect. Issues in clinical child psychology. In J. R. Lutzker (Ed.), *Handbook of child abuse research and treatment* (pp. 213–237). New York: Plenum Press.

Fantuzzo, J. W., Wray, L., Hall, R., Goins, C., & Azar, S. T. (1986). Parent and social skills training for mentally retarded mothers identified as child maltreaters. *American Journal of Mental Deficiency, 91,* 135–140.

Farber, B., & Azar, S. T. (1999). Blaming the helper. The marginalization of teachers and parents of the urban poor. *American Journal of Orthopsychiatry, 69,* 515–528.

Farber, E., McCord, D., Kinast, C., & Baum-Faulkner, D. (1984). Violence in families of adolescent runaways. *Child Abuse and Neglect, 8,* 295–299.

Farmer, E., & Owen, M. (1998). Gender and the child

protection process. *British Journal of Social Work, 28,* 545–564.

Feldman, M. A. (1998). Parents with intellectual disabilities. In J. R. Lutzker (Ed.), *Handbook of child abuse research and treatment* (pp. 401–420). New York: Plenum Press.

Feldman, R. S., Salzinger, S., Rosario, M., Alvarado, L., Caraballo, L., & Hammer, M. (1995). Parent, teacher, and peer ratings of physically abused and nonmaltreated children's behavior. *Journal of Abnormal Child Psychology, 23,* 317–334.

Fisher, P. A., Ellis, B. H., & Chamberlain, P. (1999). Early intervention foster care: A model for preventing risk in young children who have been maltreated. *Children's Services: Social Policy, Research and Practice, 2,* 159–182.

Fisher, P. A., Gunnar, M. R., Chamberlain, P., & Reid, J. B. (2000). Preventive intervention for maltreated preschool children: Impact on children's behavior, neuroendocrine activity, and foster parent functioning. *Journal of the American Academy of Child and Adolescent Psychiatry, 39,* 1356–1364.

Fox, L., Long, S. H., & Langlois, A. (1988). Patterns of language comprehension deficits in abused and neglected children. *Journal of Speech and Hearing Disorders, 53,* 239–244.

Foxx, R. M., McMorrow, M. J., & Schloss, C. (1983). Stacking the deck: Teaching social skills to retarded adults with a modified table game. *Journal of Applied Behavior Analysis, 16,* 157–170.

Fraser, M. W., Nelson, K. E., & Rivard, J. C. (1997). Effectiveness of family preservation services. *Social Work Research, 21,* 138–153.

Fraser, M. W., Pecora, P. J., & Haapala, D. A. (1997). Effectiveness of family preservation services. *Social Work Research, 21,* 138–153.

Freissthler, B. (2004). A spatial analysis of social disorganization, alcohol access, and rates of child maltreatment in neighborhoods. *Children and Youth Services Review, 26,* 803–819.

Frodi, A., & Smetana, J. (1984). Abused, neglected, and nonmaltreated preschoolers' ability to discriminate emotions in others: The effects of IP. *Child Abuse and Neglect, 8,* 459–465.

Fuller, T. L., & Wells, S. J. (2003). Predicting maltreatment recurrence among CPS cases with alcohol and other drug involvement. *Children and Youth Services Review, 25,* 553–569.

Gambrill, E. D. (1983). Behavioral intervention with child abuse and neglect. In M. Hersen, R. M. Eisler, & P. M. Miller (Eds.), *Progress in behavior modification* (Vol. 17, pp. 1–56). New York: Academic Press.

Garbarino, J. (1976). A preliminary study of some ecological correlates of child abuse: The impact of socioeconomic stress on mothers. *Child Development, 47,* 178–185.

Garbarino, J., & Sherman, D. (1980). High-risk neighborhoods and high-risk families: The human ecology of child maltreatment. *Child Development, 51,* 188–198.

Garbarino, J., & Stocking, S. H. (1980). *Protecting children from abuse and neglect.* San Francisco: Jossey-Bass.

Gardner, W., Lidz, C. W., Mulvey, E. P., & Shaw, E. C. (1996). Clinical versus actuarial prediction of violence in patients with mental illness. *Journal of Clinical Psychology, 64,* 602–609.

Garland, A., Landsverk, J., Hough, R., & Ellis-Macleod, E. (1996). Type of maltreatment as a predictor of mental health services for children in foster care. *Child Abuse and Neglect, 20,* 675–688.

Gaudin, J. M., Wodarski, J. S., Arkinson, M. K., & Avery, I. S. (1990). Remedying child neglect: Effectiveness of social network interventions. *Journal of Applied Sciences, 15,* 97–123.

Geen, R. (2004). The evolution of kinship care policy and practice. *The Future of Children, 14,* 121–149.

Gelles, R. (1996). *The book of David: How preserving families can cost children's lives.* New York Basic Books.

George, C., & Main, M. (1979). Social interactions of young abused children: Approach, avoidance and aggression. *Child Development, 50,* 306–318.

Gershater, M., Ronit, M., Lutzker, J. R., & Wesch, D. (2003). Project SafeCare: Improving health, safety, and parenting skills in families reported for, and at-risk for child maltreatment. *Journal of Family Violence, 18,* 377–386.

Grisso, T., & Appelbaum, P. S. (1992). Is it unethical to offer predictions of future violence? *Law and Human Behavior, 16,* 621–633.

Hagen, R. L., Foreyt, J. P., & Durham, T. W. (1976). The dropout problem: Reducing attrition in obesity research. *Behavior Therapy, 7,* 463–471.

Hamilton, C. E., & Browne, K. D. (1998). The repeat victimization of children: Should the concept be revised? *Aggression and Violent Behavior, 3,* 47–60.

Hansen, D. J., & Warner, J. E. (1994). Treatment adherence of maltreating families: A survey of professionals regarding prevalence and enhancement strategies. *Journal of Family Violence, 9,* 1–19.

Hart, S. N., Brassard, M. R., Binggeli, N. J., & Davidson, H. A. (2002). Psychological maltreatment. In J. E. B. Myers, L. Berliner, J. Briere, C. T. Hendrix, C. Jenny, & T. A. Reid (Eds.), *The APSAC handbook on child maltreatment* (2nd ed., pp. 79–103). Thousand Oaks, CA: Sage.

Haskett, M. E., & Myers, L. W. (1994, August). *The Parent–Child Problem-Solving Program: A description and qualitative assessment.* Paper presented at the annual meeting of the American Psychological Association, Los Angeles.

Haskett, M. E., Scott, S. S., Grant, R., Ward, C. S., & Robinson, C. (2003). Child related cognitions and affective functioning of physically abusive and comparison parents. *Child Abuse and Neglect, 27,* 663–686.

Heclos, H. H. (1997). Values underlying poverty programs in America. *The Future of Children: Children and Poverty, 7,* 141–148.

Heflinger, C. A., Simpkins, C. G., & Coombs-Orme, T.

(2000). Using the CBCL to determine the clinical status of children in state custody. *Children and Youth Services Review, 22,* 55–73.

Heitler, J. B. (1976). Preparatory techniques in initiating expressive psychotherapy with lower-class unsophisticated patients. *Psychological Bulletin, 83,* 339–352.

Hembree-Kigin, T. L., & McNeil, C. B. (1995). *Parent–child interaction therapy.* New York: Plenum Press.

Herrenkohl, R. C., Herrenkohl, E. C., Egolf, B., & Seech, M. (1979). The repetition of child abuse: How frequently does it occur? *Child Abuse and Neglect, 3,* 67–72.

Hildyard, K., & Wolfe, D. A. (2002). Child neglect: Developmental issues and outcomes. *Child Abuse and Neglect, 26,* 679–695.

Hoffman-Plotkin, D., & Twentyman, C. T. (1984). A multimodal assessment of behavioral and cognitive deficits in abused and neglected preschoolers. *Child Development, 55,* 794–802.

Holden, G. W., Buck, M. J., & Stickeis, A. M. (2000). *A four-year longitudinal study of the onset of disciplinary practices.* Unpublished manuscript, University of Texas, Austin.

Horwitz, A., Owens, P., & Simms, M. (2000). Specialized assessments for children in foster care. *Pediatrics, 106,* 59–66.

Horwitz, S. M., Balestracci, K. M., & Simms, M. D. (2001). Foster care placement improves children's functioning. *Archives of Pediatric and Adolescent Medicine, 155,* 1255–1260.

Howes, C., & Eldredge, R. (1985). Responses of abused, neglected, and non-maltreated children to the behaviors of their peers. *Journal of Applied Developmental Psychology, 6,* 261–270.

Hrdy, S. B. (1999). *Mother nature: Maternal instincts and how they shape the human species.* New York: Ballantine Books.

Hurwitz, S. M., Simms, M. D., & Farrington, R. (1994). Impact of developmental problems on young children's exits from foster care. *Journal of Developmental and Behavioral Pediatrics, 15,* 105–110.

Jaffe, P. G., Crooks, C. V., & Wolfe, D. A. (2003). Legal and policy responses to children exposed to domestic violence: The need to evaluate intended and unintended consequences. *Clinical Child and Family Psychology Review, 6,* 205–213.

Jones, R. W., & Peterson, L. W. (1993). Post-traumatic stress disorder in a child following an automobile accident. *Journal of Family Practice, 36,* 223–225.

Kaplan, S. J., Pelcovitz, D., & LaBruna, V. (1999). Child and adolescent abuse and neglect research. *Journal of the American Academy of Child and Adolescent Psychiatry, 38,* 1214–1222.

Katz, K. S., El-Mohandes, A., Johnson, D. M., Jarrett, M., Rose, A., & Cober, M. (2001). Retention of low income mothers in a parenting intervention study. *Journal of Community Health, 26,* 203–218.

Kaufman, J. (1991). Depressive disorders in maltreated children. *Journal of the American Academy of Child and Adolescent Psychiatry, 30,* 257–265.

Kaufman, J., & Cicchetti, D. (1989). The effects of maltreatment on school-aged children's socio-emotional development: Assessments in a day-camp setting. *Developmental Psychology, 25,* 516–524.

Kazdin, A. E., & Polster, R. (1973). Intermittent token reinforcement and response maintenance in extinction. *Behavior Therapy, 4,* 386–391.

Knapp, P., & Deluty, R. H. (1989). Relative effectiveness of two behavioral parent training programs. *Journal of Clinical Child Psychology, 18,* 314–322.

Knutson, J. F., & Bower, M. E. (1994). Physically abusive parenting as an escalated aggressive response. In M. Potegal & J. F. Knutson (Eds.), *The dynamics of aggression: Biological and social processes in dyads and groups* (pp. 195–225). Hillsdale, NJ: Erlbaum.

Kolko, D. J. (1992). Characteristics of child victims of physical violence: Research findings and clinical implications. *Journal of Interpersonal Violence, 7,* 244–276.

Kolko, D. J. (1996a). Clinical monitoring of treatment course in child physical abuse: Child and parent reports. *Child Abuse and Neglect, 20,* 23–43.

Kolko, D. J. (1996b). Individual cognitive behavioral treatment and family therapy for physically abused children and their offending parents: A comparison of clinical outcomes. *Child Maltreatment, 1,* 322–342.

Koverola, C., Elliot-Faust, O., & Wolfe, D. A. (1984). Clinical issues in the behavioral treatment of a child abusive mother experiencing multiple life stressors. *Journal of Clinical Child Psychology, 13,* 187–191.

Larrance, D. L., & Twentyman, C. T. (1983). Maternal attributions in child abuse. *Journal of Abnormal Psychology, 92,* 449–457.

Lewis, D. O., Shanok, S. S., Pincus, J. H., & Glaser, G. H. (1979). Violent juvenile delinquents: Psychiatric, neurological, psychological, and abuse factors. *Journal of the American Academy of Child Psychiatry, 18,* 307–319.

Lidz, C. W., Mulvey, E. P., & Gardner, W. (1993). The accuracy of predictions of violence to others. *Journal of the American Medical Association, 269,* 1007–1011.

Lieberman, A. F., Silverman, R., & Pawl, J. H. (2000). Infant–parent psychotherapy: Core concepts and current approaches. In C. H. Zeanah (Ed.), *Handbook of infant mental health* (2nd ed., pp. 472–484). New York: Guilford Press.

Lieberman, A. F., & Zeanah, C. H. (1999). Contributions of attachment theory to infant–parent psychotherapy and other interventions with infants and young children. In J. Cassidy & P. R. Shaver (Eds.), *Handbook of attachment: Theory, research, and clinical applications* (pp. 555—574). New York: Guilford Press.

Lipovsky, J. A. (1991). Posttraumatic stress disorder in children. *Family and Community Health, 14,* 42–51.

Lorber, R., Felton, D. K., & Reid, J. (1984). A social learning approach to the reduction of coercive processes in child abusive families: A molecular analysis.

Advances in Behaviour Research and Therapy, 6, 29–45.

Lorion, R. P. (1978). Research on psychotherapy and behavior change with the disadvantaged. In S. L. Garfield & A. E. Bergin (Eds.), *Handbook of psychotherapy and behavior change: An empirical analysis* (2nd ed., pp. 903–938). New York: Wiley.

Love, L. R., Kaswan, J., & Bugental, D. (1972). Differential effectiveness of three clinical interventions for different socioeconomic groupings. *Journal of Consulting and Clinical Psychology, 39,* 347–360.

Lutzker, J. R., & Bigelow, J. M. (2002). *Reducing child maltreatment: A guidebook for parent services.* New York: Guilford Press.

Lutzker, J. R., Bigelow, K. M., Doctor, R. M., Gershater, R. M., & Greene, B. F. (1998). An ecobehavioral model for the prevention and treatment of child abuse and neglect. In J. R. Lutzker (Ed.), *Handbook of child abuse research and treatment* (pp. 421–448). New York: Plenum Press.

Lutzker, J., & Rice, J. M. (1984). Project 12–Ways: Measuring outcome of a large in-home service for treatment and prevention of child abuse and neglect. *Child Abuse and Neglect, 8,* 519–524.

MacDonald, J., Brown, N., & Ellis, P. (2000). Using telephone prompts to improve initial attendance at a community mental health center. *Psychiatric Services, 51,* 812–814.

Magura, S., & Moses, B. S. (1986). *Outcome measures for child welfare services: Theory and applications.* Washington, DC: Child Welfare League of America.

Mak, A. S. (1994). Parental neglect and overprotection as risk factors in delinquency. *Australian Journal of Psychology, 46,* 107–111.

Mammen, O. K., Kolko, D. J., & Pilkonis, P. A. (2002). Negative affect and parental aggression in child physical abuse. *Child Abuse and Neglect, 26,* 407–424,

Mammen, O. K., Kolko, D. J., & Pilkonis, P. A. (2003). Parental cognitions and satisfaction: Relationship to aggressive parental behavioral in child physical abuse. *Child Maltreatment, 8,* 288–301.

Mangine, S., Royse, D., Wieche, V., & Nietzel, M. (1990). Homelessness among adults raised as foster children. *Psychological Reports, 67,* 739–745.

Mann, E., & McDermott, J. F. (1983). Play therapy for victims of child abuse and neglect. In C. E. Schaefer & K. J. O'Connor (Eds.), *Handbook of play therapy* (pp. 283–307). New York: Wiley.

Marvin, R., Cooper, G., Hoffman, K., & Powell, B. (2002). The Circle of Security Project: Attachment-based intervention with caregiver-pre-school child dyads. *Attachment and Human Development, 4,* 107—124.

Matthews, M. A. (1999). The impact of federal and state laws on children exposed to domestic violence. *The Future of Children, 9,* 50–66.

McEwen, B. S. (2001). Plasticity of the hippocampus: Adaptation to chronic stress and alleostatic load. *Annals of the New York Academy of Sciences, 933,* 265–277.

McFarlane, A. C. (1989). The treatment of post-traumatic stress disorder. *British Journal of Medical Psychology, 62,* 81–90.

McGee, R., Wolfe, D. A., & Olson, J. (1995, June). *Why me?: A content analysis of adolescents' causal attributions for their maltreatment experiences.* Paper presented at the meeting of the Canadian Psychological Association, Charlottetown, Prince Edward Island.

McGloin, J., & Widom, C. S. (2001). Resilience among abused and neglected children grown up. *Development and Psychopathology, 13,* 1021–1038.

McIntyre, A., Launsbury, K., Bernton, D., & Steel, H. (1988). Psychosocial characteristics of foster children. *Journal of Applied Developmental Psychology, 9,* 125–137.

McMahon, R. J., & Forehand, R. (1984). Parent training for the noncompliant child: Treatment outcome, generalization, and adjunctive therapy procedures. In R. F. Dangel & R. A. Polster (Eds.), *Parent training: Foundations of research and practice* (pp. 298–328). New York: Guilford Press.

McMillan, T. M. (1991). Post-traumatic stress disorder and severe head injury. *British Journal of Psychiatry, 159,* 431–433.

Melton, G. B., & Limber, S. (1989). Psychologists' involvement in cases of child maltreatment: Limits of role and expertise. *American Psychologist, 44,* 1225–1233.

Miller, L. R., & Azar, S. T. (1996). The pervasiveness of maladaptive attributions in mothers at-risk for child abuse. *Family Violence and Sexual Assault Bulletin, 12,* 31–37.

Milner, J. S. (1986). *The Child Abuse Potential Inventory: Manual* (2nd ed.). Webster, NC: Psytec.

Milner, J. S. (1993). Social information processing and physical child abuse. *Clinical Psychology Review, 13,* 275–294.

Milner, J. S. (1994). Assessing physical child abuse risk: The Child Abuse Potential Inventory. *Clinical Psychology Review, 14,* 547–583.

Milner, J. S. (2003). Social information processing in high risk and physically abusive parents. *Child Abuse and Neglect, 27,* 7–20.

Milner, J. S., & Froody, R. (1994). The impact of mitigating information on attributions for positive and negative child behavior by adults at low- and high-risk for child abusive behavior. *Journal of Social and Clinical Psychology, 13,* 335–351

Milner, J. S., Murphy, W. D., Valle, L. A., & Tolliver, R. M. (1998). Assessment issues in child abuse evaluations. In J. R. Lutzker (Ed.), *Handbook of child abuse research and treatment* (pp. 75–116). New York: Plenum Press.

Monahan, J. (1981). *The clinical prediction of violence.* Rockville, MD: National Institute of Mental Health.

Murphy, C. M., Meyer, S., & O'Leary, K. D. (1994). Dependency characteristics of partner assaultive men. *Journal of Abnormal Psychology, 103,* 729–735.

Naar-King, S., Silvern, V., Ryan, V., & Sebring, D.

(2002). Type and severity of abuse as predictors of psychiatric symptoms in adolescence. *Journal of Family Violence, 17,* 133–149.

National Research Council. (1993). *Understanding child abuse and neglect.* Washington, DC: National Academy Press.

Nayak, M. B., & Milner, J. S. (1998). Neuropsychological functioning: Comparison of mothers at high and low risk for child physical abuse. *Child Abuse and Neglect, 22,* 687–703.

Nomellini, S., & Katz, R. C. (1983). Effects of anger control training on abusive parents. *Cognitive Therapy and Research, 7,* 57–68.

Novaco, R. W. (1975). *Anger control: The development and evaluation of an experimental treatment.* Lexington, MA: Lexington Books.

Oates, R. K., Gray, J., Schweitzer, L., Kempe, R. S., & Harmon, R. J. (1995). A therapeutic preschool for abused children: The Keepsafe Project. *Child Abuse and Neglect, 19,* 1370–1386.

Olds, D., Eckenrode, J., Henderson, C. R., Kitzman, H., Powers, J., Cole, R., et al. (1997). Long-term effects of home visitation on maternal life course, child abuse and neglect, and children's arrests: 15–year follow-up of a randomized trial. *Journal of the American Medical Association, 278,* 637–643.

Olds, D., Henderson, C. R., Chamberlin, R., & Tatelbaum, R. (1986). Preventing child abuse and neglect: A randomized trial of nurse home visitation. *Pediatrics, 78,* 65–78.

Olds, D., Henderson, C. R., & Kitzman, H. (1994). Does prenatal and infancy nurse home visitation have enduring effects on qualities of parental care giving and child health at 25 to 50 months of life? *Pediatrics, 93,* 89–98.

Olds, D., Henderson, C., Eckenrode, J., Petit, L., Kitzman, J., Cole, R., et al. (1998). Reducing risks for antisocial behavior with a program of prenatal and early childhood visitation. *Journal of Community Psychology, 26,* 65–83.

O'Leary, K. D., Malone, J., & Tyree, A. (1994). Physical aggression in early marriage: Prerelationship and relationship effects. *Journal of Consulting and Clinical Psychology, 62,* 594–602.

Ovwigho, P. C., Leavitt, K. L., & Born, C. E. (2003). Risk factors for child abuse and neglect among former TANF families: Do later leavers experience greater risk? *Children and Youth Services Review, 25,* 139–163.

Parke, R. D. (1977). Socialization into child abuse: A social interactional perspective. In J. L. Tapp & F. J. Levine (Eds.), *Law, justice and the individual in society: Psychological and legal issues* (pp. 183–199). New York: Holt, Rinehart & Winston.

Patterson, G. R., & Chamberlain, P. (1988). Treatment process: A problem at three levels. In L. C. Wynne (Ed.), *State of the art in family therapy research: Controversies and recommendations* (pp. 189–223). New York: Family Process Press.

Patterson, G. R., & Chamberlain, P. (1994). A func-

tional analysis of resistance during parent training therapy. *Clinical Psychology: Science and Practice, 1,* 53–70.

Pecora, P. J. (1991). Investigating allegations of child maltreatment: The strengths and limitations of current risk assessment systems. *Child and Youth Services, 15,* 73–92.

Pelcovitz, D., Kaplan, S., Goldenberg, B., Mandel, F., Lehane, J., & Guarrera, J. (1994). Post-Traumatic Stress Disorder in physically abused adolescents. *Journal of the American Academy of Child and Adolescent Psychiatry, 33,* 305–312.

Pelton, L. H. (1994). The role of material factors in child abuse and neglect. In G. B. Melton & F. D. Barry (Eds.), *Protecting children from abuse and neglect: Foundations for a new national strategy* (pp. 131–181). New York: Guilford Press.

Peniston, E. G. (1986). EMG biofeedback-assisted desensitization treatment for Vietnam combat veterans' post-traumatic stress disorder. *Clinical Biofeedback and Health an International Journal, 9,* 35–41.

Peterson, L., Bartelstone, J., Kern, T., & Gillis, R. (1995). Parents' socialization of children's injury prevention. *Child Development, 66,* 224–235.

Peterson, L., & Brown, D. (1994). Integrating child injury and abuse–neglect research. Common histories, etiology, and solutions. *Psychological Bulletin, 116,* 295–315.

Peterson, L., Gable, S., Doyle, C., & Ewigman, B. (1997). Beyond parenting skills: Battling barriers to building bonds to prevent child abuse and neglect. *Cognitive and Behavioral Practice, 4,* 53–74.

Peterson, L., Tremblay, G., Ewigman, B., & Popkey, C. (2002). The parental daily diary: A sensitive measure of the process of change in a child maltreatment prevention program. *Behavior Modification, 26,* 627–647.

Peterson, L., Tremblay, G., Ewigman, B., & Saldana, L. (2003). Multilevel selected primary prevention of child maltreatment. *Journal of Consulting and Clinical Psychology, 71,* 601–612.

Plotkin, R. (1983). *Cognitive mediation in disciplinary action among mothers who have abused or neglected their children: Dispositional and environmental factors.* Unpublished doctoral dissertation, University of Rochester.

Prochaska, J., DiClemente, C., & Norcross, J. (1992). In search of how people change. *American Psychologist, 47,* 1102–1114.

Reid, J. B. (1985). Behavioral approaches to intervention and assessment with child abusive families. In P. H. Bornstein & A. Kazdin (Eds.), *Handbook of clinical behavior therapy with children* (pp. 772–802). Homewood, IL: Dorsey Press.

Reid, J. B., Taplin, P., & Lorber, R. (1981). A social interactional approach to the treatment of abusive families. In R. B. Stuart (Ed.), *Violent behavior: Social learning approaches to prediction, management, and treatment* (pp. 83–101). New York: Brunner/Mazel.

Reynolds, A. J., & Robertson, D. L. (2003). School based early intervention and later child maltreatment in the Chicago Longitudinal Study. *Child Development, 74,* 3–26.

Richards, D. A., & Rose, J. S. (1991). Exposure therapy for Post-Traumatic Stress Disorder: Four case studies. *British Journal of Psychiatry, 158,* 836–840.

Rieppi, R., Greenhill, L. L., Ford, R. E., Chuang, S., Wu, M., Davies, M., et al. (2002). Socioeconomic status as a moderator of ADHD treatment outcomes. *Journal of the American Academy of Child and Adolescent Psychiatry, 41*(3), 269–277.

Risley-Curtiss, C., Coombs-Orme, T., Chernoff, R., & Heisler, A (1996). Health care utilization of children entering foster care. *Research and Social Work Practice, 6,* 422–461.

Roberts, M. C., & Wright, l. (1982). Role of the pediatric psychologist as consultant to pediatricians. In J. Tuma (Ed.), *Handbook for the practice of pediatric psychology* (pp. 251–289). New York: Wiley.

Robyn, S., & Fremouw, W. J. (1996). Cognitive and affective styles of parents who physically abuse their children. *American Journal of Forensic Psychology, 14,* 63–79.

Rogosch, F., Cicchetti, D., & Aber, J. L. (1995). The role of child maltreatment in early deviations in cognitive and affective processing abilities and later peer relationship problems. *Development and Psychopathology, 7,* 591–609.

Rosenfield-Schlicter, M. D., Sarber, R. E., Bueno, G., Greene, B. F., & Lutzker, J. (1983). Maintaining accountability for an ecobehavioral treatment of one aspect of child neglect: Personal cleanliness. *Education and Treatment of Children, 6,* 153–164.

Runyon, M. K., Deblinger, E., Ryan, E. E., & Thakkar-Kolar, R. (2004). An overview of child physical abuse: Developing an integrated parent–child cognitive behavioral treatment program. *Trauma Violence, and Abuse, 5,* 65–85.

Rutter, M. (1989). Intergenerational continuities and discontinuities in serious parenting difficulties. In D. Cicchetti & V. Carlson (Eds.), *Child maltreatment: Theory and research on the causes and consequences of child abuse and neglect* (pp. 317–348). New York: Cambridge University Press.

Salzinger, S., Feldman, R. S., Hammer, M., & Rosario, M. (1993). The effects of physical abuse on children's social relationships. *Child Development, 64,* 169–187.

Salzinger, S., Kaplan, S., Pelcovitz, D., Samit, C., & Krieger, R. (1984). Parent and teacher assessment of children's behavior in child maltreating families. *Journal of the American Academy of Child Psychiatry, 23,* 458–464.

Sanders, M. (1996, November). *A media strategy for promoting parenting skills.* Paper presented at the annual meeting of the Association for Advancement of Behavior Therapy, New York.

Sanders, M. R., Pidgeon, A., Gravestock, F., Connors, M. D., Brown, S., & Young, R. (2004) Does parental attributional retraining and anger management enhance the effects of the Triple P-Positive Parenting Program with parents at-risk of child maltreatment? *Behavior Therapy, 35,* 513–535.

Sandford, D. A., & Tustin, R. D. (1974). Behavioral treatment of parental assault on a child. *New Zealand Psychologist, 2,* 76–82.

Saunders, B. E., Berliner, L., & Hanson, R. F. (Eds.). (2003). *Child physical and sexual abuse: Guidelines for treatment* (Final report, January 15, 2003). Charleston, SC: National Crime Victims Research and Treatment Center.

Schilling, R. F., & Schinke, S. P. (1984). Maltreatment and mental retardation. *Perspectives and Progress in Mental Retardation, 1,* 11–22.

Sedlak, A. J., & Broadhurst, D. D. (1996). *Third national incidence study of child abuse and neglect.* Washington, DC: U.S. Government Printing Office.

Shealy, C. N. (1995). From Boys Town to Oliver Twist: Separating fact from fiction in welfare reform and out-of-home placement of children and youth. *American Psychologist, 50,* 565–580.

Shipman, K. L., & Zeaman, J. (1999). Emotional understanding: A comparison of physically maltreating and nonmaltreating mother–child dyads. *Journal of Clinical Child Psychology, 28,* 407–417.

Skowron, E. A., & Reinemann, D. H. S. (2005). Psychological interventions for child maltreatment: A meta-analysis. *Psychotherapy: Theory, Research, Practice, and Training, 42,* 52–71.

Small, M. A., & Melton, G. B. (1994). Evaluation of child witnesses for confrontation by criminal defendants. *Professional Psychology: Research and Practice, 25,* 228–233.

Smetana, J., Kelly, M., & Twentyman, C. (1984). Abused, neglected, and nonmaltreated children's conceptions of moral and social-conventional transgressions. *Child Development, 55,* 277–287.

Smetana, J. G., Daddis, C., Toth, S. L., Cicchetti, D., Bruce, J., & Kane, P. (1999). Effects of provocation on maltreated preschoolers' understanding of moral transgressions. *Social Development, 8,* 335–348.

Sopory, P., & Dillard, J. P. (2002). The persuasive effects of metaphor: A meta-analysis. *Human Communication Research, 28,* 382–419.

Staudt, M., & Drake, B. (2002). Research on services to preserve maltreating families. *Children and Youth Services Review, 24,* 645–652.

Steele, B. F. (1975). Working with abusive parents: A psychiatric view. *Children Today, 4,* 3–5.

Stein, M. B., Hanna, C., Koverola, C., Torchia, M., & McClarty, B. (1997). Structural brain changes in PTSD: Does trauma alter neuroanatomy? *Annals of the New York Academy of Sciences, 821,* 76–82.

Steinberg, L. D., Catalano, R., & Dooley, D. (1981). Economic antecedents of child abuse and neglect. *Child Development, 52,* 975–985.

Steward, M. S., Farquhar, L. C., Dicharry, D. C., Glick, D. R., & Martin, P. W. (1986). Group therapy: A treatment of choice for young victims of child abuse.

International Journal of Group Psychotherapy, 36, 261–277.

Stovall, K. C., & Dozier, M. (2000). The development of attachment in new relationships: Single subject analyses for 10 foster infants. *Development and Psychopathology, 12,* 133–156.

Strain, P. S., Shores, R. E., & Timm, M. A. (1977). Effects of peer social initiations on the behavior of withdrawn preschool children. *Journal of Applied Behavior Analysis, 10,* 289–298.

Strain, P. S., & Timm, M. A. (1974). An experimental analysis of social interaction between a behaviorally disordered preschool child and her classroom peers. *Journal of Applied Behavior Analysis, 7,* 583–590.

Swenson, C. C., Brown, E. J., & Sheidow, A. J. (2003). Medical, legal, and mental health service utilization by physically abused children and their caregivers. *Child Maltreatment, 8,* 138–144.

Swenson, C. C., Saldana, L., Joyner, C. D., & Henggeler, S. W. (in press). *Ecological treatment for parent to child violence. Interventions for children exposed to violence.* New Brunswick, NJ: Johnson & Johnson.

Szykula, S. A., & Fleischman, M. J. (1985). Reducing out-of-home placements of abused children: Two controlled studies. *Child Abuse and Neglect, 9,* 277–284.

Terr, L. (1991). Childhood traumas: An outline and overview. *American Journal of Psychiatry, 148,* 10–20.

Tertinger, D. A., Greene, B. F., & Lutzker, J. R. (1984). Home safety: Development and validation of one component of an ecobehavioral treatment program for abused and neglected children. *Journal of Applied Behavior Analysis, 17,* 150–174.

Testa, M. F. (2001). Kinship care and permanency. *Journal of Social Service Research, 28,* 25–43.

Thompson, R. A. (1994). Social support and the prevention of child maltreatment. In G. B. Melton & F. D. Barry (Eds.), *Protecting children from abuse and neglect: Foundations for a new national strategy* (pp. 40–130). New York: Guilford Press.

Thompson, R. A., & Wilcox, B. L. (1995). Child maltreatment research: Federal support and policy issues. *American Psychologist, 50,* 789–793.

Todorov, A., & Bargh, J. A. (2002). Automatic sources of aggression. *Aggression and Violent Behavior, 7,* 53–68.

Toth, S. L., Manly, J. T., & Cicchetti, D. (1992). Child maltreatment and vulnerability to depression. *Development and Psychopathology, 14,* 97–112.

Toth, S. L., Maughan, A., Manly, J. T., Spagnola, M., & Cicchetti, D. (2002). The relative efficacy of two interventions in altering maltreated preschool children's representational models: Implications for attachment theory. *Development and Psychopathology, 16,* 877–908.

Trickett, P. K., & Kuczynski, L. (1986). Children's misbehaviors and parental discipline strategies in abusive and nonabusive families. *Developmental Psychology, 22,* 115–123.

Tymchuk, A. J. (1990). Assessing emergency responses of people with mental handicaps. *Mental Handicap, 18,* 136–142.

Tymchuk, A. J. (1992). Predicting adequacy of parenting by people with mental retardation. *Child Abuse and Neglect, 16,* 165–178.

Tymchuk, A. J. (1998). The importance of matching educational interventions to parent needs in child maltreatment. In J. R. Lutzker (Ed.), *Handbook of child abuse research and treatment* (pp. 421–448). New York: Plenum Press.

Tymchuk, A. J., Lang, C. M., Sewards, S. E., Lieberman, S., & Koo, S. (2003). Development and validation of the Home Inventory for Dangers and Safety Precautions: Continuing to address the learning needs of parents in injury prevention. *Journal of Family Violence, 18,* 241–252.

Urquiza, A. J., & McNeil, C. B. (1996). Parent–child interaction therapy: An intensive dyadic intervention for physically abusive families. *Child Maltreatment, 1,* 134–144.

U.S. Advisory Board on Child Abuse and Neglect (USABCAN). (1990). *Child abuse and neglect: Critical first steps in response to a national emergency.* Washington, DC: U.S. Government Printing Office.

U.S. Advisory Board on Child Abuse and Neglect (USABCAN). (1993). *Neighbors helping neighbors: A new national strategy for the protection of children.* Washington, DC: U.S. Government Printing Office.

U.S. Department of Health and Human Services. (2001). *Adoption and foster care analysis and former foster care parents.* Rockville, MD: Author.

van IJzendoorn, M. H., Juffer, F., & Duyvesteyn, M. G. (1994). Breaking the intergenerational cycle of insecure attachment. *Journal of Child Psychology and Psychiatry, 36,* 225–248.

Vasta, R. (1982). Physical child abuse: A dual component analysis. *Developmental Review, 2,* 164–170.

Wahler, R. G. (1980). The insular mother: Her problems in parental reinforcement control. *Journal of Applied Behavior Analysis, 2,* 159–170.

Wahler, R. G., & Dumas, J. E. (1989). Attentional problems in dysfunctional mother–child interactions: An interbehavioral model. *Psychological Bulletin, 105,* 116–130.

Watson-Perczel, M., Lutzker, J. R., Greene, B. F., & McGimpsey, B. J. (1988). Assessment and modification of home cleanliness among families adjudicated for child neglect. *Behavior Modification, 12,* 57–87.

Webster-Stratton, C. (1984). Randomized trial of two parent training programs for families with conduct-disordered children. *Journal of Consulting and Clinical Psychology, 52,* 666–678.

Webster-Stratton, C. (1994). Advancing videotape parent training: A comparison study. *Journal of Consulting and Clinical Psychology, 62,* 299–315.

Webster-Stratton, C., & Herbert, M. (1993). What really happens in parent training? *Behavior Modification, 17,* 407–456.

Wekerle, C., & Wolfe, D. A. (1993). Prevention of child physical abuse and neglect: Promising new directions. *Clinical Psychology Review, 13,* 501–540.

Wekerle, C., & Wolfe, D. A. (2003). Child maltreatment. In E. J. Mash & R. A. Barkley (Eds.), *Child psychopathology* (2nd ed., pp. 632–684). New York: Guilford Press.

Widom, C. S. (1991). Role of placement experience in mediating the criminal consequences of early childhood victimization. *American Journal of Orthopsychiatry, 61,* 195–209.

Widom, C. S. (1998). Childhood victimization. In D. P. Dohrenwend (Ed.), *Adversity, stress, and psychopathology* (pp. 81–94). Oxford: Oxford University Press.

Wodarski, J. S., Kurtz, P. D., Gaudin, J. M., & Howing, P. T. (1990). Maltreatment and the school-aged child: Major academic, socioemotional, and adaptive outcomes. *Social Work, 35,* 506–513.

Wolfe, D. A. (1985). Child-abusive parents: An empirical review and analysis. *Psychological Bulletin, 97,* 462–482.

Wolfe, D. A. (1991). *Preventing physical and emotional abuse of children.* New York: Guilford Press.

Wolfe, D. A. (1999). *Child abuse: Implications for child development and psychopathology* (2nd ed.). Thousand Oaks, CA: Sage.

Wolfe, D. A., Aragona, J., Kaufman, K., & Sandler, J. (1980). The importance of adjudication in the treatment of child abuse: Some preliminary findings. *Child Abuse and Neglect, 4,* 127–135.

Wolfe, D. A., Crooks, C. V., Lee, V., McIntyre-Smith, A., & Jaffe, P. G. (2003). The effects of exposure to domestic violence on children: A meta-analysis and critique. *Clinical Child and Family Psychology Review, 6,* 171–187.

Wolfe, D. A., Edwards, B., Manion, I., & Koverola, C. (1988). Early intervention for child abuse and neglect: A preliminary investigation. *Journal of Consulting and Clinical Psychology, 56,* 40–47.

Wolfe, D. A., Kaufman, D., Aragona, J., & Sandler, J. (1981). *The child management program for abusive parents.* Winter Park, FL: Anna.

Wolfe, D. A., & Manion, I. G. (1984). Impediments to child abuse prevention: Issues and directions. *Advances in Behaviour Research and Therapy, 6,* 47–62.

Wolfe, D. A., & McEachran, A. (1997). Child physical abuse and neglect. In E. J. Mash & L. G. Terdal (Eds.), *Assessment of childhood disorders* (3rd ed., pp. 523–568). New York: Guilford Press.

Wolfe, D. A., & Mosk, M. D. (1983). Behavioral comparisons of children from abusive and distressed families. *Journal of Consulting and Clinical Psychology, 51,* 702–708.

Wolfe, D. A., Sandler, J., & Kaufman, K. (1981). A competency-based parent training program for abusive parents. *Journal of Consulting and Clinical Psychology, 49,* 633–640.

Wolfe, D. A., Scott, K., Reitzel-Jaffe, D., Wekerle, C., Grasley, C., & Straatman, A. (2001). Development and validation of the Conflict in Adolescent Dating Relationships Inventory. *Psychological Assessment, 13,* 277–293.

Wolfe, D. A., & Wekerle, C. (1993). Treatment strategies for child physical abuse and neglect: A critical progress report. *Clinical Psychology Review, 13,* 473–500.

Wolfe, D. A., Wekerle, C., Scott, K., Straatman, A., & Grasley, C. (2004). Predicting abuse in adolescent dating relationships over one year: The role of child maltreatment and trauma. *Journal of Abnormal Psychology, 113,* 406–415.

Wolfe, D. A., Wekerle, C., Scott, K., Straatman, A., Grasley, C., & Reitzel-Jaffe, D. (2003). Dating violence prevention with at-risk youth: A controlled outcome evaluation. *Journal of Consulting and Clinical Psychology, 71,* 279–291.

Wood, W. D., & Baker, J. A. (1999). Preferences for parent education among low socioeconomic status, culturally diverse parents. *Psychology in the Schools, 36,* 239–247.

World Health Organization. (1999, March). *Report of the consultation on child abuse prevention.* Geneva: Author.

Yoshikawa, H., & Seidman, E. (2001). Multidimensional profiles of welfare and work dynamics: Development, validation, and relationship to child cognitive and mental health outcomes. *American Journal of Community Psychology, 29,* 907–936.

Zillman, D. (1979). *Hostility and aggression.* Hillsdale, NJ: Erlbaum.

Zuravin, S. J. (1991). Research definitions of child physical abuse and neglect. In R. H. Starr & D. A. Wolfe (Eds.), *The effects of child abuse and neglect: Issues and research* (pp. 100–128). New York: Guilford Press.

10

Child Sexual Abuse

Vicky Veitch Wolfe

During the past 25 years, North Americans have dramatically increased their awareness of the extent of child sexual abuse and the serious consequences of such abuse for its victims, their families, and our culture. Mental health professionals and researchers have responded to this increasingly evident problem by providing prevention and intervention services to children and their families through the mass media, the schools, the legal system, and child protective service agencies, as well as through more traditional venues such as mental health clinics and hospitals. The response has addressed prevention needs at all levels: primary, secondary, and tertiary. Primary prevention efforts have targeted schools and at-risk populations, to educate children about the risks of sexual abuse and about avenues for empowering themselves if they are approached by sexually opportunistic individuals. Secondary prevention efforts have focused on reducing "system-induced stress" when sexually abused children face the social service and justice systems. Tertiary care interventions are designed to ameliorate abuse-related sequelae and to reduce the probability of long-term effects.

Mental health inroads into developing effective prevention and intervention efforts have been remarkable, given the fact that issues related to sexual abuse have only received serious attention from mental health researchers during the past 25 years. The bulk of this chapter is organized according to primary, secondary, and tertiary interventions, with an emphasis on identification of important issues relevant to sexual abuse and strategies that have been de-

veloped to address those concerns. At the primary prevention level, basic questions about school- and parent-based personal safety skill training are addressed, including children's knowledge about personal safety training, effectiveness of various training approaches with different age and sex groups, and concerns about possible negative effects of personal safety training. Several other avenues for prevention are identified to further advance our efforts to reduce this serious societal problem. At the secondary prevention level, the path from the point of abuse disclosure through social, medical, and legal systems is discussed, along with professional policies and interventions that ease children's journeys. At the tertiary care level, several conceptual models are reviewed regarding the psychological impact of sexual abuse, including our developing knowledge of Type II or complex posttraumatic stress disorder (PTSD). Particular emphasis is placed on treatment programs that address the two primary adjustment concerns known to affect sexually abused individuals: PTSD and sexuality problems. The chapter concludes with an overview of our progress in the areas of prevention and intervention, and identifies areas in need of further development.

INCIDENCE AND PREVALENCE

Sexual abuse prevalence studies have relied primarily upon adults' retrospective reports of their childhood experiences. In a review of 19 such studies, Finkelhor (1994a) estimated that

20% of women and 5–10% of men report at least one episode of sexual abuse during their childhood. However, prevalence estimates vary considerably, depending on the definitions of sexual abuse and sampling strategies used; they range from 2% to 62% for women and 3% to 16% for men among U.S. studies, and from 3% to 29% for women and 7% to 36% for men among international studies (Finkelhor, 1994b). Nonetheless, more recent epidemiological studies have been consistent with Finkelhor's (1994a) estimates. For example, a retrospective study of 17,337 adult members of a managed care program in California revealed that 25% of women and 16% of men reported at least one episode of sexual abuse during their childhood (Dong, Anda, Dube, Giles, & Felitti, 2003). Furthermore, a sample of 3,958 women from the national Australian voter registry indicated that 20% had experienced childhood sexual abuse (Fleming, Mullen, & Bammer, 1997).

Goldman and Padayachi (2000) have outlined a number of methodological issues that account for discrepancies in prevalence estimates. Epidemiological studies have defined sexual abuse in differing ways, with three primary points of diversion: (1) definitions of sexual abuse for adolescents; (2) inclusion of noncontact sexual acts (e.g., exposure to pornography, solicitations); and (3) inclusion of coerced sexual acts by peers. The term "sexual abuse" implies a lack of consent or some level of coercion. Younger children are generally considered to lack the capacity to consent to sexual activities with older persons, and even without overt evidence of coercion, age differences of 5 or more years are considered sufficient for defining sexual activities with children as abusive. However, consent is more difficult to define for adolescents. Some studies have included cases of adolescent–adult sexual contact even without evidence of coercion if the age difference is substantial (e.g., age difference of 10 years or more, as used by Finkelhor, 1979), whereas other studies have limited adolescent cases to those that include more explicit elements of coercion (i.e., abuse of authority or physical force). Some studies have set the upper age limit among adolescents as low as 13 years of age (e.g., Mullen, Roman-Clarkson, & Walton, 1988) and others as high as 18 (e.g., Badgley et al., 1984; Wyatt, 1985). When Russell (1983) restricted her sample to those abused prior to age 14, prevalence was esti-

mated at 28%; however, when the range was extended to age 18, prevalence rose to 38%.

Including noncontact sexual activities (e.g., exhibitionism, exposure to pornography, sexual suggestions and invitations) with contact forms of abuse also greatly increases prevalence estimates. Martin, Anderson, Romans, Mullen, and O'Shea (1993) found that prevalence estimates rose from 19.7% when abuse was limited to genital contact to 25% when noncontact sexual activities were included. When Russell (1983) included noncontact sexual behaviors, her estimates rose to 48% before age 14 and 54% before age 18. Some studies limit cases to those perpetrated by individuals who are significantly older than the victims; however, other studies include all cases in which coercion was used, regardless of the age difference between the victim and perpetrator. One study demonstrated a 300% increase in prevalence when abuse perpetrated by peers was included (Roosa, Reyes, Reinholtz, & Angelini, 1998).

Although broader definitions run the risk of being overly inclusive, such definitions allow greater flexibility in interpreting epidemiological data and allow researchers to examine the impact of sexual abuse according to different definitional criteria. Long and Jackson (1990) examined several different definitions of sexual abuse, using data from a survey of college students, which produced large discrepancies in prevalence estimates. However, victims' reports of distress did not differ on the basis of definitional criteria, suggesting that broader definitions include more victims affected by their abuse.

Sampling and data collection strategies can also affect prevalence estimates. College student surveys tend to yield lower rates than more representative samples. For example, Finkelhor's (1979) college student survey yielded estimates of 19% for women and 9% of males, whereas a nationally representative sample yielded estimates of 27% for women and 16% for men (Finkelhor, Hotaling, Lewis, & Smith, 1990). Interviews, particularly those that ask about sexual abuse from a variety of perspectives (i.e., clearly defining the various forms of behaviors that constitute abuse), tend to yield higher estimates than questionnaire surveys that explicitly ask about sexual abuse, but fail to define fully the parameters of the types of acts considered abusive (e.g., Kercher & McShane, 1984; MacMillan et al., 1997;

Martin et al., 1993). Survey response rates also affect prevalence estimates. In a review of prevalence studies, Gorey and Leslie (1997) found that higher survey response rates tended to reveal lower prevalence estimates, which suggests that individuals with abuse histories are disproportionately likely to respond to anonymous surveys. Furthermore, they found a trend toward poorer participation rates among more recent studies, which raises a concern that more recent estimates of sexual abuse prevalence may be inflated. Although their review of the prevalence literature revealed rates similar to those reported by Finkelhor (1994a), when biases associated with response rates were taken into consideration, their estimates dropped to 12–17% of females and 5–8% of males.

In contrast to concerns that prevalence studies may over sample sexual abuse survivors, concerns have also been raised that retrospective surveys underestimate sexual abuse prevalence, due to high rates of underreporting and forgetting. Williams (1994) contacted women 17 years after allegations of sexual abuse were investigated and confirmed through a hospital-based service. All of the women had been 12 or younger at that time of the investigation. Despite thorough and detailed interviewing strategies, 38% of the women did not report their past abuse. Although it was likely that some women recalled their abuse but preferred not to report it, it appeared that many did not remember their abuse experience at the time they were interviewed.

Incidence data reflect the number of cases that are made known to public agencies during a specified period of time. However, incidence data grossly underestimate true rates of sexual abuse. Early estimates of official reporting among child abuse victims in general were as low as 3–6% (Russell, 1983; Timnick, 1985); however, more recent retrospective surveys estimate that between 8.7% and 12% of childhood sexual abuse was reported to police or other authorities (MacMillan, Jamieson, & Walsh, 2003; Saunders, Villeponteaux, Lipovsky, Kilpatrick, & Veronen, 1993). These increases probably reflect higher rates of disclosures and official reporting in recent years. During the 1980s and early 1990s, perhaps because of the passage of mandated reporting legislation and public awareness campaigns, reports of sexual abuse to public agencies increased dramatically (U.S. Department of

Health and Human Services, 1992–2000). Finkelhor (1994a), comparing conservative estimates of prevalence to known estimates of incidence, calculated child/adolescent disclosure rates during that period at approximately 30%.

Interestingly, during the latter half of the 1990s, reports of sexual abuse to official agencies decreased dramatically by 39% in the United States (Jones, Finkelhor, & Kopiec, 2001), and by 49% in Ontario, Canada (Trocmé, Fallon, MacLurin, & Copp, 2002). In 1990, sexual abuse reports comprised 17% of all confirmed or indicated reports of child maltreatment, whereas in 1999, sexual abuse reports comprised only 11% of such reports (U.S. Department of Health and Human Services, 2001). Surveys of child protective service administrators suggested that agency-reported declines in reported sexual abuse cases may have been due to increased caution in substantiating cases within child protective service agencies, but also the probable positive effects of prevention programs, increased prosecution, and public awareness campaigns (Jones et al., 2001). Some evidence supports the contention that at least a portion of the decline in reports reflects a true decline in the number of sexually abused children. Adult retrospective surveys from Australia and Ireland have demonstrated trends toward less abuse reported by younger, as compared to older, cohorts (Dunne, Purdie, Cook, Boyle, & Najman, 2003; McGee, Garavan de Barra, Byrne, & Conroy, 2002).

ABUSE AND VICTIM CHARACTERISTICS

Sexual abuse varies on a number of dimensions, including the acts involved, the use of coercion or force, the child's relationship to the perpetrator, and the duration and frequency of the abuse. Russell (1983) divided sexually abusive acts into three categories of severity, based on levels of sexual violation: (1) "very serious" sexual abuse (forced, unforced, and attempted vaginal, anal, or oral intercourse); (2) "serious" sexual abuse (forced or unforced digital penetration of the vagina, simulated intercourse, and fondling of genitals or breasts); and (3) "least serious" sexual abuse (forced kissing; touching clothed breasts or genitals; and intentional sexual touching of thighs, legs, buttocks, or other body parts). For incestuous abuse, 23% of cases were classified as very serious,

41% as serious, and 36% as least serious. For extrafamilial abuse, 53% of cases were categorized as very serious, 27% as serious, and 20% as least serious. Using abuse definitions similar to Russell's (1983), Vogeltanz and colleagues (1999) found that among women who reported a history of childhood sexual abuse, 57% of cases could be described as least serious, 26% as serious, and 24% as very serious. A *Los Angeles Times* poll (Timnick, 1985), which defined "coercion" as abuse that involved a weapon or forceful physical restraint, found that 15% of male victims and 19% of female victims experienced coercion. When *threat* of physical coercion is added, the rate of coercion for female victims rises to 38% (Vogeltanz et al., 1999).

Although approximately 60% of abuse occurs only once (Baker & Duncan, 1985; Finkelhor, 1979), 11% of female victims and 8% of male abuse victims are abused repeatedly over at least 1 year (Timnick, 1985). Not surprisingly, those who experience multiple episodes of abuse are more likely to report more serious forms of maltreatment. Bagley and Mallick (2000) found that only 3% of cases of one-episode abuse included vaginal or anal insertion/intercourse; for those who experienced multiple abusive events, 48% experienced vaginal insertion/intercourse, and 19% experienced anal insertion/intercourse.

Several demographic factors have been investigated as risks for sexual abuse, including age, gender, family characteristics, and racial and socioeconomic factors. Approximately 10% of sexually abused children are under age 6, with a slight increase in onset at 6–7 years, and a dramatic increase at around age 10 (33%; Bagley & Mallick, 2000; Finkelhor & Baron, 1986; Vogeltanz et al., 1999). Bagley and Mallick (2000) noted differences in onset between those who experienced one-time versus multiple abuse episodes. Among those who experienced one-time abuse, onset during preschool years was rare (3%), whereas one-time episodes were more common among girls age 11 and older (12–19%). In contrast, among those who reported multiple episodes of abuse, onset during preschool years was not uncommon (14%), but was uncommon after age 11 (5%).

Not surprisingly, girls are at higher risk for sexual abuse than boys, with girls 1.5 to 5 times more often victims than boys (Fergusson, Lynskey, & Horwood, 1996; Finkelhor, 1994a).

Sexual abuse experiences differ for boys and girls (Gordon, 1990; Watkins & Bentovim, 1992), with girls generally describing their experiences more negatively (Fischer, 1991). This may be because girls are abused by family members more often, with roughly one-third to one-half of female victims abused within the home, as compared to one-tenth to one-fifth of male victims (Fergusson et al., 1996; Finkelhor, 1994a; Vogeltanz et al., 1999). Abuse perpetrated by family members tends to be more severe. Fergusson and colleagues (1996) reported that 61.3% of abuse perpetrated by a family member included some form of intercourse, and that 71% of familial abuse involved more than one episode. From 4.5% to 6% of girls are abused by a father figure (Bagley & Mallick, 2000; Russell, 1984). Although biological fathers account for more incestuous abuse than stepfathers (more children live with fathers than with stepfathers), stepfathers are seven times more likely to abuse their stepdaughters and are more likely to commit more serious forms of abuse (Russell, 1983, 1984) In contrast, boys are more likely to be abused by someone outside the family, to be abused at a younger age, and to experience force and/or anal–genital or oral–genital contact (Gordon, 1990; Watkins & Bentovim, 1992).

Studies that have examined racial, cultural, and ethnic factors as risk factors for sexual abuse have been inconclusive (Kenny & McEachern, 2000). However, there is some evidence that sexual abuse is more common among families of lower socioeconomic status (SES) (Costello, Erkanli, Fairbank, & Angold, 2002). Nonetheless, broad cultural differences appear to be less important as risk factors than factors associated with family functioning do. Several family factors have been linked with risk of sexual abuse: unplanned pregnancy; low maternal education; parental alcohol and drug abuse; parental mental illness; harsh discipline; parent–child relationship problems; maternal death; and marital discord, separation, divorce, and maternal remarriage (Bagley & Mallick, 2000; Brown, Cohen, Johnson, & Salzinger, 1998; Dong et al., 2003; Fergusson et al., 1996; Mullen, Martin, Anderson, Romans, & Herbison, 1993; Walsh, MacMillan, & Jamieson, 2003). Several child factors have also been identified (Bagley & Mallick, 2000; Brown et al., 1998): being female, low IQ, having a disability, social isolation, and not having someone with whom one can confide. Furthermore, sexual abuse is associated with exposure to other forms of maltreatment, neglect, and domestic violence. Several studies have noted relatively high rates of physical and emotional abuse among child sexual abuse victims (Bagley & Mallick, 2000; Finkelhor & Dziuba-Leatherman, 1994; Fleming et al., 1997), as well as high rates of exposure to domestic violence (Dong et al., 2003). Risk of child sexual abuse appears to increase with the number of risk factors present. Brown and colleagues (1998) found that the chance of child sexual abuse rose from 1% when no risk factors were present to 33% when four or more risk factors were present. Bagley and Mallick (2000) found when three of more risk factors for sexual abuse were present, there was a 50% chance of sexual abuse during childhood.

Children with disabilities appear to be at heightened risk for sexual abuse, with prevalence estimates two to three times those of children without disabilities (Crosse, Kaye, & Ratnofsky, 1993; Sullivan & Knutson, 1998). Four factors have been linked to increased risk among children with disabilities (Westcott & Jones, 1999): (1) greater physical and social isolation; (2) increased dependency and lack of control over their lives and bodies, particularly in high-risk situations such as bathing, dressing, and toileting, and in situations where children are in the solitary care of individuals other than parents (e.g., residential and disability care providers, taxi drivers); (3) institutional care, with concerns raised about the level of training and qualifications for staff and insufficient efforts to assure patient safety; and (4) communication impairments that may increase risk of being selected by perpetrators, prevent reporting, and impede validation of abuse allegations. Much of the increased vulnerability in this population is among boys, particularly those between the ages of 6 and 11 (Randall, Parrila, & Sobsey, 2000; Sobsey, Randall, & Parrila, 1997; Sullivan, Brookhouser, Scanlan, Knutson, & Schulte, 1991). Sobsey and Doe (1991) found that increased contacts with disability service providers accounted for 78% of the increased risk to children with disabilities. Indeed, Sobsey and colleagues (1997) queried whether the disproportionate representation of boys among sexually abused children with disabilities is related to a tendency for their nonfamilial caregivers to be male, whereas nonfamilial caregivers of girls tend to be female.

PRIMARY PREVENTION AND PROMOTION OF EARLY DISCLOSURE

Unlike programs designed to prevent child physical abuse and neglect, where the focus has been on enhancing parenting skills (Peterson, Tremblay, Ewigman, & Saldana, 2003), child sexual abuse prevention programs have focused almost exclusively on teaching children how to recognize, avoid, and escape potentially abusive situations (Wurtele, 2002). Although schools have traditionally taught personal safety skills, the growing recognition of childhood sexual abuse in the 1980s led to an increased focus on sexual abuse prevention (Wurtele & Miller-Perrin, 1992). School-based universal delivery of prevention programs is appealing, because large numbers of children are reached at a low cost, and any stigma associated with participating is minimized because everyone is included (Wurtele, 2002).

Sexual abuse prevention programs are generally viewed as valuable and effective by educators and parents (Abrahams, Casey, & Daro, 1992; Wurtele, Kvaternic, & Franklin, 1992). By 1994, 48–85% of U.S. school districts offered child sexual abuse prevention programs (Daro, 1994). In fact, a U.S. national survey of 2,000 children between the ages of 10 and 16 revealed that 67% of children had participated in a school-based abuse or victimization prevention program at some time (Finkelhor & Dziuba-Leatherman, 1995). Similar programs have been adopted internationally. For example, by 1999, most primary schools in the Republic of Ireland had adopted a child sexual abuse program, the Stay Safe Program, with the full support of the Irish Department of Education (MacIntyre & Carr, 1999a).

School-based personal safety programs vary in many ways, but all have a central theme: Sexual abuse can be prevented if children recognize inappropriate adult behavior, react quickly to leave the situation, and tell someone about the incident (Conte, Rosen, & Saperstein, 1986). School-based prevention programs have been used with children of all grades, including children in day care and kindergarten. Programs differ in format and style, ranging from 1 to 12 or more sessions, and utilizing books and workbooks, films, enactments, and/or parental involvement (Conte et al., 1986). Program content also varies, with some programs specifically addressing sexual abuse prevention, and other programs addressing a wider array of prevention topics (e.g., prevention of physical assault by classroom bullies). Most sexual abuse prevention programs include such concepts as body ownership, the touch continuum, secrets, acting on one's own intuition, saying "No," and locating helpful people to tell. However, programs differ in the extent to which they explicitly address the sexual nature of abuse. Some programs focus on self-esteem and self-protection, avoiding direct discussion of sexual issues because of concerns about introducing children to sexuality prematurely. However, some advocate direct, explicit instruction about the sexual aspects of sexual abuse, since self-protection requires that children be able to recognize abusive situations (Finkelhor, 1986). Since at least 90% of abuse is perpetrated by individuals who are well known to the victims, some experts advocate that programs highlight this fact and teach children how to recognize and debunk the lies, manipulations, and forms of coercion that are used to gain children's compliance and secrecy (Conte et al., 1986).

Evaluation of school-based personal safety training involves several issues (Kolko, 1988; Miller-Perrin & Wurtele, 1986): (1) Do children gain new knowledge and skills, and do they retain the information over time? (2) Are some strategies more effective than others for teaching personal safety skills? (3) Are there negative effects of school-based personal safety training programs? (4) Do personal safety training programs increase rates of either actual or fabricated abuse allegations? Each of these issues is reviewed below.

Do Children Learn New Information and Skills, and Retain These over Time?

Before evaluating the effectiveness of personal safety skills programs, investigators should consider children's pretraining knowledge and skills. Even without a formal prevention program, most elementary-school-age children know that (1) they should seek help if approached sexually; (2) it is unsafe to get into a car with a stranger; (3) it is wrong for an adult to touch their private parts; and (4) it is wrong for anyone to tell them not to tell their parents about something the children did with that person (Finkelhor, Asdigian, & Dziuba-Leatherman, 1995a; Sigurdson, Strange, & Doig, 1987; D. A. Wolfe, MacPherson, Blount,

& Wolfe, 1986). However, pretraining knowledge varies with age. Wurtele and Miller-Perrin (1987) found that younger children (mean age = 6.1 years) had trouble defining sexual abuse, whereas older children (mean age = 11.3 years) usually included important concepts such as sexual contact in their definitions of sexual abuse. Older children recognized that most perpetrators are acquainted with their victims, but younger children tended to believe that perpetrators are strangers. In some cases, misconceptions are prevalent, regardless of age. For example, even older children tended to see perpetrators as deviant or "crazy," and many children believed that sexual abuse involves serious physical aggression. Most children believed that perpetrators tend to be adult or teen males, and saw victims as primarily females; however, younger boys tended to view victims as either males or females, and saw perpetrators as closer in age to themselves. Regardless of age, 20% of children could not think of ways to protect themselves against sexual abuse. When children did offer suggestions, saying "No," getting away, and telling someone were the most common.

Despite the fact that most children have some knowledge of personal safety concepts prior to training, several literature reviews have concluded that children who participate in school-based sexual abuse prevention program demonstrate statistically significant increases in knowledge and skills when compared with no-training control groups (Berrick & Barth, 1992; Finkelhor, Strapko, Willis, Holden, & Rosenberg, 1992; MacMillan, MacMillan, Offord, Griffith, & MacMillan, 1994). Based on a meta-analysis of 26 published evaluations of school-based prevention programs, Davis and Gidycz (2000) found a significant and sizable pre–post effect size (0.81, meeting the criterion of 0.80 for a large effect size). Rispens, Aleman, and Goudena (1997) also conducted a meta-analysis of personal safety programs, and included an examination of knowledge and skills retention from 1 to 6 months postintervention; they found significant retention of knowledge and skills at follow-up, with moderate effects sizes averaging 0.62.

Davis and Gidycz (2000) found that the two studies in their meta-analysis that used *in vivo* behavioral observation measures produced the largest effect sizes. Although *in vivo* strategies may more closely resemble "real-life" generalization of personal safety skills, ethical concerns limit the utility of such strategies on a routine basis. Fryer, Kraizer, and Miyoshi (1987a, 1987b) tested skill acquisition and utilization by having a "stranger" ask each child to assist him by accompanying him to his car. They found that 79% of trained children refused to accompany the stranger to the car, whereas only 53% of the untrained children refused. When the skill acquisition test was repeated 6 months later, the majority of trained children continued to refuse to accompany the stranger. More commonly, studies have evaluated knowledge and skill acquisition through vignettes, such as the What If Situations Test (WIST; Saslawsky & Wurtele, 1986). The WIST involves four vignettes describing potential encounters with adults who make sexual advances toward children. Questions are then asked to determine whether a child (1) recognizes the inappropriateness of the situation; (2) indicates that he or she would verbally refuse the advance; (3) indicates a plan to leave the situation; and (4) lists names of those whom he or she would tell about what happened.

Program effectiveness varies across student groups. Younger children learn more new information and tend to rate programs as more helpful than older children do (Davis & Gidycz, 2000; Finkelhor & Dziuba-Leatherman, 1995). Fryer and colleagues (1987a, 1987b) found that children who had a more positive self-concept prior to training were more likely to utilize their skills in an *in vivo* assessment of skill acquisition, suggesting that children must feel confident and assertive before they can muster the courage to say "no" to an adult. Girls tend to find school-based programs more interesting, more helpful, and full of more new information than boys do (Finkelhor & Dziuba-Leatherman, 1995). Changing the training format, such as using comic book heroes like Spiderman to demonstrate important concepts (Garbarino, 1987), may help make the subject more interesting to boys.

Are Some Teaching Strategies More Effective Than Others?

Programs that focus on concrete concepts and that involve modeling and behavioral rehearsal appear to be most effective in assuring knowledge and skill acquisition, as well as retention over time (Davis & Gidycz, 2000). Wurtele, Kast, Miller-Perrin, and Kondrick (1989) demonstrated that preschoolers had more difficulty learning about inappropriate touches when a "feelings-based" ("Trust your instincts") training approach was compared to a behavioral skills training approach ("Inappropriate touches are . . . "). Wurtele, Saslawsky, Miller, Marrs, and Britcher (1986) compared the effectiveness of various educational approaches for teaching personal safety skills to children. Four conditions were compared: (1) a filmed program, *Touch*; (2) a behavioral skills training program that used modeling, behavioral rehearsal, and social reinforcement; (3) a combination of the two; and (4) a no-training presentation. Behavioral skills training, alone or in combination with the film, was more effective than either the film alone or the control presentation, for both knowledge and skill acquisition.

In their national survey of children, Finkelhor and colleagues (Finkelhor, Asdigian, & Dziuba-Leatherman, 1995a, 1995b; Finkelhor & Dziuba-Leatherman, 1995) reported that 67% of children ages 10–16 indicated that they had participated in a school-based prevention program, but only 34% described programs that could be considered comprehensive in scope. Comprehensive programs were defined as having at least 9 of the following 12 components: information about sexual abuse, bullies, good and bad touch, confusing touch, incest, screaming and yelling to attract attention, telling an adult, and abuse never being a child's fault; behavioral rehearsal in class; information sheets to take home; a meeting for parents; and multiday presentations. Children who took part in more comprehensive programs were more knowledgeable about sexual victimization, reported greater use of self-protection measures when faced with threats, perceived themselves as more effective in keeping safe and minimizing their harm, and were more likely to disclose the episode to someone. Several components were particularly effective in facilitating "real-life" use of the skills taught—behavioral rehearsal, multiday presentations, and take-home information materials. In some cases, children reported that they had been exposed to several programs over their years in elementary school. Those children were more likely to report that they had used the information to help out a friend.

Despite the effectiveness of the programs in changing attitudes and behaviors, there was no evidence that the children were more capable of preventing threatening situations from becoming completed assaults. However, data were not reported as to whether those who received comprehensive training were victimized less often than those who received less comprehensive training or none at all (Gibson & Leitenberg, 2000). It is possible that children who receive comprehensive training are approached less frequently by potential perpetrators, since such children may present themselves as more assertive, suspicious, and guarded in risky situations. Evidence suggests that perpetrators tend to select children who lack confidence and self-esteem, and those they perceive as less likely to resist or tell (Elliott, Browne, & Kilcoyne, 1995).

Parental involvement in personal safety skill programs can add substantially to the learning process, particularly for preschool children. Parents can reinforce prevention concepts and skills, answer questions, and correct children's misperceptions. To avoid confusing children, it is important that parents and schools teach similar concepts. Involving parents can also reduce secrecy about the topic of sexual abuse and stimulate parent–child discussions of sexuality in general. Without some level of professional support or training, however, many parents either do not talk to their children about sexual abuse or "water down" prevention information (Elrod & Rubin, 1993; Wurtele, 1993; Wurtele, Kvaternic, et al., 1992). Parents often wait to talk to their children until they are fairly old (on average, 9 years of age; Elrod & Rubin, 1993; Finkelhor, 1986), and when they do talk to their children, they tend to emphasize risks associated with strangers, and fail to note that known adults and teenagers are also potential perpetrators.

In their survey of 10- to 16-year-olds, Finkelhor and colleagues (1995a) found that 57% reported that their parents had specifically talked to them about how to avoid sexual abuse, and that 36% had had fairly comprehensive discussions of the topic with their parents. Much of the parental instruction was prompted by children's participating in a school-based prevention program, with only 17% of the sample receiving comprehensive instruction solely from parents. Comprehensive parental discussions were defined as including at least three of four components: that perpetrators could be relatives or family friends, that abuse is never a child's fault, that children should yell or scream to attract attention, and

that they should tell an adult. Comprehensive discussions with parents were linked with greater knowledge about self-protection, more use of self-protection strategies in potentially abusive situations, and increased probability of disclosure of sexual victimizations.

Several studies have directly evaluated parent components as part of school-based personal safety programs. Wurtele and her colleagues have demonstrated that both middle- and lower-SES parents can effectively teach preschoolers the skills necessary to recognize and respond to inappropriate sexual gestures (Wurtele, Currier, Gillispie, & Franklin, 1991; Wurtele, Gillispie, Currier, & Franklin, 1992; Wurtele, Kast, & Melzer, 1992). However, parents of preschool children often require ongoing consultation and encouragement by professionals if they are to complete instruction (Wurtele, 1993). To date, only one study has actually compared parental to school-based instruction. Wurtele, Kast, and Melzer (1992) compared skill acquisition of Head Start children across four conditions: teacher-trained, parent-trained, parent- and teacher-trained, and an attention control group. Children in all three trained groups demonstrated more knowledge and skill than did the children in the attention control group. Children who received training from their parents (both parent-only and teacher and parent training) showed greater improvements in their ability to recognize inappropriate touch requests and in their personal safety skills than did children taught only by teachers.

Despite the effectiveness of parental involvement in sexual abuse prevention programs, Finkelhor and colleagues (1995a) reported that only 11% of school-based programs included a parent component. This is not surprising, since parent interest in and attendance at such programs tends to be quite poor (Tutty, 1993). Perhaps either the content or the methods of involving parents need further development. Elrod and Rubin (1993) surveyed parents and found that they most desired information on the following topics: (1) how to identify abuse; (2) how to react to signs of abuse; (3) how to get accurate information about abuse from a child without creating false allegations; and (4) how to talk with children about sex in developmentally appropriate ways.

The Committee for Children (1996) produced a 30–minute video that addresses some of these concerns, *What Do I Say Now?* The video was designed in accordance with protection motivation theory (Rogers, 1983), which posits that positive prevention attitudes and behaviors are facilitated when individuals understand the significance of a particular threat and when they believe that advocated prevention tactics can be effective. In the video, actors model how to talk to children about sexuality, teach children about safe touches, and handle a child's disclosure of sexual abuse. Burgess and Wurtele (1998) compared parents who attended a 1–hour video–discussion workshop with parents who attended a similar workshop on child safety. Parents who attended the sexual abuse prevention workshop demonstrated increased awareness of child sexual abuse risk and reported greater confidence that parent–child communication about sexual abuse would reduce their own children's risk of abuse. Furthermore, when contacted several weeks later, more of the parents who attended the sexual abuse prevention workshop reported that they had since talked with their children about sexual abuse. Like previous studies that involved parents, however, the study involved only a small number of volunteer parents; dropout was also substantial, even though transportation, child care, and flexible scheduling were offered, and the time commitment was minimal. Perhaps programs that either coincide with times when parents are attending the school for other reasons (e.g., parent–teacher conference evenings) or provide materials for home use (e.g., instructional videos) will reach a greater number of parents.

Do Programs Create Undue Fear and Worry among Participants?

Concerns have been voiced that school-based personal safety programs may have negative effects on children by creating undue fear and anxiety, contributing to their distrust of adults, and negatively affecting their attitudes toward sex. Programs that have addressed these issues have generally shown small increases in program-related fears and worries (Binder & McNiel, 1987; Garbarino, 1987; Miltenberger & Thiesse-Duffy, 1988). From their national survey of children and parents, Finkelhor and Dziuba-Leatherman (1995) found that 8% of children said they worried "a lot" and 53% said they worried "a little" following school-based personal safety programs. Furthermore,

16% of parents reported they had noticed an increase in their children's fear of adults. Children who are young, African American, and from lower-SES homes tend to report more program-related fears and worries (Finkelhor & Dziuba-Leatherman, 1995; Miller-Perrin & Wurtele, 1986). Interestingly, Finkelhor and Dziuba-Leatherman (1995) point out that fear and anxiety may actually be adaptive responses, since the children are learning about true dangers. Nevertheless, it is important that children perceive that the skills acquired as a result of training will help them cope if they are faced with a sexually abusive situation. Binder and McNiel (1987) found that children reported feeling safer and more confident in their ability to protect themselves following personal safety training. Other positive psychological effects have been noted as well, including more communication between children and their parents regarding sexuality issues, improved knowledge of genital terminology, increased body pride, and improved attitudes toward touching their own private parts (Binder & McNiel, 1987; Wurtele, 1993; Wurtele, Kast, & Melzer, 1992; Wurtele & Owens, 1997).

Do Programs Increase Rates of Either Actual or Fabricated Abuse Allegations?

School-based personal safety programs have two ultimate goals: (1) that children recognize potentially abusive situations and react in a way that enables them to avoid the abuse; and (2) that children report all inappropriate sexual advances (including sexual invitations, sexually suggestive comments, and nongenital touching, as well as more explicit sexual acts) to a responsible adult as soon as possible, whether or not more explicitly abusive behaviors occur. Finkelhor and Dziuba-Leatherman (1995) found that many children reported using skills they learned as a result of personal safety training: 25% said they had used the information from the program to help a friend; 5% said they had told an adult "no" as a result of what they had learned; and 14% said they had told an adult about something, based on information learned from the program. As noted earlier, "real-life" use of protection skills was more common among children who attended more comprehensive, multiday programs that included components such as behavioral rehearsal, take-home educational materials, and parental involvement. Despite these positive findings, there was no evidence that such prevention programs actually reduced the percentage of completed victimizations among those who experienced a threat.

Several studies have demonstrated increases in rates of reporting abuse following school-based personal safety training. Oldfield, Hays, and Megel (1996) evaluated Project Trust, an elementary-school-based victimization prevention program based on the film *Touch*, with a large sample (*n* = 1,269) of children in grades 1–6. The group that received training had a higher incidence of first-time reports of maltreatment than the control group. All maltreatment reports were independently verified, quelling concerns that abuse prevention programs might encourage false allegations of maltreatment (Goldstein, Freud, & Solnit, 1979). Kolko, Moser, and Hughes (1989) compared children who had participated in the Red Flag/Green Flag prevention program with no-training controls. Six months later, 11% of the children in the experimental condition had reported inappropriate touching, whereas no children in the control group reported abuse. MacIntyre and Carr (1999b) evaluated whether sexual abuse disclosures were affected by previous participation in Stay Safe, a school-based personal safety training program. Those who had previously been involved in a Stay Safe program were more likely to have made a purposeful disclosure of their abuse (i.e., rather than to disclose only after questioning by an adult), and were more likely to have either disclosed at school or been identified by school personnel.

To date, only one study has used adult retrospective reports to investigate the effectiveness of child sexual abuse prevention programs. Gibson and Leitenberg (2000) surveyed 825 undergraduate women about past sexual abuse and involvement in childhood sexual abuse prevention programs. Sixty-two percent reported having a "good-touch/bad-touch" type of program in either preschool or elementary school. Those who were exposed to personal safety programs were significantly less likely to report a history of sexual abuse than those who did not (8% vs. 14%). Although there were no differences between the groups with regard to disclosures of abuse during childhood, there was a trend for earlier disclosure among those who participated in the sexual abuse prevention programs.

Who Discloses Abuse?

Despite widespread efforts to encourage early disclosure, it is clear that some children and adolescents do not disclose their abuse or postpone disclosure for substantial periods of time. In Russell's (1983) epidemiological study, only a few adult survivors of childhood sexual abuse (2% of intrafamilial abuse and 6% of extrafamilial abuse) said that they had disclosed their abuse to police during childhood. More recent retrospective surveys estimate that between 8.7% and 12% of childhood sexual abuse was reported to police or other authorities (MacMillan et al., 2003; Saunders et al., 1993). A larger proportion of victims disclose abuse to family and friends, but do not disclose to authorities. Several studies estimated that approximately one-third of children disclosed their abuse to someone during their childhood or adolescence (Arata, 1998; Lamb & Edgar-Smith, 1994). Some evidence suggests even further improvements in disclosure rates. Data from the National Survey of Adolescents, which included 1,958 girls ages 12–17 years, revealed that 13% had experienced unwanted sexual contact (Kogan, 2004). Of those, 48% reported that they had disclosed their abuse to an adult. An additional 25% had not disclosed their abuse to an adult, but had revealed the abuse to a peer. Hanson and colleagues (2003), also reporting data from the National Survey of Adolescents, found that only half of those who disclosed their abuse to a relative, friend, or other confidant had also made a disclosure to an official agency.

Although disclosure rates have greatly improved, the likelihood that half to two-thirds of sexually abused children go undetected is quite concerning. Even among those who eventually disclose their abuse, fewer than 25% disclose immediately (Gomes-Schwartz, Horowitz, & Cardarelli, 1990; Kelley, Brant, & Waterman, 1993), and delays average 1.5 to 3.0 years (Oxman-Martinez, Rowe, Straka, & Thibault, 1997; Sas, Cunningham, Hurley, Dick, & Farnsworth, 1995). The most serious outcome of delayed disclosure is the risk of further abuse. Indeed, Sas et al. (1995) reported that among those who did not immediately report their abuse, 44% were abused again by the same perpetrator. Delayed disclosure also increases the risk of abuse to other children, diminishes credibility when the abuse is eventually disclosed, and impedes access to mental health services to address abuse-related sequelae (Goodman-Brown, Edelstein, Goodman, Jones, & Gordon, 2003; Myers, 1992). Furthermore, disclosures delayed by 1 month or more are associated with increased risk of developing PTSD and major depressive disorder (MDD) (Ruggiero et al., 2003).

Research suggests that a child's decision to disclose sexual abuse must be viewed within a developmental framework and with consideration of issues relevant to the abuse itself, the perpetrator, the family, and personal characteristics of the child. Some victims report that school-based personal safety programs or conversations with their parents influenced their decisions to disclose. However, children's motivations also influence disclosure, with motivations ranging from a need for protection and emotional support to feelings of anger and desire for revenge (Lamb & Edgar-Smith, 1994; Sas et al., 1995; Sorenson & Snow, 1991). In some cases, children either spontaneously talk about the abuse or consciously plan their disclosure. Other children may not feel prepared to tell, but the disclosure may be prompted by others following such clues as inappropriate sexual behaviors, changes in personality or behaviors, or detection of a sexually transmitted disease (STD), or after it becomes known that a child spent time with someone suspected of abusing others (Kelley et al., 1993; Sorenson & Snow, 1991). Approximately half of children make their initial disclosure to a parent (Berliner & Conte, 1995; Gomes-Schwartz et al., 1990; Lawson & Chaffin, 1994), but one in four children will make their initial disclosure to a peer (Henry, 1997).

Decisions to disclose sexual abuse are difficult for children, and some children will steadfastly deny abuse even when faced with compelling evidence (DiPietro, Runyan, & Frederickson, 1997; Lawson & Chaffin, 1994; Sorenson & Snow, 1991). There are many reasons why children avoid disclosure; they may fear retaliation from the perpetrator or others, may wish to avoid the stigma and family turmoil that might ensue, or may worry that they will be blamed or punished. Unfortunately, these fears are often justified, in that disclosures are often met with disbelief, do not lead to protection, and result in significant family upheaval and victim blaming (Sauzier, 1989; Sorenson & Snow, 1991). Sorenson and Snow (1991) described a child's disclosure of sexual abuse as more of a process than a specific event. Reviewing clinical records of children with confirmed allegations of sexual abuse, they reported the following: (1) 75% of victims had initially denied their abuse when first questioned by an adult; (2) 78% were initially vague and vacillated about the details of their abuse, but later provided more consistent and detailed accounts; 22% recanted the allegations at some point; and (4) 92% of those who recanted their allegations eventually reaffirmed the abuse. Recantation has been linked with a number of postdisclosure stressors, including disbelief by mothers (Elliott & Briere, 1994) and court proceedings (Gonzalez, Waterman, Kelly, McCord, & Oliveri, 1993), and has been viewed as a manifestation of PTSD avoidance (Gonzalez et al., 1993; Koverola & Foy, 1993).

Gender, age, race, and developmental status are related to children's disclosures of sexual abuse. Not surprisingly, studies indicate that boys are less likely to disclose their sexual abuse than girls (Hanson et al., 2002; Lynch, Stern, Oates, & O'Toole, 1993; Stroud, Martens, & Barker, 2000; Violatao & Genius, 1993). In addition to boys feeling very stigmatized by male-perpetrated abuse, boys may not actually define sexual acts by older girls or women as abuse (Hecht & Hansen, 1999). For both boys and girls, those who are younger than 7 and older than 14 are less likely to disclose abuse than latency-age children and young adolescents (Kogan, 2004). Adolescent boys, particularly those of African American descent, are the least likely of all victims to disclose (Hanson et al., 2002; Hecht & Hansen, 1999). Girls who experience sexual abuse after age 14 are also unlikely to disclose sexual abuse unless the perpetrator is a peer; in those cases, teen girls may confide in one of their friends (Kogan, 2004). Despite higher prevalence of sexual abuse among children with disabilities, disclosure rates are disproportionately small, and disclosures are often not reported to child protective service agencies (Kvam, 2000).

Older children are more likely to disclose their abuse in a planned and purposeful way, whereas disclosures by younger children are often prompted after an adult suspects abuse (Mian, Wehrspann, Klajner-Diamond, LeBaron, & Winder, 1986). Even after an initial disclosure, younger children are less likely than older children to disclose in the context of formal investigations (DiPietro et al., 1997), though additional interviews may aid the disclosure process (Gries, Goh, & Cavanaugh, 1996). Concerns have been raised that inflexible guidelines (e.g., universal decisions not to use anatomically correct dolls; total reliance on open-ended forms of questioning) employed in some investigations may impede disclosure for young or delayed children or those with communication problems (Saywitz, Nathanson, & Snyder, 1993).

Children and adolescents are most likely to disclose abuse if the perpetrator was a stranger, perhaps because there are fewer personal and intrafamilial costs associated with disclosure (Kogan, 2004; Stroud et al., 2000). Intrafamilial abuse, or even knowing the perpetrator, decreases the probability of immediate disclosure (Elliott & Briere, 1994; Kogan, 2004; Smith et al., 2000; Stroud et al., 2000). Many factors impede disclosure of intrafamilial abuse. Perpetrators who have more access to and authority over their victims may maintain secrecy through threats and manipulations. Offending family members often abuse their victims more frequently and over longer periods of time; the longer abuse persists, the less likely children are to disclose (Arata, 1998). Intrafamilial abuse is associated with more shame and guilt, and children often worry about the effects of disclosing intrafamilial abuse on other family members, such as mothers and siblings. Children often say they had caring and loving relationships with the perpetrators, and for some these relationships may have filled significant needs in the children's lives (Berliner & Conte, 1995; Elliott et al., 1995). Thus children often worry that the perpetrators will go to jail or hurt themselves if they disclose. Children may face familial resistance to disclosure of intrafamilial abuse, and family support plays a very significant role in the disclosure process. Lawson and Chaffin (1992) studied the willingness to disclose abuse among children diagnosed with an STD. Children were 3.5 times more likely to disclose sexual abuse when their mothers were willing to entertain the idea that the children might have been abused.

Children who experience severe forms of maltreatment (e.g., sexual penetration), physical coercion, and threats tend to have one of two reactions (Gomes-Schwartz et al., 1990). For some, the severity of the abuse facilitates disclosure, because the children may fear for their lives. However, other children may delay their disclosure until they feel safe from retribution. Paine and Hansen (2002) reported that delays in disclosure were twice as lengthy when perpetrators were violent with either the children themselves or members of their families. Kogan (2004) found that children were most likely to delay disclosures when family members had been threatened.

Future Directions for Primary Prevention

Nation and colleagues (2003) highlighted nine characteristics associated with successful primary prevention programs, drawn from prevention research in the areas of substance abuse, risky sexual behavior, school failure, and juvenile delinquency. Successful primary prevention programs tended to be theory-driven, socioculturally relevant, and comprehensive in scope. Interventions that were lengthy enough to convey important concepts and skills and that used a variety of teaching methods were more successful, as were programs that included staff training and that encouraged positive relationships among staff and participants. Timing of intervention was deemed important—not occurring so early that the information was not yet relevant, or so late that risks had already affected some participants. Finally, program evaluations were deemed important, particularly when program iterations were based on outcomes.

Research on school-based personal safety programs has addressed many of these concerns and has demonstrated success with regard to increased knowledge, skill, "real-life" skill usage to thwart victimization, and disclosure subsequent to victimizations and victimization attempts. There is also burgeoning evidence of small but significant reductions in victimizations overall. Nonetheless, the prevalence of childhood sexual abuse remains at what some have described as "epidemic" proportions (Bolen, 2003; U.S. Department of Health and Human Services, 2004). Reppucci, Woolard, and Fried (1999) advocate that primary prevention programs can only successfully address societal problems through comprehensive, multilevel efforts that target individuals, families, communities, and society at large. Likewise, some have argued for a public health approach to prevention of sexual abuse that is comprehensive and interdisciplinary, and that targets attitudes, behaviors, and social norms (Kaufman, Barber, Mosher, & Carter, 2002; McMahon & Pruett, 1999). Thus, although school-based programs are now well developed and relatively effective, it is clear that other avenues of primary prevention are underdeveloped and sorely needed if significant reductions in the prevalence of childhood sexual abuse are to be realized.

Further Development of School-Based Personal Safety Training

Within the domain of school-based primary prevention programs, several areas of growth are still needed. Current efforts focus almost solely on preschool and elementary school children, with little mention of programs for older children and adolescents. Epidemiological data reveal that sexual offenses against adolescents differ from those against younger children, and thus the information gleaned from training in earlier years may lack relevance for teens. Adolescents are more often abused by peers and are less likely to disclose their abuse, with the exception that peer-perpetrated abuse may be confided to friends. Adolescents, unfortunately, are also faced with the increased possibility that their claims of maltreatment will be questioned on the bases of consent, motivation to lie, and concerns that lifestyle issues (e.g., previous sexual relationships, drug and alcohol use, and other rule violations) damage their credibility. Thus programs designed to reach older children and adolescents will need to highlight the risks and consequences of sexual assaults by peers *and* adults, and to identify "real-life" strategies for avoiding and preventing victimization that take into account adolescents' needs to experiment, socialize with peers, and become more independent from adult supervision. Avenues of disclosure and self-protection subsequent to assault need to be discussed, along with guidance for what peers should do if a friend confides in them information about sexual abuse.

School-based personal safety programs are often criticized because they fail to teach children and parents about the modus operandi of offending juveniles and adults (Berliner, 1984; Conte et al., 1986; Kaufman et al., 2002). Several studies have investigated offending patterns (Bolen, 2000; Elliott et al., 1995; Kaufman et al., 1998). In order to obtain unsupervised access to children, perpetrators often befriend their victims and gain the trust of caregivers, sometimes offering to babysit or coach children in a sport or some other recreational activity. Some offer rides to children, and initial sexual overtures may occur in the privacy of the car. "Grooming" may precede more sexual overt acts, serving the function of desensitizing children to sexuality. Grooming behaviors can include giving drugs and alcohol, exposure to pornography, and making sexual comments and pseudosexual gestures. Sexual acts may be initiated in the course of games and may be accompanied by gifts and special attention. Because of the grooming activities and enticements, once overt sexual acts are initiated, children may feel trapped and feel that they in some way colluded in the sexual acts. Perpetrators may use threats, anger, blackmail, and bribery to insure secrecy and compliance. However, they also use "love-bargaining" strategies such as threats of rejection or trying to elicit sympathy by declaring a need for children's love and affection (Niederberger, 2002). Awareness of practices and patterns in sexual abuse can help children and parents recognize potential abusive situations either before they happen or early in the process. If parents recognize unusual aspects of an adolescent–child or adult–child relationship, they can investigate further, prohibit the relationship, or insist on appropriate boundaries.

There is very little research on personal safety training with developmentally delayed children and children with other disabilities. Tang and Lee (1999) reported a Chinese study documenting that adolescents with mild developmental delays had relatively poor knowledge of personal safety skills, which corresponded with a general lack of knowledge about sex. Given the significant risk of sexual maltreatment for this group of children, special educators may need to develop strategies for incorporating personal safety training into sex education curricula.

School-Based Programs Designed to Reduce Sexual Offending

Approximately 95% of sexual abuse is perpetrated by males (Finkelhor et al., 1990; Russell, 1983; Wyatt, 1985), and 40% of that by adolescent males (Davis & Leitenberg, 1987). Half of juveniles' offenses are committed against either friends and dates, and another 30% against acquaintances. With those figures in mind, Bolen (2003) has argued that primary prevention efforts should also be directed toward boys, adolescent males, and young men, with the goal of deterring them from sexually abusive behaviors.

Primary prevention efforts, however, are considered most effective when a relatively large proportion of those addressed have the problem, and to date it has been difficult to establish the prevalence of males who engage in sexually abusive behaviors toward children and adolescents. Nonetheless, drawing from several studies of perpetrators and victims, Bolen (2003) estimated that 10–20% of the male population is at risk of abusing a child. Research has demonstrated that a substantial proportion of men respond sexually to images of children, fantasize about having sex with children, or report that they would engage in sexual behavior with a child if there were no chance of being caught (Briere & Runtz, 1989). Furthermore, Finkelhor and Lewis (1988) reported that between 4% and 17% of adult men endorsed survey items indicating that they had engaged in sexual acts with children and adolescents that would be considered within the domain of sexual abuse.

Bolen (2000) reported that only a small, disproportionate percentage of perpetrators are ever caught (approximately 10%), with the majority identified as being either pedophilic or intrafamilial. Bolen (2003) also described a second set of perpetrators whom she labeled as "situational"; that is, they take advantage of a sexual opportunity with a child or peer (with or without coercion), but they do not necessarily see their behavior as abusive or illegal, nor do they have a special interest in children sexually. Examples include cases where male adolescents abuse a victim "for sport," engage in coerced sexual behavior in order to brag about their exploits with peers, or engage in coercive sexual acts with a sense of entitlement (as in date rape situations). Some evidence suggests that adolescent males are often unaware that coerced sexual acts with peers and sexual contacts with children are illegal, and are likewise unaware of the potential legal consequences of such (Finkelhor, 1990). Furthermore, they often fail to comprehend the impact of sexual victimization on children and young teens.

Bolen (2003) has envisioned school-based programs that are not unlike school-based personal safety programs, but are designed to reduce male sexual aggression against peers and younger children. Such programs would span preschool through high school, with a positive focus on building healthy relationships. Themes would include healthy ways of expressing masculinity, healthy boy–girl friendships and romantic relationships, and boundaries regarding coerced sexual contacts with peers and any sexual contacts with younger children. Bolen has also advocated strict enforcement of zero tolerance for any types of sexual harassment in schools. Although such a program could "stand alone" in implementation, it is possible that some of Bolen's concepts could be integrated into other school-based programs, such as those designed to prevent violence. For example, the Multisite Violence Prevention Project (2003) is a universal delivery prevention program implemented in the sixth grade. It consists of twenty 40–minute lessons designed to promote prosocial norms and behaviors, and to reduce violence and victimization.

Strategies that Place the Onus for Prevention on Caregivers and Institutions

School-based personal safety programs have been criticized because they place the onus on children to prevent abuse, even though the true responsibility for prevention should fall to caregivers and society. Forehand, Miller, Dutra, and Chance (1997) note that monitoring and supervision are fundamental to adequate parenting. Prevention programs that encourage parents and caregivers to monitor and supervise children closely in risky situations will help to minimize risks. Close monitoring of playground and neighborhood activities, as well as activities in the home, will reduce unsupervised access to children by potential perpetrators. Furthermore, close supervision of adolescents' activities will decrease the likelihood that they may inappropriately cross sexual boundaries with peers and younger children.

Although school-based personal safety training should be adapted for some populations of children with disabilities, the ability of others to avoid or defend themselves against sexual abuse is diminished by their physical, cognitive, or communication impairments (Westcott & Jones, 1999). Thus prevention strategies that focus on child protection are essential. Unfortunately, those who are in a position to care for disabled children, parents, educators, and institutional workers, have limited knowledge of important issues relevant to this population, such as responsibilities to report abuse, processes of reporting abuse, recognition of abuse, and ways of responding to abuse concerns and allegations (Orelove, Hollahan, & Myles,

2000). Moreover, police and child protection service workers often feel unprepared when required to interview children with disabilities regarding abuse concerns (Orelove et al., 2000).

As noted earlier, Sobsey and Doe (1991) attributed 78% of the increase in risk to disabled children to their increased exposure to multiple caregivers within schools and institutions. Marchant and Cross (1993) advocated establishing institutional practices that are positive for these children and that ward off potential perpetrators. In addition to the need for careful staff hiring, training, and monitoring procedures, they recommended six steps to prevent abuse of children in these settings: (1) commitment to child protection; (2) explicit practice guidelines that decrease opportunities and conditions where abuse can occur; (3) internal policies that take allegations of abuse seriously and conduct investigations in line with community standards (e.g., involvement of child protective service investigators); (4) open-door policies to parents, community agents, and adults with disabilities; (5) respect for the individuality of children with disabilities; and (6) promotion of internal awareness of abuse and abuse risk factors.

Societal-Level Interventions

Societal-level primary prevention interventions are often implemented through public education programs, incentives, and law implementation and enforcement. Mass media campaigns have been used extensively to educate the public about physical, emotional, and sexual abuse and neglect, but little has been done thus far to evaluate those efforts systematically (Daro & Donnelly, 2002), particularly with regard to sexual abuse. Media strategies have included television and radio shows, newspaper and magazine articles, public service announcements (e.g., television and radio ads, billboards, bus signs, etc.), and the Internet. The goals have primarily been to increase public awareness of child abuse and to promote healthy public attitudes toward child care and protection. Although little attention has been paid to the effectiveness of the media in addressing the problem of child abuse, Daro and Gelles (1992) provided some compelling evidence of the strength of this form of prevention. In the mid-1970s, fewer than 10% of the population was aware of the problem of child maltreatment. However, by the early 1980s, a national public opinion survey demonstrated

that more than 90% were aware that child maltreatment was a significant societal problem and were aware of some of the complexities of child maltreatment (e.g., different forms of abuse, different contributing factors, need for the public to take action to improve situation). During the intervening period of time, Prevent Child Abuse America had implemented a multimedia strategy targeting physical and emotional abuse and neglect. The survey also detected significant decreases in verbal aggression and corporal punishment as discipline strategies, as well as dramatic increases in official reports to child protective service agencies (McCurdy & Daro, 1994).

Awareness of Online Sexual Predators and Internet Prevention Strategies

The Internet, with instant messaging, e-mails, websites, and chat rooms, has greatly altered the ways that children and adolescents communicate with each other and meet new people. Unfortunately, the Internet has opened new doors to perpetrators to contact and solicit potential victims; indeed, a recent national survey documented that 20% of children and adolescents report at least one episode of sexual solicitation within a 1-year period (Mitchell, Finkelhor, & Wolak, 2003). Although research into Internet-initiated sexual abuse is in its early stages, case-based evidence suggests that those committing such abuse operate in ways similar to other perpetrators (Dombrowski, LeMasney, Ahia, & Dickson, 2004). That is, they select children and adolescents who show some level of vulnerability—either through the use of sexually suggestive nicknames on the Internet, or by presenting themselves as isolated, lonely, passive, and emotionally vulnerable. Internet perpetrators may at first present themselves as peers. Like other perpetrators, they may engage in grooming behaviors in the form of exchanges of pictures, pornography, or gifts. Once a relationship is established, online perpetrators may progress to requesting identifying information, phone numbers, and face-to-face meetings. Adolescents may be more common targets of online perpetrators, since they have greater autonomy, mobility, and sexual curiosity than children do.

Dombrowski and colleagues (2004) have described several technical strategies that can be used to reduce risk. These include installation of computer firewalls and antivirus software programs and installation of programs to monitor children's computer activities (e.g., key logger, browser history logs, chat logging, and blocking of personal information). However, they stress that psychoeducational strategies are most important, since children's computer activities are not limited to home use; they also provide a sample parent–child contract for Internet safety (see Appendix 10.1).

SECONDARY PREVENTION

Professional Reporting of Child Sexual Abuse Allegations

All states and provinces in North America require professionals to report suspected abuse to official child protection agencies; mandated reporters include mental health professionals, social workers, physicians, nurses, teachers, and other school staff (Fraser, 1986). Indeed, 56.5% of child protective service investigations are initiated by mandated reporters in hospitals, schools, day care centers, mental health centers, and social service agencies (U.S. Department of Health and Human Services, 2004). State and provincial laws vary as to the situations that require reporting (e.g., ongoing abuse, potential for abuse, past abuse even when there is no current risk of abuse), the degree of certainty necessary for mandated reporting, and sanctions for failing to report (Walters, 1995). The standard for decision making is generally "reasonable cause to believe," and beyond that, professional discretion should not play a role (Zellman & Fair, 2002). Laws for reporting child abuse override concerns about protecting patient confidentiality. Mandated reporters are protected from criminal and civil liability in all jurisdictions, unless a report is made maliciously or without probable grounds. In addition to possible legal and professional sanctions, a professional who fails to report suspected abuse may be liable for civil damages based on abuse-related injuries incurred from the point at which the professional failed to take action (*Landeros v. Flood*, 1979). However, Kalichman (1999) notes that a professional should only disclose sufficient information to protect a child and comply with reporting obligations, as release of unrelated information may also create liability problems.

Despite legal mandates, up to 40% of professionals admit that they suspected abuse at some point, but failed to report it (Zellman, 1992). Whereas 44% of professionals indicated that they consistently reported all suspicious cases, one-third were described as "discretionary reporters"; that is, they reported some but not all suspicious cases. Most individuals who fail to report suspected abuse do not lack knowledge or experience relative to child abuse (Brosig & Kalichman, 1993; Zellman & Fair, 2002). Rather, commonly cited reasons for not reporting by discretionary reporters include insufficient evidence, uncertainty of allegations, perceptions that the abuse was not sufficiently serious, adverse effects of reporting on the child or on treatment, perception that a professional could intervene more effectively than child protective services could, and negative perception of the quality of service provided by child protective services (Ashton, 1999; Delaronde, King, Bendel, & Reece, 2000; Zellman, 1992).

To date, little research has been conducted into ways to encourage professional reporting beyond professional mandates. Several states, including California, Iowa, and New York, have laws that require mandated reporters to complete a training program on reporting child abuse prior to licensure. The Iowa law requires that the training be updated every 5 years. Media campaigns have also been touted as facilitating reporting (Besharov, 1994). Several organizations have orchestrated impressive efforts to encourage reporting, including the American Professional Society on the Abuse of Children, the National Center on Child Abuse and Neglect, the National Committee for Prevention of Child Abuse, the National Resource Center on Child Sexual Abuse, the Clearinghouse of Child Abuse and Neglect Information, and the American Humane Association/ Children's Division (Besharov, 1994).

Child Sexual Abuse Investigations

Investigation Processes and Interagency Cooperation

By law, child protective services are required to investigate all bona fide reports (Van Voorhis & Gilbert, 1998), but in reality, cases are triaged in order to manage the vast number of reports. Reports that lack detail are often screened out (S. Wells, Stein, Fluke, & Downing, 1989). Thus, although mandated reporters are not intended to take the role of investigators, they should take care that the information conveyed is clear, detailed, and precise, and should consider how the information relates to child abuse legislation (Kalichman, 1999). Depending on the jurisdiction, cases may be screened out for a number of reasons (S. Wells et al., 1989), with up to half of cases closed after the initial telephone intake (Van Voorhis & Gilbert, 1998). A report is generally made to the police when the perpetrator was not a caretaker or when the offense was committed in an out-of-home placement, such as a group home, school, or residential facility. Some referrals relate to child welfare but do not reach the level of maltreatment (e.g., parental alcoholism or psychiatric problems, child truancy); in those cases, reports may be deferred to other services provided within the child welfare system's domain (e.g., parenting groups) or to other community services (e.g., day care providers, mental health and addiction services, school truancy officers). Risk assessment tools are increasingly being used to aid in child protection decisions. Leschied, Chiodo, Whitehead, Hurley, and Marshall (2003) found that risk assessment results were consistent with clinical judgments in 74–81% of cases.

Investigative interviews are often the children's entry points into the social service, mental health, and criminal justice systems. As such, a collaborative, interagency response is needed to protect children from unnecessarily redundant interviews. Among the system-induced stressors associated with child sexual abuse disclosure, having to endure multiple investigative interviews by various interviewers has repeatedly been demonstrated to have negative effects on children (Berliner & Conte, 1995; Goodman et al., 1992; Henry, 1997). To avoid the problems associated with multiple interviews and to encourage interagency cooperation, many communities conduct joint police–child protective service investigations, whereas other communities pool resources to create child abuse multidisciplinary teams. Some multidisciplinary teams have a designated workspace, whereas others meet informally to plan investigation strategies and review evidence. The National Child Advocacy Center in Huntsville, Alabama provides office space for professionals involved in investigations and treatment, comfortable interviewing rooms for children, and a Court Prep Group (Pence & Wilson, 1994; Whitcomb, 2003). There are now at least 300 such centers in the United States (Whitcomb, 2003). Saywitz, Goodman, and Lyon (2002) reported program evaluation outcome for a newly implemented multidisciplinary child interview center in California. As compared to previous cases, center cases required fewer interviews, interviewers, and interview settings, and center-based interviews were rated more positively by children.

In the United States, approximately 30% of reported maltreatment cases are substantiated, with 12% of those involving sexual abuse (Golden, 2000). Studies that have investigated sexual abuse referrals specifically indicate that about half are classified as founded, substantiated, or indicated (Jones & McGraw, 1987), with 4–8% considered false allegations or fabrications (Everson & Boat, 1989; Jones & McGraw, 1987). A fairly high percentage of cases fall into a gray area, where abuse is not substantiated, but cannot be considered fictitious either. Jones and McGraw (1987) found that investigators could not come to a reliable conclusion in 24% of cases, and that in another 17% of cases, investigators suspected the allegations were true but could not confirm them. This situation leaves victims, families, and the accused in limbo, particularly when an accused perpetrator is a family member or is someone with whom the child may have further contact. Terms such as "substantiated" or "unsubstantiated" can be imprecise, leading to misinterpretations of investigation results. Indeed, terms like "unsubstantiated" are not intended to indicate that abuse has been ruled out (Giovannoni, 1989). Jones and Seig (1988) suggested that agencies refine their classifications into five categories: "definitely true," "probably true," " possibly true," "probably false," and "definitely false."

Improving Investigative Interviews

Because of the high level of skill and specialization required in investigatory interviews with children, specially trained detectives and/or mental health professionals are generally needed to ensure that investigative interviews are effective in eliciting detailed reports from children without being suggestive or evoking false details (Martin & Besharov, 1991). Inappropriate interviewing tactics—such as repeated and leading questioning; interviewer bias; and use of bribes, threats, or other forms of coercion—negatively affect interview outcomes. Furthermore, investigative interviews must be conducted in a manner that avoids possible contamination of disclosure information; otherwise, cases are open to taint hearings (Ghetti, Alexander, & Goodman, 2002). Some jurisdictions allow defense attorneys to request pretrial taint hearings to determine whether a child's initial disclosure was influenced by inappropriate interview tactics, and to determine whether postevent questioning, comments, or other events eroded the child's memory to the point that his or her testimony at trial will be inaccurate or lack credibility.

Increased reporting and prosecution of child sexual abuse cases have led to a great expansion in research on children's memory and suggestibility and children's abilities to provide accurate, credible information when recounting events. With regard to age, two findings are clear: (1) Children's abilities to recount information improve with age (Goodman, Hirschman, Hepps, & Rudy, 1991; Peterson & Bell, 1996); and (2) young children (particularly preschoolers) are more suggestible than older children, adolescents, and adults (Ceci & Bruck, 1993; Goodman & Aman, 1991). However, these findings reflect relative differences. Young children do not necessarily have poor memories and are not necessarily highly suggestible (Eisen, Quas, & Goodman, 2001); in fact, there is considerable variation in these characteristics across individuals of all ages. Memory and suggestibility tend to vary, depending on a number of contextual factors (Saywitz et al., 2002): type of questions asked, postevent influences, type of event experienced, type of information to be recounted, conditions surrounding the interview, strength of the memory, and language used.

When children are asked to recall events, open-ended questions yield the most accurate but least detailed accounts (Goodman et al., 1991). However, free recall is not without problems. Open-ended questions about distressing or embarrassing events yield high false negatives. Furthermore, open-ended questions can result in false details (Goodman & Aman, 1991) and can be distorted if preceded by leading questions or adult-induced expectancies (Leichtman & Ceci, 1995; Poole & Lindsay, 1995; Thompson, Clarke-Stewart, & Lepore, 1997). More information is gleaned when specific questions are asked or when memory is triggered by physical cues, such as anatomically correct dolls and props associated with the events (Saywitz, Goodman, Nicholas, & Moan, 1991). However, detailed questioning can increase inaccuracies, especially if questions are posed in a yes–no format with very young children. Bruck, Ceci, and Francoeur (2000) found chance-level accuracy in responses to yes–no questions by children ages 2–4 years. In fact, Peterson and Biggs (1997) have recommended that yes–no questions should be avoided altogether for preschool-age children. Rudy and Goodman (1991), on the other hand, found that by age 4, children can answer yes–no questions reliably under some conditions, but cautioned that unelaborated and nonverbal responses suggest uncertainties (Goodman & Aman, 1991). Poole and Lamb (1998) have suggested that yes–no questions with young children be followed with open-ended questions to assure that the child has understood the questions and thoughtfully considered the answers. By age 5, however, accuracy in responding to yes–no questions about recent experiences improves dramatically to near ceiling levels (Peterson & Bell, 1996; Saywitz et al., 1991).

Saywitz and colleagues (2002) have outlined three developmental factors that affect young children's susceptibility to suggestion: (1) Young children have difficulties providing narrative accounts of events without relying on adult cues, which can be misleading; (2) young children are especially deferential to adult influences regarding perceptions and interpretation of events; and (3) young children have difficulty identifying the source of their memories (i.e., from own memories or from conversations with others). Research with young children has demonstrated that their recollections of events can be tainted by postevent interference, including exposure to suppositional questions, denigrating statements about people or acts involved in the event, false information, and distortions about the source of information (see Lyon, 1999, and Saywitz et al., 2002, for reviews). Nonetheless, other research indicates that children are typically remarkably resistant to suggestion when asked about personally relevant information, such as whether they were undressed, hit, or genitally touched (Goodman, Bottoms, Shaver, & Qin, 1995). Indeed, susceptibility to suggestion appears to occur under fairly specific circumstances (Goodman et al., 1995): (1) a preschool-age child (3–5 years of age); (2) repeated suggestions from a powerful, intimidating, or authoritative source, such as a parent; (3) suggestions about positive or neutral, rather than negative, events; (4) weak memory about the event, or long delay between the event and the recall period; and (5) the child's perception of the suggestion's plausibility.

Studies indicate that if children are taught about interview processes and expectations, and are then coached on specific skills, they provide more accurate information in subsequent interviews. Several important communication skills relevant to investigative interviews and courtroom testimony have been taught to children, including recognizing when they do not know something and responding with "I don't know," recognizing and clarifying verbose or misleading questions, answering oath-related questions, and providing detail in their responses (Dorado & Saywitz, 2001; Lyon, Saywitz, Kaplan, & Dorado, 2001; Saywitz & Moan-Hardie, 1994; Saywitz, Snyder, & Nathanson, 1999). Several interview protocols and preparation strategies have been developed to enhance investigative interviews. Two are described below.

The strategy of "narrative elaboration" was developed to help children increase the detail and relevance of information they provide without the use of leading questions (Saywitz et al., 2002). Children learn to provide independent, detailed, and forensically relevant information, using their own words, with few questions from the interviewer. Before interviewing children about a specific event, they are taught to use four forensically important topics in their recollections: participants, setting, actions, and conversations. Each topic is depicted on a cue card, using simple, unbiased stick figures and line drawings. Children then practice reporting the details of an unrelated event (e.g., their morning routine), with feedback about the level of detail and clarity in their narrative. In the subsequent interview about a specific event, an open-ended free-recall question is posed about the event; this is then followed by the display of each of the four cards and a simple question, "Does this card remind you to tell me something else?" Four studies involving children ages 4–12 have demonstrated that narrative elaboration procedures increase accurate detail in event narratives without increasing errors (Comparo, Wagner, & Saywitz, 2001; Dorado & Saywitz, 2001; Saywitz & Snyder, 1996; Saywitz, Snyder, & Lamphear, 1996). In one study, children ages 6–11 showed a 53% increase in accurate information as compared to controls (Saywitz & Snyder, 1996).

An alternative strategy is to use a structured interview protocol, such as that developed by Sternberg and colleagues (1996). Their interview protocol was developed in response to concerns that even trained interviewers move too quickly from open-ended questions to suggestive forms of questions (Aldridge & Cameron, 1999; Lamb, Sternberg, & Orbach, 2002; Warren et al., 1999). The interview protocol guides investigators toward posing more open-ended questions before opting for more specific yes–no or forced-choice questions (Saywitz et al., 2002). The interview protocol begins with rapport building, encouraging children to indicate when they do not understand something or do not know the answer to a question, and educating them about how to resist suggestive questions. The abuse-specific portion of the interview is introduced by asking a child why he or she came to the interview. If the child does not know or is unclear, a number of questions are asked that help orient the child to the topic of the interview without referring the alleged perpetrator or specifying the alleged act. If the child discloses abuse, the interviewer responds, "Tell me everything that happened to you, from the beginning to the end, as best as you can remember," followed by additional prompts such as "Tell me more about . . . " If there is a need to ask a specific question (e.g., "Where were your clothes?"), the answer (e.g., "He took them off") is followed up with another open-ended question (e.g., "Tell me everything about how they got off"). After the initial narrative is complete, the child is asked, "Did that happen one time or more than one time?" If the child indicates more than one abuse episode, the same strategy is used to gather information relevant to the last time, the first time, the best-remembered time, and any other time the child remembers.

Research indicates that this protocol promotes greater use of open-ended questions, less use of option-posing questions, and elicitation of more details in response to open-ended questions (Orbach et al., 2000; Sternberg, Lamb, Esplin, & Baradaran, 1999). Specifically, compared with 36% of children interviewed in the traditional manner, 89% made their preliminary allegations in response to open-ended prompts (Sternberg, Lamb, Orbach, Esplin, & Mitchell, 2001). However, some evidence suggests that the protocol is less effective with preschool-age and more reticent children (Hershkowitz & Elul, 1999;

Hershkowitz, Orbach, Lamb, Sternberg, & Horowitz, 2001).

Lamb (1994) reported the proceedings from an international meeting of 22 scholars concerned with child abuse investigations. Overall, the group concluded that children's recall of events can be extremely informative and accurate if the interview is free of manipulation. Six recommendations were made for eliciting the most accurate information from children:

1. An interview should occur as soon after the event as possible.
2. Multiple interviews, particularly by different interviewers, should be discouraged.
3. Leading questions should be avoided whenever possible; however, use of leading questions should not automatically be a reason to disregard a child's recollection of events.
4. For older children, narrative accounts are best elicited with open-ended questions.
5. For children under age 7, who might have difficulty answering open-ended questions, direct, developmentally sensitive questions can be used with care to avoid contamination.
6. All interviews should be videotaped, to avoid multiple interviewing and to create a record of how each interview was conducted.

Anatomically Correct Dolls

Many children do not understand the function of the investigative interview; without specific questions and/or the availability of anatomically correct dolls or other props, they may reveal very little about specific events, particularly sensitive aspects related to sexuality (Goodman et al., 1995; Saywitz et al., 1991). However, some consider such props to be excitatory, suggestive, and coercive, increasing the probability of incorrect or misleading information (Haugaard & Reppucci, 1988). Everson and Boat (1994) reported concerns that evaluators often misused anatomically correct dolls, with two particularly questionable practices: (1) premature introduction of the dolls, at times in an undressed state; and (2) reliance on doll demonstrations in lieu of verbal reports from children, which gave the impression that doll demonstrations were preferred over verbal descriptions. They also expressed concerns that some interviewers allowed children to "pretend" with the dolls, and asked suggestive questions based on the pretend play (e.g., when

a child put a doll's penis in her mouth, the interviewer said, "Whose wienie have you had in your mouth?").

Despite such concerns about anatomically correct dolls, the vast majority (92%) of mental health professionals who conduct child abuse investigations use them (Conte, Sorenson, Fogarty, & Rosa, 1991). Close to half (46%) of those who used the dolls felt that they were useful in most evaluations, and another 28% saw them as useful on a case-by-case basis (Oberlander, 1995). Anatomically correct dolls have been accepted as appropriate props in some legal jurisdictions (*Kehinde v. Commonwealth*, 1986; *People v. Rich*, 1987). Saywitz and colleagues (1991) found dolls to be particularly useful in eliciting sensitive information over and beyond the information provided from simple recall requests, particularly when paired with direct questioning about touching (e.g., pointing to the doll's body parts, including nongenital and genital parts, and asking, "Did he touch you there?"). Many other research studies support the use of props and anatomically correct dolls in helping children, particularly older children, to provide detail about genital contacts (see Goodman, Quas, Bulkley, & Shapiro, 1999).

The use of anatomically correct dolls in interviews appears to increase the probability of disclosure among children being evaluated for possible sexual abuse. Leventhal, Hamilton, Rekedal, Tebano-Micci, and Eyster (1989) examined disclosure rates of 60 children under age 7 who were first interviewed without the dolls and then with the dolls. Children were three times more likely to provide a detailed description of sexual abuse and twice as likely to name a suspected perpetrator during the interview with the dolls. Bybee and Mowbray (1993), in a retrospective analysis of investigative material concerning day care abuse, found that young children (less than 5 years of age) were more likely to make credible, explicit disclosures when interviewed with anatomically correct dolls. Whereas only 30% of those interviewed without the dolls disclosed abuse, 90% made disclosures with the dolls. For those children more than 5 years of age, 58% made disclosures when interviewed with the dolls, whereas 21% of those interviewed without the dolls made disclosures.

The use of anatomically correct dolls with very young children (ages 3–4) remains quite controversial. One of the primary reasons for using anatomically correct dolls is to give young children with limited verbal skills a communication tool. DeLoache and Marzolf (1995) found that children under 3½ years of age had difficulty using dolls to represent themselves. In fact, young children provided more correct information in direct recall without the dolls than they did when asked to demonstrate the event with the dolls. Several studies indicate that the use of anatomically correct dolls with 3-year-olds does not facilitate their ability to respond to questions about medical examinations or doctors' visits (Goodman & Aman, 1991; Ornstein, Follmer, & Gordon, 1995), and may actually increase the probability of their committing errors (Bruck, Ceci, Francoueur, & Renick, 1995; Goodman, Quas, Batterman-Faunce, Riddlesberger, & Kuhn, 1997). In contrast, Goodman, Quas, and colleagues (1997) found that when information about genital touching during a medical examination was examined separately from other exam-related details, all age groups (3- to 4-year-olds, 4-year-olds, and 7-year-olds) showed a significant increase in correct information during doll use as compared to the free-recall situation. Improvements were particularly pronounced among the 3- to 4-year-olds; 18% of these children reported genital contact during free recall, whereas 71% reported genital contact during the doll demonstration task.

Given the widespread but controversial use of anatomically correct dolls, as well as other questions about conducting investigative interviews with children, various societies have published guidelines for conducting such interviews. The American Professional Society on the Abuse of Children (APSAC, 1990) published guidelines that specifically addressed the use of dolls and props. APSAC recommended that tools be made available to assist children in communicating; these could include drawings, toys, dollhouses, tools, and puppets, as well as anatomically correct dolls. The preferred practice when using anatomically correct dolls was to have them available for identification of body parts, clarification of previous statements, or demonstrations by nonverbal or low-verbal children after there was an indication of abuse activity. In 1991, the American Psychological Association's Council of Representatives published a position paper regarding the use of anatomically correct dolls in forensic evaluations. Although it was recognized that anatomically correct dolls served a valuable purpose as a communication tool for both young and older children, the council cautioned that practitioners should videotape or otherwise carefully document their procedures and should be prepared to justify their procedures with clinical and empirical rationales and interpretations. The council also urged continued research regarding normative behavior of abused and nonabused children with the dolls, as well as further investigation of their stimulus properties.

Medical Investigations

After sexual abuse disclosure, or when abuse is suspected but not disclosed, medical examination and treatment have several important functions (Jenny, 2002): diagnosis of STDs, diagnosis and management of pregnancy, collection of forensic evidence, identification of mental health problems, medical documentation, and collaboration with multidisciplinary teams addressing child abuse.

Genital examinations of sexually abused children generally require frog-leg and/or knee–chest positioning, and most of the important clinical and forensic information can be gathered through unaided visual inspection (Atabaki & Paradise, 1999; Paradise et al., 1997). However, a small percentage of physicians (20%) use colposcopes, which provide illumination, magnification, and photography. Colposcopes have been shown to help clarify findings that are not clearly visible to the unaided eye (Adams, Phillips, & Ahmad, 1990). Videocolposcopy can also be used to record the examination and can be viewed by the patient as the examination proceeds (Palusci & Cyrus, 2001). Vaginal or anal instruments such as speculums or anoscopes are generally not required, but in some cases a Foley catheter and catheter balloon may be inserted into the vagina to help visualize hymenal structures (Starling & Jenny, 1997).

Most physical examinations of sexually abused children reveal nothing abnormal, since many sexual acts do not cause physical trauma or heal before exams take place (Adams, Harper, Knudson, & Revilla, 1994). In fact, Berenson and colleagues (2000) found that at least 90% of girls ages 3–8 years who described digital or penile penetration showed no signs of genital injury. Two factors have been found to predict abnormal genital findings: recency of the last incident, and history of blood following the assault (Adams et al., 1994). Some genital aberrations that were once thought to be consistent with a history of sexual abuse have since been found to be either fairly common among nonabused children or have other possible causes, such as infections or accidental traumas (e.g., straddle injuries; Atabaki & Paradise, 1999; Bayes & Jenny, 1990).

Adams (2001) described a series of revisions to a classification scale for evaluating medical evidence in sexual abuse investigations, with iterations to the coding system based on evolving medical findings from studies of abused and nonabused children and adolescents. The coding system yields four categorical findings based on the medical examination, each with well-defined medical anchors: "normal," "nonspecific" (findings that could be from sexual abuse but could also be from other causes), "concerning" (findings noted in children with sexual abuse histories, but alternative causes should be ruled out), and "clear evidence" (findings that have no explanation other than trauma to the hymen or perianal tissues). A second 4–point classification system provides an overall assessment of the likelihood of sexual abuse, which reflects statements from the child and laboratory and physical examination findings: "no indication of abuse," "possible abuse," "probable abuse," and "definite evidence of abuse or sexual contact." Again, each classification has well-defined anchors. Studies of earlier versions of the classification scale revealed acceptable reliability (Roberts & Moran, 1995); however, concerns have been raised that physicians' findings of medical indicators are sometimes influenced by their knowledge of children's abuse histories (Paradise, Winter, Finkel, Berenson, & Beiser, 1999). Given the sensitivity of anogenital examinations and the complexity of interpreting medical findings, extensive, specialized training and experience are often required for cases that have potential forensic implications (Makoroff, Braudley, Brandner, Myers, & Shapiro, 2002; Paradise et al., 1997).

With the exception of some postnatal infections that are transmitted *in utero* and typically detected during infancy, several STDs are strongly indicative of sexual abuse (e.g., gonorrhea, chlamydia, trichomonal vaginal infections, bacterial vaginosis, genital and anal warts, syphilis, and HIV; Jenny, 2002). Among children with identified sexual abuse, 2–7% of girls and 0–5% of boys present with an STD, most commonly chlamydia, genital warts, or gonorrhea (Siegel, Schubert, Myers, & Shapiro, 1995; Yordan & Yordan, 1992). Risk factors include multiple perpetrators, perpetra-

tor STD, sibling with an STD, prior consensual sexual contact, genital discharge, genital injury, and sexual maturity. Because of limited risk among sexual abuse victims and clearly defined risk factors, the Centers for Disease Control and Prevention (1998) recommend STD screening only for sexually abused children with specific risk factors.

Based on a national incidence study (Holmes, Resnick, Kilpatrick, & Best, 1996), approximately 32,000 pregnancies result from rape each year in the United States, and half of impregnated victims are under age 18. For adolescents, 17% of rape-related pregnancies result from incestuous abuse by a father, stepfather, or other relative. Medical counseling is often needed to help an adolescent make decisions relative to abortion versus a full-term pregnancy, and to adoption versus keeping the baby if pregnancy is chosen. Adolescents' pregnancies are often complicated, due to their age and tendencies to use drugs and alcohol. Pregnancies resulting from incest also have an increased risk of birth defects, which varies with the degree of relatedness (Jenny, 2002).

In addition to pregnancy and gynecological problems, sexually abused children are also at risk for a number of other health problems. Such children are prone to develop urinary tract infections and anal inflammations, and thus have increased rates of nocturnal and diurnal enuresis, constipation, and encopresis (Jenny, 2002). Sexually abused children also show an increased prevalence of somatic symptoms, such as headaches, abdominal and pelvic pain, and menstrual problems. Concerns have been raised that somatic symptoms among abuse and trauma victims may stem from chronic stress on the hypothalamic–pituitary–adrenal axis (Heim, Ehlert, Hanker, & Hellhammer, 1998). Concerns have also been raised that sexual abuse victims are at increased risk of developing eating disorders, particularly bulimia nervosa (Deep, Lilenfeld, Plotnicov, Pollice, & Kaye, 1999; Garfinkel et al., 1995).

EFFORTS TO REDUCE FEAR AND DISTRESS RELATED TO ANOGENITAL EXAMINATIONS

Most sexual abuse victims experience mild to moderate anticipatory anxiety and acute distress related to anogenital examinations (Lazebnik et al., 1994; Steward, Schmitz, Steward, Joye, & Reinhart, 1995; Waibel-Duncan & Sanger, 1999), and some case reports describe more extreme distress (Berson, Herman-Giddens, & Frothingham, 1993; Lawson, 1990). Lazebnik and colleagues (1994) reported that 14–16% reported a lot of pain and/or fear associated with anogenital exams, and Hogan (1996) reported that 10% of those presenting for exams required sedation. Studies indicate that parents and children generally receive little preparation for anogenital exams and often hold false beliefs that may contribute to their stress (e.g., that the examination will be painful, include an internal pelvic examination, involve needles and blood tests, and require further discussion of their allegations; Waibel-Duncan & Sanger, 1999).

Simple, time-efficient procedures may facilitate adaptation to anogenital exams. For example, children who received simple explanations of procedures and preexamination tours demonstrated increased knowledge and comfort with the procedures (Waibel-Duncan & Sanger, 1999), and a 10–minute teaching film that depicted positive coping techniques (deep breathing, guided imagery, and positive self-statements) reduced fear ratings and observed distress during examinations (Lynch & Faust, 1998). Palusci and Cyrus (2001) evaluated the effect of videocolposcopy on anogenital examination. They found that 85% of children and adolescents opted to watch videocolposcopy during the course of their examination and were rated as cooperative or enthusiastic before and during procedures. Children younger than 3, adolescent girls, and those who evidenced physical findings showed less interest in watching the videotapes, however.

Involvement with the Judicial System

About half of substantiated cases of sexual abuse result in criminal charges; however, of those, up to half are dropped or dismissed following preliminary hearings (Cross, Whitcomb, & De Vos, 1995; Martone, Jaudes, & Cavins, 1996; Stroud et al., 2000). Decisions to proceed with prosecution typically have little to do with aspects of the crime and are more often related to child, family, and offender characteristics. Prosecution is less likely when a child is young or male, when the mother does not support prosecution, and when the accused individual is a family member (Cross et al., 1995; Stroud et al., 2000). Of the cases that remain viable following preliminary hearings, most take at least 1 to 1½ years before resolution. To address the problem of excessive de-

lays, some states (e.g., Washington and California) have statutes that facilitate speedier trials when victims and/or witnesses are children (National Center for Prosecution of Child Abuse, 1993). On the whole, cases slated for trial are successful for the prosecution. Half to 85% of defendants plead guilty prior to trial, and of the small number of cases that proceed to trial, two-thirds result in guilty verdicts (Cross et al., 1995; DeJong & Rose, 1991; Martone et al., 1996; Stroud et al., 2000). Sentencing varies considerably across jurisdictions. For example, Stroud and colleagues (2000) reported that convicted perpetrators (guilty pleas and guilty verdicts) averaged 11-year jail terms, but most sentences were suspended. Parole sentences averaged just under 4 years. On the other hand, Martone and colleagues (1996) found that most perpetrators served time, with average sentences of 6.8 years. Cross and colleagues (1995) reported that 38% were incarcerated more than 1 year, 40% were incarcerated less than 1 year, and 22% were placed on probation.

Approximately 50% of cases referred for prosecution require that children testify at some legal proceeding, such as a preliminary hearing (Goodman et al., 1992); if cases proceed to trial, at least 80% of child victims testify (Cross et al., 1995). However, because of the small number of cases that proceed to trial, this accounts for only 3–4% of sexually abused children known to official agencies (Saunders, Kilpatrick, Resnick, Hanson, & Lipovsky, 1992). Nonetheless, child sexual abuse cases are the most common types of trials that involve child witnesses (Goodman et al., 1999). Most children find testifying in court to be very stressful (Lipovsky, Tidwell, Kilpatrick, Saunders, & Dawson, 1991; Sas et al., 1995). Prior to testifying, children identify a number of fears, including fears of the testimony itself, the defense attorney, and seeing the defendant; after testifying, children report that the most distressing aspects were seeing the defendant and not having their parents in the courtroom (Goodman et al., 1992). Children also fear that the defendant will retaliate and that they will not be believed.

Despite their court-related fears and anxieties, many children feel relieved after testifying in court, with subsequent reductions in anxiety and depressive symptoms (Goodman et al., 1992). Children's adjustment following court proceedings appears to relate to three factors (Goodman et al., 1992; Runyan, Everson,

Edelson, Hunter, & Coulter, 1988; Whitcomb, 2003): testifying in multiple, prolonged, or delayed proceedings; harsh direct examination or cross-examination; and maternal support or lack of it. Nonetheless, there is little evidence that participating in legal proceedings results in long-term adjustment problems, although it may delay psychological recovery from the abuse (Goodman et al., 1992; Lipovsky, 1992). In fact, some evidence suggests that children can benefit from the experience. Sas and colleagues (1995) found that 85% of children who provided courtroom testimony were positive about their involvement and reported no regrets; only 9% harbored regrets. Ninety-one percent of victims said that they would advise a friend to tell the police if a similar incident occurred; 84% said that they would call the police if they were abused again, and 80% said that they would want the case prosecuted.

As noted earlier, many cases of child sexual abuse go unprosecuted, because of concerns about the negative effects of testifying in court and concerns that the children will not be able to provide accurate, credible testimony. These issues are closely intertwined, since court-related stress can negatively affect both the accuracy of children's evidence (Saywitz & Nathanson, 1993) and jurors' perceptions of a child's credibility (Golding, Fryman, Marsil, & Yozwiak, 2003; Leippe, Manion, & Romanczyk, 1992; G. L. Wells, Tuttle, & Luus, 1989). Interventions to assist child witnesses fall into two categories: "protective" and "empowering" (Davies & Westcott, 1995). Protective interventions alter the system to reduce stress (e.g., testifying via closed-circuit television [CCTV], allowing hearsay evidence), whereas empowering interventions teach children about court processes and assist them in overcoming their anxieties.

Child-Friendly Prosecution Practices

One of the most common accommodations for child witnesses is "vertical prosecution" (Goodman et al., 1999), where one attorney follows a case from the investigation stage through the trial. Vertical prosecution expedites progression toward trial; this is important, since children's memories tend to deteriorate over time, and both parents and victims tend to become increasingly reluctant to participate with excessive delays (Whitcomb, 1992). Regular contact between the prosecutor's office and the families can reduce stress on victims and their families, which is often accomplished through victim advocates (Lipovsky & Stern, 1997). Victim advocates typically provide tours of the court prior to the trial, and then attend court with a child as a support, since a parent, who may be called as a witness, is often not allowed in the courtroom when the child testifies. These adaptations to prosecution practices are generally perceived by prosecutors and judges as helpful (Cashmore & Bussey, 1996; Goodman et al., 1999).

Closed-Circuit Television

To relieve a child of the stress of direct confrontation with a defendant, some courts have allowed the child to testify either with a screen that blocks the child's view of the defendant (but allows the defendant to view the child) or via CCTV. Of the two options, CCTV is more popular, since it appears to reduce child stress more effectively. Typically, the child testifies in a room adjacent to the courtroom, and the testimony is viewed in the courtroom via a television monitor. Often arrangements are made for two-way communication, so that the child can view the courtroom as the court views the child. Experimental studies using mock trials provide support for strategies such as CCTV that shield child victims from accused persons during the children's testimony. Peters (1990) demonstrated that the presence of defendants during questioning was associated with a decline in children's willingness to disclose incriminating information, particularly if a defendant had asked a child to keep a secret (Peters, 1990). Mock-trial experimental studies also demonstrate that testifying in a smaller private room with or without CCTV is less anxiety-producing than testifying in open court, and that lower levels of anxiety result in fewer errors of omission (i.e., providing less information) and commission (i.e., less resistance to leading questions), particularly with younger children (Saywitz & Nathanson, 1993; Tobey, Goodman, Batterman-Faunce, Orcutt, & Sachsenmaier, 1995). Moreover, when children's anxiety is less obvious, jurors tend to focus more on the relevant aspects of the testimony and less on the children's emotional state (Swim, Borgida, & McCoy, 1992).

CCTV and other strategies that protect a child from direct confrontation with an accused person have been challenged as an infringement upon the accused's right to "face-to-face" confrontation with the accuser, which is guaranteed by the "confrontation clause" of the U.S. Constitution's Sixth Amendment (and similar rights in other countries) . The confrontation clause has the following purposes: It (1) ensures that the witness provides testimony under oath; (2) requires that the witness submit to cross-examination; and (3) permits the "trier of fact" to observe the demeanor of the witness while he or she is testifying in the presence of the defendant, in order to assess the witness's credibility (Bulkley, 1988). Two issues have been debated about applying the confrontation clause with child witnesses (Gordon, 1992): (1) Does the term "confront" require an actual face-to-face encounter? (2) Does potential emotional trauma to a witness qualify as sufficient ground for an exception to the practice of requiring testimony in the presence of the accused? In *Maryland v. Craig* (1990), the U.S. Supreme Court ruled that the right to face-to-face confrontation is not absolute and that CCTV for child witnesses is permissible, because the state has a compelling interest in protecting child witnesses from emotional harm. However, the court also ruled that decisions to use CCTV must be made on a "case-by-case" basis, with the goal of protecting the welfare of a "particular" child. Furthermore, the court ruled that the reason for CCTV was the potential harm from testifying in the presence of the accused, not simply a child's fear of testifying in court. In Canada, court decisions have also allowed the use of screens and CCTV for child sexual assault witnesses, provided that a judge finds that it is "necessary in order to obtain a full and candid account of the acts complained of" (*R. v. Levogiannis,* 1993; MacKay, 2005).

As of 2002, 37 states had enacted statutes that authorized judges to allow child witnesses to testify via CCTV (National Center for Prosecution of Child Abuse, 2002). However, use of CCTV in the United States has been rare, due to concerns about possible legal challenges by the defense, financial impediments to installing and maintaining the equipment, and preferences by prosecutors to have children testify directly in the courtroom (Goodman et al., 1999; Tobey et al., 1995). Indeed, some experimental studies indicate that jurors may view children who testify via CCTV more negatively than they view those who testify in open court. Both Tobey and colleagues (1995) and Orcutt, Goodman, Tobey, Batterman-Faunce, and

Thomas (2001) found that mock jurors rated children who provided CCTV testimony as less believable, less accurate, more likely to have made up the story, less able to discern fact from fantasy, less attractive, less intelligent, and less confident. However, CCTV did not appear to influence the jurors' decisions. Neither study found differences in jurors' abilities to discern the accuracy of children's testimony when children testified via CCTV versus open court, and there was no relationship between jurors' ratings of children's believability and perceptions of the defendants' guilt. Thus current evidence suggests that CCTV does not interfere with the right of either the victim or the defendant to a fair trial. For defendants, CCTV does not enhance victim sympathy, and for victims, perceived differences in personal characteristics do not appear to affect trial outcomes in a systematic way.

Because of legal and ethical constraints, it has been difficult to evaluate the effectiveness of CCTV in the United States and Canada in actual trials. However, England and Australia are more liberal in their use of CCTV, thus allowing for real-world examination of its use in courtrooms (Davies & Westcott, 1995). Two quasi-experimental studies have evaluated the effectiveness of CCTV—one in England (Davies & Noon, 1991) and the other in Australia (Cashmore, 1992). Neither study involved random assignment to comparison groups; rather, the samples were compared to cases in other districts where CCTV was not implemented. As a result, the comparison cases differed from those with CCTV on such variables as age, gender, and reason for providing testimony. In both studies, court personnel (judges, prosecutors, defense attorneys, court clerks) were surveyed regarding their opinions about CCTV; as well, evaluations were conducted to determine whether children performed better with CCTV. Both studies found that children who provided testimony via CCTV seemed less stressed than children who testified in open court, provided more thorough accounts during their testimony, and were more resistant to leading questions. Children who wanted CCTV but were denied its use were rated as more unhappy, as less cooperative, and as providing fewer details. Despite being offered the use of CCTV, some children in Cashmore's (1992) study chose to testify in open court. No differences were found between the children who declined CCTV and those who used it. Thus children who do not opt for CCTV when it is available tend to do fine without it. Cashmore found that defense attorneys and prosecutors were equally satisfied with CCTV. In fact, defense attorneys saw an advantage to CCTV, because the children were more composed and could therefore be questioned more rigorously with less risk of an emotional breakdown.

Hearsay Evidence

Despite improvements in interviewing and courtroom procedures, in some cases children are either too young or too vulnerable to testify in court. In those cases, if the matter is to be prosecuted, hearsay evidence may be necessary. Hearsay statements are those made outside of court; as such, they are not subject to cross-examination and are therefore, according to the U.S. Constitution's Sixth Amendment, not admissible in criminal court. There are two requirements for hearsay statements to be admissible into evidence (Gordon, 1992): (1) The declarant must be unavailable to testify (e.g., deceased, unwilling, or unable to testify); and (2) there must be some compelling evidence to the "almost certain" reliability of the statements, either through a recognized exception (e.g., a dying declaration, an excited utterance) or through circumstances surrounding the making of the statements that support their reliability. For example, although a child may be too young or vulnerable to testify in court, under less stressful circumstances the child may have made statements that appear to be reliable such as during an investigative interview or during a disclosure to a parent.

The issue of hearsay in child sexual abuse cases was addressed by the U.S. Supreme Court in the case of *Idaho v. Wright* (1990). This case involved a child who was deemed too immature to testify in court; however, the child had made incriminating statements to a pediatrician, which were allowed in the lower court as an exception to the hearsay prohibition. Although the Supreme Court ruled that the child's statements were not sufficiently reliable to be submitted as evidence for the case of *Idaho v. Wright*, it did not dismiss the possibility of allowing evidence in similar cases, especially if a child makes statements spontaneously or repeatedly and if the statements are accompanied by other factors suggesting reliability (e.g., mental state, use of terminology unexpected

for a child of similar age, or lack of motive to fabricate). The Supreme Court, however, refused to specify criteria necessary for ruling when hearsay evidence may be admissible, leaving cases that use hearsay open for appeal. Child hearsay statutes vary across jurisdictions; some require that a child must be unavailable to testify, others allow hearsay only when the child can also testify, and some require corroborating evidence (Montoya, 1999). Surveys of judges reveal that close to 75% allowed exceptions to the hearsay prohibition in domestic dispute and child sexual abuse cases (Hafemeister, 1996).

The U.S. Supreme Court recently ruled in *Crawford v. Washington* (2004) that in order for "testimonial" hearsay evidence to be admissible for an "unavailable" witness, the defense must have had the opportunity to cross-examine the witness. This ruling is likely to have an impact only on trials where the child will not testify (Vieth, 2004). It is not clear what constitutes "testimonial" evidence, which reflects statements that are intended for use at trial. Thus, it is possible that information from investigative interviews might still be used in criminal trials even when the child is not available for cross-examination, since it is unclear whether such interviews would be considered testimonial (i.e., investigative interviews have multiple purposes such as child protection and mental health care, not just prosecution). Furthermore, it is possible that the ruling will not apply to a case in which the child is not available to testify as a direct result of the defendant's conduct. That is, if the child is too frightened to testify because of the sexual abuse or because of threats or admonitions toward the child, then hearsay evidence might still be used even if the child does not testify.

When provided with hearsay evidence, jurors are faced with two concerns (Warren, Nunez, Keeney, Buck, & Smith, 2002): (1) deciding whether an out-of-court statement was in fact made, and if so, whether it was accurately reported by the hearsay witness; and (2) evaluating the child's credibility without the benefit of being able to observe the child's demeanor while providing the statement and without the benefit of information gleaned from cross-examination. Laboratory research suggests that hearsay testimony is affected by complex interactions among many variables, including age of the hearsay witness, age of the victim, gender of the juror, and relationship of the hearsay witness to the victim (i.e., parent, acquaintance, professional; Golding, Alexander, & Stewart, 1999; Ross, Lindsay, & Marsil, 1999). Hearsay evidence provided by professional interviewers can be particularly persuasive to jurors, even beyond the persuasiveness of direct testimony by the children (Warren et al., 2002). In particular, testimony by professionals who provided the "gist" of their conversations with children was given more weight than testimony that was a verbatim recounting of adult questions and child answers. Essentially, "less was more." The perceived weight of "gist" testimony is cause for concern, however, since research indicates that professionals often fail to record important details of interviews (Lamb, Orbach, Sternberg, Hershkowitz, & Horowitz, 2000; Warren et al., 2002). A professional who anticipates the need to provide hearsay evidence regarding a child's report of abuse should record both his or her questions and the child's responses, and should be prepared to give both the "gist" of the interview and the verbatim details to support these conclusions.

Myers, Redlich, Goodman, Prizmich, and Imwinkelried (1999) conducted a retrospective survey of jurors with regard to adult and child hearsay witnesses. Jurors rated children's direct, in-court testimony as more influential in reaching their verdicts than adult hearsay testimony. However, in comparison to child hearsay evidence, adult evidence was viewed as more accurate, consistent, and confident, and adult testimony was seen as more complete and as less likely to have been influenced by attorneys' questions.

Videotaping Investigative Interviews and Use of Videotapes in Lieu of In-Court Testimony

There are several arguments for and against videotaping investigative interviews. Videotaping can reduce the number of times children are interviewed, preserve children's initial disclosures, document interviewing strategies, and encourage confessions from perpetrators (Myers, 1992). Videotaping encourages interviewers to use proper techniques, and can be used to refresh children's memory before they testify and used to convince nonoffending parents that the abuse occurred (Poole & Lamb, 1998). Henry (1997) found that cases where videotapes were made had fewer subsequent interviews, were less likely to require child tes-

timony in court, and were more likely to result in guilty pleas by the defendants. The 1991 Criminal Justice Act in Great Britain established that videotapes of forensic interviews are admissible in court for criminal cases involving children under the age of 14 years.

On the other hand, videotapes of interviews can be used by defense attorneys as evidence of contamination of children's stories by overemphasizing interview flaws and minor inconsistencies between videotaped disclosures and trial testimony (Myers, 1992). Experimental research indicates that jurors are more likely to find children credible and to find defendants guilty when children testify in court than when videotapes of investigative interviews are presented (Redlich, Goodman, Myers, & Qin, 1996; Swim et al., 1992).

Courtroom Preparation Programs

"Courtroom preparation programs," also known as "victim/witness assistance programs," generally include a number of educational components that acquaint children with the courtroom, court processes, and people in the courtroom (Davies & Westcott, 1995). Children often learn the meaning of taking the oath, the importance of telling the truth, and ways to respond to unfair questioning tactics. Some programs include stress management strategies such as deep breathing exercises, desensitization to courtroom fears and anxieties, and empowerment strategies to enhance motivation and confidence for courtroom testimony (Sas, Hurley, Austin, & Wolfe, 1991). A number of teaching resources have been developed to assist with court preparation, including activity booklets (e.g., Ontario Ministry of the Attorney General, 1989) and videotapes (e.g., Canadian Department of Justice, 1992; Spectrum South Productions, 1989). Doll-size courtrooms, court-related puppets and clothing, and visits to the courtroom facilitate both the educational and desensitization processes. Some programs are conducted in a group format (Sisterman Keeney, Amacher, & Kastanaskis, 1992), whereas other programs are individualized (Sas et al., 1991). All programs avoid direct discussion of the case details, in order to avoid allegations of coaching (Davies & Westcott, 1995). Compared to other courtroom innovations, preparing children for court was reported by prosecutors to be the most commonly implemented procedure and was perceived as the most effective strategy available to reduce child stress and enhance the likelihood of guilty verdicts (Goodman et al., 1999).

Unfortunately, detailed evaluations of courtroom preparation programs have been limited. Sas and colleagues (1991; Sas, Hurley, Hatch, Malla, & Dick, 1993) evaluated the Child Witness Project by comparing a basic education and support courtroom preparation program with an enhanced education, support, and stress management program. Unfortunately, the groups differed, with the children in the enhanced program having been abused more frequently and experiencing more court delays. Children in the enhanced program showed greater improvements in both general and abuse-specific fears, and prosecutors rated children from the enhanced program as better witnesses. However, the prosecutors were aware of the children's involvement in the two programs, and may have had an interest in demonstrating the effectiveness of the enhanced program (Saywitz et al., 2002). Saywitz and colleagues (2002) have advocated for experimental analogue studies to examine different courtroom preparation programs, with particular emphasis on outcome variables such as increased accuracy of testimony and reduced fear of testifying. Procedures used to improve detail and accuracy for investigative interviews (e.g., narrative elaboration, resistance to suggestive questioning) may also be effective in improving courtroom testimony.

Child Protection and Family Issues

Maternal Protection and Need for Foster Care

Regardless of whether criminal prosecution of perpetrators takes place, child protective services are often involved in child sexual abuse cases from the point of disclosure until there is no longer a risk of abuse. Child protective services tend to limit their continued involvement to cases where parents or caregivers are implicated in the abuse, or when concerns are raised that parents cannot protect the children from further harm by the perpetrators or other potential offenders. In most cases, child protective services monitor "at-risk" children in their homes through voluntary agreements or through court-imposed supervision orders. However, approximately 17% of sexually abused children go into foster care (Finkelhor,

1983). Thirty percent of children enter foster care subsequent to protection concerns related to sexual abuse. However, once in foster care, many more children disclose a history of sexual abuse. Sexually abused children who go into foster care are more likely to have come from low-SES families, to have experienced multiple abuse episodes, and to have mothers who did not support their allegations (Hunter, Coulter, Runyan, & Everson, 1990; Leifer, Shapiro, & Kassem, 1993).

Ryan, Warren, and Weincek (1991) found that a mother's role in protecting her child was a potent predictor of foster care placement. However, compared to other reasons for foster placement (e.g., neglect, physical abuse), sexually abused children tend to remain in foster care for shorter durations (approximately 8 months shorter; Lie & McMurtry, 1991). Thus, because reintegration with families is highly likely for child sexual abuse victims in foster care, efforts to resolve family problems and facilitate successful reunification are very important.

Gomes-Schwartz and colleagues (1990) described four types of maternal responses to abuse allegations: (1) a decisive, nonambiguous, protective response, with responsibility attributed to the accused; (2) ambivalent loyalties between child and perpetrator, requiring support from child protective services to assure adequate protection; (3) an immobilization response, resulting in a failure to protect the child, but moderate support and no overt blame of the child; and (4) rejection of the child, alignment with the perpetrator, and no child protective action. Most mothers are decisive, supportive, and protective in response to their children's allegations. Indeed, optimal parental support and protection subsequent to abuse allegations appear to be related to the quality of the parent–child bond (Bolen & Lamb, 2002). However, most studies reveal that some mothers do not support their children's allegations, ranging from 16% (Pierce & Pierce, 1985; Sas et al., 1995) to 50% (Tufts New England Medical Center, 1984). Belief in a child's allegations does not necessarily result in protective action, however. Pintello and Zuravin (2001) found that 20% of mothers who believed their children's allegations failed to take protective actions. On the other hand, they also found that 52% of mothers who were ambivalent about their children's allegations nonetheless took protective action. Although one might anticipate that previous involvement with child protective services might sensitize parents to concerns about abuse and neglect, this does not appear to be the case. Previous involvement with child protective services has been found to have either no relationship to parental belief and protection (Pintello & Zuravin, 2001) or a negative relationship (Bolen & Lamb, 2002).

The more seriously the abuse allegations affect a mother's lifestyle and sense of self, the less likely the mother is to believe the allegations (Elliott & Briere, 1994; Gomes-Schwartz et al., 1990; Lawson & Chaffin, 1992; Sirles & Franke, 1989). Mothers tend to have more difficulty believing allegations against their current partners, particularly when allegations are made against stepfathers and common-law partners with whom the mothers have either new, intense, or financially reliant relationships (Elliott & Briere, 1994; Everson, Hunter, Runyan, Edelsohn, & Coulter, 1989; Faller, 1984; Gomes-Schwartz et al., 1990; Leifer, Kilbane, & Grossman, 2001). When mothers are faced with the difficult choice between their spouses and their children, approximately one-fourth opt to stay with their spouses (Everson et al., 1989; Gomes-Schwartz et al., 1990). In contrast, mothers are often quite supportive when allegations occur in the midst of preexisting spousal problems or when the spouses have already separated (Faller, 1984; Sirles & Franke, 1989).

Mothers are also less likely to believe their children's allegations when alternative explanations are available (Sirles & Franke, 1989). Young children are perceived as having little sexual knowledge and little motive for making false allegations, and are therefore most often believed. As children grow older, mothers are less likely to believe their allegations, particularly when the allegations include very serious forms of abuse or when a child's story indicates that the mother was home when the abuse occurred. Sadly, children with unsupportive mothers tend to suffer more episodes of abuse and are ultimately more likely to recant their allegations (Elliott & Briere, 1994; Leifer et al., 1993). Mothers also tend to have more difficulty believing their children when their partners have substance use problems or when their partners also physically abused the children. Apparently, in these circumstances, mothers are more likely to find a reason for the children to lie about the abuse (e.g., retaliation for the physical abuse), or are more accustomed to making excuses for the partners' inappropriate behavior (Elliott & Briere, 1994).

Several treatment outcome studies have included parent components, and those are discussed in the section on tertiary care. However, these programs do not address the specific problems faced by mothers who are conflicted between their role as spouses and their role as parents. Our local child protective service agency (London–Middlesex Children's Aid Society) provides a group for nonoffending mothers who either opt to stay with their spouses or maintain plans for family reunification (A. Topham, personal communication, April 12, 2004). The group runs on a continuous basis for approximately 35 sessions per year. It combines psychoeducation and support, and addresses a number of problems facing mothers coping with incest: understanding the modus operandi of incestuous fathers (e.g., offending cycles, warning signs, grooming patterns, secrecy, manipulations of children and spouses); their maternal role as chaperone when the abused children are in the presence of the perpetrators; balancing their roles as parents and spouses; nonabused children's relationships with the perpetrators; coping with postdisclosure family changes; maternal feelings of isolation and shame; and coping with their own histories of maltreatment.

Enhancing Child Adjustment to Foster Care

Most evidence indicates that sexually abused children placed in foster care have significant adjustment problems (Dubner & Motta, 1999). In fact, two of the factors associated with foster care placement—multiple abuse experiences and nonsupportive mothers—have been shown to be significant predictors of maladjustment among sexually abused children (Goodman et al., 1992; Wolfe, Gentile, & Wolfe, 1989). However, concerns have been raised that foster placement itself has iatrogenic effects on children, due to separation from attachment figures, loss of other social supports, and changes to their environment (Melton et al., 1995). In addition, children may feel that they are being treated unjustly, since they are the ones required to leave their homes (Ghetti et al., 2002). Concerns have also been raised that foster care increases risk of further abuse (Nunno & Rindfleisch, 1991).

Gomes-Schwartz and colleagues (1990) found that placement outside the home following sexual abuse allegations was associated with poorer outcomes, both initially following disclosure and at an 18-month follow-up. However, because of the close connection between foster care and poor maternal support, it is difficult to identify whether foster care or lack of maternal support was the more powerful predictor. Leifer and Shapiro (1995) studied adjustment of African American girls subsequent to sexual abuse allegations, and found no differences between girls who remained at home and those who were placed in foster care. However, most of the girls in foster care resided in stable placements; this appears to be more common among African American children in foster care than among nonminority children, perhaps due to tendencies to place African American children with relatives (Benedict, Zuravin, & Stallings, 1996; Berrick, Barth, & Needell, 1994).

Most studies indicate that stability of placement is of paramount importance when adjustment to foster care is being evaluated (Aldgate, Colton, Chate, & Heath, 1993; Cantos, Gries, & Slis, 1996; James, Landsverk, & Slymen, 2004; Widom, 1991). James and colleagues (2004) identified four patterns of placement stability among foster children: early stability, later stability, variable pattern, and instability. Compared to other children placed in foster care, sexually abused children were overrepresented in the two extreme groups: early stability and instability. For the early-instability pattern, children settled into a stable placement within several months in care and remained in that placement for the entire 18 months of the study. These children were very unlikely to require residential placement or inpatient services, and were unlikely to be absent without leave from their placements. Half stabilized in nonrelative foster homes, and half stabilized in the homes of relatives. The unstable pattern was characterized as multiple brief placements (mean = 7.2), with no placement lasting more than 9 months. Younger children in this group tended to bounce back and forth between different kinship and nonrelative foster homes, whereas older children were more likely to experience internalizing types of problems and were more likely to have episodic stays in residential care settings. These findings suggest that the placement patterns probably reflected the children's emotional and behavioral problems, rather than agency-produced placement problems.

Sexually abused children who are not able to return to their homes may be deemed appropriate for adoption. Among foster children with special needs (those older than 3 years of age, those with physical or mental disabilities, those with psychological/emotional disorders, minority children, and those with siblings), sexual abuse victims constitute a large proportion who go on to be adopted (Leung & Erich, 2002; McNamara & McNamara, 1990). However, adopting children with a history of sexual abuse is associated with increased family stress—more so than adopting other special-needs children. Family stress increases if a child was both sexually and physically abused, and if siblings are adopted to the same home. Much of this stress may be related to the sexual behavior problems prevalent among sexually abused children. Smith, Howard, and Monroe (1998) reported a strong association between adoption disruption and child history of sexual abuse, and identified eight behavior problems that characterized sexually abused children in adoptive placements: sexual acting out, lying, tantrums, defiance, profanity, vandalism, hostility, and attachment difficulties. Of these behavior problems, sexual acting out appears to be a significant factor in adoption breakdowns (Partridge, Hornby, & McDonald, 1986; Smith et al., 1998).

On the positive side, being in foster care probably facilitates access to mental health services, particularly for sexual abuse victims (Garland, Landsverk, Hough, & Ellis-McLeod, 1996; Halfon, Berkowitz, & Klee, 1992; Harman, Childs, & Kelleher, 2000). Services most often focus on conduct, emotional, and adjustment disorders (Halfon et al., 1992). Older children are more likely to utilize mental health services, as are European American children (Blumberg, Landsverk, Ellis-McLeod, Ganger, & Culver, 1996; Garland et al., 1996; Halfon et al., 1992). Service use by nonfoster children who are nonetheless involved with child protective services was examined by Kolko, Selelyo, and Brown (1999). They found greater mental health utilization by European Americans and in cases when parental distress was high.

Although mental health services are often available to foster children, the opportunity and responsibility for rehabilitation often lie largely within their foster homes. Foster parents' sensitively and skill in dealing with child adjustment problems predicts placement success (Doelling & Johnson, 1990). Nevertheless, foster parents typically do not receive specialized training prior to receiving children into their homes, yet are expected to parent children with very serious mental health problems. Several programs have been developed to help foster parents cope with the special needs of sexually abused children (Barth, Yeaton, & Winterfelt, 1994; Treacy & Fisher, 1993). Training issues have included (1) typical development, particularly with regard to sexuality; (2) sexual abuse dynamics and sexual abuse sequelae; (3) strategies for coping with sexual abuse sequelae; (4) strategies for improving behavioral and emotional adjustment; (5) strategies for reducing the number of failed placements; and (6) building a support network among foster parents.

Improvements in foster parents' knowledge of child development and recognition of problematic behaviors have been noted with interventions as simple and time-efficient as quarterly newsletters that provide relevant information about foster care, child maltreatment, and parenting (Rich, 1996). More extensive approaches have demonstrated even more far-reaching effects. Treacy and Fisher (1993) described a five-session (10-hour) program that emphasized five steps for coping with foster children's behavior problems: (1) monitoring and observing children's behavior; (2) considering whether the behaviors are typical, atypical, or related to their past trauma; (3) considering the message conveyed by the children's behavior; (4) formulating effective parental messages for the children; and (5) setting appropriate limits and using effective discipline strategies. A follow-up evaluation indicated good satisfaction with the program, increased knowledge of sexual development, and increased comfort in coping with problems associated with past sexual abuse. The foster parents also reported feeling more competent and more satisfied in their relationships with their sexually abused foster children. Barth and colleagues (1994) reported similar results with a 10-session psychoeducational group program. They highlighted two practicalities that appeared to enhance group attendance: child care and travel expenses.

Access to and Reunification with Incestuous Relatives

In paternal and sibling abuse cases, many children continue to have contact with their incestuous relatives following disclosure, although this contact is usually supervised by a child protective service agency, a supervised access program, or a family member (Hamilton, 1997). Supervised access with an incestuous relative can serve several positive functions (Straus, 1995): It can (1) help the child gain a realistic assessment of the person and their relationship; (2) serve as a steppingstone to less restricted access; and (3) allow the child to maintain a relationship with the family member in a safe situation. On the negative side, a child may fear this relative, and visits may stimulate PTSD symptomatology. When legal proceedings are in progress, a child's access may introduce divided loyalties between wanting to please the perpetrator and following through with prosecution.

When postdisclosure access between a child and an incestuous relative is being planned, care should be taken to balance the child's need for the relationship with the child's need to manage abuse-related symptomatology. Tebbutt, Swanston, Oates, and O'Toole (1997), in their longitudinal study of abuse-related sequelae, found that contact between intrafamilial perpetrators and victims between the 18-month and 5-year follow-up period was predictive of long-term depressive symptoms. In an exploratory study, Hamilton (1997) reviewed 40 child protective service files to examine factors associated with father–child access and with positive adjustment to access. Access supervisors were more likely to note positive adjustment to access when the father (1) had admitted to the abuse, (2) emotionally supported the child, (3) abided by supervision rules, (4) was highly involved in treatment services, and (5) demonstrated positive parenting behaviors during access visits.

In accord with these findings, some therapists advocate that father–child access not occur until both the father and child have progressed far enough in therapy to be ready for an abuse clarification session. Abuse clarification requires that the father (1) accept responsibility for the sexual abuse, (2) apologize to the victim and other family members, and (3) agree to abide by a plan to assure the child's safety and security (Swenson & Hanson, 1998). The therapist for the father guides him toward preparation of a letter to the victim outlining the following: (1) his grooming of the child to initiate the abuse, (2) full admission of the abuse perpetrated, and (3) a plan to prevent further abusive behaviors.

Once the father's therapist feels that he is ready for the abuse clarification session, the child's therapist or social worker is contacted to begin preparing the child for the meeting. Child preparation includes the following: (1) a review of the rationale for an abuse clarification session (i.e., the father is to apologize and listen to what the child has to say); (2) the child and therapist make rules about the meeting (e.g., no touching, no blaming the child or the child's mother); and (3) the child prepares what he or she would like to say to the father (e.g., how the abuse made him or her feel, the effects of the abuse). The abuse clarification session is usually held in the office of the child's therapist or social worker, and progresses through the following issues: (1) clarification of the facts; (2) acceptance of responsibility by the father; (3) agreement about terms of future access; (4) discussion of a safety plan; and (5) discussion of long-term plans for the family (e.g., reunification, permanent separation, divorce).

O'Connell (1986) described a process of family reunification following the abuse clarification process that allows for contingency-based progression from access in public places, to family outings outside the home, home visits, and finally overnight visits. Specific rules are outlined at each step of increasing access that are designed to ensure child safety. For instance, rules for access in public places might strictly limit physical contact and restrict conversations related to sexuality, dating partners, and the sexual abuse. When home visits are initiated, rules might include restrictions of time alone between the victim and the perpetrator, enhanced child privacy boundaries, and strict rules about the perpetrator's nighttime behavior and dress around the child. No research has evaluated the effectiveness of such reunification strategies in terms of the numbers who seek to reunify and those who succeed in carrying out all of O'Connell's steps. Furthermore, no studies have evaluated the effects of reunification on children.

Alexander (1990) described several treatment goals important for incestuous families, particularly those that plan to reunite: (1) child protection; (2) elimination of secrecy related to the abuse; and (3) acceptance of responsibility for the abuse by the perpetrator and, where appropriate, by the nonoffending spouse (e.g., for failure to monitor, protect, and report abuse). Establishment of appropriate family system boundaries is seen as an important therapeutic goal, including physical boundaries relative to personal space and property, and boundaries between parent, marital, and sibling subsystems. Furthermore, it is deemed appropriate to dismantle other existing boundaries between the family and outside societal and social contacts (e.g., social service agencies, child contacts with peers).

Sibling Incest

Most authors who have addressed incest have focused attention on the father–daughter relationship; however, sibling incest occurs at least five times more often than parent–child abuse (Finkelhor, 1980; Smith & Israel, 1987). Although some consider sibling incest to be within the realm of sexual exploration, there is growing awareness that sibling incest can lead to serious emotional sequelae for victims (Adler & Schultz, 1995; Cyr, Wright, McDuff, & Perron, 2002; Rudd & Herzberger, 1999). Two recent clinic-based studies suggest that the psychological sequelae to brother–sister abuse can be on a par with those of father–daughter incest (Cyr et al., 2002; Rudd & Herzberger, 1999). Clinic-based studies of sibling incest reveal that from 46% to 89% of cases involve attempted or completed vaginal or anal penetration, with most victims at least 5 years younger than the offenders. In fact, Cyr and colleagues (2002) found that brothers were more likely than either fathers or stepfathers to commit penetration abuse, and Rudd and Herzberger (1999) found that brothers were more likely than fathers or stepfathers to use force. They also found that incestuous brothers often physically abused their sisters, in addition to the sexual abuse. Many such brothers have histories of conduct problems and arrests for nonsexual offenses, and have personal histories of sexual and/or physical abuse.

Sibling incest tends to occur in large, chaotic families with multiple problems (Finkelhor, 1980; Worling, 1995). Fathers often are absent or abuse alcohol, and the offending brothers have taken on a parental role (Cyr et al., 2002; Finkelhor, 1980; Rudd & Herzberger, 1999; Russell, 1986). Mothers have a disproportionate rate of childhood sexual abuse (Adler & Schultz, 1995; Cyr et al., 2002; Smith & Israel, 1987) and may fail to monitor their children closely (Rudd & Herzberger, 1999).

Incestuous adolescent siblings often receive the same types of treatment services as adolescent perpetrators in general (for reviews, see Becker, 1998; Becker & Johnson, 2001). For an adolescent sibling perpetrator, strategies must be put in place to assure the safety of the victim and other children. In many instances, this requires that the perpetrator live with a relative, in a foster home, or in a group home facility. Some group home facilities have been developed to address the special needs of incestuous adolescent siblings. As with incestuous fathers, there is little empirical guidance for reintegration of incestuous brothers back into their homes. Parents are often torn in their allegiances to the victim and the perpetrator, and the rights and needs of one often interfere with those of the other. It would appear that with some variations to developmental concerns, the strategies described by O'Connell (1986) could serve as a starting point for developing a plan for reintegrating incestuous adolescent siblings back into their homes.

Sexual Abuse Allegations within the Context of Custody and Access Disputes

Faller (1991) reported several different scenarios often observed in custody/access disputes involving sexual abuse allegations: (1) The mother separated from the father after allegations of abuse came forward (8%); (2) abuse occurred prior to the separation, but was disclosed by the child subsequent to the separation (19%); (3) abuse began after the separation and was verified after disclosure (39%); (4) allegations were made after separation because one parent overinterpreted signs of child stress or other concerns as evidence of sexual abuse (32%); and (5) deliberate fabrications were brought forward to gain advantage in custody and access proceedings (2%). Although some believe that sexual abuse allegations are commonly used as a weapon in custody and access disputes (see Faller, Corwin, & Olafson, 1993), evidence suggests that only 2% of all custody and access disputes involve such allegations (Thoennes & Tjaden, 1990). Some also argue that false allegations are more common in custody and access disputes. However, Elliott and Briere (1994) found no difference in case disposition (substantiated, unsubstantiated, or unclear) based on whether the case involved a custody dispute. Thus it is clear that allegations of sexual abuse in the course of a custody/access dispute should be investigated carefully, and investigators should carefully examine the context in which the abuse, separation, and access concerns arose.

When sexual abuse allegations are a component of a custody/access dispute, all parties (the parents, the child, and in some cases the state) have serious vested interests in the outcomes. Unlike other custody and access disputes, which may be limited to questions about primary residence and frequency of visitation, abuse allegations raise the stakes to questions such as a child's risk for further abuse, triggers of trauma-related symptoms for the child, parental alienation, and no or very restricted contact between the accused parent and the child. Whereas most custody and access disputes are resolved between the parties or with mediation, disputes that involve allegations of sexual abuse often require custody and access evaluations and/or family court appearances. Thus cases that progress to custody and access evaluations and/or family court appearances often disproportionately involve sexual abuse allegations.

Custody and access assessments in these cases are quite complex, requiring assessment expertise in custody and access issues, child sexual abuse, and sexual abuse perpetrators (Bow, Quinnell, Zaroff, & Assemany, 2002). Although guidelines exist for custody and access evaluations (e.g., American Psychological Association, 1994), sexual abuse evaluations (e.g., APSAC, 1997), and evaluations of accused perpetrators (Association for the Treatment of Sexual Abusers, 2005), no guidelines exist for assessments that involve all three concerns (Bow et al., 2002). Thus these assessments often require an individual evaluator with expertise in all three areas, a team approach, or referrals to outside experts for portions of the assessment to assure adequate coverage of all important issues. The complexities of these cases are reflected in the time commitments involved. Bow and colleagues (2002) found that most assessments required 9 weeks of involvement, with 22 hours to complete the data-gathering phase, and an additional 10 hours to write the report. Most assessments require the following (Bow et al., 2002): (1) a court order for a forensic evaluation by a neutral assessor; (2) access to all relevant records; (3) detailed accounting of the chronology of events related to the custody/access dispute and the sexual abuse allegations; (4) multiple data sources, involving at least all of the primary parties to the access dispute; (5) interviews with the child; (6) psychological testing; (7) sexual history of the alleged perpetrator;

(8) parent–child observations; and (9) information from collateral sources (e.g., police, protective services, physicians, therapists, grandparents, new spouses/partners).

TERTIARY INTERVENTIONS

Sexual Abuse Sequelae: An Overview

Past literature reviews (Kendall-Tackett, Williams, & Finkelhor, 1993; Wolfe & Birt, 1997) highlight three major findings regarding sexual abuse sequelae: (1) Sexually abused children display and report more internalizing and externalizing adjustment problems than their nonabused peers; (2) sexually abused children display a broad range of behavioral and emotional problems, some specifically linked to their sexual abuse experience and others apparently linked to the familial and other environment circumstances often associated with sexual maltreatment (e.g., parent–child relationship problems, parental adjustment problems); and (3) two problem areas—PTSD symptoms and sexuality problems—appear to represent specific effects of sexual abuse, in that they are disproportionately prevalent among sexually abused children as compared to groups of other troubled children (e.g., clinic-referred nonabused children; other children involved with child protective service agencies). Kendall-Tackett and colleagues (1993) found that from 20% to 50% of children appear to be symptom-free at the time they are assessed. However, at least 30% show clinically significant problems within the first several months following disclosure (Wolfe, Gentile, & Wolfe, 1989). Several classes of factors are thought to mediate the impact of sexual abuse on children: abuse factors, premorbid child characteristics, family functioning, and community supports and stressors (Trickett & McBride-Chang, 1995; Wolfe & Birt, 1997).

Despite evidence of general abatement of abuse-related symptoms across childhood (Kendall-Tackett et al., 1993), considerable evidence links childhood sexual abuse with adult psychological symptomatology. Two meta-analytic studies of long-term sequelae revealed consistent findings (Jumper, 1995; Neumann, Hauskamp, Pollock, & Briere, 1996). A history of childhood sexual abuse was found to be related to a number of symptom domains, including anxiety, anger, depression, revictimiza-

tion, self-mutilation, sexual problems, substance use problems, suicidal ideation/behaviors, impairment of self-concept, interpersonal problems, obsessions and compulsions, dissociation, posttraumatic stress responses, and somatization. The magnitude of the effect of a history of sexual abuse in predicting these symptoms was small to moderate (Neumann et al., 1996), and was more evident in community and epidemiological studies than in studies of more restricted populations, such as university students (Jumper, 1995; Neumann et al., 1996). Neumann and colleagues (1996) noted a particularly strong relationship between history of childhood sexual abuse and posttraumatic stress responses and revictimization.

In a subsequent meta-analytic review of the adult literature on sexual abuse survivors, Rind, Tromovitch, and Bauserman (1998) sparked a controversy by concluding that these survivors, on average, were only slightly less well adjusted than controls. Furthermore, poorer adjustment among the survivors could not be attributed to their sexual abuse history, because this history was often confounded with family dysfunction, and family dysfunction consistently accounted for more variance than abuse variables did. Rind and colleagues argued that overly inclusive definitions of sexual abuse (e.g., using age discrepancies to define abuse, rather than victim reports of coercion or negative reactions) had the effect of including individuals of vastly different experiences, including many "victims" who described their experiences as consensual and positive. They suggested that "child–adult sex" and "adolescent–adult sex" be differentiated from the terms "child sexual abuse" and "adolescent sexual abuse." This suggestion received diverse reactions, including praise from pedophilic societies, condemnation from the U.S. Congress, and considerable debate among those in the mental health fields (Sher & Eisenberg, 2002).

The issues raised by the Rind and colleagues (1998) review are complex and are not fully explored in this chapter. However, a major concern is raised with regard to the types of outcomes considered in the review. Although Neumann and colleagues (1996) considered a broad range of potential outcomes to sexual abuse, they concluded that the effects were strongest for two primary areas of impact—posttraumatic stress reactions and risk of revictimization. In contrast, Rind and colleagues did not consider revictimization in their review, and they combined posttraumatic stress responses with other anxiety symptoms. As well, they disregarded the evidence of sexual behavior problems reported by Kendall-Tackett and colleagues (1993); they stated in a subsequent paper that sexualized behavior was not a symptom, but rather reflective of a value judgment (Rind, Tromovitch, & Bauserman, 2001). This highlights a general concern that research on the impact of sexual abuse has often lacked a conceptual basis for connecting abuse to psychological outcome. That is, many studies have investigated either outcomes that are fairly pervasive among those who do not have abuse histories (e.g., hostility, locus of control, paranoia) or outcomes that are not uniquely linked to sexual abuse and have many contributing factors, including family dysfunction (e.g., depression). On the other hand, PTSD, risk of revictimization, and sexual behavior problems have clear conceptual ties to the experience of sexual abuse, and not surprisingly provide the greatest evidence for specific short- and long-term effects of sexual abuse.

With this in mind, PTSD and child sexual problem conceptualizations and research findings are explored in the following sections, followed by a review of intervention studies that address these specific concerns. Although risk of revictimization has also been identified as an effect of sexual abuse among adults, this issue has received relatively little attention among child victims. However, both PTSD and sexuality problems are likely linked with risk for revictimization. That is, sexuality problems may place children and adolescents at increased risk for sexual and other victimizations, and PTSD and associated adjustment problems may affect their ability to respond effectively when posed with a threatening situation.

PTSD Conceptualizations of Sexual Abuse Sequelae

The PTSD literature provides an important framework for conceptualizing sexual abuse sequelae. Briefly, the *Diagnostic and Statistical Manual of Mental Disorders*, fourth edition, text revision (DSM-IV-TR; American Psychiatric Association, 2000) PTSD diagnostic criteria include the following:

1. An experience of an event posing serious threat, to which the individual responds with great helplessness, fear, or horror (Criteria A1 and A2, respectively).
2. Three sets of symptoms, including *reexperiencing* aspects of the abuse (e.g., nightmares, intrusive thoughts; Criterion B; one symptom required); *avoidance* strategies that serve as a means of escape from trauma-related stimuli (Criterion C; three symptoms required); and persistent, increased autonomic *arousal* (particularly when the person is faced with trauma-related stimuli or memories of the trauma; Criterion D; two symptoms required).
3. Duration of symptoms for at least a 1-month period beyond the initial 3-month posttrauma period (Criterion E).
4. Significant interference of the symptoms with ability to function effectively at home, with friends, and/or at work or school (Criterion F).

The DSM-IV-TR supports consideration of PTSD as a possible diagnosis for child sexual abuse victims; in fact, in defining trauma, it includes "developmentally inappropriate sexual experiences with or without threatened or actual violence or injury" (p. 464). The DSM-IV-TR notes that young children may differ from older children and adults in the manifestation of PTSD symptoms. Young children may express intrusive thoughts through thematic, repetitive play. They may complain of frightening dreams, but may be unable to describe or recognize the content as trauma-related. Finally, rather than describing flashbacks, young children may reenact their trauma through play or art (American Psychiatric Association, 2000).

Despite these developmental considerations, concerns have been raised that the DSM-IV-TR diagnostic criteria are too restrictive for young children, because many of the criteria require cognitive and verbal abilities beyond their years (Scheeringa, Zeanah, Drell, & Larrieu, 1995). Scheeringa and his colleagues (Scheeringa, Peebles, Cook, & Zeanah, 2001; Scheeringa, Zeanah, Myers, & Putnam, 2003) have proposed and evaluated alternative PTSD criteria for preschool-age children, and made the following recommendations: (1) eliminating Criterion A2, since young children have difficulty reporting previously experienced emotional states; (2) reducing the number of avoidance symptoms from three to one; and (3) further clarifying how the DSM-IV-TR symptoms are manifested in preschool-age children. For example, for the Criterion C4 symptom "diminished interest in or participation in significant activities," it is noted that young children typically display this through constriction of play. DSM-IV-TR diagnostic criteria were compared with the proposed diagnostic algorithm, using a sample of 62 traumatized and 63 nontraumatized preschool children (20 months to 6 years). With the new criteria, 26% of the traumatized children met PTSD criteria, as compared to none when DSM-IV-TR criteria were used.

Research with older sexually abused children (i.e., not preschool-age children) has documented relatively high rates of PTSD symptoms via a number of assessment strategies, including parent reports (e.g., Wells, McCann, Adams, Voris, & Ensign, 1995), child reports (e.g., Dubner & Motta, 1999; Friedrich, Jaworski, Hexschl, & Bengston, 1997), social worker checklists (e.g., Mennen & Meadows, 1993), chart reviews (e.g., Kiser, Heston, Millsap, & Pruitt, 1991), and professional evaluations (e.g., Livingston, Lawson, & Jones, 1993; McLeer, Deblinger, Henry, & Orvaschel, 1992). Compared to other negative life events in childhood, such as serious accidents, natural and human-made disasters, and even physical abuse, sexual abuse appears to be particularly potent in provoking PTSD symptomatology (Bal, Crombez, Van Oost, & Debourdeaudhuij, 2003; Bal, Van Oost, Debourdeaudhuij, & Crombez, 2003; Boney-McCoy & Finkelhor, 1996; Dubner & Motta, 1999). Despite relatively high rates of negative life events among clinic-referred children in general, PTSD is more prevalent among sexual abuse victims than among other clinic-referred children and adolescents (Wolfe & Birt, 2004a). High rates of PTSD symptomatology have been demonstrated among several populations of sexually abused children, including nationally represented samples (Boney-McCoy & Finkelhor, 1996), school-based, nonclinical samples (Bal, Van Oost, et al., 2003); children identified through child protective services and clinical agencies (McLeer, Callaghan, Henry, & Wallen, 1994; Wolfe & Birt, 2004a); child witnesses awaiting criminal trials (D. A. Wolfe, Sas, & Wekerle, 1994); children abused by extrafamilial perpetrators (Ligezinska et al., 1996); and foster children (Dubner & Motta, 1999).

Between 49% and 60% of sexually abused children meet diagnostic criteria for PTSD (Dubner & Motta, 1999; Kendall-Tackett et al., 1993; Wolfe & Birt, 2004a; D. A. Wolfe et al., 1994). A number of factors have been related to the development of PTSD among these children. Sexual abuse victims who experience additional forms of maltreatment, especially physical abuse, are at particular risk for PTSD (Kiser et al., 1991; Wolfe & Birt, 2004a). Young children appear to be at greater risk for PTSD (Dubner & Motta, 1999; Wolfe & Birt, 2004a; Wolfe et al., 1989). Several studies have also linked PTSD symptoms to social support and family functioning (Boney-McCoy & Finkelhor, 1996; Kiser et al., 1991; McLeer et al., 1992) and to attributional style (Taska & Feiring, 1995; Wolfe et al., 1989). Several abuse variables have been linked with PTSD, including abuse severity (Kiser et al., 1991; D. A. Wolfe et al, 1994; Wolfe et al., 1989), coercion and force (Basta & Peterson, 1990), and relationship to the offender (McLeer et al., 1992). More recently, PTSD studies have begun to explore the role of peritraumatic reactions (i.e., thoughts, emotions, and behaviors at the time of the trauma; Criterion A2 in the DSM-IV-TR PTSD criteria) with regard to the development and intensity of PTSD symptoms. With non-abuse-related traumatic events, such as vehicle accidents and disasters, evidence suggests that peritraumatic reactions are more potent predictors of PTSD than specific trauma factors (Ehlers, Mayou, & Bryant, 2003; Shannon, Lonigan, Finch, & Taylor, 1994; Stallard, Velleman, & Baldwin, 1998). Likewise, children's recollections of peritraumatic reactions to their sexual abuse experiences appear to be more powerful predictors of PTSD than specific abuse characteristics, such as abuse severity, force, frequency, duration, and perpetrator (Wolfe & Birt, 2004b).

Conceptual Models of PTSD

Several conceptual models have been developed to account for the various symptoms that contribute to PTSD (Brewin & Holmes, 2003). Janoff-Bulman (1989), building on previous work by Horowitz (1986), suggested that PTSD reexperiencing symptoms reflect the accommodation process that occurs when one is trying to assimilate a traumatic event into one's preexisting schema. In Janoff-Bulman's "shattered assumption" theory, trauma is a challenge to usually held perceptions of the world as safe, orderly, and meaningful. Similarly, Silver, Boone, and Stones (1983) conceptualized PTSD reexperiencing symptoms as attempts to "make meaning" of the traumatic experiences. That is, reexperiencing symptoms may reflect a child's need to understand the traumatic event or may indicate that the child is missing information that may help him or her "make meaning" of the trauma. As an analogy, children may experience their abuse as a puzzle that has many missing pieces or pieces that do not fit together. Once their puzzle is "put together," their reexperiencing symptoms are likely to abate. For young children, the pieces of the puzzle may be simple and few; however, because of these children's developmental immaturity, those pieces may be quite challenging. These puzzle pieces may include questions such as "Am I safe?," "Will my parents protect me?," or "Why did he hurt me?" A young child may have great difficulty understanding that a perpetrator could have been "fun and nice" but also scary and hurtful. As children mature and have a greater capacity to understand the dynamics of sexual abuse and the complexity of interpersonal relationships, reexperiencing symptoms may reemerge and encompass new concepts (e.g., attributions of responsibility, feelings of guilt, and conflicting feelings about the perpetrator).

Ehlers and Clark (2000) have elaborated on these concepts by considering cognitive appraisals in place prior to, during, and after traumatic events. Whereas the "shattered assumptions" model suggests that those with previously positive belief systems would be most affected by trauma, research indicates that those who have experienced previous traumas are actually at greater risk of developing PTSD (Yehuda, 2004). Ehlers and Clark's cognitive model proposes that previously held beliefs about negative life events might affect reactions to events and reactions after events, accounting for why some persons develop PTSD whereas others do not. "Mental defeat," somewhat like the "learned helplessness" concept, is seen as influencing individuals' perception of their ability to influence their fate and as fostering self-perceptions of weakness, ineffectiveness, and vulnerability.

Berliner and Wheeler (1987) used Mowrer's (1960) two-factor theory (classical and instrumental conditioning) to conceptualize the persistent symptoms of anxiety and avoidance frequently observed in victims. Fear and anxiety become classically conditioned to circumstances associated with the abuse (e.g., darkness, bedtime, male caretakers), which subsequently evoke high levels of fear and physiological reactivity. Avoidance behaviors are then instrumentally maintained through negative reinforcement (i.e., avoiding circumstances associated with the trauma reduces stress reactions).

During the past decade, considerable research has linked the hyperarousal dimension of PTSD to trauma-induced alterations in neural processes (Charney, Deutch, Southwick, & Krystal, 1995). There is evidence to suggest a dose–response effect; that is, individuals who experienced more intense or more frequent exposure to traumatic events tend to show correlated increases in physiological reactivity when faced with ordinary stressors (Southwick, Yehuda, & Morgan, 1995). Repetitive "fight or flight" neural activation can lead to sensitization—a process in which decreasingly intense external stimuli are required to evoke neural activations. Infants and young children, whose brains are still developing, may be particularly vulnerable to long-term alterations of neural processes following trauma (Perry, Pollard, Blakley, Baker, & Vigilante, 1995). Essentially, the neural processing changes may cause children to be stuck in a perpetual state of fear, characterized by hyperreactivity and emotional sensitivity. Such children can move easily from mild anxiety to feeling threatened and terrorized. It is possible that these changes in physiological reactivity create changes similar to those of attention-deficit/hyperactivity disorder (ADHD). Glod and Teicher (1996) found that physically and sexually abused children with PTSD displayed activity patterns similar to those of children with ADHD (based on motion-logger actigraphs). These activity patterns were most prevalent for children who experienced abuse during the very early years of their childhood. Interestingly, ADHD is one of the most common diagnoses among children evaluated for the effects of sexual abuse and trauma (McLeer et al., 1994); however, it is also very common among other clinic-referred children without a history of abuse.

Dual-representation theory (Brewin, Dalgleish, & Joseph, 1996) provides a basis for integrating cognitive and conditioning constructs into a more parsimonious explanation of the cognitive and physiological manifestations of

PTSD. Dual-representation theory posits that memories of traumatic events are represented in two distinct memory systems associated with different brain regions. Verbally accessible memory includes aspects of trauma that can be accessed, understood, and expressed through language. However, situationally accessible memory contains sensory information and operates subconsciously. These different memory systems account for distinct aspects of PTSD. For example, verbally accessible memory may influence the intrusive-thoughts dimension of PTSD, and may operate in ways similar to those described in the model of shattered assumptions and the cognitive theory. However, situationally accessible memories are accessed through association with trauma-related triggers, and are more commonly experienced as the sensory elements of flashbacks (i.e., *feeling* as if one is reexperiencing the event); these may operate more in line with Mowrer's two-factor theory.

Type II PTSD and Complex PTSD Conceptualizations

Early efforts to conceptualize sexual abuse sequelae as PTSD were criticized for failing to account for the full range of symptoms described for sexually abused children (Finkelhor, 1990) and for adult survivors of abuse (Herman, 1992a). Terr (1987) recognized that child sexual abuse differs from many forms of trauma in that it is often repeated over long periods in secret, thereby requiring victims to adapt to their abusive situation via strategies that are either developmentally or psychologically inappropriate or damaging, particularly when these strategies are generalized beyond the abusive situation. Terr described these adaptations as psychogenic numbing, dissociation, distrust, relationship problems, suicidal ideation, rage, and "unremitting sadness." Terr (1987, 1991) has thus proposed a dual classification for trauma-related disorders: Type I disorders follow exposure to a single traumatic event, whereas Type II disorders result from multiple or long-standing experiences with extreme stress (e.g., sexual abuse). Although patients with both types of PTSD are thought to experience core PTSD symptoms (reexperiencing, avoidance, hyperarousal), those with Type II PTSD also develop atypical coping patterns and psychological symptoms that eventually become integrated into their personalities. My colleagues and I (Wolfe & Birt, 1997;

Wolfe & Gentile, 1992) have identified four areas of dysfunction beyond core PTSD symptoms that reflect the types of symptoms described by Terr (1987, 1991): (1) learned helplessness, attributional style, and depression; (2) dysfunctional coping with trauma-related circumstances and with day-to-day stressors; (3) dissociation; and (4) difficulties regulating negative emotion. These dysfunctions in turn are thought to disrupt multiple areas of functioning, but are particularly damaging to the development of social competence and interpersonal relationships.

Similar dual conceptualizations of PTSD emerged simultaneously within the adult literature (e.g., Herman, 1992b). Research with adult trauma survivors supports both an expansion of the PTSD concept to include additional sequelae, and a link between these symptom groupings and early extensive interpersonal trauma (Pelcovitz et al., 1997; Roth, Newman, Pelcovitz, van der Kolk, & Mandel, 1997; van der Kolk, Pelcovitz, et al., 1996). Seven problem areas have been identified as characteristic of victims of "extreme stress": (1) affect regulation and impulsivity; (2) regulation of attention and consciousness; (3) self-perception; (4) perception of the perpetrator; (5) relationships with others; (6) somatization; and (7) systems of meaning.

Despite considerable support for the idea of expanding the breadth of the PTSD diagnosis, the idea of an alternative diagnostic classification requires considerable study. Currently, symptom variations are often treated diagnostically and therapeutically as comorbid conditions; some patients with PTSD have concurrent diagnoses such as MDD, dissociative identity disorder, and/or borderline personality disorder (Shalev, Friedman, Foa, & Keane, 2000). This approach has considerable validity, since several of the common comorbid diagnoses have well developed conceptual underpinnings and empirically validated treatment strategies that inform the study of trauma effects. Some Type II or complex PTSD symptoms can be conceptualized as extreme manifestations of Type I PTSD symptoms, and thus may simply require refinements to descriptions of symptom criteria. For example, affect dysregulation and somatization symptoms might be considered part of the PTSD hyperarousal domain, and dissociative symptoms might be considered extreme manifestations of the avoidance domain. Finally, some symptoms of complex PTSD may be associated with conditions other than trauma, such as dysfunctional family backgrounds and premorbid propensities to cope with life stressors in ineffective ways.

DEPRESSION, LEARNED HELPLESSNESS, AND ATTRIBUTIONAL STYLE

Research strongly supports links among trauma, PTSD, and depression. Links between trauma and depression have been established in nationally representative samples of children and adolescents (Boney-McCoy & Finkelhor, 1996; Kilpatrick et al., 2003) and adults (Kessler, Sonnega, Bromet, Hughes, & Nelson, 1995). Studies also reveal high comorbidity between PTSD and mood disorders. The National Comorbidity Survey (Kessler et al., 1995) found that 49% of adults with a lifetime history of PTSD also met criteria for lifetime MDD, with MDD secondary to trauma and PTSD in 53–78% of comorbid cases. Using data from the National Survey of Adolescents, Kilpatrick and colleagues (2003) found that 47% of boys and 71% of girls with PTSD had a comorbid diagnosis of MDD. Whereas noncomorbid PTSD was related to ethnicity (higher among Hispanics and African Americans than European Americans) and age (higher among older adolescents), PTSD with comorbid MDD was related to being female; having a family history of drug and alcohol problems; and being exposed to sexual assault, physical assault, and/or family violence. Although most studies have exclusively studied links between trauma and MDD, Lizardi and colleagues (1995) found that early-onset dysthymia was more closely associated than MDD with a history of sexual and physical abuse and with poor parent–child relationships.

Studies have found higher prevalences of depressive symptoms and mood disorders among sexually abused children than among nonabused children (Boney-McCoy & Finkelhor, 1996; Brant, King, Olson, Ghaziuddin, & Naylor, 1996; Bryant & Range, 1996; Kiser et al., 1991; Koverola, Pound, Heger, & Lytle, 1993; Ligezinska et al., 1996; Runyon, Faust, & Orvaschel, 2002). As in the adult literature, sexually abused girls, as compared to boys, are more likely to present with comorbid PTSD and MDD (Runyon et al., 2002).

These findings suggest either that trauma is a risk factor for developing depression, or that those who develop PTSD subsequent to trauma have an increased risk of also developing a mood disorder. Alternatively, it is possible that among trauma victims, symptoms of depression and PTSD are so closely associated that they form one unified syndrome rather than two distinct disorders. Blanchard, Buckley, Hickling, and Taylor (1998) investigated whether the relationship between these two disorders is simply due to an overlap in symptom criteria, or whether these disorders are truly distinct when they occur subsequent to a traumatic event. Indeed, 3 of the 17 PTSD symptoms—sleep disturbance, impaired concentration, and anhedonia—constitute 3 of the 9 symptoms identified for MDD. Thus, if these symptoms are present for an individual with PTSD, only two additional symptoms are required for a diagnosis of MDD. Based on confirmatory factor analyses of data derived from adult motor vehicle accident survivors, Blanchard and colleagues found two correlated, but independent, reactions to trauma, not a single reaction. They also found that those who met criteria for PTSD and MDD were more subjectively distressed, had more social dysfunction, and lower rates of spontaneous remission than those with PTSD alone. These findings are mirrored in those of Runyon and colleagues (2002). They found that children who presented with both PTSD and MDD tended to have more serious PTSD symptoms, including more flashbacks and sleep disturbance, whereas those who presented with PTSD but without MDD were more likely to report trauma-related amnesia.

How might trauma and negative life events be responsible for increased rates of depression? The hopelessness theory of depression suggests one path. Individuals base their attributions of causes to events on three dimensions (internal–external, stable–unstable, and global–specific; Seligman et al., 1984). Individuals tend to base their causal attributions on situational factors; however, when causation is ambiguous, individuals attribute causation in their own idiosyncratic style. A self-enhancing attributional style (similar to the more familiar notion of optimism) is characterized by internal, stable, global attributions about positive events and by external, unstable, and specific attributions about negative events, and is associated with positive self-esteem and resistance to depression. A self-deprecatory attributional style (similar to pessimism) is characterized by external, unstable, specific attributions about positive events and internal, stable, global attributions about negative events, and is related to poor self-concept and depressive symptomatology (Seligman et al., 1984).

Peterson and Seligman (1983) suggest that individual differences in attributional style are shaped by life events, but also affect reactions to life events. Thus, as negative life events "pile up," an individual's attributional style is likely to change, and such changes may affect the ways the individual copes with subsequent life events (e.g., the person may respond with learned helplessness even when events are controllable). Thus we might expect that those who experience more negative life events will show a more pessimistic attributional style, and that this attributional style will then relate to depression. There is little question that depression and attributional style are related, both in the general population and among clinical populations (Joiner & Wagner, 1995; Gladstone & Kaslow, 1995). In a longitudinal study of children in grades 3 through 8, Nolen-Hoeksema, Girgus, and Seligman (1992) found a developmental progression in the prediction of depression with regard to attributional style and negative life events: In grades 3 and 4, life events, but not attributional style, predicted depression; in grades 5 and 6, attributional style predicted depression; and in grades 7 and 8, an interaction of attributional style and negative life events predicted depression. Attributional style, on the other hand, was primarily predicted by depression: When children became depressed, their attributional style worsened and remained stable even when depressive symptoms abated. Thus it is possible that negative life events affect depression during the early years, that depression affects attributional style during middle childhood, and that the "attributional scars" left from childhood depression remain stable and combine with negative life events to predict depression as children enter their "tween" years.

Investigations of attributional style and depression with sexually abused children have demonstrated findings similar to those of research on nonabused children. Several studies demonstrate a relationship between depression and attributional style among sexually abused children (Feiring, Taska, & Lewis, 1999, 2002; Mannarino & Cohen, 1996; Mannarino, Cohen, & Berman, 1994; Wolfe et al., 1989). There is some evidence that childhood physical and/or sexual abuse is associated with a more pessimistic attributional style, both among children (Cerezo & Frias, 1994) and among adult survivors (Gold, 1986). Feiring and colleagues (2002) found that attributional style moderated the link between abuse severity and depression and self-esteem during the initial postdisclosure adjustment phase. One year later, attributional style was a significant predictor of both depression and self-esteem, whereas the severity of the abuse was no longer a significant predictor. Some abuse-specific attributions have also been linked with negative outcomes. The most widely researched negative attributions are self-blame, guilt, and shame, which have been linked with depression and low self-esteem (Crouch, Smith, Ezzell, & Saunders, 1999; Feiring et al., 2002; Manion et al., 1998). Perceptions of vulnerability to future abuse and perceptions of the world as a dangerous place have also been linked with depression (Crouch et al., 1999; Hazzard, Celano, Gould, Lawry, & Webb, 1995; Mannarino & Cohen, 1996; Mannarino et al., 1994; Wolfe et al., 1989).

DYSFUNCTIONAL COPING

"Coping" has generally been defined as "any and all responses made by an individual who encounters a potentially harmful outcome" (Silver & Wortman, 1980, p. 281). Coping is typically dichotomized in terms of a bipolar dimension, such as approach versus avoidance coping or problem-focused versus emotion-focused coping. However, Causey and DeBow (1992) found support for six coping factors. Two factors are considered effective strategies (Problem Solving and Seeking Social Support), and three factors are considered ineffective reactions (Distancing, Internalizing, and Externalizing). The sixth factor relates to perception of problems as Controllable versus Uncontrollable. The distinction of Problem Solving and Seeking Social Support is particularly helpful, since several theoretical models view coping as closely linked with perceived availability of social support (Compas & Epping, 1993; Vernberg, LaGreca, Silverman, & Prinstein, 1996). The Distancing factor is also important since it corresponds conceptually to the avoidance dimension of PTSD, and the distinction of Internalizing and Externalizing emotional reactions has importance in terms of possible connections with different symptom patterns (i.e., internalizing and externalizing problems).

The Causey and DeBow (1992) method of assessing coping is also distinguished from other coping assessment strategies, in that coping is seen as context-specific; norms are available for two situations, interpersonal conflicts and academic difficulties. No one coping strategy is effective in all situations, and effective coping may depend upon matching coping strategies to the controllability or relative stress of the situation, or the appropriate or socially accepted response to the stressor. For example, when a stressor is moderate and controllable, strategies intended to alter the situation are associated with lower levels of distress and fewer negative emotions (Hubert, Jay, Saltoun, & Hayes, 1988; Hyson, 1983). However, when a person is faced with high-stress, uncontrollable stressors, coping strategies that reduce emotional distress or enable the person to avoid the stressors appear to be the most effective (Altshuler & Ruble, 1989; Band & Weisz, 1988; Spirito, Stark, & Williams, 1988). For instance, distraction is a commonly used coping strategy when stressors are perceived as uncontrollable (David & Suls, 1999).

Children's decisions to report the onset of sexual abuse may have more to do with premorbid child characteristics such as coping style than with the abuse itself (Love, Jackson, & Long, 1990). When confronted with a sexual abuse situation, a child may perceive the situation as controllable and moderately stressful and may act to stop the abuse, either by refusing to participate or by telling someone about the abuse after the first episode. However, if the child perceives the situation to be uncontrollable or if the child experiences great horror or terror, he or she may cope differently—using strategies such as distancing, repression, and avoidance, and responding with high levels of negative emotion. Indeed, emerging research on peritraumatic reactions reveals considerable variation in children's reactions to traumatic circumstances and abusive situations; in most cases, peritraumatic reactions have very little to do with variations in the traumatic event (Ehlers et al., 2003; Wolfe & Birt, 2004b). This suggests that peritraumatic responses may be linked with premorbid tendencies toward emotion-focused coping. Unfortunately, in the case of child sexual abuse, avoidant and distancing coping reactions place the child at risk for further maltreatment (Sas et al., 1995). Although premorbid coping style may predict peritrau-

matic reactions and coping at the time of the abuse, it is likely that aspects of the abusive situation will reinforce avoidant, distancing, and emotion-focused coping when the child is faced with more controllable stressors in the future.

Several studies have demonstrated a link among sexual abuse trauma; emotional distress; and ineffective coping strategies such as wishful thinking, inappropriate tension reduction strategies (eating, drinking, drug use, sex), emotion-focused coping, and avoidant coping (Bal, Crombez, et al., 2003; Bal, Van Oost, et al., 2003; Chaffin, Wherry, & Dykman, 1997; Tremblay, Hebert, & Piche, 1999). Furthermore, Bal, Crombez, and colleagues (2003) found that avoidant coping mediated the relationship between sexual abuse and psychological distress. Similar mediating effects have been demonstrated with adult sexual abuse survivors (Merrill, Thomsen, Sinclair, Gold, & Milner, 2001; Runtz & Shallow, 1997). Browne (2002) found that adolescents in foster care with sexual and/or physical abuse histories were more likely to cope with stressful situations independently, whereas their nonabused peers in foster care were more likely to seek support from peers.

DISSOCIATION

Dissociation is an ephemeral phenomenon that has been difficult to study. Because it is an intrapsychic event that affects one's ability to self-monitor internal states, dissociation is difficult to document by self-report, and only the behavioral manifestations of dissociation are observable by others. "Dissociation" has been defined as lapses in psychobiological and cognitive processing and the behavioral and cognitive manifestations of those lapses (Ogata, Sroufe, Weinfield, Carlson, & Egeland, 1997). Dissociation has also been described as a failure to integrate various aspects of oneself and one's experiences (Ogata et al., 1997), and as such, has been closely linked with "self" conceptualizations. Recent psychometric analyses have helped clarify the nature of dissociation. Waller, Putnam, and Carlson (1996) examined the factor structure of the Dissociative Experiences Scale (DES; Bernstein & Putnam, 1986) with a large sample of adults; they identified three main dissociative constructs: Amnesia, Absorption, and Depersonalization. We (Wolfe & Birt, 2002) reported similar factor structures for the parent report Child Dissociative Checklist (CDC; Putnam, Helmers, & Trickett, 1993) and a child report version of the CDC. The parent report version yielded three scales (Forgetful/Confused, Absorption, and Stable Personality), and the child report version yielded two scales (Forgetful/Confused and Absorption).[1] Both the DES Amnesia and the CDC Forgetful/Confused scales reflect lapses in memory for events that one was personally involved in. Both the DES and CDC Absorption scales reflect processes in which one becomes so engrossed in an activity that awareness of ongoing events and surroundings is lost. The DES Depersonalization scale reflects tendencies to separate aspects of one's experience of events (e.g., while remaining cognitively aware of ongoing events, one may feel disconnected from one's body or emotional reactions), whereas the Wolfe and Birt (2002) CDC Stable Personality scale included items that reflect variations in personality and behavior patterns across time and situation.

Dissociation is generally considered to fall along a continuum from typical everyday occurrences (e.g., intense thought absorption, lapses in memory when driving) to the most extreme form of dissociation, dissociative identity disorder (Ross & Joshi, 1992). Some suspect that children have a greater (or even innate) capacity to dissociate, which dissipates as more effective coping strategies develop. For instance, Perry and colleagues (1995) described infantile dissociation as occurring when a caregiver is not available to rescue an infant from fear-producing situations. If crying fails to summon support, the infant moves from a hyperaroused condition to dissociation, reflecting either a "freeze" or "surrender" response. If similar conditions recur, dissociative responses may be strengthened to the point that even a low-grade stressor evokes dissociative reactions. In a similar vein, Terr (1991) conceptualized dissociation as a coping strategy used to reduce overwhelming anxiety in situations of extreme stress. However, when intensively or repeatedly traumatized, young children may rely upon their dissociative capacities as a coping strategy, such that dissociative responses are negatively reinforced and therefore maintained as automatic reactions to stressful situations; they may become similar to habits.

Waller and colleagues (1996) proposed that pathological dissociation is not just the higher end of a dissociation continuum, but rather a distinct construct that is inherently pathological. Based on taxometric analyses of the DES (Bernstein & Putnam, 1986), Waller and colleagues identified eight items reflective of pathological dissociation, forming a scale labeled the DES-Taxon (DES-T). The eight items are finding oneself in a place and not knowing how one got there, finding new things among one's belongings that cannot be accounted for, feeling as if one is standing next to oneself, not recognizing friends or family members, other people and objects not feeling real, feeling that one's body does not belong to oneself, acting differently in different situations, and hearing voices.

Dissociation has been closely linked with chronic, overwhelming early childhood trauma—particularly with severe neglect, psychological unavailability, and sexual abuse, but also to a lesser extent with physical abuse and exposure to family violence (Briere & Runtz, 1989; Chu & Dill, 1990; Ogata et al., 1997). Parental dissociation is also a risk factor for child dissociation (Coons, 1985), perhaps because dissociation may increase parental psychological unavailability or because the parent and child may have experienced simultaneous traumas (e.g., child and spouse abuse); alternatively, parental dissociation has been linked with increased probability of child maltreatment (Egeland & Sussman-Stillman, 1996).

Although the onset of dissociative disorders is believed to occur in early childhood, dissociative disorders are rarely diagnosed in children, perhaps because our current nosologies are based more on the adult than on the child literature. Indeed, Putnam, Hornstein, and Peterson (1996) noted that most younger children do not meet the clear-cut diagnostic criteria for disorders such as dissociative identity disorder; they are more often given the diagnosis of dissociative disorder not otherwise specified. Children's dissociative symptoms are often attributed to other causes. For instance, trance-like behaviors may be misdiagnosed as truancy, conduct problems, or moodiness (Coons, 1986; McElroy, 1992). Some dissociative symptoms, such as imaginary friends, can be interpreted as typical (McElroy, 1992). Often dissociation goes undiagnosed, either because symptoms are not evident at the time of assessment (Kluft, 1985) or because other diagnoses are given, such as PTSD, MDD, schizophrenia, or borderline personality disorder (Coons, Bowman, & Milstein, 1988). Perhaps with the development of more reliable and valid tools for defining and assessing dissociation in children, diagnostic practices will improve as well.

AFFECT DYSREGULATION AND EMOTION MANAGEMENT

Emotion can be conceptualized as an "energized response to a demanding environmental stimulus" (Dodge, 1989, p. 339). Negative emotions such as fear, anger, and sadness have long been perceived as complex interactions among three response systems (i.e., the tripartite model; Lang, 1984): psychophysiological, behavioral, and cognitive. Emotion regulation reflects an individual's ability to coordinate responses across these three domains to achieve personal goals within the context of social and cultural norms (Campos, Mumme, Kermoian, & Campos, 1994; Dodge, 1989). Psychological concepts of emotions have traditionally focused on psychophysiological reactions and cognitive appraisals of internal states; behavioral correlates of emotions, such as links between anger and aggression; and environmental circumstances that give rise to socially inappropriate or problematic behavioral expressions of emotions. Campos and his colleagues (Campos, Campos, & Barrett, 1989; Campos et al., 1994) have expanded the study of emotions by focusing on the relational and communicative functions of emotion. Their functionalist perspective on emotions has fostered a growing field of research that examines how social processes shape and regulate emotional expression and emotion regulation within different contexts (e.g., parent–child and peer relationships), and how emotional development relates to psychological health.

Developmental research has identified three components of emotional competence (Shipman, Zeman, Penza, & Champion, 2000): (1) the ability to recognize emotions and communicate emotional states effectively; (2) the ability to understand the causes and consequences of emotional expressions, and the ability to respond effectively to one's own emotions, as well as to the emotional displays of others; and (3) the ability to regulate emotional expression and emotional experience within differing social and cultural contexts. Within the realm of typical social development, these skills have been linked with children's socioemotional competence and psychological adjustment (Garber, Braafladt, & Weiss, 1995; Rubin, Coplan, Fox, & Calkins, 1995). Developmental research on emotion regulation indicates that parents play a key role in children's development of emotion regulation abilities. For example, Eisenberg and colleagues (2001) assessed parent–child interactions in the context of an emotionally evocative slide show. They found that mothers who displayed more warmth, positive affect, and support toward their children were also more likely to link the emotional material on the slides to their children's personal experiences. Such interactions were thought to facilitate children's understanding of others' emotions. These parental characteristics were associated with fewer unregulated emotional displays and externalizing behaviors on the children's part.

Concerns have been raised that child sexual maltreatment, particularly abuse that occurs within the context of familial relationships, may disrupt children's emotional development—as a function of the trauma associated with the abuse, but also as a function of the dysfunctional family system in which incestuous abuse occurs (Cole & Putnam, 1992). The functionalist perspective on emotional development would suggest that atypical social contexts such as a maltreating environment result in the development of atypical emotion management strategies (Campos et al., 1994). That is, some emotion management strategies may effectively modulate affect in the abusive environment (e.g., decreased emotional awareness, suppression of emotional expression), whereas these same strategies may subsequently interfere with successful adaptation to other contexts, such as peer relationships. Though this field of research is fairly new, several studies provide convincing evidence that further research in this area is warranted. Research with physically abused children indicates that they are less able than their nonabused peers to encode and decode facial expressions, understand the dynamics behind emotionally arousing situations, or regulate emotion within peer relationships (Camras et al., 1988, 1990; Rogosch, Cicchetti, & Aber, 1995). Shields, Ryan, and Cicchetti (2001) studied a group of children who had experienced mixed forms of maltreatment (sexual abuse, physical abuse, and/or neglect) and a comparison sample during a summer camp experience. Camp counselors rated the maltreated children as more emotionally dysregulated, and peers rated them as less cooperative and more disruptive and aggressive. The relationship between maltreatment and social adjustment was partially mediated by the children's negative representations of caregivers and by their emotion regulation abilities.

One study has specifically examined emotion management skills among intrafamilially abused girls in comparison to a nonabused control group (Shipman et al., 2000). The sexually maltreated girls had poorer understanding of emotions, had more difficulty accurately appraising the causes and consequences of emotionally arousing situations, and had more negative expectations about reactions to their own emotional expressions. They were less aware of their own emotions, showed more emotion dysregulation, and failed to respond to others' emotional displays in a culturally appropriate manner. The results suggested that sexually maltreated girls may fail to attend to, process, and interpret emotional information, and that this failure then interferes with their ability to establish and maintain positive interpersonal relationships. For example, in response to questions about how to respond to negative emotional displays in others, maltreated girls were more likely to say that they would ignore the emotional displays or leave the situation. In contrast, their nonmaltreated peers were more likely to indicate that they would provide assistance or support. Thus, although avoidance strategies may protect an intrafamilially maltreated girl in the course of conflict with her parents (i.e., it might be unsafe for her to confront either the perpetrator or the nonabusing parent), similar avoidance patterns with peers may interfere with her ability to establish relationships outside the maltreatment context.

CURRENT STATUS OF THE TYPE II PTSD DEBATE FOR CHILDREN

From this review of the current literature regarding trauma and PTSD and the four associated areas of dysfunction (depression, dissociation, dysfunctional coping, and affect dysregulation), it is clear that including these constructs in a conceptualization of PTSD more generally, and of PTSD in sexually abused children specifically, is a step forward in developing a more comprehensive account of trauma-related sequelae. The question remains, however, as to whether these areas of dysfunction can be integrated into a single conceptual model that is parsimonious and empirically supported. The study by Blanchard and colleagues (1998) highlights the need to consider (1) whether each area of dysfunction is distinguishable from PTSD, and (2) whether adding the area of dysfunction to our nosology of PTSD will aid in our ability to define distinct patient groups.

Sexual Problems

Unlike most of the other problems associated with childhood sexual abuse, childhood sexuality problems have not been identified by the DSM-IV-TR as constituting a specific disorder, possibly because there was relatively little research on the topic prior to the 1990s. However, considerable research has since documented the frequencies of various sexual behaviors across childhood and adolescence, which can now serve to help delineate typical from atypical and problematic childhood sexual interests and behaviors. Sexual behaviors can be sorted into several categories (Friedrich et al., 1992): personal boundary deviations, exhibitionism, general role diversions, self-stimulation, sexual anxiety, excessive or precocious sexual interest, sexual intrusiveness, sexual knowledge, and voyeuristic behavior. For the most part, research on the sexual behaviors of children under 12 has relied on parent report, using either the Child Sexual Behavior Inventory (CSBI; Friedrich, 1997) or the Sexual Problems scale of the Child Behavior Checklist (CBCL; Achenbach, 1991). More recently, studies of preschool-age children have also surveyed day care providers (e.g., Sandnabba, Santtila, Wannäs, & Krook, 2003); however, it appears that parents have more opportunities to observe sexual behaviors than day care providers, and thus parent report estimates tend to be higher (Larsson & Svedin, 2002).

Surveys conducted in the United States, Sweden, and Finland reveal that some sexual behaviors are fairly common in children, whereas other behaviors are quite rare. Studies further reveal that frequencies of behaviors vary with age (Friedrich, Fisher, Broughton, Houston, & Shafran, 1998). For example, among preschoolers, 44% of girls and 60% of males engage in genital self-touching, up to 44% of boys and girls touch women's breasts, and 27% of boys and girls try to look at people when they are nude. Among children ages 6–9, it is still fairly common for boys and girls to engage in genital self-touching (40% and 21%, respectively) and to try to look at people when they are nude (20% for both genders). From ages 10 to 12, common sexual behaviors include interest in looking at nudity in pictures or on TV (8.5% to 15% for boys and girls), and both genders show increased interest in the opposite sex (24–29%). Most sexual behaviors decrease across the span of childhood, including genital self-touching, attempts to look at people when they are nude, and touching women's breasts; however, interest in looking at nudity in media (TV, pictures) and interest in the opposite sex tends to increase with age. Several behaviors are unusual regardless of age—particularly overt sexual acts that involve others, such as invitations to engage in sexual acts, French kissing, oral–genital contact, touching animal genitalia, undressing playmates, making sexual sounds, pretend sexual play, and trying to have sexual intercourse. Other unusual sexual behaviors across all childhood ages are drawings that include sex parts, pretending that toys are having sex, and inserting objects in the vagina or rectum.

Chaffin, Letourneau, and Silovsky (2002) have defined child sexual problem behaviors by the following conditions: Such a behavior (1) occurs at greater frequency than developmentally expected; (2) interferes with child's development; (3) occurs with coercion, intimidation, or force; (4) associated with emotional distress; (5) occurs between children of divergent ages or developmental abilities; and (6) repeatedly recurs in secrecy after intervention by caregivers. Research has clearly linked child sexual behavior problems to a history of child sexual abuse. Kendall-Tackett and colleagues (1993) estimated that approximately one-quarter of sexually abused children display such problems. However, the link between sexual behavior problems and child sexual abuse appears to be strongest among preschool-age children. Johnson (1988) reported that 72% of 4- to 6-year-olds with sexual behavior problems had a history of being sexually abused, compared with 42% of 7- to 10-year-olds and 35% of 11- to 12-year-olds. Numerous studies have documented sexual behavior differences between sexually abused children and their nonabused peers (see Friedrich, 1993, for a review). More recently, Friedrich and colleagues (2001) demonstrated differences on the CSBI between sexually abused children and both normative and psychiatric controls. Caution is needed, however, in making assumptions that sexual behavior problems inevitably reflect a history of child sexual abuse. Drach, Wientzen, and Ricci (2001) found no relationship between child sexual behavior problems and confirmation of sexual abuse concerns among children presenting for forensic child abuse investigations.

In the Friedrich and colleagues (2001) study, sexual behavior problems were related to several sexual abuse characteristics: penetration, abuse by a family member, multiple perpetrators, and frequent and longer-term abuse. Family sexuality and child life stress (i.e., events such as parental separations, illnesses, and foster care) also contributed to predictions of sexual behavior problems. Others have linked child sexual problems to child characteristics such as impulsivity, aggression, poor interpersonal skills, and lack of empathy for others (Johnson & Feldmeth, 1993; Rasmussen, Burton, & Christopherson, 1992). Several parental characteristics have also been identified: poor monitoring, family violence, life stress, and poor parent–child attachment (Pithers, Gray, Busconi, & Houchens, 1998; Rasmussen et al., 1992).

Evidence suggests that problematic sexual behaviors during childhood may lead to sexual offending during adolescence, and concerns have been raised that adolescent offending often predates adult offending. Burton (2000) surveyed adjudicated adolescents about their histories of childhood sexual behavior problems and sexual offending. Of those adjudicated for sexual offenses, 45% admitted to sexual offending prior to age 12. For the entire sample (adjudicated adolescents with an admitted history of sexual offending, whether their index offense was sexual assault or not), 47% reported a history of childhood sexual problems. Those with continuous offending (those who began sexual offending in childhood and continued offending during adolescence) had committed more sexual offenses and had engaged in more serious sexual offenses than those whose acts were limited to either childhood or adolescence. Continuously offending adolescents also had more extensive sexual abuse histories. Although it is widely believed that many adult perpetrators of sexual abuse began offending during adolescence, it is not clear how many offending adolescents go on to commit offenses as adults (Prentky & Knight, 1993; Worling, 1998). However, one study demonstrated that 37% of untreated, violent adolescents who committed sexual offenses went on to commit similar offenses as adults (Rubinstein, Yeager, Goodstein, & Lewis, 1993).

Sexual abuse victims are also at significant risk for other sexual problems during adolescence. They tend to be younger when they begin consensual sexual activities, and younger when they have their first consensual sexual intercourse experience (Miller, Monson, & Norton, 1995; Noll, Trickett, & Putnam, 2000; Wyatt, 1985). Up to 66% of pregnant teens report a history of childhood sexual abuse (Boyer & Fine, 1991; Gershenson et al., 1989). In a study of women engaging in prostitution, approximately 60% reported a history of childhood sexual abuse prior to entering prostitution, and 73% indicated that they began their prostituting while they were still minors (Fraser, 1985). In a longitudinal investigation with sexual abuse victims, both childhood sexual abuse and neglect were linked with subsequent prostitution (Widom & Kuhns, 1996). Furthermore, a history of sexual abuse has been related to unsafe sexual decision making and poor HIV-preventive communication skills (Brown, Kessel, Lourie, Ford, & Lipsitt, 1997).

Based on a longitudinal study of female sexual abuse victims, Noll and colleagues (2000) identified three trajectories for sexual development among adolescents/young women who had been sexually abused at least 7 years earlier. Those who had been abused by their biological fathers, as compared to other sexual abuse survivors, tended to be more preoccupied with sex, felt more pressure to have sex, were less effective in their birth control practices, and were more likely to have given birth at least once. These young women reported more male friends and fewer female friends than the other young women, fewer nonpeer male relationships (fathers, grandfathers, etc.), and low satisfaction with male nonpeers. Concerns were raised that those who experienced abuse by their fathers were predisposed to be overly sexual in their relationships with boys, perhaps due to socialization within the father–daughter relationship. In contrast, those who were abused by multiple, nonparental family members and who experienced physical coercion showed less sexual preoccupation, had more negative attitudes toward sex, felt little pressure to engage in sex, and reported more responsible birth control use. Young women who had experienced abuse by one nonparental family member showed no differences from the comparison group in sexual attitudes and behaviors.

Psychotherapy for Sexual Abuse Victims and Their Families

Most longitudinal studies of sexual abuse victims demonstrate significant abatement of symptoms over time (Kendall-Tackett et al., 1993; Oates, O'Toole, Lynch, Stern, & Cooney,

1994; Sas et al., 1993). However, these trends toward symptom abatement appear to stop as time passes. In their 5-year follow-up of an Australian sample of sexually abused children, Tebbutt and colleagues (1997) found no symptom abatement between their 18-month and 5-year follow-up periods. Despite general improvement in symptomatology, a high percentage of sexually abused children continue to show clinically significant symptoms at various assessment points during their childhood (Jumper, 1995; Neumann et al., 1996). Furthermore, between 10% and 33% of sexually abused children show more symptoms over time, including some who were symptom-free at the initial assessment (Kendall-Tackett et al., 1993; Oates et al., 1994). Chronicity of abuse appears to be the only abuse-related variable that consistently relates to duration of symptoms (Famularo, Kinscherff, & Fenton, 1990; Oates et al., 1994). Maternal support and maternal coping have also been related to duration of symptoms (Everson et al., 1989; Goodman et al., 1992). Involvement in therapy does not necessarily relate to symptom abatement (Oates et al., 1994). However, abuse-specific treatment programs show evidence of treatment-related symptom reductions (Finkelhor & Berliner, 1995; Kendall-Tackett et al., 1993).

These longitudinal findings, combined with research on abuse sequelae, highlight the need for sexual abuse treatment and outcome studies of such treatment to assure the following three characteristics (Beutler, Williams, & Zetzer, 1994; Finkelhor & Berliner, 1995):

1. The treatment protocol should address symptoms known to relate to sexual abuse (e.g., PTSD or sexuality problems) or factors known to exacerbate or attenuate sexual abuse sequelae (e.g., social support/family dysfunction, attributional concerns, coping deficits).
2. Participants in treatment research must show clinically significant abuse-related symptoms that are quantified through psychometrically sound assessment tools.
3. The research design must include random assignment to appropriate comparison groups, to control for the passage of time and placebo effects. Because of ethical concerns about withholding treatment, random assignment to treatments that are "standard" in the community is recommended (e.g., nondirective play therapy or standard group therapy for children).

Availability and Utilization of Mental Health Services for Sexual Abuse Victims

Results from a recent national survey of child crime victims revealed that approximately 20% of children who experienced a serious physical or sexual assault received treatment (Kopiec, Finkelhor, & Wolak, 2004). However, only 51% of the parents who had considered the possibility of counseling for their children actually followed through and obtained services. Factors associated with a family's obtaining services were as follows: (1) The perpetrator was known to the victim; (2) the child seemed sad; (3) someone had advised the caregiver that the child should receive counseling; and (4) the family had health insurance. In half of the cases where children received counseling, caregivers had not considered or sought the treatment service provided to their children. In those cases, counseling was most often provided at school, particularly if the assault had occurred at the school and if there was a perception that the victim was at fault to some degree. Of all the assault victims who received counseling, 41% received services at school. Indeed, school psychologists and school guidance counselors are the major providers of mental health care to children and adolescents in the United States (Burns et al., 1995; Leif et al., 1996).

Horowitz, Putnam, and Noll (1997) reported utilization of mental health services among female sexual abuse victims, all of whom had been abused by a family member. Although 98.5% had some therapy experience, there was considerable variation in the duration of treatment and the number of sessions. Whereas a third were involved in treatment for less than 1 year, another third were engaged in therapy for over 2 years. Almost all received individual counseling, half participated in group therapy, and 60.5% were involved in some form of family counseling. Services were primarily provided through sexual assault centers, but 17% received services at a psychiatric hospital, 12% were treated at school, and 7% received residential treatment. Most girls received between 9 and 25 therapy sessions. Family therapy was more common among those whose perpetrator was either a biological father or a sibling. Although 43% of children were reported by their caregivers as having a negative attitude about therapy prior to their first appointment, 60% of those with such an attitude changed their minds and had a positive attitude after commencing therapy. Higher scores on measures of depression and a history of more frequent abuse were related to more involvement in therapy. As is true of those receiving psychotherapy services in general, minorities received the fewest number of therapy sessions.

Developing a Treatment Plan

Sexually abused children are often referred for treatment simply because of their abuse history, because their caregivers expect that the abuse caused psychological damage, or because the caregivers hope to prevent problems "down the road." However, sexual abuse is an event, not a psychological disorder (Berliner, 1997); therefore, the treatment needs of individual children vary widely. Sexually abused children also present for psychotherapy at a number of points in the postdisclosure process. In some cases, referrals are made fairly soon after disclosure, and the families may be in a crisis situation. In other cases, children may be referred because their behavioral and emotional problems have hit a crisis point (e.g., school and foster placements are in jeopardy, or concerns are raised about the need for inpatient or residential treatment). In many cases, children are referred when they enter foster care, and thus the children are coping not only with abuse issues, but also adjusting to a new home, a new school, and separation from their parents. In short, it is important to clarify the presenting problems and consider each child's overall mental health needs, as well as the child's needs that are specific to the sexual abuse.

Before delving into the clinical assessment, it is important to do some general "housekeeping" tasks. As with all clinical cases, it is important to review rules and limits of confidentiality with both the child and caregivers. In most jurisdictions, there are three limits to patient confidentiality: (1) when there is evidence of eminent harm to self or others; (2) when there is evidence of past child abuse that has not already been disclosed, or when there is evidence of significant risk of child abuse; and (3) when a judge issues a court order for clinical records. Whereas most clinical cases have a relatively low risk of requiring clinicians to disclose information without patient and caregiver consent, the risk is clearly higher for sexually abused children and their families. Not only are these families often already involved with child protective services, there may be ongoing or foreseeable legal proceedings in the form of criminal prosecutions, child welfare proceedings, civil suites, and custody and access matters. In our clinic, parents/caregivers and older children are asked to sign a form indicating that they are aware of the limits of confidentiality. It is also important to clarify legal and personal preferences regarding how information shared by one family member will be shared or not shared with other parties. When a child's parents are separated or divorced, it is important to clarify custody and access arrangements and to make sure that both parents and the child are aware of the noncustodial parent's rights to clinical information about the child. These rights differ across jurisdictions, so clinicians should keep abreast of current legislation.

As soon as possible in the assessment process, it is important to have parents/caregivers and older children sign the appropriate consent forms to allow communication with other involved parties, such as child protective services, schools, and lawyers. Intervention plans may include consulting with social workers, schools, and caregivers, and may also include home and school behavioral programs to help establish routines and more positive parent–child interactions. If plans are in place for a child to testify in legal proceedings, it is often wise for the clinician to communicate with prosecutors, to advise them of his or her involvement and inform them of treatment plans. In some cases, clinicians may need to assure prosecutors that their therapeutic procedures will in no way be suggestive or leading with regard to the children's ability to recall events for criminal proceedings. As noted earlier in this chapter, some communities have programs to prepare children for court; however, if such a program is not available, it may be appropriate to consider how the stress of testifying in court will be addressed in the course of therapeutic involvement. Parents who are highly traumatized or who suffer from mental health problems may need to be referred for their own counseling.

If custody and access issues (related either to the abuse or to other circumstances) are outstanding care should be taken to clarify one's role as a psychotherapist, not a custody/access evaluator, and to suggest an independent assessor or mediator to address those issues. Parents are often under the mistaken belief that clinicians' opinions about custody and access arrangements will play an important role in legal decision making. However, because therapists are generally not in a position to make an unbiased judgment about such matters (usually only one parent accompanies a child to counseling when parents are separated or divorced), ethical and professional guidelines generally prohibit clinicians from providing a legal opinion about such matters.

Once "housekeeping" items are addressed, the assessment process can begin. Adequate assessment is required to assure that a treatment plan matches a child's needs. Although the issue of matching presenting problems to type of intervention appears to be fundamental to effective mental health interventions, a surprising number of sexual abuse treatment outcome evaluation programs have failed to match presenting problems with the intervention offered (Beutler et al., 1994; Finkelhor & Berliner, 1995). The problem is magnified in clinical service programs. A survey of programs offering services to sexually abused children and their families revealed that fewer than half utilized standardized or program-specific assessment tools on a regular basis, and that even fewer programs (26%) integrated assessment into the therapeutic process at points before, during, and after treatment (Keller, Cicchinelli, & Gardner, 1989).

Given the wide array of symptoms linked to sexual abuse, the assessment process should be thorough (multimethod, multisymptom, and multi-informant). Assessment strategies should include parent and child reports (and school reports when appropriate and available). When observational assessments (observations of family interactions, play during nondirective play therapy sessions, and behaviors and conversational content during interviews and art sessions) are possible, they can facilitate the interpretations of more standardized assessments (Crittenden, 1996). The assessment protocol should include measures that tap both global (general personality and adjustment problems) and abuse-specific (PTSD Type I and II problems) difficulties. The assessment process should also explore known mediators of abuse-specific sequelae (e.g., attributional and coping style, family relationships). A full exploration of assessment issues is beyond the scope of this chapter; the interested reader should consult Wolfe and Birt (1997).

Our clinic has established a core assessment protocol that includes parent and child reports of the following: child and family demographics and background, child developmental history, and child life events. It also includes measures of current child trauma symptoms (Children's Impact of Traumatic Events Scale–II, parent report and child report versions; Wolfe, 2002); child depression (Children's Depression Inventory; Kovacs, 1999) and overall adjustment (Achenbach System of Empirically Based Assessment [ASEBA]; Achenbach & Rescorla, 2001a, 2001b); child coping (Self-Report Coping Scale; Causey & DuBow, 1992); family adjustment (Family Adaptability and Cohesion Scale–IV; Olson, Goral, & Tiesel, 2002); and parental adjustment (Brief Symptom Inventory; Derogatis, 1993). Clinicians can also administer the Draw-A-Person (with inquiry) as an alternative child assessment strategy, which serves as an icebreaker and provides a standard opportunity to observe a child's behavior in less structured circumstances. As needed, additional assessment tools are administered—including more detailed family assessment measures (e.g., the Family Relations Test; Bene & Anthony, 1957); the CDC, parent report and child report versions (Putnam et al., 1993; Wolfe & Birt, 2002); and teacher-completed adjustment measures, such as the ASEBA Teacher's Report Form (Achenbach & Rescorla, 2001a, 2001b). Psychologists with the team provide feedback to clinicians about the assessment results, and the standard assessment battery serves as our clinic database. Thus we are able to utilize assessment information on a case-by-case basis, and we have the information available for making programmatic decisions.

Once a thorough assessment has been conducted, a clinician needs to triage clinical needs according to those that should be addressed within the realm of the clinician's services and the priorities of those services, and needs that can be served by different agencies (e.g., courtroom preparation programs, groups in the community or at school, individual therapy for a parent). For many sexually abused children and their families, the abuse and its aftermath represent one of many sets of stressors. Treating multiproblem, high-stress families requires good patient–therapist communication about therapeutic process and expectations, the most important being regular attendance. Indeed, multiproblem families tend to have difficulties with regular attendance, so therapists often need to structure therapy to facilitate attendance. McNeil and Herschell (1998) provide several suggestions: (1) Establish convenient, regularly scheduled appointment times that coincide with the availability of transportation and care for other children in the family; (2) establish service contracts that outline responsibilities and consequences for attending and missing scheduled appointments; (3) create a therapeutic environment that is positive, warm, and supportive, and that both the child and parent enjoy; (4) try to provide therapeutic assistance early in the clinical process, so that the family comes to value therapy, and assure that families understand the value of each session in reaching specified therapeutic goals; and (5) avoid "putting out fires" that are not related to treatment goals, by reminding family members of alternative resources for addressing their concerns and reminding them of the need to address "one problem at a time" if sustainable process is to be made.

Because of the heterogeneous needs of sexually abused children and their families, a "modular" treatment approach may be the most effective strategy for developing individualized treatment plans and for evaluating therapeutic effectiveness. That is, specific programs and techniques need to be developed and evaluated that address the particular abuse-specific sequelae exhibited by particular children. Clinicians can then prioritize treatment goals and can systematically utilize proven interventions in a goal-oriented fashion. Particular abuse-specific goals should be established and monitored on a regular basis. Friedrich (1996) has described a goal attainment process that allows for continuous monitoring of therapeutic progress. Goals are individually established, with acceptable and desirable outcomes denoted. In our clinic, specific goals are set following assessment, with a time-limited service plan designed to address specific goals. At the end of each "unit" of treatment (usually about 10 sessions), goal attainment is evaluated, and decisions are made regarding the need for further treatment.

With this in mind, treatment for sexually abused children, particularly those with Type II PTSD, often requires three components: stabilization, abuse-specific treatment, and social reintegration. Although one might conceptualize these components as occurring in phases, the exigencies of particular cases more often govern the order and pace of therapy across the three domains. The central goal of the stabilization component is to facilitate positive, stable home and school environments, and to address any ongoing stressors that are likely to disrupt abuse-specific treatment. Parents often need generic guidance about ways to manage common child behavioral difficulties, as well as guidance about how to respond to emotional displays and behavioral patterns that relate specifically to the abuse. Likewise, children often need to learn the foundations of coping and stress management, in order to address both ongoing stressors and stressors specific to the sexual trauma.

Abuse-specific interventions are those that address symptoms specifically linked to trauma and abuse—primarily PTSD and sexuality problems, but also abuse-related attributions and dissociation. Several forms of cognitive-behavioral therapy have been developed that focus on trauma-related exposures, narrative integrations, affect regulation, social support, and cognitive reframing. Terr (2003), in a moving and insightful case study, highlighted three interrelated components of trauma work: abreaction (full emotional expression of the traumatic event), context (understanding the experience), and correction (finding ways that would have prevented the trauma and/or ways of preventing similar traumas in the future).

Once abuse-specific goals are met, consideration should be given to a need for a third component of treatment, social reintegration. Many sexually abused children not only present with Type II PTSD and sexuality problems, but may also lack social competence, due to their impoverished social environments and due to the stressors associated with the abuse disclosure (Kinard, 2002). They may have lacked opportunities to develop their recreational skills, and thus have difficulties fitting in with their peers at recess and after school. They may lack interpersonal skills and self-confidence in social situations. Although most of these children benefit from joining sports teams and Scout troops, many lack confidence in their abilities, feel uncomfortable socially, and have difficulty regulating their affect in typical peer activities such as competitive games. For this reason, we have developed a group we call Winners. Winners takes a positive psychology perspective, focusing on the building of positive self-esteem, affect regulation skills, optimistic thinking, goal setting and attainment, and interpersonal skills within the recreational contexts of playing games and gym activities. The goals of Winners are to help children develop the confidence to engage in esteem-building activities with peers, build trust in interpersonal relationships with staff and peers, and learn how to utilize affect regulation skills in the context of peer interactions. Many of the Winners components mirror concepts taught in the Resourceful Adolescent Program (Shochet et al., 2001), but are modified for use with younger children. We generally encourage parents to follow up Winners by encouraging their children to join sports teams and to participate in community activities .

Interventions Designed to Reduce PTSD Type I and II Symptoms

Trauma-Focused Psychotherapy for Children and Their Families

In line with both cognitive and conditioning theories, effective treatment of a child's PTSD symptoms requires that the child be exposed to elements of the trauma; preferably, this exposure should include the child providing verbal descriptions of important trauma details. Not only does exposure to distressing memories help the desensitization process, but telling the story helps the child "make sense" of his or her abuse experiences. Research with several different types of traumas has demonstrated that exposure to memories of the trauma is probably the essential element of effective PTSD treatments (van der Kolk, McFarlane, & van der Hart, 1996). Cognitive and cognitive-behavioral therapy, systematic desensitization, stress inoculation, and eye movement desensitization and reprocessing all include elements of exposure and all have demonstrated effectiveness with adult trauma victims.

Foa and Riggs (1993) note that fear-related aspects of trauma memories tend to be more disorganized than other memories, and that this disorganization probably affects a victim's ability to process fear-related information. Perhaps fear-related memories elicit avoidance responses to such an extent that the victim never fully thinks through the entire sequence of his or her memories of the trauma. Rothbaum and Foa (1996) suggest that adult victims derive long-term benefits from therapies that involve prolonged exposure, in part because the process permits a reevaluation of the meaning represented in the memories. Furthermore, repeatedly recalling the memories makes it possible to give structure and organization to the memories.

Two problems arise in translating these exposure-based therapy concepts to children, particularly for those who are quite young. First, many child victims are seen for therapy simultaneously with legal proceedings. Many children have never fully disclosed their abuse, and information revealed in therapy may require further disclosure through legal channels. If a child will be a witness in a criminal proceeding, great caution and careful documentation are needed to assure that processes designed to help a child "make meaning" of his or her experiences do not in some way "lead" or influence further disclosures (i.e., disclosures following leading statements or questions). Careful communication between the therapist and the prosecutor may assure that the process of treatment does not interfere with prosecution.

The second and more common problem with therapy geared toward exposure and "making meaning" relates to the second set of symptom criteria for PTSD, avoidance symptoms. The two most commonly reported avoidance symptoms are that a child "avoids people, places, and situations that remind [him or her] of the trauma" and "avoids thoughts associated with the trauma" (Wolfe & Birt, 2004a). Most children find talking about their past abuse experiences stressful and are quite skillful at avoiding activities that require them to remember or discuss their abuse openly. In fact, avoidance is the likely key to why trauma victims fail to process the emotional aspects of their trauma adequately.

Highly avoidant children may need to be "eased" into discussions of the abuse, once they feel comfortable with their therapists. Most therapies for sexually abused children include avenues for expressing trauma-related feelings and thoughts through both verbal and nonverbal means, such as play, art, and/or drama. Considerable debate has developed regarding the advantages of traditional nondirective play therapy and more directive, goal-oriented play approaches (Rasmussen & Cunningham, 1995). Nondirective play therapy provides a warm, supportive environment for children to resolve their own problems with minimal direction from therapists. Such therapy also helps build therapist–child rapport and allows a child to use play as a medium of expression. The primary disadvantage of this approach lies with the assumption that sexually abused children can "make meaning" of their abuse without external interventions or "corrections." Terr (1991) noted that traumatized children may repeatedly reenact trauma-related themes without apparent resolution. Interpretations and/or corrections are seen as necessary for a child to progress and move forward.

For example, for a child who repeatedly reenacts themes of vulnerability, a therapist might add elements to the play reenactments—themes of external protection (e.g., the mother arrives in time to foil an abuse attempt) or themes of self-efficacy (e.g., the child manages to divert the perpetrator's attention while the child dials 911 to report abusive behavior). Some traumatized children may be so avoidant of trauma-related issues that they limit their play to highly structured activities that allow little self-expression. Thus the children have little opportunity to explore their experiences via the play environment. A more directive play therapist might create an environment for such a child that encourages exploration of abuse-related issues, perhaps through games or activities that address abuse issues directly. Rasmussen and Cunningham (1995) note several other factors that may inhibit sexually abused children from working on their traumas via nondirective play therapy: demands for secrecy by a perpetrator; lack of assertiveness or a belief that children should not talk to adults about sexual abuse; a desire to please the therapist and therefore not to talk about negative life events; and cognitive misattributions or distortions (e.g., children's beliefs that they did something wrong or that a perpetrator will know what happens in the playroom setting).

As an alternative, the play environment can be used to help children understand their abuse via planned activities and experiences. Educational materials can be helpful in assisting children to make meaning of their abuse. The movie *Good Things Can Still Happen* (National Film Board of Canada, 1992) is an entertaining and insightful film designed to help children understand the linkage between symptoms and past abuse. Cunningham and MacFarlane (1991) have developed a number of activities suitable for working individually with children in a structured playroom atmosphere, including a PTSD workbook that involves information, art activities, self-expression, and coping activities. The Rainbow

Game (Rainbow House, Children's Resource Center, 1989) is a board game that includes a number of psychological techniques of self-expression and desensitization (e.g., word association, thematic apperception cards); it also prompts children to solve problems related to uncomfortable situations that place them at risk for abuse, or family- and peer-related problems. Davis and Sparks (1988) have developed a series of therapeutic stories that can be used to introduce such concepts as trauma, empowerment, and healing, as well as issues of secrecy and disclosure.

Eventually, it is important that children be able to talk about their abuse experiences with their therapists (Terr, 2003). However, young children may not be accustomed to providing details in their narratives about life events, or may minimize the sexual aspects of their stories (Saywitz et al., 1991). Saywitz's narrative elaboration procedure (Saywitz & Nathanson, 1993) may be helpful in assisting children to describe their abuse by providing children with cues for information they can include in their stories, without being suggestive. In line with the idea that traumatic memories are processed and stored through different channels, the retelling process should address both verbal accounts of the events, as well as emotional reexperiencing (Terr, 2003). However, as noted earlier, children from dysfunctional homes may have difficulty identifying and describing emotions, and therefore may have difficulty describing their feelings at the time of the abuse. Indeed, they may either avoid emotional expression altogether or have great difficulty regulating the affect associated with the retelling process. Emotional charts can help children identify emotions associated with the abuse, and gentle questioning can help children elaborate on their emotional states and process their feelings. Children might be prompted to elaborate on what it was about the situation that created their emotions and how they coped with their emotions. In the course of exposure sessions, children can use previously taught affect regulation strategies, such as deep breathing and relaxation skills to cope and gain a sense of mastery with regard to their memories of abuse.

Friedrich's (1990) Traumatic Events Interview process, drawn from the work of Eth and Pynoos (1985), provides a good example of a clinical strategy for promoting effective, therapeutic verbal accounts of traumatic experiences. After the therapist "sets the stage" for the child to tell his or her story (e.g., by letting the child know that the therapist has talked with other children who have had similar experiences, creating an expectation that the events need to be described, and/or asking the child to tell the story through drawing), a process of "revivification" can occur, in which the child is encouraged to discuss the details of the abuse and his or her emotional reactions and sensory experiences at the time. To facilitate the retelling, the child is encouraged to recall the worst moments and to explore nightmares that provide clues as to troubling aspects of the trauma. The child is also asked to "make meaning" of the events—that is, to describe his or her understanding of why it happened. The therapist's role at the end of the interview process is to facilitate the story's cohesion and to help the child articulate dialectical emotional reactions (e.g., fear vs. anger, relief vs. guilt). Aspects of the story that reflect positive personal qualities of the victim can be emphasized, such as the child's bravery and wisdom at the time of the trauma and in the present accounting of the events. The interview can end with a discussion of what the child has learned about him- or herself and the abuse as a result of the interview.

Considerable research supports the idea that writing about one's traumatic experiences can be therapeutic (Lepore, Greenberg, Bruno, & Smyth, 2002). Pennebaker, Kiecolt-Glaser, and Glaser (1988) brought attention to this strategy by asking university freshmen to write about their deepest thoughts and feelings relevant to stressful life events, and then following them over the course of their first year at the university. Students in the experimental condition, as compared to those in the control condition, demonstrated both mental and physical health benefits. Lepore and colleagues (2002) suggest that writing about a traumatic event helps desensitize reactivity to stressful stimuli and helps to restructure trauma-related cognitions. Thus one strategy to facilitate children's exposure to and processing of trauma-related memories is to have children write their stories. In our clinic, we have adapted our writing strategy from a book, *Bobby's Story* (Mars, 1999). Bobby is a young child in foster care, and children relate circumstances in their own lives to those experienced by Bobby. Cohen, Deblinger, Mannarino, and Steer (2004) describe a similar process, which they refer to as creating "trauma narratives."

The purpose of creating trauma narratives, as used in our clinic, is to facilitate children's exposure to both the verbally accessible and emotional aspects of the trauma, to facilitate the process of "making meaning" of the traumatic circumstances, and to facilitate the development of a sense of optimism and agency for their future. Some children choose to write the material by hand, whereas others prefer to produce their books on a computer. Details of their stories can be illustrated by using their own drawings, by inserting pictures from magazines, and by inserting images and clip art from graphics programs or from the Internet. Some children prefer to type the material themselves, whereas others prefer to dictate their accounts while the therapist types. Typically a book takes several weeks and even months to complete. Book materials are often reviewed prior to adding new materials, thus providing additional exposure experiences and helping a child to integrate various components of his or her story. The final product is a keepsake that chronicles the child's experiences, documents his or her interpretation of events, and typically ends with the positive aspects of the current situation and a future orientation.

Children begin the writing process by introducing themselves, and describing themselves with regard to their interests, family members, school situation, and other defining characteristics of who they are. This sets a stage to bolster the children's sense of self and the "here and now," and to provide a positive first experience in writing their stories. The children are then encouraged to explore various aspects of the events that were associated with the trauma, usually addressing less traumatic aspects first and then moving toward more difficult aspects. This often takes the form of a chronological account, but not always. Therapists can prompt the children to provide important details, with the idea of promoting expression of increasingly emotionally evocative material. Once the details of the events are produced, children are encouraged to examine how the trauma has affected their lives, and how they have coped. Generally, most children continue to have trauma symptoms at the time their books are being written. Children can use their books to write about those symptoms and their current efforts toward overcoming their problems.

Deblinger and Heflin (1996) described the use of a multicomponent intervention that included a "gradual exposure" intervention (i.e.,

systematic desensitization and prolonged exposure), along with sessions that addressed personal safety training; feelings related to the abuse; relaxation and coping skills; and relationships among thoughts, feelings, and behaviors. For the gradual exposure component, children were encouraged to confront feared stimuli, including their thoughts and memories of the abuse, in a graduated fashion: They were initially encouraged to endure low-level anxiety-provoking stimuli before moving on to confront more distressing stimuli. Children were provided with alternative methods for confronting and addressing abuse-related issues, including openly discussing the abuse, reading, doll play, drawing, writing, poetry, and singing. Therapists initiated discussions of abuse-related issues by reviewing factual information regarding sexual abuse, such as prevalence and information about sexual abuse and perpetrators. Children were then encouraged to describe their least distressing abuse-related memories, followed by increasingly stressful aspects of the abuse. By the end of treatment, the children were expected to confront abuse reminders and discuss abuse-related memories without experiencing significant distress.

Deblinger and Heflin (1996) also described a three-part group program for parents of sexually abused children: (1) coping skills training; (2) training in gradual exposure and in ways to assist children with their gradual exposure therapy; and (3) training in behavior management strategies for assisting children with abuse-related sequelae. The coping skills component was designed to assist parents in coping with their own emotional responses to the sexual abuse disclosure. The coping skills sessions had three goals: (1) educating parents about sexual abuse; (2) helping parents express their emotions in healthy ways; and (3) teaching them effective coping skills. Information about the ways perpetrators engage children and the reasons why children do not disclose abuse is often helpful in debunking parents' dysfunctional thoughts about their own feelings of guilt and responsibility, or their attributions of blame toward the children. Cognitive strategies were used to address dysfunctional thoughts that were either inaccurate, nonproductive (e.g., preoccupation with anger toward a perpetrator), or pessimistic.

Gradual exposure sessions focused on three issues: (1) being able to confront and cope with abuse-related discussions; (2) being able to talk to children directly about the sexual abuse experience; and (3) ways to teach their children about sex and personal safety skills. Open lines of communication were encouraged, and training was based on the principles described by Faber and Mazlish (1980). Parents were taught how to maintain open communication about the abuse as their children matured by encouraging questions about the abuse and sex, reinforcing children's efforts to share their problems with the parents, and encouraging children to express their feelings in effective and appropriate ways.

For the behavior management component, parents learned about the ways that children develop behavioral and emotional problems, particularly problems resulting from sexual abuse. Various behavior management strategies were reviewed, including use of positive reinforcement and praise, principles of differential attention, use of effective instructions, and use of time out. Two specific issues were addressed: sleep problems (sleeping alone, dealing with nightmares) and inappropriate sexual behaviors (masturbation, sexual behavior with peers).

Deblinger, Lippmann, and Steer (1996) examined the effectiveness of the parent and child components with a sample of 100 boys and girls ages 7–13. Four conditions were compared: child-only treatment, parent-only treatment, combined parent–child treatment, and community care. Compared to a community control group and the mother-only training group, children who participated in the gradual exposure treatment displayed fewer parent-reported and child-reported PTSD symptoms at the end of treatment. Improvements in PTSD scores were evident at 6– and 9-month and at 1- and 2-year follow-ups (Deblinger, Steer, & Lippmann, 1999).

Mothers assigned to the parent-only or the combined parent–child treatment, as compared to the child-only treatment or the community control group, described significantly greater decreases in their children's externalizing behaviors and greater improvement in their own parenting skills; their children described significantly greater decreases in their self-reported levels of depression. These findings are particularly encouraging, since some researchers have found that externalizing problems and sexual behavior problems are more resistant to change than some of the other problems related to child sexual abuse (Lanktree & Briere, 1995; Nelki & Waters, 1988).

In a more recent, multisite study, Cohen and colleagues (2004) described a similar parent–child intervention, trauma-focused cognitive-behavioral therapy (TF-CBT). The child program included the following elements: expression of feelings; coping skills; recognizing relationships between thoughts, feelings, and behaviors; gradual exposure; cognitive processing of the abuse experiences; and psychoeducation about child abuse and body safety. The gradual exposure component was enhanced for the study by having the children create trauma narratives, typically in the form of illustrated books. The program also included three joint parent–child sessions designed to optimize communication, to have parents and children review personal safety and healthy sexuality, and to have them review the trauma narrative together. TF-CBT was compared to child-centered therapy (CCT), a parent–child intervention designed to foster a more trusting relationship. Children in the TF-CBT condition showed greater improvement on measures of PTSD, depression, and total behavior problems. They also showed more improvements in interpersonal trust, perceived credibility, and shame. Parents in the TF-CBT condition reported more improvement in their own depression, abuse-related distress, parental support, and parenting practices. More than twice the number of children in the CCT condition continued to meet PTSD criteria fully at posttreatment.

Two programs have developed and evaluated cognitive-behavioral treatments for preschool-age children. Treatments that specifically address preschool-age sexual abuse victims are particularly important for two reasons: (1) Approximately one-third of sexual abuse cases involve a child under age 6; and (2) preschoolers, as compared to adolescents and children, tend to show a higher prevalence of sexually inappropriate behaviors (Friedrich, Urquiza, & Beilke, 1986) and greater fears and PTSD symptoms (Wolfe et al., 1989). Because of the age of these young victims, nonoffending parents need to play a central role in their treatment. Cohen and Mannarino (1996b) developed and evaluated the Cognitive-Behavioral Treatment for Sexual Abuse Program (CBT-SAP), which provided individual therapy to sexually abused children and their nonoffending parents. The program for parents included the following components: attributions of responsibility, emotional support, behavior management, legal issues, and coping with parents' own past abuse. The children's program included the following components: personal safety skill training, feelings about the perpetrator, regressive behaviors, and inappropriate sexual behaviors. Intervention strategies included cognitive reframing, thought stopping, positive imagery, contingency management, and problem solving. Pre–post comparisons of treatment efficacy, compared with a nonspecific therapy approach, demonstrated superior effectiveness of the CBT-SAP on the following variables: the CBCL Internalizing and Externalizing scales, the CSBI, and the Weekly Behavior Record (21 common preschool behavior problems). For the CSBI and the CBCL, preintervention problem scores all fell into the clinical range; at postintervention, all scores from the CBT-SAP group averaged in the nonclinical range. Analyses were conducted to examine factors related to treatment outcome for the CBT-SAP and control groups. In both cases, parental distress related to the abuse was the only variable that added significantly to the prediction equation (Cohen & Mannarino, 1996a). Many of the treatment gains persisted at a 1-year follow-up assessment, and the CBT-SAP group continued to be superior in functioning to the controls (Cohen & Mannarino, 1997).

Deblinger, Stauffer, and Steer (2001) described an 11–session, 2–hour cognitive-behavioral program with parent and child components. The parent component mirrored that from the Deblinger and Heflin (1996) program. The children's group focused on communicating and expressing feelings and personal safety skills (including a behavioral rehearsal component), within the context of other age-appropriate preschool activities such as crafts, singing songs, and reading stories. As compared to a comparison group (parents participated in a self-help group; children took part in the play and personal safety skill group without the behavioral rehearsal portion), mothers in the cognitive-behavioral group were less emotionally upset about their children's sexual abuse, and the children in this group demonstrated better knowledge of personal safety skills. However, the groups improved equally on PTSD symptoms.

Building on the therapeutic strategies of Cohen and Mannarino (1996b) and Deblinger and Heflin (1996), King and colleagues (2000) developed two cognitive-behavioral programs,

one for children and the other involving children and nonoffending mothers. Both programs included 20 child sessions, but the family component had an additional 20 parent sessions that addressed similar issues to those covered in the Cohen and Mannarino (1996b) and Deblinger and Heflin (1996) interventions. As compared to a wait-list control condition, children in both treatment programs showed significantly greater reductions in all three domains of PTSD symptomatology, but those receiving the family component did not evidence greater improvements than those receiving the child-only treatment component. However, the sample size was fairly small.

Psychopharmacological Interventions for PTSD

Alterations to neural processes may account for concerns that PTSD anxieties are particularly resistant to extinction. Nonetheless, some treatment outcome studies with adult combat veterans have demonstrated reductions in physiological reactivity as a result of exposure-based cognitive-behavioral treatments (Boudewyns & Hyer, 1990; Bowen & Lambert, 1986). Adult patients with PTSD are particularly likely to misuse drugs and alcohol, perhaps in an attempt to self-medicate their physiological symptoms (Davidson & van der Kolk, 1996). Furthermore, evidence suggests that both adolescent and adult survivors of child sexual abuse are at increased risk for misusing drugs and alcohol (Peters et al., 2003; see Simpson & Miller, 2002, for a review). For example, Rohsenow, Corbett, and Devine (1988) found that a high percentage of adolescents presenting to residential substance use programs had a history of childhood sexual abuse (71–90% of females and 42% of males).

As remedies for these psychophysiological effects, psychopharmacological approaches have been used both independently and as adjuncts to psychotherapeutic treatment approaches for PTSD. In their review of psychopharmacological treatments for adult PTSD, Albucher and Liberzon (2002) recommended selective serotonin reuptake inhibitors (SSRIs) as the first line of pharmacological treatment, citing evidence from several large controlled trials that various SSRI medications can be effective in treating all three PTSD symptom domains. However, they caution that most studies have had relatively high dropout rates ranging from 13% to 64%, perhaps due to unpleasant medication effects (though these are seen as less prevalent than the side effects of other antidepressant medications) or due to a tendency for patients with PTSD in general to drop out of treatment prematurely. Albucher and Liberzon also noted some evidence for the effectiveness of adrenergic agents (e.g., propranolol, clonidine) for treating hyperarousal symptoms, alone or in combination with other medications, particularly during the early stages of PTSD immediately following trauma exposure. Both propranolol and clonidine have been evaluated with children. Famularo, Kinscherff, and Fenton (1988) reported use of propranolol with child victims of physical and/or sexual abuse, and noted improvements of symptoms related to hypervigilance and hyperarousal. Terr (1997) described using propranolol as an adjunct to systematic desensitization for a young trauma victim. Harmon and Riggs (1997) described using clonidine to treat PTSD symptoms among traumatized preschool children. Positive effects were noted for aggression, impulsivity, emotional lability, hyperarousal, hypervigilance, generalized anxiety, oppositionality, insomnia, and nightmares.

Despite limited empirical guidance for use of medications to treat PTSD symptoms with child and adolescent patients (Cohen, Berliner, & Mannarino, 2003), a survey of child psychiatrists (Cohen, Mannarino, & Rogal, 2001) revealed that 95% used SSRIs to treat PTSD with their child patients, and many others used adrenergic agents, tricyclic antidepressants, anticonvulsants, and antipsychotics. Cohen and colleagues (2003) noted that SSRIs are often selected because adult research supports their efficacy, they have demonstrated effectiveness with other childhood anxiety disorders, and they have fewer unfavorable side effects. At this point, however, no medication has received approval by the U.S. Food and Drug Administration (FDA) for PTSD with child and adolescent patients, including SSRIs. Furthermore, the FDA issued a public health advisory in October 2004 warning that SSRI antidepressants increased the risk of suicidality in children and adolescents with MDD and other psychiatric conditions (U.S. FDA, 2004b). The FDA directed manufacturers to include a Patient Medication Guide and a boxed warning on products regarding the increased risk of suicidality. Recommendations were made to physicians to monitor patients closely, and a schedule was suggested of weekly contacts for the first 4 weeks, biweekly contacts for the subsequent month, and a 12-week follow-up if a patient continued on the medication (FDA, 2004a).

Interventions Addressing Dissociative Symptoms

As noted earlier, dissociation may serve an adaptive function during the traumatic experience by reducing the stress associated with the abuse. However, generalization of dissociative symptoms outside of the abusive situation can become habit-like and can interfere with a child's ability to function interpersonally and academically. As noted earlier, dissociation tends to take three forms: (1) failure to monitor and attend to one's environment, resulting in memory difficulties and forgetfulness; (2) increased absorption into narrow ranges of experience (e.g., being totally engrossed in one's thoughts, play activities, or television programs); and (3) poorly integrated aspects of oneself, perhaps laying the seeds for eventual development of dissociative identity disorder.

In my own limited experience with dissociative children, triggers for the attentional and absorption aspects of dissociative behaviors tend to be ordinary stressors, such as interpersonal or familial stressors, academic pressures, or boredom. Dissociative tendencies are quite notable when children are in the classroom, and may take the form of dawdling, procrastination, passive noncompliance, and intellectual slowness. The "automatic" nature of dissociation in response to stress or other triggers has a resemblance to other habits and stress-related responses, and thus may require treatment components such as those used to address habit disorders. Components of treatment of habit disorders include increasing one's awareness of the habit, self- or other-monitoring, and developing of an alternative or competing response (Azrin & Nunn, 1973). Gil (1991) and James (1989) describe similar strategies for addressing dissociative behavior by providing a label that the child and therapist can use to communicate about the dissociation. The child is then helped to identify situations when he or she dissociates and to develop alternative responses. Gil suggests that the therapist in the playroom environment ask the child to act "as if" he or she is dissociating, which allows the therapist to gain an understanding of the child's dissociative behavior. Collaborative work with teachers and caregivers is essential, since children are unlikely to exhibit dissociative behaviors during structured therapy sessions. Teachers and caregivers can be taught to label the dissociative behaviors for these children and to provide positive instruction and rewards for on-task or alternative behaviors. Because of the "habitual" nature of dissociative behaviors, problems may recur during times of high stress, and booster sessions may be required to assure that the habit does not recur.

With regard to the third form of dissociation, poorly integrated aspects of self, little treatment literature is available for children and adolescents. However, a general guideline for treatment of all child abuse victims is to facilitate personal development in all domains, rather than restricting therapeutic involvement to factors associated with the abuse. In other words, it is important to assure that sexually abused children are progressing well socially, emotionally, interpersonally, and academically, not just that they show reduced PTSD and/or sexuality problems. When this is done, child sexual abuse victims are more likely to develop a sense of self that is well rounded and integrated, not fragmented and dominated by trauma-related sequelae.

Interventions to Address Sexual Behavior Problems for Children under Age 12

A number of programs have been developed to address sexual behavior problems for children under age 12 (see Araji, 1997, for an overview of different treatment programs). Chaffin and colleagues (2002) reviewed two unpublished randomized clinical trials of fairly intensive treatment programs that included both parents and children (Bonner, Walker, & Berliner, 1993; Pithers & Gray, 1993). Although both studies demonstrated reductions in problematic sexual behaviors, neither study demonstrated improvements over less structured comparison treatments. Once sexualized behaviors are identified, most parents will be warned about the importance of monitoring their children when they are with other children, whether it is part of the specific treatment protocol or not. Thus, with high levels of parental monitoring, it may be difficult to assess fully whether children's propensities to engage in sexualized behaviors with peers are suppressed due to fewer opportunities or due to the additive effects of child and parent therapy. This may account for the failure to find group treatment differences, particularly with time-limited programs.

Most sexual behavior treatment programs include both parent and child components. Chaffin and colleagues (2002) highlighted 10 areas often included in parent components: (1) the importance of supervision; (2) arranging for supervision when the child is away from home (e.g., day care, teachers); (3) privacy and sexual behavior rules; (4) distinguishing typical from atypical sexual behaviors; (5) maintaining a nonsexual home environment; (6) communication with children around sexual issues; (7) guidance in implementing behavioral management strategies; (8) guidance in how to support child development of self-control; (9) parent–child communication skills; and (10) appropriate physical and emotional nurturance with children. Seven areas were identified for work with children: (1) acknowledging the sexual behaviors (not a priority with preschool children); (2) rules about sexual behaviors; (3) age-appropriate sex education; (4) impulse- and self-control strategies; (5) sexual abuse prevention/personal safety skills; (6) social skill development; and (7) emotion regulation and coping skills.

In my own practice, depending on the types and frequency of sexualized behaviors reported, parents are often strongly urged to monitor their children's peer play 100% of the time, and are encouraged to arrange for appropriate monitoring of peer interactions in other settings (e.g., day care programs; schools; camps; and unstructured activities with friends, relatives, and neighbors). This can be quite onerous for parents and children alike, and care is needed to assure that the children are not stigmatized by the supervision process. The unfortunate reality is that very few parents are able to achieve the 100% supervision goal, and without monitoring, children may find ways to engage covertly (and perhaps coercively) in sexually inappropriate behaviors with peers. In addition to the potential negative impact of such behaviors on their peers, the social consequences can include being ostracized—if not by the peers, certainly by their parents. Indeed, recurrent sexualized behaviors can have serious implications for both school and home placements. Whereas the parent and child treatment components described by Chaffin and colleagues (2002) are important to successful treatment, it is often difficult to gauge treatment success while the supervision process is in effect. In my own work with these families, I usually work toward gradually lifting supervision once treatment has been successful in addressing relevant sexual behavior risk factors and the child has demonstrated no inappropriate peer-related sexual behavior for a significant period of time. For example, parents may at first have a rule that children must be within visual range when playing with their peers; this can then be loosened to allow play in nearby rooms (with doors open) or outdoors, with frequent monitoring. The process can continue until it is clear that with less intensive supervision, the children are able to refrain from engaging in sexualized behaviors.

Children who present with these problems are often highly sexualized in their presentation and in their interactions with others, which raises concerns that sexuality plays an overly predominant role in their sense of self-worth and value to others. Therefore, as a concomitant intervention, it is important to establish a strategy to help sexualized children develop an alternative sense of self—through positive relationships and achievements at home and school, with adults and children, and in sports, arts, and/or academics. By so doing, children are less likely to attempt to engage other children in sexual behaviors, because they have more socially appropriate interests and skills (e.g., playing soccer and other school-year games, doing art and craft projects together, and talking about interests such as books and music). The balance between supervision and age-appropriate peer activities can be difficult to achieve, but both should hold high priority. Research with adolescent and adult perpetrators has consistently linked offending and relapse to deficits in social skills (Lakey, 1994).

Treatment for Offending Adolescents

Approximately 20% of individuals charged for sexual offenses in North American are adolescents (Federal Bureau of Investigation, 1993; Statistics Canada, 1997). By 1995, over 600 specialized treatment programs were available for adolescent perpetrators (Freeman-Longo, Bird, Stevenson, & Fiske, 1995). Treatment programs often include concurrent groups and individual and family therapy (e.g., Worling & Curwen, 2000), and many utilize cognitive-behavioral strategies, social skills training, sex education, values clarification, cognitive restructuring, covert sensitization, and arousal

satiation (e.g., Becker, 1990). The National Adolescent Perpetrator Network (1988) identified 19 issues that should be addressed in the treatment of offending juveniles: (1) accepting responsibility; (2) identification of offense patterns; (3) ability to disrupt the cycle of offending; (4) personal victimization in terms of sexual, physical, and emotional abuse, and neglect; (5) empathy for the victim; (6) power and control issues; (7) reduction of deviant sexual arousal; (8) development of a positive sexual identify for oneself; (9) understanding the effects of offending on self and others; (10) family issues that trigger offending; (11) "thinking errors" linked with offending; (12) identification and expression of feelings; (13) appropriate social relationships with peers; (14) trust in adults; (15) addictive, compulsive qualities linked with offending; (16) substance use and offending; (17) skill deficits that interfere with successful functioning; (18) relapse prevention; and (19) restitution and reparations to the victim and community.

Despite the proliferation of treatment programs for offending adolescents, outcome evaluations have been limited. Ethical concerns are raised about random assignment to nontreatment programs, particularly when suitable alternative treatments are not available. Program evaluations have primarily been limited to follow-up evaluations of recidivism rates, which are quite unreliable in terms of detecting true rates of posttreatment offending. Worling and Curwen (2000) evaluated a specialized community-based treatment program by comparing those who remained in treatment for at least 1 year to a mixed group of adolescent perpetrators who received preassessment only, refused treatment, or dropped out early. Follow-up ranged from 2 to 10 years. Recidivism was 5% for the treatment group and 18% for the comparison sample, with recidivism predicted by sexual interest in children.

Summary of Tertiary Interventions

Research has indicated two symptoms areas relatively prevalent among sexually abused children: PTSD and sexuality problems. The PTSD literature has grown substantially in recent years, and has included significant conceptual advances in our thinking about the disorder. Indeed, these theoretical advances have helped hone our concepts about risk for developing PTSD and our concepts about the underlying dynamics of each of the three primary PTSD symptom domains. Recent theoretical advances have also broadened our perspective of trauma sequelae beyond the symptoms described by the DSM-IV-TR PTSD symptom criteria. Specifically, some have called for alterations of existing nosologies to account for adjustment problems linked with exposure to multiple traumatic events, including depression and related cognitive constructs, dissociation, affect regulation problems, and coping deficits. Each of these concerns has bearing on overall adjustment, with particular concerns about interpersonal adjustment.

Evidence-based, multicomponent PTSD programs have been developed for use with sexually abused children and their families. Although the focus of the treatments tends to be on the exposure elements, the programs include other important elements (e.g., improved understanding of emotions, affect regulation skills, cognitive and attributional concerns, and improved parent–child relationships). The creation of trauma narratives as an exposure technique is a particularly important clinical advance. Future research is needed to evaluate the effectiveness of the various components to the treatment programs. Moreover, in addressing problems in line with a Type II conceptualization of PTSD, future research is needed to identify appropriate treatment goals and adjunctive therapy components to address such issues as coping, cognitive style, positive sense of self, self-efficacy, and interpersonal relationship skills.

The field has also progressed significantly in our understanding of what distinguishes typical from atypical childhood sexual behaviors. Sexual behavior problems are increasingly being recognized as significant clinical concerns that warrant further research. Several treatment protocols have been developed to address sexualized behavior in children; however, initial efforts to validate treatment approaches have not demonstrated effectiveness beyond that of control groups. However, these studies highlight the path toward further development of both treatment strategies and treatment outcome research methods with this population. Given the serious implications of sexualized behaviors among children, this area of investigation should be given a high priority. Treatment outcome research is quite limited with adolescents. However, this group has a very high potential for serious adjustment problems that have implications for lifelong negative out-comes. Indeed, adolescent adjustment subsequent to sexual abuse is the likely bridge between childhood sequelae and adult adjustment problems.

FUTURE DIRECTIONS

There are many areas of good news for those who work with sexually abused children, and many areas of growth ahead. We are beginning to witness signs that prevention efforts may be paying off in the form of reduced sexual abuse prevalence rates. Comprehensive, universally delivered school-based personal safety training programs are widely implemented across North America; these appear to be effective in teaching skills that truly help children avoid potentially abusive situations, and when abuse does occur, the skills taught appear to help children know the avenues for reporting the abuse and stopping its recurrence. The new interest in including parental components in school-based personal safety is a very positive step. Training programs that include parental components not only improve children's personal safety training skills, but are also likely to help parents become more proactive in assuring their children's protection from potential perpetrators. Indeed, there is a growing awareness of the need for prevention efforts that place less onus on children to protect themselves and greater emphasis on strategies for creating a safer society. Other societal changes have also helped toward this end—increased awareness by professionals of mandated reporting laws, improved abuse investigation practices, increased prosecution, better recognition of the problem of offending adolescents, and improved treatments for offending adolescents and adults. New directions for prevention include greater emphasis on preventing sexual aggression through school-based programs similar to the violence prevention programs now being evaluated. Despite these advances, sexual abuse continues at epidemic proportions. The recognition of the prevalence of sexual abuse and the broad scope of its effects has led some to suggest that sexual abuse should be considered a public health concern. Indeed, recognizing sexual abuse as a public health concern will help sustain and invigorate both public and professional efforts toward eliminating this serious threat to our children's safety and mental health.

Despite current prevention efforts, approximately 70% of child sexual abuse goes undetected (Finkelhor, 1994a). Unfortunately, our current prevention efforts fail to reach many of the children who are most seriously affected (i.e., children abused by family members over long period of time; Sas et al., 1995). Many children fail to disclose abuse because they are concerned about the effects of disclosure. Children are often threatened with violence toward them or toward loved ones if they tell; they are also often led to believe that they will not be believed, that they will go to jail or foster care, or that people will think bad things about them. Most prevention programs do not teach children about the role of child protective services and the process that occurs following disclosure of sexual abuse. Children may need to know that concerted efforts will be made to assure their safety following abuse disclosures; moreover, they may need to be educated about the lies that perpetrators use to ensure their silence (Conte et al., 1986). Many children either are unaware of the role of child protective services or hold negative misperceptions. Whereas police often conduct public relations campaigns to inform the public of their roles, perhaps child protective services should do the same through school- and media-based initiatives that inform children of their roles and put a friendly face on these services.

Even when children disclose sexual abuse and abuse is confirmed, prosecution occurs in only 50% of cases. Sexual abuse cases involving children under the age of 6 are typically not prosecuted, leaving a large proportion of children particularly vulnerable. Even when prosecution is successful in obtaining convictions, it is questionable whether judicial sentencing results in jail or probation terms sufficient to protect the public, either by assuring adequate treatment for perpetrators or by keeping these individuals away from children. Initiatives to inform the public when known perpetrators live in neighborhoods (Megan's Law, 1994; Pam Lychner Sexual Offender Tracking and Identification Act, 1996) and laws keeping those with repeat offenses incarcerated (*Kansas v. Hendricks*, 1997) are important for reducing risks to children.

Twenty years ago, one of the major concerns regarding children's disclosure of sexual abuse was the effect of "system-induced trauma." These systemic stressors included multiple investigative interviews, frightening and often in-

effective legal proceedings, and fragmented child protective service efforts, often due to concerns about the reliability of children's abuse reports. Among the premier accomplishments of the past 20 years have been improvements in our understanding of children's memories and their abilities to recall stressful events without influence of suggestion. Innovations that empower children to tell their stories, such as narrative elaboration training, hold great potential for improvements in investigation, prosecution, and mental health. Great strides have also been made toward "child-friendly" prosecution practices that alter prosecution strategies and empower children in their role as witnesses.

The past decade has witnessed increased sophistication in our understanding of the effects of sexual abuse on children and adolescents, and the impact of such abuse during adult years. There is growing recognition not only that childhood abuse may cause stress and emotional harm, but that abuse has the potential to disrupt typical developmental processes (e.g., one's sense of hope and optimism, one's ability to cope with stress, one's sense of self, and one's ability to form positive and meaningful emotional relationships with others). With our greater understanding of the mechanisms that underlie the short- and long-term effects of abuse, our capacity to identify important treatment goals and intervention strategies is improving. Research on peritraumatic reactions suggests that children's reactions to the stress of the abusive situation may have a significant role in the eventual development of PTSD. This suggests that children who are better able to regulate their affect and who utilize social supports to help them cope are not only more likely to react effectively in the moment of the traumatic event, but are also less likely to develop PTSD down the road. Schools have begun to implement universal delivery programs designed to prevent depression and other mental health problems. A good example is the Resourceful Adolescent Program developed by Shochet and colleagues (2001) for adolescents in grade 8. This program focuses on building several domains of effective coping, including affect regulation, positive thinking, and interpersonal relationships skills. It is likely that these skills will not only help reduce rates of depression, but will also have a positive impact on children's ability to cope with day-to-day stressors and with major traumatic circumstances such as sexual abuse. However, these programs are generally not implemented until the latter years of elementary school or at the entrance to high school. Developmentally sensitive modifications of these programs for earlier grades are needed.

As research into PTSD with children and adolescents develops, there is growing recognition that diagnostic criteria developed with adult trauma victims in mind are not necessarily "one size fits all." Indeed, because of developmental differences in cognition, language, emotion regulation, and dependency, many of the DSM-IV-TR diagnostic criteria are inappropriate for young children; without modifications to these, we are likely to miss identifying some children who are clearly symptomatic as a result of abuse. Alternative criteria for Type I PTSD, as well as developmentally informed criteria related to Type II or complex PSTD, are needed. Furthermore, attention to defining developmentally inappropriate sexual behavior problems is needed. When the dimensions of these abuse-related problems are further clarified, mental health interventions can be developed to address these concerns. Indeed, now that PTSD has been identified as a primary outcome of child sexual abuse, effective programs to treat it have been developed and empirically validated. Of particular note is the collaborative work of Deblinger and her colleagues and of Cohen and Mannarino. Innovations in gradual exposure techniques, paired with treatment components that address emotions, thoughts, behaviors, and relationships, provide important guidance for mental health therapists who are "in the trenches" providing services to children.

Technological advances, particularly neurological imaging capabilities, will undoubtedly advance our understanding of the effects of sexual abuse. Of particular note are some recent findings reported by De Bellis (2001) regarding the impact of maltreatment on children's brains, and the links between these brain effects and decreased intellectual performance. Whereas research with adult trauma victims has revealed some specific areas of brain atrophy associated with trauma and PTSD (see Yehuda & McFarlane, 1997, for a comprehensive review of psychobiology issues with adult trauma victims), findings with children and adolescents suggest more global brain atrophy. Indeed, these findings are likely to spark a new direction in research that focuses on the cogni-

tive and academic impact of child maltreatment and trauma.

ACKNOWLEDGMENTS

I would like to acknowledge the editorial assistance of my colleagues at the Child and Adolescent Centre, with special appreciation of the contributions by Jennifer Nachshen (who assisted with the literature review) and by Lorrie Vandersluis (who provided clerical assistance).

NOTE

1. It appeared that children were less able to coherently report symptoms associated with Stable Personality, though parent report did reveal a Stable Personality construct.

REFERENCES

Abrahams, N., Casey, K., & Daro, D. (1992). Teachers' knowledge, attitudes, and beliefs about child abuse and its prevention. *Child Abuse and Neglect, 16*, 229–238.

Achenbach, T. M. (1991). *Manual for the Child Behavior Checklist/4—18 and 1991 Profile*. Burlington: University of Vermont, Department of Psychiatry.

Achenbach, T. M., & Rescorla, L. A. (2001a). *Mental health practitioners' guide to the Achenbach System of Empirically Based Assessment (ASEBA)* (2nd ed.). Burlington: University of Vermont, Research Center for Children, Youth, and Families.

Achenbach, T. M., & Rescorla, L. A. (2001b). *Manual for the ASEBA School-Age Forms & Profiles*. Burlington: University of Vermont, Research Center for Children, Youth, & Families.

Adams, J. A. (2001). Evolution of a classification scale: Medical evaluation of suspected child sexual abuse. *Child Maltreatment, 6*, 31–36.

Adams, J. A., Harper, K., Knudson, S., & Revilla, J. (1994). Examination findings in legally confirmed child sexual abuse: It's normal to be normal. *Pediatrics, 94*, 310–317.

Adams, J. A., Phillips, P., & Ahmad, M. (1990). The usefulness of colposcopic photographs in the evaluation of suspected child sexual abuse. *Adolescent Pediatric Gynecology, 3*, 75–82.

Adler, N. A., & Schultz, J. (1995). Sibling incest offenders. *Child Abuse and Neglect, 19*, 811–819.

Albucher, R. C., & Liberzon, I. (2002). Psychopharmacological treatment in PTSD: A critical review. *Journal of Psychiatric Research, 36*, 355–367.

Aldgate, J., Colton, M., Chate, D., & Heath, A. (1992). Educational attainment and stability in long term foster care. *Children and Society, 6*, 91–103.

Aldridge, J., & Cameron, S. (1999). Interviewing child witnesses: Questioning techniques and the role of training. *Applied Developmental Science, 3*, 136–147.

Alexander, P. C. (1990). Interventions with incestuous families. In S. W. Henggeler & C. M. Borduin (Eds.), *Family therapy and beyond: A multisystemic approach to treating the behavior problems of children and adolescents* (pp. 324–344). Pacific Grove, CA: Brooks/Cole.

Altshuler, J., & Ruble, D. (1989). Developmental changes in children's awareness of strategies of coping with uncontrollable events. *Child Development, 60*, 1337–1349.

American Professional Society on the Abuse of Children (APSAC). (1990). *Psychosocial evaluation of suspected sexual abuse in children* (2nd ed.). Charleston, SC: Author.

American Psychiatric Association (2000). *Diagnostic and statistical manual of mental disorders* (4th ed., text rev.). Washington, DC: Author.

American Psychological Association. (1994). Guidelines for child custody evaluations in divorce proceedings. *American Psychologist, 49*, 677–680.

Araji, S. (1997). *Sexually aggressive children: Coming to understand them.* Thousand Oaks, CA: Sage.

Arata, C. M. (1998). To tell or nor to tell: Current functioning of child sexual abuse survivors who disclosed their victimization. *Child Maltreatment, 3*, 63–71.

Ashton, V. (1999). Worker judgments of seriousness about and reporting of suspected child maltreatment. *Child Abuse and Neglect, 23*, 539–548.

Association for the Treatment of Sexual Abusers. (2005). *ATSA practice standards and guidelines for the evaluation, treatment, and management of adult male sexual abusers.* Beaverton, OR: Author.

Atabaki, S., & Paradise, J. E. (1997). The medical evaluation of the sexually abused child: Lessons from a decade of research. *Pediatrics, 104*, 178–186.

Azrin, N., & Nunn, R. G. (1973). Habit-reversal: A method of eliminating nervous habits and tics. *Behaviour Research and Therapy, 11*, 619–628.

Badgley, R. F., Allard, H. A., McCormick, N., Proudfoot, P., Fortin, D., Ogilvie, D., et al. (1984). *Sexual offenses against children and youth* (Vols. 1–2). Ottawa: Canadian Government Publishing Centre.

Bagley, C. C., & Mallick, K. (2000). Prediction of sexual, emotional, and physical maltreatment and mental health outcomes in a longitudinal cohort of 290 adolescent women. *Child Maltreatment, 5*, 218–226.

Baker, A. W., & Duncan, S. P. (1985). Child sexual abuse: A study of prevalence in Great Britain. *Child Abuse and Neglect, 9*, 457–467.

Bal, S., Crombez, G., Van Oost, P., & Debourdeaudhuij, I. (2003). The role of social support in well-being and coping with self-reported stressful events in adolescents. *Child Abuse and Neglect, 27*, 1377–1395.

Bal, S., Van Oost, P., Debourdeaudhuij, I., & Crombez, G. (2003). Avoidant coping as a mediator between self-reported sexual abuse and stress-related symptoms in adolescents. *Child Abuse and Neglect, 27*, 883–897.

Band, E., & Weisz, J. (1988). How to feel better when it feels bad: Children's perspectives on coping with everyday stress. *Developmental Psychology, 24*, 247–253.

Barth, R. P., Yeaton, J., & Winterfelt, N. (1994). Psychoeducational groups with foster parents of sexually abused children. *Child and Adolescent Social Work Journal, 11*, 405–424.

Basta, S., & Peterson, R. (1990). Perpetrator status and the personality characteristics of molested children. *Child Abuse and Neglect, 14*, 555–566.

Bayes, J., & Jenny, C. (1990). Genital and anal conditions confused with child sexual abuse trauma. *American Journal of Diseases of Children, 144*, 1319–1322.

Becker, J. V. (1990). Treating adolescent sexual offenders. *Professional Psychology: Research and Practice, 21*, 362–365.

Becker, J. V. (1998). What we know about the characteristics and treatment of adolescents who have committed sexual offenses. *Child Maltreatment, 3*, 317–329.

Becker, J. V., & Johnson, B. R. (2001). Treating juvenile sex offenders. In J. B. Ashford & D. Bruce (Eds.), *Treating adult and juvenile offenders with special needs* (pp. 273–289). Washington DC: American Psychological Association.

Bene, E., & Anthony, J. (1957). *Manual for the Family Relations Test.* London: National Foundation for Education Research.

Benedict, M. A., Zuravin, S., & Stallings, R. R. (1996). Adult functioning of children who lived in kin vs. non-relative family foster home. *Child Welfare, 75*, 529–549.

Berenson, A. B., Chacko, M. R., Wiemann, C. M., Mishaw, C. O., Friedrich, W. N., & Grady, J. J. (2000). A case–control study of anatomic changes resulting from sexual abuse. *American Journal of Obstetrics and Gynecology, 192*, 820–834.

Berliner, L. (1997). Trauma-specific therapy for sexually-abused children. In D. Wolfe, R. McMahon, & R. Peters (Eds.), *Child abuse: New directions in prevention and treatment across the lifespan* (pp. 157–176). Thousand Oaks, CA: Sage.

Berliner, L., & Conte, J. (1995). The process of victimization: The victims' perspective. *Child Abuse and Neglect, 14*, 29–40.

Berliner, L., & Wheeler, J. R. (1987). Treating the effects of sexual abuse on children. *Journal of Interpersonal Violence, 2*, 415–434.

Bernstein, E., & Putnam, F. W. (1986). Development, reliability and validity of a dissociation scale. *Journal of Nervous and Mental Disease, 174*, 727–735.

Berrick, J. D., & Barth, R. (1992). Child sexual abuse prevention: Research review and recommendations. *Social Work Research and Abstracts, 28*, 6–15.

Berrick, J. D., Barth, R. P., & Needell, B. (1994). A comparison of kinship foster homes and foster family homes: Implications for kinship care as family preservation. *Children and Youth Services Review, 16*, 33–63.

Berson, N. L., Herman-Giddens, M. E., & Frothingham, T. E. (1993). Children's perceptions of genital examinations during sexual abuse evaluations. *Child Welfare, 62,* 41–49.

Besharov, D. J. (1994). Responding to child sexual abuse: The need for a balanced approach. *The Future of Children, 4,* 135–155.

Beutler, L. E., Williams, R. E., & Zetzer, H. A. (1994). Efficacy of treatment for victims of child sexual abuse. *The Future of Children, 4,* 156–175.

Binder, R. L., & McNiel, D. E. (1987). Evaluation of a school-based sexual abuse prevention program: Cognitive and emotional effects. *Child Abuse and Neglect, 11,* 497–506.

Blanchard, E. B., Buckley, T. C., Hickling, E., & Taylor, A. E. (1998). Posttraumatic stress disorder and comorbid major depression: Is the correlation an illusion? *Journal of Anxiety Disorders, 12,* 21–37.

Blumberg, E., Landsverk, J., Ellis-MacLeod, E., Ganger, W., & Culver, S. (1996). Use of the public mental health system by children in foster care: Client characteristics and service use patterns. *Journal of Mental Health Administration, 23,* 389–405.

Bolen, R. (2000). Extrafamilial child sexual abuse: A study of perpetrator characteristics and implications for prevention. *Violence against Women, 6,* 1137–1169.

Bolen, R. (2003). Child sexual abuse: Prevention or promotion? *Social Work, 48,* 174–185.

Bolen, R. M., & Lamb, J. L. (2002). Guardian support of sexually abused children: A study of its predictors. *Child Maltreatment, 7,* 265–276.

Boney-McCoy, S., & Finkelhor, D. (1996). Is youth victimization related to trauma symptoms and depression after controlling for prior symptoms and family relationships?: A longitudinal, prospective study. *Journal of Consulting and Clinical Psychology, 64,* 1406–1416.

Bonner, B. L., Walker, C. E., & Berliner, L. (1993). *Children with sexual behavior problems: Assessment and treatment.* Washington, DC: Administration for Children, Youth, and Families, U.S. Department of Health and Human Services.

Boudewyns, P. A., & Hyer, L. (1990). Physiological response to combat memories and preliminary treatment outcome in Vietnam veteran PTSD patients treated with direct therapeutic exposure. *Behavior Therapy, 21,* 63–87.

Bow, J. N., Quinnell, F. A., Zaroff, M., & Assemany, A. (2002). Assessment of sexual abuse allegations in child custody cases. *Professional Psychology: Research and Practice, 33,* 566–575.

Bowen, G. R., & Lambert, J. A. (1986). Systematic desensitization therapy with posttraumatic stress disorder cases. In C. R. Figley (Ed.), *Trauma and its wake* (Vol. 2, pp. 280–291). New York: Brunner/Mazel.

Boyer, D., & Fine, D. (1991). Sexual abuse as a factor in adolescent pregnancy and child maltreatment. *Family Planning Perspectives, 24,* 4–11.

Brant, E. F., King, C. A., Olson, E., Ghaziuddin, N., & Naylor, M. (1996). Depressed adolescents with a history of sexual abuse: Diagnostic comorbidity and suicidality. *Journal of the American Academy of Child and Adolescent Psychiatry, 34,* 34–41.

Brewin, C. R., Dalgleish, T., & Joseph, S. (1996). A dual representation theory of posttraumatic stress disorder. *Psychological Review, 103,* 670–686.

Brewin, C. R., & Holmes, E. A. (2003). Psychological theories of post traumatic stress disorder. *Clinical Psychology Review, 23,* 339–376.

Briere, J., & Runtz, M. (1989). University males' sexual interest in children: Predicting potential indices of "pedophilia" in a nonforensic sample. *Child Abuse and Neglect, 13,* 65–75.

Brosig, C. L., & Kalichman, S. (1992). Child abuse reporting decisions: Effects of statutory wording of reporting requirements. *Professional Psychology: Research and Practice, 23,* 486–492.

Brown, J., Cohen, P., Johnson, J., & Salzinger, S. (1998). A longitudinal analysis of risk factors for child maltreatment: Findings of a 17-year prospective study of officially recorded and self-reported child abuse and neglect. *Child Abuse and Neglect, 22,* 1065–1978.

Brown, L. K., Kessel, S. M., Lourie, K. J., Ford, H., & Lipsitt, L. (1997). Influence of sexual abuse on HIV-related attitudes and behaviors in adolescent psychiatric inpatients. *Journal of the American Academy of Child and Adolescent Psychiatry, 36,* 316–322.

Browne, D. (2002). Coping alone: Examining the prospects of adolescent victims of child abuse placed in foster care. *Journal of Youth and Adolescence, 31,* 57–66.

Bruck, M., Ceci, S. J., & Francoeur, E. (2000). Children's use of anatomically detailed dolls to report genital touching in a medical examination: Developmental and gender comparisons. *Journal of Experimental Psychology: Applied, 6,* 74–83.

Bruck, M., Ceci, S., Francoeur, E., & Renick, A. (1995). Anatomically detailed dolls do not facilitate preschoolers' reports of a pediatric examination involving genital touching. *Journal of Experimental Psychology: Applied, 1,* 95–109.

Bryant, S., & Range, L. (1996). Suicidality in college women who report multiple versus single types of maltreatment by parents: A brief report. *Journal of Child Sexual Abuse, 4,* 87–94.

Bulkley, J. (1988). Legal proceedings, reforms, and emerging issues in child sexual abuse cases. *Behavioral Sciences and the Law, 6,* 153–180.

Burgess, E. S., & Wurtele, S. K. (1998). Enhancing parent–child communication about sexual abuse: A pilot study. *Child Abuse and Neglect, 22,* 1167–1175.

Burns, B., Costello, E., Angold, A., Tweed, D., Stangl, D., Farmer, E., et al. (1995). Children's mental health service use across service sectors. *Health Affairs, 14,* 147–159.

Burton, D. L. (2000). Were adolescent sexual offenders children with sexual problems? *Sexual Abuse: A Journal of Research and Treatment, 12,* 37–48.

Bybee, D., & Mowbray, C. (1993). An analysis of allegations of sexual abuse in a multi-victim day-care centre case. *Child Abuse and Neglect, 17,* 767–783.

Campos, J., Campos, R. G., & Barrett, K. C. (1989). Emergent themes in the study of emotional development and emotion regulation. *Developmental Psychology, 25,* 394–402.

Campos, J., Mumme, D., Kermoian, R., & Campos, R. (1994). A functionalist perspective on the nature of emotion. In N. A. Fox (Ed.), The development of emotion regulation: Biological and behavioral considerations. *Monographs of the Society for Research in Child Development, 59*(2–3, Serial No. 240), 284–303.

Camras, L. A., Ribordy, S., Hill, J., Martino, S., Sachs, V., Spaccarelli, S., et al. (1988). Recognition and posing of emotional expressions by abused children and their mothers. *Developmental Psychology, 24,* 776–781.

Camras, L., Ribordy, S., Hill, J., Martino, S., Sachs, V., Spaccarelli, S., et al. (1990). Maternal facial behavior and the recognition and production of emotional expression by maltreated and nonmaltreated children. *Developmental Psychology, 26,* 304–312.

Canadian Department of Justice. (1992). *Kids in court in the Northwest Territories.* Ottawa: Author.

Cantos, A. L., Gries, L. T., & Slis, V. (1996). Correlates of therapy referral in foster children. *Child Abuse and Neglect, 20,* 921–931.

Cashmore, J. (1992). *The use of close circuit television for child witnesses in the ACT.* Sydney: Australian Law Reform Commission.

Cashmore, J., & Bussey, K. (1996). Judicial views of witness competence. *Law and Human Behavior, 20,* 331–324.

Causey, D. L., & DeBow, E. F. (1992). Development of a self-report coping measure for elementary school children. *Journal of Clinical Child Psychology, 21,* 47–59.

Ceci, S., & Bruck, M. (1993). Suggestibility of the child witness: An historical review and synthesis. *Psychological Bulletin, 113,* 403–439.

Centers for Disease Control and Prevention. (1998). Guidelines for treatment of sexually transmitted diseases. *Morbidity and Mortality Weekly Report, 47,* 111–116.

Cerezo, M. A., & Frias, D. (1994). Emotional and cognitive adjustment in abused children. *Child Abuse and Neglect, 18,* 923–932.

Chaffin, M., Letourneau, E., & Silovsky, J. F. (2002). Adults, adolescents, and children who sexually abuse children: A developmental perspective. In J. E. B. Myers, L. Berliner, J. Briere, C. T. Hendrix, C. Jenny, & T. A. Reid (Eds.), *The APSAC handbook on child maltreatment* (2nd ed., pp. 205–232). Thousand Oaks, CA: Sage.

Chaffin, M., Wherry, J. N., & Dykman, R. (1997). School-age children's coping with sexual abuse: Abuse stresses and symptoms associated with four coping strategies. *Child Abuse and Neglect, 21,* 227–240.

Charney, D. S., Deutch, A. Y., Southwick, S. M., & Krystal, J. H. (1995). Neural circuits and mechanisms of post-traumatic stress disorder. In M. J. Friedman, D. S. Charney, & A. Y. Deutch (Eds.), *Neurobiological and clinical consequences of stress: From normal adaptation to PTSD* (pp. 271–287). Philadelphia: Lippincott-Raven.

Chu, J. A., & Dill, D. L. (1990). Dissociative symptoms in relation to childhood physical and sexual abuse. *American Journal of Psychiatry, 147,* 887–892.

Cohen, J. A., Berliner, L., & Mannarino, A. P. (2003). Psychosocial and pharmacological interventions for child crime victims. *Journal of Traumatic Stress, 16,* 175–186.

Cohen, J. A., Deblinger, E., Mannarino, A. P., & Steer, R. A. (2004). A multisite, randomized controlled trial for children with sexual abuse-related PTSD symptoms. *Journal of the American Academy of Child and Adolescent Psychiatry, 43,* 393–402.

Cohen, J. A., & Mannarino, A. P. (1996a). Factors that mediate treatment outcome of sexually abused preschool children. *Journal of the American Academy of Child and Adolescent Psychiatry, 34,* 1402–1410.

Cohen, J. A., & Mannarino, A. P. (1996b). A treatment outcome study for sexually abused preschool children: Initial findings. *Journal of the American Academy of Child and Adolescent Psychiatry, 35,* 42–50.

Cohen, J. A., & Mannarino, A. P. (1997). A treatment study for sexually abused preschool children: Outcome during a one-year follow-up. *Journal of the American Academy of Child and Adolescent Psychiatry, 36,* 1228–1235.

Cohen, J. A., Mannarino, A. P., & Rogal, S. S. (2001). Treatment practices for childhood posttraumatic stress disorder. *Child Abuse and Neglect, 25,* 123–136.

Cole, P. M., & Putnam, F. W. (1992). Effect of incest on self and self functioning: A developmental psychopathology perspective. *Journal of Consulting and Clinical Psychology, 60,* 174–184.

Committee for Children (Producer). (1996). *What do I say now?: How to help protect your child from sexual abuse* [Film]. (Available from Committee for Children, 2203 Airport Way South, Suite 500, Seattle, WA 98134-2027)

Comparo, L., Wagner, J., & Saywitz, K. (2001). Interviewing children about real and fictitious events: Revisiting the narrative elaboration procedure. *Law and Human Behavior, 25,* 63–80.

Compas, B. E., & Epping, J. E. (1993). Stress and coping in children and families: Implications for children coping with disaster. In C. Saylor (Ed.), *Children and Disasters* (pp. 11–28). New York: Plenum Press.

Conte, E. J., Sorenson, E., Fogarty, L., & Rosa, J. D. (1991). Evaluating children's reports of sexual abuse: Results from a survey of professionals. *American Journal of Orthopsychiatry, 61,* 428–437.

Conte, J., Rosen, C., & Saperstein, L. (1986). An evaluation of a program to prevent the sexual victimization of young children. *Child Abuse and Neglect, 9,* 319–328.

Coons, P. M. (1985). Children of parents with multiple

personality disorder. In R. P. Kluft (Ed.), *Childhood antecedents of multiple personality disorder* (pp. 151–165). Washington, DC: American Psychiatric Press.

Coons, P. M., Bowman, E. S., & Milstein, V. (1988). Multiple Personality Disorder: A clinical investigation of 50 cases. *Journal of Nervous and Mental Disease, 176,* 519–527.

Costello, E. J., Erkanli, A., Fairbank, J. A., & Angold, A. (2002). The prevalence of potentially traumatic events in childhood and adolescence. *Journal of Traumatic Stress, 15,* 99–112.

Crawford v. Washington, 541 U.S. 36, 124 S. Ct. 1354 (2004).

Crittenden, P. A. (1996). Research on maltreating families: Implications for intervention. In J. Briere, J. Bulkley, C. Jenny, & T. Reid (Eds.), *The APSAC handbook on child maltreatment* (pp. 158-174). Thousand Oaks, CA: Sage.

Cross, T. P., Whitcomb, D., & De Vos, E. (1995). Criminal justice outcomes of prosecution of child sexual abuse: A case flow analysis. *Child Abuse and Neglect, 19,* 1431–1442.

Crosse, S. B., Kaye, E., & Ratnofsky, A. C. (1993). *A report on the maltreatment of children with disabilities.* (Contract No. 105-89-11639). Rockville, MD: Westat, Inc., National Centre on Child Abuse and Neglect.

Crouch, J. L., Smith, D. W., Ezzell, C. W., & Saunders, B. E. (1999). Measuring reactions to sexual trauma among children: Comparing the Children's Impact of Traumatic Events Scale and the Trauma Symptom Checklist for Children. *Child Maltreatment, 4,* 255–263.

Cunningham, C., & MacFarlane, K. (1991). *When children molest children: Group treatment strategies for young sexual abusers.* Orwell, VT: Safer Society Press.

Cyr, M., Wright, J., McDuff, P., & Pevron, A. (2002). Intrafamilial sexual abuse: Brother–sister incest does not differ from father–daughter and stepfather–stepdaughter incest. *Child Abuse and Neglect, 26,* 957–973.

Daro, D. A. (1994). Prevention of child sexual abuse. *The Future of Children, 4,* 198–223.

Daro, D. A., & Donnelly, A. C. (2002). Child abuse prevention: Accomplishments and challenges. In J. E. B. Myers, L. Berliner, J. Briere, C. T. Hendrix, C. Jenny, & T. A. Reid (Eds.), *The APSAC handbook on child maltreatment* (2nd ed., pp. 431–448). Thousand Oaks, CA: Sage.

Daro, D., & Gelles, R. (1992). Public attitudes and behaviors with respect to child abuse prevention. *Journal of Interpersonal Violence, 7,* 517–531.

David, J., & Suls, J. (1999). Coping efforts in daily life: Role of Big Five traits and problem appraisals. *Journal of Personality, 67,* 265–294.

Davidson, J. R. T., & van der Kolk, B. A. (1996). The psychopharmacological treatment of posttraumatic stress disorder. In B. A. van der Kolk, A. C.

McFarlane, & L. Weisaeth (Eds.), *Traumatic stress: The effects of overwhelming experience on mind, body, and society* (pp. 510–524). New York: Guilford Press.

Davies, G., & Noon, E. (1991). *An evaluation of the live link for child witnesses.* London: Home Office.

Davies, G., & Westcott, H. (1995). The child witness in the courtroom: Empowerment or protection? In M. Zaragoza, J. Graham, G. Hall, R. Hirschman, & Y. Ben-Porath (Eds.), *Memory and testimony in the child witness* (pp. 199–213). Thousand Oaks, CA: Sage.

Davis, G. E., & Leitenberg, H. (1987). Adolescent sexual offenders. *Psychological Bulletin, 101,* 417–427.

Davis, M. K., & Gidycz, C. A. (2000). Child sexual abuse prevention programs: A meta-analysis. *Journal of Clinical Child Psychology, 29,* 257–265.

Davis, N., & Sparks, T. (1988). *Therapeutic stories to heal children* (rev. ed.). Oxon Hill, MD: Psychological Associates.

De Bellis, M. D. (2001). Developmental traumatology: The psychobiological development of maltreated children and its implications for research, treatment, and policy. *Development and Psychopathology, 13,* 539–564.

Deblinger, E., & Heflin, A. F. (1996). *Treating sexually abused children and their nonoffending parents: A cognitive-behavioral approach.* Thousand Oaks, CA: Sage.

Deblinger, E., Lippmann, J., & Steer, R. A. (1996). Sexually abused children suffering posttraumatic stress symptoms: Initial treatment outcome findings. *Child Maltreatment, 1,* 310–321.

Deblinger, E., Stauffer, L. B., & Steer, R. A. (2001). Comparative efficacies of supportive and cognitive behavioral group therapies for young children who have been sexually abused and their nonoffending mothers. *Child Maltreatment, 6,* 332–343.

Deblinger, E., Steer, R. A., & Lippmann, J. (1999). Two-year follow-up study of cognitive behavioral therapy for sexually abused children suffering post-traumatic stress symptoms. *Child Abuse and Neglect, 23,* 1371–1378.

Deep, A., Lilenfeld, L. R., Plotnicov, K. H., Pollice, C., & Kaye, W. H. (1999). Sexual abuse in eating disorder subtypes and control women: The role of comorbid substance dependence in bulimia. *International Journal of Eating Disorders, 25,* 1–10.

DeJong, A. R., & Rose, M. (1991). Legal proof of child sexual abuse in the absence of physical evidence. *Pediatrics, 88,* 506–511.

Delaronde, S., King, G., Bendel, R., & Reece, R. (2000). Opinions among mandated reporters toward child maltreatment reporting policies. *Child Abuse and Neglect, 27,* 901–910.

DeLoache, J. S., & Marzolf, D. P. (1995). The use of dolls to interview young children: Issues of symbolic representation. *Journal of Experimental Child Psychology, 60,* 1–19.

Derogatis, L. (1993). *The Brief Symptom Inventory*

(BSI): *Administration, scoring, and procedures manual* (3rd ed.). Minneapolis, MN: National Computer Systems.

DiPietro, E. K., Runyan, D., & Frederickson, D. D. (1997). Predictors of disclosure during medical evaluation for suspected sexual abuse. *Journal of Child Sexual Abuse, 6*, 133–142.

Dodge, K. (1989). Coordinating responses to aversive stimuli: Introduction to a special section on the development of emotion regulation. *Developmental Psychology, 25*, 339–342.

Doelling, J. L., & Johnson, H. H. (1990). Predicting success in foster placement: The contribution of parent–child temperament characteristics. *American Journal of Orthopsychiatry, 60*, 585–593.

Dombrowski, S. C., LeMasney, J. W., Ahia, C. E., & Dickson, S. A. (2004). Protecting children from online sexual predators: Technological, psychoeducational, and legal considerations. *Professional Psychology: Research and Practice, 35*, 65–73.

Dong, M., Anda, R. F., Dube, S. R., Giles, W. H., & Felitti, V. J. (2003). The relationship of exposure to childhood sexual abuse to other forms of abuse, neglect, and household dysfunction during childhood. *Child Abuse and Neglect, 27*, 625–639.

Dorado, J., & Saywitz, K. J. (2001). Interviewing preschoolers from low- and middle-SES communities: A test of the narrative elaboration recall improvement techniques. *Journal of Clinical Child Psychology, 30*, 566–578.

Drach, K. M., Wientzen, J., & Ricci, L. R. (2001). The diagnostic utility of sexual behavior problems in diagnosing sexual abuse in a forensic child abuse evaluation clinic. *Child Abuse and Neglect, 25*, 489–503.

Dubner, A., & Motta, R. (1999). Sexually and physically abused foster children and posttraumatic stress disorder. *Journal of Consulting and Clinical Psychology, 67*, 367–373.

Dunne, M. P., Purdie, D. M., Cook, M. D., Boyle, F. M., & Najman, J. M. (2003). Is child sexual abuse declining?: Evidence from a population-based survey of men and women in Australia. *Child Abuse and Neglect, 27*, 141–152.

Egeland, B., & Sussman-Stillman, A. (1996). Dissociation as a mediator of child abuse across generations. *Child Abuse and Neglect, 20*, 1123–1132.

Ehlers, A., & Clark, D. M. (2000). A cognitive model of posttraumatic stress disorder. *Behaviour Research and Therapy, 38*, 319–345.

Ehlers, A., Mayou, R. A., & Bryant, B. (2003). Cognitive predictors of posttraumatic stress disorder in children: Results of a prospective longitudinal study. *Behaviour Research and Therapy, 41*, 1–10.

Eisen, M. L., Quas, J. A., & Goodman, G. S. (2001). *Memory and suggestibility in the forensic interview.* Mahwah, NJ: Erlbaum.

Eisenberg, N., Losoya, S., Guthrie, I., Murphy, B., Shepard, S., Padgett, S., et al. (2001). Parental socialization of children's dysregulated expression of emotion and externalizing problems. *Journal of Family Psychology, 15*, 183–205.

Elliott, D. M., & Briere, J. (1994). Forensic sexual abuse evaluations of older children: Disclosures and symptomatology. *Behavioral Sciences and the Law, 12*, 261–277.

Elliott, M., Browne, K., & Kilcoyne, J. (1995). Child sexual abuse prevention: What offenders tell us. *Child Abuse and Neglect, 19*, 579–594.

Elrod, J. M., & Rubin, R. H. (1993). Parental involvement in sexual abuse prevention education. *Child Abuse and Neglect, 17*, 527–538.

Eth, S., & Pynoos, R. S. (1985). Psychiatric interventions with children traumatized by violence. In E. Benedek & D. Schetky (Eds.), *Emerging issues in child psychiatry and the law* (pp. 285–309). New York: Norton.

Everson, M., & Boat, B. (1989). False allegations of sexual abuse of children and adolescents. *Journal of the American Academy of Child and Adolescent Psychiatry, 28*, 230–235.

Everson, M., & Boat, B. (1994). Putting the anatomical doll controversy in perspective: An examination of major doll uses and relative criticisms. *Child Abuse and Neglect, 18*, 113–129.

Everson, M., Hunter, W., Runyan, D., Edelsohn, G., & Coulter, M. (1989). Maternal support following disclosure of incest. *American Journal of Orthopsychiatry, 59*, 197–207.

Faber, A., & Mazlish, E. (1980). *How to talk so kids will listen and listen so kids will talk.* New York: Avon.

Faller, K. (1991). Possible explanations for sexual abuse allegations in divorce. *American Journal of Orthopsychiatry, 61*, 86–91.

Faller, K. C. (1984). Is the child victim of sexual abuse telling the truth? *Child Abuse and Neglect, 8*, 473–481.

Faller, K. C., Corwin, D. L., & Olafson, E. (1993). Research on false allegations of sexual abuse in divorce. *APSAC Advisor, 6*, 6–10.

Famularo, R., Kinscherff, R., & Fenton, T. (1988). Propranolol treatment of childhood posttraumatic stress disorder, acute type. *American Journal of Diseases of Children, 142*, 1244–1247.

Famularo, R., Kinscherff, R., & Fenton, T. (1990). Symptom differences in acute and chronic presentation of childhood post-traumatic stress disorder. *Child Abuse and Neglect, 14*, 349–444.

Federal Bureau of Investigation. (1993). *Uniform crime reports for the United States.* Washington, DC: U.S. Department of Justice.

Feiring, C., Taska, L., & Lewis, M. (1999). Age and gender differences in children and adolescents adaptation to sexual abuse. *Child Abuse and Neglect, 23*, 115–128.

Feiring, C., Taska, L., & Lewis, M. (2002). Adjustment following sexual abuse discovery: The role of shame and attributional style. *Developmental Psychology, 38*, 79–92.

Fergusson, D., Lynskey, M., & Horwood, J. (1996). Childhood sexual abuse and psychiatric disorder in young adulthood: I. Prevalence of sexual abuse and factors associated with sexual abuse. *Journal of the American Academy of Child and Adolescent Psychiatry, 34*, 1355–1364.

Finkelhor, D. (1979). *Sexually victimized children*. New York: Free Press.

Finkelhor, D. (1980). Sex among siblings: A survey on prevalence, variety, and effects. *Archives of Sexual Behavior, 9*, 171–194.

Finkelhor, D. (1983). Removing the child—prosecuting the offender in cases of sexual abuse: Evidence from the National Reporting System for Child Abuse and Neglect. *Child Abuse and Neglect, 7*, 195–205.

Finkelhor, D. (1986). Prevention: A review of programs and research. In D. Finkelhor, S. Araji, L. Baron, A. Browne, S. Peters, & G. Wyatt (Eds.), *A sourcebook on child sexual abuse* (pp. 224–254). Beverly Hills, CA: Sage.

Finkelhor, D. (1990). Early and long term effects of child sexual abuse: An update. *Professional Psychology: Research and Practice, 21*, 325–330.

Finkelhor, D. (1994a). Current information on the scope and nature of child sexual abuse. *The Future of Children, 4*, 31–53.

Finkelhor, D. (1994b). The international epidemiology of child sexual abuse. *Child Abuse and Neglect, 18*, 409–417.

Finkelhor, D., Asdigian, N., & Dziuba-Leatherman, J. (1995a). The effectiveness of victimization prevention instruction: An evaluation of children's responses to actual threats and assaults. *Child Abuse and Neglect, 19*, 141–153.

Finkelhor, D., Asdigian, N., & Dziuba-Leatherman, J. (1995b). Victimization prevention programs for children: A follow-up. *American Journal of Public Health, 85*, 1684–1689.

Finkelhor, D., & Baron, L. (1986). High risk children. In D. Finkelhor, S. Araji, L. Baron, A. Browne, S. Peters, & G. Wyatt (Eds.), *A sourcebook on child sexual abuse* (pp. 60–88). Beverly Hills, CA: Sage.

Finkelhor, D., & Berliner, L. (1995). Research on the treatment of sexually abused children: A review and recommendations. *Journal of the American Academy of Child and Adolescent Psychiatry, 34*, 1408–1423.

Finkelhor, D., & Dziuba-Leatherman, J. (1994). Victimization of children. *American Psychologist, 49*, 173–183.

Finkelhor, D., & Dziuba-Leatherman, J. (1995). Victimization prevention programs: A national survey of children's exposure and reactions. *Child Abuse and Neglect, 19*, 129–139.

Finkelhor, D., Hotaling, G., Lewis, I. A., & Smith, C. (1990). Sexual abuse in a national survey of adult men and women: Prevalence, characteristics, and risk factors. *Child Abuse and Neglect, 14*, 19–28.

Finkelhor, D., & Jones, L. M. (2003). Putting together evidence on declining trends in sexual abuse: A complex puzzle. *Child Abuse and Neglect, 27*, 133–135.

Finkelhor, D., & Lewis, I. A. (1988). An epidemiological approach to the study of child molestation. *Annals of the New York Academy of Sciences, 528*, 64–78.

Finkelhor, D., Strapko, N., Willis, D., Holden, E., & Rosenberg, M. (1992). *Prevention of child maltreatment: Developmental and ecological perspectives* (pp. 150–167). Oxford: Wiley.

Fischer, G. J. (1991). Is lesser severity of child sexual abuse a reason more males report having liked it? *Annals of Sex Research, 2*, 131–139.

Fleming, J., Mullen, P., & Bammer, G. (1997). A study of potential risk factors for sexual abuse in childhood. *Child Abuse and Neglect, 21*, 49–58.

Foa, E. B., & Riggs, D. S. (1993). Posttraumatic stress disorder in rape victims. In M. B. Riba & A. Tasman (Eds.), *American Psychiatric Press review of psychiatry* (Vol. 12, pp. 272–303). Washington, DC: American Psychiatric Press.

Forehand, R., Miller, D. S., Dutra, R., & Chance, M. W. (1997). Role of parenting in adolescent deviant behavior: Replication across and within two ethnic groups. *Journal of Consulting and Clinical Psychology, 65*, 1036–1041.

Fox, R. E. (1991). Proceedings of the American Psychological Association, Incorporated, for the year 1990: Minutes of the annual meeting of the Council of Representatives. *American Psychologist, 46*, 689–726.

Fraser, B. (1986). A glance at the past, a gaze at the present, a glimpse at the future: A critical analyses of the development of child abuse reporting statutes. *Journal of Juvenile Law, 10*, 641–686.

Fraser, P. (1985). *Pornography and prostitution in Canada*. Ottawa: Government of Canada.

Freeman-Longo, R. E., Bird, S., Stevenson, W. F., & Fiske, J. A. (1995). *1994 nationwide survey of treatment programs and models*. Brandon, VT: Safer Society Press.

Friedrich, W. N. (1990). *Psychotherapy with sexually abused children and their families*. New York: Norton.

Friedrich, W. N. (1993). Sexual victimization and sexual behavior in children: A review of recent literature. *Child Abuse and Neglect, 17*, 59–66.

Friedrich, W. N. (1996). An integrated model of psychotherapy for abused children. In J. Briere, L. Berliner, J. Bulkley, C. Jenny, & T. Reid (Eds.), *The APSAC handbook on child maltreatment* (pp. 104–118). Thousand Oaks, CA: Sage.

Friedrich, W. N. (1997). *Child Sexual Behavior Inventory: Professional manual*. Odessa, FL: Psychological Assessment Resources.

Friedrich, W. N., Fisher, J., Broughton, D., Houston, M., & Shafran, C. R. (1998). Normative sexual behavior in children: A contemporary sample. *Pediatrics, 101*, E9.

Friedrich, W. N., Fisher, J. L., Dittner, C. A., Acton, R., Berliner, L., Butler, J., et al. (2001). Child Sexual Behavior Inventory: Normative, psychiatric, and sexual abuse comparisons. *Child Maltreatment, 6*, 37–49.

Friedrich, W. N., Grambsch, P., Damon, L., Hewitt, S. K., Koverola, C., Lang, R. A., et al. (1992). Child

Sexual Behavior Inventory: Normative and clinical comparisons. *Psychological Assessment, 4*, 303–311.

Friedrich, W. N., Jaworski, T. M., Hexschl, J. E., & Bengston, B. S. (1997). Dissociative and sexual behaviors in children and adolescents with sexual abuse and psychiatric histories. *Journal of Interpersonal Violence, 12,* 155–171.

Friedrich, W. N., Urquiza, A. J., & Beilke, R. L. (1986). Behavior problems in sexually abused young children. *Journal of Pediatric Psychology, 11,* 47–57.

Fryer, G. E., Kraizer, S. K., & Miyoshi, T. (1987a). Measuring actual reduction of risk to child abuse: A new approach. *Child Abuse and Neglect, 11,* 173–179.

Fryer, G. E., Kraizer, S. K., & Miyoshi, T. (1987b). Measuring children's retention of skills to resist stranger abduction: Use of the simulation technique. *Child Abuse and Neglect, 11,* 181–185.

Garbarino, J. (1987). Children's responses to a sexual abuse prevention program: A study of the Spiderman comic. *Child Abuse and Neglect, 11,* 143–148.

Garber, J., Braafladt, N., & Weiss, B. (1995). Affect regulation in depressed and nondepressed children and young adolescents. *Development and Psychopathology, 7,* 93–115.

Garfinkel, P. E., Lin, E., Goering, P., Spegg, C., Goldbloom, D. S., Kennedy, S., et al. (1995). Bulimia nervosa in a Canadian community sample: Prevalence and comparison of subgroups. *American Journal of Psychiatry, 152,* 1052–1058.

Garland, A. F., Landsverk, J. L., Hough, R. L., & Ellis-MacLeod, E. (1996). Type of maltreatment as a predictor of mental health service use for children in foster care. *Child Abuse and Neglect, 20,* 675–688.

Gershenson, H., Musick, J., Ruch-Ross, H., Magee, V., Rubino, K.,& Rosenberg, D. (1989). The prevalence of coercive sexual experience among teenage mothers. *Journal of Interpersonal Violence, 4,* 204–219.

Ghetti, S., Alexander, K. W., & Goodman, G. S. (2002). Legal involvement in child sexual abuse cases: Consequences and interventions. *International Journal of Law and Psychiatry, 25,* 235–251.

Gibson, L. E., & Leitenberg, H. (2000). Child sexual abuse prevention programs: Do they decrease the occurrence of child sexual abuse? *Child Abuse and Neglect, 24,* 1115–1125.

Gil, E. (1991). *The healing power of play: Working with abused children.* New York: Guilford Press.

Giovannoni, J. (1989). Substantiated and unsubstantiated reports of child maltreatment. *Children and Youth Services, 11,* 299–318.

Gladstone, R., & Kaslow, N. (1995). Depression and attributions in children and adolescents: A meta-analytic review. *Journal of Abnormal Child Psychology, 23,* 597–606.

Glod, C. A., & Teicher, M. H. (1996). Relationship between early abuse, posttraumatic stress disorder, and activity levels in prepubertal children. *Journal of the American Academy of Child and Adolescent Psychiatry, 34,* 1384–1393.

Gold, E. (1986). Long-term effects of sexual victimization in childhood: An attributional approach. *Journal of Consulting and Clinical Psychology, 54,* 471–475.

Golden, O. (2000). The federal response to child abuse and neglect. *American Psychologist, 55,* 1050–1053.

Golding, J. M., Alexander, M. C., & Stewart, T. L. (1999). The effect of hearsay witness age in a child sexual assault trial. *Psychology, Public Policy, and Law, 5,* 420–438.

Golding, J. M., Fryman, H. M., Marsil, D. F., & Yozwiak, J. A. (2003). Big girls don't cry: The effect of child witness demeanor on juror decisions in a child sexual abuse trial. *Child Abuse and Neglect, 27,* 1311–1321.

Goldman, J. D. G., & Padayachi, U. K. (2000). Some methodological problems in estimating incidence and prevalence in child sexual abuse research. *Journal of Sex Research, 37,* 305–314.

Goldstein, J., Freud A., & Solnit, A. J. (1979). *Before the best interests of the child.* New York: Free Press.

Gomes-Schwartz, B., Horowitz, J. M., & Cardarelli, A. P. (1990). *Child sexual abuse: The initial effects.* Newbury Park, CA: Sage.

Gonzalez, L. S., Waterman, J., Kelly, R., McCord, J., & Oliveri, M. K. (1993). Children's patterns of disclosures and recantations of sexual and ritualistic abuse allegations in psychotherapy. *Child Abuse and Neglect, 17,* 281–289.

Goodman, G. S., & Aman, C. J. (1991). Children's use of anatomically detailed dolls to recount an event. *Child Development, 61,* 1859–1871.

Goodman, G. S., Bottoms, B., Shaver, P. R., & Qin, J. (1995, March). *Factors affecting children's susceptibility versus resistance to false memory.* Paper presented at the biennial meeting of the Society for Research in Child Development, Indianapolis, IN.

Goodman, G. S., Hirschman, J. E., Hepps, D., & Rudy, L. (1991). Children's memory for stressful events. *Merrill–Palmer Quarterly, 37,* 109–158.

Goodman, G. S., Quas, J. A., Batterman-Faunce, J., Riddlesberger, M., & Kuhn, J. (1997). Children's reactions to and memory for a stressful event: Influences of age, anatomical dolls, knowledge, and parental attachment. *Applied Developmental Science, 1,* 54–75.

Goodman, G. S., Quas, J. A., Bulkley, J., & Shapiro, C. (1999). Innovations for child witnesses: A national survey. *Psychology, Public Policy, and Law, 5,* 255–281.

Goodman, G. S., Taub, E. P., Jones, D. P. H., England, P., Port, L. K., Rudy, L., et al. (1992). Testifying in criminal court: Emotional effects on child sexual assault victims. *Monographs of the Society for Research in Child Development, 57*(6), 1–163.

Goodman-Brown, T. B., Edelstein, R. S., Goodman, G. S., Jones, D. P. H., & Gordon, D. S. (2003). Why children tell: A model of children's disclosure of sexual abuse. *Child Abuse and Neglect, 27,* 525–540.

Gordon, M. A. (1990). The family environment of sexual abuse: An examination of the gender effect. *Journal of Family Violence, 5,* 321–332.

Gordon, M. A. (1992). Recent Supreme Court rulings on child testimony in sexual abuse cases. *Journal of Child Sexual Abuse, 1,* 61–73.

Gorey, K. M., & Leslie, D. R. (1997). The prevalence of child sexual abuse: Integrative review adjustment for potential response and measurement biases. *Child Abuse and Neglect, 21,* 391–398.

Gries, L. T., Goh, D. S., & Cavanaugh, J. (1996). Factors associated with disclosure during child sexual abuse assessment. *Journal of Child Sexual Abuse, 5,* 1–18.

Hafemeister, T. J. (1996). Protecting child witnesses: Judicial efforts to minimize trauma and reduce evidentiary barriers. *Violence and Victims, 11,* 71–92.

Halfon, N., Berkowitz, G., & Klee, L. (1992). Mental health service utilization by children in foster care in California. *Pediatrics, 89,* 1238–1244.

Hamilton, L. (1997). *Contact between sexually abused children and their incestuous fathers: Implications for child post-disclosure adjustment.* Unpublished senior honors thesis, University of Western Ontario, London, ON, Canada.

Hanson, R., F., Kievit, L. W., Saunders, B. E., Smith, D. W., Kilpatrick, D. G., Resnick, H., et al. (2003). Correlates of adolescent reports of sexual assault: Findings from the National Survey of Adolescents. *Child Maltreatment, 8,* 261–272.

Harman, J. S., Childs, G. E., & Kelleher, K. J. (2000). Mental health care utilization and expenditures by children in foster care. *Archives of Pediatric and Adolescent Medicine, 154,* 1114–1117.

Harmon, R., & Riggs, P. (1997). Clonidine for posttraumatic stress disorder in preschool children. *Journal of the American Academy of Child and Adolescent Psychiatry, 35,* 1247–1249.

Haugaard, J., & Reppucci, N. (1988). *The sexual abuse of children.* San Francisco: Jossey-Bass.

Hazzard, A., Celano. M., Gould, J., Lawry, W., & Webb, C. (1995). Predicting symptomatology and self-blame among child sex abuse victims. *Child Abuse and Neglect, 19,* 707–714.

Hecht, D., & Hansen, D. (1999). Adolescent victims and intergenerational issues in sexual abuse. In V. Van Hasselt & M. Hersen (Eds.), *Handbook of psychological approaches with violent criminal offenders: Contemporary strategies and issues* (pp. 303–328). New York: Plenum Press.

Heim, C., Ehlert, U., Hanker, J. P., & Hellhammer, D. H. (1998). Abuse-related posttraumatic stress disorder and alternations of the hypothalamic–pituitary–adrenal axis in women with chronic pelvic pain. *Psychosomatic Medicine, 60,* 309–318.

Henry, J. (1997). System intervention trauma to child sexual abuse victims following disclosure. *Journal of Interpersonal Violence, 12,* 499–512.

Herman, J. L. (1992a). Complex PTSD: A syndrome in survivors of prolonged and repeated trauma. *Journal of Traumatic Stress, 5,* 377–391.

Herman, J. L. (1992b). *Trauma and recovery.* New York: Basic Books.

Hershkowitz, I., & Elul, A. (1999). The effects of investigative utterances on Israeli children's reports of physical abuse. *Applied Developmental Science, 3,* 28–33.

Hershkowitz, I., Orbach, Y., Lamb, M. E., Sternberg, K. J., & Horowitz, D. (2001). The effects of mental context reinstatement on children's accounts of sexual abuse. *Applied Cognitive Psychology, 15,* 235–248.

Hogan, M. (1996). Oral midazolam for pediatric nonacute sexual abuse examinations. *Child Maltreatment, 1,* 361–363.

Holmes, M. M., Resnick, H. S., Kilpatrick, D. G., & Best, C. L. (1996). Rape-related pregnancy: Estimates and descriptive characteristics from a national sample of women. *American Journal of Obstetrics and Gynecology, 175,* 320–324.

Horowitz, L. A., Putnam, F. W., & Noll, J. G. (1997). Factors affecting utilization of treatment services by sexually abused girls. *Child Abuse and Neglect, 21,* 35–48.

Horowitz, M. (1986). *Stress response syndromes* (2nd ed.) Northvale, NJ: Aronson.

Hubert, N., Jay, S., Saltoun, M., & Hayes, M. (1988). Approach–avoidance and distress in children undergoing preparation for painful medical procedures. *Journal of Clinical Child Psychology, 17,* 194–202.

Hunter, W. M., Coulter, M. L., Runyan, D. K., & Everson, M. D. (1990). Determinants of placement for sexually abused children. *Child Abuse and Neglect, 14,* 407–417.

Hyson, M. (1983). Going to the doctor: A developmental study of stress and coping. *Journal of Child Psychology and Psychiatry, 24,* 247–259.

Idaho v. Wright, 110 S. Ct. 3139 (1990).

James, B. (1989). *Treating traumatized children.* Lexington, MA: Lexington Books.

James, S., Landsverk, J., & Slymen, D. J. (2004). Placement movement in out-of-home care: Patterns and predictors. *Children and Youth Services Review, 26,* 185–206.

Janoff-Bulman, R. (1989). Assumptive words and the stress if traumatic events: Applications of the schema construct. *Social Cognition, 7,* 113–136.

Jenny, C. (2002). Medical issues in child sexual abuse. In J. E. B. Myers, L. Berliner, J. Briere, C. T. Hendrix, C. Jenny, & T. A. Reid (Eds.), *The APSAC handbook on child maltreatment* (2nd ed., pp. 235–247). Thousand Oaks, CA: Sage.

Johnson, T. C. (1988). Child perpetrators—children who molest other children: Preliminary findings. *Child Abuse and Neglect, 13,* 571–585.

Johnson, T. C., & Feldmeth, J. R. (1993). Sexual behaviors: A continuum. In E. Gil & T. C. Johnson (Eds.), *Sexualized children: Assessment and treatment of sexualized children and children who molest* (pp. 41–52). Rockville, MD: Launch Press.

Joiner, T. E., & Wagner, K. D. (1995). Attributional style and depression in children and adolescents: A meta-analytic review. *Clinical Psychology Review,* 15, 777–798.

Jones, D. P. H., & McGraw, J. M. (1987). Reliable and fictitious accounts of sexual abuse of children. *Journal of Interpersonal Violence,* 2, 27–45.

Jones, D. P. H., & Seig, A. (1988). Child sexual abuse allegations in custody or visitation cases: A report of 20 cases. In B. Nicholson & J. Bulkley (Eds.), *Sexual abuse allegations in custody and visitation cases* (pp. 22–36). Washington, DC: American Bar Association.

Jones, L. M., Finkelhor, D., & Kopiec, K. (2001). Why is sexual abuse declining?: A survey of state child protection administrators. *Child Abuse and Neglect,* 25, 1139–1158.

Jumper, S. A. (1995). A meta-analysis of the relationship of child sexual abuse to adult psychological adjustment. *Child Abuse and Neglect,* 19, 715–728.

Kalichman, S. C. (1999). *Mandated reporting of suspected child abuse: Ethics, law, and policy* (2nd ed.). Washington, DC: American Psychological Association.

Kansas v. Hendricks, W. L. 338555 (June 23, 1997).

Kaufman, K., Barber, M., Mosher, H., & Carter, M. (2002). Reconceptualizing child sexual abuse as a public health concern. In P. A. Schewe (Ed.), *Preventing violence in relationships: Interventions across the life span* (pp. 27–54). Washington, DC: American Psychological Association.

Kaufman, K., Holmberg, J., Orts, K., McCrady, F., Rotzien, A., Daleiden, E., & Hilliker, D. (1998). Factors influencing sexual offenders' modus operandi: An examination of victim–offender relatedness and age. *Child Maltreatment,* 3, 349–361.

Kehinde v. Commonwealth, 1 Va. App. 342, 338 S.E. 2d 356 (1986).

Keller, R. A., Cicchinelli, L. F., & Gardner, D. M. (1989). Characteristics of child sexual abuse treatment programs. *Child Abuse and Neglect,* 13, 361–368.

Kelley, S. J., Brant, R., & Waterman, J. (1993). Sexual abuse of children in day care centers. *Child Abuse and Neglect,* 17, 71–89.

Kendall-Tackett, K. A., Williams, L. M., & Finkelhor, D. (1993). Impact of sexual abuse on children: A review and synthesis of recent empirical studies. *Psychological Bulletin,* 13, 164–180.

Kenny, M., & McEachern, A. (2000). Racial, ethnic, and cultural factors of childhood sexual abuse: A selected review of the literature. *Clinical Psychology Review,* 20, 905–922.

Kercher, G., & McShane, M. (1984). The prevalence of child sexual victimization in an adult sample of Texas residents. *Child Abuse and Neglect,* 8, 495–502.

Kessler, R., Sonnega, A., Bromet, E., Hughes, M., & Nelson, C. (1995). Posttraumatic stress disorder in the National Comorbidity Survey. *Archives of General Psychiatry,* 52, 1048–1060.

Kilpatrick, D. G., Ruggiero, K. J., Acierno, R., Saunders, B. E., Resnick, H. S., & Best, C. L. (2003). Violence and risk of PTSD, major depressive disor-der, substance abuse/dependence, and comorbidity: Results from the National Survey of Adolescents. *Journal of Consulting and Clinical Psychology,* 71, 692–700.

Kinard, E. M. (2002). Participation in social activities: Maternal ratings of maltreated and nonmaltreated children. *American Journal of Orthopsychiatry,* 72, 118–127.

King, N. J., Tonge, B. J., Mullen, P., Myerson, N., Heyne, D., Rollings, S., et al. (2000). Treating sexually abused children with posttraumatic stress symptoms: A randomized clinical trial. *Journal of the American Academy of Child and Adolescent Psychiatry,* 39, 1347–1355.

Kiser, L. J., Heston, J., Millsap, P. A., & Pruitt, D. B. (1991). Physical and sexual abuse in childhood: Relationship with post-traumatic stress disorder. *Journal of the American Academy of Child and Adolescent Psychiatry,* 30, 776–783.

Kluft, R. P. (1985). Introduction: Multiple personality disorder in the 1980's. In R. P. Kluft (Ed.), *Childhood antecedents of multiple personality* (pp. xiii–xiv). Washington, DC: American Psychiatric Press.

Kogan, S. M. (2004). Disclosing unwanted sexual experiences: results from a national sample of adolescent women. *Child Abuse and Neglect,* 28, 1–19.

Kolko, D. J. (1988). Educational programs to promote awareness and prevention of child sexual victimization: A review and methodological critique. *Clinical Psychology Review,* 8, 195–209.

Kolko, D. J., Moser, J., & Hughes, J. (1989). Classroom training in sexual victimization awareness and prevention skills: An extension of the Red Flag/Green Flag People program. *Journal of Family Violence,* 4, 25–45.

Kolko, D. J., Selelyo, J., & Brown, E. J. (1999). The treatment histories and service involvement of physically and sexually abusive families: Description, correspondent, and clinical correlates. *Child Abuse and Neglect,* 23, 459–476.

Kopiec, K., Finkelhor, D., & Wolak, J. (2004). Which juvenile crime victims get mental health treatment? *Child Abuse and Neglect,* 28, 45–59.

Kovacs, M. (1999). *The Children's Depression Inventory.* Tonawanda, NY: Multi-Health Systems.

Koverola, C., & Foy, D. (1993). Post traumatic stress disorder symptomatology in sexually abused children: Implications for legal proceedings. *Journal of Child Sexual Abuse,* 2, 21–35.

Koverola, C., Pound, J., Heger, A., & Lytle, C. (1993). Relationship of child sexual abuse to depression. *Child Abuse and Neglect,* 17, 390–400.

Kvam, M. H. (2000). Is sexual abuse of children with disabilities disclosed?: A retrospective analysis of child disability and the likelihood of sexual abuse among those attending Norwegian hospitals. *Child Abuse and Neglect,* 24, 1073–1084.

Lakey, J. F. (1994). The profile and treatment of male adolescent sex offenders. *Adolescence,* 29, 755–761.

Lamb, M. E. (1994). The investigation of child sexual

abuse: An interdisciplinary consensus statement. *Journal of Child Sexual Abuse, 3,* 93–106.

Lamb, M. E., Orbach, Y., Sternberg, K. J., Hershkowitz, I., & Horowitz, D. (2000). Accuracy of investigators' verbatim notes of their forensic interviews with alleged child abuse victims. *Law and Human Behavior, 24,* 699–708.

Lamb, M. E., Sternberg, K. J., & Orbach, Y. (2002). Is ongoing feedback necessary to maintain the quality of investigative interviews with allegedly abused children? *Applied Developmental Science, 6,* 35–41.

Lamb, S., & Edgar-Smith, S. (1994). Aspects of disclosure: Mediators of outcome of childhood sexual abuse. *Journal of Interpersonal Violence, 19,* 307–326.

Landeros v. Flood, 17 Cal. 3d 399 (1979).

Lang, P. J. (1984). Cognition in emotion: Concept and action. In C. E. Izard, J. Kagan, & R. B. Zajonc (Eds.), *Emotions, cognitions, and behavior* (pp. 192–228). New York: Cambridge University Press.

Lanktree, C., & Briere, J. (1995). Outcome of therapy for sexually abused children: A repeated measures study. *Child Abuse and Neglect, 19,* 1145–1156.

Larsson, I., & Svedin, C. G. (2002). Teachers' and parents' reports on 3- to 6-year-old children's sexual behavior: A comparison. *Child Abuse and Neglect, 26,* 247–266.

Lawson, L. (1990). Preparing sexually abused girls for genital evaluation. *Issues in Comprehensive Pediatric Nursing, 13,* 155–164.

Lawson, L., & Chaffin, M. (1992). False negatives in sexual abuse disclosure interviews: Incidence and influence of caretaker's belief in abuse in cases of accidental abuse discovery by diagnosis of STD. *Journal of Interpersonal Violence, 7,* 532–542.

Lazebnik, R., Zimet, G. D., Egvert, J., Anglin, T. M., Williams, P., Bunch, D. L., et al. (1994). How children perceive the medical evaluation for suspected sexual abuse. *Child Abuse and Neglect, 18,* 739–745.

Leichtman, M., & Ceci, S. (1995). Effects of stereotypes and suggestions on preschoolers' reports. *Developmental Psychology, 31,* 568–578.

Leif, P. J., Alegria, M., Cohen, P., Goodman, S. H., Horwitz, S. M., Hoven, C. W., et al. (1996). Mental health service use in the community and schools: Results from the four-community MECA study. *Journal of the American Academy of Child and Adolescent Psychiatry, 35,* 889–897.

Leifer, M., Kilbane, T., & Grossman, G. (2001). A three-generational study comparing the families of supportive and unsupportive mothers of sexually abused children. *Child Maltreatment, 64,* 353–364.

Leifer, M., & Shapiro, J. P. (1995). Longitudinal study of the psychological effects of sexual abuse in African American girls in foster care and those who remain home. *Journal of Child Sexual Abuse, 4,* 27–44.

Leifer, M., Shapiro, J. P., & Kassem, L. (1993). The impact of maternal history and behavior upon foster placement and adjustment in sexually abused girls. *Child Abuse and Neglect, 17,* 755–766.

Leippe, M. R., Manion, A. P., & Romanczyk, A. (1993). Discernability or discrimination?: Understanding jurors' reactions to accurate and inaccurate child and adult eyewitnesses. In G. S. Goodman & B. L. Bottoms (Eds.), *Child victims, child witnesses: Understanding and improving testimony* (pp. 469–201). New York: Guilford Press.

Lepore, S. J., Greenberg, M. A., Bruno, M., & Smyth, J. M. (2002). Expressive writing and health: Self-regulation of emotion-related experience, physiology, and behavior. In S. J. Lepore & J. M. Smyth (Eds.), *The writing cure: How expressive writing promotes health and emotional wellbeing* (pp. 99–117). Washington, DC: American Psychological Association.

Leschied, A. W., Chiodo, D., Whitehead, P. C., Hurley, D., & Marshall, L. (2003). The empirical basis of risk assessment in child welfare: The accuracy of risk assessment and clinical judgment. *Child Welfare, 82,* 527–540.

Leung, P., & Erich, S. (2002). Family functioning of adoptive children with special needs: Implications of familial supports and child characteristics. *Children and Youth Services Review, 24,* 799–816.

Leventhal, J. M., Hamilton, J., Rekedal, S., Tebano-Micci, A., & Eyster, C. (1989). Anatomically correct dolls used in interviews of young children suspected of having been sexually abused. *Pediatrics, 84,* 900–906.

Lie, G., & McMurtry, S. L. (1991). Foster care for sexually abused children: A comparative study. *Child Abuse and Neglect, 15,* 111–121.

Ligezinska, M., Firestone, P., Manion, I. G., McIntyre, J., Ensom, R., & Wells, G. (1996). Children's emotional and behavioral reactions following disclosures of extrafamilial sexual abuse: Initial effects. *Child Abuse and Neglect, 20,* 111–125.

Lipovsky, J. (1992). Assessment and treatment of post-traumatic stress disorder in child survivors of sexual assault. In D. Foy (Ed.), *Treating PTSD* (pp. 113–141). New York: Guilford Press.

Lipovsky, J., & Stern, P. (1997). Preparing children for court: A multidisciplinary view. *Child Maltreatment, 2,* 150–163.

Lipovsky, J., Tidwell, R., Kilpatrick, D., Saunders, B., & Dawson, V. (1991, November). *Children as witnesses in criminal court: Is the process harmful?* Paper presented at the 25th annual meeting of the Advancement of Behavior Therapy, New York.

Livingston, R., Lawson, L., & Jones, J. (1993). Predictors of self-reported psychopathology in children abused repeatedly by a parent. *Journal of the American Academy of Child and Adolescent Psychiatry, 32,* 948–953.

Lizardi, H., Klein, D. N., Ouimette, P. C., Riso, L. R., Anderson, R. L., & Donaldson, S. K. (1995). Reports of the childhood early home environment in early-onset dysthymia and episodical major depression. *Journal of Abnormal Psychology, 194,* 132–139.

Long, P. J., & Jackson, J. L. (1990, November). *Defining childhood sexual abuse.* Poster presented at the 24th annual meeting of the Association for Advancement of Behavior Therapy, San Francisco.

Love, L. C., Jackson, J. L., & Long, P. J. (1990, November). *Childhood sexual abuse: Correlates of active termination.* Poster presentation at the 24th annual meeting of the Association for Advancement of Behavior Therapy, San Francisco.

Lynch, D. L., Stern, A. E., Oates, K., & O'Toole, B. I. (1993). Who participates in child sexual abuse research? *Journal of Child Psychology and Psychiatry, 34,* 935–944.

Lynch, L., & Faust, J. (1998). Reduction of distress in children undergoing sexual abuse medical examination. *Journal of Pediatrics, 133,* 296–299.

Lyon, T. D. (1999). The new wave of suggestibility research: A critique. *Cornell Law Review, 84,* 1004–1087.

Lyon, T. D., Saywitz, K., Kaplan, D. L., & Dorado, J. S. (2001). Reducing maltreated children's reluctance to answer hypothetical oath-taking competency questions. *Law and Human Behavior, 25,* 81–92.

MacIntyre, D., & Carr, A. (1999a). Evaluation of the effectiveness of the Stay Safe primary prevention program for child sexual abuse. *Child Abuse and Neglect, 23,* 1307–1325.

MacIntyre, D., & Carr, A. (1999b). Helping children to the other side of silence: A study of the impact of the Stay Safe Programme on Irish children's disclosures of sexual victimization. *Child Abuse and Neglect, 23,* 1327–1340.

MacKay, R. (2005). Bill C-2: An act to amend the Criminal Code (Protection of Children and Other Vulnerable Persons) and the Canadian Evidence Act. Ottawa, ON, Canada: Library of Parliament Information and Research Service.

MacMillan, H. L., Fleming, J. E., Trocme, N., Boyle, M. H., Wong, M., Racine, Y. A., et al. (1997). Prevalence of child physical and sexual abuse in the community: Results from the Ontario Health Supplement. *Journal of the American Medical Association, 278,* 131–135.

MacMillan, H. L., Jamieson, E., & Walsh, C. A. (2003). Reported contact with child protection services among those reporting child physical and sexual abuse: Results from a community survey. *Child Abuse and Neglect, 27,* 1397–1408.

MacMillan, H. L., MacMillan, J. H., Offord, D. R., Griffith, L., & MacMillan, A. (1994). Primary prevention of child sexual abuse: A critical review. Part II. *Journal of Child Psychology and Psychiatry, 35,* 857–876.

Makoroff, R. L., Brauley, J. L., Brandner, A. M., Myers, D. A., & Shapiro, R. A. (2002). Genital examinations for alleged sexual abuse of prepubertal girls: Findings by pediatric emergency medicine physicians compared with child abuse trained physicians. *Child Abuse and Neglect, 26,* 1235–1242.

Manion, I., Firestone, P., Cloutier, P., Ligezinska, M., McIntyre, J., & Ensom, R. (1998). Child extrafamilial sexual abuse: Predicting parent and child functioning. *Child Abuse and Neglect, 22,* 1285–1304.

Mannarino, A., & Cohen, J. (1996). Abuse-related attributions and perceptions of general attributions, and locus of control in sexually abused girls. *Journal of Interpersonal Violence, 11,* 162–180.

Mannarino, A., Cohen, J., & Berman, S. R. (1994). The Children's Attributions and Perceptions Scale: A new measure of sexual abuse-related factors. *Journal of Clinical Child Psychology, 23,* 204–211.

Marchant, R., & Cross, M. (1993). Places of safety?: Institutions, disabled children and abuse. In *Abuse and children who are disabled* [Training resource pack]. Nottingham, UK: Ann Craft Trust, University of Nottingham, Centre for Social Work.

Mars, B. L. (1999). *Bobby's story: A feelings workbook.* Washington, DC: Child Welfare League of America.

Martin, J., Anderson, J. Romans, S., Mullen, P., & O'Shea, M. (1993). Asking about child sexual abuse: Methodological implications of a two stage survey. *Child Abuse and Neglect, 17,* 383–392.

Martin, S. E., & Besharov, D. J. (1991). *Police and child abuse: New policies for expanded responsibilities.* Washington, DC: U. S. Department of Justice, Office of Justice Programs, National Institute of Justice.

Martone, M., Jaudes, P. K., & Cavins, M. K. (1996). Criminal prosecution of child sexual abuse cases. *Child Abuse and Neglect, 20,* 457–464.

Maryland v. Craig, 110 S. Ct. 3157; 47 Cr.L. 2258, U.S. Sup. Ct. (1990).

McCurdy, K., & Daro, D. (1994). Current trends in child abuse reporting and fatalities. *Journal of Interpersonal Violence, 9,* 1–8.

McElroy, L. P. (1992). Early indicators of pathological dissociation in sexually abused children. *Child Abuse and Neglect, 16,* 833–846.

McGee, H., Garavan de Barra, M., Byrne, J., & Conroy, R. (2002). *The SAVI report: Sexual abuse and violence in Ireland. A national study of Irish experiences, beliefs, and attitudes concerning sexual violence.* Dublin: Liffey.

McLeer, S. V., Callaghan, M., Henry, D., & Wallen, J. (1994). Psychiatric disorders in sexually abused children. *Journal of the American Academy of Child and Adolescent Psychiatry, 33,* 313–319.

McLeer, S. V., Deblinger, E., Henry, D., & Orvaschel, H. (1992). Sexually abused children at high risk for post-traumatic stress disorder. *Journal of the American Academy of Child and Adolescent Psychiatry, 31,* 875–879.

McMahon, P. M., & Pruett, R. C. (1999). Child sexual abuse as a public health issue: Recommendations of an expert panel. *Sexual Abuse, 11,* 257–266.

McNamara, J., & McNamara, B. H. (Eds.). (1990). *Adoption and the sexually abused child.* Portland: Human Services Development Institute, University of Southern Maine.

McNeil, C. B., & Herschell, A. D. (1998). Treating multi-problem, high stress families: Suggested strategies for practitioners. *Family Relations, 47,* 259–262.

Megan's Law, P.L. 104-145, 110 Stat. 1345 (1994).

Melton, G., Goodman, G. S., Kalichman, S. C., Levine, M., Saywitz, K., & Koocher, G. P. (1995). Empirical research on child maltreatment and the law. *Journal of Clinical Child Psychology, 24,* 47–77.

Mennen, F. E., & Meadows, D. (1993). The relationship of sexual abuse to symptom levels in emotionally disturbed girls. *Child and Adolescent Social Work Journal, 10,* 319–328.

Merrill, L. L., Thomsen, C. J., Sinclair, B. B., Gold, S. R., & Milner, J. S. (2001). Predicting the impact of child sexual abuse on women: The role of abuse severity, parental support, and coping strategies. *Journal of Consulting and Clinical Psychology, 69,* 992–1006.

Mian, M., Wehrspann, W., Klajner-Diamond, H., LeBaron, D., & Winder, C. (1986). Review of 125 children 6 years of age and under who were sexually abused. *Child Abuse and Neglect, 4,* 223–229.

Miller, B. C., Monson, B. H., & Norton, M. C. (1995). The effects of forced sexual intercourse on white female adolescents. *Child Abuse and Neglect, 19,* 1289–1301.

Miller-Perrin, C., & Wurtele, S. (1986). The child sexual abuse prevention movement: A critical analysis of primary and secondary approaches. *Clinical Psychology Review, 8,* 313–329.

Miltenberger, R., & Thiesse-Duffy, E. (1988). Evaluation of home-based programs for teaching personal safety skills to children. *Journal of Applied Behavior Analysis, 21,* 81–87.

Mitchell, K. J., Finkelhor, D., & Wolak, J. (2003). The exposure of youth to unwanted sexual material on the Internet: A national survey of risk, impact, and prevention. *Youth and Society, 34,* 330–358.

Montoya, J. (1999). Child hearsay statutes: At once over-inclusive and under-inclusive. *Psychology, Public Policy, and Law, 5,* 304–322.

Mowrer, O. H. (1960). *Learning theory and behavior.* New York: Wiley.

Mullen, P. E., Martin, J. L., Anderson, J. C., Romans, S. E., & Herbison, G. P. (1993). Childhood sexual abuse and mental health in adult life. *British Journal of Psychiatry, 163,* 721–732.

Mullen, P. E., Roman-Clarkson, S. E., & Walton, V. A. (1988). Impact of sexual and physical abuse on women's mental health. *Lancet, i,* 841–845.

Multisite Violence Prevention Project. (2004). The Multisite Violence Prevention Project: Background and overview. *Journal of Preventive Medicine, 26,* 3–11.

Myers, J. E. B. (1992). *Legal issues in child abuse and neglect.* Newbury Park, CA: Sage.

Myers, J. E. B., Redlich, A. D., Goodman, G. S., Prizmich, L. P., & Imwinkelried, E. (1999). Jurors' perceptions of hearsay in child sexual abuse cases. *Psychology, Public Policy, and Law, 5,* 388–419.

Nation, M., Crusto, C., Wandersman, A., Kumpfer, K. L., Seybolt, D., Morrissey-Kane, E., et al. (2003). What works in prevention: Principles of effective prevention programs. *American Psychologist, 58,* 449–456.

National Adolescent Perpetrator Network. (1988). The revised report from the National Task Force on Juvenile Sexual Offending. *Juvenile and Family Court Journal, 44,* 1–120.

National Center for Prosecution of Child Abuse. (1993). *Legislation regarding special procedures for child victims/witnesses in criminal child abuse cases.* Washington, DC: Author.

National Center for Prosecution of Child Abuse. (2002). *Legislation regarding the use of closed-circuit television testimony in criminal child abuse proceedings.* Washington, DC: Author.

National Film Board of Canada (Producer). (1992). *Good things can still happen* [Film]. Montreal: Producer.

Nelki, J. S., & Waters, J. (1988). A group for sexually abused young children: Unraveling the web. *Child Abuse and Neglect, 13,* 369–377.

Neumann, D. A., Hauskamp, B. M., Pollock, V. E., & Briere, J. (1996). The long-term sequelae of childhood sexual abuse in women: A meta-analytic review. *Child Maltreatment, 1,* 6–16.

Niederberger, J. M. (2002). The perpetrator's strategy as a crucial variable: A representative study of sexual abuse of girls and its sequelae in Switzerland. *Child Abuse and Neglect, 26,* 55–71.

Nolen-Hoeksema, S., Girgus, J. S., & Seligman, M. (1992). Predictors and consequences of childhood depressive symptoms: A 5-year longitudinal study. *Journal of Abnormal Psychology, 101,* 405–422.

Noll, J. G., Trickett, P. K., & Putnam, F. W. (2000). Social network constellation and sexuality of sexually abused and comparison girls in childhood and adolescence. *Child Maltreatment, 5,* 323–337.

Nunno, M., & Rindfleisch, N. (1991). The abuse of children in out of home care. *Children and Society, 5,* 295–305.

Oates, R. K., O'Toole, B. I., Lynch, D. L., Stern, A., & Cooney, G. (1994). Stability and change in outcomes for sexually abused children. *Journal of the American Academy of Child and Adolescent Psychiatry, 33,* 945–953.

Oberlander, L. B. (1995). Psycholegal issues in child sexual abuse evaluations: A survey of forensic mental health professionals. *Child Abuse and Neglect, 19,* 475–490.

O'Connell, M. A. (1986). Reuniting incest offenders with their families. *Journal of Interpersonal Violence, 1,* 374–386.

Ogata, J. R., Sroufe, L. A., Weinfield, N. S., Carlson, E. A., & Egeland, B. (1997). Development and the fragmented self: Longitudinal study of dissociative symptomatology in a nonclinical sample. *Development and Psychopathology, 9,* 855–879.

Oldfield, D., Hays, B. J., & Megel, M. E. (1996). Evaluation of the effectiveness of Project Trust: An elementary school-based victimization prevention strategy. *Child Abuse and Neglect, 20,* 821–832.

Olson, D., Gorall, D., & Tiesel, J. (2002). *Family Inventories Package*. Minneapolis, MN: Life Innovations.

Ontario Ministry of the Attorney General. (1989). *What's my job in court?* Toronto: Author.

Orbach, Y., Hershkowitz, I., Lamb, M. E., Sternberg, K. J., Esplin, P. W., & Horowitz, D. (2000). Assessing the value of structured protocols for forensic interviews of alleged child abuse victims. *Child Abuse and Neglect, 6*, 733–752.

Orcutt, H. K., Goodman, G. S., Tobey, A. E., Batterman-Faunce, J. M., & Thomas, S. (2001). Detecting deception in children's testimony: Factfinders' abilities to reach the truth in open court and closed-circuit trials. *Law and Human Behavior, 25*, 339–372.

Orelove, F. F., Hollahan, D. J., & Myles, K. T. (2000). Maltreatment of children with disabilities: Training needs for a collaborative response. *Child Abuse and Neglect, 24*, 185–194.

Ornstein, P. A., Follmer, A., & Gordon, B. N. (1995). *The influence of dolls and props on young children's recall of pediatric examinations*. Paper presented at the biennial meeting of the Society for Research in Child Development, Indianapolis, IN.

Oxman-Martinez, J., Rowe, W. S., Straka, S. M., & Thibault, Y. (1997). La baisse d'abuse sexuels. *Revue Québeçoise de Psychologie, 18*, 77–90.

Paine, M. L., & Hansen, D. J. (2002). Factors influencing children to disclose sexual abuse. *Clinical Psychology Review, 22*, 271–295.

Palusci, V. J., & Cyrus, T. A. (2001). Reaction to videocolposcopy in the assessment of child sexual abuse. *Child Abuse and Neglect, 25*, 1535–1546.

Pam Lychner Sexual Offender Tracking and Identification Act, P.L. No. 103-236, 110 Stat. 3093 (1996).

Paradise, J. E., Finkel, M. A., Beiser, A. S., Berenson, A. B., Greenberg, D. B., & Winter, M. R. (1997). Assessments of girls' genital findings and the likelihood of sexual abuse: Agreement among physicians self-rated as skilled. *Archives of Pediatrics and Adolescent Medicine, 15*, 883–891.

Paradise, J. E., Winter, M. R., Finkel, M. A., Berenson, A. B., & Beiser, A. S. (1999). Influence of the history on physicians' interpretations of girls' genital findings. *Pediatrics, 103*, 980–986.

Partridge, S., Hornby, H., & McDonald, T. (1986). *Legacies of loss, visions of gains: An inside look at adoption disruption*. Portland: Human Services Development Institute, University of Southern Maine.

Pelcovitz, D., van der Kolk, B., Roth, S., Mandel, F., Kaplan, S., & Resnick, P. (1997). Development of a criteria set and a Structured Interview for Disorders of Extreme Stress (SIDES). *Journal of Traumatic Stress, 10*, 3–16.

Pence, D., & Wilson, C. (1994). Reporting and investigating child sexual abuse. *The Future of Children, 4*, 70–83.

Pennebaker, J. W., Kiecolt-Glaser, J. K., & Glaser, R. (1988). Disclosure of traumas and immune function: Health implications for psychotherapy. *Journal of Consulting and Clinical Psychology, 56*, 230–245.

People v. Rich, 520 N.Y.S. 2d 911 (1987).

Perry, B. D., Pollard, R. A., Blakley, T. L., Baker, W. L., & Vigilante, D. (1995). Child trauma, the neurobiology of adaptation, and use dependent development of the brain: How states become traits. *Infant Mental Health Journal, 16*, 271–291.

Peters, D. (1990). Confrontational stress and children's testimony: Some experimental findings. In S. Ceci (Chair), *Do children lie? Narrowing the uncertainties*. Symposium conducted at the meeting of the American Psychology and Law Society, Williamsburg, VA.

Peters, R., Tortolero, S., Addy, R., Markham, C., Escobar-Shaves, S., Fernandez-Esquer, M., et al. (2003). The relationship between sexual abuse and drug use: Findings from Houston's Safer Choices 2 program. *Journal of Drug Education, 33*, 49–59.

Peterson, C., & Bell, M. (1996). Children's memory for traumatic injury. *Child Development, 6*, 3045–3070.

Peterson, C., & Biggs, M. (1997). Interviewing children about trauma: Problems with "specific" questions. *Journal of Traumatic Stress, 10*, 279–290.

Peterson, C., & Seligman, M. E. P. (1983). Learned helplessness and victimization. *Journal of Social Issues, 39*, 103–106.

Peterson, L., Tremblay, G., Ewigman, B., & Saldana, L. (2003). Multilevel selected primary prevention of child maltreatment. *Journal of Consulting and Clinical Psychology, 71*, 601–612.

Pierce, R., & Pierce, L. H. (1985). Analysis of sexual abuse hotline reports. *Child Abuse and Neglect, 9*, 37–45.

Pintello, D., & Zuravin, S. (2001). Intrafamilial child sexual abuse: Predictors of postdisclosure maternal belief and protective action. *Child Maltreatment, 6*, 344–352.

Pithers, W. D., & Gray, A. (1993). *Pre-adolescent sexual abuse research project*. Washington, DC: National Center on Child Abuse and Neglect.

Pithers, W. D., Gray, A., Busconi, A., & Houchens, P. (1998). Caregivers of children with sexual behavior problems: Psychological and familial functioning. *Child Abuse and Neglect, 22*, 129–141.

Poole, D. A., & Lamb, M. E. (1998). *Investigative interviews of children: A guide for helping professionals*. Washington, DC: American Psychological Association.

Poole, D. A., & Lindsay, D. S. (1995). Interviewing preschoolers: Effects of nonsuggestive techniques, parental coaching, and leading questions on reports of nonexperienced events. *Journal of Experimental Child Psychology, 60*, 129–154.

Prentky, R. A., & Knight, R. A. (1993). Age of onset of sexual assault: Criminal and life history correlates. In G. C. Nagayama Hall, R. Hirschman, J. R. Graham, & M. S. Zaragoza (Eds.). *Sexual aggression: Issues in etiology, assessment, and treatment* (pp. 43–62). Washington, DC: Taylor & Francis.

Putnam, F. W., Helmers, K., & Trickett, P. K. (1993). Development, reliability, and validity of a child dissociation scale. *Child Abuse and Neglect, 19, 645–656.*

Putnam, F. W., Hornstein, N., & Peterson, G. (1996). Clinical phenomenology of child and adolescent dissociative disorders: Gender and age effects. *Child and Adolescent Psychiatric Clinics of North America, 5,* 351–360.

R. v. Khan, 79 C. R. 3d 1 (1990).

R. v. Levogiannis, 4 S.C.R. 475, 1993 Can.L.II 47 (S.C.C.) (1993).

Rainbow House, Children's Resources Center. (1989). *Rainbow Game.* Warner Robins, GA: Author.

Randall, W., Parrila, R., & Sobsey, D. (2000). Gender, disability status, and risk for sexual abuse in children. *Journal of Developmental Disabilities, 7,* 1–15.

Rasmussen, L. A., Burton, J., & Christopherson, B. (1992). Precursors to offending and the trauma outcome process in sexually reactive children. *Journal of Child Sexual Abuse, 1,* 33–48.

Rasmussen, L. A., & Cunningham, C. (1995). Focused play therapy and nondirective play therapy: Can they be integrated? *Journal of Child Sexual Abuse, 4,* 1–20.

Redlich, A., Goodman, G. S., Myers, J. E. B., & Qin, J. (1996, June). *Jurors' perceptions of children's evidence in child sexual abuse cases: Effects of videotaped testimony and hearsay.* Poster presented at the annual meeting of the American Psychological Association, San Francisco.

Reppucci, N. D., Wolland, J. L., & Fried, C. S. (1999). Social, community, and preventive interventions. *Annual Review of Psychology, 50,* 387–418.

Rich, H. (1996). The effects of a health newsletter for foster parents on their perceptions of the behavior and development of foster children. *Child Abuse and Neglect, 20,* 437–445.

Rind, B., Tromovitch, P., & Bauserman, R. (1998). A meta-analytic examination of assumed properties of child sexual abuse using college samples. *Psychological Bulletin, 124,* 22–53.

Rind, B., Tromovitch, P., & Bauserman, R. (2001). The validity and appropriateness of methods, analyses, and conclusions in Rind et al. (1998): A rebuttal of victimological critique from Ondersma et al. (2001) and Dallam et al. (2001). *Psychological Bulletin, 127,* 734–758.

Rispens, J., Aleman, A., & Goudena, P. (1997). Prevention of child sexual abuse victimization: A meta-analysis of school programs. *Child Abuse and Neglect, 21,* 975–987.

Roberts, I., & Moran, K. (1995). Inter-rater reliability in the medical diagnosis of child sexual abuse. *Journal of Pediatric Child Health, 31,* 290–291.

Rogers, R. W. (1983). Preventive health psychology: An interface of social and clinical psychology. *Journal of Social and Clinical Psychology, 1,* 120–127.

Rogosch, F. A., Cicchetti, D., & Aber, J. L. (1995). The role of child maltreatment in early deviations in cognitive and affective processing abilities and later peer relationship problems. *Development and Psychopathology, 7,* 591–609.

Rohsenow, D., Corbett, R., & Devine, D. (1988). Molested as children: A hidden contribution to substance abuse? *Journal of Substance Abuse Treatment, 5,* 13–18.

Roosa, M. W., Reyes, L., Reinholtz, C., & Angelini, P. J. (1998). Measurement of women's child sexual abuse experiences: An empirical demonstration of the impact of choice of measure on estimates of incidence rates and relationships with pathology. *Journal of Sex Research, 35,* 225–240.

Ross, C., & Joshi, S. (1992). Schneiderian symptoms and childhood trauma in the general population. *Comprehensive Psychiatry, 33,* 269–273.

Ross, D. F., Lindsay, R. C. L., & Marsil, D. F. (1999). The impact of hearsay testimony on conviction rates in trials of child sexual abuse: Toward balancing the rights of defendants and child witnesses. *Psychology, Public Policy, and Law, 5,* 439–455.

Roth, S., Newman, E., Pelcovitz, D., van der Kolk, B., & Mandel, F. (1997). Complex PTSD in victims exposed to sexual and physical abuse: Results from the DSM-IV field trial for posttraumatic stress disorder. *Journal of Traumatic Stress, 10,* 539–555.

Rothbaum, B. O., & Foa, E. B. (1996). Cognitive-behavioral therapy for posttraumatic stress disorder. In B. A. van der Kolk, A. C. McFarlane, & L. Weisaeth (Eds.), *Traumatic stress: The effects of overwhelming experience on mind, body, and society* (pp. 491–509). New York: Guilford Press.

Rubin, K. H., Coplan, R. J., Fox, N. A., & Calkins, S. (1995). Emotionality, emotion regulation, and preschoolers' social adaptation. *Development and Psychopathology, 7,* 49–62.

Rubinstein, M., Yeager, C. A., Goodstein, C., & Lewis, D. O. (1993). Sexually assaultive male juveniles: A follow-up. *American Journal of Psychiatry, 150,* 262–265.

Rudd, J. M., & Herzberger, S. D. (1999). Brother–sister incest, father–daughter incest: A comparison of characteristics and consequences. *Child Abuse and Neglect, 23,* 915–928.

Rudy, L., & Goodman, G. (1991). Effects of participation on children's reports: Implications for children's testimony. *Developmental Psychology, 27,* 1–26.

Ruggiero, K. J., Smith, D. W., Hanson, R. F., Resnick, H. S., Saunders, B. E., Kilpatrick, D. G., et al. (2003). Is disclosure of childhood rape associated with mental health outcome? Results from the National Women's Study. *Child Maltreatment, 9,* 62–77.

Runtz, M. G., & Shallow, J. R. (1997). Social support and coping strategies as mediators of adult adjustment following child maltreatment. *Child Abuse and Neglect, 21,* 211–226.

Runyan, D., Everson, M., Edelson, G., Hunter, M., & Coulter, M. L. (1988). Impact of legal interventions on sexually abused children. *Journal of Pediatrics, 113,* 647–653.

Runyon, M. K., Faust, J., & Orvaschel, H. (2002). Differential symptom pattern of post-traumatic stress disorder (PTSD) in maltreated children with and without concurrent depression. *Child Abuse and Neglect, 26,* 39–53.

Russell, D. E. (1983). The incidence and prevalence of interfamilial and extra familial sexual abuse of female children. *Child Abuse and Neglect, 7,* 133–146.

Russell, D. E. H. (1984). The prevalence and seriousness of incestuous abuse: Stepfathers vs. biological fathers. *Child Abuse and Neglect, 8,* 15–22.

Russell, D. E. H. (1986). *The secret trauma: Incest in the lives of girls and women* (rev. ed.). New York: Basic Books.

Ryan, P., Warren, B. L., & Weincek, P. (1991). Removal of the perpetrator versus removal of the victim in cases of intrafamilial child sexual abuse. In D. D. Knutson & J. L. Miller (Eds.), *Abused and battered: Social and legal responses of family violence* (pp. 123–133). Hawthorne, NY: Aldine de Gruyter.

Sandnabba, N. K., Santtila, P., Wannäs, M., & Krook, K. (2003). Age and gender specific sexual behaviors in children. *Child Abuse and Neglect, 27,* 579–605.

Sas, L., Hurley, P., Austin, G., & Wolfe, D. (1991). *Reducing system-induced trauma for child sexual abuse victims through court preparation, assessment, and follow-up* (Final report to the National Welfare Grants Division, Health and Welfare Canada, Project No. 4555-1-125). Ottawa: Health and Welfare Canada.

Sas, L., Hurley, P., Hatch, A., Malla, S., & Dick, T. (1993). *Three years after the verdict: A longitudinal study of the social and psychology adjustment of child witnesses referred to the Child Witness Project.* London, ON, Canada: London Family Court Clinic.

Sas, L. D., Cunningham, A. H., Hurley, P., Dick, T., & Farnsworth, A. (1995). *Tipping the balance to tell the secret: Public discovery of child sexual abuse.* London, ON, Canada: Family Court Clinic.

Saslawsky, D., & Wurtele, S. (1986). Educating children about sexual abuse: Implications for pediatric intervention and possible prevention. *Journal of Pediatric Psychology, 11,* 235–245.

Saunders, B., Kilpatrick, D., Resnick, H., Hanson, R., & Lipovsky, J. (1992). *Epidemiological characteristics of child sexual abuse: Results from Wave II of the National Women's Study.* Paper presented at the San Diego Conference on Responding to Child Maltreatment, San Diego, CA.

Saunders, B., Villeponteaux, L., Lipovsky, J., Kilpatrick, D., & Veronen, L. (1993). Child sexual abuse as a risk factor for mental disorders among women: A community survey. *Journal of Interpersonal Violence, 7,* 189–204.

Sauzier, M. (1989). Disclosure of child sexual abuse: For better or for worse? *Psychiatric Clinics of North America, 12,* 455–569.

Saywitz, K. J., Goodman, G., & Lyon, T. (2002). Interviewing children in and out of court: Current research and practice implications. In J. E. B. Myers, L.

Berliner, J. Briere, C. T. Hendrix, C. Jenny, & T. A. Reid (Eds.), *The APSAC handbook on child maltreatment* (2nd ed., pp. 349–377). Thousand Oaks, CA: Sage.

Saywitz, K. J., Goodman, G., Nicholas, E., & Moan, S. (1991). Children's memories of a physical examination involving genital touch: Implications for reports of child sexual abuse. *Journal of Consulting and Clinical Psychology, 59,* 682–691.

Saywitz, K. J., & Moan-Hardie, S. (1994). Reducing the potential for distortion of childhood memories. *Consciousness and Cognition, 3,* 257–293.

Saywitz, K. J., & Nathanson, R. (1993). Children's testimony and their perceptions of stress in and out of the courtroom. *Child Abuse and Neglect, 17,* 613–622.

Saywitz, K. J., Nathanson, R., & Snyder, L. (1993). Credibility of child witnesses: The role of communicative competence. *Topics in Language Disorders, 13,* 59–78.

Saywitz, K. J., & Snyder, L. (1996). Narrative elaboration: Test of a new procedure for interviewing children. *Journal of Consulting and Clinical Psychology, 64,* 1347–1357.

Saywitz, K. J., Snyder, L., & Lamphear, V. (1996). Helping children tell what happened: A follow-up study of the narrative elaboration procedure. *Child Maltreatment, 1,* 200–212.

Saywitz, K. J., Snyder, L., & Nathanson, R. (1999). Facilitating the communicative competence of the child witness. *Applied Developmental Science, 3,* 58–68.

Scheeeinga, M. S., Peebles, C. D., Cook, C. A., & Zeanah, C. H. (2001). Toward establishing procedural, criterion, and discriminant validity for PTSD in early childhood. *Journal of the American Academy of Child and Adolescent Psychiatry, 40,* 52–60.

Scheeringa, M. S., Zeanah, C. H., Drell, M. J., & Larrieu, J. A. (1995). Two approaches to the diagnosis of posttraumatic stress disorder in infancy and early childhood. *Journal of the American Academy of Child and Adolescent Psychiatry, 35,* 191–200.

Scheeringa, M. S., Zeanah, C. H., Myers, L., & Putnam, F. W. (2003). New findings on alternative criteria for PTSD in preschool children. *Journal of the American Academy of Child and Adolescent Psychiatry, 42,* 561–570.

Seligman, M., Peterson, C., Kaslow, N., Tanenbaum, R., Alloy, L., & Abramson, L. (1984). Attributional style and depressive symptoms among children. *Journal of Abnormal Psychology, 93,* 235–238.

Shalev, A. Y., Friedman, M. J., Foa, E. B., & Keane, T. M. (2000). Integration and summary. In E. B. Foa, T. M. Keane, & M. J. Friedman (Eds.), *Effective treatments for PTSD: Practice guidelines from the International Society for Traumatic Stress Studies* (pp. 359–379). New York: Guilford Press.

Shannon, M. P., Lonigan, C. J., Finch, A. J., Jr., & Taylor, C. M. (1994). Children exposed to disaster: I. Epidemiology of post-traumatic symptoms and symptom profiles. *Journal of the American Academy of Child and Adolescent Psychiatry, 33,* 80–93.

Sher, K. J., & Eisenberg, N. (2002). Publication of Rind et al. (1998): The editors' perspective. *American Psychologist, 57*, 206–210.

Shields, A., Ryan, R. M., & Cicchetti, D. (2001). Narrative representations of caregivers and emotion dysregulation as predictors of maltreated children's rejection by peers. *Developmental Psychology, 37*, 321–337.

Shipman, K., Zeman, J., Penza, S., & Champion, K. (2000). Emotion management skills in sexually maltreated girls: A developmental psychopathology perspective. *Development and Psychopathology, 12*, 47–62.

Shochet, I. M., Dadds, M. R., Holland, D., Whitefield, K., Harnett, P. H., & Osgarby, S. M. (2001). The efficacy of a universal school-based program to prevent adolescent depression. *Journal of Clinical Child Psychology, 30*, 303–315.

Siegel, R. M., Schubert, C. J., Myers, P. A., & Shapiro, R. A. (1995). The prevalence of sexually transmitted diseases in children and adolescents evaluated for sexual abuse in Cincinnati: Rationale for limited STD testing in prepubertal girls. *Pediatrics, 87*, 1090–1094.

Sigurdson, E., Strange, M., & Doig, T. (1987). What do children know about preventing sexual assault? How can their awareness be increased? *Canadian Journal of Psychiatry, 32*, 551–557.

Silver, R. L., Boone, C., & Stones, M. H. (1983) Searching for meaning and misfortune: Making sense of incest. *Journal of Social Issues, 39*, 81–102.

Silver, R. L., & Wortman, C. (1980). Coping with undesirable life events. In J. Garber & M. Seligman (Eds.), *Human helplessness: Theory and applications* (pp. 279–340). New York: Academic Press.

Simpson, T. L., & Miller, W. R. (2002). Concomitance between childhood sexual and physical abuse and substance use problems: A review. *Clinical Psychology Review, 22*, 27–77.

Sirles, E. A., & Franke, P. J. (1989). Factors influencing mothers' reactions to intrafamilial sexual abuse. *Child Abuse and Neglect, 13*, 131–139.

Sisterman Keeney, K., Amacher, E., & Kastanaskis, J. (1992). The court prep group: A vital part of the court process. In H. Dent & R. Flin (Eds.), *Children as witnesses* (pp. 201–210). Chichester, UK: Wiley.

Smith, D. W., Letourneau, E. J., Saunders, B. E., Kilpatrick, D. G., Resnick, H. S., & Best, C. L. (2000). Delay in disclosure of childhood rape: Results from a national survey. *Child Abuse and Neglect, 24*, 273–287.

Smith, H., & Israel, E. (1987). Sibling incest: A study of the dynamics of 25 cases. *Child Abuse and Neglect, 11*, 101–108.

Smith, S., Howard, J. A., & Monroe, A. D. (1998). An analysis of child behavior problems in adoptions in difficulty. *Journal of Social Science Research, 24*, 61–84.

Sobsey, D., & Doe, T. (1991). Patterns of sexual abuse and assault. *Sexuality and Disability, 9*, 243–259.

Sobsey, D., Randall, W., & Parrila, R. K. (1997). Gender differences in abused children with and without disabilities. *Child Abuse and Neglect, 21*, 707–720.

Sorenson, T., & Snow, B. (1991). How children tell: The process of disclosure in child sexual abuse. *Child Welfare, 70*, 3–15.

Southwick, S. M., Yehuda, R., & Morgan, C. A. (1995). Clinical studies of neurotransmitter alterations in post-traumatic stress disorder. In M. J. Friedman, D. S. Charney, & A. Y. Deutch (Eds.), *Neurobiological and clinical consequences of stress: From normal adaptation to post-traumatic stress disorder* (pp. 335–349). Philadelphia: Lippincott-Raven.

Spectrum South Productions. (1989). *Taking the stand for kids who testify.* (Available from Victim Witness Assistance Program of the 13th Circuit Solicitors Office, Suite 101, Courthouse Annex, Greenville, SC 20601)

Spirito, A., Stark, L., & Williams, C. (1988). Development of a brief coping checklist for use with pediatric populations. *Journal of Pediatric Psychology, 13*, 555–574.

Stallard, P., Velleman, R., & Baldwin, S. (1998). Prospective study of posttraumatic stress disorder in children involved in road traffic accidents. *British Medical Journal, 317*, 1619–1623.

Starling, S. P., & Jenny, C. (1997). Forensic examination of adolescent female genitalia: The Foley catheter technique. *Archives of Pediatric and Adolescent Medicine, 151*, 102–103.

Statistics Canada. (1997). *Canadian crime statistics, 1996.* Ottawa: Statistics Canada, Canadian Centre for Justice Statistics.

Sternberg, K. J., Lamb, M. E., Esplin, P. W., & Baradaran, L. (1999). Using a scripted protocol to guide investigative interviews: A pilot study. *Applied Developmental Science, 3*, 70–76.

Sternberg, K. J., Lamb, M. E., Hershkowitz, I., Esplin, P. W., Redlich, A., & Sunshine, N. (1996). The relation between investigative utterance types and the informativeness of child witnesses. *Journal of Applied Developmental Psychology, 17*, 439–451.

Sternberg, K. J., Lamb, M. E., Orbach, Y., Esplin, P. W., & Mitchell, S. (2001). Use of structured investigative protocol enhances young children's response to free-recall prompts in the course of forensic interviews. *Journal of Applied Psychology, 86*, 997–1105.

Steward, M., Schmitz, M., Steward, D., Joye, N., & Reinhart, M. (1994). Children's anticipation of and response to colposcopic examination. *Child Abuse and Neglect, 19*, 997–1005.

Straus, R. B. (1995). Supervised visitation and family violence. *Family Law Quarterly, 29*, 229–252.

Stroud, D. D., Martens, S. L., & Barker, J. (2000). Criminal investigation of child sexual abuse: A comparison of cases referred to the prosecutor to those not referred. *Child Abuse and Neglect, 24*, 689–700.

Sullivan, P. M., Brookhauser, P. E., Scanlan, J. M., Knutson, J. F., & Schulte, L. E. (1991). Patterns of physical and sexual abuse of communicatively handicapped children. *Annals of Otology, Rhinology, and Laryngology, 100,* 188–194.

Sullivan, P. M., & Knutson, J. F. (1998). The association between child maltreatment and disabilities in a hospital-based epidemiological study. *Child Abuse and Neglect, 22,* 271–288.

Swenson, C. C., & Hanson, R. F. (1998). Sexual abuse of children: Assessment, research, and treatment. In J. R. Lutzker (Ed.), *Handbook on research and treatment in child abuse and neglect* (pp. 475–499). New York: Plenum Press.

Swim, J., Borgida, E., & McCoy, K. (1992). Videotaped versus in-court witness testimony: Does protecting the child witness jeopardize due process? *Journal of Applied Social Psychology, 23,* 603–631.

Tang, C., & Lee, Y. (1999). Knowledge on sexual abuse and self-protection skills: A study on female Chinese adolescents with mild mental retardation. *Child Abuse and Neglect, 23,* 269–279.

Taska, L., & Feiring, C. (1995). *Children's adaptation to sexual abuse: The role of shame and attribution.* Poster presented at the annual meeting of the Association for Advancement of Behavior Therapy, Washington, DC.

Tebbutt, J., Swanston, H., Oates, R. K., & O'Toole, B. I. (1997). Five years after child sexual abuse: Persisting dysfunction and problems of prediction. *Journal of the American Academy of Child and Adolescent Psychiatry, 35,* 330–339.

Terr, L. C. (1987). *Severe stress and sudden shock: The connection.* Sam Hibbs Award Lecture presented at the annual convention of the American Psychiatric Association, Chicago.

Terr, L. C. (1991). Childhood traumas: An outline and overview. *American Journal of Psychiatry, 148,* 10–20.

Terr, L. C. (1997, August 25–29). *The long-term effects of childhood trauma.* Workshop presented at the Cape Cod Institute, Cape Cod, MA.

Terr, L. C. (2003). "Wild child": How three principles of healing organized 12 years of psychotherapy. *Journal of the American Academy of Child and Adolescent Psychiatry, 42,* 1401–1409.

Thoennes, N., & Tjaden, P. (1990). The extent, nature, and validity of sexual abuse allegations in custody and visitation disputes. *Child Abuse and Neglect, 14,* 151–163.

Thompson, W. C., Clarke-Stewart, A., & Lepore, S. J. (1997). What did the janitor do?: Suggestive interviewing and the accuracy of children's accounts. *Law and Human Behavior, 21,* 405–426.

Timnick, L. (1985, August 25). 22% in survey were child abuse victims. *Los Angeles Times,* pp. 1, 34.

Tobey, A. E., Goodman, G. S., Batterman-Faunce, J. M., Orcutt, H. K., & Sachsenmaier, T. (1995). Balancing the rights of children and defendants: The effects of closed-circuit television in children' accuracy and jurors perceptions. In M. S. Zaragoza, J. R., Graham, G. C. N. Hall, R. Hirschman, & Y. S. Ben-Porath (Eds.), *Memory and testimony in the child witness* (pp. 214–239). Thousand Oaks: Sage.

Treacy, E. C., & Fisher, C. B. (1993). Foster parenting the sexually abused: A family life education program. *Journal of Child Sexual Abuse, 2,* 47—63.

Tremblay, C., Hebert, M., & Piche, C. (1999). Coping strategies and social support as mediators of consequence in child sexual abuse victims. *Child Abuse and Neglect, 23,* 929–945.

Trickett, P. K., & McBride-Chang, C. (1995). The developmental impact of different forms of child abuse and neglect. *Developmental Review, 15,* 311–337.

Trocmé, N., Fallon, B., MacLurin, B., & Copp, B. (2002). *The changing face of child welfare investigations in Ontario: Ontario incidence studies of reported child abuse and neglect (OIS 1993/1998).* Toronto: Centre of Excellence for Child Welfare, Faculty of Social Work, University of Toronto.

Tufts New England Medical Center, Division of Child Psychiatry. (1984). *Sexually exploited children: Service and research project* (Final report for the Office of Juvenile Justice and Delinquency Prevention). Washington, DC: U.S. Department of Justice.

Tutty, L. M. (1993). Are child sexual abuse prevention programs effective?: A review of the research. *Revue Sexologique, 1,* 93–114.

U.S. Department of Health and Human Services. (1992–2000). *Child maltreatment 1990–1998: Reports from the states to the National Child Abuse and Neglect Data System.* Washington, DC: Author.

U.S. Department of Health and Human Services. (2001). *Trends in the well-being of America's children and youth 2001.* Washington, DC: Author.

U.S. Department of Health and Human Services. (2004). *Child maltreatment 2002: Reports from the States to the National Child Abuse and Neglect Data Systems—National statistics on child abuse and neglect.* Washington, DC: Author.

U.S. Food and Drug Administration (FDA). (2004). *FDA public health advisory October 15, 2004: Suicidality in children and adolescents being treated with antidepressant medications.* Retrieved from www.fda.gov/cder/drug/antidepressants/SSRIPHA200410.htm

van der Kolk, B. A., McFarlane, A., & van der Hart, O. (1996). A general approach to the treatment of posttraumatic stress disorder. In B. A. van der Kolk, A. C. McFarlane, & L. Weisaeth (Eds.), *Traumatic stress: The effects of overwhelming experience on mind, body, and society* (pp. 510–524). New York: Guilford Press.

van der Kolk, B. A., Pelcovitz, D., Roth, S., Mandel, F., McFarlane, A., & Herman, J. (1996). Dissociation, somatization, and affect dysregulation: The complexity of adaptation to trauma. *American Journal of Psychiatry, 153*(Festschrift Suppl.), 83–93.

Van Voorhis, R., & Gilbert, N. (1998). The structure and performance of child abuse reporting systems. *Children and Youth Services Review, 20,* 207–221.

Vernberg, E. M., LaGreca, A. M., Silverman, W., & Prinstein, M. J. (1996). Prediction of posttraumatic stress symptoms in children after Hurricane Andrew. *Journal of Abnormal Psychology, 105,* 237–248.

Vieth, V. I. (2004). Keeping the balance true: Admitting child hearsay in the wake of *Crawford v. Washington*, *Update Newsletter, 16*(12). Retrieved from www.ndaa-apri.org/apri/programs/ncpca/update_express_march_2004.html

Violatao, C., & Genius, M. (1993). Problems of research in male child sexual abuse: A review. *Journal of Child Sexual Abuse, 2*, 33–54.

Vogeltanz, N. D., Wilsnack, S. C., Harris, T. R., Wilsnack, R. W., Wonderlich, S. A., & Kristjanson, A. F. (1999). Prevalence and risk factors for childhood sexual abuse in women: National survey findings. *Child Abuse and Neglect, 23*, 579–592.

Waibel-Duncan, M. K., & Sanger, M. (1999). Understanding and reacting to the anogenital exam: Implications for patient preparation. *Child Abuse and Neglect, 23*, 281–286.

Waller, N., Putnam, F. W., & Carlson, E. B. (1996). Types of dissociation and dissociative types: A taxometric analysis of dissociative experiences. *Psychological Methods, 1*, 300–321.

Walsh, C., MacMillan, H. L., & Jamieson, E. (2003). The relationship between parental substance abuse and child maltreatment: Findings from the Ontario Health Supplement. *Child Abuse and Neglect, 27*, 1409–1425.

Walters, D. (1995). Mandatory reporting of child abuse: Legal, ethical, and clinical implications within a Canadian context. *Canadian Psychology, 36*, 163–182.

Warren, A. R., Nunez, Z., Keeney, J. M., Buck, J. A., & Smith, B. (2002). The believability of children and their interviewers' hearsay testimony: When less is more. *Journal of Applied Psychology, 87*, 846–857.

Warren, A. R., Woodall, C. E., Thomas, M., Nunno, M., Keeney, J. M., Larson, S. M., et al. (1999). Assessing the effectiveness of a training program for interviewing child witnesses. *Applied Developmental Science, 3*, 128–135.

Watkins, B., & Bentovim, A. (1992). The sexual abuse of male children and adolescents: A review of current research. *Journal of the American Academy of Child and Adolescent Psychiatry, 33*, 197–248.

Wells, G. L., Tuttle, J. W., & Luus, C. A. E. (1989). The perceived credibility of child witnesses: What happens when they use their own words. In S. J. Ceci, D. F. Ross, & M. P. Toglia (Eds.), *Perspectives in children's testimony* (pp. 23–36). New York: Springer-Verlag.

Wells, R. D., McCann, J., Adams, J., Voris, J., & Ensign, J. (1995). Emotional, behavioral, and physical symptoms reported by parents of sexually abused, nonabused, and allegedly abused prepubescent females. *Child Abuse and Neglect, 19*, 155–164.

Wells, S., Stein, T., Fluke, J., & Downing, J. (1989). Screening in child protective services. *Social Work, 34*, 45–48.

Westcott, H. L., & Jones, D. P. H. (1999). Annotation: The abuse of disabled children. *Journal of Child Psychology and Psychiatry, 40*, 497–506.

Whitcomb, D. (1992). *When the victim is a child* (2nd ed.). Washington, DC: National Institute of Justice.

Whitcomb, D. (2003). Legal interventions for child victims. *Journal of Traumatic Stress, 16*, 149–157.

Widom, C. S. (1991). The role of placement experiences in mediating the criminal consequences of early childhood victimization. *American Journal of Orthopsychiatry, 61*, 195–209.

Widom, C. S., & Kuhns, J. B. (1996). Childhood victimization and subsequent risk for promiscuity, prostitution, and teenage pregnancy: A prospective study. *American Journal of Public Health, 86*, 1607–1612.

Williams, L. M. (1994). Recall of childhood trauma: A prospective study of women's memories of child sexual abuse. *Journal of Consulting and Clinical Psychology, 62*, 1167–1176.

Wolfe, D. A., MacPherson, T., Blount, R., & Wolfe, V. V. (1986). Evaluation of a brief intervention for educating school children in awareness of physical and sexual abuse. *Child Abuse and Neglect, 10*, 5–92.

Wolfe, D. A., Sas, L., & Wekerle, C. (1994). Factors associated with the development of post-traumatic stress disorder among child victims of sexual abuse. *Child Abuse and Neglect, 18*, 37–50.

Wolfe, V. V. (2002). *The Children's Impact of Traumatic Events Scale II (CITES-II)*. Unpublished assessment instrument. (Available from V. V. Wolfe, Child and Adolescent Centre, London Health Sciences Centre, 346 South St., London, Ontario N6A 4G5, Canada)

Wolfe, V. V., & Birt, J. (1997). Child sexual abuse. In E. J. Mash & L. G. Terdal (Eds.), *Assessment of childhood disorders* (3rd ed., pp. 569–623). New York: Guilford Press.

Wolfe, V. V., & Birt, J. (November, 2002). Parent- and child-reported dissociative symptoms: Relationship to peritraumatic experiences. In N. Rodriguez (Chair), *Peritraumatic dissociation and posttraumatic stress disorder in traumatized children and adolescents*. Symposium conducted at the meeting of the International Society for Traumatic Stress Studies, Baltimore.

Wolfe, V. V., & Birt, J. (2004a). *The Children's Impact of Traumatic Events Scale—Revised (CITES-R): Scale structure, internal consistency, discriminant validity, and PTSD diagnostic patterns*. Manuscript submitted for publication.

Wolfe, V. V., & Birt, J. (2004b). *The Children's Peritraumatic Experiences Questionnaire: A measure to assess DSM-IV PTSD Criterion A2*. Manuscript submitted for publication.

Wolfe, V. V., & Gentile, C. C. (1992). Psychological assessment of sexually abused children. In W. O'Donahue & J. H. Ger (Eds.), *The sexual abuse of children: Vol. 2. Clinical issues* (pp. 143–187). Hillsdale, NJ: Erlbaum.

Wolfe, V. V., Gentile, C. C., & Wolfe, D. A. (1989). The impact of sexual abuse on children: A PTSD formulation. *Behavior Therapy, 20*, 215–228.

Worling, J. (1995). Adolescent sibling-incest offenders: Differences in family and individual functioning when compared to adolescent nonsibling offenders. *Child Abuse and Neglect, 19*, 633–643.

Worling, J., & Curwen, T. (2000). Adolescent sexual offender recidivism: Success of specialized treatment and implications for risk prediction. *Child Abuse and Neglect, 24,* 965–982.

Worling, J. A. (1998). Adolescent sexual offender treatment at the SAFE-T Program. In W. L. Marshall, Y. M. Fernandez, S. M. Hudson, & T. Ward (Eds.), *Sourcebook for treatment programs for sexual offenders* (pp. 353–366). New York: Plenum Press.

Wurtele, S. K. (1993). The role of maintaining telephone contact with parents during the teaching of a personal safety program. *Journal of Child Sexual Abuse, 2,* 65–82.

Wurtele, S. K. (2002). School-based child sexual abuse prevention. In P. A. Schewe (Ed.), *Preventing violence in relationships: Interventions across the life span* (pp. 9–54). Washington, DC: American Psychological Association.

Wurtele, S. K., Currier, L. L., Gillispie, E. I., & Franklin, C. F. (1991). An efficacy of a parent-implemented program for teaching preschoolers body safety skills. *Behavior Therapy, 22,* 69–83.

Wurtele, S. K., Gillispie, E. I., Currier, L. L., & Franklin, C. F. (1992). A comparison of teachers vs. parents as instructors of a personal safety program for preschoolers. *Child Abuse and Neglect, 16,* 127–137.

Wurtele, S. K., Kast, L. C., & Melzer, A. (1992). Sexual abuse prevention education for young children: A comparison of teachers and parents as instructors. *Child Abuse and Neglect, 16,* 865–876.

Wurtele, S. K., Kast, L. C., Miller-Perrin, C. L., & Kondrick, P. A. (1989). A comparison of programs for teaching personal safety skills to preschoolers. *Journal of Consulting and Clinical Psychology, 57,* 505–511.

Wurtele, S. K., Kvaternic, M., & Franklin, C. F. (1992). Sexual abuse prevention for preschoolers: A survey of parents' behaviors, attitudes, and beliefs. *Journal of Child Sexual Abuse, 1,* 113–128, 505–511.

Wurtele, S. K., & Miller-Perrin, C. L. (1987). An evaluation of side effects associated with participation in a child sexual abuse prevention program. *Journal of School Health, 57,* 228–231.

Wurtele, S. K., & Miller-Perrin, C. L. (1992). *Preventing child sexual abuse: Sharing the responsibility.* Lincoln: University of Nebraska Press.

Wurtele, S. K., & Owens, J. (1997). Teaching personal safety skills to young children: An investigation of age and gender across five studies. *Child Abuse and Neglect, 21,* 805–814.

Wurtele, S. K., Saslawsky, D., Miller, C., Marrs, S., & Britcher, J. (1986). Teaching personal safety skills for potential prevention of sexual abuse: A comparison of treatments. *Journal of Consulting and Clinical Psychology, 54,* 688–692.

Wyatt, G. E. (1985). The sexual abuse of Afro-American and White-American women in childhood. *Child Abuse and Neglect, 9,* 507–519.

Yehuda, R. (2004). Risk and resilience in posttraumatic stress disorder. *Journal of Clinical Psychiatry, 65,* 29–36.

Yehuda, R., & McFarlane, A. C. (1997). Psychobiology of posttraumatic stress disorder. *Annals of the New York Academy of Sciences, 821,* 1–55.

Yordan, E. E., & Yordan, R. A. (1992). Sexually transmitted diseases and human immunodeficiency virus screen in a population of sexually abused girls. *Adolescent Pediatric Gynecology, 5,* 1878–1891.

Zellman, G. L. (1992). The impact of case characteristics on child abuse reporting decisions. *Child Abuse and Neglect, 16,* 57–74.

Zellman, G. L., & Fair, C. (2002). Preventing and reporting abuse. In J. E. B. Myers,, L. Berliner, J. Briere, C. T. Hendrix, C. Jenny, & T. A. Reid (Eds.), *The APSAC handbook on child maltreatment* (2nd ed., pp. 449–476). Thousand Oaks, CA: Sage.

Child's Responsibilities

I, _____ , have read this contract with my mom/dad/legal guardian, _____ , and I understand the rules of Internet use in my home. I will keep this contract clearly posted by my computer. If I should run into any problems while surfing the Internet or while in a chat room, I will contact my parents and abide by the rules listed in this contract.

- I will never give out my home telephone number or address over the Internet.
- I will not give out any information about my family, such as where my parents work and the names of my brothers and sisters
- I will not use my real name in chat rooms and will always use a "nickname."
- I will not tell a stranger on the Internet where I go to school.
- I will never meet someone I have talked to on the Internet unless my parents approve and come with me to the meeting.
- I will never send pictures of my family or me over the Internet without my parents' permission.
- I will not talk to anyone over the Internet who makes me feel uncomfortable; I will tell my parents right away when this happens.
- I will tell my parents if anyone is threatening me or using bad language.
- I will always keep in mind while talking to people on the Internet that they are strangers and some strangers can be bad.
- I will obey my parents' rules about being on the Internet, including obtaining their permission to sign on and download material.

Parents' Responsibilities

I, _____ , will supervise my child while he or she is on the Internet to ensure that my child is using this tool responsibly and not endangering him- or herself by communicating inappropriately with strangers he or she may meet over the Internet.

- I will not use this contract as a way to control every action taken by my child on the Internet.
- I will respect my child's need for a degree of privacy while speaking to friends on the Internet.
- I will spend time with my child and learn about what interests him or her on the Internet.
- I will be aware of the procedure for contacting my online provider for advice, should someone appear to be bothering my child. I will also contact the Cyber Tip Line at (800) 843-5678 or www.cybertipline.com if I suspect someone has been soliciting my child for sex or sending pornographic material to my child.
- I will teach my child to use judgment while online, and I will ensure that my child is educated about the hazards of Internet use and how to use the Internet safely.

Parent's Signature: _____

Child's Signature: _____

Date: _____

Note. From Dombrowski et al. (2004). Copyright 2004 by the American Psychological Association. Adapted by permission.

VI

PROBLEMS OF ADOLESCENCE

□ 11 □

Adolescent Substance Use Problems

Laura MacPherson, Kevin Frissell, Sandra A. Brown, and Mark G. Myers

OVERVIEW OF ADOLESCENT SUBSTANCE USE PROBLEMS

History

Adolescent use and misuse of psychoactive substances are not new phenomena, despite increasing attention to the issue. However, it was not until the early 1970s, with the growing prevalence of illicit drug use, that public attention focused on this issue. Prior to the 1970s, alcohol and tobacco were the psychoactive substances predominantly used by adolescents. The late 1960s and early 1970s saw increased acceptance by youths of various other drugs, most notably marijuana. With the increased acceptance and availability of psychoactive substances, the prevalence of experimental and problematic use of alcohol and drugs during adolescence likewise increased. Concern regarding youth substance use and misuse provoked the emergence of school-based substance use prevention programs in the 1970s, as well as several surveys of youth alcohol and drug use: the National Household Survey on Drug Abuse, which began in 1971 and is repeated every 2–3 years; and the Monitoring the Future Study, an annual survey of high school students initiated in 1975. Recently published data from the Monitoring the Future Study (Johnston, O'Malley, & Bachman, 2003) detail trends in youth alcohol and drug use over the 27 years from 1975 to 2002. Within this time frame, the prevalence of alcohol and drug use among high school seniors peaked in 1979 (88.1% and 54.2% annual prevalence for alcohol and illicit drug use, respectively) and reached a low in 1992 (72.7% and 27.1%). However, since 1992 there has been an increasing trend in the annual prevalence of illicit drug use through the 1990s and early 2000s, whereas the annual prevalence of alcohol use has remained moderately stable (Johnston et al., 2003; Substance Abuse and Mental Health Services Administration, 2003). The bulk of our current knowledge regarding the etiology and progression of substance use is derived from information generated in the past two and a half decades and forms the empirical basis for interventions designed for youths.

In the late 1970s and early 1980s, adolescent-specific treatment of substance use emerged (e.g., Woltzen et al., 1986) based on prevalent adult models of alcohol and drug treatment (e.g., the disease model of addiction, also known as the "Minnesota model"; Laundergan, 1982). Until the 1980s, the majority of adolescents had been treated within adult treatment settings, with little attention provided to critical developmental issues and differences between adolescent and adult addiction (Beschner & Friedman, 1985). The 1980s saw a proliferation of adolescent treatment programs in response to the public perception of "epidemic" drug use by youths. These adolescent-specific programs included developmentally specific components, such as family, peer group, and recreation therapies, and school consultation (e.g., Joanning, Quinn, Thomas, & Mullen, 1992; Liddle & Dakof, 1995; Obermeier & Henry, 1985). As health care costs and restrictions increased throughout the 1990s, inpatient services decreased. It is not currently known whether these costs and restrictions have influenced adolescent treatment development. However, it is possible that current realities in health care coverage may threaten the continued development of more comprehensive and developmentally appropriate treatments (Winters, Latimer, & Stinchfield, 1999).

Despite improvements in attention to adolescent issues, adolescent treatment facilities have typically based their programs on the disease model of addiction, which was developed for adults with alcohol dependence (Institute of Medicine, 1990). To date, this Minnesota model remains the most widely implemented strategy in treating adolescent substance abuse (e.g., Hoffman, Mee-Lee, & Arrowhead, 1993). A disadvantage of this relatively unitary approach to addiction is that dependent adolescents represent a heterogeneous population with diverse problems and needs. Current approaches to adolescent substance treatment also suffer from a paucity of knowledge regarding what constitutes effective treatment and the processes whereby teens succeed or fail following treatment (Brown, Mott, & Myers, 1990). The appropriateness of existing models of treatment for adolescent substance misuse has generally received limited empirical attention, and treatment outcome research lags behind adult research in this area (e.g., Kaminer, Burleson, Blitz, Sussman, & Rounsaville, 1998).

Nature

At the simplest level, a "substance use problem" can be defined as a pathological involvement with alcohol and/or drugs (Bukstein & Kaminer, 1994). A description of the nature of such problems among adolescents rests largely on examination of substance involvement's effects on functioning across various life domains, and to a lesser extent reflects absolute levels of involvement with alcohol and other drugs (i.e., quantity and frequency of use). The results of youth substance involvement are most frequently expressed in deterioration in interpersonal relationships; elevations in accident and injury rates; increases in family conflict; declines in academic functioning; higher levels of negative affect (e.g., depression, anxiety); and involvement in various antisocial behaviors (theft, property destruction, truancy, etc.). The diverse nature of adolescent substance use is evident in the difficulties in ascertaining the direction of causality. For example, for some teens substance involvement may escalate in response to certain difficulties (e.g., negative affect, psychiatric disorders, environmental stressors), ultimately exacerbating the original problem. Alternately, increased involvement with alcohol and other drugs by "normally" functioning youths may precipitate deterioration in psychosocial functioning (e.g., school problems, withdrawal and isolation, legal problems). For yet others, substance use is embedded within a matrix of deviant behaviors and attitudes—a phenomenon described as the "problem behavior" syndrome (Donovan & Jessor, 1985; Jessor & Jessor, 1977).

The context of adolescent alcohol and drug use must be considered in describing the nature of this involvement. For example, youth substance involvement differs by ethnicity and cultural background. In general, European American, Hispanic, and Native American youths show the highest rates of alcohol and drug involvement, with African American and Asian adolescents typically reporting the lowest rates, although there are important differences across gender and class of substance (Wallace et al., 2003). Some evidence suggests that ethnic differences in vulnerability to substance involvement reflect variability in exposure to risk factors (such as early initiation of use) and protective factors (such as family bonding) (e.g., Epstein, Botvin, Griffin, & Diaz, 2001; Galaif & Newcomb, 1999; Mahaddian, Bentler, & Newcomb, 1988). For example, Mahaddian and colleagues (1988) examined the relationships between 10 risk factors and substance involvement among European American, Hispanic, African American, and Asian adolescents. European American and Hispanic youths had similar levels of risk for substance involvement and exposure to the risk factors. However, for European Americans low religious commitment and early alcohol use were the principal risk factors, while for Hispanics deviance was the dominant risk. African American and Asian adolescents had lower exposure to risk factors than European American and Hispanic youths. For African Americans, poor family relationships constituted the single most important risk; among Asians, low religiosity, poor self-esteem, poor family relationships, and sensation seeking were important factors. A study examining early initiation of substance use by European American and African American fifth graders (Catalano et al., 1993) found similar patterns, in that ethnic differences emerged in exposure to risk factors. The African American children exhibited more aggression and delinquency and reported more deviant siblings, whereas the European American children endorsed higher intentions to use substances and reported less parental use of family management strategies. The influence of protective factors has been examined to a lesser extent, although preliminary evidence suggests that school and family connectedness, and parental support and monitoring, serve to attenuate the influence of risk factors related to substance use (Epstein et al., 2001; Sale, Sambrano, Springer, & Turner, 2003; Wills & Yaeger, 2003).

Ethnic differences in the relationship between risk and protective factors for substance use remain to be examined among adolescents. However, in adult populations, some ethnic differences in protective factors have been examined, such as variants of the gene coding for the enzyme that metabolizes acetaldehyde (ALDH2), a metabolite of alcohol (Wall, Shea, Chan, & Carr, 2001). Among adults, a genetic variant of ALDH2 that acts as a protective factor for alcohol use disorders is more prevalent among certain Asian populations, and it is likely that this genetic variant also acts as a protective factor among adolescents of Asian decent. Furthermore, in relation to smoking behavior, data suggest that genetic polymorphisms within dopaminergic pathways (e.g., SLC6A3) act as protective factors for lower likelihood of smoking and late initiation of smoking (Lerman et al., 1999; Sabol et al., 1999), and may differ in prevalence across African Americans and European Americans. Thus it is apparent that ethnic and cultural differences play a role in the divergent trajectories of substance involvement observed for youths of different ethnicities. Although factors influencing the likelihood of substance misuse do not appear to vary substantially by ethnicity, ethnic differences are apparent in the extent of exposure to or presence of these risk factors.

Another important contextual consideration is the observed increase in experimentation and involvement with substances during adolescence, which for some youths reflects "normative" behavior (e.g., Kaminer, 1999; Shedler & Block, 1990). Despite the concerns regarding youth substance involvement, there appears to be a discontinuity in school-based samples,

such that youth alcohol problems do not consistently predict adult alcohol dependence (e.g., Blane, 1976; Newcomb & Bentler, 1988; Newcomb, Schier, & Bentler, 1993; Rohde, Lewinsohn, Kahler, Seeley, & Brown, 2001). However, early initiation of alcohol use, in comparison to experience of alcohol-related problems, is predictive of adult alcohol use disorders (Grant & Dawson, 1997). It has also been reported that 80% of adults who smoke began smoking before age 18 (U.S. Department of Health and Human Services, 1994), and that 71% of adults who smoke daily began daily smoking by age 18 (Fiore et al., 2000). Heavy drug use during adolescence has been found to be associated with a variety of negative consequences during early adulthood, including impaired social relationships as well as physical and psychological disturbances (Duncan et al., 1997; Newcomb & Bentler, 1988).

Regarding comorbidity of mental health disorders, adolescent rates of comorbid substance use and other Axis I disorders in treatment samples have varied from 50% (Abrantes, Brown, & Tomlinson, 2004; Grilo, Becker, Walker, & Levy, 1995) to 82% (Stowell & Estroff, 1992). Adolescents with substance use disorders are more likely to have disruptive behavior disorders (Fergusson, Lynskey, & Horwood, 1993; Lewinsohn, Hops, Roberts, Seeley, & Andrews, 1993; Rhode, Lewinsohn, & Seeley, 1996), with conduct disorder (CD) the most frequently co-occurring disorder (Greenbaum, Foster-Johnson, & Petrila, 1996; Kandel et al., 1999). Adolescent substance use disorders also co-occur at higher rates with mood disorders and to a lesser extent with anxiety disorders (Kandel et al., 1999; Rohde, Lewinsohn, & Seeley, 1996). Moreover, some studies have noted a greater prevalence of Axis II psychopathology, such as Cluster B traits (e.g., borderline personality disorder features), among adolescents with substance use disorders (Grilo et al., 1995); adolescent substance use disorders were found in one study to predict Axis II pathology in young adulthood (Lewinsohn, Rhode, Seeley, & Klein, 1997).

Research has indicated that adolescents with comorbid psychopathology are more likely to relapse, and progress to relapse more rapidly, than their noncomorbid peers during the first 6 months after treatment (Tomlinson, Brown, & Abrantes, 2004). Comorbid adolescents have been found to relapse in contexts similar to those for relapse in both comorbid adults and noncomorbid adolescents (Anderson, Frissell, & Brown, in press). For both types of adolescents, relapse occurs frequently in social pressure situations, but comorbid adolescents relapse most frequently in situations involving temptations and urges as well as negative affect. Disruptive disorders and anxiety symptoms, although not depressive disorders, have been associated with specific types of relapse situations (Anderson et al., in press). In addition, for adolescents, the severity of psychiatric diagnosis and the severity of substance use symptoms interact. For example, severity of depressive disorders is associated with more withdrawal symptoms; individuals with severe externalizing disorders tend to demonstrate more substance dependence symptoms; and the severity of attention-deficit/hyperactivity disorder (ADHD) symptoms is related to higher prevalence of alcohol dependence (Abrantes et al., 2004).

Regarding clinical course following treatment, information has become available from longitudinal studies indicates that adolescents return to substance use following treatment at rates similar to those of adults (Brown, Myers, Mott, & Vik, 1994; Brown, Vik, & Creamer, 1989), and that these teens evidence continued difficulties as they enter early adulthood (Brown, 1993; Chung et al., 2003). However, there is variation in clinical course among adolescents, with multiple substance use trajectories emerging as teens make the transition from adolescence to young adulthood (e.g., Brown, D'Amico, McCarthy, & Tapert, 2001). Specifically, subgroups of youths either increase their substance use over time, maintain high levels of use, decrease use over time following an initial period of heavy use, abstain, or maintain low levels of use over a four year period. It has also been demonstrated that comorbid psychopathology plays a role in the clinical course of adolescent substance abuse (Tomlinson et al., 2004). Thus the available empirical evidence demonstrates the important role that development plays in the onset, maintenance, and course of adolescent substance misuse.

Prevention

Given the normative nature of substance use in adolescence, and the association between early initiation of substance use and future development of substance use problems, it is not surprising that much research over the past several decades has focused on the prevention of youth substance use. Such investigations have produced a wealth of data related to the efficacy of traditional didactic educational approaches, and more recently cognitive-behavioral and motivation enhancement (ME) prevention programs, for youths. In general, traditional didactic educational prevention programs have been shown to be ineffective in preventing and reducing substance use and related negative consequences for youths. For example, Drug Abuse Resistance Education (DARE) is a widely implemented prevention program for youths. It is designed to provide information on negative aspects of substance use; to enhance self-esteem, social skills, general decision-making skills, and peer pressure resistance skills; and to increase institutional bonding (e.g., with police officers), in order to postpone or prevent the initiation of substance use (Dukes, Stein, & Ullman, 1997). Studies evaluating outcomes of the DARE program, including meta-analyses, have shown that throughout 10 years of follow-up, DARE appears to increase knowledge about substances and positive social skills. However, the program does not prevent or postpone the initiation of substance use (Dukes et al., 1997; Ennett, Tobler, Ringwalt, & Flewelling, 1994; Lynam et al., 1999), although one study found that DARE resulted in reduced use of amphetamines/barbiturates, LSD, cocaine, and inhalants for males at a 6-year follow-up (Dukes et al., 1997). Critiques of the DARE program point to possible explanations for the program's ineffectiveness, including the program's traditional didactic format (which mirrors classroom instruction) and the program's focus on negative consequences of substance use (D'Amico & Fromme, 2001). Furthermore, it has been hypothesized that programs such as DARE that advocate abstinence may undermine prevention efforts by inciting rebellious attitudes in youths who are just beginning to experiment with substances, thus potentially increasing the likelihood that they will continue to engage in the substance use (Marlatt & Witkiewitz, 2002). Among adolescents who have more experience with substances and their effects, interventions that advocate no use may actually increase substance use, because these youths reject the message of intervention (Brown & Kreft, 1998). These propositions are supported by the prevention literature, which shows that alternative prevention programs—ones that are more interactive, are more adaptive to personal needs, and focus on altering the positive reinforcements of substance use generally—have more favorable outcomes (Brown, 2001; D'Amico & Fromme, 2001; Marlatt & Witkiewitz, 2002; Tobler & Stratton, 1997).

Evidence for the efficacy of alternative prevention approaches comes from research on ME and programs that implement cognitive-behavioral prevention components. Concordant with the research reviewed in this chapter on efficacious treatments for substance use disorders, research generally supports the efficacy of these alternative approaches to substance abuse prevention. Furthermore, research investigating level of prevention "dose" generally indicates that brief interventions for the prevention of substance use and related problems result in positive outcomes equivalent to those of more lengthy interventions (Baer et al., 1992). The tactic of meeting the individual at his or her personal stage of substance involvement is a key element of ME strategies, which are brief, client-centered approaches that help the clients to resolve ambivalence regarding substance use behaviors (Lawendowski, 1998; Miller & Rollnick, 2002). Research supports the efficacy of ME strategies for those at risk of experiencing substance use problems and future substance dependence (Obert, Rawson, & Miotto, 1997). Those at risk may not recognize their drug or alcohol use as problematic, and thus many fail to seek treatment (Brown, 1993). A brief, single-session ME intervention with heavy-drinking college students resulted in significant reductions in frequency and quantity of alcohol consumed, as well as in negative alcohol-related consequences; 43% of intervention participants had resolved their risk-taking behavior at a 4-year follow-up, compared to 33% of controls (Baer, Kivlahan, Blume, McKnight, & Marlatt, 2001). In addition, a series of studies of adolescents receiving brief ME interventions for smoking and alcohol use in a hospital setting evidenced reductions in tobacco use and alcohol-related risk behaviors and injuries (Colby et al., 1998; Monti et al., 1999). Results also indicated that younger adolescents who smoked evidenced more positive effects than older ones did (Colby et al., 1998). Furthermore, findings from a meta-analysis of ME studies for substance-abusing adults and youths indicated that ME strategies are effective, producing significant effect sizes in the moderate to high

range (Dunn, Deroo, & Rivara, 2001). Thus ME interventions seem to hold promise as a prevention approach for reducing substance use and related consequences for youths who have not yet progressed to significant levels of substance-related impairment.

Cognitive-behavioral prevention approaches—programs that incorporate components addressing social influence, substance outcome expectancies, and skills training to enhance peer resistance, as well as communication and coping skills—show promise in the prevention of substance use and related problems (Brown, 2001; Johnson, Amatetti, Funkhouser, & Johnson, 1988). In particular, perceptions of substance-use-related social norms are consistent predictors of substance use (Lilja, Wilhelmsen, Larsson, & Hamilton, 2003), and addressing the inaccuracy of these perceptions has been applied and investigated as an avenue of prevention. Adolescents who currently drink are significantly more likely than those who formerly drank or do not drink at all to overestimate the extent of their friends' alcohol use and to underestimate the level of abstinence in their peer group (Feldman, Harvey, Holowaty, & Shortt, 1999). Several studies of interventions for youths that challenge social norms demonstrate the potential efficacy of such an approach in reducing binge drinking, the belief that heavy drinking is normative (Donaldson, Graham, & Hansen, 1994; Haines & Spear, 1996), substance-related risk taking behaviors such as drinking and driving (D'Amico & Fromme, 2001; Shope, Elliott, Raghunathan, & Waller, 2001), and strength of beliefs regarding the acceptability of drug use (Donaldson et al., 1994).

Cognitive-behavioral strategies that address substance use outcome expectancies and/or skills training in an interactive manner have also shown promise in the prevention of substance use and related problems for both early and late adolescents. For example, a moderation-oriented intervention approach that incorporated skills training and addressed substance outcome expectancies among college students was effective at a 1-year follow-up in reducing weekly alcohol use, peak blood alcohol concentrations, and driving after consuming four or more drinks (Kivlahan, Marlatt, Fromme, Coppel, & Williams, 1990). Other interactive prevention programs focusing on life skills, including social skills, resisting peer pressure, and personal responsibility, resulted in less substance use (i.e., alcohol, marijuana, tobacco) for middle-school-age adolescents (Botvin, Baker, Dusenbury, Tortu, & Botvin, 1990) and less alcohol use for high-school-age adolescents (Peleg, Neumann, Friger, Peleg, & Sperber, 2001), compared to their respective control groups. The Alcohol Misuse Prevention Study focused on increasing high school students' alcohol misuse knowledge and refusal skills in order to decrease rates of alcohol use and related risk behaviors (Shope, Copeland, Maharg, & Dielman, 1996). This intervention was successful in increasing alcohol misuse prevention knowledge and reducing alcohol misuse among program participants, compared to a no-treatment control group. Furthermore, an interactive multiple-component cognitive-behavioral intervention for adolescents—including skills training, discussions of stress-specific coping skills, identification of high-risk situations, social support, and alternatives to substance use—was effective in reducing alcohol, cannabis, and other drug use (Wagner, Brown, Monti, Myers, & Waldron, 1999). A program specifically designed to alter risk perception of alcohol-related activities among high school students resulted in fewer drinking and driving behaviors (i.e., drinking and driving, riding with a drinking driver) among program participants, compared to those not participating (Sheehan et al., 1996).

More recently, a model of substance use prevention has been advocated that stems from an ME framework and is designed to facilitate substance use self-change among youths (Brown, 2001). A basic assumption of this model is that prevention programs that are interactive, focus on specific concerns of youths, present convenient options for obtaining prevention content, and are packaged in delivery modalities consonant with youth preferences will attract voluntary participation of youths with heterogeneous background characteristics (e.g., varying levels of substance involvement; age, gender, and ethnic variability) and will be effective at promoting change attempts and reducing substance use. In an ongoing study of a secondary intervention program to facilitate self-change of adolescent alcohol consumption among high school students (Brown, 2001; Brown, Anderson, Schulte, Sintov, & Frissell, 2005), youths who self-select into the prevention program voluntarily choose to participate in one of three intervention formats (i.e., group, individual, or Internet). Intervention foci are similar across formats and include cognitive-behavioral strategies described above, including normative challenges, discussions of alcohol outcome expectancies, coping skills training, evaluation of personal substance-related consequences, alternative reinforcement/behaviors to substance use, and communication skills. To optimize the developmental appropriateness of the program, intervention delivery (i.e., formats, presentation of intervention content, advertisements) has been developed in collaboration with input from youths representative of those targeted for intervention. Furthermore, specific content addressed in intervention sessions is garnered from youth participants. Outcomes of this prevention model are currently under investigation; however, preliminary results are favorable. Approximately 10% of youths at participating high schools self-select into the program; participants are diverse in terms of background and substance use characteristics; and increases in alcohol use over time are less pronounced for participants than for the total school population (Brown, 2001; Brown et al., 2005). Future analyses will determine the impact of this prevention model on facilitating alcohol change attempts and producing positive outcomes for alcohol use.

Current Definitions

The diagnoses of substance abuse and substance dependence in adolescents still rely on criteria that were originally developed for adults and that provide no distinctions between adult and adolescent features of the disorders. The *Diagnostic and Statistical Manual of Mental Disorders*, fourth edition, text revision (DSM-IV-TR; American Psychiatric Association, 2000) defines psychoactive substance dependence as repeated use resulting in physiological dependence and compulsive substance-taking behavior. A DSM-IV-TR diagnosis of substance dependence requires evidence of at least three of seven specified criteria within a 12-month period. The first two criteria reflect physical consequences of use—tolerance (continued use leading to lesser subjective effects from the same quantity of the substance) and withdrawal (unpleasant behavioral, physiological, and cognitive symptoms that occur as concentrations of the substance in the individual's system diminish). The remaining five criteria focus on preoccupation with use, involvement in obtaining the substance, failure to control use, and impaired psychosocial functioning as a consequence of use.

In contrast to substance dependence, DSM-IV-TR defines psychoactive substance abuse as a milder form of substance involvement that, though producing negative consequences, does not meet dependence criteria. Substance abuse is defined as a pattern of maladaptive use resulting in clinically significant impairment or distress; the diagnosis requires that one of four symptoms be evident within a 12-month period. Again, this diagnosis focuses on negative social, legal, and/or interpersonal consequences of substance involvement, and does not include symptoms of physical dependence (i.e., tolerance and withdrawal). In the past several years, an increasing number of studies have examined the reliability and validity of existing classification systems as they apply to adolescents (Bukstein & Kaminer, 1994; Harrison, Fulkerson, & Beebe, 1998; Lewinsohn, Rohde, & Seeley, 1996; Martin, Kaczynski, Maisto, Bukstein, & Moss, 1995; Stewart & Brown, 1995). However, few studies have attempted to produce an alternative definition of youth substance use disorders (e.g., Clark, 2004; Martin, Langenbucher, Kaczynski, & Chung, 1996).

Although the DSM criteria are often used with adolescents, several of the existing criteria are not appropriate for teens (Martin et al., 1995; Stewart & Brown, 1995). For example, substance-using adolescents typically do not exhibit the types of consequences that correspond with the extensive history of involvement commonly found for adults, such as medical complications and a progression of the disorder (Blum, 1987; Brown, Mott, & Stewart, 1992; Clark, Kirisci, & Tarter, 1999; Deas, Riggs, Langenbucher, Goldman, & Brown, 2000; Kaminer, 1991; Langenbucher et al., 2000). Furthermore, adolescents seen in clinical settings are typically involved with multiple drugs, resulting in patterns of withdrawal and dependence symptoms that are more complex than those associated with the DSM-based diagnostic classification (Stewart & Brown, 1995). In particular, adolescents display fewer physiological withdrawal symptoms, but more affective distress. Results of a study of DSM-IV alcohol abuse and dependence symptoms and five exploratory domains of problems typical for adolescents (Martin et al., 1995) provided some support for the utility of the DSM-IV definition of alcohol dependence. The domains of

blackouts, passing out, risky sexual behavior, craving, and declining school grades were found to be specific to a diagnosis of adolescent alcohol abuse. However, in the Stewart and Brown (1995) investigation, the presentations for tolerance, withdrawal, and medical problems were found to differ between adults and adolescents. In addition, other research suggests that adolescents with alcohol use disorders make the transition from abuse to dependence more rapidly, and are less likely to experience blackouts or withdrawal, than are adults (Clark, Kirisci, et al., 1999; Deas et al., 2000; Langenbucher et al., 2000). Further complicating the issue of diagnosis, some studies report that symptoms of abuse and dependence tend to cluster together and are best represented by a single dimension (e.g., Fulkerson, Harrison, & Beebe, 1999). Finally, concerns remain regarding the specificity of adult-derived DSM-IV-TR symptoms in discriminating between typical and pathological substance use among youths. For instance, research has suggested (1) that certain symptoms, such as tolerance, are likely to occur in both problematic and nonproblematic use among youths (Martin et al., 1995); and (2) that the DSM-IV criteria of tolerance, and of consuming a greater amount or for a longer period of time than intended, are the most common alcohol dependence symptoms among adolescents (Chung, Martin, Armstrong, & Labouvie, 2002). This type of research highlights the need for specific considerations in the definition of substance abuse and dependence for adolescents.

Theoretical Formulation

The prevalent conceptualization of addictive behaviors in youths emerge from a biobehavioral perspective, which acknowledges the contribution of biological, psychological, and social-environmental factors to the emergence of alcohol and drug use problems (e.g., Donovan, 1988) in the context of related developmental factors and characteristics (Cicchetti & Rogosch, 1999; Price & Lento, 2001). As articulated in current developmental psychopathology–focused conceptualizations of substance use, these biobehavioral factors can influence an individual's trajectory toward or away from progression into substance use disorders, depending on the individual's developmental level (Price & Lento, 2001). In addition, there exists an ongoing, dynamic progression in the relationships between social-environmental risk and protective factors and the individual's personal characteristics (e.g., genetic predispositions, neurodevelopment, cognitions, emotions). That is, there is a mutual, transactional process in which external factors influence the development of an individual's features and characteristics, and vice versa (Cicchetti & Rogosch, 1999; Price & Lento, 2001).

Within this biobehavioral model, treatment is often conceptualized from a cognitive-behavioral perspective based on a social learning theory understanding of substance misuse (e.g., Abrams & Niaura, 1987; Marlatt & Gordon, 2005; Monti, Abrams, Kadden, & Cooney, 1989; Waldron & Kaminer, 2004). Although a cognitive-behavioral perspective acknowledges the contributions of multiple domains to the emergence of alcohol and drug use problems, it centers on the influence of environmental forces and of learned beliefs and behaviors. Modeling by family members, peers, and society is a critical influence in the emergence of alcohol and drug use behaviors. In particular, beliefs regarding the effects of substances evolve through observations of alcohol and drug use in the context of family, peers, and society/culture (Christiansen, Goldman, & Inn, 1982; Goldman, Brown, & Christiansen, 1987). Beliefs formed early in life regarding the effects of alcohol and drug use are important, in that they predict onset and escalation of substance involvement during adolescence (Christiansen, Roehling, Smith, & Goldman, 1989; Goldman, Darkes, & Del Boca, 1999). Expectations that use of alcohol or other drugs will facilitate social interactions, provide relief from stress, promote acceptance within the peer group, and/or produce the positive feelings associated with being "high" appear to be involved in decisions regarding substance involvement (Fromme & D'Amico, 2000; Goldman, Brown, Christiansen, & Smith, 1991; Smith, Goldman, Greenbaum, & Christiansen, 1995). Adolescents at greater risk for developing substance use problems are typically those who have limited abilities for managing negative mood states, hold more positive beliefs about substances, are exposed to adult substance-using models, are involved with deviant peer groups, are unskilled in appropriate social interactions, have difficulties experiencing positive feelings without alcohol and drug use, and/or are ineffective in managing social

pressures for substance involvement (e.g., Bentler, 1992; Chassin & Ritter, 2001; Pandina & Schuele, 1983). This perspective on the development of adolescent substance misuse is consistent with skills-based approaches to substance abuse treatment (e.g., Monti et al., 1989), family-based approaches (e.g., Donohue & Azrin, 2001), ME approaches (Brown, 2001), and cognitive-behavioral treatment for adolescents (e.g., Kaminer, Burleson, Blitz, Sussman, & Rounsaville, 1998). This conceptualization of adolescent substance use problems implies that effective treatment for such problems must consider youth perceptions/motivations, must include skills for managing and changing the circumstances associated with substance use, and must provide sources of reinforcement that can serve as alternatives to alcohol and drug use.

Etiologies

Within the developmental psychopathology perspective described above, multiple biobehavioral risk factors have been identified that precede, interact with, and increase the likelihood of developing substance use problems. These risk factors have been variously described, but can be conceptualized broadly as intrapersonal and environmental/contextual. At the intrapersonal level, risk factors include biological liability (family history of substance misuse), individual temperament and psychopathology, and personal attitudes and beliefs regarding substance use. Extensive research demonstrates that children who have parents with alcohol or drug problems are at increased risk of substance misuse, emotional difficulties, and other problem behaviors (e.g., Bennett, Wolin, & Reiss, 1988; Chassin, Fora, & King, 2004; Chassin, Rogosch, & Barrera, 1991; Knop, Teasdale, Schulsinger, & Goodwin, 1985; McMorris, Tyler, Whitbeck, & Hoyt, 2002; Moos & Billings, 1982; Ohannessian et al., 2004; Russell, 1990). Children with an alcohol-abusing parent are found to have poorer emotional, behavioral, and cognitive functioning than children of nonalcoholic parents (e.g., Tarter & Edwards, 1988).

Specifically related to the genetic transmission of alcohol/drug dependence, the level of response to the effects of alcohol is a heritable trait, and research has found that a low level of this response (e.g., body sway) is predictive of later development of alcohol problems

(Schuckit, 1994, 1998). Conversely, high reactivity, related to aldehyde dehydrogenase status, inhibits the emergence of alcohol abuse and dependence (Wall et al., 2001). Research on genetic factors in addictive disorders is increasingly suggesting multiple genetically related risks, which interact with environmental and developmental factors to promote or inhibit substance involvement (e.g., Rose, Chassin, Presson, & Sherman, 1996; Walden, McGue, Iacono, Burt, & Elkins, 2004). Substantial advances have been made in research on the genetics of proneness to nicotine and other drug dependence, implicating multiple systems such as neurotransmitters (e.g., Carmelli, Swan, Robinette, & Fabsitz, 1992; Swan & Carmelli, 1997).

Various temperamental factors, which are presumed to be largely inherited (Tarter & Edwards, 1988), have been found to be predictive of substance use problems. Most notably, poor impulse control and high sensation-seeking tendencies have been associated with greater substance involvement (Baker & Yardley, 2002; Cloninger, 1987; Donohew et al., 1999; Shedler & Block, 1990). In addition, externalizing disorders (e.g., CD) are associated with greater lifetime risk for substance dependence (Grilo, Becker, Fehon, Edell, & McGlashan, 1996; Kandel et al., 1999; Robins & Price, 1991; Vaillant, 1983). These observations suggest that the concordance between various undercontrolled behaviors is partly explained by common genetic influences (McGue, 1994; Slutske et al., 2002). Such findings are consistent with developmental hypotheses (e.g., Sher, 1991, 1994) that substance use and other conduct problems share similar etiological characteristics, such as deficits in self-regulation of affect (e.g., temperament) and socialization (e.g., deviant peer group).

Although comorbidity of other Axis I disorders with substance use disorders has been identified in large population-based studies (e.g., Kandel et al, 1999; Rohde et al., 1996), the relative sequencing of onset of these disorders is important for identifying the extent to which one increases risk for the other. CD has been shown to particularly increase risk for both the onset and progression of substance use disorders (e.g., Caspi, Moffitt, Newman, & Silva, 1996; Clark, Kirisci, & Moss, 1998; Clark, Parker, & Lynch, 1999; Sung, Erkanli, Angold, & Costello, 2004); for example, some

studies suggest that severity of delinquent behavior may lead to increased severity of substance use, but not vice versa (Fagan, Weiss, & Cheng, 1990; Hammersley, Forsyth, & Lavelle, 1990). Other studies, however, indicate that CD may also occur secondary to a substance use disorder (Brown, Gleghorn, Schuckit, Myers, & Mott, 1996). The extent to which ADHD affords increased risk for substance use disorders likewise continues to be debated, with some studies finding that an ADHD diagnosis predicts subsequent substance use disorders (Gittelman, Mannuzza, Shenker, & Bonagura, 1985; Mannuzza, Klein, Bessler, Malloy, & LaPadula, 1998) and accelerates the speed of transition from substance abuse to dependence (Wilens, Biederman, & Spencer, 1999). Other findings suggest that the greater prevalence of CD symptomatology in youths with ADHD may partially account for the increased risk of substance use disorder development (Biederman et al., 1997), with recent research indicating that comorbid diagnoses of ADHD and CD predict a greater extent of substance use in young adulthood than an ADHD diagnosis alone does (Barkley, Fischer, Smallish, & Fletcher, 2004). Finally, a number of studies have noted a relationship between adolescent depression and substance use problems, with onset of depression predating substance use disorders (Burke, Burke, & Rae, 1994; Deas-Nesmith, Campbell, & Brady, 1998; Rohde, Lewinsohn, & Seeley, 1991).

Within the domain of environmental influences, nonbiological familial factors play a role in the development of adolescent substance use and misuse. Alcohol- and/or drug-misusing parents model substance use behaviors that play a role in forming children's beliefs and attitudes concerning the anticipated effects of substance use (i.e., expectancies) (Bandura, 1977). Significantly, adolescents with an alcohol-abusing parent are found to anticipate more reinforcement from alcohol than do those with no parental alcohol misuse (Brown, Creamer, & Stetson, 1987). This latter point is particularly relevant, since children who hold heightened expectancies for the positive effects of use (e.g., for managing negative emotions or facilitating social interactions) are at greater risk for later developing alcohol-related problems (Smith & Goldman, 1994). In addition, parental substance misuse often increases the availability and accessibility of alcohol and drugs for children.

Other family factors also influence the likelihood of adolescent substance misuse. Parenting style has been found to be related to adolescent substance use problems. For example, parental hostility and lack of warmth have been found to be related to both problematic alcohol use (Johnson & Pandina, 1991) and drug use (Shedler & Block, 1990). A more recent study suggests that the influence of parenting style on alcohol use is mediated by self-regulation and perceived drinking control, indicating that environmental and intrapersonal factors interact with each other to influence the likelihood of substance misuse (Patock-Peckman, Cheong, Balhorn, & Nagoshi, 2001). Substance use is also found to increase with greater familial stress and conflict, as well as with reduced parental monitoring (e.g., Baer, Garmezy, McLaughlin, & Pokorny, 1987; Brown, 1989; Jacob & Leonard, 1994; Wills & Yaeger, 2003). Conversely, certain family factors operate to protect adolescents from problematic substance use. For example, greater parental support and control, higher level of parental education, and greater parental religiosity predict lower adolescent alcohol use (Stice, Barrera, & Chassin, 1993; Vakalahi, 2001). In sum, parental substance abuse and dependence, as well as characteristics of family interactions, influence the development of adolescent substance use and problems.

Peer relations play an important role in the initiation and progression of adolescent substance use (Barnes, Farrell, & Banerjee, 1994). Modeling of substance use within the peer group provides immediate access to substances, encourages youths to engage in these behaviors, and peers then provide reinforcement for conformity (Costa, Jessor, & Turbin, 1999) as well as maladaptive coping (Richter, Brown, & Mott, 1991). Also, difficult interactions with peers, particularly during early and middle adolescence, create social anxiety, perceived pressure to drink/use, and increased interpersonal conflict (e.g., Hundleby & Mercer, 1987); these factors enhance the appeal of substance use through expectations that alcohol or drug use will provide relief from social stress or reduce social tension by providing a common behavioral activity. Moreover, peer influences interact with family factors to determine substance use risk. For example, affiliations with deviant peers who model substance use and other risky behaviors are more likely for teens whose parents themselves misuse substances or are less

involved in monitoring their children (Patterson, DeBaryshe, & Ramsey, 1989).

In summary, there are multiple sources of risk for adolescent substance abuse. Risks appear to aggregate into three primary pathways: (1) deviance proneness, (2) stress and negative affect, and (3) reinforcement from substance use effects. Whereas deviance proneness has been a dominant focus in the literature (e.g., Donovan & Jessor, 1985), studies of reinforcement from substance use effects have highlighted both biological features and cognitive features (e.g., Goldman et al., 1991; Schuckit, 1998). Chassin and her colleagues (Chassin et al., 1991; Colder & Chassin, 1993) have articulated a pathway whereby children from alcoholic families experience higher levels of negative affect related to increased stress and temperamental emotionality. The relation between negative affect and substance use is in turn influenced by peer use. Models such as this one provide examples of the interplay among biological, cognitive, and environmental influences in the development of substance use problems, and highlight the complexities inherent in the development of these early problems.

ASSESSMENT

Basic Considerations

Assessment of adolescent substance use problems considers the biological, psychological, and social factors influencing the clinical presentation (Donovan & Marlatt, 1988; Vik, Brown, & Myers, 1997). Consideration of the multiple influences on the development and progression of substance involvement is essential to treatment planning (Brown, 1993). Thus each of the following areas should be evaluated: (1) substance involvement characteristics (e.g., use, context, consequences); (2) intrapersonal factors (e.g., coping/social skills, comorbid psychopathology, antisocial tendencies); (3) environmental factors (e.g., family functioning, social support, cultural influences, life stress, peer substance use); and (4) functioning in major life domains (e.g., physical health, academics, interpersonal relations, extracurricular activities/hobbies) (Meyers et al., 1999; Tapert, Stewart, & Brown, 1999). To the extent possible, a broad-spectrum assessment should be conducted, including adolescent self-reports (e.g., clinical interview, self-administered structured questionnaires, and self-monitoring), reports from significant others (e.g., parents, teachers); and objective measures (e.g., neuropsychological/academic functioning, toxicology screens). Although an ideal assessment includes all possible sources of data, the reality of clinical practice often dictates that reports from the adolescent and family members and toxicology screens are the only sources of information.

Sequential assessment is typically recommended: initial screening, followed by diagnosis (including comorbid psychopathology), and then by an assessment of problems and deficits in the domains of functioning affected by substance use (to determine the appropriate level and intensity of intervention). In cases where available information clearly indicates problematic substance involvement (e.g., previous history of treatment, drug-related arrests), screening becomes less important, and the clinician can proceed with a broader-based assessment to identify problem domains. A thorough substance use assessment also serves the important dual purposes of (1) providing baseline information, which can be used for assessing progress during the course of treatment; and (2) enhancing motivation for entering treatment and adhering to the selected intervention strategy (Miller & Rollnick, 2002).

As adolescent problems are, substance misuse is embedded within the developmental context. Developmental changes during adolescence are accompanied by normative increases in negative affect, substance experimentation, and other risky behaviors. The biological changes accompanying puberty precipitate behavioral and emotional changes that are difficult to separate from the effects of alcohol and drug use (Brown et al., 1990). Thus the developmental tasks of adolescence in general and the individual adolescent's stage of development are critical factors to consider in developing an accurate clinical picture.

Further complicating assessment is the heterogeneous nature of adolescent substance use problems (Meyers et al., 1999). Substance-misusing youths vary in the types of substances they use, the frequency and intensity of their use, their beliefs regarding effects and consequences of use, the motivations underlying their use, and the nature of factors that precipitate and accompany their use. Thus flexibility is needed in determining the optimal intervention strategy for each youth. This latter point is consistent with evidence that multiple pathways exist for the successful resolution of adolescent substance misuse (Brown, 1993, 2001).

Instruments for Assessment of Substance Misuse

With the introduction of psychometrically validated instruments, standardized assessment has become more feasible and is strongly recommended. Employment of standardized assessment procedures offers various advantages over individual clinicians' judgment, such as providing a basis for comparing and validating clinical decisions, and protecting against the introduction of rater bias (Henly & Winters, 1989). Standardized instruments have the additional advantage of providing a time-efficient means for gathering large quantities of information. Data gathered from standardized instruments can help inform the clinical interview, during which the clinician can clarify previously obtained information and can verify the accuracy of responses. Although direct observation of adolescent substance use behavior is unrealistic, observation and rating of in-session behavior can provide valuable information regarding cognitive, affective, and interpersonal functioning. Finally, information regarding intellectual and academic functioning is particularly useful. Since neuropsychological deficits and learning disabilities are often observed among adolescents with substance use problems (Tapert & Brown, 2000; Weinberg, 2001) and may interact with adolescents' use of coping skills to remain abstinent following treatment (Tapert, Brown, Myers, & Granholm, 1999), this information is essential to selecting appropriate intervention strategies and determining the need for educational compensation or remediation. Table 11.1 lists several standardized instruments for assessing adolescent substance misuse.

For screening purposes, the Personal Experience Screening Questionnaire (PESQ; Winters, 1991, 1992) is recommended for its theoretical and psychometric strengths. This measure is brief, includes response bias scales that indicate invalid responding, and provides cutoffs and normative values for determining substance problem severity. At this time, the normative sample for the PESQ contains few minority subjects, and thus results from minority respondents must be interpreted with caution.

TABLE 11.1. Measures of Adolescent Alcohol and Other Drug Involvement

Measure	Description
	Screening measures
Adolescent Drinking Inventory: Drinking and You (Harrell & Wirtz, 1989)	A 24-item questionnaire designed for use by clinicians without specialized training in substance use assessment. Utilizes a multidimensional conceptualization of adolescent drinking and has been shown to possess good psychometric properties.
Rutgers Alcohol Problem Index (RAPI; White & Labouvie, 1989)	A 23-item measure assessing drinking-related problems. The RAPI includes DSM-III-R criteria required for a diagnosis of alcohol abuse. Initial work supports validity; however, further work is needed to establish psychometric properties.
Drug and Alcohol Problem Quick Screen (Schwartz & Wirth, 1990)	A 30-item scale designed to detect adolescent substance misuse, from which a 14-item short form has also been developed. Intended for use in primary care settings; however, this measure has not been independently validated, and data have not been published on clinical samples.
Personal Experience Screening Questionnaire (PESQ; Winters, 1991)	A 40-item questionnaire designed to identify adolescents in need of a drug use assessment referral. The PESQ includes a problem severity scale, two response distortion scales, and a supplemental information section on substance use and psychosocial functioning history. The PESQ has demonstrated excellent psychometric properties with both nonclinical and clinical populations.
	Multidimensional measures
Personal Experience Inventory (PEI; Winters & Henly, 1989a)	A self-administered interview that includes 276 items divided into five sets of scales: basic scales (i.e., substance involvement), clinical scales, validity scales, personal adjustment scales, and family and peer environment scales. The PEI is intended to provide information for identifying problems, planning treatment, and evaluating outcome. This measure has been comprehensively and rigorously evaluated and has been shown to have adequate reliability and validity.
Drug Use Screening Inventory—Revised (DUSI-R; Kirisci, Mezzich, & Tarter, 1995; Tarter, Laird, Bukstein, & Kaminer, 1992)	A 159-item self-administered questionnaire that profiles substance use involvement in conjunction with the severity of disturbance in ten domains of everyday functioning. The DUSI-R yields a needs assessment and diagnostic summary intended to inform treatment planning. Available work shows that the DUSI-R possesses adequate psychometric properties.
Customary Drinking and Drug Use Record (CDDR; Brown, Creamer, & Stetson, 1987; Brown et al., 1998)	A structured interview with 143 items, the CDDR gathers information about ages at onset of use; frequency of cigarette, alcohol, and drug use; alcohol and drug withdrawal; DSM-III-R psychoactive substance dependence symptoms (excluding nicotine); and life problems related to alcohol and drug use. The lifetime version of the CDDR obtains lifetime information regarding use of alcohol and other drugs. This structured clinical interview has good reliability and validity for clinical samples of substance-misusing teens (Brown et al., 1998; Stewart & Brown, 1995).
Structured Clinical Interview for Adolescents (SCI; Brown, Vik, & Creamer, 1989)	A structured interview designed to provide demographic and background information that can inform both research and clinical decision making. The SCI elicits information regarding academic, interpersonal, and psychosocial functioning, including previous treatment for alcohol or other mental health problems, peer substance involvement, motivation for entering treatment, and motivation and efficacy for reducing substance use. In addition, it includes a comprehensive assessment of familial history of alcohol and drug misuse. Several studies indicate that the SCI has adequate psychometric characteristics.

(continued)

TABLE 11.1. *(continued)*

Measure	Description
	Multidimensional measures *(cont.)*
Teen Addiction Severity Index (T-ASI; Kaminer, Bukstein, & Tarter, 1991; Kaminer, Wagner, Plummer, & Seifer, 1993)	An adaptation of the Addiction Severity Index (McLellan et al., 1980). This semistructured interview yields seven measures: substance involvement, academic functioning, employment status, family relationships, peer/social status, legal status, and psychiatric disturbance. Limited data suggest adequate reliability for the T-ASI.
Adolescent Diagnostic Interview (ADI; Winters & Henly, 1989a)	A comprehensive structured interview designed to yield DSM-III-R diagnoses for psychoactive substance abuse. In addition to substance use diagnoses, the ADI provides a global rating of functioning, an assessment of severity of psychosocial stressors, and a rating of cognitive functioning. The ADI is thus designed to provide detailed diagnostic information relevant to treatment planning for substance-misusing youths. Validity of diagnosis has been demonstrated for white adolescents.

Several multidimensional assessment instruments are currently available. These provide information on various domains of functioning consistent with a biobehavioral conceptualization of adolescent substance misuse. The Personal Experience Inventory (PEI; Winters & Henly, 1989b; Winters, Stinchfield, & Henly, 1996) is a well-validated self-report measure with normative data available. The PEI consists of several subscales assessing problem severity, drug and alcohol use history, and psychosocial adjustment, but does not provide a formal diagnosis. The Drug Use Screening Inventory—Revised (DUSI-R; Kirisci, Mezzich, & Tarter, 1995; Tarter, Laird, Bukstein, & Kaminer, 1992), assesses substance use involvement and severity of impairment for 10 domains of functioning (e.g., school adjustment, social skills, family functioning). The DUSI-R is unique in that it is designed to facilitate the application of assessment findings to treatment planning by providing a needs assessment, domain severity scores, and a diagnostic summary. Reports have supported the validity and reliability of the DUSI-R (e.g., Kirisci et al., 1995). Also available is a semistructured interview measure, the Teen Addiction Severity Index (T-ASI; Kaminer, Bukstein, & Tarter, 1991; Kaminer, Wagner, Plummer, & Seifer, 1993), which is an adolescent-specific version of the widely used Addiction Severity Index (McLellan, Luborsky, O'Brien, & Woody, 1980). The T-ASI assesses seven domains of functioning, including substance use, school, employment, family, peer/social, legal, and psychiatric. Although available information is limited at this time, it

suggests that the T-ASI possesses adequate psychometric properties. Another adolescent version of the Addiction Severity Index has also recently been developed by creators of the original instrument (the Comprehensive Addiction Severity Index for Adolescents; Meyers, McLellan, Jaeger, & Pettinati, 1995). This measure assesses risk factors, symptomatology, and consequences of substance involvement across seven primary areas of functioning: academics, alcohol/drug use, family relationships, peer relationships, legal issues, psychiatric difficulties, and recreation. Initial examination of the reliability and validity of this measure has provided preliminary evidence for its psychometric utility (Meyers et al., 1995, 1998).

Finally, the Structured Clinical Interview (SCI; Brown, Creamer, & Stetson, 1987; Brown et al., 1989), which assesses lifetime and current functioning in major life domains in relation to adolescent substance involvement, is typically used in conjunction with the Customary Drinking and Drug Use Record (CDDR; Brown, Creamer, & Stetson, 1987; Brown et al., 1998). The latter is a psychometrically sound instrument allowing diagnosis and onset dates for differential diagnosis purposes; it also provides a detailed evaluation of involvement with alcohol and various drug types, as well as of withdrawal/dependence and consequences of substance involvement.

In addition to measures that provide an indication of the severity of substance use and its consequences, several instruments have been developed to evaluate specific features of adolescent substance involvement. For example, the Inventory of Drug Taking Situations (IDTS; Annis & Graham, 1985; Turner, Annis, & Sklar, 1997) is a 50-item self-report questionnaire that evaluates the frequency of use in diverse situations. The IDTS includes situations in eight domains, including conflict, social pressure, pleasant social situations, positive emotions, negative emotions, physical discomfort, testing personal control, and urges/temptations. The questionnaire is scored to provide a profile of use across the eight areas, and as such allows identification of settings or circumstances associated with frequent substance use which can then be targeted in the course of treatment. A companion measure to the IDTS that may assist in the process of identifying relapse risk situations is the Drug Taking Confidence Questionnaire (DTCQ; Annis & Martin, 1985). This questionnaire, identical in item content domains to the IDTS, measures self-efficacy for abstaining in each situation. Another useful measure is the Adolescent version of the Alcohol Expectancy Questionnaire (AEQ-A; Christiansen & Goldman, 1983). This self-administered questionnaire measures anticipated effects of alcohol in seven domains (global positive changes, social and physical pleasure, cognitive and motor enhancement, sexual enhancement, cognitive and behavioral deterioration, arousal, and relaxation/tension reduction). Numerous studies support the concurrent and predictive validity of the AEQ-A (see Brown, Christiansen, & Goldman, 1987; Christiansen et al., 1989), which can characterize aspects of alcohol use that are of particular importance to the adolescent. This information can be used for targeting areas for which alternative means of reinforcement must be developed, and for selecting interventions designed to modify or alter alcohol-related beliefs (Brown, 1993; Smith & Goldman, 1994). Measures also exist to examine adolescents' expected outcomes of engaging in other substance use, such as the Short Smoking Consequences Questionnaire for tobacco (Myers, McCarthy, MacPherson, & Brown, 2003), the Marijuana Effect Expectancy Questionnaire (MEEQ; Aarons, Brown, Stice, & Coe, 2001), and the Stimulant Effect Expectancy Questionnaire (SEEQ; Aarons et al., 2001), all of which have been psychometrically tested with adolescents. Finally, a recently developed measure of adolescents' beliefs regarding the expected outcomes of ceasing alcohol use (Metrik, McCarthy, Frissell, MacPherson, & Brown, 2004) is a useful tool in identifying anticipated benefits and problems of ceasing alcohol use.

Assessment of Domains Related to Substance Misuse

Several domains that are influenced by and/or contributing to adolescent substance misuse are important to consider in the assessment process. A particularly useful measurement package is the Achenbach System for Empirically Based Assessment (ASEBA; Achenbach & Rescorla, 2001; McConaughy, 2001), which includes the Child Behavior Checklist (CBCL), the Teacher's Report Form (TRF), and the Youth Self-Report (YSR). The CBCL is a parent self-report instrument that assesses a variety of behavior problems and social competence. The CBCL includes three Social Competence scales (Activities, Social, and School) and eight Behavior Problem scales (e.g., Attention Problems, Withdrawn, Depressed, and Aggressive Behavior), with adolescent normative data available for a variety of clinical populations. Additionally, the ASEBA may also produce six DSM-oriented scales (e.g., Affective Problems, Conduct Problems). The TRF is designed to be completed by teachers, and elicits information regarding academic performance, adaptive functioning, and behavioral and emotional problems. The majority of the TRF items (99 out of the total 122 items) are identical to those on the CBCL, thus allowing for comparison of these behaviors in different settings. Finally, the YSR is a self-report form worded in the first person with items that overlap substantially with the CBCL and TRF. Comparison across these sources of information highlights convergence and divergence in perceptions of problems between the adolescent and adults. The multiple sources of information can be particularly useful to the clinician in determining the degree to which an adolescent is likely to be open to intervention for particular problem areas. In addition, information from the CBCL and/or the related measures can be utilized to identify areas for intervention and is especially well suited for assessing progress and treatment outcome (McConaughy, 2001).

Another measure of adolescent behavioral functioning is the Behavior Assessment System for Children, Second Edition (BASC-2; Reynolds & Kamphaus, 2004). This scale has only been recently published, but the original

BASC (Reynolds & Kamphaus, 1994) has satisfactory psychometric properties for use with adolescents and includes a normative reference sample for interpreting scores. Convergent validity has also been preliminarily established (Merydith, 2001).

A formal diagnostic assessment for the presence of additional psychiatric conditions is recommended, because of the high rates of comorbid psychopathology found among substance-misusing youths (e.g., Abrantes et al., 2004; Crowley & Riggs, 1995; Kandel et al., 1999; Rohde et al., 1996). This assessment can be conducted in the course of the clinical interview or can utilize structured procedures based on DSM criteria, such as the Diagnostic Interview Schedule for Children—Version IV (DISC-IV; Costello, Edelbrock, Dulcan, Kalas, & Klaric, 1987; Shaffer, Fisher, Lucas, Dulcan, & Schwab-Stone, 2000) and the Schedule for Affective Disorders and Schizophrenia for School-Age Children—Present and Lifetime Version (K-SADS-PL; Kaufman et al., 1997; Puig-Antich & Orvaschel, 1987).

Finally, the issue of tobacco use is one that is often overlooked in the course of substance use treatment, yet represents a significant problem among youths with other substance use disorders (Myers & Brown, 1996). Examinations of clinical samples of substance-abusing teens reveal rates of smoking three to four times higher than those in the general adolescent population, persistent cigarette smoking following substance use treatment regardless of alcohol or drug use outcome, and smoking-related health problems among these youths (Myers & Brown, 1994; Upadhyaya, Deas, Brady, & Kruesi, 2002). Failure to assess and treat nicotine use in the context of other substance involvement may inadvertently reinforce tobacco use, because adolescents may perceive this failure as tacit approval of tobacco use (Myers, 1999). At this time, it is premature to recommend that adolescents be required to abstain from tobacco products in the course of treatment for substance misuse, although a controlled study of a smoking cessation intervention in the context of alcohol and drug treatment among adults reported higher rates of abstinence from alcohol and drugs among patients who were randomly assigned to the smoking intervention, compared to those who received treatment as usual (Bobo, McIlvain, Lando, Walker, & Leed-Kelly, 1998). However,

it is important for this issue to be addressed and for adolescents to receive a clear message that tobacco use is discouraged.

Unfortunately, information about cigarette smoking is not elicited on many of the standardized measures of adolescent substance use (e.g., the PEI, the PESQ), with the exception of the CDDR. Tobacco assessment should include age at first use of cigarettes and other tobacco products (e.g., chewing tobacco), onset of regular/weekly use, and current pattern of tobacco use (e.g., days per week of use, times cigarettes or other tobacco products are used per day, and most recent use of tobacco products). Brief measures are available to assess level of nicotine dependence among youth, such as the modified Fagerström Tolerance Questionnaire (Prokhorov, Koehly, Pallonen, & Hudmon, 1998).

Formulating Treatment Recommendations

Case formulation rests on detailing the functions served by substance use for the adolescent, identifying areas of needed intervention and goals for treatment, and outlining intervention options. It is important to conceptualize the data in a manner that permits identification of the factors promoting and maintaining adolescent substance use; anticipates obstacles to behavior change; and identifies improvements and strengths (personal, familial, environmental) that will facilitate youth change efforts as well as maintenance of gains. The case formulation should include detailed feedback to the teen; a list of youth- and adult-identified problems; and evaluation of motivation for change of critical behaviors, contexts within which use frequently occurs, and available resources for maintaining behavior change.

Case formulation begins with generating personalized feedback on the teen's substance involvement relative to normative samples, and providing a comprehensive problem list that outlines the relationship of substance use to youth- and adult-defined presenting problems and symptoms. A critical issue in determining an appropriate intervention approach is the presence of concomitant psychopathology. Information from the assessment must be adequate to permit the clinician to determine the presence of conditions other than substance misuse; to evaluate the course of such problems; and to estimate the degree to which they precede, are independent of, or follow from the substance use. A timeline sequencing substance use and other mental health symptomatology is especially helpful in clarifying the nature of the relationship between substance use and other psychopathology (Brown, Inaba, et al., 1994). Conditions that predate the onset of substance use, or for which symptoms exist during periods of protracted abstinence, provide evidence for an independent disorder. Because substance effects can mimic or produce symptoms consistent with major psychiatric disorders, the clinician should exercise caution in inferring the presence of a comorbid condition if such symptoms are assessed while the adolescent is still involved in substance use or during the first 3 weeks of withdrawal (Brown & Schuckit, 1988).

Next, the adolescent's motivation for changing substance use patterns and related behaviors is critical to designing appropriate treatment for each teen (e.g., Hester & Miller, 1988; Miller & Rollnick, 2002). Evaluating motivation of youths in substance abuse treatment is especially important, because these youths generally enter treatment because of external pressures or influences (Brown, 1993; Cady, Winters, Jordon, Solberg, & Stinchfield, 1996), and because motivation for change varies by substance and is typically related to adverse consequences (Brown & Ramo, in press). Consideration of motivation for change is essential to engaging the adolescent in the treatment process and collaboratively developing acceptable short-term treatment goals to which the adolescent will adhere.

The provision of feedback from the assessment to the adolescent and his or her family, and the manner in which the feedback is delivered, are important for engagement and compliance with initial treatment recommendations. Miller and Rollnick (2002) emphasize the value of personalized feedback for persuading clients of the necessity for behavior change. To this end, it is useful to (1) provide a complete description of assessment findings in a manner that assures comprehension by the adolescent and his or her family; (2) avoid confrontational approaches, which increase resistance; (3) attend to and reflect reactions to assessment information; (4) request feedback from the adolescent and family; (5) anticipate possible strong emotional reactions; and (6) comprehensively summarize the feedback session and solicit additional input from the adolescent and family.

TREATMENT

Overview

Given the heterogeneity of substance-abusing youths entering treatment and the limited empirical evidence on outcomes of diverse interventions for these youths, no single intervention approach is recommended for adolescents. Instead, treatment programs typically incorporate multiple components designed to address the domains of functioning affected by substance involvement. Intervention should address the specific problems identified by and for each adolescent and be sensitive to developmental stages and needs of the individual. This client–treatment matching strategy suggests an approach to treatment that is (1) flexible and can be adapted to meet the particular needs and developmental stage of each client; (2) diverse, to reflect the heterogeneity and preferences of adolescents; and (3) sensitive to concomitant problems (e.g., other psychopathology, family issues) (Brown, 2001). To this end, we subscribe to a cognitive-behavioral intervention as the core intervention for adolescent substance use and abuse. This can be employed as the sole treatment or can be incorporated within a multicomponent intervention program (e.g., family, etc.). The intervention to be described below focuses on deficits commonly associated with adolescent substance involvement, and is based on a body of research that identifies predictors and correlates of successful outcome following treatment for adolescent substance use problems (e.g., Brown et al., 2001; Kelly, Myers, & Brown, 2000; Kypri, McCarthy, Coe, & Brown, 2004; Latimer, Winters, Stinchfield, & Traver, 2000). The intervention is described here as an individual-focused intervention; however, these techniques are readily translated into a group format.

Empirical Evidence for Treatment Efficacy

Current programs generally advertise a broad range of therapeutic components and incorporate age-appropriate elements to address school, peer, family, legal, health and other issues (e.g., depression, anxiety). These programs are usually based on the medical/disease model of addiction that was developed within the field of adult alcoholism, and empirical evidence for this model's efficacy for adolescents is only recently emerging. Recent studies of substance-misusing adolescents indicate that Twelve-Step attendance is associated with lower rates of use following treatment (Kelly, Myers, & Brown, 2002). Initial studies of treatment outcome for substance-abusing and substance-dependent youths were primarily descriptive and based on data gathered in the 1970s (e.g., Hubbard, Cavanaugh, Graddock, & Rachel, 1983; Sells & Simpson, 1979) on older adolescent participants in adult treatment programs. Despite the lack of specificity of these earlier programs for youths, treatment appeared to reduce hard drug use among teens, but had a more limited impact on levels of alcohol and marijuana use. These early naturalistic evaluations of adolescents are similar to recent reports, with better outcomes for use of drugs other than alcohol and tobacco (Brown et al., 2001; Yih-Ing et al., 2001).

More recently, family-based interventions have received increased attention because of consistent evidence for the role of family factors in adolescent substance use (for reviews, see Deas & Thomas, 2001; Waldron, 1997). In particular, multicomponent family approaches that are integrative (i.e., that also incorporate nonfamily issues) are found to be effective in reducing both substance use and problem behaviors (for reviews, see Deas & Thomas, 2001; Liddle & Dakof, 1995). These integrative approaches incorporate traditional family systems efforts to change the interactional patterns within the family that serve to maintain substance use behaviors. Integrative family therapy approaches also draw on other psychotherapeutic techniques to address adolescent peer relationships, school functioning, and legal issues.

For example, Szapocznik and colleagues (Coatsworth, Santisteban, McBride, & Szapocznik, 2001; Santisteban et al., 2003; Szapocznik, Kurtines, Foote, Perez-Vidal, & Hervis, 1983, 1986) have published several efficacy reports of brief strategic family therapy (BSFT), which focuses on interactional patterns within the family system and between family members and other systems in the environment. These researchers have demonstrated that BSFT is effective in engaging families in therapy, reducing adolescent substance involvement, and improving family relations when either the family (conjoint family therapy) or only the adolescent ("one-person family therapy") is seen in treatment (Coatsworth et al., 2001; Santisteban et al., 2003; Szapocznik et

al., 1983, 1986, 1988). In addition, multidimensional family therapy, developed by Liddle and colleagues (1992), focuses on both adolescent substance involvement, conduct problems, and intrapersonal and extrafamilial factors in treating substance use problems. Adolescents receiving multidimensional family therapy have shown greater reductions in drug use at the end of treatment and at a 1-year follow-up than participants in comparison interventions. Other integrative family approaches with efficacy results for adolescent substance abuse include family systems therapy (Joanning et al., 1992), brief family therapy (Lewis, Piercy, Sprenkle, & Trepper, 1990), and multisystemic therapy (Henggeler et al., 1991). With few exceptions (e.g., Henggeler, Clingempeel, Brondino, & Pickrel, 2002), studies of these integrative family approaches have provided consistent empirical support for their utility in treating adolescent substance abuse (Deas & Thomas, 2001).

Cognitive-behavioral approaches have also shown considerable success as treatments for youths. For example, structural behavioral treatments were found to result in better outcomes (in terms of substance use, family relations, and emotional and behavior problems) than a supportive counseling program (Azrin, Donohue, Besalel, Kogan, & Acierno, 1994). The core components of this behavioral program included stimulus control, urge control, and contracting (e.g., Kaminer, Burleson, & Goldberg, 2002). Other cognitive-behavioral treatments for adolescent substance use have incorporated components such as problem-solving skills, peer refusal skills, and communication skills, and have found support for these approaches (Waldron & Kaminer, 2004; Waldron, Slesnick, Brody, Turner, & Peterson, 2001).

Unfortunately, studies of pharmacological treatment of substance use disorders among adolescents are rare and are extremely limited (Lifrak, Alterman, O'Brien, & Volpicelli, 1997). Furthermore, research regarding the efficacy of nicotine replacement therapies for adolescents who smoke has not provided support for their use with this population (Hurt et al., 2000; Smith et al., 1996), although current Centers for Disease Control and Prevention guidelines suggest their use for nicotine-dependent adolescents (Fiore et al., 2000). Rather, research to date has focused on how pharmacological treatment of a comorbid condition affects substance use. Studies examining the relationship between treatment of mood disorders and substance use outcomes among adolescents provide preliminary evidence that intervening with these comorbid conditions may be effective in reducing not only symptoms of the mood disorders, but substance use as well (Deas & Thomas, 2001). Nevertheless, due to the paucity of studies of pharmacological treatments for substance-misusing adolescents, it is premature to broadly recommend pharmacotherapy for this population.

In the absence of any clear evidence regarding optimal approaches to adolescent substance use treatment, interventions must be based on the following: sensitivity to adolescent development issues; incorporation of the relevant research literature (e.g., risk factors, predictors of clinical course); a comprehensive conceptualization of adolescent substance use; and a focus on problem behaviors and mental health disorders common among youths with substance use disorders (Brown, 2001; Chung et al., 2003; Liddle & Dakof, 1995).

Empirical Evidence for Predictors and Correlates of Clinical Course

Evidence for the utility of cognitive-behavioral interventions for adolescent substance use comes largely from studies investigating clinical samples of adolescents treated for substance use problems. In the realm of family factors, poorer treatment outcome is found to be related to greater lifetime exposure to familial substance misuse, less expressiveness by family members, and lower family support as perceived by the adolescents (e.g., Brown et al., 1990). In the broader domain of social resources, more satisfaction with social supports and a greater proportion of nonusing peers in an adolescent's social network are predictive of less alcohol and drug use following treatment (Richter et al., 1991; Vik, Grizzle, & Brown, 1992), as is family involvement in Twelve-Step meetings (Myers & Brown, 1994). Personal characteristics such as lower self-esteem, more delinquent-type behaviors, and other mental health disorders have also been associated with poorer treatment outcome (Brown et al., 1996; Myers, Brown, & Mott, 1995; Richter et al., 1991; Tomlinson et al., 2004). Persistence in some type of formal treatment (e.g., aftercare, Twelve-Step, etc.) is associated with better outcome for both adolescents (e.g., Winters,

Stinchfield, Opland, Weller, & Latimer, 2000) and adults (e.g., Project MATCH Research Group, 1997). For example, participation in Twelve-Step groups following substance abuse treatment appears to have modest salutary effects for adolescents, primarily by maintaining motivation for abstinence (Kelly et al., 2000). A broader array of skills for coping with situations presenting common temptations for substance use is also predictive of better outcomes for substance-abusing youths (Myers & Brown, 1994, 1996; Myers, Brown, & Mott, 1993).

Viewed in concert, this pattern of findings suggest that intervention strategies targeted at improving personal resources (e.g., improving coping skills, increasing social support, maintaining involvement in treatment) and reducing environmental risks facilitate posttreatment success for adolescents with alcohol and other drug problems. Specifically, studies of coping with relapse risk suggest that behavioral strategies specific to managing substance use temptations, utilization of abstaining social resources, and awareness of the negative consequences of alcohol and drug use are important aspects of successful outcome for these adolescents.

As for the clinical course following treatment, adolescents with less posttreatment alcohol and drug use have been found to improve on measures of emotional, interpersonal, familial, academic, vocational, and recreational functioning (e.g., Brown, Myers, et al., 1994). A noteworthy finding is that improvement in some domains (e.g., school grades, family relations) occurs more slowly than in others (e.g., depression, school attendance). Of note, a minority of adolescents who return to alcohol or drug use shortly after treatment are later able to maintain stable abstinence. More recent longitudinal research on youths after treatment indicates several common substance use trajectories (Brown et al., 2001; Chung et al., 2003). Specifically, in the several years following treatment these youths either increased their substance use over time, maintained high levels of use, decreased use over time following an initial period of heavy use, abstained, or maintained low levels of use. Furthermore, adolescents who maintained total or near-total abstinence demonstrated better interpersonal, occupational, and educational functioning than did adolescents who continued regular substance involvement. Several independent longitudinal investigations using semiparametric analytic techniques confirm these adolescent posttreatment substance use trajectories (Chung et al., 2003) and highlight the heterogeneity in long-term patterns of adolescent substance involvement. Across studies, trajectories involving long-term reductions in use are associated with improvements in psychosocial functioning (e.g., interpersonal conflict, family cohesion) and neurocognitive functioning. When considering treatment, the clinician is cautioned to hold realistic expectations for the time course of progress and the likely variability in improvement across domains of youth functioning.

Cognitive-Behavioral Skills Training: Overview and Rationale

The selection of a cognitive-behavioral intervention is consistent with the evidence reviewed above for the importance of social resources, coping skills, substance-related attitudes, self-esteem, and family relations as predictors of adolescent treatment outcome. Based on such findings and the underlying biobehavioral theoretical perspective, the intervention outlined in Table 11.2 and described below focuses on identifying the role occupied by alcohol and drug use in the life of the adolescent (i.e., by conducting a functional analysis of substance use behavior), and centers on motivating the youth to employ strategies to alter his or her substance use and related behaviors.

Because adolescents are in treatment for many problems, family issues may be of partic-

ular salience in the therapy of adolescent substance misuse. Previous research provides evidence for the important role of the family in the outcome of treatment for adolescent substance use problems, in that reestablishment of positive family relations appears to play a significant role in successful treatment outcome, particularly for younger teens (Brown, 1993). In addition, family functioning improves following persistent offspring abstinence (Donohue & Azrin, 2001; Stewart & Brown, 1994). In general, we recommend that family structure, family functioning, and parenting be assessed, and that such issues be integrated into the course of treatment. Whether family involvement consists of an additional family intervention above and beyond the individual or group intervention, or is limited to inclusion in the regular course of treatment with the teen, treatment should be based on the needs and characteristics of each family. Depending on the presence of parental alcohol and drug misuse or other psychopathology, and on family members' motivation for change, the intervention approach may vary markedly.

Our description of the present intervention focuses primarily on the adolescent. In this context, the initial stages of intervention consist of ME and strategies (e.g., social skills training and affect regulation) designed to improve functioning in inter- and intrapersonal domains. The focus during this initial portion of the intervention is on motivation for change and coping skills, rather than on substance use per se.

Strategies for preventing relapse are introduced later in the intervention and focus more specifically on situations and circumstances surrounding previous substance use. Relapse prevention is considered a particularly important component of this intervention. "Relapse" is conceptualized as a process of returning to problematic substance use, rather than as a discrete event; consequently, single occurrences of alcohol or drug use ("lapses" or "slips") are considered learning opportunities rather than failure experiences. This model identifies situations in which substance use previously occurred, and that tax or exceed the adolescent's coping resources, as representing high risk for relapse. The probability of a lapse in a given situation is related to personal motivation to sustain an abstinent lifestyle, the extent to which substance use was previously employed to manage similar circumstances, the availabil-

---

TABLE 11.2. Cognitive-Behavioral Skills Training Outline

1. Core sessions
   - Motivation enhancement (ME)
   - Introduction of functional analysis
   - Cognitive-behavioral skills training modules

2. Interpersonal skills
   - Assertiveness
   - Giving and receiving criticism; expressing feelings
   - Dealing with conflict (anger and frustration)

3. Managing negative emotions

4. Relapse prevention
   - Rationale/identifying high-risk situations
   - Coping with high-risk situations
   - Refusal skills
   - Goal setting/alternative activities

ity of effective coping and affect regulation strategies, and the individual's belief in his or her ability to cope successfully with such situations (self-efficacy; Brown & Ramo, in press).

Finally, strategies for maintenance of behavior change must be planned in accordance with clinical course for adolescents. Youths evidence high rates of relapse in the initial months following treatment (Brown et al., 1990), with the first 6 months representing the period of greatest risk (e.g., Brown, 1993). In addition, this period poses the greatest stress for youths, and reports of anxiety and depression are prevalent. Thus continued intervention contacts appear to be critical to maintaining treatment gains during this period.

Session Structure

Each session within this intervention contains similar elements and proceeds in a similar sequence: motivation evaluation and ME; review and discussion of previous material and assignments; introduction of new material; practice (i.e., role plays) of new skills; and, finally, selection of skill enhancement assignments.

Given the emergence of independence and need for autonomy during adolescence, it is important for the clinician to solicit feedback from the adolescent about the perceived helpfulness and relevance of all material covered in sessions. In particular, attention should be given to the teen's understanding and appraisal of session material and assignments, in order to anticipate and identify barriers to compliance and to determine optimal directions of cooperation. This collaborative strategy is helpful in engaging the youth; reducing resistance; and tailoring treatment to the pace, ability, and motivation of each adolescent.

Introduction of new material is preceded by discussion of a rationale, which should conform with the motivational and functional analysis. Comprehension and acceptance of the rationale are enhanced when the clinician can provide examples relevant to the adolescent's personal experience and facilitate the adolescent's generation of personal examples. Also helpful are handouts that outline each topic area and provide concrete, teen-specific examples relevant to assignments. In general, new material should be introduced briefly and should be made personally relevant to the adolescent. When new skills are being taught, it is useful for the clinician to model

the skill, and then to engage the adolescent in a role play.

ME and skill enhancement assignments are important, since these provide an opportunity to clarify youth goals and practice skills *in situ*. Input from the adolescent is important in deciding the details and extent of each assignment. It is generally best to limit the amount of "homework" assigned in order to minimize problems with compliance, since skill enhancement assignments are often perceived as "school-like." In addition, possible barriers to completion (e.g., time constraints, frequency of target situations) should be expected, evaluated, and discussed prior to jointly defining practice exercises. It is particularly important to select assignments that can be successfully executed, build on motivation for abstinence, and result in success (so as to enhance self-efficacy).

Core Sessions

The core sessions of the present intervention are designed to engage the adolescent, to jointly define and prioritize treatment goals and areas for intervention, and to introduce the functional analysis framework that is employed throughout treatment. Although the core sessions are presented at the outset of treatment, the specific skills training modules are designed to be flexible and can be introduced to correspond with the identified needs, goals, and developmental stage of each adolescent.

Motivation Enhancement

Since youths typically enter substance use treatment at the request of someone else (e.g., parents, school or legal authority), motivation is a particularly important issue to address at the outset of therapy. The role of motivation in changing addictive behaviors has been afforded much attention, in part because of the difficulty of engaging and retaining individuals in substance use treatment (e.g., Miller & Rollnick, 2002; Miller, Turner, & Marlatt, 2001). For example, among adolescents, ME techniques have been shown to be effective in reducing alcohol use and related problems with adolescents presenting at hospital emergency departments in smoking cessation (Colby et al., 1998; Myers et al., 2003), and ME is a mechanism whereby support groups promote abstinence

(Kelly et al., 2000; Monti et al., 1999). Motivation is believed to fluctuate over time, and thus it must be constantly monitored among youths. Strategies to reduce client resistance highlight personal motivation and are particularly important in the case of adolescents, who are often rebellious and unconventional by nature or have not yet made a personal commitment to change their substance involvement. To this end, an adolescent must be involved in the process of goal setting and identifying problem areas in order to reduce resistance; compliance and motivation will be improved to the extent that the adolescent has a sense of partnership and control in the treatment process.

A client–treatment matching approach is considered useful for enhancing motivation and compliance (e.g., Brown, 2001; Hester & Miller, 1988). A key principle of this approach is that interventions matched to the adolescent's cognitive style and ability will improve outcomes—an important consideration, given the variability in adolescent cognitive development (Brown & Ramo, in press). Providing choices as to the content of specific intervention components is also important for increasing an adolescent's motivation and personal commitment for change (Brown, 2001). A collaborative approach may additionally serve to maintain focus (e.g., motivation to reduce certain problems) and reduce resistance to treatment. Within a skills training intervention, the adolescent can be given choices about specific domains to be addressed and particular techniques and strategies to be employed. In addition, decisions about the extent to which additional elements (e.g., family therapy, intervention for other problem areas) may enhance goal attainment can be made in collaboration with the adolescent and family.

Hester and Miller (1988) have proposed adolescent-specific factors to consider in tailoring an intervention:

1. Severity of substance involvement.
2. Other concurrent psychopathology.
3. Quality of support systems: home, family relationships, community resources, school, and peer relationships.
4. Severity of deviant or antisocial behaviors.
5. Personal characteristics: aggression, impulsivity, self-esteem.
6. Social skills and functioning.
7. Physical health.
8. Academic status.

The client–treatment matching process is based on assessment results and includes negotiating goals of treatment; selecting the intensity of intervention (e.g., inpatient vs. outpatient, frequency of sessions); choosing the modality of intervention (e.g., family therapy, group therapy, individual therapy, etc.); determining maintenance strategies (i.e., identifying and implementing supports for a substance-free lifestyle); and providing posttreatment evaluation and contact (Miller, 1989).

For adolescents, substance use treatment goals should address the various problems identified, rather than focusing exclusively on substance use (Brown, 2001). It is possible that assessment results may contradict an adolescent's perceptions of problems, and thus may lead to resistance. Therefore, an ME approach may be particularly important when problems identified by the adolescent differ from those perceived by the parents and the clinician. For instance, first testing adolescent-identified goals or concerns may increase his or her openness to continued intervention. Conversely, failure by the teen to achieve a self-identified goal will serve as evidence for the relevance of other problems identified during the assessment. Often, negotiating for a "trial of abstinence" allows the teen an opportunity to have a positive therapeutic experience and makes potential impediments to lengthening abstinence more salient.

Finally, the process of client–treatment matching should include consideration of important individual characteristics, such as gender, ethnicity, and concomitant psychopathology. For example, several studies have found that girls have higher rates of physical and sexual abuse, and are more likely than boys to report the use of alcohol to relieve emotional discomfort or stress (Thompson & Wilsnack, 1984; Windle & Barnes, 1988). In one study, girls obtained higher scores on use of drugs to manage emotional discomfort, as well as on sensitivity to the emotional effects of drug use (Opland, Winters, & Stinchfield, 1995). Thus, in intervening with a female adolescent, it may be valuable to pay particular attention to the use of substances for emotional management and to incorporate affect regulation techniques (Opland et al., 1995).

Ethnic differences must also be considered in the process of treatment planning and intervention. For example, African American and Hispanic adolescents have been found to be less likely than European American youths to seek treatment for substance use problems (Dembo & Shern, 1982; Windle, Miller-Tutzauer, Barnes, & Welte, 1991), and Hispanics were found in one study to have poorer rates of retention (de Leon, Melnick, Schoket, & Jainchill, 1993). Other authors have suggested that minority involvement in addiction treatment is detrimentally influenced by the perception of Twelve-Step fellowships as exclusive, by misconceptions regarding the principles underlying these self-help groups, and by concerns regarding racism (Smith, Buxton, Bilal, & Seymour, 1993). Acculturative differences between parents and children may further complicate issues regarding treatment matching, in that interventions that may seem relevant to more acculturated youths may not appear to be culturally appropriate to their parents. Sensitivity to cultural differences in discussion and presentation of the intervention plan may enhance engagement and participation in treatment. For example, in certain cultures labels such as "alcoholism" are considered pejorative and may provoke discontinuation of treatment, and thus should be avoided. Similarly, the emphasis on privacy of personal and family problems is a cultural value for many Asian Americans, and consequently individual or family formats are preferred to group treatment modalities. For some African Americans, community-based resources such as churches can serve as adjuncts to treatment in lieu of Twelve-Step groups, which may be perceived as Eurocentric. The work of Szapocznik and colleagues in tailoring and empirically testing their theoretically driven BSFT (Szapocznik, Hervis, & Schwartz, in press) with Hispanic families of substance-using adolescents (Santisteban et al., 2003) is an important example of matching a treatment model (family therapy) to an ethnic group's unique cultural values (i.e., familism). In addition, results of this study indicated that families randomly assigned to BSFT reported greater improvements in adolescents' deviant behaviors, substance use, and family functioning (Santisteban et al., 2003).

Given variability in adherence to cultural biases, it is imperative that clinicians assess cultural values directly and not assume that a single approach to treatment will be appropriate for all clients of a given ethnicity or cultural background. In general, it is important to keep in mind that broad ethnic groupings (i.e., African American, Hispanic, Asian) include varied and heterogeneous subgroups. Moreover, since risk factors vary by ethnic origin, it is important that assessment findings be interpreted and explained in reference to the appropriate group and subgroup. To this end, the clinician must pay particular attention to the presence and influence of particular risk factors that may vary by group or subgroup (e.g., family structure, substance involvement within the home/family and within the community). It may be useful to be forthright and elicit the client's concerns about cultural issues/differences from the onset, thereby providing an opportunity to address and discuss these issues.

As noted earlier, additional psychopathology is common among adolescents treated for alcohol and drug problems. CD, mood disorders, and ADHD are typically the most frequently observed concomitant disorders (e.g., Bukstein, Glancy, & Kaminer, 1992; Greenbaum et al., 1996; Kandel et al., 1999). To the extent that additional psychopathology has been identified during the assessment phase, such problems must be addressed in the course of treatment. For example, referral for pharmacotherapy evaluation may be appropriate. Although little is known about the incremental value of medication for concomitant psychopathology among substance-misusing adolescents, psychoactive medication is commonly prescribed in substance use treatment settings and may be useful to the extent that such medication has been proven effective for the comorbid condition. For example, recent preliminary reports suggest the utility of pharmacotherapy for both ADHD and mood disorders when these co-occur with substance use disorders (Riggs, Thompson, Mikulich, Whitmore, & Crowley, 1996). In addition, a recent meta-analysis of the literature on stimulant treatment of ADHD suggests that if such treatment continues into adolescence, risk for subsequent substance use disorder is reduced (Wilens, Faraone, Biederman, & Gunawardene, 2003). Also, given the high incidence of disruptive behaviors among substance-misusing adolescents (e.g., Brown et al., 1996), it may be fruitful to incorporate behavioral interventions focused on these problems, including conflict resolution, communication skills interventions, and multiple-systems interventions that may be helpful for youths with CD (e.g., Forgatch & Patterson, 1989; Robin & Foster, 1989). The reader is referred to other chapters in this volume that address treatment for relevant comorbid disorders.

Introduction of Functional Analysis

A functional analysis of alcohol and drug use (e.g., McCrady, 2001) forms the framework of the intervention and is based on a conceptualization of alcohol and drug use as a learned behavior. From this perspective, the functions served by alcohol and drug use in the life of an addicted individual must be identified in order for appropriate intervention strategies to be selected and implemented. The functional analysis thus serves as a tool for identifying the stimuli, reinforcement contingencies, cognitions, affective states, and behaviors that maintain alcohol and drug involvement; thus it helps target the particular strategies and skill domains to be selected for inclusion during the course of treatment.

After the rationale for the functional analysis is provided, the "behavior chain" (see Figure 11.1) is introduced as the tool used in a functional analysis. The behavior chain (consisting of triggers, thoughts, feelings, behaviors, and consequences [positive and negative]) is best presented in graphic form on a flipchart or chalk board. Also, the adolescent should be provided with behavior chain worksheets (Figure 11.1) to complete for different precipitants (triggers) of use. First discussed are the antecedents to behavior: triggers, thoughts, and feelings. A "trigger" is broadly defined as a circumstance that increases the probability of substance use. A trigger can be a person, place, or thing that has previously been associated with adolescent substance use (e.g., social situations, offers of alcohol and/or drugs by peers,

arguments with friends or family members). Once the concept has been introduced, personal examples are elicited.

Following the discussion of triggers, it is usually best to introduce the feelings component of the chain, even though thoughts immediately follow in the behavior chain diagram. Youths may be unfamiliar with the notion that thoughts can lead to feelings, but may be more adept at identifying and labeling affective states. An adolescent is asked to generate a list of emotions he or she has experienced in response to the triggers previously identified (e.g., an argument may result in anger and frustration; offers of alcohol and drugs may elicit a desire to use [urges or craving]). The idea that thoughts can cause feelings is next addressed in the context of Beck's concept of "automatic thoughts," which are cognitions that enter consciousness without effort and escape awareness (Beck, Rush, Shaw, & Emery, 1979). An adolescent-identified trigger is then selected, and the adolescent is asked to identify some thoughts related to the resulting feeling (e.g., an argument with parents may result in thoughts such as "I wish they'd get off my back" or "What's the big deal?"). Because the adolescent may initially have difficulty with this task, the clinician must be able to provide examples of thoughts associated with different types of situations. It is also valuable to examine the role of drug-use-specific thoughts that may serve to motivate use. For example, Beck, Wright, Newman, and Liese (1993) describe three types of "addictive beliefs" about drugs that develop serve to maintain addiction and

Trigger $\rightarrow$	Thought $\rightarrow$	Feeling $\rightarrow$	Behavior $\rightarrow$	Consequences	
				Positive	Negative
1. Gathering with friends, offered drugs	"I'll feel left out if I don't use." "They'll think I'm stupid if I say no."	Anxious, uncomfortable	Use drugs	Feel comfortable with peers; have a good time; enjoy high	Guilt; feel like failure; hangover; spent money; punishment; loss of privileges; parents upset
2. Argument with parents	"They don't listen or understand." "I'm sick of being blamed for everything."	Angry, frustrated	Use drugs	Forget about argument; feel relaxed; feel less angry	Parents more angry; problems not addressed

FIGURE 11.1. Sample behavior chain worksheet.

increase risk for relapse: "anticipatory" beliefs, or expected positive consequences ("It'll be fun at the party"); negative reinforcement or "relief-oriented" beliefs ("Using will get rid of my cravings," "If I use, I won't feel so stressed"); and "permissive" beliefs, which justify or rationalize use ("I can't focus without using," "I can control my use—there's no problem"). These types of thoughts should be discussed as motivating substance use, and the adolescent asked to generate examples relevant to each type of addictive belief. It should also be pointed out that thoughts in response to a trigger can be either positive or negative (i.e., automatic thoughts are not necessarily "bad"). In order to establish comprehension of the antecedent portion of the behavior chain (triggers, thoughts, and feelings), completion of several examples representing different types of triggers, thoughts, and feelings is recommended.

Discussion of the next link in the chain, behavior, follows presentation of the antecedents. Consistent with a focus on substance use, alcohol and/or drug use behaviors are always noted on the chain in order to highlight the relationship between specific triggers and use, and later to specify adaptive alternative behaviors to use of alcohol and drugs. An outline of the consequences of alcohol and/or drug use behaviors constitutes the next task to be completed. Consistent with an ME approach, the positive consequences resulting from use are discussed first (e.g., use following an argument may provide relief from anger and frustration; use in response to social pressure may facilitate social comfort). Acknowledging the positive consequences emphasizes factors that reinforce and maintain substance use; it also builds credibility with skeptical adolescents, who expect adults to focus only on negative outcomes. Subsequent to positive consequences, negative consequences for each trigger identified, beginning with those most proximal, are addressed. For example, alcohol or drug use when an adolescent is angry after an argument may lead to temporary relief, but the same negative feelings may eventually return. A more distal consequence is that use to relieve emotions results in avoidance of the issues underlying conflict, thereby assuring that the real issues are never addressed or changed. In the case of substance use in social contexts, intoxication may alter interactions (e.g., being belligerent, behaving foolishly, risky/sexual behavior) and can thus impair relationships. The adolescent should be encouraged to generate as many personal consequences as possible, and then to elaborate on personal negative consequences, including the long-term effects of substance use (e.g., discomfort interacting with others when not intoxicated, as a result of not having learned or used adaptive social skills; not being involved in rewarding activities, because of neglect of alternative activities; parental anger and punishment).

Attention to the balance between positive and negative consequences is a useful motivational strategy (i.e., do the overall negative consequences of use outweigh the positives?). This approach can be used to monitor current motivation and to maintain or enhance motivation for change—an issue of particular importance, since motivation for abstinence tends to fluctuate over time. A written record of the negative consequences of substance use by the adolescent is an effective strategy for providing a concrete reminder of personal motives for change. The clinician is advised to avoid confrontation and refrain from imposing the opinion, but rather to highlight the adolescent's perception of consequences as primary.

Next discussed is the use of the behavior chain worksheet for identifying means by which to break the chain that leads to alcohol and drug use. Each link in the chain is a potential point where change can occur. For example, the ultimate behavior of alcohol or drug use can be disrupted by avoiding or altering certain triggers. Examination and reframing of perceptions or thoughts in reaction to a trigger may serve to avert emotions that can precipitate use. Finally, alternative means can be learned for managing the feelings that precede alcohol or drug use. Highlighting these multiple options provides choices for the adolescent.

In order to enhance the validity of the behavior chain, the clinician and adolescent should generate concrete examples of how alcohol and drug use behaviors can be influenced by acting on each link in the chain. Based on the previously agreed-upon areas for intervention, the adolescent can then be assigned to complete several behavior chain worksheets for the first area chosen to be addressed. In order to motivate and engage the adolescent, the clinician must project optimism and confidence in the feasibility of this approach. It should be clarified that the behavior chain framework can accommodate a large range of strategies and tools, from which the adolescent can select those best matched to his or her individual needs and abilities. Overall, the introduction of the behavior chain should serve to illustrate how this framework will be used throughout treatment to help identify new skills, strategies, and behaviors for changing the old substance use behaviors or other problem behaviors.

Cognitive-Behavioral Skills Training Modules

The several topics below are typically included in cognitive-behavioral intervention for substance-involved adolescents. Selection and sequencing of specific modules are based on the identified problem areas, targets of change identified by each adolescent, and negotiated treatment goals. The amount of time devoted to each topic is determined by the needs, interests and abilities of each adolescent. The skills modules are organized into three domains: interpersonal skills, managing negative emotions, and relapse prevention.

Interpersonal Skills

ASSERTIVENESS

Effective assertive behavior is relevant to important social development during adolescence and is generally introduced first. The utility of assertive behavior for improving interpersonal relationships serves as the rationale for this module: Good relationships help decrease conflict and the resulting negative emotions, and increase self-efficacy, thereby reducing the likelihood of alcohol and drug use to manage feelings and resist use pressures. Beginning with a general discussion of assertiveness, the clinician should have the adolescent describe his or her understanding of the concept and contrast this with aggressiveness and passivity. After clarifying the meaning and value of assertiveness and discussing concrete examples, the clinician outlines basic individual rights. Providing the adolescent with a list of rights and asking for examples of how these rights might be violated are helpful at this point. Personal examples should be elicited (and/or provided from the clinician's observation and knowledge of the client) of situations where the adolescent had his or her rights violated and instances where he or she violated the rights of others. Individual rights should be highlighted. That is, every person has the following rights:

1. To make his or her own decisions.
2. To have and express his or her own feelings.
3. To have and express his or her own thoughts, beliefs, and opinions.
4. To decide whether to agree to or decline a request.
5. To be healthy and safe, and not to be abused (physically, emotionally, or sexually).

The presentation of assertiveness and personal rights is followed by a discussion of passive and aggressive behaviors. Once personal passive and aggressive behaviors have been identified, the adolescent is asked to prioritize problems with assertiveness; these are then examined, using the behavior chain to demonstrate their negative consequences. Next, the following guidelines for assertive behavior are reviewed, with a focus on those pertinent to the previously completed behavior chains:

1. You can only control your own behavior, not that of others. You can ask others to change their behavior, but they have the right to refuse.
2. It is important to know in advance what you want in a particular situation.
3. Communicate clearly and specifically what it is you want.
4. Pay attention to body language; avoid presenting a passive or aggressive posture.
5. The timing of assertive behavior is important. In particular, make sure you're calm and composed when making a request or having a discussion with someone.
6. It is important to use "I" statements, and avoid words such as "should" and "never."
7. When criticizing, address the *behavior* you don't like, rather than characteristics of the *person*.
8. To provide constructive feedback, use the "sandwich" technique: Start with something positive about the issue/person, follow this with criticism/feedback, then end with a positive comment.
9. Be willing to compromise; plan ahead of time what you're willing and unwilling to negotiate.

After these assertive guidelines are reviewed, the behavior chains are reworked, substituting assertive for passive or aggressive behaviors. The different consequences that result from assertive behavior should be emphasized by role plays of assertive behaviors, which are repeated until the teen demonstrates improved performance and confidence.

Practicing assertive skills in situations that engender success is critical. To this end, initial assignments must be focused on relatively nonthreatening situations for which success is highly likely. The adolescent should be asked to complete a number of behavior chains for triggers relevant to assertive behaviors drawn from daily experiences.

GIVING AND RECEIVING CRITICISM; EXPRESSING FEELINGS

Given the importance of mastering the affective lability of adolescence, the next module focuses on situations in which the adolescent has had difficulty expressing positive or negative feelings appropriately or accepting or providing criticism. Personal examples are reviewed and need not be substance-related. In the event that the adolescent has difficulty providing examples, reference can be made to interpersonal conflict items endorsed on the IDTS (Annis & Graham, 1985). Family and school examples abound in this domain and can be useful content in the parent and family components of the intervention as well.

The adolescent completes a behavior chain worksheet for each example, followed by a discussion of how the antecedents and behavior could be changed to produce a more positive outcome. When reviewing alternative behaviors, the clinician should refer to the guidelines for assertive behavior. Discussion of the behavior chain and alternative behaviors is followed by a role play of the alternative behaviors, starting with less threatening situations. The importance of planning and rehearsal prior to entering the situation should be emphasized: What is the teen's goal, and what behaviors will be most likely to achieve that goal? Completion of behavior chains for triggers relevant to situations involving the expression of criticism and other feelings drawn from the adolescent's daily experiences is suggested.

DEALING WITH CONFLICT (ANGER AND FRUSTRATION)

The next module begins with having the adolescent identify recent conflict situations (arguments, fights). Conflicts with friends and peers are examined separately from family conflict situations. A behavior chain worksheet is completed for each trigger, including the antecedents and behaviors that led to anger and/or

frustration. Next, the adolescent is asked to identify links in the chain that can be altered to avoid the previous consequences. Of particular importance are identifying thoughts (perceptions and beliefs about what occurred in the situation) and behaviors that were ineffective in these conflicts, and using the assertive behavior guidelines to generate alternative thoughts and behaviors in response to triggers. Role plays of the alternative behaviors aid skill development and diminish the uncomfortable affective arousal prevalent in these situations.

The adolescent should be guided in selecting a minor, frequently occurring conflict situation for initial practice. It is often helpful to identify a recent unresolved conflict situation that the adolescent can attempt to address (after practicing in the session). For future sessions, the adolescent can be assigned to identify additional ongoing conflict situations or anticipated conflicts. Family-related conflicts may be more effectively addressed in the context of a family session, particularly when it is judged that behavior change on the part of the adolescent will be insufficient to alter well-established family patterns of such conflicts.

Managing Negative Emotions

The next skills training domain concentrates on skills and strategies for managing other negative emotional states, such as depression, anxiety, and anger, which are common during adolescent development. Because negative affect increases with the transition through puberty and is frequently associated with substance use, effective means for managing such emotions are particularly important. As a general rule, it is valuable to characterize the experience of negative affect as a typical part of everyday life, and to point out that it can occur even in situations where the teen has responded or behaved appropriately (e.g., one can't control other people's behavior).

Once relevant negative emotions and corresponding trigger situations have been identified (based on previous assessment information, the IDTS, etc.), the behavior chain is employed to detail the thoughts and behaviors that contribute to and exacerbate the emotions. The selection of specific strategies for managing negative emotions should depend on the situational triggers and the adolescent's level of cognitive ability. Matching strategies to cognitive style is particularly important in this context, since some adolescents are more comfortable with concrete behavioral strategies than with cognitive approaches (and vice versa). Youths may perceive alcohol and/or drug use as an effective means for managing negative emotions. As such, it is particularly important to assess these beliefs (e.g., with the AEQ-A) to enhance the adolescent's confidence in the utility of the selected mood management techniques, and to boost his or her self-efficacy for successfully implementing alternative strategies.

A menu of cognitive and behavioral strategies from which the teen selects skills most relevant to his or her trigger situations and personal style is helpful, as negative affect can emerge across a variety of circumstances. Strategies for managing such feelings as anger, frustration, anxiety, depression, and boredom should be selected in accordance with identified triggers and clinical judgment regarding the particular needs of each adolescent. Although a detailed outline of strategies for adolescent mood management is beyond the scope of this chapter, several excellent sources describe specific techniques that are easily incorporated within the present framework (e.g., Burns, 1989, 1999; Clarke, Lewinsohn, & Hops, 1990).

Once mood management strategies have been selected in collaboration with the adolescent, the behavior chain is used to illustrate how these strategies function. For example, the clinician can say, "Progressive muscle relaxation is a skill that helps you feel less stressed and anxious. If you feel less stressed, you'll be less likely to use alcohol/drugs to calm yourself," or "Being involved in enjoyable activities will help you feel better when you're down and make it less likely that you'll use to deal with being depressed or bored," or "Learning to think differently about situations where you get upset can reduce these feelings and help you feel more in control." The adolescent's comprehension of how the selected strategies will help him or her manage unpleasant feelings is essential to motivate compliance. In session, practice and rehearsal are particularly valuable for enhancing compliance with these strategies.

The adolescent should be assisted in identifying upcoming situations that may precipitate negative emotions. Specific strategies are then prescribed for practice. Having the adolescent perform daily mood ratings (e.g., a daily rating of anxiety level on a 1–10 scale) can help identify particular emotions to be targeted, and is also useful in providing feedback as to the effectiveness of the strategies employed.

Relapse Prevention

RATIONALE/IDENTIFYING HIGH-RISK SITUATIONS

The discussion of relapse prevention for adolescents starts with defining "relapse" as a process of returning to problematic alcohol and drug use, rather than a single, all-or-none event (Marlatt & Gordon, 2005). It is important to clarify that a single occasion of use (a "slip" or "lapse") does not represent a failure or an inevitable return to problematic use; rather, one's reaction to a lapse plays a large role in what happens next. Because of the high rate of lapses following treatment for adolescent substance misuse, it is critical that such an event be perceived as a learning experience rather than a failure. If the youth perceives recovery from alcohol and drugs as a process during which setbacks may occur, he or she can prepare for feelings (e.g., guilt and failure in the event of a lapse) and use the episode to learn to avoid future lapses. Discussion of a lapse is intended to increase the adolescent's awareness of potential relapse risks and to facilitate planning for such an event. It must be emphasized that discussion of this issue in no way implies permission to use! In the course of discussing this topic, it is imperative to elicit feedback and reactions from the adolescent regarding the described process of relapse and the meaning of a lapse.

The concepts of "high-risk situations" and "coping" are introduced following the discussion of relapse. Because many of the triggers discussed in previous sessions represent relapse risk situations, the concept of high-risk situations should be easily comprehended by the adolescent. Although some such situations are common among adolescents (e.g., being at a party where alcohol and/or drugs are being used; Brown et al., 1989), unique risks must also be identified to enhance preparedness and vigilance. The rationale for relapse prevention training rests on the notion that preparation and the availability of specific coping skills are necessary tools for reducing the probability of lapses in high-risk situations. It is helpful to elicit from the adolescent his or her own experiences (if any) at successfully managing temptations to use alcohol and/or drugs. Success experiences in this realm are important for building the adolescent's self-efficacy for relapse risk situations.

Adolescents often underestimate the difficulty of coping with relapse risk situations (e.g., Myers & Brown, 1990a); thus examples of likely high-risk situations are valuable. Typical adolescent high-risk situations include social situations, direct or indirect social pressure, and family conflict (Brown et al., 1989). Additional situations previously identified as triggers during the course of treatment or endorsed on the IDTS (Annis & Graham, 1985) can be utilized as examples. An adolescent's responses to the DTCQ regarding his or her confidence in abstaining can serve to identify situations perceived as particularly difficult to manage. It is important to convey that it is also important to be prepared to manage less common situations associated with past use, as well as unanticipated events. Behavior chain worksheets completed during the course of treatment are a good source for illustrating the broad range of situations that increase risk for relapse. Once high-risk situations are identified, a discussion of perceived risk (why might a situation be difficult or easy to handle?) and adolescent-generated strategies for managing the circumstances can develop. Feedback as to the likely accuracy of these perceptions is valuable at this point, along with an emphasis on the importance of being prepared for the unexpected (e.g., unanticipated physiological arousal, shift in cognitions).

The adolescent should be assigned to generate two lists of potential high-risk situations: those that are likely to be encountered in the present, and more distal (future) risks. The particular approach taken with regard to relapse will also depend on external constraints (e.g., probation drug testing, etc.). Clear discussions of the impact of these external factors need to take place with the teen and parents early in the therapeutic process. Behavior chain worksheets, including coping strategies for avoiding lapses (alternative behaviors), should be completed for a number of the situations (the exact number should be based on negotiation with the adolescent). Asking the adolescent to generate coping strategies can aid clinical assessment of abilities and identification of coping efforts the adolescent perceives as useful. An additional useful exercise is to have the adolescent monitor socially sanctioned pressures to use substances via a log of images (e.g., television, magazines, newspapers, movies, adult discussions, etc.) designed to promulgate the use of alcohol and other drugs. The exercise also helps the adolescent identify previously unrecognized cues for substance involvement.

COPING WITH HIGH-RISK SITUATIONS

Having identified a variety of high-risk situations, the adolescent is assisted in determining which are likely to pose the greatest and most immediate risk for relapse. Considerations include the following: (1) Has the adolescent previously been successful in managing a given type of situation? (2) How skilled is the adolescent in the strategies required to manage a particular situation? (3) What is the adolescent's self-efficacy for avoiding use in a given situation? (4) How realistic is the adolescent's estimate of difficulty for each situation? A review of upcoming events can serve to identify and prioritize particularly risky situations to be worked on in sessions. Once a list of high-risk situations is completed, a behavior chain worksheet is completed to evaluate each identified situation in detail and to specify alternative behaviors for altering and/or managing the specific circumstances involved.

Planning and rehearsal of coping strategies are especially important for managing likely high-risk situations. Once a risk situation is encountered, there is little time to think through alternatives; therefore, at least one strategy perceived as effective and feasible by the adolescent must be identified and rehearsed for each type of situation. In-session work should thus focus on planning and rehearsing coping alternatives. Strategies discussed will be dictated by the type of situation targeted (e.g., mood management strategies for negative affect, assertive skills for conflict situations, etc.). Avoiding high-risk situations is a useful strategy that is recommended early in treatment, but is unlikely to be effective if used exclusively over the long term. It is helpful to engage the adolescent in a detailed discussion of how each plan will be executed, how the adolescent and others may react in the situation, and how the adolescent perceives his or her self-efficacy for executing the coping efforts. This discussion serves to anticipate and identify potential barriers to coping. Finally, because of the high frequency of adolescent lapses, it is important to outline a plan of action in the case of a slip, particularly when difficult situations are imminent. Providing the adolescent with a concrete plan that includes clearly specified steps to be followed can decrease the likelihood of a protracted relapse following a slip. A "slip management plan" can include such strategies as contacting the clinician, calling a nonusing friend, attending a support group meeting, discarding any alcohol or drugs in the adolescent's possession, or leaving the use situation. This plan should be reinforced by drawing up, together with the adolescent, a "relapse recovery plan" contract that is then signed by the adolescent. Of course, actions to be taken and requirements based on external contingencies must also be considered. Regardless of external factors, repeated slips need to be dealt with aggressively in treatment, as use compromises the teen's cognitive abilities and affective motivation for successful treatment participation and places the teen at risk for negative consequences (e.g., risky sexual behavior, driving under the influence, etc.).

Practice of coping skills outside the therapeutic setting is assigned following in-session practice. Initial practice must be planned for situations presenting low risk, with subsequent inclusions of more difficult circumstances. The primary goals of practice assignments in this phase of treatment is to build coping skills and self-efficacy for managing high-risk situations. To facilitate success, it may be useful to have a support person (e.g., a nonusing peer, a parent) accompany the adolescent in high-risk situations. The use of avoidance and reliance on support persons should be gradually faded out in the later stages of treatment.

REFUSAL SKILLS

Discussion of refusal skills is particularly important, since adolescents commonly experience lapses in social situations with ample models of alcohol and/or drug use. The prominent role of peer modeling in reinforcement of alcohol and drug use is recognized as a critical difficulty for youths maintaining abstinence. The extent of this difficulty is evident, as the prevalence of alcohol and drug involvement increases throughout adolescence (Johnston et al., 2003). In this context, abstinence is behavior at odds with the reality of many adolescent social environments.

Particularly helpful in refusing substance offers are the review and rehearsal of assertiveness skills. In addition to behavioral skills, cognitive factors are important for drug refusal. It is helpful to evaluate adolescent perception of the meaning of refusals of peer substance offers. For example, likelihood of refusal may

rest on the adolescent's beliefs about how he or she is perceived and accepted by others. The forces of social influence can be countered by discussing the adolescent's concerns regarding peer acceptance, and by examining the accuracy of these perceptions (e.g., cognitive techniques of reframing or examining "irrational" thoughts). Before assigning refusal practice in "real-life" situations, the clinician must ascertain that the adolescent will be able to manage such situations successfully, and (at least initially) has a supportive peer present.

GOAL SETTING/ALTERNATIVE ACTIVITIES

A major concern for many substance misusing adolescents is the fear that life will be dull and uninteresting in the absence of drugs and alcohol. Therefore, identifying and developing enjoyable, non-substance-use-related activities are critical aspects of relapse prevention. Other benefits of rewarding and enjoyable pursuits include enhancing self-esteem, developing a sense of autonomy, developing a nonusing peer group, and altering identity development (which is critical during adolescence). Since research demonstrates that involvement in alternative activities accompanies the successful resolution of substance use problems for adults and teens alike (Brown, 1993), this is a particularly useful component of intervention.

By the time substance-abusing adolescents enter treatment, they generally have limited hobbies or extracurricular activities. It is therefore useful to systematically explore activities an adolescent was involved in before the onset of substance use; new areas of potential interest (i.e., hobbies, recreational activities, sports, social activities, jobs); and possible volunteer activities, which place the teen in a position of responsibility and respect. As the first step, it is helpful to generate a menu or list of potential activities. The clinician can facilitate the selection of activities by "brainstorming" specific examples for different types or domains of activities. The adolescent can rank activities based on his or her personal interest and, with the clinician, develop a plan for how each activity will be pursued. A focus on making detailed, concrete plans and on identifying potential barriers is important to facilitate youth follow-through. The clinician should assist the adolescent in setting specific, attainable goals (e.g., "Goal: Join group X by next month. Steps to complete: (1) Call to get information,

(2) arrange transportation, (3) attend a meeting," etc.). It is important that the selected activities, goals, and plan of action be realistic, attainable, and perceived as feasible by the adolescent.

Evaluating Progress and Treatment Outcome

Success is evaluated by improvement in identified problem areas and substance involvement. Ongoing assessment of progress should include each area addressed during the course of treatment. At a minimum, scales and measures initially used to identify problem areas and affective states during assessment should be readministered at the end of treatment. As suggested earlier, the CBCL and its self-report version for youths, the YSR, can be utilized throughout the treatment process to evaluate improvement and identify remaining problem areas. Screening measures such as the PEI may prove helpful in assessing substance use status and changes in peers following treatment. Systematic evaluation of progress and treatment outcome is strongly recommended, as it provides feedback to the adolescent, furnishes the clinician with objective evidence for the efficacy of intervention, and assists both client and clinician in anticipating new or continued problems.

Maintenance of Behavior Change

Maintenance of behavior change for youths is greatly assisted by continued clinical contact following the completion of treatment. Because the initial 6 months following treatment represent the time of greatest risk for relapse, relapse prevention efforts should be maintained during this period. Follow-up contacts can consist of office visits or phone calls, scheduled with gradually decreasing frequency. Such contacts provide opportunity for the clinician to assess the maintenance of behavior change and quickly intervene in the case of lapses or relapses, to address any problems that have occurred, and evaluate the emergence of new clinical symptoms (e.g., depression, anxiety). A flexible approach is recommended to facilitate the variety of pathways to sustained abstinence for adolescents (Brown, 1993). Consistent therapist support is important, even when adolescents initiate activities that vary from those traditionally recommended (as long as these are consistent with treatment goals).

Prompt attention to lapse and relapse events is critical. Adolescents differ from adults in that they more often lapse on substances other than their previous "drug of choice" (Brown, Tapert, Tate, & Abrantes, 2000), and as many as one-quarter of initial lapses do not result in full-blown relapse (Brown, 1993). Thus rapid attention to lapses can interrupt the process of relapse and obstruct a return to chronic problematic drug and/or alcohol use. As previously noted, lapses can be considered opportunities for learning and should be reviewed and discussed in a nonjudgmental fashion. Behavior chain worksheets should be employed to examine the reasons underlying a return to substance use and help temper the feelings of guilt and failure that often accompany such an episode. Review of lapse episodes should also be used to highlight the importance of vigilance, preparation, and motivation in the face of high-risk situations.

Finally, treatment outcome can be enhanced by therapist support for nontraditional efforts at maintaining abstinence. Affiliation with traditional support systems for abstinence (Alcoholics Anonymous/Narcotics Anonymous, recovery support groups) is a strong predictor of long-term abstinence following adolescent treatment (Brown, 1993; Kelly et al., 2002). However, some adolescents successfully utilize alternative supports or efforts, which are equally effective in promoting long-term abstinence (Brown, 1993). For example, younger adolescents not involved in traditional recovery organizations may maintain abstinence through increased family involvement. A supportive family unit with increased structure and activities may provide adequate support for continued abstinence by improving family cohesion and communication. Early individuation by older adolescents represents another nontraditional avenue for success. Adolescents who succeed in maintaining abstinence by this path often have parents with severe alcohol or drug dependence, and are able to achieve abstinence by gaining independence from their families without involvement in the traditional recovery community. These adolescents usually become involved in activities that provide substance-free structured environments (e.g., work, extracurricular activities), and that enhance independence and self-esteem. Although only a subgroup of adolescents utilize these alternative pathways to abstinence, strategies such as these are important for teens who have a difficult time identifying with traditional abstinence-focused support groups or do not perceive them as personally helpful.

Problems in Implementation

Youths can appear to be difficult clients, because they seldom enter treatment of their own accord and are facing the challenging demands of adolescent development in addition to their addiction. As discussed throughout the chapter, issues regarding motivation for change, resistance to treatment, and poor compliance with the intervention are of great importance. Another difficult issue encountered in treating adolescent substance use problems is that of continued alcohol and drug use during the course of treatment. Strategies for the detection of substance use (e.g., random toxicology screens) and contingencies in response to episodes of use must be outlined in detail and agreed upon at the outset of treatment, although contingencies may be renegotiated as treatment progresses. A further factor complicating the therapeutic decision-making process is confidentiality, which is an issue common to all therapeutic settings in which minors are treated, either independently or in concert with parents and other family members. Although no uniform recommendation is made here, due to the considerable variability in circumstances that may lead an adolescent to treatment, the agreements between therapist and adolescent and between therapist and family must be clearly outlined, preferably in the first session. In situations in which adolescent drug use is to be automatically reported (e.g., drug screens, teen reports, etc.), consequences should be explicitly specified. Even in such situations, confidentiality regarding other information emerging in treatment should be clearly differentiated.

Motivation for and Compliance with Treatment

Adolescent development is a critical consideration when one is designing interventions for enhancing motivation and reducing resistance to treatment. Motivation for change is a critical issue in the treatment of addictive behaviors, and as such should be assessed and addressed throughout the course of treatment. To this end, several developmental issues must be kept in mind. For example, although they are expected to behave as adults, adolescents usually have less control over day-to-day events or external stressors in their lives, and as a consequence may feel powerless or helpless. Challenge of authority is part of the growth process for youth identity and autonomy. Thus engaging the adolescent in a collaborative fashion and involving him or her in the process of treatment planning and decision making are particularly important to reduce resistance and enhance compliance (i.e., the adolescent should enter the treatment process with a sense of "ownership").

Adolescents with substance use problems generally present with a wide range of neurocognitive abilities, and many have comorbid mental health problems. Attentional difficulties are fairly common, as are minor memory deficits in drug withdrawal. Thus intervention content must be carefully matched to the cognitive level and abilities of each adolescent. Information should be presented in manageable quantities, and in language that is appropriate for the adolescent's level of comprehension. Presenting too much information or failing to ensure that material is comprehended will lead to frustration and will diminish motivation and compliance. It is important to keep in mind that techniques developed for adults may be inappropriate for use with adolescents. The clinician must be sensitive to this issue and not make any a priori assumptions regarding the appropriateness of materials. In evaluating whether a particular technique will be effective, feedback must be sought from the adolescent regarding acceptability of the material, its perceived helpfulness, and his or her willingness to try each exercise. Feedback should be elicited in a sensitive manner that does not diminish the adolescent, but seeks to optimize the intervention activities for the individual.

Since tasks that appear "school-like" are often met with resistance, compliance with between-session assignments can be problematic. Assignments should be referred to as "exercises" or "skill-building activities" rather than as "homework." In order to reduce resistance, tasks that focus on activities and behaviors rather than on reading and writing are generally assigned. It is often helpful to go over an assignment in detail during the session, in order to identify potential obstacles or difficulties that may impede compliance. The adolescent should make a commitment to attempt this task at the close of each session, or the activity should be youth-modified to bring it into acceptable range. In addition, beginning the session with a review of the previous assignment informs the therapist of new issues and reinforces the youth's efforts and compliance. Feedback from the adolescent should be elicited as to how helpful the task was and how much it was liked or disliked. This information can then be used to modify subsequent tasks if necessary, and to clarify problems regarding resistance and barriers to compliance.

Substance Use during the Course of Treatment

Because the traditional goal of treatment for substance use problems is complete abstinence from psychoactive substances, issues of continued use, lapse, and relapse must be addressed and agreed upon at the outset of intervention. Agreement must be reached as to the means by which substance use will be monitored, as well as the consequences of repeated lapses or continued use.

By contrast, consideration of nicotine has been only inconsistently targeted in alcohol and drug treatment programs. Given that tobacco use is prevalent among youths in treatment (Myers & Brown, 1994) and represents the leading cause of death among adults previously treated for alcohol problems (Hurt et al., 1996), this is an issue that should also be addressed in the course of treatment. Providing a youth with smoking cessation materials (e.g., those available from the American Lung Association or the U.S. Department of Health and Human Services; Fiore et al., 2000, is a booklet of clinical guidelines for smoking cessation) encourages the youth to consider cessation of nicotine and can be incorporated into standard treatment if the teen is so motivated.

Substance use can be monitored through a variety of methods, including self-report by the adolescent, parent report, and urine toxicology screening. Urine screening is commonly employed because it is an objective indicator of use, can serve as a deterrent to use, and may encourage honest reporting by the adolescent. The urine-screening procedure is best presented as a standard procedure required of all individuals treated for substance misuse. The adolescent must be provided with a rationale for the employment of urine screens, with an emphasis on accountability and rewards for sustained abstinence. The procedure can also be framed as a means of protection, since continued alcohol and/or drug use may lead to the adverse consequences and problems that precipitated treatment.

Urine screens can be administered routinely, at random intervals, or at the clinician's discretion. Regular (e.g., weekly, semiweekly, or monthly) urine screens may be perceived as less intrusive than random testing and should be linked to the youth's goals and reinforcing consequences. When relatively infrequent urine testing is selected, the clinician must reserve the right to request testing when evidence suggests unacknowledged alcohol and/or drug use by the adolescent. The clinician should provide examples of the circumstances that may motivate such a request (e.g., behavioral withdrawal symptoms, atypical mood changes, family reports of unusual behavior), and should clarify that if such a circumstance arises, the underlying reasons will be fully discussed with the adolescent. Additional issues pertaining to urine toxicology screening include the cost of the procedure, impact on the therapeutic relationship, access to the results by other persons (e.g., parents), and appropriate and inappropriate reactions on the part of parents. In particular, parents should be discouraged from displaying a punitive response in the case of a positive urine screen. Rather, they should be encouraged to perceive isolated instances of use as an opportunity for learning, which should be discussed with the adolescent in a supportive and appropriate manner. Negative screens should be highlighted and linked to graduated privileges for the youth.

A basic intervention rule is that the adolescent must not arrive at a session under the influence of alcohol or drugs. It must be made clear that no useful work can be accomplished if the adolescent is intoxicated during sessions. If such an event does occur, the clinician must carefully assess the situation and decide on appropriate action. For example, is the adolescent in any danger? Can the teen be sent home safely? What modifications should be made to the intervention? Such an occurrence should be followed by a makeup session scheduled as soon as is feasible in order to process the event.

Given that abstinence is the goal of treatment, the expectation that the adolescent not use alcohol or drugs during the course of treatment should be made explicit. In reality, especially in outpatient settings, absolute abstinence throughout the course of treatment is often difficult to achieve. As discussed above, lapse experiences represent powerful learning opportunities. However, continued alcohol and drug use by the adolescent may also indicate that the selected course and modality of treatment are not effective. Thus it is incumbent upon the clinician to clearly define the consequences of individual and repeated use episodes. In general, treatment proceeds with the understanding that lapses may occur, but that open and honest discussion of any such lapses is a condition for continued treatment. Denial of use in the face of objective evidence, or a pattern of continued use that does not diminish with time, indicates the need for intervention modifications and perhaps a more intensive level of treatment (e.g., inpatient or residential).

CASE EXAMPLE

Tim, a 16-year-old high school sophomore, was brought to treatment by his mother and father after being placed in juvenile detention by police for possession of a controlled substance. His parents were extremely distressed by their son's downward spiral of social withdrawal, depression, and irresponsible behavior over the preceding year. Recently, Tim had failed to come home on a number of occasions; he had started missing school regularly; and his previously good grades had deteriorated remarkably. Despite their efforts to speak with him of their concerns, Tim remained sullen and uncommunicative. Consequently, the parents increasingly threatened more serious disciplinary action, but found it difficult to carry out their punishments for fear of further alienating their son. In particular, Tim's father, who was a computer software salesman, had become increasingly angry with his son. His preference was to have their son leave home until he "stopped using drugs and cleaned up his act." In contrast, Tim's mother was frightened to have him leave home, for fear he would choose to live with his drug-using friends and become involved in more deviant behavior. Furthermore, she felt much empathy for her son's distress, as well as guilt that perhaps her employment or attention to her older (college-age) son might somehow be responsible for Tim's current difficulties.

After a brief meeting with Tim and his parents, Tim was interviewed separately while his parents were asked to complete several self-report measures (e.g., the CBCL). He clearly had no wish to be in treatment and felt that his parents and school officials were unfair to him. His friends, who Tim felt cared about him deeply, likewise thought that his parents were punitive and considered their substance involvement "normal" for males their age. Tim initially did not disclose his level of use, but acknowledged experimenting with alcohol, marijuana, cocaine, and methamphetamines. (He did report smoking cigarettes regularly, but he did not want his parents to know about this.) When queried, he stated that he used no more than his peers, and that he did not think his drug use was a problem, as he was still attending school and had never failed a class. From his perspective, kids who couldn't handle their drug use started stealing for their habit and dropped out of school. He was not like those "problem users"; he was "not an addict."

Following some discussion of the circumstances that brought him to treatment, including probation-mandated abstinence, Tim agreed to come to treatment to placate his parents and show the judge he was wrong. It was explained to Tim that, with the exception of the results of urine toxicology screens (required as part of his probation), all other material in the sessions would be held in confidence unless the therapist was legally required by law to release information. After some discussion, Tim agreed to participate in therapy in order to appease the legal system and diminish the conflict at home. Although he clearly underestimated the difficulties of not using during the upcoming week, he agreed that for 1 week he would avoid his usual friends, and that he would generate a list of recreational or special things to be used in the future as rewards for abstinence and compliance. Tim also agreed to complete several self-report questionnaires before the next session, in 2 days. The therapist offered to discuss at the next session the possibility of writing a letter to school officials indicating that Tim had started treatment. Finally, the Hamilton Rating Scale for Depression was completed to assess the severity of Tim's current depressive symptoms.

At the end of the initial session, the therapist–teen contract was discussed with the parents, and a contract was negotiated between the parents and therapist that was to be honored regardless of Tim's behavior over the next several days. Tim's parents agreed to make a list of things they liked about their son and to specify potential family rewards for Tim's efforts at an alcohol- and drug-free lifestyle. Tim and his parents were then informed about the usual affective, cognitive, and physiological withdrawal symptoms from stimulants and depressants, so as to prepare them for the experiences likely to occur over the next few days and weeks. All parties agreed to meet in 2 days to complete the assessment and treatment-planning process.

At the second session, following a brief discussion of withdrawal symptoms and current family relations, Tim's list of special recreational activities and rewards was reviewed. It was expanded to include low-cost small rewards and substantive rewards for major goals he might set and accomplish himself. Tim's parents presented their list of positive things about their son, and the family activity list was reviewed. All agreed to one family activity, which Tim selected.

Following this, the SCI (Brown, Creamer, et al., 1987), the CDDR (Brown et al., 1998), and the DISC-IV (Shaffer et al., 2000) were completed with Tim. The SCI made it clear that although Tim was still in school, his previously good grades had deteriorated, substance involvement was prevalent among his closest friends, and he currently engaged in few extracurricular activities. Although his parents never used drugs other than cigarettes and were currently abstaining from alcohol, there was a substantial family history of alcohol dependence among both maternal and paternal relatives. Based on Tim's responses to the CDDR, he met criteria for DSM-defined marijuana, stimulant, and nicotine dependence, and had a history of alcohol abuse and experimentation with inhalants and hallucinogens. His preferred drug was methamphetamine, which he obtained from his friends, and its use was related to several life problems (legal, school, family). His use of stimulants was usually followed by alcohol consumption, although he did not consider alcohol a problem.

Not surprisingly, Tim appeared less depressed than when previously seen. With encouragement, he acknowledged anger at his parents, the police, and school officials, and reported feeling "tense" most of the time. Since Tim had difficulty articulating details regarding the topography of his drug use, he was asked to complete the IDTS, which indicated use across both interpersonal and intrapersonal situations. He also completed the AEQ-A, the MEEQ, and the SEEQ, to determine salient dimensions of reinforcement associated with his drug involvement. Tim agreed to have a teacher to whom he felt connected complete the TRF version of the CBCL and gave the therapist permission to contact the teacher, pending parental agreement.

Although the assessment process was not yet complete, motivational interviewing strategies were used to ascertain self-identified concerns for Tim, regardless of his perception of their relation to his substance involvement. Clearly, Tim was motivated to reduce family conflict and sustain his success in school, but he was concerned about the social consequences of changing his drug involvement. However, he was also embarrassed by his recent arrest and was determined not to be stereotyped because of his drug-related arrest and probation. The therapist empathized with his concerns and encouraged him to begin to explore ways in which he could accomplish his personal goals.

At the close of the session, a joint discussion was held with Tim and his parents to review the family activity, select a family activity for the upcoming week, and provide the parents an opportunity to discuss their current concerns and efforts to support their son. The previous contracts were renewed until the third session. The therapist described the next session as their planning session, in which the therapist would provide detailed feedback from the assessment process and in which each family member would discuss goals and concerns. The closing expectation was that all family members would be actively engaged in the therapeutic process to accomplish both personal and mutually agreed-upon goals.

A review of the teen, parent, and teacher assessment data indicated no major psychopathology independent of Tim's substance involvement. However, results of the CBCL and TRF did suggest less than optimal social competence. Results of the DISC-IV indicated that Tim did not meet criteria for other Axis I psychopathology; however, he did endorse some subthreshold symptoms of social anxiety and depression. The IDTS and expectancy questionnaires indicated that Tim used substances predominantly in social contexts, and that the greatest anticipated reinforcement for use involved enhanced comfort in social interactions and diminished stress related to such situations.

The third session began with all family members present. The therapist reported negative results of the toxicology screen sent since the last session, and congratulated Tim on his continued success in this area. Assessment feedback was next provided to Tim and his parents about the lack of major psychopathology independent of Tim's substance involvement, but a number of symptoms and life problems appearing secondary to his substance involvement. The findings of social difficulties were next discussed in the context of typical developmental changes of adolescence. In particular, since peer relations become a salient focus in middle adolescence, difficulties in this area may raise anxiety across many settings, leaving the teen with less than optimal confidence for mastering social relations in general. Following a discussion of this issue with Tim, and with the therapist modeling, the parents were able to verbalize a new appreciation for Tim's social concerns. A general agreement was reached that increasing Tim's social comfort and competence was an important objective for therapy.

Tim's parents were given feedback regarding "normal" parental responses when an adolescent is experiencing the difficulties of the type Tim had been displaying. The parents confirmed their frustrations and fears regarding Tim's behavior. In particular, although they believed he was at an age at which more independence in decision making and activities should be unfolding, they felt considerable ambivalence about granting him increasing independence, given his recent difficulties. Since the issue of independence was a primary source of conflict for Tim and his parents, all agreed that the goal of increasing independence was important and that concrete steps needed to be taken in the therapeutic process to ensure that this typical developmental transition could unfold, contingent on positive behaviors (a list of which was generated).

Finally, when the therapist asked whether Tim wanted to discuss drug-related issues, Tim indicated that he preferred to deal with these privately with the therapist. He did acknowledge to his parents, however, that he had experimented with marijuana, alcohol, methamphetamine, inhalants, and hallucinogens. Tim's right to deal with this privately was discussed, along with the advantages and disadvantages for the family. His parents arrived at a decision to respect and support his wishes for privacy, so long as they were kept informed of the results from the mandated toxicology screens. The parents agreed that for 1 month they would discuss with Tim only concerns about his behavior, and would discuss their personal concerns regarding drug-related matters (e.g., the family history of alcohol and drug problems) primarily with the therapist. There was a clear understanding that all of the contracts would be reviewed and could be renegotiated if problems arose or if the family members' wishes changed. After some discussion of possible consequences of any future drug use by Tim, his parents agreed to have three discussions at home of the advantages and disadvantages of each consequence, and to have this be a topic for the family portion of the session the following week.

The therapist then met with Tim privately and shared with him detailed results of the substance components of the assessment. Tim acknowledged "feeling dependent on stimulants, marijuana, or alcohol" in social situations, but had never considered cigarettes a problem. He was enthusiastic about wanting to improve his social skills and management of situations where he felt anxious about interpersonal matters. He acknowledged fears about losing important male relationships and social activities if he chose not to use with his friends. This opportunity was used to introduce and conduct a functional analysis of his substance involvement with friends. Based on Tim's previous statements, the behavior chain was outlined by the therapist, with Tim filling in and refining all components (e.g., triggers, thoughts, feelings, behaviors, short-term and long-term consequences). A role-playing exercise was conducted to help Tim develop a strategy to manage social pressures during the upcoming week. Finally, given Tim's positive response to the functional analysis approach, he selected a second risk situation and agreed to conduct his own functional analysis, which would be discussed in the next session.

The fourth session began the structured cognitive-behavioral skills training program with the initiation of assertiveness training. Following a review of the functional analysis of a second social pressure situation for use, the rationale for assertive skills was introduced, and Tim chose to focus on this area. Assertion was introduced through a discussion of Tim's understanding of the concept and by generating examples of passive, assertive, and aggressive responses to a generic social offer of marijuana. These responses were used to compare and counteract characteristics of each form of behavior, and to discuss individual rights and general guidelines for deciding on assertive behaviors. With the aid of handouts and worksheets, a nonthreatening situation was identified (i.e., asking for more information about homework). Tim agreed to do a functional analysis of this situation and make at least one assertive clarification request for homework at school each day. The session closed with a brief family discussion of the previous week's family activity, selection of a new activity, and the therapist's role-playing how to assertively request a clarification from Tim's parents. A discussion of concrete consequences, should Tim experience a lapse, was also held. It was agreed that a lapse would result in immediate family discussion with the therapist and loss of an independence reward. Subsequent sessions continued with a review of previous material, progression to the next content area (e.g., criticism, conflict management, dealing with negative emotions, etc.), and role plays for each. At the end of each session a family discussion was held, reviewing family activities, planning a new activity, and discussing aspects of Tim's behavior that merited either a personal reward or an "independence" reward.

On two occasions the parents were seen independently to discuss Tim's progress, their concerns, and improvement/issues regarding family relations. At the ninth session, the first half of the session was devoted to a discussion of a lapse, in which Tim's parents confronted him upon returning home from an outing with friends and smelled alcohol on his breath. Although Tim had not been subject to a random urinanalysis that week, he acknowledged having had one beer with his friends. Tim preferred to discuss the details privately, but listened to his parents' feelings, including disappointment, fear, and reduced trust. Two independence privileges were taken away (i.e., seeing these friends in an unsupervised context and use of the car for 3 weeks). The parents then agreed not to discuss the incident again; however, the next level of consequences was discussed in case a second use episode should occur. When discussing this event individually with the therapist, Tim initially focused on his anger at his parents and their lack of trust in him. However, in response to motivational interviewing techniques used by the therapist, Tim acknowledged the previously agreed-upon consequences for substance use and, subsequently, his difficulties in managing the social situation in which drinking had occurred. Since resistance to social pressure from a date had not been a previously evaluated situation, a functional analysis was conducted in the session, and assertive responses were generated and

role-played. The therapist discussed the lapse as a learning opportunity, and Tim self-generated several new high-risk situations he had experienced in the previous 2 weeks. He chose to generate his own functional analysis and come to the next session with assertive responses and acceptable coping strategies that could be employed. The therapist and Tim reviewed his general progress in therapy, including markedly improved relations with his parents up to this point, increasing self-confidence in social situations, decreased anxiety, and relative success in staying off alcohol and other substances (except for nicotine). The concept of relapse prevention was discussed, and Tim agreed that he needed a social context with peers in which drug use was discussed. Since he displayed considerable resistance to Alcoholics Anonymous or Narcotics Anonymous, a school-based group was selected. This program, while using the Twelve-Step model, had the advantage of being available on a daily basis at school and would not require involving his parents in transportation (which was a salient issue to him, given the loss of driving privileges).

In order to maintain Tim's motivation, the therapist at one point agreed to a meeting with Tim's counselor at school, and on another occasion met with his probation officer. After several relapse prevention sessions, the focus in therapy shifted for both Tim and his parents with his resumption of extracurricular activities. For the parents, this demonstrated his progress in increasing responsibility; for Tim, it provided increasing opportunities for independence, as well as a gradual transition in his social support network to include more nonusing peers. Finally, to help facilitate a transition in Tim's image of himself as lacking social competence, he agreed to volunteer at a senior citizen program run by the city. In this context, in which no one knew of his former substance involvement, he was treated with considerable respect and appreciation. He was also able to practice many competence exercises prior to employing them in peer interactions.

Therapy was reduced to biweekly sessions after 3 months and then to monthly sessions for an additional 6 months. Near the end of therapy, Tim felt confident enough that he was able to discuss his former use with his parents; they were able both to empathize with his experience and to congratulate him on his success in changing his drug use and becoming more responsible. Consequently, it was easier for them to support his increasing independence. The family members continued to have a family activity or family night at least once per week, to maintain their mutual progress in therapy as well. Tim was last known to have successfully completed his probationary period, plus 1 additional year of abstinence beyond that, before he left home to begin college.

CONCLUSION

As is obvious, there are numerous pathways to substance misuse for youths. Multiple intrapersonal and environmental risk factors have been identified that precede substance use and misuse, and increase the likelihood of developing substance use problems. Similarly, multiple trajectories exist for substance-misusing adolescents following treatment. Current research indicates that those who continue to abstain from substance use following treatment, or who decrease their use over time, evidence better psychosocial functioning outcomes. Preliminary empirical evidence suggests that better substance use outcomes for adolescents are associated with treatment completion and participation in self-help group attendance following treatment.

The various risks and resources also influence decisions about optimal forms of intervention for adolescents and their families. Until recently, adolescent treatment for substance misuse has primarily evolved from existing adult treatment modalities, and has been mainly based on a disease model of substance misuse. Little empirical evidence exists for the disease model's efficacy when applied to adolescents. Consequently, important developmental issues specific to adolescents have only recently been applied to treatment of adolescent substance misuse. With the exception of emergent research on family-based and cognitive-behavioral interventions, little treatment outcome research is available to guide the design of developmentally appropriate interventions for substance-misusing adolescents.

Using a biobehavioral model of substance misuse, we have presented a developmentally appropriate intervention to treat adolescent substance misuse that is easily applied and has the flexibility to address the heterogeneity of adolescent substance use problems, intrapersonal and environmental risks, and concomit-

ant problems (e.g., family issues). The treatment detailed in this chapter is cognitive-behavioral and incorporates important components targeting issues of motivation. Although the treatment as described is individual-based, it can also be easily extended to a group format. When the treatment process includes cognitive and behavioral intervention strategies that provide the opportunity for success experiences for youths, and when non-substance-related reinforcers are included in their lives, teens are able to benefit from the therapeutic process. Given the critical role that developmental factors play in the value of various activities and rewards, it is critical to have adolescents play an active role in determining the content of the techniques used to facilitate their transition out of a substance-misusing lifestyle. Finally, decisions regarding the type and intensity of family involvement vary with the resources and limitations that parents bring to this context.

In future directions, as innovative approaches to adolescent substance misuse treatment continue to be developed and empirically examined, it is our hope that such efforts will ultimately establish a solid basis for best practices in treating adolescent addiction.

REFERENCES

Aarons, G. A., Brown, S. A., Stice, E., & Coe, M. T. (2001). Psychometric evaluation of the Marijuana and Stimulant Effect Expectancy Questionnaires for adolescents. *Addictive Behaviors, 26,* 219–236.

Abrams, D. B., & Niaura, R. S. (1987). Social learning theory. In H. T. Blane & K. E. Leonard (Eds.), *Psychological theories of drinking and alcoholism* (pp. 181–226). New York: Guilford Press.

Abrantes, A., Brown, S. A., & Tomlinson, K. (2004). Psychiatric comorbidity among inpatient substance abusing adolescents. *Journal of Child and Adolescent Substance Abuse, 13,* 83–101.

Achenbach, T. M., & Rescorla, L. A. (2001). *Manual for the ASEBA school-age forms and profiles: An integrated system of multi-informant assessment.* Burlington: University of Vermont, Research Center for Children, Youth, and Families.

American Psychiatric Association. (2000). *Diagnostic and statistical manual of mental disorders* (4th ed., text rev.). Washington, DC: Author.

Anderson, K. A., Frissell, K. C., & Brown, S. A. (in press). Context of first post-treatment use for substance abusing adolescents with comorbid psychopathology. *Journal of Child and Adolescent Substance Abuse.*

Annis, H. M., & Graham, J. M. (1985). *Inventory of Drug Taking Situations*. Toronto: Addiction Research Foundation.

Annis, H. M., & Martin, G. (1985). *Drug Taking Confidence Questionnaire*. Toronto: Addiction Research Foundation.

Azrin, N. H., Donohue, B., Besalel, V. A., Kogan, E. S., & Acierno, R. (1994). Youth drug abuse treatment: A controlled outcome study. *Journal of Child and Adolescent Substance Abuse, 3,* 1–16.

Baer, J. S., Kivlahan, D. R., Blume, A. W., McKnight, P., & Marlatt, G. A. (2001). Brief intervention for heavy-drinking college students: 4-year follow-up and natural history. *American Journal of Public Health, 91,* 1310–1316.

Baer, J. S., Marlatt, G. A., Kivlahan, D. R., Fromme, K., Larimer, M. E., & Williams, E. (1992). An experimental test of three methods of alcohol risk reduction with young adults. *Journal of Consulting and Clinical Psychology, 60,* 974–979.

Baer, P. E., Garmezy, L. B., McLaughlin, R. J., & Pokorny, A. D. (1987). Stress, coping, family conflict, and adolescent alcohol use. *Journal of Behavioral Medicine, 10,* 449–466.

Baker, J. R., & Yardley, J. K. (2002). Moderating effect of gender on the relationship between sensation seeking-impulsivity and substance use in adolescents. *Journal of Child and Adolescent Substance Abuse, 12,* 27–43.

Bandura, A. (1977). *Social learning theory*. Englewood Cliffs, NJ: Prentice-Hall.

Barkley, R. A., Fischer, M., Smallish, L., & Fletcher, K. (2004). Young adult follow-up of hyperactive children: Antisocial activities and drug use. *Journal of Child Psychology and Psychiatry, 45*(2), 195–211.

Barnes, G. M., Farrell, M. P., & Banerjee, S. (1994). Family influences on alcohol abuse and other problem behaviors among black and white adolescents in a general population sample. *Journal of Research on Adolescence, 4,* 183–201.

Beck, A. T., Rush, A. J., Shaw, B. F., & Emery, G. (1979). *Cognitive therapy of depression*. New York: Guilford Press.

Beck, A. T., Wright, F. D., Newman, C. F., & Liese, B. S. (1993). *Cognitive therapy of substance abuse*. New York: Guilford Press.

Bennett, L. A., Wolin, S. J., & Reiss, D. (1988). Cognitive, behavioral, and emotional problems among school-age children of alcoholic parents. *American Journal of Psychiatry, 145,* 185–190.

Bentler, P. M. (1992). Etiologies and consequences of adolescent drug use: Implications for prevention. *Journal of Addictive Diseases, 11,* 47–61.

Beschner, G. M., & Friedman, A. S. (1985). Treatment of adolescent drug abusers. *International Journal of the Addictions, 20,* 971–993.

Biederman, J., Wilens, T., Mick, E., & Faraone, S. V. (1997). Is ADHD a risk factor for psychoactive substance use disorders?: Findings from a 4-year prospective follow-up study. *Journal of the American Academy of Child and Adolescent Psychiatry, 36,* 21–29.

Blane, H. (1976). Middle-aged alcoholics and young drinkers. In, H. Blane & M. Chafetz (Eds.), *Youth, alcohol, and social policy* (pp. 5–38). New York: Plenum Press.

Blum, R. W. (1987). Adolescent substance abuse: Diagnostic and treatment issues. *Pediatric Clinics of North America, 34,* 523–537.

Bobo, J. K., McIlvain, H. E., Lando, H. A., Walker, R. D., & Leed-Kelly, A. (1998). Effect of smoking cessation counseling on recovery from alcoholism: Findings from a randomized community intervention trial. *Addiction, 93,* 877–887.

Botvin, G. J., Baker, E., Dusenbury, L., Tortu, S., & Botvin, E. M. (1990). Preventing adolescent drug abuse through a multimodal cognitive-behavioral approach: Results of a three year study. *Journal of Consulting and Clinical Psychology, 58,* 437–446.

Brown, J. H., & Kreft, I. G. G. (1998). Zero effects of drug prevention programs: Issues and solutions. *Evaluation Review, 22*(1), 3–14.

Brown, S. A. (1989). Life events of adolescents in relation to personal and parental substance abuse. *American Journal of Psychiatry, 146,* 484–489.

Brown, S. A. (1993). Recovery patterns in adolescent substance abuse. In J. S. Baer, G. A. Marlatt, & R. J. McMahon (Eds.), *Addictive behaviors across the lifespan: Prevention, treatment and policy issues* (pp. 161–183). Newbury Park, CA: Sage.

Brown, S. A. (2001). Facilitating change for adolescent alcohol problems: A multiple options approach. In E. F. Wagner & H. B. Waldron (Eds.), *Innovations in adolescent substance abuse interventions* (pp. 169–187). New York: Elsevier.

Brown, S. A., Anderson, K. G., Schulte, M. T., Sintov, N. D., & Frissell, K. C. (2005). Facilitating youth self-change through school based intervention. *Addictive Behaviors, 30,* 1797–1810.

Brown, S. A., Christiansen, B. A., & Goldman, M. S. (1987). The Alcohol Expectancy Questionnaire: An instrument for the assessment of adolescent and adult alcohol expectancies. *Journal of Studies on Alcohol, 48,* 483–491.

Brown, S. A., Creamer, V. A., & Stetson, B. A. (1987). Adolescent alcohol expectancies in relation to personal and parental drinking patterns. *Journal of Abnormal Psychology, 96,* 117–121.

Brown, S. A., D'Amico, E. J., McCarthy, D. M., & Tapert, S. F. (2001). Four-year outcomes from adolescent alcohol and drug treatment. *Journal of Studies on Alcohol, 62,* 381–388.

Brown, S. A., Gleghorn, A., Schuckit, M., Myers, M. G., & Mott, M. A. (1996). Conduct disorder among adolescent substance abusers. *Journal of Studies on Alcohol, 57,* 314–324.

Brown, S. A., Inaba, R., Gillin, J. C., Stewart, M. A., Schuckit, M. A., & Irwin, M. R. (1994). Alcoholism and affective disorder: Clinical course of depressive symptomatology. *American Journal of Psychiatry*, *152*, 45–52.

Brown, S. A., Mott, M. A., & Myers, M. G. (1990). Adolescent drug and alcohol treatment outcome. In R. R. Watson (Ed.), *Prevention and treatment of drug and alcohol abuse* (pp. 373–403). Clifton, NJ: Humana Press.

Brown, S. A., Mott, M. A., & Stewart, M. A. (1992). Adolescent alcohol and drug abuse. In C. E. Walker & M. C. Roberts (Eds.), *Handbook of clinical child psychology* (2nd ed., pp. 677–693). New York: Wiley.

Brown, S. A., Myers, M. G., Lippke, L. F., Tapert, S. F., Stewart, D. G., & Vik, P. (1998). Psychometric evaluation of the Customary Drinking and Drug Use Record (CDDR): A measure of adolescent alcohol and drug involvement. *Journal of Studies on Alcohol, 59*, 427–438.

Brown, S. A., Myers, M. G., Mott, M. A., & Vik, P. (1994). Correlates of successful outcome following treatment for adolescent substance abuse. *Journal of Applied and Preventive Psychology, 3*, 61–73.

Brown, S. A., & Ramo, D. E. (in press). Clinical course of youth following treatment for alcohol and drug problems. In H. Liddle & C. Rowe (Eds.), *Treating adolescent substance abuse: State of the science*. New York: Cambridge University Press.

Brown, S. A., & Schuckit, M. A. (1988). Changes in depression among abstinent alcoholics. *Journal of Studies on Alcohol, 49*, 412–417.

Brown, S. A., Tapert, S. F., Tate, S. R., & Abrantes, A. M. (2000). The role of alcohol in adolescent relapse and outcome. *Journal of Psychoactive Drugs, 32*, 107–115.

Brown, S. A., Vik, P. W., & Creamer, V. A. (1989). Characteristics of relapse following adolescent substance abuse treatment. *Addictive Behaviors, 14*, 291–300.

Bukstein, O. G., Glancy, L. J., & Kaminer, Y. (1992). Patterns of affective comorbidity in a clinical population of dually diagnosed adolescent substance abusers. *Journal of American Academy of Child and Adolescent Psychiatry, 31*, 1041–1045.

Bukstein, O., & Kaminer, Y. (1994). The nosology of adolescent substance abuse. *American Journal of Addictions, 3*, 1–13.

Burke, J. D., Burke, K. C., & Rae, D. S. (1994). Increased rates of drug abuse and dependence after onset of mood or anxiety disorders in adolescence. *Hospital and Community Psychiatry, 45*, 451–455.

Burns, D. D. (1989). *Feeling good: The new mood therapy*. New York: Signet.

Burns, D. D. (1999). *The feeling good handbook*. New York: Penguin Putnam.

Cady, M. M., Winters, K. C., Jordan, D. A., Solberg, K. B., & Stinchfield, R. D. (1996). Motivation to change as a predictor of treatment outcome for adolescent substance abusers. *Journal of Child and Adolescent Substance Abuse, 5*, 73–91.

Carmelli, D., Swan, G. E., Robinette, D., & Fabsitz, R. (1992). Genetic influence on smoking: A study of male twins. *New England Journal of Medicine, 327*, 829–833.

Caspi, A., Moffitt, T. E., Newman, D. L., & Silva, P. A. (1996). Behavioral observations at age 3 predict adult psychiatric disorders: Longitudinal evidence from a birth cohort. *Archives of General Psychiatry, 53*, 1033–1039.

Catalano, R., Hawkins, J. D., Krenz, C., Gillmore, M., Morrison, D., Wells, E., et al. (1993). Using research to guide culturally appropriate drug abuse prevention. *Journal of Consulting and Clinical Psychology, 61*, 804–811.

Chassin, L., Fora, D. B., & King, K. M. (2004). Trajectories of alcohol and drug use dependence from adolescence to adulthood: The effects of familial alcoholism and personality. *Journal of Abnormal Psychology, 113*, 483–498.

Chassin, L., & Ritter, J. (2001). Vulnerability to substance use disorders in childhood and adolescence. In R. E. Ingram & J. M. Price (Eds.), *Vulnerability to psychopathology: Risk across the lifespan* (pp. 107–134). New York: Guilford Press.

Chassin, L., Rogosch, F., & Barrera, M. (1991). Substance use and symptomatology among adolescent children of alcoholics. *Journal of Abnormal Psychology, 100*, 449–463.

Christiansen, B. A., & Goldman, M. S. (1983). Alcohol-related expectancies versus demographic/background variables in the prediction of adolescent drinking. *Journal of Consulting and Clinical Psychology, 51*, 249–257.

Christiansen, B. A., Goldman, M. S., & Inn, A. (1982). Development of alcohol-related expectancies in adolescents: Separating pharmacological from social-learning influences. *Journal of Consulting and Clinical Psychology, 50*, 336–344.

Christiansen, B. A., Roehling, P. V., Smith, G. T., & Goldman, M. S. (1989). Using alcohol expectancies to predict adolescent drinking behavior after one year. *Journal of Consulting and Clinical Psychology, 57*, 93–99.

Chung, T., Martin, C. S., Armstrong, T. D., & Labouvie, E. W. (2002). Prevalence of DSM-IV alcohol diagnoses and symptoms in adolescent community and clinical samples. *Journal of the American Academy of Child and Adolescent Psychiatry, 41*, 546–554.

Chung, T., Martin, C. S., Grella, C. E., Winters, K. C., Abrantes, A. M., & Brown, S. A. (2003). Course of alcohol problems treated in adolescents. *Alcoholism: Clinical and Experimental Research, 27*, 253–261.

Cicchetti, D., & Rogosch, F. A. (1999). Psychopathology as a risk for adolescent substance use disorders: A developmental psychopathology perspective. *Journal of Clinical Child Psychology, 28*, 355–365.

Clark, D. B. (2004). The natural history of adolescent alcohol use disorders. *Addiction, 99*(Suppl.), 5–22.

Clark, D. B., Kirisci, L., & Moss, H. B. (1998). Early adolescent gateway drug use in sons of fathers with substance use disorders. *Addictive Behaviors, 23*, 561–566.

Clark, D. B., Kirisci, L., & Tarter, R. E. (1999). Adolescent versus adult onset and the development of substance use disorders in males. *Drug and Alcohol Dependence, 49,* 115–121.

Clark, D. B., Parker, A., & Lynch, K. (1999). Psychopathology and substance-related problems during early adolescence: A survival analysis. *Journal of Clinical Child Psychology, 28,* 333–341.

Clarke, G., Lewinsohn, P., & Hops, H. (1990). *Leader's manual for adolescent groups: Adolescent Coping with Depression Guide.* Eugene, OR: Castalia.

Cloninger, C. R. (1987). Neurogenetic adaptive mechanisms in alcoholism. *Science, 236,* 410–416.

Coatsworth, J. D., Santisteban, D. A., McBride, C. K., & Szapocznik, J. (2001). Brief strategic family therapy versus community control: Engagement, retention, and an exploration of the moderating role of adolescent symptom severity. *Family Process, 40,* 313–332.

Colby, S. M., Monti, P. M., Barnett, N. P., Rohsenow, D. J., Weissman, K., Spirito, A., et al. (1998). Brief motivational interviewing in a hospital setting for adolescent smoking: A preliminary study. *Journal of Consulting and Clinical Psychology, 66,* 574–578.

Colder, C. R., & Chassin, L. (1993). The stress and negative affect model of adolescent alcohol use and the moderating effects of behavioral undercontrol. *Journal of Studies on Alcohol, 54,* 326–333.

Costa, F. M., Jessor, R., & Turbin, M. S. (1999). Transition into adolescent problem drinking: The role of psychosocial risk and protective factors. *Journal of Studies on Alcohol, 60*(4), 480–490.

Costello, A. J., Edelbrock, C., Dulcan, M. K., Kalas, R., & Klaric, S. (1987). *Diagnostic Interview Schedule for Children (DISC).* Pittsburgh, PA: Western Psychiatric Institute and Clinic, University of Pittsburgh School of Medicine.

Crowley, T. J., & Riggs, P. D. (1995). Adolescent substance use disorder with conduct disorder and comorbid conditions. In E. Rahdert & D. Czechowicz (Eds.), *Adolescent drug abuse: Clinical assessment and therapeutic interventions* (DHHS Publication No. 95-3908, NIDA Research Monograph 156, pp. 49–112). Washington, DC: U.S. Government Printing Office.

D'Amico, E. J., & Fromme, K. (2001). Brief prevention for adolescent risk-taking behavior. *Addiction, 97,* 563–574.

Deas, D., Riggs, P., Langenbucher, J., Goldman, M., & Brown, S. (2000). Adolescents are not adults: Developmental considerations in adolescent alcohol users. *Alcoholism: Clinical and Experimental Research, 24,* 232–237.

Deas, D., & Thomas, S. E. (2001). An overview of controlled studies of adolescent substance abuse treatment. *American Journal on Addictions, 10,* 178–189.

Deas-Nesmith, D., Campbell, S., & Brady, K. (1998). Substance use disorders in an adolescent inpatient psychiatric population. *Journal of the National Medical Association, 90,* 233–238.

de Leon, G., Melnick, G., Schoket, D., & Jainchill, N. (1993). Is the therapeutic community culturally relevant?: Findings on race/ethnic differences in retention in treatment. *Journal of Psychoactive Drugs, 25,* 77–86.

Dembo, R., & Shern, D. (1982). Relative deviance and the processes of drug involvement among inner-city youths. *International Journal of the Addictions, 17,* 1373–1399.

Donaldson, S. I., Graham, J. W., & Hansen, W. B. (1994). Testing the generalizability of intervening mechanism theories: Understanding the effects of adolescent drug use prevention interventions. *Journal of Behavioral Medicine, 17,* 195–218.

Donohew, R. L., Hoyle, R. H., Clayton, R. R., Skinner, W. F., Colon, S. E., & Rice, R. E. (1999). Sensation seeking and drug use by adolescents and their friends: Models for marijuana and alcohol. *Journal of Studies on Alcohol, 60,* 622–631.

Donohue, B., & Azrin, N. (2001). Family behavior therapy. In E. F. Wagner & H. B. Waldron (Eds.), *Innovations in adolescent substance abuse interventions* (pp. 205–225). New York: Elsevier.

Donovan, D. M. (1988). Assessment of addictive behaviors: Implications of an emerging biopsychosocial model. In D. M. Donovan & G. A. Marlatt (Eds.), *Assessment of addictive behaviors* (pp. 3–48). New York: Guilford Press.

Donovan, D. M., & Marlatt, G. A. (Eds.). (1988). *Assessment of addictive behaviors.* New York: Guilford Press.

Donovan, J. E., & Jessor, R. (1985). Structure of problem behavior in adolescence and young adulthood. *Journal of Consulting and Clinical Psychology, 53,* 890–904.

Dukes, R. L., Stein, J. A., & Ullman, J. B. (1997). Long-term impact of Drug Abuse Resistance Education (D.A.R.E.). *Evaluation Review, 21,* 483–500.

Duncan, T. E., Duncan, S. C., Alpert, A., Hops, H., Stoolmiller, M., & Muthen, B. (1997). Latent variable modeling of longitudinal and multilevel substance data. *Multivariate Behavioral Research, 32,* 275–318.

Dunn, C., Deroo, L., & Rivara, F. P. (2001). The use of brief interventions adapted from motivational interviewing across behavioral domains: A systematic review. *Addiction, 96,* 1725–1742.

Ennett, S. T., Tobler, N. S., Ringwalt, C. L., & Flewelling, R. L. (1994). How effective is drug abuse resistance education?: A meta-analysis of Project DARE outcome evaluations. *American Journal of Public Health, 84*(9), 1394–1401.

Epstein, J. A., Botvin, G. J., Griffin, K. W., & Diaz, T. (2001). Protective factors buffer effects of risk factors on alcohol use among inner-city youth. *Journal of Child and Adolescent Substance Abuse, 11,* 77–90.

Fagan, J., Weiss, J. G., & Cheng, Y. (1990). Delinquency and substance use among inner-city students. *Journal of Drug Issues, 20,* 351–402.

Feldman, L., Harvey, B., Holowaty, P., & Shortt, L.

(1999). Alcohol use beliefs and behaviors among high school students. *Journal of Adolescent Health, 24,* 48–58.

Fergusson, D. M., Lynskey, M. T., & Horwood, L. J. (1993). The effect of maternal depression on maternal ratings of child behavior. *Journal of Abnormal Child Psychology, 21,* 245–269.

Fiore, M. C., Bailey, W. C., Cohen, S. J., Dorfmanm S. F., Goldstein, M. Q., Gritz, E. R., et al. (2000). *Treating tobacco use and dependence: Clinical practice guidelines.* Rockville, MD: U.S. Department of Health and Human Services, Public Health Service.

Forgatch, M. S., & Patterson, G. R. (1989). *Parents and adolescents living together: Part 2. Family problem solving.* Eugene, OR: Castalia.

Fromme, K., & D'Amico, E. J. (2000). Measuring adolescent alcohol outcome expectancies. *Psychology of Addictive Behaviors, 14,* 206–212.

Fulkerson, J. A., Harrison, P. A., & Beebe, T. J. (1999). DSM-IV substance abuse and dependence: Are there really two dimensions of substance use disorders in adolescents? *Addiction, 94,* 495–506.

Galaif, E. R., & Newcomb, M. D. (1999). Predictors of polydrug use among four ethnic groups: A 12-year longitudinal study. *Addictive Behaviors, 24*(5), 607–631.

Gittelman, R., Mannuzza, S., Shenker, R., & Bonagura, N. (1985). Hyperactive boys almost grown up: I. Psychiatric status. *Archives of General Psychiatry, 42,* 937–947.

Goldman, M. S., Brown, S. A., & Christiansen, B. A. (1987). Expectancy theory: Thinking about drinking. In H. T. Blane & K. E. Leonard (Eds.), *Psychological theories of drinking and alcoholism* (pp. 173–220). New York: Guilford Press.

Goldman, M. S., Brown, S. A., Christiansen, B. A., & Smith, G. T. (1991). Alcoholism and memory: Broadening the scope of expectancy research. *Psychological Bulletin, 110,* 137–146.

Goldman, M. S., Darkes, J., & Del Boca, F. K. (1999). Expectancies' mediation of biopsychosocial risk for alcohol use and alcoholism. In E. I. Kirsch (Ed.), *How expectancies shape experience* (pp. 233–262). Washington DC: American Psychological Association.

Grant, B. F., & Dawson, D. A. (1997). Age at onset of alcohol use and its association with DSM-IV alcohol abuse and dependence: Results from the National Longitudinal Alcohol Epidemiologic Survey. *Journal of Substance Abuse, 9,* 103–110.

Greenbaum, P. E., Foster-Johnson, L., & Petrila, A. (1996). Co-occurring addictive and mental disorders among adolescents: Prevalence research and future directions. *American Journal of Orthopsychiatry, 66,* 52–60.

Grilo, C. M., Becker, D. F., Fehon, D. C., Edell, W. S., & McGlashan, T. H. (1996). Conduct disorder, substance use disorders, and coexisting conduct and substance use disorders in adolescent inpatients. *American Journal of Psychiatry, 153,* 914–920.

Grilo, C. M., Becker, D. F., Walker, M. L., & Levy, K. N.

(1995). Psychiatric comorbidity in adolescent inpatients with substance use disorders. *Journal of the American Academy of Child and Adolescent Psychiatry, 34*(8), 1085–1091.

Haines, M., & Spear, S. F. (1996). Changing the perception of the norm: A strategy to decrease binge drinking among college students. *Journal of American College Health, 45,* 134–140.

Hammersley, R., Forsythe, R., & Lavelle, T. (1990). The criminality of new drug users in Glasgow. *British Journal of Addiction, 85,* 1583–1594.

Harrell, A. V., & Wirtz, P. W. (1989). Screening for adolescent problem drinking: Validation of a multidimensional instrument for case identification. *Psychological Assessment: A Journal of Consulting and Clinical Psychology, 1,* 61–63.

Harrison, P. A., Fulkerson, J. A., & Beebe, T. J. (1998). DSM-IV substance use disorder criteria for adolescents: A critical examination based on a statewide school survey. *American Journal of Psychiatry, 155,* 486–492.

Henggeler, S. W., Borduin, C. M., Melton, G. B., Mann, B. J., Smith, L. A., Hall, J. A., et al. (1991). Effects of multisystemic therapy on drug use and abuse in serious juvenile offenders: A progress report from two outcome studies. *Family Dynamics Addiction Quarterly, 1,* 40–51.

Henggeler, S. W., Clingempeel, W. G., Brondino, M. J., & Pickrel, S. G. (2002). Four-year follow-up of multisystemic therapy with substance-abusing and substance-dependent juvenile offenders. *Journal of the American Academy of Child and Adolescent Psychiatry, 41,* 868–874.

Henly, G. A., & Winters, K. C. (1989). Development of psychosocial scales for the assessment of adolescents involved with alcohol and drugs. *International Journal of the Addictions, 24,* 973–1001.

Hester, R. K., & Miller, W. R. (1988). Empirical guidelines for optimal client-treatment matching. In E. R. Rahdert & J. Grabowski (Eds.), *Adolescent drug abuse: Analyses of treatment research* (DHHS Publication No. ADM 88–1523, NIDA Research Monograph No. 77, pp. 27–38). Washington, DC: U.S. Government Printing Office.

Hoffman, N., Mee-Lee, D., & Arrowhead, A. (1993). Treatment issues in adolescent substance abuse and addictions: Options, outcome, effectiveness, reimbursement, and admission criteria. *Adolescent Medicine: Stare of the Art Reviews, 4,* 371–390.

Hubbard, R. L., Cavanaugh, E. R., Graddock, S. G., & Rachel, J. V. (1983). *Characteristics, behaviors and outcomes for youth in TOPS study* (Report submitted to National Institute on Drug Abuse, Contract No. 271–79–3611). Research Triangle Park, NC: Research Triangle Institute.

Hundleby, J. D., & Mercer, G. W. (1987). Family and friends as social environments and their relationship to young adolescents' use of alcohol, tobacco, and marijuana. *Journal of Marriage and the Family, 49,* 151–164.

Hurt, R. D., Croghan, G. A., Beede, S. D., Wolter, T. D., Croghan, I. T., & Patten, C. A. (2000). Nicotine patch therapy in 101 adolescent smokers. *Archives of Pediatric Adolescent Medicine, 154,* 31–37.

Hurt, R. D., Offord, K. P., Croghan, I. T., Gomez-Dahl, L., Kottke, T. E., Morse, R. M., et al. (1996). Mortality following inpatient addictions treatment: Role of tobacco use in a community-based cohort. *Journal of the American Medical Association, 275,* 1097–1103.

Institute of Medicine. (1990). *Broadening the base of treatment for alcohol problems.* Washington, DC: National Academy Press.

Jacob, T., & Leonard, K. E. (1994). Family and peer influences in the development of adolescent alcohol abuse. In R. Zucker, G. Boyd, & J. Howard (Eds.), *The development of alcohol problems: Exploring the biopsychosocial matrix of risk* (DHHS Publication No. ADM 94-3495, NIAAA Research Monograph No. 26, pp. 123–156). Washington, DC: U.S. Government Printing Office.

Jessor, R., & Jessor, S. L. (1977). *Problem behavior and psychosocial development: A longitudinal study of youth.* New York: Academic Press.

Joanning, H., Quinn, W., Thomas, F., & Mullen, R. (1992). Treating adolescent drug abuse: A comparison of family systems therapy, group therapy, and family drug education. *Journal of Marital and Family Therapy, 18,* 345–356.

Johnson, E. M., Amatetti, S., Funkhouser, J. E., & Johnson, S. (1988). Theories and models supporting prevention approaches to alcohol problems among youth. *Public Health Reports, 103,* 578–586.

Johnson, V., & Pandina, R. J. (1991). Effects of the family environment on adolescent substance use, delinquency and coping styles. *American Journal of Alcohol and Drug Abuse, 17,* 71–88.

Johnston, L. D., O'Malley, P. M., & Bachman, J. G. (2003). *Monitoring the Future national survey results on drug use, 1975–2002: Vol. 1. Secondary school students* (NIH Publication No. 03-5375). Rockville, MD: National Institute on Drug Abuse.

Kaminer, Y. (1991). Adolescent substance abuse. In R. J. Frances & S. I. Miller (Eds.), *Clinical textbook of addictive disorders* (pp. 320–346). New York: Guilford Press.

Kaminer, Y. (1999). Addictive disorders in adolescents. *Addictive Disorders, 22,* 275–288.

Kaminer, Y., Bukstein, O. G., & Tarter, R. E. (1991). The Teen Addiction Severity Index: Rationale and reliability. *International Journal of the Addictions, 26,* 219–226.

Kaminer, Y., Burleson, J. A., Blitz, C., Sussman, J., & Rounsaville, B. J. (1998). Psychotherapies for adolescent substance abusers: A pilot study. *Journal of Nervous and Mental Disease, 186,* 684–690.

Kaminer, Y., Burleson, J. A., & Goldberg, R. (2002). Cognitive-behavioral coping skills and psychoeducation therapies for adolescent substance abuse. *Journal of Nervous and Mental Disease, 190,* 737–745.

Kaminer, Y., Wagner, E. F., Plummer, B. A., & Seifer, R. (1993). Validation of the Teen Addiction Severity Index (T-ASI): Preliminary findings. *American Journal on Addictions, 2,* 250–254.

Kandel, D. B., Johnson, J. G., Bird, H. R., Weissman, M. M., Goodman, S. H., Lahey, B. B., et al. (1999). Psychiatric comorbidity among adolescent with substance use disorders: Findings from the MECA study. *Journal of the American Academy of Child and Adolescent Psychiatry, 38,* 693–699.

Kaufman, J., Birmaher, B., Brent, D., Rao, U., Flynn, C., Moreci, P., et al. (1997). Schedule for Affective Disorders and Schizophrenia for School-Age Children—Present and Lifetime Version (K-SADS-PL): Initial reliability and validity data. *Journal of the American Academy of Child and Adolescent Psychiatry, 36,* 980–988.

Kelly, J. F., Myers, M. G., & Brown, S. A. (2000). A multivariate process model of adolescent 12-step attendance and substance use outcome following inpatient treatment. *Psychology of Addictive Behaviors, 14,* 376–389.

Kelly, J. F., Myers, M. G., & Brown, S. A. (2002). Do adolescents affiliate with 12-step groups?: A multivariate process model of effects. *Journal of Studies on Alcohol, 63,* 293–304.

Kirisci, L., Mezzich, A., & Tarter, R. E. (1995). Norms and sensitivity of the adolescent version of the Drug Use Screening Inventory. *Addictive Behaviors, 20,* 149–157.

Kivlahan, D. R., Marlatt, G. A., Fromme, K., Coppel, D. B., & Williams, E. (1990). Secondary prevention with college drinkers: Evaluation of an alcohol skills training program. *Journal of Consulting and Clinical Psychology, 58,* 805–810.

Knop, J., Teasdale, T. W., Schulsinger, F., & Goodwin, D. W. (1985). A prospective study of young men at high risk for alcoholism: School behavior and achievement. *Journal of Studies on Alcohol, 46,* 273–278.

Kypri, K., McCarthy, D. M., Coe, M. T., & Brown, S. A. (2004). Transition to independent living and substance involvement of treated and high risk youth. *Journal of Child and Adolescent Substance Abuse, 13,* 85–100.

Langenbucher, J., Martin, C., Labouvie, E., Sanjuan, P., Bavly, L., & Pollock, N. (2000). Toward the DSM-IV: A withdrawal-gate model of alcohol abuse and dependence. *Journal of Consulting and Clinical Psychology, 68,* 799–809.

Latimer, W. W., Winters, K. C., Stinchfield, R., & Traver, R. E. (2000). Demographic, individual, and interpersonal predictors or adolescent alcohol and marijuana use following treatment. *Psychology of Addictive Behaviors, 14,* 162–173.

Laundergan, J. C. (1982). *Easy does it: Alcoholism treatment outcomes, Hazelden, and the Minnesota model.* Minneapolis, MN: Hazelden Foundation.

Lawendowski, L. A. (1998). A motivational intervention for adolescent smokers. *Preventive Medicine, 27,* A39–A46.

Lerman, C., Caporaso, N. E., Audrain, J., Main, D., Bauman, E. D., Lockshin, B., et al. (1999). Evidence suggesting the role of specific genetic factors in cigarette smoking. *Health Psychology, 18,* 14–20.

Lewinsohn, P. M., Hops, H., Roberts, R. E., Seeley, J. R., & Andrews, J. A. (1993). Adolescent psychopathology: I. *Journal of Abnormal Psychology, 102,* 133–144.

Lewinsohn, P. M., Rohde, P., & Seeley, J. R. (1996). Alcohol consumption in high school adolescents: Frequency of use and dimensional structure of associated problems. *Addiction, 91,* 375–390.

Lewinsohn, P. M., Rohde, P., Seeley, J. R., & Klein, D. N. (1997). Axis II psychopathology as a function of Axis I disorders in childhood and adolescence. *Journal of the American Academy of Child and Adolescent Psychiatry, 36,* 1752–1759.

Lewis, R. A., Piercy, F. P., Sprenkle, D. H., & Trepper, T. S. (1990). Family-based interventions for helping drug-abusing adolescents. *Journal of Adolescent Research, 5,* 82–95.

Liddle, H. A., & Dakof, G. A. (1992). *Effectiveness of family-based treatment for adolescent substance use.* Paper presented at the annual conference of the Society for Psychotherapy Research, Pittsburgh, PA.

Liddle, H. A., & Dakof, G. A. (1995). Family-based treatment for adolescent drug use: State of the science. In E. Rahdert & D. Czechowicz (Eds.), *Adolescent drug abuse: Clinical assessment and therapeutic interventions* (DHHS Publication No. ADM 95-3908, NIDA Research Monograph No. 156, pp. 218–254). Washington, DC: U.S. Government Printing Office.

Liddle, H. A., Dakof, G. A., Diamond, G., Holt, M., Aroyo, J., & Watson, M. (1992). The adolescent module in multidimensional family therapy. In G. W. Lawson & A. W. Lawson (Eds.), *Adolescent substance abuse: Etiology, treatment, and prevention* (pp. 165–186). Gaithersburg, MD: Aspen.

Lifrak, P. D., Alterman, A. I., O'Brien, C. P., & Volpicelli, J. R. (1997). Naltrexone for alcoholic adolescents. *American Journal of Psychiatry, 154,* 439–441.

Lilja, J., Wilhelmsen, B. U., Larsson, S., & Hamilton, D. (2003). Evaluation of drug use prevention programs directed at adolescents. *Substance Use and Misuse, 38,* 1831–1863.

Lynam, D. R., Milich, R., Zimmerman, R., Novak, S. P., Logan, T. K., Martin, C., et al. (1999). Project DARE: No effects at 10-year follow-up. *Journal of Consulting and Clinical Psychology, 67,* 590–593.

Mahaddian, E., Bentler, P. M., & Newcomb, M. D. (1988). Risk factors for substance use: Ethnic differences among adolescents. *Journal of Substance Abuse, 1,* 11–24.

Mannuzza, S., Klein, R. G., Bessler, A., Malloy, P., & LaPadula, M. (1998). Adult psychiatric status of hyperactive boys grown up. *American Journal of Psychiatry, 155*(4), 493–498.

Marlatt, G. A., & Gordon, J. A. (Eds.). (2005). *Relapse prevention: Maintenance strategies in the treatment of addictive behaviors* (2nd ed.). New York: Guilford Press.

Marlatt, G. A., & Witkiewitz, K. (2002). Harm reduction approaches to alcohol use: Health promotion, prevention, and treatment. *Addictive Behaviors, 27,* 867–886.

Martin, C. S., Kaczynski, N. A., Maisto, S. A., Bukstein, O. M., & Moss, H. B. (1995). Patterns of DSM-IV alcohol abuse and dependence symptoms in adolescent drinkers. *Journal of Studies on Alcohol, 56,* 672–680.

Martin, C. S., Langenbucher, J. W., Kaczynski, N. A., & Chung, T. (1996). Staging in the onset of DSM-IV alcohol abuse and dependence symptoms in adolescent drinkers. *Journal of Studies on Alcohol, 57,* 549–558.

McConaughy, S. H. (2001). The Achenbach System of Empirically Based Measurement. In J. J. W. Andrews, D. H. Saklofske, & H. L. Janzen (Eds.), *Handbook of psychoeducational assessment: Ability, achievement, and behavior in children* (pp. 289–324). San Diego, CA: Academic Press.

McCrady, B. S. (2001). Alcohol use disorders. In D. H. Barlow (Ed.), *Clinical handbook of psychological disorders* (3rd ed., pp. 376–434). New York: Guilford Press.

McGue, M. (1994). Why developmental psychology should find room for behavioral genetics. In C. A. Nelson (Ed.), *Minnesota Symposia on Child Psychology: Vol. 27. Threats to optimal development: Integrating biological, psychological, and social risk factors* (pp. 105–119). Hillsdale, NJ: Erlbaum.

McLellan, A. T., Luborsky, L., O'Brien, C. P., & Woody, G. E. (1980). An improved evaluation instrument for substance abuse patients: The Addiction Severity Index. *Journal of Nervous and Mental Disease, 168,* 26–33.

McMorris, B. J., Tyler, K. A., Whitbeck, L. B., & Hoyt, D. R. (2002). Familial and "on-the-street" risk factors associated with alcohol use among homeless and runaway adolescents. *Journal of Studies on Alcohol, 63,* 34–43.

Merydith, S. P. (2001). Temporal stability and convergent validity of the Behavior Assessment System for Children. *Journal of School Psychology, 39,* 253–265.

Metrik, J., McCarthy, D. M., Frissell, K. C., MacPherson, L., & Brown, S. A. (2004). Adolescent alcohol reduction and cessation expectancies. *Journal of Studies on Alcohol, 65,* 217–226.

Meyers, K., Hagan, T. A., Zanis, D., Webb, A., Frantz, J., Ring-Kurtz, S., et al. (1999). Critical issues in adolescent substance use assessment. *Drug and Alcohol Dependence, 55,* 235–246.

Meyers, K., McLellan, A. T., Jaeger, J. L., & Pettinati, H. M. (1995). The development of the Comprehensive Addiction Severity Index for Adolescents (CASI-A): An interview for assessing multiple problems of adolescents. *Journal of Substance Abuse Treatment, 12,* 181–193.

Meyers, K., Webb, A., Randall, M., McDermott, P., Mulvaney, F., Tucker, W., et al. (1998). *Psychometric properties of the Comprehensive Addiction Severity Inventory (CASI).* Paper presented at the 60th Annual Scientific Meeting of the College on Problems of Drug Dependence (CPDD), Scottsdale, AZ.

Miller, E. T., Turner, A. P., & Marlatt, G. A. (2001). The harm reduction approach to the secondary prevention of alcohol problems in adolescents and young adults: Considerations across a developmental spectrum. In P. M. Monti, S. M. Colby, & T. A. O'Leary (Eds.), *Adolescents, alcohol, and substance abuse: Reaching teens through brief interventions* (pp. 58–79). New York: Guilford Press.

Miller, W. R. (1989). Matching individuals with interventions. In R. K. Hester & W. R. Miller (Eds.), *Handbook of alcoholism treatment approaches* (pp. 261–272). New York: Pergamon Press.

Miller, W. R., & Rollnick, S. (Eds.). (2002). *Motivational interviewing: Preparing people for change* (2nd ed.). New York: Guilford Press.

Monti, P. M., Abrams, D. B., Kadden, R. M., & Cooney, N. L. (1989). *Treating alcohol dependence: A coping skills training guide.* New York: Guilford Press.

Monti, P. M., Colby, S. M., Barnett, N. P., Spirito, A., Rohsenow, D. J., Myers, M., et al. (1999). Brief intervention for harm reduction with alcohol-positive older adolescents in a hospital emergency department. *Journal of Consulting and Clinical Psychology, 67,* 989–994.

Moos, R. H., & Billings, A. G. (1982). Children of alcoholics during the recovery process: Alcoholic and matched control families. *Addictive Behaviors, 7,* 155–163.

Myers, M. G. (1999). Smoking interventions with adolescent substance abusers. *Journal of Substance Abuse Treatment, 16,* 289–298.

Myers, M. G., & Brown, S. A. (1990). Coping and appraisal in relapse risk situations among substance abusing adolescents following treatment. *Journal of Adolescent Chemical Dependency, 1,* 95–116.

Myers, M. G., & Brown, S. A. (1994). Smoking and health in substance abusing adolescents: A two year followup. *Pediatrics, 93,* 561–566.

Myers, M. G., & Brown, S. A. (1996). The Adolescent Relapse Coping Questionnaire: Psychometric validation. *Journal of Studies on Alcohol, 57,* 40–46.

Myers, M. G., Brown, S. A., & Mott, M. A. (1993). Coping as a predictor of adolescent substance abuse treatment outcome. *Journal of Substance Abuse, 5,* 15–29.

Myers, M. G., Brown, S. A., & Mott, M. A. (1995). Preadolescent conduct disorder behaviors predict relapse and progression of addiction for alcohol and drug abusing adolescents. *Alcoholism: Clinical and Experimental Research, 19,* 1528–1536.

Myers, M. G., McCarthy, D. M., MacPherson, L., & Brown, S. A. (2003). Constructing a short form of the smoking consequences questionnaire with adoles-cent and young adults. *Psychological Assessments, 15*(2), 163–172.

Newcomb, M. D., & Bentler, P. M. (1988). *Consequences of adolescent drug use.* Beverly Hills, CA: Sage.

Newcomb, M. D., Schier, L. M., & Bentler, P. M. (1993). Effects of adolescent drug use on adult mental health: A prospective study of a community sample. *Experimental and Clinical Psychopharmacology, 1,* 215–241.

Obermeier, G., & Henry, P. (1985). Inpatient treatment of adolescent alcohol and polydrug abusers. *Seminars in Adolescent Medicine, 1,* 293–301.

Obert, J. L., Rawson, R. A., & Miotto, K. (1997). Substance abuse treatment for "hazardous users": An early intervention. *Journal of Psychoactive Drugs, 29,* 291–298.

Ohannessian, C. M., Hesselbrock, V. M., Kramer, J., Kuperman, S., Bucholz, K. K., Schuckit, M. A., et al. (2004). The relationship between parental alcoholism and adolescent psychopathology: A systematic examination of parental comorbid psychopathology. *Journal of Abnormal Child Psychology, 32,* 519–533.

Opland, E., Winters, K., & Stinchfield, R. (1995). Gender differences in drug-abusing adolescents. *Psychology of Addictive Behaviors, 9,* 167–175.

Pandina, R. J., & Schuele, J. A. (1983). Psychosocial correlates of alcohol and drug use of adolescent students and adolescents in treatment. *Journal of Studies on Alcohol, 44,* 950–973.

Patterson, G. R., DeBaryshe, B. D., & Ramsey, E. (1989). A developmental perspective on antisocial behavior. *American Psychologist, 44,* 329–335.

Patock-Peckham, J. A., Cheong, J., Balhorn, M. E., & Nagoshi, C. T. (2001). A social learning perspective: A model of parenting styles, self-regulation, perceived drinking control, and alcohol use and problems. *Alcoholism: Clinical and Experimental Research, 25,* 1284–1292.

Peleg, A., Neumann, L., Friger, M., Peleg, R., & Sperber, A. D. (2001). Outcomes of a brief alcohol abuse prevention program for Israeli high school students. *Journal of Adolescent Health, 28,* 263–269.

Price, J. M., & Lento, J. (2001). The nature of child and adolescent vulnerability: History and definitions. In R. E. Ingram & J. M. Price (Eds.), *Vulnerability to psychopathology: Risk across the lifespan* (pp. 20–38). New York: Guilford Press.

Project MATCH Research Group. (1997). Matching alcoholism treatments to client heterogeneity: Project MATCH posttreatment drinking outcomes. *Journal of Studies on Alcohol, 58*(1), 7–23.

Prokhorov, A. V., Koehly, L. M., Pallonen, U. E., & Hudmon, K. S. (1998). Adolescent nicotine dependence measured by the modified Fagerstrom Tolerance Questionnaire at two time points. *Journal of Child and Adolescent Substance Abuse, 7,* 35–47.

Puig-Antich, J., & Orvaschel, H. (1987). *Schedule for Affective Disorders and Schizophrenia for School-*

Age Children: Epidemiologic Version and Present Episode version. Pittsburgh, PA: Western Psychiatric Institute and Clinic.

Reynolds, C., & Kamphaus, R. (1994). *Behavior Assessment System for Children*. Circle Pines, MN: American Guidance Service.

Reynolds, C., & Kamphaus, R. (2004). *BASC-2: Behavior Assessment System for Children, Second Edition*. Circle Pines, MN: American Guidance Service.

Richter, S. S., Brown, S. A., & Mott, M. A. (1991). The impact of social support and self-esteem on adolescent substance abuse treatment outcome. *Journal of Substance Abuse, 3*, 371–385.

Riggs, P. D., Thompson, L. L., Mikulich, S. K., Whitmore, E. A., & Crowley, T. J. (1996). An open trial of pemoline in drug-dependent delinquents with attention-deficit hyperactivity disorder. *Journal of the American Academy of Child and Adolescent Psychiatry, 35*, 1018–1024.

Robin, A. L., & Foster, S. L. (1989). *Negotiating parent–adolescent conflict: A behavioral–family systems approach*. New York: Guilford Press.

Robins, L. N., & Price, R. K. (1991). Adult disorders predicted by childhood conduct problems: Results from the NIMH Epidemiologic Catchment Area project. *Psychiatry, 54*, 116–132.

Rohde, P., Lewinsohn, P. M., Kahler, C. W., Seeley, J. R., & Brown, R. A. (2001). Natural course of alcohol use disorders from adolescence to young adulthood. *Journal of the American Academy of Child and Adolescent Psychiatry, 40*, 83–90.

Rohde, P., Lewinsohn, P. M., & Seeley, J. R. (1991). Comorbidity of unipolar depression: II. Comorbidity with other mental disorders in adolescents and adults. *Journal of Abnormal Psychology, 100*, 214–222.

Rohde, P., Lewinsohn, P. M., & Seeley, J. R. (1996). Psychiatric comorbidity with problematic alcohol use in high school students. *Journal of the American Academy of Adolescent and Child Psychiatry, 35*, 101–109.

Rose, J. S., Chassin, L., Presson, C. C., & Sherman, S. J. (1996). Demographic factors in adult smoking status: Mediating and moderating influences. *Psychology of Addictive Behaviors, 10*(1), 28–37.

Russell, M. (1990). Prevalence of alcoholism among children of alcoholics. In M. Windle & J. S. Searles (Eds.), *Children of alcoholics: Critical perspectives* (p. 9–38). New York: Guilford Press.

Sabol, S. Z., Nelson, M. L., Fisher, C., Gunzerath, L., Brody, C. L., Hu, S., et al. (1999). A genetic association for cigarette smoking behavior. *Health Psychology, 18*, 7–13.

Sale, E., Sambrano, S., Springer, J. F., & Turner, C. W. (2003). Risk, protection, and substance use in adolescents: A multi-site model. *Journal of Drug Education, 33*, 91–105.

Santisteban, D. A., Coatsworth, J. D., Perez-Vidal, A., Kurtines, W. M., Schwartz, S. J., LaPierre, A., et al. (2003). Efficacy of brief strategic family therapy in modifying Hispanic adolescent behavior problems and substance use. *Journal of Family Psychology, 17*, 121–133.

Sells, S. B., & Simpson, D. D. (1979). Evaluation of treatment outcome for youths in the Drug Abuse Reporting Program (DARP): A followup study. In G. M. Beschner & A. S. Friedman (Eds.), *Youth drug abuse: Problems, issues and treatment* (pp. 571–628). Lexington, MA: Lexington Books.

Schuckit, M. A. (1994). Low level of response to alcohol as a predictor of future alcoholism. *American Journal of Psychiatry, 151*(2), 184–189.

Schuckit, M. A. (1998). Biological, psychological, and environmental predictors of the alcoholism risk: A longitudinal study. *Journal of Studies on Alcohol, 59*, 485–494.

Schwartz, R. H., & Wirth, P. W. (1990). Potential substance abuse: Detection among adolescent patients: Using the Drug and Alcohol Problem (DAP) Quick Screen, a 30–item questionnaire. *Clinical Pediatrics, 29*, 38–43.

Shaffer, D., Fisher, P., Lucas, C. P., Dulcan, M. K., & Schwab-Stone, M. E. (2000). NIMH Diagnostic Interview Schedule for Children Version IV (NIMH DISC-IV): Description, differences from previous versions, and reliability of some common diagnoses. *Journal of the American Academy of Child and Adolescent Psychiatry, 39*, 28–38.

Shedler, J., & Block, J. (1990). Adolescent drug use and psychological health: A longitudinal inquiry. *American Psychologist, 45*, 612–630.

Sheehan, M., Schonfeld, C., Ballard, R., Schofield, F., Najman, J., & Siskind, V. (1996). A three year outcome evaluation of a theory based drink driving education program. *Journal of Drug Education, 26*, 295–312.

Sher, K. J. (1991). *Children of alcoholics: A critical appraisal of theory and research*. Chicago: University of Chicago Press.

Sher, K. J. (1994). Individual-level risk factors. In R. Zucker, G. Boyd, & J. Howard (Eds.), *The development of alcohol problems: Exploring the biopsychosocial matrix of risk* (DHHS Publication No. ADM 94-3495, NIAAA Research Monograph No. 26, pp. 77–108). Washington, DC: U. S. Government Printing Office.

Shope, J. T., Copeland, L. A., Maharg, R., & Dielman, T. E. (1996). Effectiveness of a high school alcohol misuse prevention program. *Alcoholism: Clinical and Experimental Research, 20*, 791–798.

Shope, J. T., Elliott, M. R., Raghunathan, T. E., & Waller, P. F. (2001). Long-term follow-up of a high school alcohol misuse prevention program's effect on students' subsequent driving. *Alcoholism: Clinical and Experimental Research, 25*, 403–410.

Slutske, W. S., Heath, A. C., Madden, P. A. F., Bucholz, K. K., Statham, D. J., & Martin, N. G. (2002). Personality and genetic risk for alcoholism. *Journal of Abnormal Psychology, 111*, 124–133.

Smith, D. E., Buxton, M. E., Bilal, R., & Seymour, R. B.

(1993). Cultural points of resistance to the 12-step recovery process. *Journal of Psychoactive Drugs, 25,* 97–108.

Smith, G. T., & Goldman, M. S. (1994). Alcohol expectance theory and the identification of high-risk adolescents. *Journal of Research on Adolescence, 4,* 229–247.

Smith, G. T., Goldman, M. S., Greenbaum, P. E., & Christiansen, B. A. (1995). Expectancy for social facilitation from drinking: the divergent paths of high-expectancy and low-expectancy adolescents. *Journal of Abnormal Psychology, 104,* 32–40.

Smith, T. A., House, R. F., Croghan, I. T., Gauvin, T. R., Colligan, R. C., Offord, K. P., et al. (1996). Nicotine patch therapy in adolescent smokers. *Pediatrics, 98,* 659–667.

Stewart, D. G., & Brown, S. A. (1995). Withdrawal and dependency symptoms among adolescent alcohol and drug abusers. *Addiction, 90,* 627–635.

Stewart, M. A., & Brown, S. A. (1994). Family functioning following adolescent substance abuse treatment. *Journal of Substance Abuse, 5,* 327–339.

Stice, E., Barrera, M., & Chassin, L. (1993). Relation of parental support and control to adolescents' externalizing symptomatology and substance use: A longitudinal examination of curvilinear effects. *Journal of Abnormal Child Psychology, 21,* 609–629.

Stowell, R. J., & Estroff, T. W. (1992). Psychiatric disorders in substance-abusing adolescent inpatients: A pilot study. *Journal of the American Academy of Child and Adolescent Psychiatry, 35,* 1036–1040.

Substance Abuse and Mental Health Services Administration. (2003). *Results from the 2002 National Survey on Drug Use and Health: National findings* (Office of Applied Studies, NHSDA Series H-22, DHHS Publication No. SMA 03-3836). Rockville, MD: Author.

Sung, M., Erkanli, A., Angold, A., & Costello, E. J. (2004). Effects of age at first substance use and psychiatric comorbidity on the development of substance use disorders. *Drug and Alcohol Dependence, 75,* 287–299.

Swan, G. E., & Carmelli, D. (1997). Behavior genetic investigations of cigarette smoking and related issues in twins. In K. Blum & E. P. Noble (Eds.), *Handbook of psychiatric genetics* (pp. 387–406). Boca Raton, FL: CRC Press.

Szapocznik, J., Hervis, O., & Schwartz, S. (in press). *Brief strategic family therapy.* Rockville, MD: National Institute on Drug Abuse.

Szapocznik, J., Kurtines, W. A., Foote, F., Perez-Vidal, A., & Hervis, O. (1983). Conjoint versus one-person family therapy: Some evidence for the effectiveness of conducting family therapy through one person. *Journal of Consulting and Clinical Psychology, 51,* 889–899.

Szapocznik, J., Kurtines, W. A., Foote, F., Perez-Vidal, A., & Hervis, O. (1986). Conjoint versus one-person family therapy: Further evidence for the effectiveness of conducting family therapy through one person

with drug abusing adolescents. *Journal of Consulting and Clinical Psychology, 54,* 395–397.

Szapocznik, J., Perez-Vidal, A., Brickman, A. L., Foote, F., Santisteban, D., Hervis, O., et al. (1988). Engaging adolescent drug abusers and their families in treatment: A strategic structural systems approach. *Journal of Consulting and Clinical Psychology, 56,* 552–557.

Tapert, S. F., & Brown, S. A. (2000). Substance dependence, family history of alcohol dependence and neuropsychological functioning in adolescence. *Addiction, 95,* 1043–1053.

Tapert, S. F., Brown, S. A., Myers, M. G., & Granholm, E. (1999). The role of neurocognitive abilities in coping with adolescent relapse to alcohol and drug use. *Journal of Studies on Alcohol, 60,* 500–508.

Tapert, S. F., Stewart, D. G., & Brown, S. A. (1999). Drug abuse in adolescence. In A. J. Goreczny & M. Hersen (Eds.), *Handbook of pediatric and adolescent health psychology* (pp. 161–178). Boston: Allyn & Bacon.

Tarter, R. E., & Edwards, K. (1988). Psychological factors associated with the risk for alcoholism. *Alcoholism: Clinical and Experimental Research, 12,* 471–480.

Tarter, R. E., Laird, S. B., Bukstein, O. G., & Kaminer, Y. (1992). Validation of the Drug Use Screening Inventory: Preliminary findings. *Psychology of Addictive Behaviors, 6,* 233–236.

Thompson, K. M., & Wilsnack, R. W. (1984). Drinking and drinking problems among female adolescents: Patterns and influences. In S. C. Wilsnack & L. J. Beckman (Eds.), *Alcohol problems in women: Antecedents, consequences, and intervention.* New York: Guilford Press.

Tobler, N. S., & Stratton, H. H. (1997). Effectiveness of school-based drug prevention programs: A meta-analysis of the research. *Journal of Primary Prevention, 18,* 71–128.

Tomlinson, K. L., Brown, S. A., & Abrantes, A. (2004). Psychiatric comorbidity and substance use treatment outcomes of adolescents. *Psychology of Addictive Behaviors, 18*(2), 160–169.

Turner, N. E., Annis, H. M., & Sklar, S. M. (1997). Measurement of antecedents to drug and alcohol use: Psychometric properties of the Inventory of Drug-Taking Situations (IDTS). *Behaviour Research and Therapy, 35,* 465–483.

Upadhyaya, H. P., Deas, D., Brady, K. T., & Kruesi, M. (2002). Cigarette smoking and psychiatric comorbidity in children and adolescents. *Journal of the American Academy of Child and Adolescent Psychiatry, 41,* 1294–1305.

U.S. Department of Health and Human Services. (1994). *Preventing tobacco use among young people: A report of the Surgeon General.* Washington, DC: U.S. Government Printing Office.

Vaillant, G. E. (1983). *The natural history of alcoholism.* Cambridge, MA: Harvard University Press.

Vakalahi, H. F. (2001). Adolescent substance use and

family-based risk and protective factors: A literature review. *Journal of Drug Education, 31,* 29–46.

Vik, P. W., Brown, S. A., & Myers, M. G. (1997). Assessment of adolescent substance use problems, In E. J. Mash & L. G. Terdal (Eds.), *Assessment of childhood disorders* (3rd ed., pp. 717–748). New York: Guilford Press.

Vik, P. W., Grizzle, K., & Brown, S. A. (1992). Social resource characteristics and adolescent substance abuse relapse. *Journal of Adolescent Chemical Dependency, 2,* 59–74.

Wagner, E. S., Brown, S. A., Monti, P., Myers, M. G., & Waldron, H. B. (1999). Innovations in adolescent substance abuse and prevention. *Alcoholism: Clinical and Experimental Research, 23,* 236–249.

Walden, B., McGue, M., Iacono, W. G., Burt, S. A., & Elkins, I. (2004). Identifying shared environmental contributions to early substance use: The respective roles of peers and parents. *Journal of Abnormal Psychology, 113,* 440–450.

Waldron, H. B. (1997). Adolescent substance abuse and family therapy outcome: A review of randomized trials. *Advances in Clinical Child Psychology, 19,* 199–234.

Waldron, H. B., & Kaminer, Y. (2004). On the learning curve: Emerging evidence supporting cognitive-behavioral therapies for adolescent substance abuse. *Addiction, 99*(Suppl. 2). 93–105.

Waldron, H. B., Slesnick, B., Brody, J. L., Turner, C. W., & Peterson, T. R. (2001). Treatment outcomes for adolescent substance abuse at 4- and 7-month assessments. *Journal of Consulting and Clinical Psychology, 69,* 802–813.

Wall, T. L., Shea, S. H., Chan, K. K., & Carr, L. G. (2001). A genetic association with the development of alcohol and other substance use behavior in Asian Americans. *Journal of Abnormal Psychology, 110,* 173–178.

Wallace, J. M., Jr., Bachman, J. G., O'Malley, P. M., Schulenberg, J. E., Cooper, S. M., & Johnston, L. D. (2003). Gender and ethnic differences in smoking, drinking and illicit drug use among American 8th, 10th and 12th grade students, 1976–2000. *Addiction, 98,* 225–234.

Weinberg, N. Z. (2001). Risk factors for adolescent abuse. *Journal of Learning Disabilities, 34,* 343–363.

White, H. R., & Labouvie, E. W. (1989). Towards the assessment of adolescent problem drinking. *Journal of Studies on Alcohol, 50,* 30–37.

Wilens, T. E., Biederman, J., & Spencer, T. J. (1999). Attention-deficit/hyperactivity disorder in youth. In R. L. Hendren (Ed.), *Disruptive behavior disorders in children and adolescents* (pp. 1–45). Washington, DC: American Psychiatric Press.

Wilens, T. E., Faraone, S. V., Biederman, J., & Gunawardene, S. (2003). Does stimulant therapy of attention-deficit/hyperactivity disorder beget later substance abuse?: A meta-analytic review of the literature. *Pediatrics, 111,* 179–185.

Wills, T. A., & Yaeger, A. M. (2003). Family factors and adolescent substance use: Models and mechanisms. *Current Directions in Psychological Science, 12,* 222–226.

Windle, M., & Barnes, G. M. (1988). Similarities and differences in correlates of alcohol consumption and problem behaviors among male and female adolescents. *International Journal of the Addictions, 23,* 707–728.

Windle, M., Miller-Tutzauer, C., Barnes, G. M., & Welte, J. (1991). Adolescent perceptions of helpseeking resources for substance abuse. *Child Development, 62,* 79–189.

Winters, K. C. (1991). *The Personal Experience Screening Questionnaire.* Los Angeles: Western Psychological Services.

Winters, K. C. (1992). Development of an adolescent alcohol and other drug abuse screening scale: Personal Experience Screening Questionnaire. *Addictive Behaviors, 17,* 479–490.

Winters, K. C., & Henly, G. A. (1989a). *The Adolescent Diagnostic Interview.* Los Angeles: Western Psychological Services.

Winters, K. C., & Henly, G. A. (1989b). *The Personal Experience Inventory.* Los Angeles: Western Psychological Services.

Winters, K. C., Latimer, W. L., & Stinchfield, R. D. (1999). Adolescent treatment. In P. J. Ott, R. E. Tarter, & R. T. Ammerman (Eds.), *Sourcebook on substance abuse: Etiology, epidemiology, assessment, and treatment* (pp. 350–361). Boston: Allyn & Bacon.

Winters, K. C., Stinchfield, R. D., & Henly, G. A. (1996). Convergent and predictive validity of scales measuring adolescent substance abuse. *Journal of Child and Adolescent Substance Abuse, 5,* 37–55.

Winters, K. C., Stinchfield, R. D., Opland, E., Weller, C., & Latimer, W. W. (2000). The effectiveness of the Minnesota Model approach in the treatment of adolescent drug abusers. *Addiction, 95,* 601–611.

Woltzen, M. C., Filstead, W. J., Anderson, C. O. L., Anderson, S., Twadell, S., Sisson, C., et al. (1986). Clinical issues central to the residential treatment of alcohol and substance misusers. *Advances in Adolescent Mental Health, 2,* 271–282.

Yih-Ing, H., Grella, C. E., Hubbard, R. L., Hsieh, S. C., Fletcher, B. W., Brown, B. S., et al. (2001). An evaluation of drug treatments for adolescents in 4 US cities. *Archives of General Psychiatry, 58,* 689–695.

Eating Disorders

Lisa Terre, Walker S. Carlos Poston II, and John P. Foreyt

Anorexia nervosa (AN) and bulimia nervosa (BN) are complex disorders that are often perplexing to therapists and difficult to manage. The purpose of this chapter is to review the history, nature, etiology, and treatment of these disorders, as well as to provide a brief introduction to the proposed diagnostic category of binge-eating disorder (BED).

Individual psychotherapy, inpatient approaches, outpatient programs, and specific therapeutic techniques and components are presented. Throughout the chapter, we emphasize that treatment of these disorders is enhanced when psychologists work collaboratively with other health professionals on multidisciplinary teams in comprehensive, multicomponent treatment programs. Although the last decade has been marked by important advances in our understanding of eating disorders, a solid empirical base is just beginning to emerge. For this reason, we believe that many treatments for eating disorders should still be considered experimental at the present time. As Ben-Tovim (2003) has recently noted, "the absence of authoritative evidence for treatment effectiveness makes it increasingly hard to protect resource intensive treatments in anorexia and bulimia nervosa, and existing theories of the causation of the disorders are too non-specific to generate effective programs of prevention" (p. 65). Commenting specifically on the empirical support for the management of child and adolescent eating disorders, Gowers and Bryant-Waugh (2004) have concluded that "the evidence base for effective interventions is surprisingly weak" (p. 63).

However, with the increasing research and clinical interest in these disorders, we hope that more of the methods described in this chapter will be empirically established in the near future, and that new approaches will emerge.

HISTORY

Cases of self-inflicted starvation and weight loss have a long recorded history, dating back at least to the 4th century A.D. (Lacey, 1982). For instance, there is some suggestion that Princess Margaret of Hungary may have suffered from AN in the 11th century (Halmi, 1982). Devotional literature of the Middle Ages is also punctuated with numerous inspirational accounts of pious women who, by virtue of spiritual power, were reported to have existed on very little food over extended time periods (Bell, 1985; Halmi, 1982; Hammond, 1879; Lacey, 1982).

Richard Morton's account in 1694 is generally credited as the first clinical description of AN. He detailed the case of a patient in a state of "nervous consumption" characterized by decreased appetite, amenorrhea, food aversion, emaciation, and hyperactivity, who died 3 months after refusing medication (Powers & Fernandez, 1984). The disorder garnered further recognition when Sir William Gull coined the term "anorexia nervosa" in 1874 to describe a condition beginning in adolescence, predominantly among females, characterized by a "morbid mental state," with metabolic sequelae associated with prolonged starvation and calorie depletion, if not treated in a timely way. Laseque (1873) independently described the cognitive/perceptual body image distortions associated with the disorder, as well as the family's role (Strober, 1986). The accounts of Gull and Laseque provoked a debate on the benefits and disadvantages of family involvement in treatment, with some arguing that successful intervention required the patient's separation from the family environment (Playfair, 1888), whereas others claimed that removal from the family home constituted unnecessary cruelty and expense (Myrtle, 1888).

Views changed when, in 1914, Simmonds described a malnourished patient in poor health, who subsequently was found on autopsy to have a pituitary lesion. Consequently, in the following 10–20 years, AN tended to be seen as a medical disorder caused by pituitary abnormalities. Then, with the spread of psychoanalytic thought in the 1940s and 1950s, AN became increasingly differentiated from the medically based "Simmonds disease" and was reconceptualized as a psychiatric disorder characterized by an excessive drive for thinness, including purgative behaviors; body image disturbance; and denial of illness rooted in unconscious conflicts around oral-sadistic impulses, oral impregnation, and regressive fantasies (Sheehan & Summers, 1949; Stunkard, 1993).

The prevailing psychoanalytic viewpoint was challenged by the clinical studies of Hilde Bruch (1973), whose work stimulated a major rethinking of AN and its treatment to emphasize faulty developmental learning experiences, particularly discrimination of internal states and body boundaries, perceptions of ineffectiveness, and lack of autonomy. Treatment consequently was aimed at promoting patients' self-efficacy and autonomy. More recently, Minuchin, Rosman, and Baker (1978) conceptualized AN as a family disorder and further advanced understanding and treatment by centering on structural aspects of the family, such as boundaries, roles, alliances, and methods of conflict resolution.

By contrast to AN, it is difficult to make judgments regarding historical accounts of bulimic behavior, except in the case of the binge-eating/purging type of AN. In early Roman times, "vomitoria" (public places where people went to vomit) were described, and Seneca, a Stoic philosopher who lived about 65 A.D., wrote, "Men eat to vomit and vomit to eat" (quoted in Lowenberg, Todhunter, Wilson, Savage, & Lubawski, 1974, p. 45). The public nature of the vomiting, however, is not consistent with the secretiveness of the purging (and bingeing) included in current conceptualizations of BN. The Babylonian Talmud (see Kaplan & Garfinkel, 1984), written about 400 A.D., describes bulimia as a symptom of various illnesses. Gull (1874) mentioned that a patient with AN had an occasional "voracious" appetite. Janet (1919) noted the occurrence of a cluster of symptoms, including vomiting, bulimia, and mood lability, in one group of patients with AN (e.g., Kaplan & Garfinkel, 1984; Lowenberg et al., 1974; Stunkard, 1993). Binswanger's (1958) classic account of Ellen West presented a detailed picture of extreme binge–purge cycles, laxative abuse, and dramatic vomiting in a woman who was not, but wished to be, underweight.

Given that binge eating also may occur in the absence of purging or other inappropriate compensatory behaviors, the *Diagnostic and Statistical Manual of Mental Disorders*, fourth edition, text revision (DSM-IV-TR; American Psychiatric Association [APA], 2000) has proposed BED as a tentative diagnostic category worthy of further study. The nature and current status of AN, BN, and BED are discussed below.

Similar to etiological perspectives on AN, conceptualizations of BN and BED have emphasized family relationships and transitions (Schwartz, Barrett, & Saba, 1985). In the last few years, however, the field of eating disorders generally has shifted attention beyond the immediate family to encompass broader societal and cultural factors (e.g., Crisp, Palmer, & Kalucy, 1976; Iancu, Spivak, Ratzoni, Apter, & Weizman, 1994; Keel & Klump, 2003; Malson & Swann, 1999; Markey, 2004; Schwartz, Thompson, & Johnson, 1982; Wildes, Emery, & Simons, 2001; Wilfley & Rodin, 1995). Most significant is the observation that the incidence of eating disorders appears to be on the rise (Iancu et al., 1994; Jones, Fox, Babigian, & Hutton, 1980; Wilfley & Rodin, 1995; Willi & Grossman, 1983); the increase corresponds to heightened social pressures, particularly for women, toward increasing thinness (Keel & Klump, 2003; Malson & Swann, 1999; Schwartz et al., 1982; Steiner et al., 2003; Wilfley & Rodin, 1995).

Biological theories have also reappeared. These focus on the hormonal changes accompanying puberty (Garfinkel & Garner, 1982; Leibowitz, 1983; Strober, 1986) and on differences in central nervous system (CNS) and neurotransmitter functioning (Bailer & Kaye, 2003; Brambilla, 2001; Braun & Chouinard, 1992; Brewerton, 1995; Chowdhury et al., 2003; Kaye & Weltzin, 1991; Wolfe, Metzger, & Jimerson, 1997; Wurtman & Wurtman, 1984). Statistical relationships between eating and mood disorders in first-degree relatives have been used to argue for a genetic component to both types of disorders (Hudson, Pope, Jonas, & Yurgelun-Todd, 1983; Steiger, Stotland, Ghadirian, & Whitehead, 1995). Although additional preliminary support for the potential role of genetic etiological factors has been reported for both AN and BN (Fichter & Noegel, 1990; Holland, Sicotte, & Treasure, 1988; Hsu, Chesler, & Santhouse, 1990; Jacobi, Hayward, deZwann, Kraemer, & Agras, 2004; Treasure & Holland, 1995), the data strongly suggest complex gene–environment interactions and genetically based vulnerabilities to psychopathology, rather than simple gene–behavior models (Holland et al., 1988; Jacobi et al., 2004; Kendler, 2001; Kendler et al., 1991; Strober, 1991, 1995). Moreover, some of the very preliminary genetic data available for eating disorders tend to be overinterpreted, as is the case in much of the behavioral genetics literature on psychological disorders (Bulik, Sullivan, Wade, & Kendler, 2000; Kendler, 2001; Poston & Winebarger, 1996).

NATURE OF THE DISORDERS

Definitions and Occurrence

AN and BN are currently recognized by specific sets of symptoms, according to the DSM-IV-TR (APA, 2000). The diagnostic criteria for AN are presented in Table 12.1.

The central characteristic of AN is a "drive for thinness" involving weight loss beyond the point of social desirability, attractiveness, and good health. Despite very low weights, individuals with AN deny that they are too thin and instead declare themselves "too fat." Secondary to this weight loss and near-starvation are preoccupation with food, amenorrhea, and a variety of psychological and physiological disturbances. In addition to curtailing food intake, high levels of exercise and purging may be used as weight control strategies (APA, 2000).

TABLE 12.1. DSM-IV-TR Criteria for Anorexia Nervosa (AN)

A. Refusal to maintain body weight at or above a minimally normal weight for age and height (e.g., weight loss leading to maintenance of body weight less than 85% of that expected; or failure to make expected weight gain during period of growth, leading to body weight less than 85% of that expected).

B. Intense fear of gaining weight or becoming fat, even though underweight.

C. Disturbance in the way in which one's body weight or shape is experienced, undue influence of body weight or shape on self-evaluation, or denial of the seriousness of the current low body weight.

D. In postmenarcheal females, amenorrhea, i.e., the absence of at least three consecutive menstrual cycles. (A woman is considered to have amenorrhea if her periods occur only following hormone, e.g., estrogen, administration.)

Specify type:

Restricting Type: during the current episode of Anorexia Nervosa, the person has not regularly engaged in binge-eating or purging behavior (i.e., self-induced vomiting or the misuse of laxatives, diuretics, or enemas)

Binge-Eating/Purging Type: during the current episode of Anorexia Nervosa, the person has regularly engaged in binge-eating or purging behavior (i.e., self-induced vomiting or the use of laxatives, diuretics, or enemas)

Note. From American Psychiatric Association (2000, p. 589). Copyright 2000 by the American Psychiatric Association. Reprinted by permission.

As shown in Table 12.1, AN in the DSM-IV-TR is divided into two specific types: the binge-eating/purging type and the restricting type. Those meeting diagnostic criteria for AN, binge-eating/purging type, would most likely have been diagnosed with AN and BN as concurrent disorders under DSM-III-R criteria (Woodside, 1995).

By contrast, the salient characteristic of BN is an excessive intake of food (usually high in calories) over a relatively short period of time, accompanied by "recurrent inappropriate compensatory behavior in order to prevent weight gain" (APA, 2000, p. 594). Such compensatory behaviors may take various forms as the diagnostic criteria indicate. Because those with BN usually regard their binge eating as shameful and "out of control," this behavior typically occurs in secret. The DSM-IV-TR diagnostic criteria for BN are presented in Table 12.2. Because a substantial proportion of individuals with BN and AN either present with a history of the other disorder or develop time-limited symptoms of the other disorder (APA, 1996; Fairburn & Harrison, 2003; Walsh & Devlin, 1998), AN and BN are sometimes considered to occur on a continuum of severity (APA,

TABLE 12.2. DSM-IV-TR Criteria for Bulimia Nervosa (BN)

A. Recurrent episodes of binge eating. An episode of binge eating is characterized by both of the following:

  (1) eating, in a discrete period of time (e.g., within any 2-hour period), an amount of food that is definitely larger than most people would eat during a similar period of time and under similar circumstances
  (2) a sense of lack of control over eating during the episode (e.g., a feeling that one cannot stop eating or control what or how much one is eating)

B. Recurrent inappropriate compensatory behavior in order to prevent weight gain, such as self-induced vomiting; misuse of laxatives, diuretics, enemas, or other medications; fasting; or excessive exercise.

C. The binge eating and inappropriate compensatory behaviors both occur, on average, at least twice a week for 3 months.

D. Self-evaluation is unduly influenced by body shape and weight.

E. The disturbance does not occur exclusively during episodes of Anorexia Nervosa.

Specify type:

  Purging Type: during the current episode of Bulimia Nervosa, the person has regularly engaged in self-induced vomiting or the misuse of laxatives, diuretics, or enemas

  Nonpurging Type: during the current episode of Bulimia Nervosa, the person has used other inappropriate compensatory behaviors, such as fasting or excessive exercise, but has not regularly engaged in self-induced vomiting or the misuse of laxatives, diuretics, or enemas

Note. From American Psychiatric Association (2000, p. 594). Copyright 2000 by the American Psychiatric Association. Reprinted by permission.

1996; Strober, Freeman, Lampert, Diamond, & Kaye, 2000; Wilson & Pike, 2001).

BED is included in the "Criteria Sets and Axes Provided for Further Study" appendix of the DSM-IV-TR. Inclusion in this appendix is intended to provide researchers and clinicians with the guidance necessary to evaluate the reliability, validity, and utility of the proposed diagnostic categories. As with BN, the salient characteristic of BED is an excessive intake of food (usually high in calories) over a relatively short period of time. The key distinction between this proposed syndrome and BN is the absence of inappropriate compensatory behaviors as described in Table 12.2. BED has been of particular interest to researchers studying the eating behaviors of obese populations (Brody, Walsh, & Devlin, 1994; Cooper, Fairburn, & Hawker, 2003; Stunkard & Allison, 2003) and of populations engaging in binge eating without a focus on weight control (Pike et al., 2001; Woodside, 1995). The research criteria for BED are presented in Table 12.3.

Peak age at onset may be somewhat earlier in AN than in BN. Specifically, AN tends to begin in adolescence, generally between the ages of 14 and 18 (APA, 2000; Bulik, 2002; Halmi, Casper, Eckert, Goldberg, & Davis, 1979), whereas the mean age of onset for BN is 17–19 (Agras & Kirkley, 1986; APA, 2000; Bulik, 2002; Fairburn & Cooper, 1982; Mehler, 2003a; Mitchell, Hatsukami, Eckert, & Pyle, 1985). Both disorders occur in females approximately 90% of the time (APA, 2000; Fairburn & Harrison, 2003; Halmi, 1974, 1982; Hay & Leonard, 1979; Ricciardelli & McCabe, 2004). AN has been most frequently noted in upper socioeconomic groups, although there have been indications of a somewhat less unequal socioeconomic distribution in recent years (Eckert, 1985; McClelland & Crisp, 2001; Wildes et al., 2001).

Although women's lifetime prevalence of AN is often estimated at roughly 0.5% (APA, 2000), epidemiological studies have reported ranges between 0.2% and 1.3% in female samples (Hoek, 1995; Hoek & van Hoeken, 2003; Wakeling, 1996; Woodside, 1995). BN is somewhat more prevalent than AN, with estimates varying between 1% and 3% (APA, 2000; Hoek, 1995; Hoek & van Hoeken, 2003; Hsu, 1996). However, broadening the criteria to include clinically significant levels of bulimic behaviors increases the prevalence considerably. Depending on the restrictiveness of the di-

TABLE 12.3. DSM-IV-TR Research Criteria for Binge-Eating Disorder (BED)

A. Recurrent episodes of binge eating. An episode of binge eating is characterized by both of the following:

    (1) eating, in a discrete period of time (e.g., within any 2-hour period), an amount of food that is definitely larger than most people would eat in a similar period of time under similar circumstances

    (2) a sense of lack of control over eating during the episode (e.g., a feeling that one cannot stop eating or control what or how much one is eating)

B. The binge-eating episodes are associated with three (or more) of the following:

    (1) eating much more rapidly than normal

    (2) eating until feeling uncomfortably full

    (3) eating large amounts of food when not feeling physically hungry

    (4) eating alone because of being embarrassed by how much one is eating

    (5) feeling disgusted with oneself, depressed, or very guilty after overeating

C. Marked distress regarding binge eating is present.

D. The binge eating occurs, on average, at least 2 days a week for 6 months.

    Note: The method of determining frequency differs from that used for Bulimia Nervosa; future research should address whether the preferred method of setting a frequency threshold is counting the number of days on which binges occur or counting the number of episodes of binge eating.

E. The binge eating is not associated with the regular use of inappropriate compensatory behaviors (e.g., purging, fasting, excessive exercise) and does not occur exclusively during the course of Anorexia Nervosa or Bulimia Nervosa.

Note. From American Psychiatric Association (2000, p. 787). Copyright 2000 by the American Psychiatric Association. Reprinted by permission.

agnostic criteria utilized (Edwards & Kerry, 1993; Hoek & van Hoeken, 2003), between 4% and 19% of all young women may engage in clinically significant levels of bulimic behavior (Halmi, Falk, & Schwartz, 1981; Kaltiala-Heino, Rissanen, Rimpela, & Rantanen, 1999; Pyle et al., 1983; Strangler & Printz, 1980).

Rates of AN and BN seem to be on the rise, particularly in younger age groups (APA, 1996; Ash & Piazza, 1995; Edwards & Kerry, 1993; Jones et al., 1980; Mehler, 2003a; Willi & Grossman, 1983). However, it is unclear whether these increases reflect better screening and earlier detection efforts or represent an actual upsurge in rates (Fairburn & Harrison, 2003; Fombonne, 1995; Gowers & Bryant-Waugh, 2004; Pawluck & Gorey, 1998; Rosen, 2003). There are preliminary suggestions that patients with early/childhood-onset AN may not differ significantly from those with adolescent-onset AN in terms of psychopathology and key diagnostic features (Cooper, Watkins, Bryant-Waugh, & Lask, 2002; Watkins & Lask, 2002). However, because the current diagnostic criteria have been criticized as being insufficiently sensitive to developmental issues (Powers & Santana, 2002a; Robin, Gilroy, & Dennis, 1998), and because children may present symptoms somewhat differently from their adolescent counterparts (Powers & Santana, 2002a; Robin et al., 1998; Rosen, 2003), there is some concern that the current nosology may underestimate eating disorders in prepubescent youths (Robin et al., 1998). In addition, prepubertal gender differences may be less pronounced (Robin et al., 1998; Robb & Dadson, 2002). Young participants in certain professional or recreational subcultures emphasizing conformance to rigid weight standards, such as dancers and some athletes, may be at particularly high risk for disordered eating (Bettle, Bettle, Neumarker, & Neumarker, 1998; Byrne & McLean, 2001; Hulley & Hill, 2001; Powers & Santana, 2002a; Ricciardelli & McCabe, 2004; Robb & Dadson, 2002). Indeed, the medical literature commonly refers to the "female athlete triad" to mean the combination of osteoporosis, amenorrhea, and eating disorders (Daluiski, Rahbar, & Meals, 1997; Seidenfeld & Rickert, 2001). Although research on the natural history of AN and BN is just beginning to emerge (Brewerton, 2002; Steiner & Lock, 1998), there is some indication that symptoms of disordered eating early in life may heighten risk at later developmental levels (Kotler, Cohen, Davies, Pine, & Walsh, 2001). Yet there is a clear need for additional prospective research in young populations to clarify the natural course of eating problems, as well as age-related changes in their manifestations (Brewerton, 2002; Steiner & Lock, 1998; Terre, 1993).

As noted above, BED is a proposed category intended for further study. Accordingly, the specific epidemiological contours of the disorder are just beginning to take shape. Nevertheless, preliminary estimates indicate that the prevalence of BED may range from less than 1% to approximately 4% in community samples and perhaps as much as 50% among patients at obesity clinics (APA, 2000; Hoek & van Hoeken, 2003; Striegel-Moore & Franko, 2003; Walsh & Devlin, 1998). By comparison to both AN and BN, BED seems to emerge a bit later, typically in late adolescence or early adulthood, and to be somewhat more equally represented across genders and among ethnically diverse groups (APA, 2000, Fairburn & Harrison, 2003; Pike, Dohm, Striegel-Moore, Wilfley, & Fairburn, 2001; Striegel-Moore et al., 2003; Striegel-Moore & Franko, 2003; Walsh & Devlin, 1998). Because BED is not punctuated by the compensatory behaviors associated with AN and BN, obesity is a common comorbidity (deZwaan, 2001; Dingemans, Bruna, & van Furth, 2002; Fairburn & Harrison, 2003; Pike et al., 2001; Stunkard & Allison, 2003; Walsh & Devlin, 1998). There are some suggestions that binge-eating problems may be more common than anticipated among children and adolescents in obesity treatment programs (Decaluwe, Braet, & Fairburn, 2003).

Associated Psychological and Medical Conditions

Psychological

A relationship between eating disorders and other psychological conditions has frequently been noted. Among the most commonly reported Axis I and II comorbidities are mood, anxiety, substance use, and personality disorders (APA, 1996, 2000; deZwaan, 2001; Dingemans et al., 2002). However, because the bulk of these findings are based on cross-sectional studies yielding correlational data, the precise nature of these relationships is difficult to unravel. For instance, it has been suggested that some of these associated disorders (e.g., mood problems) may be the results of severe caloric restriction and/or compensatory behaviors (APA, 1996; O'Brien & Vincent, 2003), or may be artifacts of commonly used self-report methodologies that may tend to overestimate certain types of psychopathology (O'Brien & Vincent, 2003). Nevertheless, in a therapeutic context, these commonly co-occurring conditions make the assessment and management of eating disorders much more complex, as has been frequently discussed

elsewhere (e.g., deZwann, 2001; Gowers & Bryant-Waugh, 2004; Haas & Clopton, 2003; Kotler, Boudreau, & Devlin, 2003; O'Brien & Vincent, 2003; Rosenvinge, Martinussen, & Ostensen, 2000). (For excellent reviews on psychological comorbidity, see, e.g., O'Brien & Vincent, 2003; Rosenvinge et al., 2000.)

Medical

Numerous medical complications in multiple body systems have been identified in patients with eating disorders. Some of these include metabolic and structural brain abnormalities, such as reversible brain atrophy and gray matter volume deficits, altered serotonin activity, and changes in cerebral blood flow (Drevelengas, Chourmouzi, Pitsavas, Charitandi, & Boulogianni, 2001; Frank et al., 2001; Hirano, Tomura, Okane, Watarai, & Tashiro, 1999; Lambe, Katzman, Mikulis, Kennedy, & Zipursky, 1997; Rastam et al., 2001; Roser et al., 1999). Various cardiac irregularities have also been observed, including both structural and functional abnormalities (Eidem, Cetta, Webb, Graham, & Jay, 2001; Mont et al., 2003; Panagiotopoulos, McCrindle, Hick, & Katzman, 2000; Swenne, 2000; Swenne & Larsson, 1999). Dental and dermatological abnormalities range from dental erosion and skin lesions on the hands of patients who purge to gingival changes, alopecia, and other mucocutaneous signs in patients with AN (Daluiski et al., 1997; Hediger, Rost, & Itin, 2000; Schulze et al., 1999; Strumia, Varotti, Manzato, & Gualandi, 2001; Studen-Pavlovich & Elliott, 2001). Endocrinological manifestations of eating disorders are varied, but may consist of osteopenia and osteoporosis, as well as a variety of metabolic irregularities (Golden, 2003; Levine, 2002; Mehler, 2003b; Seidenfeld & Rickert, 2001; Slupik, 1999; Stoving, Hangaard, Hansen-Nord, & Hagen, 1999). Although amenorrhea is among the diagnostic criteria for AN, a wide variety of other gynecological complications may occur (Key, Mason, Allan, & Lask, 2002; Rome, 2003; Seidenfeld & Rickert, 2001). A myriad of gastrointestinal problems are often associated with eating disorders. For example, difficulties with gastric capacity, gastric emptying, and gastrointestinal peptide release, as well as occult gastrointestinal bleeding, have all been reported (Anderson, Shaw, & McCargar, 1997; Baranowska, Radzikowska, Wasilewska-Dziubinska, Roguski, & Borowiec, 2000;

Ferron, 1999; Jeejeebhoy, 1998). The vast majority of these medical comorbidities subside with nutrition (e.g., Abella et al., 2002; APA, 1996; Drevelengas et al., 2001; McLoughlin et al., 2000; Mont et al., 2003). However, some, such as growth stunting (Lantzouni, Frank, Golden, & Shenker, 2002; Modan-Moses et al., 2003) and long-term fracture risk (Lucas, Melton, Crowson, & O'Fallon, 1999), may present continuing challenges even after an average weight is attained. Finally, "the mortality rates associated with AN . . . are higher than for any other psychiatric disorder" (Agras, 2001, p. 372), with an aggregate mortality rate of approximately 5.6% per decade, including both suicide and death secondary to medical complications (Agras, 2001). Taken together, these comorbidities highlight the importance of a biopsychosocial approach to the assessment and management of patients with eating disorders (Caruso & Klein, 1998; Kreipe & Birndorf, 2000).

Adding to the health and personal toll associated with eating disorders are the related socioeconomic outcomes. For example, based on a comparison of treatment costs for eating disorders to those for other psychiatric conditions, Agras (2001) concluded that the therapy expenditures for AN exceed those for schizophrenia, and that the costs of treating BN and BED are at least comparable to and perhaps in excess of those attributable to obsessive–compulsive disorder (Agras, 2001). BED's link with overweight and obesity further heightens risk for additional medical complications (e.g., hypertension, Type 2 diabetes, dyslipidemia), thereby adding to its social and economic impact (Terre, Poston, & Foreyt, 2005). In addition, the discrimination and stigmatization attendant to overweight and obesity are well known (see Terre et al., 2005, for a review). Hence eating disorders are associated with substantial personal and societal burden.

Differential Diagnosis

A variety of psychiatric disorders may be associated with changes in weight and/or eating behavior. However, they should not all be considered eating disorders, despite some suggestions that eating disorders are simply variants of the others (Garfinkel, 1995; Garfinkel & Kaplan, 1986). For example, in conversion disorders, schizophrenia, and mood disorders, changes in appetite and attitudes toward food are sometimes evident. These disorders usually can be distinguished from AN by the absence of an intense drive for thinness, a disturbed body image, and an increased activity level, which are specific indicators for AN (Woodside, 1995). Although individuals with AN and schizophrenia both may avoid specific foods, this avoidance generally occurs in very different contexts. Those with AN may refuse foods due to concerns about caloric content, whereas those with schizophrenia may avoid foods for reasons that are unrelated to fear of weight gain per se but consistent with broader disturbances in reality testing that characterize psychotic disorders, such as a belief that the food is "poisoned" (APA, 2000; First, Frances, & Pincus, 2002). Similarly, even though body dysmorphic disorder (BDD) centers on an appearance preoccupation and depression may be associated with weight loss, these disorders usually are not characterized by a fear of becoming "fat" despite being underweight, which is the hallmark of AN (APA, 2000; First et al., 2002). Likewise, overeating in depressive disorders occurs in the broader context of other mood symptoms and typically does not include the compensatory behaviors characteristic of BN (APA, 2000; First et al., 2002). As noted above, the diagnostic process is complicated by the fact that eating disorders are often comorbid with several others, most notably mood, anxiety, substance use, and personality disorders (APA, 1996, 2000).

Further hindering the classification process is the number of different labels for eating disorders that have been popularized in recent years. Among those currently in use are "anorexia nervosa" (APA, 2000; Casper, Eckert, Halmi, Goldberg, & Davis, 1980), "bulimia" (Mitchell & Pyle, 1982), "bulimia nervosa" (APA, 2000; Russell, 1979), "bulimarexia" (Boskind-Lodahl & White, 1978), "binge eating" (Abraham & Beumont, 1982), "binge–purge syndrome" (Hawkins, Fremouw, & Clement, 1984), "self-induced vomiting" (Rich, 1978), "dietary chaos syndrome" (Palmer, 1979), "psychogenic vomiting" (Rosenthal, Webb, & Wruble, 1980), and "laxative abuse syndrome" (Oster, Materson, & Rogers, 1980). The validity of each as a separate syndrome or entity has not been established, and the interrelationships between these possible diagnostic entities are not well known. Of these, only AN and BN are currently listed as diagnoses in the DSM-IV-TR (APA, 2000). As noted previously, BED is listed as a diagnostic category worthy of further study.

An additional problem inherent in the study of the eating disorders contained in the DSM-IV-TR is the continuing evolution of the diagnostic categories. The approximate 16–47% overlap between AN and BN (Casper et al., 1980; Theander, 1970), as assessed via the diagnostic criteria contained in the DSM-III-R (APA, 1987), resulted in the creation of two "types" of AN in the DSM-IV and DSM-IV-TR. Specifically, those individuals who previously would have been concurrently diagnosed with AN and BN would most likely qualify for the diagnosis of AN, binge-eating/purging type. Average-weight and underweight persons with binge eating tend to be similar on a number of demographic, clinical, and psychometric variables and to differ from those with AN who do not binge (Garner, Garfinkel, & O'Shaughnessy, 1983). Moreover, compared to their counterparts who do not engage in binge eating, individuals with AN who binge have long been described as more likely to have problems with mood, impulsive behavior, and self-control, such as affective lability, shoplifting, alcohol and other substance misuse, self-mutilation, and sexual activity (Garfinkel, Moldofsky, & Garner, 1980); may be more extroverted (Beumont, 1977); have histories of obesity both personally and in their families; show greater childhood maladjustment; have higher rates of familial alcoholism and affective illness; and experience greater conflict and negativity in family relationships (Strober, 1986). Accordingly, the binge-eating/purging subtype of AN has often been viewed as more difficult to treat and as associated with poorer outcomes (Garfinkel et al., 1980). However, more recent evidence on the differences between the restricting and binge-eating/purging subtypes has been mixed, with some studies lending support to the distinction (e.g., Fassino, Amianto, Gramaglia, Facchini, & Daga, 2004; Vervaet, van Heeringen, & Audenaert, 2004) and others casting doubt on it (e.g., Eddy et al., 2002; Pryor, Wiederman, & McGilley, 1996). For instance, the frequently reported "crossover rate" between restricting AN and binge-eating/purging AN (e.g., Eddy et al., 2002) as well as between AN and BN (e.g., Agras, Walsh, Fairburn, Wilson, & Kramer, 2000; Fairburn, Cooper, & Shafran, 2003), is often cited as evidence for a single shared eating disorder psychopathology in which restricting AN is only one "phase" (Eddy et al., 2002; Fairburn et al., 2003). Clearly, additional work is warranted in this area.

ETIOLOGY

Given that eating disorders generally begin during the adolescent years, most etiological theories are set against the backdrop of adolescence and its concomitants. In addition, culturally defined norms and influences, personality factors, and affective difficulties are often considered important causal factors (Iancu et al., 1994; Markey, 2004; Polivy & Herman, 2004; Striegel-Moore, 1995). The transition between childhood and adolescence involves numerous biopsychosocial changes requiring adaptation. These include shifts in body appearance and functioning; identity development; and the reorganization of social roles, supports, and family relationships, with escalating responsibility for independent functioning. These demands for readjustment and increasing maturity may interact with emerging competencies and predispositions in such a way as to lower the threshold for emotional distress and dysfunction (Steiner et al., 2003; Terre & Burkhart, 1996; Terre & Ghiselli, 1997). Indeed, there is some evidence that women with eating disorders may be especially sensitive to achievement-relevant concerns (Narduzzi & Jackson, 2000). Other factors (e.g., culture, family, negative life events, and personality traits, as discussed below) may exacerbate or ameliorate the potential difficulties inherent in negotiating this developmental transition (Bulik, 2002; Fornari & Dancyger, 2003; Terre & Ghiselli, 1997).

Cultural Influences

Even the briefest literature review on eating disorders illustrates the etiological significance typically accorded to societal factors. Specifically, it is theorized that the traditional definition of femininity has much to do with the development of eating disorders (Gilbert & Thompson, 1996; Iancu et al., 1994; Wilfley & Rodin, 1995). From this perspective, social norms shape women's motivational priorities by defining femininity and self-worth in terms of body size (Bulik, 2002; Striegel-Moore, 1995; Williamson, 1998). Because a woman's interpersonal relationships may be disproportionately influenced by the approximation of her physical appearance to that of the feminine cultural ideal (which currently is extremely thin), women may be more vulnerable than their male counterparts to developing a preoccupation with weight and fear of becoming "fat" (Iancu et al., 1994; Lee, 1995;

Wiederman & Pryor, 2000). By contrast to their female counterparts, men may experience more social pressure to increase muscle mass than to become smaller and thinner (Ricciardelli & McCabe, 2004; Robb & Dadson, 2002). From a feminist perspective, women experiencing eating disorders may be especially sensitive to coercive pressures to conform to socially derived notions of beauty and femininity, which currently are skewed toward unrealistic thinness (Schwartz, Chambliss, Brownell, Blair, & Billington, 2003). The persistence and pervasiveness of these messages (e.g., across different mass media categories) can have a corrosive impact on a young woman's emerging sense of competence. These social influences also reinforce and maintain the equation of thinness with self-worth and success (Fairburn, Shafran, & Cooper, 1999; Gilbert & Thompson, 1996; Williamson, 1998). In short, "the central role of beauty in female identity and in women's interpersonal relationships serves to channel women's identity concerns into preoccupation with shape and weight" (Striegel-Moore, 1993, p. 162). Against this backdrop, eating disorders may evolve in some women under the interactive influence of additional developmental stressors at the societal, familial, and individual levels (e.g., pressures for women to achieve in multiple domains of accomplishment, in the context of contradictory cultural messages regarding women's proper roles in Western culture, family attitudes about weight and dieting, individual body-relevant experiences/attitudes, and personality factors) (Bulik, 2002; Fairburn & Harrison, 2003; Gilbert & Thompson, 1996; Heinberg, 1996; Steiner et al., 2003; Striegel-Moore, 1993, 1995).

However, results of cross-cultural studies have challenged the adequacy of etiological models based on the "culture of thinness" (Gilbert & Thompson, 1996, p. 185) concept to completely explain the development of eating disorders. Based on a review of cross-cultural studies, Lee (1995) concluded that the feminist perspective may be somewhat ethnocentric. Specifically, in non-Western cultures, AN often occurs in individuals who do not manifest the "fat phobia" that is so characteristic of AN in Western samples (Lee, 1995; Ngai, Lee, & Lee, 2000; Simpson, 2002). These cross-cultural findings raise the possibility that the application of culturally flexible diagnostic criteria may enhance both the validity and utility of the eating disorder categories (Lee, 1995) by focusing more attention on the factors of etiological significance in each culture (Simpson, 2002). Some of the assumptions inherent in feminist etiological frameworks have also been questioned by the results of other research reporting similarities between men and women with AN on a variety of clinical indices and familial aggregation patterns (e.g., Strober, Freeman, Lampert, Diamond, & Kaye, 2001; Woodside et al., 2001).

An important contribution to this cultural controversy was recently offered in a review on AN and BN as culture-bound syndromes (Keel & Klump, 2003). This review highlighted several areas of distinctiveness between the two disorders, including historical evidence preceding formal recognition of the disorders, epidemiological shifts since formal recognition, and cross-cultural epidemiology. Based on these results, Keel and Klump (2003) concluded:

> BN may be a culture-bound syndrome, influenced by weight concerns, anonymous access to large quantities of food, and a motivation to prevent the effects of binge eating on weight through the use of inappropriate compensatory behavior. Conversely . . . weight concerns can influence the incidence of AN but . . . whatever cultural influences contribute to the etiology of AN, they are not particularly limited in their distribution across history or cultures. (p. 763)

As these authors point out, the extent to which subsequent research will support the notion of BN (but not AN) as a culture-bound syndrome remains an open empirical question. The issue of the distinctiveness of eating disorders is further discussed later in the present chapter.

Psychosocial Influences

Concern about body weight, and fairly reasonable weight control efforts and dieting, tend to precede the development of eating disorders (Beumont, Booth, Abraham, Griffiths, & Turner, 1983; Walsh & Devlin, 1998; Woodside, 1995). However, the precise etiological role of dieting in the development of eating disorders remains controversial (Fairburn, Cooper, Doll, & Welch, 1999; Fairburn, Welch, Doll, Davies, & O'Connor, 1997; Halmi, 1997; Howard & Porzelius, 1999). Given the widespread recognition that the etiology of eating disorders is complicated, an exclusive focus on one factor such as dieting may be misleading (Steiner et al., 2003). Hence, although dieting figures prominently in many comprehensive etiological models as one of many important factors (e.g., Fairburn & Harrison, 2003; Halmi, 2002), it is generally conceptualized as insufficient as a complete explanation for these complex disorders (e.g., Fairburn et al., 1999; Wilson & Pike, 2001).

Similarly, current research on the role of personality in the development of eating disorders also emphasizes the multifaceted nature of eating disorders and casts doubt on the likelihood of identifying one single causative factor (Leon, Fulkerson, Perry, & Early-Zald, 1995; Strober, 1991, 1995). Over the years, individuals with AN have been described as exhibiting constrictive, conforming, obsessive characteristics (Sohlberg & Strober, 1994; Vitousek & Manke, 1994); perfectionistic standards (Halmi et al., 2000; Tyrka, Waldron, Graber, & Brooks-Gunn, 2002); social inhibition, compliance, and emotional constraint (Wonderlich, 1995); and "self-hate guilt" (Berghold & Lock, 2002). Cloninger (1986, 1988), using a three-dimensional personality model, asserted that individuals with AN tend to be low in novelty seeking, high in harm avoidance, and high in reward dependence. Research on the personality traits associated with BN has revealed less consistent patterns. For instance, patients with BN have been characterized as manifesting poor impulse control, chronic depression, acting-out behaviors, and low frustration tolerance (Wonderlich, 1995), as well as affective lability, difficult temperament, and inhibition (Vitousek & Manke, 1994). In one of the few longitudinal studies to date, Vohs, Bardone, Joiner, Abramson, and Heatherton (1999) reported that perfectionistic standards predicted bulimic behavior in women who considered themselves overweight, but only in the context of low-self esteem. Finally, populations with eating disorders have been described as experiencing greater than typical rates of personality disorders, personality-disorder-related symptoms (Vitousek & Manke, 1994; Wonderlich, 1995), chronic low self-esteem (Silverstone, 1992), and poor introceptive awareness (Leon et al., 1995).

Recently, studies have examined information-processing patterns in AN and BN. Although findings are just beginning to emerge, to date they have been somewhat inconsistent. For instance, some researchers have found alexithymia, deficits in emotional processing, and some attentional biases to be associated with AN (Dobson & Dozois, 2004; Zonnevijlle-Bender, van Goozen, Cohen-Kettenis, van Elburg, & van Engeland, 2002), whereas others (Mendlewicz, Nef, & Simon, 2001) have reported no specific AN-related deficits in cognition or attention in emotional Stroop and word recognition testing. Results relevant to BN have also been difficult to interpret conclusively. However, two recent reviews have raised the possibilities (1) that BN may be associated with attentional biases (Dobson & Dozois, 2004); and (2) that in terms of emotion and threat processing, bulimic behavior may serve as a cognitive avoidance strategy against unpleasant self-awareness but not necessarily food-related information, which may explain some of the inconsistencies noted above (Ainsworth, Waller, & Kennedy, 2002). Clearly, there is a need for additional research in this area.

There are also reports suggesting that eating disorders may be triggered by traumatic separations, losses, and other adversities (Garner, Garfinkel, Schwartz, & Thompson, 1980; Hodes & Le Grange, 1993; Jacobi et al., 2004; Johnson, Cohen, Kasen, & Brook, 2002; Kalucy, Crisp, & Harding, 1977; Strober, 1981). These have included family discord and divorce, parental death, dysfunctional parental behavior, separations from the family of origin (e.g., for college or summer vacation), parental illness, sibling or parental pregnancy, and numerous other types of family difficulties (Beumont, Abraham, Argall, George, & Glaun, 1978; Jacobi et al., 2004; Johnson et al., 2002; Kalucy, Crisp, & Harding, 1977; Theander, 1970). Imagined or actual instances of personal failure have been noted to precede AN as well (Dally, 1969; Halmi, 1974; Rowland, 1970).

Specific traumas, such as childhood sexual abuse, have been suggested as potential etiological factors in the development of eating disorders (Everill & Waller, 1995; Jacobi et al., 2004; Wonderlich, Brewerton, Jocic, Dansky, & Abbott, 1997; Waller, 1998). However, results of studies examining the associations between eating disorders and sexual abuse have produced mixed results. For example, some investigators have found higher reported rates of childhood sexual abuse in those with BN than in populations without eating disorders (Rorty, Yager, & Rossotto, 1994). Yet a recent meta-analytic review on the relationship between child sexual abuse and eating disorders

(Smolak & Murnen, 2002) concluded that although there was a small positive relationship overall, results varied according to the specific methodology employed. Moreover, sexual abuse is not an eating-disorder-specific risk factor, but is more often associated with increased risk for general psychiatric disturbance (Fairburn & Harrison, 2003; Jacobi et al., 2004; Vize & Cooper, 1995; Welch & Fairburn, 1994). Therefore, it is possible that sexual abuse may exert an indirect influence on the development of eating disorders by virtue of its relationship with other risk factors. For instance, Waller (1998) reported that abuse history in a sample of women with eating disorders was correlated with less perceived personal control, and that among the abused women, external locus of control was related to greater severity of eating disorders. Taken together, findings to date suggest that childhood sexual abuse is not a primary or specific risk factor for eating disorders. Rather, if abuse is a factor of etiological significance in eating disorders, it is probably part of a complex interaction with other risk factors that still is not well understood (Jacobi et al., 2004; Vize & Cooper, 1995).

Although the majority of women do not develop eating disorders (Ben-Tovim, 2003; Bulik, 2002), any etiological theory must account for the fact that AN and BN occur predominantly in women. Adolescence is a time of transition for males as well as females, but fewer males develop eating disorders. As discussed above, the converging social influences reinforcing the equation of thinness with feminine self-worth and success may constitute gender-linked risk factors for AN and BN. However, this assumption of gender-specific risk does not seem as compelling in the case of BED, where the gender disparity is much less marked (Robb & Dadson, 2002). Hence it is unlikely that gender differences in the internalization of cultural values completely account for the risk of eating disorders (Ben-Tovim, 2003; Kaye, 1999).

Neurobiological/Genetic Influences

Some physiological conditions may serve as predisposing factors in certain individuals, and these factors then may be compounded by societal contingencies for weight control, particularly in females. The relative efficacy of antidepressants in the treatment of BN (see "Treatment," below) has led to the development of a serotonin hypothesis (Brewerton, 1995; Ericsson, Poston, & Foreyt, 1996; Kaye & Weltzin, 1991; Weltzin, Fernstrom, & Kaye, 1994). Specifically, given the research linking serotonin to carbohydrate consumption and binge eating in both animals and humans, BN may be associated with lower endogenous levels of CNS serotonin (Brambilla, 2001; Jimerson et al., 1997). In an effort to compensate for this deficiency, individuals with BN may consume foods high in tryptophan and relatively low in protein (such as those found in a typical high-carbohydrate meal). Hence binge eating may serve as a form of mood regulation and self-medication, which can be ameliorated by the higher levels of serotonin brought about by the use of antidepressant medications (Advokat & Kutlesic, 1995; Craighead & Agras, 1991; Wolfe et al., 1997). Based in part on the relative ineffectiveness of medication interventions designed to raise the levels of serotonin available to the CNS in the treatment of AN (Advokat & Kutlesic, 1995), the serotonergic hypothesis also suggests that AN may be associated with overactivity in CNS serotonergic activity (Brewerton, 1995). This overactivity subsequently leads to decreased food intake with associated weight loss. Taken together, these data suggest that serotonin dysregulation may play an important role in the etiology or maintenance of eating disorders (Brewerton, 1995; Jacobi et al., 2004; Kaye, 1999).

Disruptions in other neurotransmitter systems have also been implicated in the etiology of eating disorders (Mauri et al., 1996). Some studies have found alterations in noradrenergic and peptide neuromodulator activity in patients with BN. For example, there are some reports (Brambilla, 2001; Kaye et al., 1990) of reduced levels of norepinephrine and serotonin metabolites in the cerebrospinal fluid of patients with BN.

Finally, it has been proposed that eating disorders are neuropsychological disorders, with some studies showing differences between patients with eating disorders and controls in brain metabolic functions and hemispheric activity (Braun & Chouinard, 1992; Chowdhury et al., 2003; Maggia & Bianchi, 1998). Although the data from these studies suggest that neurotransmitter dysregulation and neuropsychological dysfunctions may play a role in the etiology or maintenance of eating disorders, they do not point to a definitive causal role. It is possible that these neurochemical changes occur as *results* of eating-disordered behavior and are not actually causal (Bailer & Kaye, 2003; Kaye & Weltzin, 1991). Specifically, these neurotransmitter derangements may be the consequence of extremes in dietary intake and purging or other compensatory behaviors. As such, they may be more important in the maintenance of eating-disordered behaviors that hinder recovery (Bailer & Kaye, 2003; Kaye & Weltzin, 1991). Another problem with this area of research is that many of these neurotransmitter and neuropeptide modulator alterations are not specific to BN or to eating disorders in general. For example, similar alterations in serotonin regulation have been found in depression, impulsivity, substance use disorders, and obsessive–compulsive disorder (Jarry & Vaccarino, 1996; Weltzin et al., 1994). Furthermore, decreased levels of cholecystokinin have been found in both patients with BN and patients with panic disorder (Brambilla et al., 1993; Lydiard et al., 1993). Due to this lack of disorder-related specificity, it has been suggested that dysregulation in serotonin and other neurotransmitter systems may be a common pathway for many disorders, rather than a specific mechanism in eating disorders (Ericsson et al., 1996). A final criticism of the physiological research is that it is often based on small and potentially biased clinical samples, and that it suffers from methodological problems. Gillberg (1994) noted that many findings in the eating disorder literature, particularly in the area of etiology, lack replication and are based on potentially biased and nonrepresentative samples. In addition, some of these studies suffer from methodological and statistical shortcomings. For example, the Kaye and colleagues (1990) study cited earlier, which found differences between patients with BN and controls in cerebrospinal fluid levels of norepinephrine and serotonin metabolites, was based on a small sample (27 patients with BN and 14 control patients). The investigators also computed multiple *t*-tests without correcting for potential alpha inflation. In a study of cerebral hemispheric glucose metabolism, differences were found between patients with BN and controls (Wu et al., 1990). The authors noted that the patterns of metabolism were also different from those found in studies of patients with AN and depression (Wu et al., 1990). Unfortunately, this study too suffered from a very small sample size (eight patients

with BN and eight matched controls), and the investigators again performed multiple comparisons without correcting for alpha inflation. If the data from these two studies had applied the Bonferroni correction, or some other method to control alpha inflation (e.g., multivariate analysis), it is questionable whether any of the findings would have remained statistically significant (Ross & Pam, 1995).

Several prenatal, perinatal, and early childhood complications have been investigated as possible risk factors for eating disorders. For instance, Watkins, Willoughby, Waller, Serpell, and Lask (2002) posit a "temperature at conception" hypothesis, based on data indicating that early-onset AN may be associated with spring and early summer births. Perinatal difficulties—such as very preterm birth (≤ 32 weeks), particularly among girls with low birthweight for gestational age; birth trauma (Cnattingius, Hultman, Dahl, & Sparen, 1999); and pediatric infectious disease or postinfectious process (Powers & Santana, 2002a; Sokol, 2000; Sokol et al., 2002)—have also been linked with AN. Because this is a relatively new line of research, these findings, although tantalizing, are best viewed as preliminary pending further replication.

Various other etiological influences have been investigated, including genetic risk factors. Yet, despite the general consensus that eating disorders have some familial component (Bulik et al., 2000; Costa, Brennen, & Hochgeschwender, 2002; Waters & Kendler, 1995) that perhaps accounts for as much as 50% or more of the variance (Jacobi et al., 2004; Klump, Kaye, & Strober, 2001), no specific genetic loci have yet been identified with certainty (e.g., Anonymous, 2001; Costa et al., 2002; Jacobi et al., 2004). Unraveling genetic and environmental influences is complicated for a variety of reasons, ranging from the relatively low prevalence of AN and BN to difficulties inherent in genetic analyses and their interpretation (Bulik et al., 2000; Costa et al., 2002; Jacobi et al., 2004; Karwautz et al., 2001; Kendler, 2001; Klump, Miller, Keel, McGue, & Iacono, 2001; Waters & Kendler, 1995). For instance, as Kendler (2001) points out, "traits or disorders do not have a *true* heritability. Rather, all heritability estimates are specific to a population with its range of environmental exposures. Whether any heritability estimate can be extrapolated to other populations or similar populations with different environments is an empirical question" (p. 1008; emphasis in original). Hence the specific contributions of genetic versus environmental influences to eating disorders are unclear at present (Bulik et al., 2000; Jacobi et al., 2004; Kendler, 2001).

In sum, efforts to explain the etiology of eating disorders have focused on a wide variety of possible influences and mechanisms, with a particular emphasis on biological and genetic factors in recent years. As noted above, an overemphasis on physiological mechanisms creates a false and outdated dichotomy between mind and body, which is inconsistent with more contemporary biopsychosocial approaches. It is doubtful that the occurrence of these complex disorders will be explained without an understanding of the many relevant interacting dimensions, including physiological, societal, familial, psychiatric, and psychological influences (Ericsson et al., 1996; Fairburn & Harrison, 2003; Walsh & Devlin, 1998). Furthermore, it is highly probable that no narrow definition of the psychological dimension will suffice. Our behavioral–systems view thus includes a recognition and assessment of cognitive factors, emotional regulation, coping skills, and behavioral–environmental contingencies. Consideration of these multiple interacting factors holds promise for advancing our understanding of the etiological mechanisms involved in these disorders.

ASSESSMENT

A detailed review of assessment instruments is beyond the scope of the present chapter (for a thorough discussion, see, e.g., Foreyt & Mikhail, 1997). Nevertheless, several general points are worth noting as a prelude to our focal discussion on intervention.

Given the complex nature of eating disorders, comprehensive, multimodal assessment is required (APA, 1996; Devlin, 1996; Foreyt & McGavin, 1988; Foreyt & Mikhail, 1997; Lee & Miltenberger, 1997; Tobin, Johnson, Steinberg, Staats, & Baker Dennis, 1991). Figure 12.1 illustrates the range of factors that currently seem relevant to these disorders. Accordingly, assessment should extend beyond eating behavior per se to include (1) self-regulation, particularly mood/affective regulation (including the identification and expression of feelings); (2) social competence and

interpersonal relationships; (3) personal identity, self-esteem, and sexual identity; (4) distorted beliefs and cognitions; (5) psychological comorbidities such as mood, anxiety, personality, and substance use disorders, as well as the history of other psychological problems and treatment; and (6) family functioning, especially when the patient is a child or adolescent (APA, 1996; Fairburn et al., 2003; Foreyt & Mikhail, 1997; Weltzin & Bolton, 1998; Williamson, Duchmann, Barker, & Bruno, 1998; Williamson, Zucker, Martin, & Smeets, 2001).

Assessment of the Family Environment

The family is perhaps the most critical context for the inculcation and development of interpersonal roles and skills. Typically, as children grow, mature, and seek increasing independence, family roles shift accordingly; this results in exposure to expanded spheres of social influence, as well as opportunities to experiment with new roles and activities. Although the family continues to provide a secure base, its influence is increasingly replaced with other sources of stress and support as a youth makes the transition from middle adolescence to young adulthood (Terre & Burkhart, 1996; Terre & Ghiselli, 1997). To the extent that eating disorders may interfere with this normative developmental process (e.g., by increasing parental concern and involvement in children's lives to levels consistent with those more appropriate at younger ages), eating problems "may represent a failed attempt to manage developmental tasks of adolescence" (Lock, Le Grange, Agras, & Dare, 2001, p. 5).

The question remains, however, why some youths seem to have exceptional difficulty negotiating this developmental transition while others do not (e.g., Bulik, 2002; Fornari & Dancyger, 2003). In an effort to answer this question, considerable attention has focused on the families of girls with eating disorders. There is some suggestion that family characteristics and interaction patterns, such as parental overprotectiveness, indirect communication styles (especially around emotional-laden material), and certain conflict resolution strategies, may differentiate families whose adolescents develop eating disorders from those who do not (Casper & Troiana, 2001; Hodes & Le Grange, 1993; Johnson & Pure, 1986; Laliberte, Boland, & Leichner, 1999; Shoebridge & Gowers, 2000; Williamson et al.,

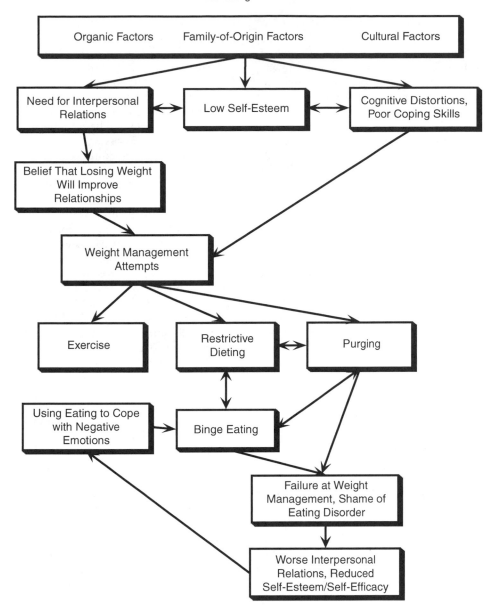

FIGURE 12.1. The vicious cycle of eating disorders.

1998). Other research points to early attachment and parent–child bonding difficulties (Leung, Thomas, & Waller, 2000; Ward et al., 2001), as well as to parental/family eating- and weight-relevant behaviors such as dieting, family history of dysfunctional eating, and family disparagement and/or teasing about a child's appearance (Fairburn & Harrison, 2003), as possible factors of significance.

Although far from definitive, these research findings have stimulated efforts to include family characteristics in the routine evaluation of young patients with eating disorders (Hodes & Le Grange, 1993; Johnson & Pure, 1986), especially when the patient is younger than 18 and is still residing in the family home (APA, 1996; Lock et al., 2001; Williamson et al., 1998; Woodside, 1995). Depending on the family constellation (e.g., a single parent, adoptive or foster parents), the definition of "family" may extend beyond sheer consanguity to include other caregiving household members (Lock et al., 2001). In addition to the variables highlighted above, other aspects of family functioning commonly assessed include parental perceptions of the onset and details of the child's disordered eating, factors associated with problem onset, associated changes in the child's behavior, biopsychosocial developmental history, broader family difficulties, and family impact of the child's eating disorder, as well as parental knowledge and expectations relevant to adolescence (Lock et al., 2001; Strober & Yager, 1985; Weltzin & Bolton, 1998; Williamson et al., 1998; Woodside, 1995). Of course, this information should be assessed with great sensitivity and with a clear recognition that family members often feel responsible for their child's disorder (e.g., Lock et al., 2001). Because it will be important for the clinician to establish a working alliance with the family that enhances their participation (Gowers & Bryant-Waugh, 2004; Lock et al., 2001; Strober & Yager, 1985; Weltzin & Bolton, 1998; Woodside, 1995), it is widely recommended that the clinician take "an agnostic view of the cause of the illness that holds the family not guilty from the perspective of treatment" (Lock et al., 2001, p. 26).

Assessment of Relationships and Environment Outside the Family

As discussed previously, during adolescence the family's influence gradually becomes eclipsed by that of other external sources of support (e.g., teachers, peers, colleagues), which gain ascendancy as youths become increasingly mobile, independent, and involved in the world around them. These extrafamilial experiences provide critical opportunities for acquiring the key skills and competencies (e.g., social competence, identity formation) that undergird healthy adult functioning (Terre & Burkhart, 1996; Terre & Ghiselli, 1997). To the extent that eating disorders are marked by difficulties in negotiating this normative developmental process, these disorders may hinder timely psychosocial development. Indeed, there are data to suggest that individuals with AN and BN may have serious interpersonal difficulties. Of 102 consecutive patients seen by Crisp, Hsu, Harding, and Hartshorn (1980), 23 were excessively shy, and 43 had few or no friends during childhood. These difficulties may persist even after eating disorder symptoms improve. A review of 700 outcome studies (Schwartz & Thompson, 1981) found that only 47% of those with AN had married or were maintain-

ing active partnerships. Patients with BN reported that their problems with eating and weight interfered "a great deal" with their social relationships (94%) and school or job performance (84%) (Leon, Carroll, Chernyk, & Finn, 1985). Bulimic behavior also may be associated with decreased social contact (Johnson & Larson, 1982). These findings highlight the importance of assessing the level and extent of patients' social functioning.

Medical Assessment

All patients with eating disorders should undergo medical assessment. Clearly, a complete review of the medical assessment of AN and BN is beyond the scope of this chapter. For such, the reader is referred to excellent comprehensive reviews by Caruso and Klein (1998), Kreipe and Birndorf (2000), McGilley and Pryor (1998), Mehler (2001), Mitchell (1985, 1986a, 1986b), Kaplan and Garfinkel (1993), Powers and Santana (2002b), and Walsh, Wheat, and Freund (2000).

A standard medical assessment typically includes physical examination, standard laboratory tests, multiple-channel chemistry analysis, complete blood count, and urinalysis. In addition, endocrinological/metabolic, cardiovascular, renal, gastrointestinal, musculoskeletal, dermatological, hematological, and pulmonary systems usually are reviewed (APA, 1996; McGilley & Pryor, 1998; Mehler, 2001; Woodside, 1995). The clinician should be alert to complaints of weakness, tiredness, constipation, and depression; these can be produced by electrolyte abnormalities (McGilley & Pryor, 1998; Mehler, 2001; Webb & Gehi, 1981), which are complications of vomiting and purgative abuse. The medical assessment is used, along with other measures, to determine whether hospitalization is necessary. Hospitalization is useful for nutritional rehabilitation and general medical care (e.g., APA, 1996). A complete review of criteria for inpatient treatment is beyond the scope of the present chapter. (For more thorough discussions, see, e.g., Andersen, 1986; Andersen, Bowers, & Evans, 1997; Lock et al., 2001; Powers, 1984; and Williamson et al., 2001.)

TREATMENT

The treatment of eating disorders is an area of ongoing study, with the scientific merit of many approaches remaining to be explored and established. We review approaches that have and have not been rigorously examined, in the hope that future research will be conducted to validate and refine the methods of experienced clinicians. Treatments include individual approaches (various forms of individual psychotherapy, as well as psychopharmacology); family therapy; group psychotherapy; and intensive programs involving all of the preceding plus training in coping skills, assertiveness, women's issues, and nutritional education. Treatment can take place in inpatient settings, outpatient settings, or both. Team approaches are becoming increasingly popular. The primary elements in each of these modalities, along with adjunctive techniques, are reviewed. Table 12.4 outlines the organization of the treatment overview.

The approaches and techniques described below are designed specifically for the treatment of AN, BN, and BED. However, some have been used with other target problems as well. Although ongoing research in these areas is extensive, more and better studies of the comparative efficacy of these techniques, either combined or used separately, continue to be warranted. We advocate the use of multi-component, multidisciplinary approaches to the treatment of eating disorders. For expository purposes, various components of these programs have been highlighted here. Yet readers should not assume that any of these components represents an entire treatment, unless explicitly stated. Future research will be needed to refine the use of these techniques. Moreover, the numerous ethical issues surrounding assessment and treatment of patients with eating disorders have yet to be resolved (e.g., Bartholomew & Paxton, 2003; Draper, 2000; English, 2002; MacDonald, 2002; Robb et al., 2002; Watson, Bowers, & Andersen, 2000). Clinicians should not attempt to treat patients with eating disorders without specific training in these disorders.

Psychosocial Therapies: General Issues

Most types of psychotherapy have been utilized with patients who have eating disorders, including individual and group interventions from behavioral, cognitive-behavioral, psychodynamic, and interpersonal perspectives. This section discusses general issues relevant to psychological interventions in eating disorders.

In individual psychotherapy, we believe that the cornerstones of the treatment, both philosophically and pragmatically, are flexibility and sensitivity. It is important to tailor the therapeutic program to the patient's specific timing, pacing, and stylistic needs. Specifically, treatments for eating disorders must be designed to integrate psychosocial interventions, medical management, and the appropriate dietary and rehabilitative services, as well as psychiatric medications when warranted (Weltzin & Bolton, 1998; Williamson et al., 1998; Yager, 1995). In addition, the therapist must have the sensitivity and skill necessary to forge a positive therapeutic alliance that will provide a secure base from which the patient can actively engage and persist in treatment (Fairburn, Marcus, & Wilson, 1993; Gowers & Bryant-Waugh, 2004; Lock et al., 2001; Weltzin & Bolton, 1998; Williamson et al., 1998; Wilson & Pike, 2001). In this regard, building trust is key, particularly when the patient is ambivalent about treatment or perceives family pressure to participate (Bruch, 1985; Gowers & Bryant-

TABLE 12.4. Overview of Treatment Modalities

   I. Psychosocial therapies: General issues

  II. Inpatient approaches

 III. Multicomponent outpatient treatment programs

 IV. Psychotherapy techniques and therapeutic approaches
    A. Behavioral therapies and techniques
       1. Exposure plus response prevention
       2. Operant conditioning
       3. Response delay
       4. Self-monitoring
       5. Social skills training
       6. Stimulus control
       7. Systematic desensitization
    B. Cognitive and cognitive-behavioral techniques
    C. Supportive–expressive therapy
    D. Interpersonal psychotherapy
    E. Body image work
    F. Family therapy
    G. Feminist approaches
    H. Group therapy
    I. Physical therapy
    J. Psychoeducational approaches

  V. Pharmacological treatment

 VI. Combined modalities: Integrating pharmacological and psychological treatments

Waugh, 2004; Levenkron, 1983; Wilson & Pike, 2001).

Because treatment is often long-term and may involve periodic relapses, the therapist must respond flexibly to changes in each patient's level of functioning and maturity (Goodsitt, 1985, 1997). Although developmentally appropriate levels of autonomy should be encouraged, the therapist should not overestimate patients' abilities for self-sufficiency, which may be discordant with their chronological age in some cases (Lock et al., 2001).

As noted previously, the therapist should take care to provide a rationale that does not blame the patient or the patient's family for the disorder (Bruch, 1985; Goodsitt, 1997). For instance, Lock and colleagues (2001) acknowledge family members' past life accomplishments and encourage them to draw on these strengths to address the eating problem.

Other important aspects of therapy include (1) conducting a thorough initial assessment and continuing to gather information throughout treatment, ranging from data on weight and amounts of food consumed to broader information about social and family functioning (Fairburn, Marcus, et al., 1993; Lock et al., 2001; Wilson & Pike, 2001); (2) providing the patient with an understanding of the treatment approach and realistic expectations about treatment outcome (Fairburn, Marcus, et al., 1993; Williamson et al., 1998; Wilson & Pike, 2001); and (3) educating the patient regarding the physiology and psychology of disordered eating (Fairburn, Marcus, et al., 1993; Lock et al., 2001; Wilson & Pike, 2001).

Inpatient Approaches

Hospitalization is not so much an approach as it is a setting in which many therapeutic techniques and procedures can be conducted under close supervision. Indications for hospitalization may include a variety of factors extensively discussed by others (Andersen, 1986; Andersen et al., 1997; APA, 1996; Fairburn, Marcus, et al., 1993; Fichter, 1995; Lock et al., 2001; Powers, 1984; and Williamson et al., 1998, 2001), such as the following:

• Weight 15–25% below average or more, particularly if accompanied by evidence of dehydration or malnutrition.
• Serious medical instabilities and metabolic abnormalities (e.g., hypokalemic alkalosis from bulimic complications).
• Psychiatric emergencies (e.g., clinical depression and/or suicidal thoughts, intents, or gestures).
• Nonresponsiveness to outpatient treatment.

Most hospital programs are multidisciplinary and have many therapeutic components, including outpatient therapy and follow-up services. Psychiatry, psychology, nursing, dietetics, occupational therapy, and physical therapy, as well as social and general medicine services, may be involved in an integrated team approach to treatment (Breiner, 2003; Cummings et al., 2001; Kohn & Golden, 2001). There are many excellent eating disorders treatment programs in North America, some of which are free-standing facilities and some of which are operated within university medical schools.[1]

Each member of the interdisciplinary team contributes to the patient's care within his or her scope of practice. Yet a review of different treatment programs makes clear that professional roles are not neatly dictated by discipline. That is, programs take different approaches to the question of which professions or disciplines are represented on the team and what roles various professionals play. However, the following description represents a common configuration of multidisciplinary treatment team members and their roles:

1. Psychiatrists usually prescribe and monitor psychotropic medications, conduct intake evaluations, and in some cases may provide individual and family therapy. Given the structure and tradition of hospitals, psychiatrists also tend to occupy administrative and directorial positions (Powers & Powers, 1984).
2. Psychologists normally provide psychological evaluations; take responsibility for the psychological aspects of treatment plans; and conduct individual, group, and family therapy. The psychologist typically develops behavioral management contracts when these are part of treatment. However, because a patient's reactions to the program may have an adverse impact on the patient's relationship with the professional administering the program, Powers and Powers (1984) recommend a clear differentiation between the staff member implementing the behavioral management program and

the psychotherapist seeking to establish a therapeutic alliance with the patient.

3. A medical consultant or consulting team is needed to obtain careful medical histories; to conduct physical examinations, laboratory screening, and possibly neurological assessments as a part of the evaluation process; and to provide ongoing medical monitoring of patients' physical stability (Lock et al., 2001; Powers & Powers, 1984; Williamson et al., 1998).

4. The nursing staff ordinarily monitors patients' routine medical signs and symptoms, implements treatment plans, and supervises meals (including the prevention of food refusal and purging) (American Dietetic Association, 2001; Cummings et al., 2001; King & Turner, 2000; Powers & Powers, 1984; Williamson et al., 1998). Because members of the nursing staff often have the most day-to-day interaction with patients, adequate preparation, continuing education, and team support are key factors in enhancing nurses' satisfaction with these professional responsibilities (King & Turner, 2000).

5. Dietitians and nutritionists usually take responsibility for the nutrition component of the treatment plan—for instance, by helping assess and educate patients about nutrition, energy balance, and meal planning (American Dietetic Association, 2001; Cummings et al., 2001). In the past, there was often a tendency to emphasize "good" versus "bad" foods, and in many ways this reinforced patients' dichotomous thinking (Beumont, Beumont, Touyz, & Williams, 1997; Kalucy, Gilchrist, McFarlane, & McFarlane, 1985). However, the American Dietetic Association's recent positions underscore the importance of "individualized guidance and a meal plan that provides a framework for meals and snacks and food choices (but not a rigid diet)" (American Dietetic Association, 2001, p. 813), as well as a "lifelong commitment to healthful lifestyle behaviors emphasizing sustainable and enjoyable eating practices and daily physical activity" (Cummings, Parham, & Strain, 2002, p. 1145).

For patients with AN, refeeding tends to begin with a diet of 1,000–1,600 calories per day, which is gradually increased to 3,000–3,600 calories per day (Anzai, Lindsey-Dudley, & Bidwell, 2002; APA, 1996; Williamson et al., 1998). It is important to develop a consensus at the outset of treatment among the patient, fam-

ily, and treatment team about the timing and pace of refeeding. Patient involvement in meal planning is also encouraged (Breiner, 2003; Cummings et al., 2001). It is common to set limits on the duration of meals, after which time patients may be given a supplement or liquid meal (Anzai et al., 2002; Breiner, 2003; Imbierowicz et al., 2002; Powers, 1984). There is general agreement that nasogastric tube feedings are rarely required with most patients (Andersen et al., 1997; APA, 1996; Powers, 1984; Robb et al., 2002), consistent with the general philosophy of care emphasizing patient–team collaboration (Breiner, 2003; Cummings et al., 2001; Matusevich, Garcia, Gutt, de la Parra, & Finkelsztein, 2002).

Tuschen and Bents (1995) have described an intensive inpatient treatment for BN, developed at the University of Marburg in Germany. This program begins with a comprehensive psychological and medical assessment designed to obtain both global and specific measures of functioning. After a comprehensive cognitive preparation phase, the program begins exposure therapy with cognitive intervention. Specifically, each patient's day is very structured, and during the course of treatment each patient is repeatedly exposed to "forbidden" food, binge food and binge triggers, actual total body shape, and actual body weight. Cognitive interventions are relatively nonconfrontational, and consist of the facilitation of cognitive dissonance and the development of skills to adaptively utilize and reduce the dissonance. Finally, this inpatient protocol puts a special emphasis on relapse prevention and self-management.

Goal Weights

During inpatient weight stabilization of patients with AN, it is important to establish reasonable weight goals and predictable weight gain milestones, broken down into achievable weekly targets—usually between 1 and 3 pounds per week (APA, 1996; Weltzin & Bolton, 1998). However, as Williamson and colleagues (1998) point out, decisions about specific goal weights are complex and must be tailored to the unique needs of each patient considering such factors as "medical necessity, the patient's beginning height/weight ratio and body composition, weight history, anticipated length of stay, and the patient's fear of weight gain/tolerance of increases in food consumption" (p. 422). Given the matrix of biopsychosocial dynamics involved, these kinds of decisions are best formulated from a multidisciplinary perspective (APA, 1996; Matusevich et al., 2002; Williamson et al., 1998) .

Special Problems

Special problems that may complicate inpatient treatment have been discussed in detail by Garfinkel, Garner, and Kennedy (1985), Gowers and Bryant-Waugh (2004), Fichter (1995), Williamson and colleagues (1998), Weltzin and Bolton (1998), and Woodside (1995). Some of these are summarized below.

1. Patients may not be completely convinced that their weight and eating behaviors are sufficiently serious to require treatment and hospitalization. Consequently, they may be either overtly resistant to or more subtly ambivalent about cooperating with the treatment protocol. Families may further exacerbate this situation—for instance, by minimizing patient symptoms, supporting patient resistance, and/ or yielding to patient requests for premature discharge, particularly in highly enmeshed families where parent–child separation may be difficult, or in situations where family members experience significant levels of guilt and/or fear of being blamed for the patient's dysfunction. Adding to this matrix of dynamics is the staff, whose members may experience considerable frustration in the context of patient and/or family treatment noncompliance. Staff members' reactions to patients and families may either help or hinder the treatment process.

2. Inherent in any hospitalization is some loss of autonomous functioning and control. For some patients, this loss of control may be especially threatening and may bring preexisting concerns about competence, self-control, and self-sufficiency to the surface. Accordingly, some patients may be prone to interpret inpatient treatment as an effort by others to control rather than to help them.

3. Serious comorbid conditions, such as severe depression and medical problems, may hinder treatment. For this reason, it is important that staff members be well trained in the treatment of eating disorders and prepared for these complications.

4. Some patients may be especially responsive to the inadvertent reinforcement contingencies in some units, whereby the most seriously ill patients receive the most staff attention. In such a context, illness behavior could be increased unintentionally.

5. Interactions among patients with different eating disorders may not always be harmonious, particularly when some patients with medical emergencies (such as those with AN) may require more staff time and attention.

Indications for inpatient admission have been considered previously in this chapter. General problems with admission to a hospital have been described by Kalucy and colleagues (1985). In addition, several recent discussions detail admission criteria at different levels of care (e.g., Anzai et al., 2002; Cummings et al., 2001).

Over the last 10–15 years, the length of hospitalization has been trending downward (Anzai et al., 2002; APA, 1996; Wiseman, Sunday, Klapper, Harris, & Halmi, 2001), with lengths of stay calculated in days rather than months. Despite considerable variability, typical durations of hospitalization range from fewer than 7 days to 26 days (Anzai et al., 2002; Kaczynski, Denison, Wiknertz, Ryno, & Hjalmers, 2000; Striegel-Moore, Leslie, Petrill, Garvin, & Rosenheck, 2000; Wiseman et al., 2001). In the context of shorter hospital stays, inpatient treatment increasingly emphasizes stabilization of the patient's immediate medical condition (APA, 1996; Fennig, Fennig, & Roe, 2002; Lock et al., 2001; Patel, Pratt, & Greydanus, 2003; Weltzin & Bolton, 1998; Williamson et al., 1998; Wiseman et al., 2001). However, the APA (1996) still recommends that patients with AN be discharged only "when they are medically stable and weight has been restored to a suitable level, behavioral symptoms have been substantially controlled, sufficient work with psychological and family factors has been undertaken assuring that aftercare treatment will be focused on relevant areas, and a targeted aftercare plan has been formulated and can be implemented" (p. 62). Similarly, the APA's guidelines for discharging patients with BN emphasize "substantial control of binge–purge cycles, laxative abuse, and other disabling symptoms," and add that discharge should occur only "when a targeted aftercare plan has been formulated and can be implemented" (1996, p. 64).

In an effort to address patient needs more efficiently in the context of diminishing inpatient resources, an increasing number of programs have developed continuum models providing a broader spectrum of services emphasizing continuity across levels of care (Anzai et al., 2002; Cummings et al., 2001; Fennig et al., 2002; Grigoriadis, Kaplan, Carter, & Woodside, 2001). In these comprehensive treatment programs, patients typically are carefully evaluated and then assigned to one of several levels of care on the basis of well-articulated biopsychosocial criteria. For instance, Williamson and colleagues (1998) detailed a three-level model including inpatient, partial day hospital, and outpatient treatment. More recently, Cummings and colleagues (2001) have described a program with five continua of care, consisting of inpatient hospitalization, partial hospitalization, day treatment, intensive outpatient treatment, and outpatient services. In these comprehensive programs, results of the initial assessment guide patients to the least restrictive alternative that is appropriate in each case. In cases where inpatient treatment is initially indicated, patients can make the transition to less intensive care as soon as is warranted (e.g., Cummings et al., 2001; Williamson et al., 1998).

Multicomponent Outpatient Treatment Programs

Intensive, multicomponent outpatient treatment programs are becoming increasingly popular for the treatment of AN, BN, and BED (Agras et al., 1994; Lacey, 1985; Mitchell, Hatsukami, Goff, et al., 1985; Weltzin & Bolton, 1998; Wooley & Kearney-Cooke, 1986). These programs typically combine educational seminars with group, individual, family, and body image therapy, incorporating many of the themes discussed above and utilizing many of the techniques outlined below. These approaches may also be utilized in conjunction with pharmacological interventions (Yager, 1994). Nevertheless, the bulk of the treatment outcome research tends to center on specific strategies. For that reason, we discuss the evidence for specific psychotherapy techniques and treatment components below.

Psychotherapy Techniques and Therapy Components

Comparisons of therapeutic processes and techniques have failed to identify a clear choice among approaches that works best *for all eating disorders*. Specifically, reviews of the literature tend to find that behavioral, cognitive,

cognitive-behavioral, and interpersonal therapeutic approaches perform significantly better than either no treatment or pharmacological interventions alone (Richards et al., 2000; Wilson & Fairburn, 1993). Yet there is no consistent, clear-cut pattern of differential performance among the above-mentioned theoretical approaches in the scientific literature *for all eating disorders*. In fact, reviews of the literature indicate that almost every type of therapeutic technique has been attempted with eating disorders, and that virtually all have shown some efficacy (APA, 1996; Garner & Garfinkel, 1985, 1997; Richards et al., 2000).

One major exception is in the treatment of BN, where (as detailed below) cognitive-behavioral therapy (CBT) is currently recommended as the empirically supported *initial* treatment of choice, given that interpersonal psychotherapy (IPT) yields slower results (Agras et al., 2000; Chambless et al., 1998; Dalle-Grave, Ricca, & Todesco, 2001; Fairburn & Harrison, 2003; Thompson-Brenner, Glass, & Westen, 2003; Wilson, 1999; Wilson & Pike, 2001). A brief discussion of these and several other commonly used therapeutic interventions follows.

Behavioral Therapies and Techniques

EXPOSURE PLUS RESPONSE PREVENTION

There has been some controversy about the role of exposure plus response prevention (ERP) procedures in the treatment of bulimic behaviors. Rosen and Leitenberg (1982) initially hypothesized that vomiting is a response to overeating that decreases anxiety related to fear of gaining weight. As a result, the individual learns that vomiting after eating leads to anxiety reduction. Rosen and Leitenberg proposed that binge eating might not occur if an individual with BN were prevented from vomiting afterward. Although some research has supported the use of ERP procedures (Gray & Hoage, 1990; Kennedy, Katz, Neitzert, Ralveski, & Mendlowitz, 1995; Leitenberg, Rosen, Gross, Nudelman, & Vara, 1988; Williamson, Prather, et al., 1989; Wilson, Rossiter, Kleinfield, & Lindholm, 1986), several of these studies lacked adequate controls and had small samples. A controlled study by Agras, Schneider, Arnow, Raeburn, and Telch (1989) found that ERP procedures added no benefit to, and indeed potentially detracted from, the efficacy of CBT. Despite suggestions that the Agras and colleagues study suffered from methodological problems, such as not allowing for adequate ERP practice (Leitenberg & Rosen, 1989), more recent research attempting to address these problems has not demonstrated benefit from adding ERP procedures to CBT (Carter, McIntosh, Joyce, Sullivan, & Bullik, 2003; Wilson, Eldredge, Smith, & Niles, 1991). In a study comparing ERP alone to CBT alone, 1-year follow-up data indicated that patients assigned to the ERP-alone condition experienced significantly greater relapse, whereas patients in the CBT-alone group maintained or slightly improved their scores on measures of bulimia-specific psychopathology and more general measures of psychological functioning (Cooper & Steere, 1995). Other research (e.g., Bulik, Sullivan, Carter, McIntosh & Joyce, 1998; Carter et al., 2003) has also raised questions about the benefits of ERP over and above those associated with CBT alone. Notwithstanding Leitenberg and Rosen's (1989) contention that ERP procedures are designed to supplement CBT or other treatments and not to replace them, the role of ERP procedures in the treatment of bulimic behaviors is currently unclear.

OPERANT CONDITIONING TECHNIQUES

Operant conditioning techniques have been used to facilitate weight gain in hospital settings. These techniques use positive and negative contingencies (e.g., social praise, recreational activities, visiting privileges, hospital rewards, bed rest, and/or earlier or later discharge) in association with a performance criterion such as eating or weight gain (Bachrach, Erwin, & Mohr, 1965; Griffiths et al., 1998; Lang, 1965; Leitenberg, Agras, & Thompson, 1968; Steinhausen, 1995b; Williamson et al., 1998). In the case of AN, this criterion is generally a predetermined weight or weight increase. Given that the use of operant techniques presupposes the ability to control the environmental contingencies, this approach has been used primarily in inpatient settings. Although this type of contingency management can produce initial and rapid weight gains, these procedures have not been shown to be more effective than other treatments in terms of extended weight maintenance, including simpler hospital programs with discharge contingent on weight gains (Garfinkel, Moldofsky, & Garner, 1977). Research utilizing operant approaches suggests that in terms of treatment efficacy, they are not

superior to CBT techniques (e.g., Wilson & Fairburn, 1993). These findings are consistent with the more traditional assertion that operant conditioning techniques are helpful when part of a comprehensive treatment program, but inadequate when used alone (Bemis, 1978; Steinhausen, 1995b). In addition, a study comparing the efficacy of behavior therapy, IPT, and CBT found very high rates of attrition/withdrawal and poorer outcomes among patients receiving the behavior therapy intervention (Fairburn, Jones, Peveler, Hope, & O'Connor, 1993).

RESPONSE DELAY

Response delay procedures are based on the theory that impulses are more easily delayed than resisted. It is hypothesized that during the delay period, the event sequence will be altered, thereby causing the urge to subside, become more manageable, and ultimately yield to resistance efforts. The delay tactic can involve allowing some predetermined length of time to pass or engaging in some alternative activity (Garner, Vitousek, & Pike, 1997). For instance, a client with BN may choose to wait 20 minutes before bingeing or, alternatively, may call a friend, walk the dog, or take a leisurely bath. It is important that the activity be selected ahead of time and involve something of the client's choice that is experienced as pleasurable, esteem-building, and/or self-nurturing. Garner and Bemis (1985) recommend that some clients (particularly those who have not yet made a commitment to stop vomiting) prepare a "mnemonic card" listing prebinge delay tactics for consultation on those occasions when urges to binge seem irresistible. Response delay strategies are commonly included in multicomponent behavioral programs. As such, they are presently considered one well-accepted strategy routinely incorporated into broader treatment packages, which may explain the dearth of current research specifically focused on response delay per se.

SELF-MONITORING TECHNIQUES

Self-monitoring techniques are generally recognized as helpful, particularly when patients binge. Although formats differ, patients are typically encouraged to record the context and parameters of their binge eating; associated and preceding thoughts, feelings, and events; and the presence or absence of others (Fairburn, Marcus, et al., 1993; Wilson &

Pike, 2001). Fairburn (1980) described elaborate self-monitoring in conjunction with cognitive techniques in the treatment of four women with BN who engaged in vomiting. The self-monitoring was used as a vehicle for the clients and therapist to explore options for increasing self-control over eating and decreasing food avoidance. Utilizing similar methods, Agras and colleagues (1989) compared the effectiveness of self-monitoring alone to that of a complete CBT package (including self-monitoring). Although self-monitoring alone was effective, the CBT package significantly outperformed it. These results suggest that, although important, self-monitoring should be viewed as one meaningful component of CBT, and not as a "treatment" in and of itself.

SOCIAL SKILLS TRAINING

Social skills training has been used to help correct the deficits in social competencies, assertiveness, interpersonal communication, and basic problem-solving capabilities frequently observed in those with eating disorders. Social skills training was used in one study to modify the social isolation and interpersonal anxiety associated with AN (Pillay & Crisp, 1981). In the study, one group of hospitalized patients with AN received social skills training, and another group was placed in a placebo condition. At a 1-year follow-up, the social skills group did not differ significantly from the placebo-treated group in terms of weight, but these patients were less likely to terminate treatment and reported a more rapid decrease in their levels of anxiety, depression, and fear of negative evaluation. Fichter (1995) recommended incorporating the typical targets of social skills training interventions into inpatient interventions for AN to enhance overall effectiveness and generalization of treatment. Currently, it is common for social skills to be addressed within the broader context of comprehensive treatment packages (e.g., Williamson et al., 1998). As such, little current research has focused specifically on the value added by social skills training.

STIMULUS CONTROL STRATEGIES

Stimulus control strategies are used routinely in the multicomponent treatment of eating disorders to minimize or neutralize environmental cues that lead to inappropriate eating (e.g., Cooper et al., 2003; Fairburn, Marcus, et al., 1993). These strategies include reducing household binge triggers (e.g., favorite "binge foods"), structuring the environment to promote healthful eating practices (e.g., by replacing countertop candy with fresh fruit), and avoiding high-risk eating situations (e.g., "all you care to eat" buffets). Stimulus control procedures were evaluated in a single-case study by Viens and Hranchuk (1993), which found that stimulus control procedures emphasizing minimal therapist contact, in the absence of cognitive therapy, were successful in reducing vomiting frequency in a 35-year-old female patient with BN. Of course, no strong conclusions can be drawn about the efficacy or generalizability of these procedures from this case study. Given that stimulus control procedures are ubiquitous in CBT programs, these strategies should be further evaluated in larger, controlled investigations to assess their specific contribution to the overall efficacy of comprehensive treatment programs.

SYSTEMATIC DESENSITIZATION

Systematic desensitization has been used to decrease anxiety related to fears of gaining weight and/or being criticized (Hallsten, 1965; Lang, 1965; Ollendick, 1979), self-deprecating thoughts (Monti, McCrady, & Barlow, 1977), and changes in physical appearance concomitant with weight gain (Schnurer, Rubin, & Roy, 1973). Unfortunately, in recent years, little attention has focused on systematic desensitization in the treatment of eating disorders.

Cognitive/Cognitive-Behavioral Techniques

Cognitive retraining or restructuring techniques combat distorted body image, erroneous beliefs and assumptions, and misinterpretations of environmental "messages" (Beck, 1976). Individuals with AN or BN may be especially prone to evaluate their self-worth in terms of shape and weight. Based on an overgeneralization and incorporation of very real social pressures (discussed above), such individuals may hold a variety of dysfunctional beliefs, such as equating overweight with unworthiness, weakness, and a dismal future, as well as the corollary that being thin means that one is worthy, is strong, and will realize all one's dreams (Fairburn, Cooper, & Cooper, 1986; Fairburn, Marcus, et al., 1993; Fairburn, Shafran, et al., 1999; Tuschen & Bents, 1995). Therapy consequently involves questioning these social values, identifying the ways patients may apply them in their lives, and learning to challenge them (Pike, Loeb, & Vitousek, 1996). Common categories of cognitive distortions, and procedures for facilitating CBT of eating disorders, have been detailed by many others (e.g., Fairburn, Marcus, et al., 1993; Fernandez, 1984; Garner, 1986; Garner & Bemis, 1982; Pike et al., 1996; Wilson & Pike, 2001).

As noted in the introduction to the section on psychotherapy techniques, CBT has been well established as an empirically supported treatment for BN (Anderson & Maloney, 2001; Dalle-Grave et al., 2001; Fairburn & Harrison, 2003; Thompson-Brenner et al., 2003; Wilson, 1999; Wilson & Pike, 2001). Research utilizing approaches that combine cognitive and behavioral interventions (i.e., CBT) has demonstrated meaningful levels of clinical improvement (Mitchell, Hoberman, Peterson, Mussell, & Pyle, 1996; Pike et al., 1996). In a study of 50 patients with BN, CBT was found to be mildly superior to supportive–expressive treatment on measures of vomiting frequency, but the results were much stronger when other symptoms were examined (e.g., concern about eating and weight, depression, and self-esteem) (Garner et al., 1993). CBT techniques, and CBT techniques used in combination with pharmacological interventions, tend to be superior to pharmacological interventions alone in reducing the primary symptoms of BN (e.g., Agras, 1997; Casper, 2002; Crow & Mitchell, 1996a, 1996b; Goldbloom et al., 1997; Mitchell, deZwaan, & Roerig, 2003).

CBT also seems promising in the treatment of AN (Bowers, 2001; Serfaty, Turkington, Heap, Ledsham, & Jolley, 1999; Wilson & Fairburn, 1993) as well as of BED (Ricca, Mannucci, Zucchi, Rotella, & Faravelli, 2000; Wilfley & Cohen, 1997; Wilfley et al., 2002). Finally, as discussed below, recent studies of CBT approaches indicate that IPT may perform similarly well, but IPT may take longer to be effective (Fairburn & Harrison, 2003; Fairburn, Jones, et al., 1993; Fairburn et al., 2003; Wilfley et al., 2002).

Supportive–Expressive Therapy

Supportive–expressive therapy, originally developed as a brief psychoanalytic approach (Luborsky, 1984), has also been applied in the treatment of eating disorders. Supportive-expressive therapy posits that eating disorder symptoms disguise underlying interpersonal problems. Therapy is nondirective and interpretive, with a focus on listening to the patient, promoting expression of feelings, and identifying problems and solutions. A primary task during therapy is to explore the past in order to illuminate interpersonal difficulties and establish core conflictual relationship themes that underlie eating disorder symptoms. As noted earlier, supportive–expressive therapy was found to be slightly less effective than CBT in reducing the frequency of self-induced vomiting, but CBT was significantly more effective in ameliorating dysfunctional attitudes about eating and weight, depression, poor self-esteem, and general psychological distress (Garner et al., 1993).

Interpersonal Psychotherapy

IPT is focused on helping the client "recognize and alter maladaptive interpersonal interactions" (Gillies, 2001, p. 314). For the treatment of BN, IPT has been found to be as effective as CBT, but IPT appears to work somewhat more slowly (Agras et al., 2000; Fairburn et al., 1995, 2003; Garner et al., 1993; Wilfley et al., 2002). Commenting on this temporal pattern, several writers (e.g., Agras, 1991; Wilson & Pike, 2001) have discussed the possibility that IPT may address secondary mechanisms (e.g., dissatisfaction with social relationships, difficulties in social functioning, negative affect, and low self-esteem) implicated in the development and maintenance of BN. However, Wilson and Pike (2001) have cautioned that "the absence of a statistically significant difference between CBT and IPT over follow-up may be more a function of their differential posttreatment status (a regression-toward-the-mean effect) than any delayed 'catch-up' property of IPT" (p. 339). Research on the efficacy of IPT for patients with BED who have not responded to CBT has not found it effective (Agras et al., 1995), suggesting that patients benefiting from CBT may not be significantly different from those who benefit from IPT (e.g., Agras et al., 1995). Clearly, this issue deserves further investigation.

Body Image Work

Body image work helps patients become more aware and accepting of their bodies. Photographs, videotapes, various types of role playing, cognitive restructuring, movement, expressive art, and guided imagery therapies are often employed. Wooley and Kearney-Cooke (1986) discussed the use of a combination of such techniques. More recently, Rosen, Reiter, and Orosan (1995) evaluated a body-image-oriented form of CBT with patients diagnosed with BDD. They found that patients treated with CBT experienced significant decreases in their body image disturbance, compared to no-treatment controls. In addition, remission was achieved in 82% of treated patients at termination and 77% of cases at follow-up (Rosen et al., 1995). Although these cognitive-behavioral methods are integrated routinely into current treatment programs for eating disorders (e.g., Fairburn, Marcus, et al., 1993; Weltzin & Bolton, 1998; Williamson et al., 1998), few current empirical investigations have focused specifically on body image work. More research on the additive value of body image work would be helpful in guiding decisions about incorporating these approaches into broader multicomponent treatment packages.

Family Therapy

Family therapy ranges from supportive, informational counseling to more intensive work focused on changing a family's structural and/or functional patterns. Family therapy has been used as a treatment by itself (e.g., Minuchin et al., 1978) and as an element of multi-component treatment packages (e.g., Dare & Eisler, 1997; Strober & Yager, 1985). As a primary treatment, family therapy generally encourages a patient with AN to disengage gradually from the family, progress toward adolescence and adulthood, and realign family roles and boundaries along more developmentally appropriate and adaptive lines (e.g., Lock et al., 2001). The agenda of family therapy as an element of a treatment package (Wooley & Kearney-Cooke, 1986) includes helping the patient find a way to achieve age-appropriate separation from the family without the feared loss of all family connectedness; express personal needs and feelings clearly; and enhance communication between the parents, so that the patient is not needed as a facilitator (Wooley & Kearney-Cooke, 1986).

Dare and Eisler (1995) reviewed several studies focusing on the differential utility of family versus individual supportive therapy for the treatment of eating disorders. Summarizing the results, these authors reported that adolescents receiving family intervention for AN outperformed those receiving individual treatment on measures of maintained body weight at a 5-year follow-up. Russell, Szmukler, Dare, and Eisler (1987), in a controlled trial, found that family therapy was superior to individual supportive therapy in patients whose eating disorders started before age 19 and whose eating disorders were not chronic. Crisp and colleagues (1991) also found family therapy to be an important component of their combined therapy in a study of 90 patients with AN. Their study compared the efficacy of four treatment modalities: inpatient treatment; outpatient individual therapy coupled with family psychotherapy plus dietary counseling; outpatient group family therapy plus dietary counseling; and no treatment. Both of the treatment protocols that included family therapy were found to be superior to the no-treatment condition on measures of weight gain, return of menstruation, and aspects of social and sexual adjustment. By contrast, an evaluation of behavioral–family systems therapy (BFST; see below) for AN with adolescent females found that family therapy and ego-oriented individual therapy, which focuses on improving a patient's ego strength, coping skills, and individuation from the family, were equivalent in producing improvements in eating attitudes, body dissatisfaction, interoceptive awareness, depression, and family conflict (Robin, Siegel, Koepke, Moye, & Tice, 1994; Robin, Siegel, & Moye, 1995). In addition, many of these improvements were maintained 1 year after treatment termination. In fact, the only difference in outcome between the two therapy approaches was that BFST produced greater changes in body mass index. Similarly, few differences were found in a study that compared family therapy to separate counseling for the patient and parents (Le Grange, Eisler, Dare, & Russell, 1992). Clearly, as Gillberg (1994) has suggested, more research is needed to clarify the role and benefits of family therapy in the treatment of eating disorders.

The paucity of controlled evaluations notwithstanding, family involvement is considered a key component of comprehensive treatment for an eating disorder, especially when the patient is a legal minor or still resides with the family of origin (Lemmon & Josephson, 2001; Lock et al., 2001; Weltzin & Bolton, 1998; Williamson et al., 1998). A recent manualized, family-based intervention for AN (Lock et al., 2001) has shown preliminary promise in the treatment of adolescents and may inspire more systematic research in this area (Lock & Le

Grange, 2001) . In a recent study of 34 families, Krautter and Lock (2004) reported that both adolescents and their families perceived the treatment to be effective and acceptable.

Another family approach to treating AN, BFST, combines components of behavior modification, cognitive therapy, and family systems therapy (e.g., Robin, Bedway, Siegel, & Gilroy, 1996). As discussed above, comparisons of BFST with ego-oriented individual therapy (e.g., Robin et al., 1994) have found generally equivalent efficacy in adolescent females, with a majority of patients in the BFST group attaining their target weights by a 1-year follow-up (Robin et al., 1999). These preliminary data suggest that BFST may be a potentially efficacious treatment for adolescents and their families. It is hoped that these results will encourage additional larger-scale, controlled investigations.

Feminist Approaches to Treatment

Although the definition of a "feminist approach," with respect to psychological interventions, is continually evolving and somewhat difficult to articulate, a brief description of the ideas that fall under the umbrella of the term is warranted. Wooley (1995) has discussed the importance of considering the social and cultural context of patients with eating disorders. Feminist therapists attempt to broaden the focus from blaming the individual with an eating disorder to examining the pathological social factors beyond the patient. By contrast to traditional techniques (which may be rooted in many of the same cultural biases and pressures that contribute to women's eating problems), feminist approaches are designed to empower patients, in order to minimize the risk of revictimization in the course of treatment (Striegel-Moore, 1995). They also consider the potential impact of sexual abuse on the development of eating disorders in children (Kearney-Cooke & Striegel-Moore, 1994) and adults (Everill & Waller, 1995). Unfortunately, these approaches have rarely been subjected to empirical testing.

Group Therapy

GROUP APPROACHES FOR AN

Compared to group approaches for patients with BN or BED, group therapy has traditionally been much less common in the treatment of AN (Hall, 1985). However, group work may be beneficial for those patients whose medical conditions have been stabilized. For instance, Williamson and colleagues (1998) described several group therapy protocols for young patients with AN, including a body image group, a meal-planning/nutritional education group, a family group, and an adolescent group. More recently, several other group treatments for AN have shown potential promise, such as a group CBT program with four phases (motivation, day patient, outpatient, and separation; Gerlinghoff, Gross, & Backmund, 2003), as well as an 8-week nutrition and behavior change group conducted by a multidisciplinary team (Waisberg & Woods, 2002). Several authors have detailed specific factors relevant to the group treatment of eating disorders, including group size, composition, climate (e.g., Polivy & Federoff, 1997; Tasca, Flynn, & Bissada, 2002), structure through various treatment stages (Gerlinghoff et al., 2003; Hall, 1985), and members' readiness to change (Gusella, Butler, Nichols, & Bird, 2003).

GROUP APPROACHES FOR BN

Experiential group therapy has been advocated for the treatment of average-weight women with BN. This type of therapy may incorporate a feminist perspective, taking the position that eating disorders are caused in part by the conflicting role demands placed on women. From this perspective, BN is considered to be "related to the struggle to achieve a perfect, stereotypic female image in which women surrender most of their self-defining powers to others" (White & Boskind-White, 1981, p. 501). Treatment consequently questions these standards (Boskind-Lodahl & White, 1978). In an early report (Boskind-Lodahl & White, 1978), of 12 of 13 women who completed treatment, 4 ceased bingeing, 6 reduced the frequency and length of their binges, and 2 had no change. Follow-up 1 year later suggested that the successes had been maintained. A similar treatment procedure was followed with a separate sample of 14 women (White & Boskind-White, 1981). Six months after treatment, 3 of the women reported a cessation of binges, 7 reported reduced frequency and decreased duration of binges, and 4 reported little change in binges. All of the 10 women who found the treatment helpful in reducing their binge behavior also reported that they no longer engaged in purge behavior, despite a high frequency of purges prior to treatment. Unfortunately, as a group, these studies suffer from being statistically underpowered, which is a problem plaguing research on all too many of these approaches to eating disorders.

Both CBT and IPT (discussed above as empirically supported treatments) have been delivered in group formats. Both approaches have shown efficacy in group settings for patients with BN and BED (e.g., Leung, Waller, & Glyn, 2000; Wilfley et al., 2002).

Physical Therapy

Moderate exercise (walking, stretching) is thought to promote a healthy distribution of weight gain and a balanced view of physical activity as part of a healthy lifestyle (Andersen, 1986; Carraro, Cognolato, & Bernardis, 1998; Duesund & Skarderud, 2003). As such, lifestyle activity is often included as one facet of multicomponent treatment packages. For instance, adjunctive exercise has been shown to enhance extended CBT for BED (Pendleton, Goodrick, Poston, Reeves, & Foreyt, 2002). There is also some preliminary evidence that adapted physical activity/graded exercise may be a valuable component in comprehensive interventions for AN (Andersen, 1986; Carraro et al., 1998; Duesund & Skarderud, 2003). However, the exact role of graded exercise in the treatment of AN remains unclear. For instance, Thien, Thomas, Markin, and Birmingham (2000) reported that although inclusion of a graded exercise program had a beneficial impact on compliance, it did not affect body composition in the short term. Hence a more fine-grained exploration of graded exercise programs is merited.

Psychoeducational Approaches

Based on the idea that maladaptive beliefs and behaviors develop as the result of erroneous or insufficient information, psychoeducational approaches have been viewed as an important part of treatment for eating disorders (Olmsted & Kaplan, 1995). Psychoeducation typically consists of providing information to patients about the nature of their disorders and methods for overcoming them, with the intention of promoting attitudinal and behavior change. In addition, psychoeducational programs tend to focus on a coaching model of treatment. That is, because the patient is empowered with information and methods, the locus of change is

within the patient (Garner, 1997; Olmsted & Kaplan, 1995). Psychoeducational programs cover a wide range of topics, depending on the treatment population and professionals involved. For eating disorders, topics may include the multidimensional etiology of AN, BN, and BED; the negative consequences of dieting; nutritional information; set-point theory; the effects of starvation on behavior; the cultural context of eating disorders; body image and self-esteem issues; cognitive and behavior change strategies; medical complications; and relapse prevention—just to name a few (Garner, 1997; Olmsted & Kaplan, 1995). Finally, psychoeducational programs most often are provided to patients (and in some cases family members) in group formats that facilitate interaction and support.

Johnson, Connors, and Stuckey (1983) and Connors, Johnson, and Stuckey (1984) treated two groups of 10 women with BN over a 12-week period. Therapy included didactic presentations as well as group process interventions. The didactic presentations focused on challenging beliefs about the value of thinness and distorted ideas about food, weight, and dieting. Participants also were taught to reduce bingeing and purging by means of behavioral strategies, and to "normalize" eating by means of self-monitoring and self-graduated goal setting. Binge–purge episodes were reduced by 70% at posttreatment and at a 6-month follow-up. Three participants had ceased bingeing, eight had reduced their frequency by more than 50%, six had reduced their frequency by between 30% and 50%, and three patients were unchanged. Olmsted and colleagues (1991) utilized a sequential cohort design to compare the relative effectiveness of an 18-week CBT intervention for BN with that of a 4-week (five-session) group psychoeducational protocol. CBT was found to be significantly more effective for the most seriously ill patients (32% of the sample who reported bingeing more than 42 times in the month prior to treatment) on measures of vomiting frequency. For less severely ill patients, no significant difference on measures of vomiting frequency between CBT and the psychoeducational intervention was detected. A similar but less robust finding was reported for scores on the Drive for Thinness and Maturity Fears scales included in this study. More recently, Geist, Heinmaa, Stephens, Davis, and Katzman (2000) found that family therapy and family group psychoeducation were both associated with weight restoration in adolescents with AN. Taken together, this pattern of results highlights the relative effectiveness of psychoeducational interventions for the delivery of efficient and cost-effective treatment of eating disorders for some patients (e.g., Stice & Ragan, 2002; Wiseman, Sunday, Klapper, Klein, & Halmi, 2002).

Innovative Methods of Treatment Delivery

Increasingly, new technologies are being used in the management of eating disorders, including computer-based methods of learning to eat and recognize satiety (Bergh, Brodin, Lindberg, & Sodersten, 2002), adjunctive e-mail in the outpatient treatment of AN (Bailey, Yager, & Jenson, 2002; Yager, 2001), and the delivery of family therapy for AN via telehealth (Goldfield & Boachie, 2003). Although many of the issues surrounding the use of these approaches have yet to be fully explored and resolved (Bailey et al., 2002; Goldfield & Boachie, 2003), these innovative methods deserve more systematic investigation.

Psychosocial Treatments: Conclusions

Despite the vast array of psychosocial treatments potentially available for the treatment of eating disorders, none address all symptoms of all eating disorders in all patients. For example, although CBT substantially improves symptoms of BN and BED, not all patients may benefit (Agras et al., 1995; Fairburn et al., 2003; Thompson-Brenner et al., 2003). In fact, as noted above, the evidence for many psychosocial therapies is weak or equivocal at this time, especially in the case of interventions with children and adolescents. As Gowers and Bryant-Waugh (2004) point out, "the gaps in the knowledge base regarding effective treatments in child and adolescent eating disorders suggest that almost any adequately powered well-conducted trial would add to knowledge" (p. 78). Across developmental levels, patients with eating disorders appear to have high rates of relapse, regardless of the treatment modality (Fisher, 2003; Keller, Herzog, Lavori, Bradburn, & Mahoney, 1992; Steinhausen, 1995b, 2002). This suggests that current psychosocial treatments are not adequate, and that future efforts should focus on optimizing empirically supported treatments, evaluating other existing therapies, and developing new approaches (e.g., Ben-Tovim, 2003; Gowers &

Bryant-Waugh, 2004). For example, Fairburn and colleagues (2003) have offered a new "transdiagnostic" theory and treatment for eating disorders, which address key maintenance processes such as clinical perfectionism, core low self-esteem, mood intolerance, and interpersonal difficulties, in an effort to optimize CBT. In addition, existing therapies that have shown promise in the treatment of other disorders (e.g., motivation enhancement and dialectical behavioral therapies) recently have been applied to eating disorders with some preliminary success (see Kotler et al., 2003, for an excellent review). Efforts such as these, as well as up-and-coming theories and strategies, are essential to advancing the state of the science.

Pharmacological Treatment

Anorexia Nervosa

Pharmacological treatment has typically been explored as one component of multicomponent programs for AN. The medications used have included neuroleptic antidepressants (Hoffman & Halmi, 1993) and antianxiety medications. For example, Garfinkel and Walsh (1997) suggested that small amounts of a benzodiazepine (e.g., lorezapam) before meals may be helpful for some highly anxious patients with AN. Andersen and colleagues (1997) have argued that the use of medications to stimulate appetite is misguided, in that appetite is not disturbed in patients with AN. They refrain from using antidepressant medications until patients have attained average weight, and then use them only if a patient meets the criteria for major depressive disorder. More recently, other drugs such as olanzapine (an atypical neuroleptic) have been explored in preliminary case, retrospective, and open-label studies with very small numbers of participants as possibly promoting weight gain among patients with AN (Malina et al., 2003; Mehler et al., 2001; Powers, Santana, & Bannon, 2002). Reports on the use of citalopram (Fassino et al., 2002) and tramadol (Mendelson, 2001) have also been published. Although these results have seemed promising, interpretation of these findings is difficult until more controlled studies with larger numbers of participants have been reported.

The current consensus, based on the accumulation of empirical results to date, seems to have coalesced around the view that pharmacological treatments are not generally effective in the acute treatment of patients with AN, although they may be helpful in mitigating relapse after healthy weight has been achieved in some patients within the broader context of a comprehensive treatment program (Attia, Mayer, & Killory, 2001; Casper, 2002; Kotler & Walsh, 2000; Krueger & Kennedy, 2000; Mitchell et al., 2003; Zhu & Walsh, 2002).

Bulimia Nervosa

Pharmacological treatments for BN have been associated with more positive outcomes than those for AN; antidepressants have been associated most consistently with the short-term amelioration of binge-eating and purging behaviors (Casper, 2002; Mitchell et al., 2003). However, pharmacotherapy has generally not been linked with durable long-term improvements without psychotherapy, and it has not been shown to be more effective than CBT alone (Casper, 2002; Fairburn & Harrison, 2003; Mitchell et al., 2003; Zhu & Walsh, 2002).

Various types of antidepressants, as well as the anticonvulsant medication phenytoin sodium, have been explored in the treatment of binge eating. Mitchell, Raymond, and Specker (1993) reviewed the efficacy of antidepressants as reported in 12 different double-blind controlled trials. In the seven studies of tricyclic antidepressants reviewed, significant reductions in binge eating and/or vomiting were noted when compared to placebo. The reduction in binge eating ranged from 47% to 91%. Antidepressant medications typically used included releasing agents and reuptake inhibitors, such as imipramine, amitriptyline, desipramine, and fenfluramine; the last of these was withdrawn from the market in September 1997, along with dexfenfluramine, due to potentially serious side effects such as valvular heart disease (Centers for Disease Control and Prevention, 1997; Connolly et al., 1997; U.S. Food and Drug Administration, 1997).

In conjunction with the serotonin etiological theory discussed earlier in this chapter, the selective serotonin reuptake inhibitor (SSRI) fluoxetine has also shown efficacy in the treatment of BN. Advocat and Kutlesic (1995) describe the serotonin hypothesis in the following way: "Bulimia nervosa is the behavioral expression of functional underactivity of serotonin . . . in the central nervous system" (p. 61).

They review two studies utilizing fluoxetine. Both studies, using small samples, reported significant short-term improvement in bingeing and vomiting, along with good long-term maintenance of gains. Patients treated with fluoxetine for 16 weeks demonstrated significant reductions in binge-eating and vomiting episodes, compared to patients treated with a placebo (Goldstein, Wilson, Thompson, Potvin, & Rampey, 1995). Fluoxetine treatment alone has produced results similar to the combination of psychodynamically oriented supportive psychotherapy and fluoxetine (Walsh et al., 1997). When compared to CBT, however, fluoxetine alone produced poorer outcomes and the combination of both was only marginally better than CBT alone (Goldbloom et al., 1997; Walsh et al., 1997).

Another partial serotonin agonist, ipsapirone, was evaluated in an open pilot study with 17 patients. The investigators found that symptoms of BN improved greatly during the 4 weeks of treatment, but since this was not a "blinded" or placebo-controlled study, it can only be concluded that ipsapirone may be a promising pharmacological intervention (Geretsegger, Greimel, Roed, & Hesselink, 1995).

Monoamine oxidase (MAOI) antidepressants have been used because of data suggesting a link between BN and mood disorders (Hudson, Laffer, & Pope, 1982; Mitchell et al., 1993; Walsh et al., 1982). Results have been mixed. Russell (1979) reported that these antidepressants failed to have an effect on eating behavior. By contrast, Walsh and colleagues (1982) noted dramatic improvement in both mood and eating behavior in six women meeting the DSM-III-R criteria for BN as well as atypical depression (Liebowitz, Quitkin, & Stewart, 1981). Unfortunately, there was no control group, the sample size was small, the method for measuring improvement was not specified, and follow-up data were not presented. In addition, Walsh and colleagues (1988), and Kennedy and colleagues (1988) using MAOIs, found reductions in bingeing behaviors comparable to those typically found with tricyclic antidepressant medications. However, given the side effects typically associated with MAOIs, they should not be considered as the first line of treatment for BN.

Desipramine, a tricyclic, has fewer side effects than the MAOIs. An advantage of desipramine is that it does not require that patients be placed on diets with rigid restrictions. Furthermore, in one study using a double-blind, placebo-controlled, partial crossover trial, desipramine hydrochloride reduced binge frequency by 91%, whereas the placebo group showed a 19% increase in binge frequency (Hughes, Wells, Cunningham, & Ilstrup, 1984). Of the 22 patients on the drug, 15 attained complete abstinence from bingeing and purging after 6 weeks of treatment. However, questions about the endurance of these improvements remain to be fully explored (e.g., Gowers & Bryant-Waugh, 2004; Mitchell et al., 2003). Moreover, because tricyclic antidepressants may have potentially adverse side effects, individuals (especially youths) who are prescribed these drugs should be carefully monitored, and medication should be discontinued when problems arise (e.g., Diler & Avci, 2002; Gorman & Kent, 1999; Srinivasan, Ashok, Vaz, & Yeragani, 2004; Tingelstad, 1991).

Anticonvulsant medications, such as phenytoin sodium, have been used in the treatment of eating disorders, based on the hypothesis that binge eating may be a symptom of epileptic convulsions. Abnormal electroencephalograms have been found in some individuals with compulsive eating disorders (Green & Rau, 1974; Rau & Green, 1975). Treatment successes as high as 90% have been reported with phenytoin (Green & Rau, 1974). However, the criteria for improvement were unclear, and there were no controls for placebo effects. Wermuth, Davis, Hollister, and Stunkard (1977) used a double-blind crossover study with phenytoin and a placebo ($n = 19$). Although binge frequency was significantly reduced during the phenytoin phase compared to placebo, improvement continued during the placebo phase. Overall, only 40% of participants experienced marked or moderate improvement. Other studies (Weiss & Levitz, 1976; Greenway, Dahms, & Bray, 1977) on the effects of anticonvulsant medication on compulsive eating indicated a lack of response to medication. With further study, Green and Rau (1977) concluded that a neurophysiological element is evident in some, but not all, compulsive eating. However, much more research is needed in this area. (For excellent reviews on pharmacotherapy for eating disorders, see Barbarich, Kaye, & Jimerson, 2003; Gowers & Bryant-Waugh, 2004; and/or Mitchell et al., 2003.)

In sum, recent reviews of the extant literature have concluded that antidepressants generally have been shown useful in the short-term treatment of BN, with various types of antidepressants appearing roughly comparable (Bacaltchuk, Hay, & Mari, 2000). However, pharmacotherapy alone has been associated with substantial relapse and less overall effectiveness than CBT (Bacaltchuk et al., 2000; Casper, 2002; Fairburn & Harrison, 2003; Mitchell et al., 2003; Zhu & Walsh, 2002).

Combined Modalities: Integrating Pharmacology and Psychology

Newer research in the treatment of eating disorders has focused on the efficacy of combining pharmacological and psychological interventions (Crow & Mitchell, 1996a, 1996b; Mitchell, Peterson, Myers, & Wonderlich, 2001; Mitchell et al., 2003). However, the cumulative results to date raise questions about whether medications (e.g., antidepressants) enhance treatment effects over and above those associated with CBT alone, especially over the long run when medication is withdrawn (Gowers & Bryant-Waugh, 2004; Mitchell et al., 2003).

For instance, Agras and colleagues (1992) compared the antidepressant desipramine alone to CBT alone, and the combination of CBT and antidepressant medication, in the treatment of BN. In this study, 71 participants were randomly assigned to one of the following groups: desipramine withdrawn at 16 weeks; desipramine withdrawn at 24 weeks; combined treatment (medication withdrawn at either 16 or 24 weeks); and 15 sessions of CBT. In general, CBT and the antidepressant–CBT combination both outperformed medication alone on measures of binge eating and purging. Most interestingly, the results of this study suggested that continued use of CBT prevented relapse in subjects withdrawn from medication at 16 weeks.

In a study combining group-administered CBT with tricyclic antidepressant medication, subjects in the combined condition showed a 51% abstinence rate in bulimic behaviors, compared to a 16% abstinence rate in the medication-only condition (Mitchell et al., 1990). By contrast, in a study of the treatment of binge eating as a method of facilitating weight loss in obese patients, the use of desipramine did not lead to greater improvements in binge-eating symptoms than CBT alone did. Neither CBT nor the combination of CBT with desipramine improved overall weight loss at the end of treatment or follow-up (Agras et al., 1994).

These contradictory findings suggest that the value of augmenting CBT with drug treatment for patients with BN or BED is still unclear and should be further studied (Agras, 1997; Crow & Mitchell, 1994; Fairburn & Harrison, 2003; Mitchell et al., 2003). Given the paucity of research focused on young samples, empirically supported conclusions about adjunctive pharmacotherapy with children and adolescents are premature at present (Gowers & Bryant-Waugh, 2004).

Prediction of Outcome

With the notable exception of the empirical support for CBT and IPT, there are very few data suggesting that different treatments have better or worse outcomes, and few differential outcome data based on treatment and symptom characteristics. For the most part, treatment effectiveness has been explored in relationship to *patient*, not *treatment*, characteristics.

Several writers (e.g., Eckert, 1985; Steinhausen, 2002) have reviewed prognostic indicators in AN. Favorable long-term prognosis has been related to early age at onset of illness (Halmi, 1974; Halmi, Brodland, & Rigas, 1975; Hsu, Crisp, & Harding, 1979; Morgan & Russell, 1975; Pierloot, Wellens, & Houben, 1975; Sturzenberger, Cantwell, Burroughs, Salkin, & Green, 1977; Theander, 1970). Poor outcomes have been associated with longer duration of illness and previous hospitalizations (Garfinkel et al., 1977; Howard, Evans, Quintero-Howard, Bowers, & Andersen, 1999; Hsu et al., 1979; Morgan & Russell, 1975; Pierloot et al., 1975; Seidensticher & Tzagournis, 1968; Steinhausen, Boyadjieva, Grigoriu-Serbanescu, Seidel, & Winkler Metzke, 2000; Zipfel, Lowe, Reas, Deter, & Herzog, 2000); very low weight during illness (Dally, 1969; Hsu et al., 1979; Morgan & Russell, 1975; Zipfel et al., 2000); and the presence of bulimic symptoms, such as vomiting and laxative abuse (Fichter & Quadflieg, 1999; Garfinkel et al., 1977; Halmi, 1974; Halmi et al., 1975; Hsu et al., 1979; Ostuzzi, Didonna, & Micciolo, 1999; Steinhausen, 2002; Zipfel et al., 2000).

Less commonly mentioned negative prognosticators include overestimation of body size (Garfinkel et al., 1977; Kalucy, Crisp, Lacy, &

Harding, 1977); premorbid personality and family relationship difficulties (Dally, 1969; Hsu et al., 1979; Morgan & Russell, 1975; Steinhausen, 2002); depressive and obsessive–compulsive symptoms (Halmi, Brodland, & Loney, 1973; Nilsson, Gillberg, Gillberg, & Rastam, 1999; Rastam, Gillberg, & Wentz, 2003; Signorini, Bellini, Pasanisi, Contaldo, & De Filippo, 2003; Steinhausen, 2002; Wentz, Gillberg, Gillberg, & Rastam, 2001); high rates of physical complaints (Halmi et al., 1973); and neuroticism (Dally, 1969; Pierloot et al., 1975; Steinhausen, 2002). Although some research has suggested that lower socioeconomic status may be associated with a less favorable outcome (Garfinkel et al., 1977; Halmi et al., 1973; Hsu et al., 1979; Seidensticher & Tzagournis, 1968), others (e.g., Steinhausen, 2002) raise questions about the predictive value of socioeconomic factors.

Research focusing on the 10-year follow-up of a sample of 76 severely ill females with AN suggested that the disorder can be variable in course, chronicity, and outcome (Eckert, Halmi, Marchi, Grove, & Crosby, 1995). At the 10-year follow-up, 23.7% of the sample had no diagnosis; 35.5% were diagnosed with eating disorder not otherwise specified; 22.4% met diagnostic criteria for BN; 9.2% met diagnostic criteria for AN; 2.65% met diagnostic criteria for both AN and BN; and 6.6% of the sample had died. In addition, the patients in this sample with AN were found to live alone and remain single longer than typical. Furthermore, participants in this sample, when married, had fewer than expected offspring relative to age- and sex-matched populations. Finally, this group appeared to have had a higher than expected level of induced abortions. Wonderlich, Fullerton, Swift, and Klein (1994), in a 5-year outcome study of 30 patients with eating disorders, found that those with personality disorders did not differ consistently in the amount of symptomatic change over time from those without personality disorders. Steinhausen (1995a), in a review of 68 outcome studies on AN conducted from 1953 to 1989, concluded that early age of onset, histrionic personality, conflict-free parent–child relationships, short interval between onset and treatment, short duration of inpatient treatment without readmission, and high socioeconomic status/education were favorable prognostic indicators. Unfavorable prognostic indicators included vomiting and other bulimic symptoms, high loss of weight, chronicity, and premorbid developmental and/or clinical abnormalities. In an updated review, Steinhausen (2002) concluded that the outcome of AN had not improved significantly over the second half of the 20th century, with fewer than half of patients recovering fully, approximately 33% showing some improvement, and 20% continuing to struggle with AN.

Several reviews on the outcome of patients with BN have been published. For instance, Hsu (1995) suggested that the most common difficulty at follow-up is subsyndromal bulimia, followed by full BN. In general, after CBT, approximately 50% of patients with BN were asymptomatic at 2- to 10-year follow-up. Average-weight patients with bulimia did not tend to develop AN, and their rate of obesity was found to be lower than that of the general population. Herzog and colleagues (1993) found percentage of body weight increase and type of eating disorder to be the only variables associated with outcome during a 1-year follow-up. Specifically, patients diagnosed with BN tended to fare better than those diagnosed with either AN or both BN and AN (by DSM-III-R criteria). With respect to body weight, each 10% increase in percentage of body weight was associated with an 18% increase in hazard. More recently, a review of women diagnosed with BN between 1981 and 1987 (Keel, Mitchell, Miller, Davis, & Crow, 1999) concluded that symptom duration at baseline and substance use history were unfavorable prognostic indicators.

Rorty, Yager, and Rossotto (1993) examined the factors that former patients with BN felt were especially instrumental in their recovery. Responses from 40 female participants suggested several such factors, including a sense of being "fed up" with the disorder, the desire to have a better life, the importance/difficulty of cognitive change, and the development of empathic and caring relationships with others. Factors perceived by the former patients as making recovery more difficult included lack of understanding by important others, insufficient acknowledgment or activity by therapists, and the sabotage of the healing process by family members or others.

Although not focused specifically on treatment outcome, a recent study on the natural course of BN and BED in community women (Fairburn, Cooper, Doll, Norman, & O'Connor, 2000) highlighted the differential outcome of these two disorders. Over a 5-year period, the majority of those with BED were considered to have recovered; the course of those with BN was more variable, punctuated by higher relapse rates and marked by less positive overall outcome.

In considering treatment outcome data, it is worth noting that several concerns have been raised about the conceptualization and assessment of recovery represented in the current literature. For instance, Windauer, Lennerts, Talbot, Touyz, and Beumont (1993) have stressed the importance of validating outcome measures on which conclusions of "cure" are based. Jarmon and Walsh (1999) raised similar questions and further recommend increased science-practice integration in the development of improved methodologies for assessing outcomes.

CONCLUSIONS

This chapter has reviewed the considerable controversy and complexity surrounding the treatment of the eating disorders (i.e., AN, BN, and BED). The field currently is one of intense activity and interest. Yet few questions about these disorders have been answered definitively. It is now time for a comprehensive view of eating disorders—one that recognizes the interplay among biological, social, behavioral, and psychological factors. The importance of cultural factors (such as the changing nature of women's roles) is increasing at the same time that biological factors (such as neurological functioning) are being explored. The *Zeitgeist* encourages clinicians to incorporate recognition of these different spheres in their treatment of clients with eating disorders.

Although eating disorders are very complex and multifactorial, much of the current research suffers from significant deficiencies that makes it difficult to determine the value or importance of many potential etiologies and treatments (e.g., Ben-Tovim, 2003; Gowers & Bryant-Waugh, 2004; Keel & Mitchell, 1997). Accordingly, several issues deserve further attention in future research.

Issue 1: Are Eating Disorders Distinct Disorders?

Although nosological or syndromal classification is the standard in mental health in general and for eating disorders in particular, some have suggested that eating disorders may not be distinct disorders. For example, it is well known that patients with eating disorders experience a high frequency of comorbid psychological conditions, including mood, anxiety, and substance use disorders (Braun & Chouinard, 1992; Cooper, 1995; Holderness, Brooks-Gunn, & Warren, 1994; Wilson, 1995). Among the reasons for this high frequency of co-occurrence are overlap in symptoms for the different syndromes, poor interrater reliability of many psychiatric diagnostic categories, and the common biological pathways that have been implicated in these disorders (Brewerton, 1995; Jarry & Vaccarino, 1996; Kaye, Weltzin, Hsu, & Bulik, 1991; van Praag, 1993). For example, some Axis I disorders have kappa coefficients below .70, indicating less than adequate reliability (Kirk & Kutchins, 1992). In addition, the neurotransmitter serotonin is thought to play a role in the etiology or maintenance of eating disorders, substance use disorders, depression, and obsessive–compulsive disorder; this suggests a common physiological mechanism, even though they all are supposed to be distinct disorders (Brewerton, 1995). Also, many of the cognitive and behavioral features of each of these disorders are observationally and phenomenologically similar and seem to elicit the same physiological reward mechanisms. Finally, none of these disorders has a distinct and reliable biological marker that is not shared by one of the mentioned comorbid conditions (Gillberg, 1994; Jarry & Vaccarino, 1996). Based on this evidence, some investigators have concluded that eating disorders may be addictions or may exist on a continuum with obsessive–compulsive disorder (Gold, 1993; Jarry & Vaccarino, 1996; Parham, 1995).

Yet discontinuities between eating disorders and other disorders have also been highlighted in recent years. For instance, as discussed above, the frequency with which co-occurring medical and mood symptoms resolve with increased and/or better-regulated food intake runs counter to the assumption that eating disorders simply represent atypical forms of other conditions (APA, 1996). Moreover, several studies suggest that AN and BN may share specific familial liability that is distinct from that involved in other comorbid problems, such as major depressive disorder and substance dependence (Kaye, Strober, Stein, & Gendall, 1999; Lilenfeld et al., 1998; Strober,

Lampert, Morrell, Burroughs, & Jacobs, 1990; Strober et al., 2000). Further buttressing arguments for the separation of eating from other disorders such as substance dependence is the evidence that the central features of addiction (e.g., tolerance and withdrawal) do not apply to food (Goodrick, 2000; Haddock & Dill, 2000; Wilson, 1991, 1995, 2000; see Poston & Haddock, 2000, for detailed discussions of food as a drug). Finally, "the fact that eating disorders do not evolve into other conditions lends support to the distinctiveness of the diagnostic category as a whole" (Fairburn & Harrison, 2003, p. 409). Hence recent evidence provides at least some support for the divergence of eating disorders from several other psychiatric conditions.

Issue 2: Are We Focusing on the Wrong Areas?

In spite of a voluminous literature on the etiology of eating disorders, with a particular focus on physiological and personality factors, the results of treatment outcome studies for eating disorders are less than satisfying. Patients with eating disorders appear to have high relapse rates, experience their disorders for long periods of time, and often suffer from several other comorbid psychiatric conditions (Ben-Tovim, 2003; Fairburn & Harrison, 2003; Keller et al., 1992; Kirschenbaum & Fitzgibbon, 1995). The continued emphasis on internal-defect models, rather than a focus on social and cultural risk factors, is puzzling (Bulik et al., 2000; Pate, Pumariega, Hester, & Garner, 1992; Striegel-Moore, 1995), given that "no study has found genetic effects alone to account for liability to eating disorders or traits" (Bulik et al., 2000, p. 17). Indeed, research has consistently reaffirmed the role of individual-specific environmental factors (Bulik et al., 2000; Jacobi et al., 2004) and the importance of complicated gene–environment transactions, in which polygenic diatheses may be protean in their manifestation across different environmental contexts (Bulik et al., 2000; Jacobi et al., 2004; Kendler, 2001). If we are to generate the new perspectives necessary to effectively prevent and treat eating disorders (discussed above), there is a clear need for truly integrated biopsychosocial perspectives highlighting which aspects of the environment may be particularly hazardous or "toxic" (e.g., Horgen & Brownell, 2002) for which individuals (Bulik et al., 2000; Jacobi et al., 2004; Kendler, 2001).

Issue 3: What Are We Missing?

There are several deficiencies in the eating disorder literature that merit attention. First, there is a strong need for epidemiological research with culturally diverse populations and in different countries (Gillberg, 1994; Keel & Klump, 2003; Pate et al., 1992; Study Group on Anorexia Nervosa, 1995; Wildes et al., 2001). For example, many of the conclusions drawn about the etiology and treatment outcome of eating disorders have been based on work with potentially biased samples (e.g., clinic-based, inpatient, and ethnically homogeneous groups). In addition, there still exists relatively little systematic epidemiological research focused on cross-cultural groups and children, although it is increasing (Gowers & Bryant-Waugh, 2004; Jacobi et al., 2004; Pate et al., 1992). It therefore is premature to debate whether the prevalence of eating disorders is increasing or becoming epidemic, because our prevalence estimates are based all too often on nonrepresentative samples (Gillberg, 1994; Gowers & Bryant-Waugh, 2004).

Another problem in the science of eating disorders is the lack of prospective and replication studies, adequate sampling and sample sizes, and appropriate analyses in both determinant and treatment outcome studies (e.g., Ericsson et al., 1996). Some studies of biological determinants suffer from small sample sizes and uncorrected statistical analyses, which lead to illusory biological differences. There is very little replication of these findings or of potentially important and useful results that may have come from more controlled studies (Gillberg, 1994). Finally, it is possible that some of the lack of reproducibility or reliability of findings lies in the narrow nosological classification system currently in favor. A system of functional classification may help to alleviate this problem by making the psychological dysfunction the elementary unit of analysis, rather than a broader and potentially less reliable syndrome (van Praag, 1993). In fact, many biological variables that have low diagnostic specificity when syndromes are considered can be related very strongly to specific psychopathological dimensions—for instance, serotonin disturbance as a moderator for disturbed aggression regulation, because low serotonin has been found to play a role in suicidal behavior, eating disorders, and aggression (van Praag, 1993).

Future research should focus on these issues in order to adequately address the problem of eating disorders.

Issue 4: Treatment and Prevention Needs

One of the most significant issues in the treatment of eating disorders is the growing recognition that a narrow behavioral focus on the disordered eating may not address important core issues that may play a role in the etiology and maintenance of eating disorders. Primary in this area is a recognition that dysfunctional interpersonal relationships and sociocultural pressures may be at the heart of eating disorders. Thus there is a need to determine whether focusing on interpersonal relationships might be more effective than a sole focus on disordered eating per se. Although IPT did not lead to further improvements in patients who did not respond to CBT (Agras et al., 1995), Wilfley and colleagues (1993) found that IPT was as effective as CBT for nonpurging BN. It is worth noting in this regard that Fairburn and colleagues (2003) have developed a new transdiagnostic theory and treatment strategy, broadening the focus of CBT to include interpersonal difficulties as one of several additional treatment modules.

Because eating disorders are associated with poor body image and low self-esteem, research should also focus on determining whether exercise can play a role in treatment. Higher levels of physical fitness are associated with positive mental health, enhanced self-esteem, reduced anxiety, and improved body image in women (Grilo, Brownell, & Stunkard, 1993; Salusso-Deonier & Schwarzkopf, 1991). Exercise may improve eating control through changes in endogenous opioid channels (Brewerton, Lydiard, Laraia, Shook, & Ballenger, 1992). These changes may facilitate improvements in mood and enhanced feelings of energy, which may help reduce eating dyscontrol associated with negative affect. Given preliminary research (discussed in the section on physical activity above) suggesting that appropriate exercise may benefit patients with eating disorders, additional work in this area is of paramount importance.

Medications are frequently promoted as a primary treatment modality, due to the tendency to view eating disorders as caused by biological deficiencies. This occurs despite the weak evidence for a biological etiology, and the fact that eating disorders occur disproportionately in women and in cultures emphasizing thinness as a value for women. Although the rewarding effects of eating can be inhibited by opiate antagonists (Marrazzi, Markham, Kinzie, & Luby, 1995), and although binge eating and vomiting can be reduced through the administration of SSRIs (Goldstein et al., 1995), medications do not address many patients' problems of social isolation and perceived lack of nurturance from interpersonal relationships. Indeed, use of prescription medications for the treatment of eating disorders may inappropriately replace needed therapy, because the provider and patient desire quick and easy solutions. Further research is crucial to evaluate whether and to what extent medications add to the effectiveness of empirically supported psychological approaches, as well as to determine how such medication regimens can be administered in controlled, ethical ways.

Public health measures are vital to help prevent the development of eating disorders. Unfortunately, there is a serious dearth of information about effective prevention programming; this is in part due to the complex nature of eating disorders, which frustrates efforts to untie the Gordian knot of associated risk and protective factors (Fairburn, 1995; Huon, Braganza, Brown, Ritchie, & Roncolato, 1998; Piran, 1999; Steiner et al., 2003). Additional research on cultural factors that may predispose some women to develop eating disorders, as well as on strategies for helping women resist unhealthy social pressures, is imperative (Battle & Brownell, 1996; Foreyt, Poston, & Goodrick, 1996; Piran, 1999; Steiner et al., 2003). Moreover, there is a clear need for targeted prevention efforts for high-risk populations, such as athletes and women with a family history of eating disorders. For example, an extended prevention program in a residential ballet school focused on changing the sociocultural climate—including peer relations, faculty–student interactions, the inculcation of healthy habits and systemwide norms (Piran, 1999)—has shown preliminary promise in preventing "even harsh external pressures, from being internalized and resulting in potentially self-destructive patterns of behavior" (Piran, 1999, p. 88). Other innovative efforts to target high-risk women have included Internet-based psychoeducational self-help programs (Zabinski et al., 2001) and multistage models for reaching high-risk women within college campus communities (e.g., Schwitzer, Bergholz, Dore, & Salimi, 1998).

However, the optimal combination, sequencing, and targeting of preventive efforts have yet to be identified (for a recent review, see, e.g., Stice & Shaw, 2004). Indeed, there are indications that some preventive interventions may be associated with unintended negative consequences. For instance, Mann and colleagues (1997) found that combining primary and secondary prevention efforts not only was ineffective in ameliorating dysfunctional eating, but resulted in a small increase in symptoms. Reflecting on these results, the authors reasoned that reducing the stigma of eating disorders during the intervention may have "normalized" these behaviors from the perspective of participants (Mann et al., 1997). Similarly, given that obesity poses serious health risks to an increasing proportion of the population (Terre et al., 2005), it will be challenging to titrate a broad public health message to motivate the initiation and maintenance of healthful weight control practices without promoting the maladaptive excesses associated with cultural pressures toward thinness.

By comparison to the emphasis on risk factors, the relative neglect of health-related competencies continues to represent a strategic oversight, considering that certain healthful practices (e.g., regular, appropriate exercise) may attenuate some of the factors associated with disordered eating, including stress and other negative mood states (Terre, 1993). Hence there is an important need for a more balanced focus in both research and preventive intervention efforts (Steiner et al., 2003; Terre, 1993). Although there will always be a role for treatment at the tertiary level, primary prevention efforts hold considerable promise for truly addressing and reducing the tremendous social impact of eating disorders.

ACKNOWLEDGMENTS

Thanks to Jill K. McGavin and Allen A. Winebarger for their contributions to earlier editions of this chapter. Preparation of this chapter was partially supported by grants from the National Institutes of Health, National Institute of Diabetes and Digestive and Kidney Diseases (1RO1-DK064284 and 5UO1-DK57177-05), and the Agency for Healthcare Research and Quality (3RO1-HSO-11282-02S1).

NOTE

1. Some of the more prominent programs that provide inpatient treatment, partial hospitalization, and/or outpatient treatment include The Renfro Center in Philadelphia; Remuda Ranch in Wickenberg, Arizona; Laureate in Tulsa, Oklahoma; Rogers Memorial Hospital in Oconomowoc, Wisconsin; Stanford University Medical School; University of Iowa Medical School; University of New Mexico Medical School; Yale University Medical School; the Neuropsychiatric Institute at the University of California, Los Angeles; Toronto General Hospital and the University of Toronto; University of Cincinnati Medical Center; and the University of Minnesota Medical School.

REFERENCES

Abella, E., Feliu, E., Granada, I., Milla, F., Oriol, A., Ribera, J., et al. (2002). Bone marrow changes in anorexia nervosa are correlated with the amount of weight loss and not with other clinical findings. *American Journal of Clinical Pathology, 118*(4), 582–588.

Abraham, S. F., & Beumont, P. J. V. (1982). How patients describe bulimia or binge eating. *Psychological Medicine, 12,* 625–635.

Advokat, C., & Kutlesic, V. (1995). Pharmacotherapy of the eating disorders: A commentary. *Neuroscience and Biobehavioral Reviews, 19,* 59–66.

Agras, W. S. (1991). Nonpharmacologic treatments of bulimia nervosa. *Journal of Clinical Psychiatry, 52*(10, Suppl.), 29–33.

Agras, W. S. (1997). The treatment of bulimia nervosa. *Drugs of Today, 33,* 405–411.

Agras, W. S. (2001). The consequences and costs of the eating disorders. *Psychiatric Clinics of North America, 24*(2), 371–379.

Agras, W. S., & Kirkley, B. G. (1986). Bulimia: Theories of etiology. In K. D. Brownell & J. P. Foreyt (Eds.), *Handbook of eating disorders: Physiology, psychology, and treatment of obesity, anorexia, and bulimia* (pp. 367–378). New York: Basic Books.

Agras, W. S., Rossiter, E. M., Arnow, B., Schneider, J. A., Telch, C. F., Raeburn, S. D., et al. (1992). Pharmacologic and cognitive-behavioral treatment for bulimia nervosa: A controlled comparison. *American Journal of Psychiatry, 149,* 82–87.

Agras, W. S., Schneider, J. A., Arnow, B., Raeburn, S. D., & Telch, C. F. (1989). Cognitive-behavioral and response-prevention treatments for bulimia nervosa. *Journal of Consulting and Clinical Psychology, 57,* 215–221.

Agras, W. S., Telch, C. F., Arnow, B., Eldredge, K., Detzer, M. J., Henderson, J., et al. (1995). Does interpersonal therapy help patients with binge eating disorder who fail to respond to cognitive-behavioral therapy? *Journal of Consulting and Clinical Psychology, 63,* 356–360.

Agras, W. S., Telch, C. F., Arnow, B., Eldredge, K., Wilfley, D. E., Raeburn, S. D., et al. (1994). Weight loss, cognitive-behavioral, and desipramine treatments in binge eating disorder: An additive design. *Behavior Therapy, 25,* 225–238.

Agras, W. S., Walsh, B. T., Fairburn, C. G., Wilson, G. T., & Kraemer, H. C. (2000). A multicenter comparison of cognitive-behavioral therapy and interpersonal psychotherapy for bulimia nervosa. *Archives of General Psychiatry, 57,* 459–466.

Ainsworth, C., Waller, G., & Kennedy, F. (2002). Threat processing in women with bulimia. *Clinical Psychology Review, 22*(8), 1155–1178.

American Dietetic Association. (2001). Position of the American Dietetic Association: Nutrition intervention in the treatment of anorexia nervosa, bulimia nervosa, and eating disorders not otherwise specified (EDNOS). *Journal of the American Dietetic Association, 101*(7), 810–819.

American Psychiatric Association (APA). (1987). *Diagnostic and statistical manual of mental disorders* (3rd ed., rev.). Washington, DC: Author.

American Psychiatric Association (APA). (1996). *Practice guidelines.* Washington, DC: Author.

American Psychiatric Association (APA). (2000). *Diagnostic and statistical manual of mental disorders text revision* (4th ed., text rev.). Washington, DC: Author.

Andersen, A. E. (1986). Inpatient and outpatient treatment of anorexia nervosa. In K. D. Brownell & J. P. Foreyt (Eds.), *Handbook of eating disorders: Physiology, psychology, and treatment of obesity, anorexia, and bulimia* (pp. 333–352). New York: Basic Books.

Andersen, A. E., Bowers, W., & Evans, K. (1997). Inpatient treatment of anorexia nervosa. In D. M. Garner & P. E. Garfinkel (Eds.), *Handbook of treatment for eating disorders* (2nd ed., pp. 327–353). New York: Guilford Press.

Anderson, D., & Maloney, K. (2001). The efficacy of cognitive-behavioral therapy on the core symptoms of bulimia nervosa. *Clinical Psychology Review, 21*(7), 971–988.

Anderson, L., Shaw, J., & McCargar, L. (1997). Physiological effects of bulimia nervosa on the gastrointestinal tract. *Canadian Journal of Gastroenterology, 11*(5), 451–459.

Anonymous. (2001). Deriving behavioural phenotypes in an international, multi-centre study of eating disorders. *Psychological Medicine, 31*(4), 635–645.

Anzai, N., Lindsey-Dudley, K., & Bidwell, R. (2002). Inpatient and partial hospital treatment for adolescent eating disorders. *Child and Adolescent Psychiatric Clinics of North America, 11*(2), 279–309.

Ash, J. B., & Piazza, E. (1995). Changing symptomatology in eating disorders. *International Journal of Eating Disorders, 18,* 27–38.

Attia, E., Mayer, L., & Killory, E. (2001). Medication

response in the treatment of patients with anorexia nervosa. *Journal of Psychiatric Practice, 7*(3), 157–162.

Bachrach, A. J., Erwin, W. J., & Mohr, P. J. (1965). The control of eating behavior in an anorexic by operant conditioning techniques. In L. Ullmann & L. Krasner (Eds.), *Case studies in behavior modification* (pp. 153–163). New York: Holt, Rinehart & Winston.

Bailer, U., & Kaye, W. (2003). A review of neuropeptide and neuroendocrine dysregulation in anorexia and bulimia nervosa. *Current Drug Targets–CNS and Neurological Disorders, 2*(1), 53–59.

Bailey, R., Yager, J., & Jenson, J. (2002). The psychiatrist as clinical computerologist in the treatment of adolescents: Old barks in new bytes. *American Journal of Psychiatry, 159*(8), 1298–1304.

Balcaltchuk, J., Hay, P., & Mari, J. (2000). Antidepressants versus placebo for the treatment of bulimia nervosa: A systematic review. *Australian and New Zealand Journal of Psychiatry, 34*(2), 310–317.

Baranowska, B., Radzikowska, M., Wasilewska-Dziubinska, E., Roguski, K., & Borowiec, M. (2000). Disturbed release of gastrointestinal peptides in anorexia nervosa and in obesity. *Diabetes, Obesity and Metabolism, 2*(2), 99–103.

Barbarich, N., Kaye, W., & Jimerson, D. (2003). Neurotransmitter and imaging studies in anorexia nervosa: New targets for treatment. *Current Drug Targets—CNS and Neurological Disorders, 2*, 61–62.

Bartholomew, T., & Paxton, S. (2003). General practitioners' perspectives regarding competence and confidentiality in an adolescent with suspected anorexia nervosa: Legal and ethical considerations. *Journal of Law and Medicine, 10*(3), 308–324.

Battle, E. K., & Brownell, K. D. (1996). Confronting a rising tide of eating disorders and obesity: Treatment vs. prevention and policy. *Addictive Behaviors, 21*, 755–765.

Beck, A. (1976). *Cognitive therapy and the emotional disorders.* New York: International Universities Press.

Bell, R. M. (1985). *Holy anorexia.* Chicago: University of Chicago Press.

Bemis, K. M. (1978). Current approaches to the etiology and treatment of anorexia nervosa. *Psychological Bulletin, 85*, 593–617.

Ben-Tovim, D. (2003). Eating disorders: Outcome, prevention and treatment of eating disorders. *Current Opinion in Psychiatry, 16*, 65–69.

Bergh, C., Brodin, U., Lindberg, G., & Sodersten, P. (2002). Randomized controlled trial of a treatment for anorexia and bulimia nervosa. *Proceedings of the National Academy of Sciences USA, 99*(14), 9486–9491.

Berghold, K., & Lock, J. (2002). Assessing guilt in adolescents with anorexia nervosa. *American Journal of Psychotherapy, 56*(3), 378–390.

Bettle, N., Bettle, O., Neumarker, U., & Neumarker, K. (1998). Adolescent ballet school students: Their quest for body weight change. *Psychopathology, 31*(3), 153–159.

Beumont, P. J. V. (1977). Further categorization of patients with anorexia nervosa. *Australian and New Zealand Journal of Psychiatry, 11*, 223–226.

Beumont, P. J. V., Abraham, S. F., Argall, W. J., George, C. W., & Glaun, D. E. (1978). The onset of anorexia nervosa. *Australian and New Zealand Journal of Psychiatry, 12*, 145–149.

Beumont, P. J. V., Beumont, C. C., Touyz, S. W., & Williams, H. (1997). Nutritional counseling and supervised exercise. In D. M. Garner & P. E. Garfinkel (Eds.), *Handbook of treatment for eating disorders* (2nd ed., pp. 178–187). New York: Guilford Press.

Beumont, P. J. V., Booth, A. L., Abraham, S. F., Griffiths, D. A., & Turner, T. R. (1983). A temporal sequence of symptoms in patients with anorexia nervosa: A preliminary report. In P. L. Darby, P. E. Garfinkel, D. M. Garner, & D. V. Coscina (Eds.), *Anorexia nervosa: Recent developments in research* (pp. 129–136). New York: Liss.

Binswanger, L. (1958). The case of Ellen West. In R. May, E. Angel, & H. F. Ellenberger (Eds.), *Existence: A new dimension in psychiatry and psychology* (pp. 236–363). New York: Basic Books.

Boskind-Lodahl, M., & White, W. C. (1978). The definition and treatment of bulimarexia in college women: A pilot study. *Journal of the American College Health Association, 27*, 84–86.

Bowers, W. (2001). Basic principles for applying cognitive-behavioral therapy to anorexia nervosa. *Psychiatric Clinics of North America, 24*(2), 293–303.

Brambilla, F. (2001). Aetiopathogenesis and pathophysiology of bulimia nervosa: Biological bases and implications for treatment. *CNS Drugs, 15*(2), 119–136.

Brambilla, F., Bellodi, L., Perna, G., Barberi, A., Panerai, A., & Sacerdote, P. (1993). Lymphocyte cholecystokinin concentrations in panic disorder. *American Journal of Psychiatry, 150*, 1111–1113.

Braun, C. M. J., & Chouinard, M. J. (1992). Is anorexia nervosa a neuropsychological disease? *Neuropsychology Review, 3*, 171–212.

Breiner, S. (2003). An evidence-based eating disorder program. *Journal of Pediatric Nursing, 18*(1), 75–80.

Brewerton, T. D. (1995). Toward a unified theory of serotonin dysregulation in eating and related disorders. *Psychoneuroendocrinology, 20*(6), 561–590.

Brewerton, T. D. (2002). Bulimia in children and adolescents. *Child and Adolescent Psychiatric Clinics of North America, 11*(2), 237–256.

Brewerton, T. D., Lydiard, R. B., Laraia, M. T., Shook, J. E., & Ballenger, J. C. (1992). CSF beta-endorphin and dynorphin in bulimia nervosa. *American Journal of Psychiatry, 149*, 1086–1090.

Brody, M. L., Walsh, B. T., & Devlin, M. (1994). Binge eating disorder: Reliability and validity of a new diagnostic category. *Journal of Consulting and Clinical Psychology, 62*, 381–386.

Bruch, H. (1973). *Eating disorders: Obesity, anorexia nervosa and the person within*. New York: Basic Books.

Bruch, H. (1985). Four decades of eating disorders. In D. M. Garner & P. E. Garfinkel (Eds.), *Handbook of psychotherapy for anorexia nervosa and bulimia* (pp. 7–18). New York: Guilford Press.

Bulik, C. (2002). Eating disorders in adolescents and young adults. *Child and Adolescent Psychiatric Clinics of North America, 11*(2), 201–218.

Bulik, C., Sullivan, P., Carter, F., McIntosh, V., & Joyce, P. (1998). The role of exposure with response prevention in the cognitive-behavioural therapy for bulimia nervosa. *Psychological Medicine, 28*(3), 611–623.

Bulik, C., Sullivan, P., Wade, T., & Kendler, K. (2000). Twin studies of eating disorders: A review. *International Journal of Eating Disorders, 27*(1), 1–20.

Byrne, S., & McLean, N. (2001). Eating disorders in athletes: A review of the literature. *Journal of Science and Medicine in Sport, 4*(2), 145–159.

Carraro, A., Cognolato, S., & Bernardis, A. (1998). Evaluation of a programme of adapted physical activity for ED patients. *Eating and Weight Disorders, 3*(3), 110–114.

Carter, F., McIntosh, V., Joyce, P., Sullivan, P., & Bulik, C. (2003). Role of exposure with response prevention in cognitive-behavioral therapy for bulimia nervosa: Three-year follow-up results. *International Journal of Eating Disorders, 33*(2), 127–135.

Caruso, D., & Klein, H. (1998). Diagnosis and treatment of bulimia nervosa. *Seminars in Gastrointestinal Disease, 9*(4), 176–182.

Casper, R. C. (2002). How useful are pharmacological treatments in eating disorders? *Psychopharmacology Bulletin, 36*(2), 88–104.

Casper, R. C., Eckert, E. D., Halmi, K. A., Goldberg, S. C., & Davis, J. M. (1980). Bulimia: Its incidence and clinical importance in patients with anorexia nervosa. *Archives of General Psychiatry, 37*, 1030–1040.

Casper, R. C., & Troiani, M. (2001). Family functioning in anorexia nervosa differs by subtype. *International Journal of Eating Disorders, 30*(3), 338–342.

Centers for Disease Control and Prevention. (1997). Cardiac valvulopathy associated with fenfluramine or dexfenfluramine: U.S. Department of Health and Human Services interim public health recommendations, November 1997. *Morbidity and Mortality Weekly Report, 46*, 1061–1066.

Chambless, D., Baker, M., Baucom, D., Beutler, L., Calhoun, K., Crits-Cristoph, P., et al. (1998). Update on empirically validated therapies II. *The Clinical Psychologist, 51*(1), 3–16.

Chowdhury, U., Gordon, I., Lask, B., Watkins, B., Watt, H., & Christie, D. (2003). Early-onset anorexia nervosa: Is there evidence of limbic system imbalance? *International Journal of Eating Disorders, 33*(4), 388–396.

Cloninger, C. R. (1986). A unified biosocial theory of

personality and its role in the development of anxiety states. *Psychiatric Development, 3*, 167–226.

Cloninger, C. R. (1988). A unified biosocial theory of personality and its role in the development of anxiety states: A reply to commentaries. *Psychiatric Development, 2*, 83–120.

Cnattingius, S., Hultman, C., Dahl, M., & Sparen, P. (1999). Very preterm birth, birth trauma, and the risk of anorexia nervosa among girls. *Archives of General Psychiatry, 56*(7), 634–638.

Connolly, H. M., Crary, J. L., McGoon, M. D., Hensrud, D. D., Edwards, B. S., Edwards, W. D., et al. (1997). Valvular heart disease associated with fenfluramine–phentermine. *New England Journal of Medicine, 337*, 581–588.

Connors, M. E., Johnson, C. L., & Stuckey, M. K. (1984). Treatment of bulimia with brief psychoeducational group therapy. *American Journal of Psychiatry, 141*, 1512–1516.

Cooper, P. J. (1995). Eating disorders and their relationship to mood and anxiety disorders. In K. D. Brownell & C. G. Fairburn (Eds.), *Eating disorders and obesity: A comprehensive handbook* (pp. 159–164). New York: Guilford Press.

Cooper, P. J., & Steere, J. (1995). A comparison of two psychological treatments for bulimia nervosa: Implications for models of maintenance. *Behaviour Research and Therapy, 33*, 875–885.

Cooper, P. J., Watkins, B., Bryant-Waugh, R., & Lask, B. (2002). The nosological status of early onset anorexia nervosa. *Psychological Medicine, 32*(5), 873–880.

Cooper, Z., Fairburn, C. G., & Hawker, D. M. (2003). *Cognitive-behavioral treatment of obesity: A clinician's guide*. New York: Guilford Press.

Costa, J., Brennen, M., & Hochgeschwender, U. (2002). The human genetics of eating disorders: Lessons from the leptin/melanocortin system. *Child and Adolescent Psychiatric Clinics of North America, 11*(2), 387–397.

Craighead, L. W., & Agras, W. S. (1991). Mechanisms of action in cognitive-behavioral and pharmacological interventions for obesity and bulimia nervosa. *Journal of Consulting and Clinical Psychology, 59*, 115–125.

Crisp, A. H., Hsu, L. K., Harding, B., & Hartshorn, J. (1980). Clinical features of anorexia nervosa: A study of a consecutive series of 102 female patients. *Journal of Psychosomatic Research, 24*, 179–191.

Crisp, A. H., Norton, K., Gowers, S., Halek, C., Bowyer, C., Yeldham, D., et al. (1991). A controlled study of the effect of therapies aimed at adolescent and family psychopathology in anorexia nervosa. *British Journal of Psychiatry, 159*, 325–333.

Crisp, A. H., Palmer, R. L., & Kalucy, R. S. (1976). How common is anorexia nervosa?: A prevalence study. *British Journal of Psychiatry, 218*, 549–554.

Crow, S. J., & Mitchell, J. E. (1994). Rational therapy of eating disorders. *Drugs, 48*, 372–379.

Crow, S. J., & Mitchell, J. E. (1996a). Pharmacological

treatments for eating disorders. In J. K. Thompson (Ed.), *Body image, eating disorders, and obesity: An integrative guide for assessment and treatment* (pp. 345–360). Washington, DC: American Psychological Association.

Crow, S. J., & Mitchell, J. E. (1996b). Integrating cognitive therapy and medications in treating bulimia nervosa. *Psychiatric Clinics of North America, 19,* 755–760.

Cummings, M., Waller, D., Johnson, C., Bradley, K., Leatherwood, D., & Guzzetta, C. (2001). Developing and implementing a comprehensive program for children and adolescents with eating disorders. *Journal of Child and Adolescent Psychiatric Nursing, 14*(4), 167–178.

Cummings, S., Parham, E., & Strain, G. (2002). Position of the American Dietetic Association: Weight management. *Journal of the American Dietetic Association, 102*(8), 1145–1155.

Dalle-Grave, R., Ricca, V., & Todesco, T. (2001). The stepped-care approach in anorexia nervosa and bulimia nervosa: Progress and problems. *Eating and Weight Disorders, 6*(2), 81–89.

Dally, P. D. (1969). *Anorexia nervosa.* New York: Grune & Stratton.

Daluiski, A., Rahbar, B., & Meals, R. (1997). Russell's sign: Subtle hand changes in patients with bulimia nervosa. *Clinical Orthopaedics and Related Research, 343,* 107–109.

Dare, C., & Eisler, I. (1995). Family therapy and eating disorders. In K. D. Brownell & C. G. Fairburn (Eds.), *Eating disorders and obesity: A comprehensive handbook* (pp. 318–323). New York: Guilford Press.

Dare, C., & Eisler, I. (1997). Family therapy for anorexia nervosa. In D. M. Garner & P. E. Garfinkel (Eds.), *Handbook of treatment for eating disorders* (2nd ed., pp. 307–324). New York: Guilford Press.

Decaluwe, V., Braet, C., & Fairburn, C. (2003). Binge eating in obese children and adolescents. *International Journal of Eating Disorders, 33*(1), 78–84.

Devlin, M. J. (1996). Assessment and treatment of binge-eating disorder. *Psychiatric Clinics of North America, 19,* 761–772.

deZwaan, M. (2001). Binge eating disorder and obesity. *International Journal of Obesity and Related Metabolic Disorders, 25*(Suppl. 1), S51–S55.

Diler, R., & Avci, A. (2002). Selective serotonin reuptake inhibitors in children and adolescents. *Swiss Medical Weekly, 132*(33–34), 470–477.

Dingemans, A. E., Bruna, M. J., & van Furth, E. F. (2002). Binge eating disorder: A review. *International Journal of Obesity and Related Metabolic Disorders, 26*(3), 299–307.

Dobson, K., & Dozois, D. (2004). Attentional biases in eating disorders: A meta-analytic review of Stroop performance. *Clinical Psychology Review, 23,* 1001–1022.

Draper, H. (2000). Anorexia nervosa and respecting a refusal of life-prolonging therapy: A limited justification. *Bioethics, 14*(2), 120–133.

Drevelengas, A., Chourmouzi, D., Pitsavas, G., Charitandi, A., & Boulogianni, G. (2001). Reversible brain atrophy and subcortical high signal on MRI in a patient with anorexia nervosa. *Neuroradiology, 43*(10), 838–840.

Duesund, L., & Skarderud, F. (2003). Use the body and forget the body: Treating anorexia nervosa with adapted physical activity. *Clinical Child Psychology and Psychiatry, 8*(1), 53–72.

Eckert, E. D. (1985). Characteristics of anorexia nervosa. In J. E. Mitchell (Ed.), *Anorexia nervosa and bulimia: Diagnosis and treatment* (pp. 3–28). Minneapolis: University of Minnesota Press.

Eckert, E. D., Halmi, K. A., Marchi, P., Grove, W., & Crosby, R. (1995). Ten-year follow-up of anorexia nervosa: Clinical course and outcome. *Psychological Medicine, 25,* 143–156.

Eddy, K., Keel, P., Doer, D., Delinsky, S., Franko, D., & Herzog, D. (2002). Longitudinal comparison of anorexia nervosa subtypes. *International Journal of Eating Disorders, 31*(2), 191–201.

Edwards, M. D., & Kerry, I. (1993). Obesity, anorexia, and bulimia. *Clinical Nutrition, 77,* 899–909.

Eidem, B., Cetta, F., Webb, J., Graham, L., & Jay, M. (2001). Early detection of cardiac dysfunction: Use of the myocardial performance index in patients with anorexia nervosa. *Journal of Adolescent Health, 29*(4), 267–270.

English, A. (2002). The health of adolescent girls: Does the law support it? *Current Women's Health Reports, 2*(6), 442–449.

Ericsson, M., Poston, W. S., & Foreyt, J. P. (1996). Common biological pathways in eating disorders and obesity. *Addictive Behaviors, 21,* 733–743.

Everill, J. T., & Waller, G. (1995). Reported sexual abuse and eating psychopathology: A review of the evidence for a causal link. *International Journal of Eating Disorders, 18,* 1–11.

Fairburn, C. G. (1980). Self-induced vomiting. *Journal of Psychosomatic Research, 24,* 193–197.

Fairburn, C. G. (1995). The prevention of eating disorders. In K. D. Brownell & C. G. Fairburn (Eds.), *Eating disorders and obesity: A comprehensive handbook* (pp. 289–293). New York: Guilford Press.

Fairburn, C. G., & Cooper, P. J. (1982). Self-induced vomiting and bulimia nervosa: An undetected problem. *British Medical Journal, 284,* 1153–1155.

Fairburn, C. G., Cooper, Z., & Cooper, P. J. (1986). The clinical features and maintenance of bulimia nervosa. In K. D. Brownell & J. P. Foreyt (Eds.), *Handbook of eating disorders: Physiology, psychology, and treatment of obesity, anorexia, and bulimia* (pp. 389–404). New York: Basic Books.

Fairburn, C. G., Cooper, Z., Doll, H., Norman, P., & O'Connor, M. (2000). The natural course of bulimia nervosa and binge eating disorder in young women. *Archives of General Psychiatry, 57*(7), 659–665.

Fairburn, C. G., Cooper, Z., Doll, H., & Welch, S. (1999). Risk factors for anorexia nervosa: Three integrated case–control comparisons. *Archives of General Psychiatry, 56*(5), 468–476.

Fairburn, C. G., Cooper, Z, & Shafran, R. (2003). Cognitive behaviour therapy for eating disorders: A "transdiagnostic" theory and treatment. *Behaviour Research and Therapy, 41,* 509–528.

Fairburn, C. G., & Harrison, P. J. (2003). Eating disorders. *Lancet, 361,* 407–416.

Fairburn, C. G., Jones, R., Peveler, R. C., Hope, R., & O'Connor, M. (1993). Psychotherapy and bulimia nervosa: Longer-term effects of interpersonal psychotherapy, behavior therapy, and cognitive behavior therapy. *Archives of General Psychiatry, 50,* 419–428.

Fairburn, C. G., Marcus, M. D., & Wilson, G. T. (1993). Cognitive-behavioral therapy for binge eating and bulimia nervosa: A comprehensive treatment manual. In C. G. Fairburn & G. T. Wilson (Eds.), *Binge eating: Nature, assessment, and treatment* (pp. 361–404). New York: Guilford Press.

Fairburn, C. G., Norman, P. A., Welch, S. L., O'Connor, M. E., Doll, H. A., & Peveler, R. C. (1995). A prospective study of outcome in bulimia nervosa and the long-term effects of three psychological treatments. *Archives of General Psychiatry, 52,* 304–312.

Fairburn, C. G., Shafran, R., & Cooper, Z. (1999). A cognitive behavioural theory of anorexia nervosa. *Behaviour Research and Therapy, 37*(1), 1–13.

Fairburn, C. G., Welch, S., Doll, H., Davies, B., & O'Connor, M. (1997). Risk factors for bulimia nervosa: A community-based case–control study. *Archives of General Psychiatry, 54*(6), 509–517.

Fassino, S., Amianto, F., Gramaglia, C., Facchini, F., & Daga, G. (2004). Temperament and character in eating disorders: Ten years of studies. *Eating and Weight Disorders, 9*(2), 81–90.

Fassino, S., Leombruni, P., Daga, G., Brustolin, A., Migliaretti, G., Cavallo, F., et al. (2002). Efficacy of citalopram in anorexia nervosa: A pilot study. *European Neuropsychopharmacology, 12*(5), 453–459.

Fennig, S., Fennig, S., & Roe, D. (2002). Physical recovery in anorexia nervosa: Is this the sole purpose of a child and adolescent medical–psychiatric unit? *General Hospital Psychiatry, 24*(2), 87–92.

Fernandez, R. C. (1984). Disturbance in cognition: Implications for treatment. In P. S. Powers & R. C. Fernandez (Eds.), *Current treatment of anorexia nervosa and bulimia* (pp. 133–142). Basel, Switzerland: Karger.

Ferron, S. (1999). Occult gastrointestinal bleeding with anorexia nervosa. *American Journal of Psychiatry, 156*(5), 801.

Fichter, M. M. (1995). Inpatient treatment of anorexia nervosa. In K. D. Brownell & C. G. Fairburn (Eds.), *Eating disorders and obesity: A comprehensive handbook* (pp. 336–343). New York: Guilford Press.

Fichter, M. M., & Noegel, R. (1990). Concordance for bulimia nervosa in twins. *International Journal of Eating Disorders, 9,* 255–263.

Fichter, M. M., & Quadflieg, N. (1999). Six-year course and outcome of anorexia nervosa. *International Journal of Eating Disorders, 26*(4), 359–385.

First, M., Frances, A., & Pincus, H. (2002). *DSM-IV-TR handbook of differential diagnosis.* Washington, DC: American Psychiatric Publishing.

Fisher, M. (2003). The course and outcome of eating disorders in adults and in adolescents: A review. *Adolescent Medicine State of the Art Reviews, 14*(1), 149–158.

Fombonne, E. (1995). Anorexia nervosa: No evidence of an increase. *British Journal of Psychiatry, 166,* 462–471.

Foreyt, J. P., & McGavin, J. K. (1988). Anorexia and bulimia. In E. J. Mash & L. G. Terdal (Eds.), *Behavioral assessment of childhood disorders* (2nd ed., pp. 776–805). New York: Guilford Press.

Foreyt, J. P., & Mikhail, C. (1997). Anorexia and bulimia nervosa. In E. J. Mash & L. G. Terdal (Eds.), *Assessment of childhood disorders* (3rd ed., pp. 683–716). New York: Guilford Press.

Foreyt, J. P., Poston, W. S., & Goodrick, G. K. (1996). Future directions in obesity and eating disorders. *Addictive Behaviors, 21,* 767–778.

Fornari, V., & Dancyger, I. (2003). Psychosexual development and eating disorders. *Adolescent Medicine State of the Art Reviews, 14*(1), 61–75.

Frank, G., Kaye, W., Weltzin, T., Perel, J., Moss, H., McConaha, C., et al. (2001). Altered response to meta-chlorophenylpiperazine in anorexia nervosa: Support for a persistent alteration of serotonin activity after short-term weight restoration. *International Journal of Eating Disorders, 30*(1), 57–68.

Garfinkel, P. E. (1995). Classification and diagnosis of eating disorders. In K. D. Brownell & C. G. Fairburn (Eds.), *Eating disorders and obesity: A comprehensive handbook* (pp. 125–134). New York: Guilford Press.

Garfinkel, P. E., & Garner, D. M. (1982). *Anorexia nervosa: A multidimensional perspective.* New York: Brunner/Mazel.

Garfinkel, P. E., Garner, D. M., & Kennedy, S. (1985). Special problems of inpatient management. In D. M. Garner & P. E. Garfinkel (Eds.), *Handbook of psychotherapy for anorexia nervosa and bulimia* (pp. 344–362). New York: Guilford Press.

Garfinkel, P. E., & Kaplan, A. S. (1986). Anorexia nervosa: Diagnostic conceptualizations. In K. D. Brownell & J. P. Foreyt (Eds.), *Handbook of eating disorders: Physiology, psychology, and treatment of obesity, anorexia, and bulimia* (pp. 266–282). New York: Basic Books.

Garfinkel, P. E., Moldofsky, H., & Garner, D. M. (1977). The outcome of anorexia nervosa: Significance of clinical features, body image and behavior modification. In R. A. Vigersky (Ed.), *Anorexia nervosa* (pp. 315–330). New York: Raven Press.

Garfinkel, P. E., Moldofsky, H., & Garner, D. M. (1980). The heterogeneity of anorexia nervosa: Bulimia as a distinct subgroup. *Archives of General Psychiatry, 37,* 1036–1040.

Garfinkel, P. E., & Walsh, B. T. (1997). Drug therapies. In D. M. Garner & P. E. Garfinkel (Eds.), *Handbook of treatment for eating disorders* (2nd ed., pp. 373–380). New York: Guilford Press.

Garner, D. M. (1986). Cognitive therapy for anorexia nervosa. In K. D. Brownell & J. P. Foreyt (Eds.), *Handbook of eating disorders: Physiology, psychology, and treatment of obesity, anorexia, and bulimia* (pp. 301–327). New York: Basic Books.

Garner, D. M. (1997). Psychoeducational principles in treatment. In D. M. Garner & P. E. Garfinkel (Eds.), *Handbook of treatment for eating disorders* (2nd ed., pp. 145–177). New York: Guilford Press.

Garner, D. M., & Bemis, K. M. (1982). A cognitive behavioral approach to anorexia nervosa. *Cognitive Therapy and Research, 6,* 123–150.

Garner, D. M., & Bemis, K. M. (1985). Cognitive therapy for anorexia. In D. M. Garner & P. E. Garfinkel (Eds.), *Handbook of psychotherapy for anorexia nervosa and bulimia* (pp. 107–146). New York: Guilford Press.

Garner, D. M., & Garfinkel, P. E. (Eds.). (1985). *Handbook of psychotherapy for anorexia nervosa and bulimia.* New York: Guilford Press.

Garner, D. M., & Garfinkel, P. E. (Eds.). (1997). *Handbook of treatment for eating disorders* (2nd ed.). New York: Guilford Press.

Garner, D. M., Garfinkel, P. E., & O'Shaughnessy, M. (1983). Clinical and psychometric comparison between bulimia in anorexia nervosa and bulimia in normal weight women. In *Understanding anorexia nervosa and bulimia: Report of Fourth Ross Conference on Medical Research* (pp. 6–14). Columbus, OH: Ross Laboratories.

Garner, D. M., Garfinkel, P. E., Schwartz, D., & Thompson, M. (1980). Cultural expectations of thinness in women. *Psychological Reports, 47,* 483–491.

Garner, D. M., Rockert, W., Davis, R., Garner, M. V., Olmsted, M. P., & Eagle, M. (1993). Comparison of cognitive-behavioral and supportive–expressive therapy for bulimia nervosa. *American Journal of Psychiatry, 150,* 37–46.

Garner, D. M., Vitousek, K. M., & Pike, K. M. (1997). Cognitive-behavioral therapy for anorexia nervosa. In D. M. Garner & P. E. Garfinkel (Eds.), *Handbook of treatment for eating disorders* (2nd ed., pp. 94–144). New York: Guilford Press.

Geist, R., Heinmaa, M., Stephens, D., Davis, R., & Katzman, D. (2000). Comparison of family therapy and family group psychoeducation in adolescents with anorexia nervosa. *Canadian Journal of Psychiatry, 45*(2), 173–178.

Geretsegger, C., Greimel, K. V., Roed, I. S., & Hesselink, J. M. K. (1995). Ipsapirone in the treatment of bulimia nervosa: An open pilot study. *International Journal of Eating Disorders, 17,* 359–363.

Gerlinghoff, M., Gross, G., & Backmund, H. (2003). Eating disorder therapy concepts with a preventive goal. *European Child and Adolescent Psychiatry, 12*(Suppl. 1), 72–77.

Gilbert, S., & Thompson, J. K. (1996). Feminist explanations of the development of eating disorders: Common themes, research findings, and methodological issues. *Clinical Psychology: Science and Practice, 3*(3), 183–202.

Gillberg, C. (1994). Whither research in anorexia and bulimia nervosa? *British Journal of Hospital Medicine, 51,* 209–215.

Gillies, L. (2001). Interpersonal psychotherapy for depression and other disorders. In D. Barlow (Ed.), *Clinical handbook of psychological disorders: A step-by-step manual* (3rd ed., pp. 309–331). New York: Guilford Press.

Gold, M. S. (1993). Are eating disorders addictions? In E. Ferrari, F. Brambilla, & S. B. Solerte (Eds.), *Primary and secondary eating disorders: A psychoneuroendocrine and metabolic approach* (pp. 455–463). New York: Pergamon Press.

Goldbloom, D. S., Olmsted, M., Davis, R., Clewes, J., Heinmaa, M., Rockert, W., et al. (1997). A randomized controlled trial of fluoxetine and cognitive behavior therapy for bulimia nervosa: Short term outcome. *Behaviour Research and Therapy, 35,* 803–811.

Golden, N. (2003). Osteopenia and osteoporosis in anorexia nervosa. *Adolescent Medicine State of the Art Reviews, 14*(1), 97–108.

Goldfield, G., & Boachie, A. (2003). Delivery of family therapy in the treatment of anorexia nervosa using telehealth. *Telemedicine Journal and E-Health, 9*(1), 111–114.

Goldstein, D. J., Wilson, M. G., Thompson, V. L., Potvin, J. H., & Rampey, A. H. (1995). Long-term fluoxetine treatment of bulimia nervosa: Fluoxetine Bulimia Nervosa Research Group. *British Journal of Psychiatry, 166,* 660–666.

Goodrick, G. K. (2000). Inability to control eating; Addiction to food or normal response to abnormal environment? In W. S. C. Poston & C. Haddock (Eds.), *Food as a drug* (pp. 123–140). New York: Haworth Press.

Goodsitt, A. (1985). Self psychology and the treatment of anorexia nervosa. In D. M. Garner & P. E. Garfinkel (Eds.), *Handbook of psychotherapy for anorexia nervosa and bulimia* (pp. 55–82). New York: Guilford Press.

Goodsitt, A. (1997). Eating disorders: A self-psychological perspective. In D. M. Garner & P. E. Garfinkel (Eds.), *Handbook of treatment for eating disorders* (2nd ed., pp. 205–228). New York: Guilford Press.

Gorman, J., & Kent, J. (1999). SSRIs and SMRIs: Broad spectrum of efficacy beyond major depression. *Journal of Clinical Psychiatry, 60*(Suppl. 4), 33–38.

Gowers, S., & Bryant-Waugh, R. (2004). Management of child and adolescent eating disorders: The current evidence base and future directions. *Journal of Child Psychology and Psychiatry, 45*(1), 63–83.

Gray, J. J., & Hoage, C. M. (1990). Bulimia nervosa: A group behavior therapy with exposure plus response prevention. *Psychological Reports, 66,* 667–674.

Green, R. S., & Rau, J. H. (1974). Treatment of compulsive eating disturbances with anti-convulsant medication. *American Journal of Psychiatry, 131,* 428–432.

Green, R. S., & Rau, J. H. (1977). The use of diphenylhydantoin in compulsive eating disorders: Further studies. In R. A. Vigersky (Ed.), *Anorexia nervosa* (pp. 377–382). New York: Raven Press.

Greenway, F. L., Dahms, W. T., & Bray, G. A. (1977). Phenytoin as a treatment of obesity associated with compulsive eating. *Current Therapeutic Research, 21,* 338–342.

Griffiths, R., Gross, G., Russell, J., Thornton, C., Beaumont, P., Schotte, D., et al. (1998). Perception of bed rest by anorexic patients. *International Journal of Eating Disorders, 23*(4), 443–447.

Grigoriadis, S., Kaplan, A., Carter, J., & Woodside, B. (2001). What treatments patients seek after inpatient care: A follow-up of 24 patients with anorexia nervosa. *Eating and Weight Disorders, 6*(3), 115–120.

Grilo, C. M., Brownell, K. D., & Stunkard, A. J. (1993). The metabolic and psychological importance of exercise in weight control. In A. J. Stunkard & T. A. Wadden (Eds.), *Obesity: Theory and therapy* (2nd ed., pp. 253–273). New York: Raven Press.

Gull, W. W. (1874). Anorexia nervosa (apepsia hysterica, anorexia hysterica). *Transactions of the Clinical Society of London, 7,* 22–28.

Gusella, J., Butler, G., Nichols, L., & Bird, D. (2003). A brief questionnaire to assess readiness to change in adolescents with eating disorders: Its applications to group therapy. *European Eating Disorders Review, 11,* 58–71.

Haas, H., & Clopton, J. (2003). Comparing clinical and research treatments for eating disorders. *International Journal of Eating Disorders, 33,* 412–420.

Haddock, C., & Dill, P. (2000). The effects of food on mood and behavior: Implications for the addictions model of obesity and eating disorders. In W. S. C. Poston & C. Haddock (Eds.), *Food as a drug* (pp. 17–47). New York: Haworth Press.

Hall, A. (1985). Group therapy for anorexia nervosa. In D. M. Garner & P. E. Garfinkel (Eds.), *Handbook of psychotherapy for anorexia nervosa and bulimia* (pp. 213–239). New York: Guilford Press.

Hallsten, E. A. (1965). Adolescent anorexia nervosa treated by desensitization. *Behaviour Research and Therapy, 3,* 87–91.

Halmi, K. A. (1974). Anorexia nervosa: Demographic and clinical features in 94 cases. *Psychosomatic Medicine, 36,* 18–25.

Halmi, K. A. (1982). Pragmatic information on the eating disorders. *Psychiatric Clinics of North America, 5,* 371–377.

Halmi, K. A. (1997). Models to conceptualize risk factors for bulimia nervosa. *Archives of General Psychiatry, 54*(6), 507–508.

Halmi, K. A. (2002). Eating disorders in females: Genetics, pathophysiology, and treatment. *Journal of Pediatric Endocrinology and Metabolism, 15*(Suppl. 5), 1379–1386.

Halmi, K. A., Brodland, G., & Loney, J. (1973). Prognosis in anorexia nervosa. *Annals of Internal Medicine, 78,* 907–909.

Halmi, K. A., Brodland, G., & Rigas, C. (1975). A follow-up study of 79 patients with anorexia nervosa: An evaluation of prognostic factors and diagnostic criteria. *Life History Research in Psychopathology, 4,* 290–298.

Halmi, K. A., Casper, R. C., Eckert, E. C., Goldberg, S. C., & Davis, J. M. (1979). Unique features associated with age of onset of anorexia nervosa. *Psychiatric Research, 1,* 290–215.

Halmi, K. A., Falk, J. R., & Schwartz, E. (1981). Binge eating and vomiting: A survey of a college population. *Psychological Medicine, 11,* 697–706.

Halmi, K. A., Sunday, S., Strober, M., Kaplan, A., Woodside, B., Fichter, M., et al. (2000). Perfectionism in anorexia nervosa: Variation by clinical subtype, obsessionality, and pathological eating behavior. *American Journal of Psychiatry, 157*(11), 1799–1805.

Hammond, W. A. (1879). *Fasting girls: Their physiology and pathology.* New York: Putnam.

Hawkins, R. C., II, Fremouw, W. J., & Clement, P. F. (Eds.). (1984). *The binge–purge syndrome: Diagnosis, treatment and research.* New York: Springer.

Hay, G. G., & Leonard, J. C. (1979). Anorexia nervosa in males. *Lancet, ii,* 574–575.

Hediger, C., Rost, B., & Itin, P. (2000). Cutaneous manifestations in anorexia nervosa. *Journal Suisse de Médecine, 130*(16), 565–575.

Heinberg, L. J. (1996). Theories of body image disturbance: Perceptual, developmental, and sociocultural factors. In J. K. Thompson (Ed.), *Body image, eating disorders, and obesity: An integrative guide for assessment and treatment* (pp. 27–47). Washington, DC: American Psychological Association.

Herzog, D. B., Sacks, N. R., Keller, M. B., Lavori, P. W., von Ranson, K. B., & Gray, H. M. (1993). Patterns and predictors of recovery in anorexia nervosa and bulimia nervosa. *Journal of the American Academy of Child and Adolescent Psychiatry, 32,* 835–842.

Hirano, H., Tomura, N., Okane, K., Watarai, J., & Tashiro, T. (1999). Changes in cerebral blood flow in bulimia nervosa. *Journal of Computer Assisted Tomography, 23*(2), 280–282.

Hodes, M., & Le Grange, D. (1993). Expressed emotion in the investigation of eating disorders: A review. *International Journal of Eating Disorders, 13,* 279–288.

Hoek, H. W. (1995). The distribution of eating disorders. In K. D. Brownell & C. G. Fairburn (Eds.), *Eating disorders and obesity: A comprehensive handbook* (pp. 207–211). New York: Guilford Press.

Hoek, H. W., & van Hoeken, D. (2003). Review of the prevalence and incidence of eating disorders. *International Journal of Eating Disorders, 34*(4), 383–396.

Hoffman, L., & Halmi, K. (1993). Psychopharmacology in the treatment of anorexia nervosa and bulimia nervosa. *Psychiatric Clinics of North America, 16,* 767–778.

Holderness, C. C., Brooks-Gunn, J., & Warren, M. P. (1994). Comorbidity of eating disorders and substance abuse: Review of the literature. *International Journal of Eating Disorders, 16,* 1–34.

Holland, A. J., Sicotte, N., & Treasure, J. (1988). Anorexia nervosa: Evidence for a genetic basis. *Journal of Psychosomatic Research, 32,* 561–571.

Horgen, K., & Brownell, K. (2002). Confronting the toxic environment: Environmental and public health actions in a world crisis. In T. A. Wadden & A. J. Stunkard (Eds.), *Handbook of obesity treatment* (pp. 95–106). New York: Guilford Press.

Howard, C., & Porzelius, L. (1999). The role of dieting in binge eating disorder: Etiology and treatment implications. *Clinical Psychology Review, 19*(1), 25–44.

Howard, W., Evans, K., Quintero-Howard, C., Bowers, W., & Andersen, A. (1999). Predictors of success or failure of transition to day hospital treatment for inpatients with anorexia nervosa. *American Journal of Psychiatry, 156*(11), 1697–1702.

Hsu, L. K. (1995). Outcome of bulimia nervosa. In K. D. Brownell & C. G. Fairburn (Eds.), *Eating disorders and obesity: A comprehensive handbook* (pp. 238–244). New York: Guilford Press.

Hsu, L. K. (1996). Epidemiology of the eating disorders. *Psychiatric Clinics of North America, 19,* 681–700.

Hsu, L. K., Chesler, B. E., & Santhouse, R. (1990). Bulimia nervosa in eleven sets of twins: A clinical report. *International Journal of Eating Disorders, 9,* 275–282.

Hsu, L. K., Crisp, A. H., & Harding, B. (1979). Outcome of anorexia nervosa. *Lancet, 1,* 61–65.

Hudson, J. I., Laffer, P. S., & Pope, H. G. (1982). Bulimia related to effective disorder by family history and response to the dexamethasone suppression test. *American Journal of Psychiatry, 139,* 685–687.

Hudson, J. I., Pope, H. G., Jonas, J. M., & Yurgelun-Todd, D. (1983). Family history study of anorexia nervosa and bulimia. *British Journal of Psychiatry, 142,* 133–138.

Hughes, P. L., Wells, L. A., Cunningham, C. J., & Ilstrup, D. M. (1984, May 9). *Treating bulimia with desipramine: A double-blind placebo-controlled study.* Paper presented at the annual meeting of the American Psychiatric Association, Los Angeles.

Hulley, A., & Hill, A. (2001). Eating disorders and health in elite women distance runners. *International Journal of Eating Disorders, 30*(3), 312–317.

Huon, G., Braganza, C., Brown, L., Ritchie, J., & Roncolato, W. (1998). Reflections on prevention in dieting-induced disorders. *International Journal of Eating Disorders, 23*(4), 455–458.

Iancu, I., Spivak, B., Ratzoni, G., Apter, A., & Weizman, A. (1994). The sociocultural theory in the development of anorexia nervosa. *Psychopathology, 27,* 29–36.

Imbierowicz, K., Braks, K., Jacoby, G., Geiser, F., Conrad, R., Schilling, G., et al. (2002). High-caloric supplements in anorexia treatment. *International Journal of Eating Disorders, 32*(2), 135–145.

Jacobi, C., Hayward, C., deZwaan, M., Kraemer, H., & Agras, W. S. (2004). Coming to terms with risk factors for eating disorders: Application of risk terminology and suggestions for a general taxonomy. *Psychological Bulletin, 130*(1), 19–65.

Janet, P. (1919). *Les obsessions et la psychasthenie.* Paris: Alcan.

Jarmon, M., & Walsh, S. (1999). Evaluating recovery from anorexia nervosa and bulimia nervosa: Integrating lessons learned from research and clinical practice. *Clinical Psychology Review, 19*(7), 773–788.

Jarry, J. L., & Vaccarino, F. J. (1996). Eating disorder and obsessive–compulsive disorder: Neurochemical and phenomenological commonalities. *Journal of Psychiatry and Neuroscience, 21,* 36–48.

Jeejeebhoy, K. (1998). Nutritional management of anorexia. *Seminars in Gastrointestinal Disease, 9*(4), 183–188.

Jimerson, D. C., Wolfe, B. E., Metzger, E., Finkelstein, D., Cooper, T., & Levine, J. (1997). Decreased serotonin function in bulimia nervosa. *Archives of General Psychiatry, 54*(6), 529–534.

Johnson, C., Connors, M., & Stuckey, M. (1983). Short-term group treatment of bulimia: A preliminary report. *International Journal of Eating Disorders, 2,* 199–208.

Johnson, C., & Larson, R. (1982). Bulimia: Analysis of moods and behavior. *Psychosomatic Medicine, 44,* 341–353.

Johnson, C., & Pure, D. L. (1986). Assessment of bulimia: A multidimensional model. In K. D. Brownell & J. P. Foreyt (Eds.), *Handbook of eating disorders: Physiology, psychology, and treatment of obesity, anorexia, and bulimia* (pp. 405–449). New York: Basic Books.

Johnson, J., Cohen, P., Kasen, S., & Brook, J. (2002). Childhood adversities associated with risk for eating disorders or weight problems during adolescence or early adulthood. *American Journal of Psychiatry, 159,* 394–400.

Jones, D. J., Fox, M. M., Babigian, H. M., & Hutton, H. E. (1980). The epidemiology of anorexia nervosa in Monroe County, New York: 1960–1976. *Psychosomatic Medicine, 42,* 551–558.

Kaczynski, J., Denison, H., Wiknertz, A., Ryno, L., & Hjalmers, N. (2000). Structured care program yielded good results in severe anorexia nervosa. *Lakartidningen, 97*(22), 2734–2737.

Kaltiala-Heino, R., Rissanen, A., Rimpela, M., & Rantanen, P. (1999). Bulimia and bulimic behaviour in middle adolescence: More common than thought? *Acta Psychiatrica Scandinavica, 100*(1), 33–39.

Kalucy, R. S., Crisp, A. H., & Harding, B. (1977). A study of 56 families with anorexia nervosa. *British Journal of Medical Psychology, 50,* 381–395.

Kalucy, R. S., Crisp, A. H., Lacey, J. H., & Harding, B. (1977). Prevalence and prognosis in anorexia nervosa. *Australian and New Zealand Journal of Psychiatry, 11,* 251–257.

Kalucy, R. S., Gilchrist, P. N., McFarlane, C. M., & McFarlane, A. C. (1985). The evolution of a multitherapy orientation. In D. M. Garner & P. E. Garfinkel (Eds.), *Handbook of psychotherapy for anorexia nervosa and bulimia* (pp. 458–487). New York: Guilford Press.

Kaplan, A. S., & Garfinkel, A. H. (1984). Bulimia in the Talmud. *American Journal of Psychiatry, 141,* 721.

Kaplan, A. S., & Garfinkel, P. E. (1993). *Medical issues and the eating disorders: The interface.* New York: Brunner/Mazel.

Karwautz, A., Rabe-Hesketh, S., Hu, X., Zhao, J., Sham, P., Collier, D., et al. (2001). Individual-specific risk factors for anorexia nervosa: A pilot study using a discordant sister-pair design. *Psychological Medicine, 31*(2), 317–329.

Kaye, W. H. (1999). The new biology of anorexia and bulimia nervosa: Implications for advances in treatment. *European Eating Disorders Review, 7*(3), 157–161.

Kaye, W. H., Ballenger, J. C., Lydiard, B., Stuart, G. W., Laraia, M. T., O'Neil, P., et al. (1990). CSF monoamine oxidase levels in normal-weight bulimia: Evidence for abnormal noradrenergic activity. *American Journal of Psychiatry, 147,* 225–229.

Kaye, W., Strober, M., Stein, D., & Gendall, K. (1999). New directions in treatment research of anorexia and bulimia nervosa. *Biological Psychiatry, 45*(10), 1285–1292.

Kaye, W. H., & Weltzin, T. E. (1991). Neurochemistry of bulimia nervosa. *Journal of Clinical Psychiatry, 52,* 21–28.

Kaye, W. H., Weltzin, T. E., Hsu, L. K. G., & Bulik, C. M. (1991). An open trial of fluoxetine in patients with anorexia nervosa. *Clinical Psychiatry, 52,* 464–471.

Kearney-Cooke, A., & Striegel-Moore, R. (1994). Treatment of childhood sexual abuse in anorexia nervosa and bulimia nervosa: A feminist psychodynamic approach. *International Journal of Eating Disorders, 15,* 305–319.

Keel, P. K., & Klump, K. L. (2003). Are eating disorders culture-bound syndromes?: Implications for conceptualizing their etiology. *Psychological Bulletin, 129*(5), 747–769.

Keel, P. K., & Mitchell, J. E. (1997). Outcome in bulimia nervosa. *American Journal of Psychiatry, 154,* 313–321.

Keel, P. K., Mitchell, J. E., Miller, K. B., Davis, T. L., & Crow, S. J. (1999). Long-term outcome of bulimia nervosa. *Archives of General Psychiatry, 56*(1), 63–69.

Keller, M. B., Herzog, D. B., Lavori, P. W., Bradburn, I. S., & Mahoney, E. M. (1992). The naturalistic history of bulimia nervosa: Extraordinary high rates of chronicity, relapse, recurrence, and psychosocial morbidity. *International Journal of Eating Disorders, 12,* 1–9.

Kendler, K. S. (2001). Twin studies of psychiatric illness. *Archives of General Psychiatry, 58,* 1005–1014.

Kendler, K. S., MacLean, C., Neale, M., Kessler, R., Heath, A., & Eaves, L. (1991). The genetic epidemiology of bulimia nervosa. *American Journal of Psychiatry, 148,* 1627–1637.

Kennedy, S. H., Katz, R., Neitzert, C. S., Ralveski, E., & Mendlowitz, S. (1995). Exposure with response prevention treatment of anorexia nervosa–bulimic subtype and bulimia nervosa. *Behaviour Research and Therapy, 33,* 685–689.

Kennedy, S. H., Piran, N., Warsh, J. J., Prendergast, P., Mainprize, E., Whynot, C., et al. (1988). A trial of isocarboxazid in the treatment of bulimia nervosa. *Journal of Clinical Psychopharmacology, 8,* 391–396.

Key, A., Mason, H., Allan, R., & Lask, B. (2002). Restoration of ovarian and uterine maturity in adolescents with anorexia nervosa. *International Journal of Eating Disorders, 32*(3), 319–325.

King, S., & Turner, D. (2000). Caring for adolescent females with anorexia nervosa: Registered nurses' perspective. *Journal of Advanced Nursing, 32*(1), 139–147.

Kirk, S. A., & Kutchins, H. (1992). *The selling of DSM: The rhetoric of science in psychiatry.* New York: Aldine de Gruyter.

Kirschenbaum, D. S., & Fitzgibbon, M. L. (1995). Controversy about the treatment of obesity: Criticisms or challenges? *Behavior Therapy, 26,* 43–68.

Klump, K., Kaye, W., & Strober, M. (2001). The evolving genetic foundations of eating disorders. *Psychiatric Clinics of North America, 24*(2), 215–225.

Klump, K., Miller, K., Keel, P., McGue, M., & Iacono, W. (2001). Genetic and environmental influences on anorexia nervosa syndromes in a population-based twin sample. *Psychological Medicine, 31*(4), 737–740.

Kohn, M., & Golden, N. (2001). Eating disorders in children and adolescents: Epidemiology, diagnosis and treatment. *Paediatric Drugs 3*(2), 91–99.

Kotler, L., Boudreau, G., & Devlin, M. (2003). Emerging psychotherapies for eating disorders. *Journal of Psychiatric Practice, 9*(6), 431–441.

Kotler, L., Cohen, P., Davies, M., Pine, D., & Walsh, B. (2001). Longitudinal relationships between childhood, adolescent, and adult eating disorders. *Journal of the American Academy of Child and Adolescent Psychiatry, 40*(12), 1434–1440.

Kotler, L., & Walsh, B. (2000). Eating disorders in children and adolescents: Pharmacological therapies. *European Child and Adolescent Psychiatry, 9*(Suppl. 1), I108–I116.

Krautter, T., & Lock, J. (2004). Is manualized family-based treatment for adolescent anorexia nervosa acceptable to patients?: Patient satisfaction at the end of treatment. *Journal of Family Therapy, 26*(1), 66–82.

Kreipe, R., & Birndorf, S. (2000). Eating disorders in adolescents and young adults. *Medical Clinics of North America, 84*(4), 1027–1049.

Krueger, S., & Kennedy, S. (2000). Psychopharmaco-therapy of anorexia nervosa, bulimia nervosa and binge-eating disorder. *Journal of Psychiatry and Neuroscience, 25*(5), 497–508.

Lacey, J. H. (1982). Anorexia nervosa and a bearded female saint. *British Medical Journal, 285,* 1816–1817.

Lacey, J. H. (1985). Time-limited individual and group treatment for bulimia. In D. M. Garner & P. E. Garfinkel (Eds.), *Handbook of psychotherapy for anorexia nervosa and bulimia* (pp. 431–457). New York: Guilford Press.

Laliberte, M., Boland, F., & Leichner, P. (1999). Family climates: Family factors specific to disturbed eating and bulimia nervosa. *Journal of Clinical Psychology, 55*(9), 1021–1040.

Lambe, E., Katzman, D., Mikulis, D., Kennedy, S., & Zipursky, R. (1997). Cerebral gray matter volume deficits after weight recovery from anorexia nervosa. *Archives of General Psychiatry, 54*(6), 537–542.

Lang, P. J. (1965). Behavior therapy with a case of anorexia nervosa. In L. P. Ullmann & L. Krasner (Eds.), *Case studies in behavior modification* (pp. 217–221). New York: Holt, Rinehart & Winston.

Lantzouni, E., Frank, G., Golden, N., & Shenker, R. (2002). Reversibility of growth stunting in early onset anorexia nervosa: A prospective study. *Journal of Adolescent Health, 31*(2), 162–165.

Laseque, C. (1873). On hysterical anorexia. *Medical Times Gazette, 2,* 265–266.

Lee, M. I., & Miltenberger, R. G. (1997). Functional assessment and binge eating: A review of the literature and suggestions for future research. *Behavior Modification, 21,* 159–171.

Lee, S. (1995). Self-starvation in context: Towards a culturally sensitive understanding of anorexia nervosa. *Social Science and Medicine, 41,* 25–36.

Le Grange, D., Eisler, I., Dare, C., & Russell, G. F. M. (1992). Evaluation of family treatments in adolescent anorexia nervosa: A pilot study. *International Journal of Eating Disorders, 12,* 347–357.

Leibowitz, S. F. (1983). Hypothalamic catecholamine systems controlling eating behavior: A potential model for anorexia nervosa. In P. L. Darby, P. E. Garfinkel, D. M. Garner, & D. V. Coscina (Eds.), *Anorexia nervosa: Recent developments in research* (pp. 221–229). New York: Liss.

Leitenberg, H., Agras, W. S., & Thompson, L. E. (1968). A sequential analysis of the effect of selective positive reinforcement in modifying anorexia nervosa. *Behaviour Research and Therapy, 6,* 211–218.

Leitenberg, H., & Rosen, J. (1989). Cognitive-behavioral therapy with and without exposure plus response prevention in treatment of bulimia nervosa: Comments on Agras, Schneider, Arnow, Raeburn, and Telch. *Journal of Consulting and Clinical Psychology, 57,* 776–777.

Leitenberg, H., Rosen, J., Gross, J., Nudelman, S., & Vara, L. S. (1988). Exposure plus response-prevention treatment of bulimia nervosa. *Journal of Consulting and Clinical Psychology, 56,* 535–541.

Lemmon, C., & Josephson, A. (2001). Family therapy for eating disorders. *Child and Adolescent Psychiatric Clinics of North America, 10*(3), 519–542.

Leon, G. E., Carroll, K., Chernyk, B., & Finn, S. (1985). Binge eating and associated habit patterns within college student and identified bulimic populations. *International Journal of Eating Disorders, 4,* 43–57.

Leon, G. R., Fulkerson, J. A., Perry, C. L., & Early-Zald, M. B. (1995). Prospective analysis of personality and behavioral vulnerabilities and gender influences in the later development of disordered eating. *Journal of Abnormal Psychology, 104,* 140–149.

Leung, N., Thomas, G., & Waller, G. (2000). The relationship between parental bonding and core beliefs in anorexic and bulimic women. *British Journal of Clinical Psychology, 39*(Pt. 2), 205–213.

Leung, N., Waller, G., & Glyn, T. (2000). Outcome of group cognitive-behavior therapy for bulimia nervosa: The role of core beliefs. *Behaviour Research and Therapy, 38*(2), 145–156.

Levenkron, S. (1983). *Treating and overcoming anorexia nervosa.* New York: Warner Books.

Levine, R. (2002). Endocrine aspects of eating disorders in adolescents. *Adolescent Medicine State of the Art Reviews, 13*(1), 129–143.

Liebowitz, M. R., Quitkin, F., & Stewart, J. W. (1981). Phenelzine and imipramine in atypical depression. *Psychopharmacological Bulletin, 17,* 159–161.

Lilenfeld, L., Kaye, W., Greeno, C., Merikangas, K., Plotnicov, K., Pollice, C., et al. (1998). A controlled family study of anorexia nervosa and bulimia nervosa: Psychiatric disorders in first-degree relatives and effects of proband comorbidity. *Archives of General Psychiatry, 55*(7), 603–610.

Lock, J., & Le Grange, D. (2001). Can family-based treatment of anorexia nervosa be manualized? *Journal of Psychotherapy Practice and Research, 10*(4), 253–261.

Lock, J., Le Grange, D., Agras, W., & Dare, C. (2001). *Treatment manual for anorexia nervosa: A family-based approach.* New York: Guilford Press.

Lowenberg, M., Todhunter, E., Wilson, E., Savage, J., & Lubawski, J. (1974). *Food and man* (2nd ed.). New York: Wiley.

Luborsky, I. (1984). *Principles of psychoanalytic psychotherapy: A manual for supportive–expressive treatment.* New York: Basic Books.

Lucas, A., Melton, L., Crowson, C., & O'Fallon, W. (1999). Long-term fracture risk among women with anorexia nervosa: A population-based cohort study. *Mayo Clinic Proceedings, 74*(10), 972–977.

Lydiard, R. B., Brewerton, T. D., Fossey, M. D., Laraia, M. T., Stuart, G., Beinfeld, M. C., et al. (1993). CSF cholecystokinin octapeptide in patients with bulimia nervosa and in normal comparison subjects. *American Journal of Psychiatry, 150,* 1099–1101.

MacDonald, C. (2002). Treatment resistance in anorexia nervosa and the pervasiveness of ethics in clinical decision making. *Canadian Journal of Psychiatry, 47*(3), 267–270.

Maggia, G., & Bianchi, B. (1998). Differential hemispheric involvement in anorexia nervosa. *Eating and Weight Disorders, 3*(3), 100–109.

Malina, A., Gaskill, J., McConaha, C., Frank, G., LaVia, M., Scholar, L., et al. (2003). Olanzapine treatment of anorexia nervosa: A retrospective study. *International Journal of Eating Disorders, 33*(2), 234–237.

Malson, H., & Swann, C. (1999). Prepared for consumption: (Dis)orders of eating and embodiment. *Journal of Community and Applied Social Psychology, 9*, 397–405.

Mann, T., Nolen-Hoeksema, S., Huang, K., Burgard, D., Wright, A., & Hanson, K. (1997). Are two interventions worse than none?: Joint primary and secondary prevention of eating disorders in college females. *Health Psychology, 16*(3), 215–225.

Markey, C. N. (2004). Culture and the development of eating disorders: A tripartite model. *Eating Disorders: The Journal of Treatment and Prevention, 12*(2), 139–156.

Marrazzi, M. A., Markham, K. M., Kinzie, J., & Luby, E. D. (1995). Binge eating disorder: Response to naltrexone. *International Journal of Obesity, 19*, 143–145.

Matusevich, D., Garcia, A., Gutt, S., de la Parra, & Finkelsztein, C. (2002). Hospitalization of patients with anorexia nervosa: A therapeutic proposal. *Eating and Weight Disorder, 7*, 196–201.

Mauri, M. C., Rudelli, R., Somaschini, E., Roncoroni, L., Papa, R., Mantero, M., et al. (1996). Neurobiological and psychopharmacological basis in the therapy of bulimia and anorexia. *Progress in Neuro-Psychopharmacology and Biological Psychiatry, 20*, 207–229.

McClelland, L., & Crisp, A. (2001). Anorexia nervosa and social class. *International Journal of Eating Disorders, 29*(2), 150–156.

McGilley, B., & Pryor, T. (1998). Assessment and treatment of bulimia nervosa. *American Family Physician, 57*(11), 2743–2750.

McLoughlin, D., Wassif, W., Morton, J., Spargo, E., Peters, T., & Russell, G. (2000). Metabolic abnormalities associated with skeletal myopathy in severe anorexia nervosa. *Nutrition, 16*(3), 192–196.

Mehler, C., Wewetzer, C., Schulze, U., Warnke, A., Theisen, F., & Dittman, R. (2001). Olanzapine in children and adolescents with chronic anorexia nervosa: A study of five cases. *European Child and Adolescent Psychiatry, 10*(2), 151–157.

Mehler, P. S. (2001). Diagnosis and care of patients with anorexia nervosa in primary care settings. *Annals of Internal Medicine, 134*(11), 1048–1059.

Mehler, P. S. (2003a). Bulimia nervosa. *New England Journal of Medicine, 349*(9), 875–881.

Mehler, P. S. (2003b). Osteoporosis in anorexia nervosa: Prevention and treatment. *International Journal of Eating Disorders, 33*(2), 113–126.

Mendelson, S. (2001). Treatment of anorexia nervosa with tramadol. *American Journal of Psychiatry, 158*(6), 963–964.

Mendlewicz, L., Nef, F., & Simon, Y. (2001). Selective handling of information in patients suffering from restrictive anorexia in an emotional Stroop test and a word recognition test. *Neuropsychobiology, 44*(2), 59–64.

Minuchin, S., Rosman, B. L., & Baker, L. (1978). *Psychosomatic families: Anorexia nervosa in context.* Cambridge, MA: Harvard University Press.

Mitchell, J. E. (1985). Medical complications. In J. E. Mitchell (Ed.), *Anorexia nervosa and bulimia: Diagnosis and treatment* (pp. 48–77). Minneapolis: University of Minnesota Press.

Mitchell, J. E. (1986a). Anorexia nervosa: Medical and physiological aspects. In K. D. Brownell & J. P. Foreyt (Eds.), *Handbook of eating disorders: Physiology, psychology, and treatment of obesity, anorexia, and bulimia* (pp. 247–265). New York: Basic Books.

Mitchell, J. E. (1986b). Bulimia: Medical and physiological aspects. In K. D. Brownell & J. P. Foreyt (Eds.), *Handbook of eating disorders: Physiology, psychology, and treatment of obesity, anorexia, and bulimia* (pp. 379–388). New York: Basic Books.

Mitchell, J. E., deZwaan, M., & Roerig, J. (2003). Drug therapy for patients with eating disorders. *Current Drug Targets–CNS and Neurological Disorders, 2*(1), 17–29.

Mitchell, J. E., Hatsukami, D., Eckert, E. D., & Pyle, R. L. (1985). Characteristics of 275 patients with bulimia. *American Journal of Psychiatry, 142*, 482–485.

Mitchell, J. E., Hatsukami, D., Goff, G., Pyle, R. L., Eckert, E., & Davis, L. E. (1985). Intensive outpatient group treatment for bulimia. In D. M. Garner & P. E. Garfinkel (Eds.), *Handbook of psychotherapy for anorexia nervosa and bulimia* (pp. 240–256). New York: Guilford Press.

Mitchell, J. E., Hoberman, H. N., Peterson, C. B., Mussell, M., & Pyle, R. L. (1996). Research on the psychotherapy of bulimia nervosa: Half empty or half full? *International Journal of Eating Disorders, 20*, 219–229.

Mitchell, J. E., Peterson, C. B., Myers, T., & Wonderlich, S. (2001). Combining pharmacotherapy and psychotherapy in the treatment of patients with eating disorders. *Psychiatric Clinics of North America, 24*(2), 315–323.

Mitchell, J. E., & Pyle, R. L. (1982). The bulimic syndrome in normal weight individuals: A review. *International Journal of Eating Disorders, 1*, 61–73.

Mitchell, J. E., Pyle, R. L., Eckert, E. D., Hatsukami, D., Pomeroy, C., & Zimmerman, R. (1990). A comparison study of anti-depressants and structured group therapy in the treatment of bulimia nervosa. *Archives of General Psychiatry, 47*, 149–157.

Mitchell, J. E., Raymond, N., & Specker, S. (1993). A review of the controlled trials of pharmacotherapy and psychotherapy in the treatment of bulimia nervosa. *International Journal of Eating Disorders, 14*, 229–247.

Modan-Moses, D., Yaroslavsky, A., Novikov, I., Segev, S., Toledano, A., Miterany, E., et al. (2003). Stunting of growth as a major feature of anorexia nervosa in male adolescents. *Pediatrics, 111*(2), 270–276.

Mont, L., Castro, J., Herreros, B., Pare, C., Azqueta, M., Magrina, J., et al. (2003). Reversibility of cardiac abnormalities in adolescents with anorexia nervosa after weight recovery. *Journal of the American Academy of Child and Adolescent Psychiatry, 42*(7), 808–813.

Monti, P. M., McCrady, B. S., & Barlow, D. H. (1977). Effect of positive reinforcement, informational feedback and contingency contracting on a bulimic anorexic female. *Behavior Therapy, 8*, 258–263.

Morgan, H. G., & Russell, G. F. M. (1975). Value of family background and clinical features as predictors of long-term outcome in anorexia nervosa: Four-year follow-up study of 41 patients. *Psychological Medicine, 5*, 355–371.

Morton, R. (1694). *Phthisiologica: Or a treatise of consumptions*. London: S. Smith & B. Walo.

Myrtle, A. S. (1888). Letters to the editor. *Lancet, i*, 899.

Narduzzi, K., & Jackson, T. (2000). Personality differences between eating-disordered women and a nonclinical comparison sample: A discriminant classification analysis. *Journal of Clinical Psychology, 56*(6), 699–710.

Ngai, E., Lee, S., & Lee, A. (2000). The variability of phenomenology in anorexia nervosa. *Acta Psychiatrica Scandinavica, 102*(4), 314–317.

Nilsson, E., Gillberg, C., Gillberg, I., & Rastam, M. (1999). Ten-year follow-up of adolescent-onset anorexia nervosa: Personality disorders. *Journal of the American Academy of Child and Adolescent Psychiatry, 38*(11), 1389–1395.

O'Brien, K., & Vincent, N. (2003). Psychiatric comorbidity in anorexia and bulimia nervosa: Nature, prevalence, and causal relationships. *Clinical Psychology Review, 23*(1), 57–74.

Ollendick, T. H. (1979). Behavioral treatment of anorexia nervosa: A five-year study. *Behavior Modification, 3*, 124–135.

Olmsted, M. P., Davis, R., Rockert, W., Irvine, J. J., Eagle, M., & Garner, D. M. (1991). Efficacy of a brief group psychoeducational intervention for bulimia nervosa. *Behaviour Research and Therapy, 29*, 71–83.

Olmsted, M. P., & Kaplan, A. S. (1995). Psychoeducation in the treatment of eating. In K. D. Brownell & C. G. Fairburn (Eds.), *Eating disorders and obesity: A comprehensive handbook* (pp. 299–305). New York: Guilford Press.

Oster, J. R., Materson, B. J., & Rogers, A. I. (1980). Laxative abuse syndrome. *American Journal of Gastroenterology, 74*, 451–458.

Ostuzzi, R., Didonna, F., & Micciolo, R. (1999). One-year weight follow-up in anorexia nervosa after inpatient psycho-nutritional rehabilitative treatment. *Eating and Weight Disorders, 4*(4), 194–197.

Palmer, R. L. (1979). The dietary chaos syndrome: A useful new term? *British Journal of Medical Psychology, 52*, 187–190.

Panagiotopoulos, C., McCrindle, B., Hick, K., & Katzman, D. (2000). Electrocardiographic findings in adolescents with eating disorders. *Pediatrics, 105*(5), 1100–1105.

Parham, E. S. (1995). Compulsive eating: Applying a medical addiction model. In T. B. VanItallie, A. P. Simonpoulos, S. P. Gullo, & W. Futterweit (Eds.), *Obesity: New directions in assessment and management* (pp. 185–194). Philadelphia: Charles Press.

Pate, J. E., Pumariega, A. J., Hester, C., & Garner, D. M. (1992). Cross-cultural patterns in eating disorders: A review. *Journal of the American Academy of Child and Adolescent Psychiatry, 31*, 802–809.

Patel, D., Pratt, H., & Greydanus, D. (2003). Treatment of adolescents with anorexia nervosa. *Journal of Adolescent Research, 18*(3), 244–260.

Pawluck, D., & Gorey, K. (1998). Secular trends in the incidence of anorexia nervosa: Integrative review of population-based studies. *International Journal of Eating Disorders, 23*(4), 347–352.

Pendleton, V. R., Goodrick, G. K., Poston, W. S., Reeves, R. S., & Foreyt, J. P. (2002). Exercise augments the effects of cognitive-behavioral therapy in the treatment of binge eating. *International Journal of Eating Disorders, 31*(2), 172–184.

Pierloot, R., Wellens, W., & Houben, M. (1975). Elements of resistance to a combined medical and psychotherapeutic program in anorexia nervosa. *Psychotherapy and Psychosomatics, 36*, 101–107.

Pike, K., Dohm, F., Striegel-Moore, R., Wilfley, D., & Fairburn, C. (2001). A comparison of black and white women with binge eating disorder. *American Journal of Psychiatry, 158*(9), 1455–1460.

Pike, K. M., Loeb, K., & Vitousek, K. (1996). Cognitive-behavioral therapy for anorexia nervosa and bulimia nervosa. In J. K. Thompson (Ed.), *Body image, eating disorders, and obesity: An integrative guide for assessment and treatment* (pp. 253–302). Washington, DC: American Psychological Association.

Pillay, M., & Crisp, A. H. (1981). The impact of social skills training within an established in-patient treatment program for anorexia nervosa. *Journal of Psychiatry, 139*, 533–539.

Piran, N. (1999). Eating disorders: A trial of prevention in a high risk school setting. *Journal of Primary Prevention, 20*(1), 75–90.

Playfair, W. S. (1888). Note on the so-called anorexia nervosa. *Lancet, i*, 817.

Polivy, J., & Federoff, I. (1997). Group psychotherapy. In D. M. Garner & P. E. Garfinkel (Eds.), *Handbook of treatment for eating disorders* (2nd ed., pp. 462–475). New York: Guilford Press.

Polivy, J., & Herman, C. P. (2004). Sociocultural idealization of thin female body shapes. *Journal of Social and Clinical Psychology, 23*(1), 1–6.

Poston, W. S. C., & Haddock, C. (Ed.). (2000). *Food as a drug*. New York: Haworth Press.

Poston, W. S. C., & Winebarger, A. A. (1996). The misuse of behavioral genetics in prevention research, or for whom the "bell curve" tolls. *Journal of Primary Prevention, 17*, 133–147.

Powers, P. S. (1984). Multidisciplinary approach to treatment and evaluation. In P. S. Powers & R. C. Fernandez (Eds.), *Current treatment of anorexia nervosa and bulimia* (pp. 166–179). Basel, Switzerland: Karger.

Powers, P. S., & Fernandez, R. C. (1984). Introduction. In P. S. Powers & R. C. Fernandez (Eds.), *Current treatment of anorexia nervosa and bulimia* (pp. 10–17). Basel, Switzerland: Karger.

Powers, P. S., & Powers, H. P. (1984). Inpatient treatment of anorexia nervosa. *Psychosomatics, 25*, 512–527.

Powers, P. S., & Santana, C. A. (2002a). Childhood and adolescent anorexia nervosa. *Child and Adolescent Psychiatric Clinics of North America, 11*(2), 219–235.

Powers, P. S., & Santana, C. A. (2002b). Eating disorders: A guide for the primary care physician. *Primary Care: Clinics in Office Practice, 29*(1), 81–98.

Powers, P. S., Santana, C. A., & Bannon, Y. S. (2002). Olanzapine in the treatment of anorexia nervosa: An open label trial. *International Journal of Eating Disorders, 32*(2), 146–154.

Pryor, T., Wiederman, M., & McGilley, B. (1996). Clinical correlates of anorexia nervosa subtypes. *International Journal of Eating Disorders, 19*(4), 371–379.

Pyle, R. L., Mitchell, J. E., Eckert, E. E., Halverson, P., Neuman, P., & Goff, G. (1983). The incidence of bulimia in freshmen college students. *International Journal of Eating Disorders, 2*, 75–85.

Rastam, M., Bjure, J., Vestergren, E., Uvebrant, P., Gillberg, I., Wentz, E., et al. (2001). Regional cerebral blood flow in weight-restored anorexia nervosa: A preliminary study. *Developmental Medicine and Child Neurology, 43*(4), 239–242.

Rastam, M., Gillberg, C., & Wentz, E. (2003). Outcome of teenage-onset anorexia nervosa in a Swedish community-based sample. *European Child and Adolescent Psychiatry, 12*(Suppl. 1), I78–I90.

Rau, J. H., & Green, R. S. (1975). Compulsive eating: A neuropsychologic approach to certain eating disorders. *Comprehensive Psychiatry, 16*, 223–231.

Ricca, V., Mannucci, E., Zucchi, T., Rotella, C., & Faravelli, C. (2000). Cognitive-behavioural therapy for bulimia nervosa and binge eating disorder: A review. *Psychotherapy and Psychosomatics, 69*(6), 287–295.

Ricciardelli, L. A., & McCabe, M.P. (2004). A biopsychosocial model of disordered eating and the pursuit of muscularity in adolescent boys. *Psychological Bulletin, 130*(2), 179–205.

Rich, C. L. (1978). Self-induced vomiting: Psychiatric considerations. *Journal of the American Medical Association, 239*, 2688–2689.

Richards, P., Baldwin, B., Frost, H., Clark-Sly, J., Berrett, M., & Hardman, R. (2000). What works for treating eating disorders?: Conclusions of 28 outcome reviews. *Eating Disorders, 8*, 189–206.

Robb, A., & Dadson, M. (2002). Eating disorders in males. *Child and Adolescent Psychiatric Clinics of North America, 11*, 399–418.

Robb, A., Silber, T., Orrell-Valente, J., Valadez-Meltzer, A., Ellis, N., Dadson, M., et al. (2002). Supplemental nocturnal nasogastric refeeding for better short-term outcome in hospitalized adolescent girls with anorexia nervosa. *American Journal of Psychiatry, 159*(8), 1347–1353.

Robin, A. L., Bedway, M., Siegel, P., & Gilroy, M. (1996). Therapy for adolescent anorexia nervosa: Addressing cognitions, feelings, and the family's role. In E. D. Hibbs & P. S. Jensen (Eds.), *Psychosocial treatments for child and adolescent disorders: empirically based strategies for clinical practice* (pp. 239–259). Washington, DC: American Psychological Association.

Robin, A. L., Gilroy, M., & Dennis, A. (1998). Treatment of eating disorders in children and adolescents. *Clinical Psychology Review, 18*(4), 421–446.

Robin, A. L., Siegel, P. T., & Moye, A. (1995). Family versus individual therapy for anorexia: Impact on family conflict. *International Journal of Eating Disorders, 17*, 313–322.

Robin, A. L., Siegel, P. T., Koepke, T., Moye, A. W., & Tice, S. (1994). Family therapy versus individual therapy for adolescent females with anorexia nervosa. *Journal of Developmental and Behavioral Pediatrics, 15*, 111–116.

Robin, A. L., Siegel, P., Moye, A., Gilroy, M., Dennis, A., & Sikand, A. (1999). A controlled comparison of family versus individual therapy for adolescents with anorexia nervosa. *Journal of the American Academy of Child and Adolescent Psychiatry, 38*(12), 1482–1489.

Rome, E. (2003). Eating disorders. *Obstetrics and Gynecology Clinics of North America, 30*(2), 353–377.

Rorty, M., Yager, J., & Rossotto, E. (1993). Why and how do women recover from bulimia nervosa?: The subjective appraisals of forty women recovered for a year or more. *International Journal of Eating Disorders, 14*, 249–260.

Rorty, M., Yager, J., & Rossotto, E. (1994). Childhood sexual, physical, and psychological abuse in bulimia nervosa. *American Journal of Psychiatry, 151*, 1122–1126.

Rosen, D. S. (2003). Eating disorders in children and young adolescents: Etiology, classification, clinical features, and treatment. *Adolescent Medicine State of the Art Reviews, 14*(1), 49–59.

Rosen, J. C., & Leitenberg, H. (1982). Bulimia nervosa: Treatment with exposure and response prevention. *Behavior Therapy, 13*, 117–124.

Rosen, J. C., Reiter, J., & Orosan, P. (1995). Cognitive-behavioral body image therapy for body dysmorphic disorder. *Journal of Consulting and Clinical Psychology, 63,* 263–269.

Rosenthal, R. H., Webb, W. L., & Wruble, L. D. (1980). Diagnosis and management of persistent psychogenic vomiting. *Psychosomatics, 21,* 722–730.

Rosenvinge, J., Martinussen, M., & Ostensen, E. (2000). The comorbidity of eating disorders and personality disorders: A meta-analytic review of studies published between 1983 and 1998. *Eating and Weight Disorders, 5*(2), 52–61.

Roser, W., Bubl, R., Buergin, D., Seelig, J., Radue, E., & Rost, B. (1999). Metabolic changes in the brain of patients with anorexia and bulimia nervosa as detected by proton magnetic resonance spectroscopy. *International Journal of Eating Disorders, 26*(2), 119–136.

Ross, C. A., & Pam, A. (1995). *Pseudoscience in biological psychiatry.* New York: Wiley.

Rowland, C. V., Jr. (1970). Anorexia nervosa: A survey of the literature and review of 30 cases. *International Psychiatric Clinics, 7,* 37–137.

Russell, G. F. M. (1979). Bulimia nervosa: An ominous variant of anorexia nervosa. *Psychological Medicine, 9,* 429–448.

Russell, G. F. M., Szmukler, G. I., Dare, C., & Eisler, I. (1987). An evaluation of family therapy in anorexia nervosa and bulimia nervosa. *Archives of General Psychiatry, 44,* 1047–1056.

Salusso-Deonier, C. J., & Scharzkopf, R. J. (1991). Sex differences in body cathexis associated with exercise involvement. *Perceptual and Motor Skills, 73,* 139–145.

Schnurer, A. T., Rubin, R. R., & Roy, A. (1973). Systematic desensitization of anorexia nervosa seen as a weight phobia. *Journal of Behavior Therapy and Experimental Psychiatry, 4,* 149–153.

Schulze, U., Pettke-Rank, C., Kreienkamp, M., Hamm, H., Brocker, E., Wewetzer, C., et al. (1999). Dermatologic findings in anorexia and bulimia nervosa of childhood and adolescence. *Pediatric Dermatology, 16*(2), 90–94.

Schwartz, D. M., & Thompson, M. G. (1981). Do anorectics get well?: Current research and future needs. *American Journal of Psychiatry, 138,* 319–323.

Schwartz, D. M., Thompson, M. G., & Johnson, C. L. (1982). Anorexia nervosa and bulimia: The sociocultural context. *International Journal of Eating Disorders, 1,* 20–36.

Schwartz, M. B., Chambliss, H., Brownell, K., Blair, S., & Billington, C. (2003). Weight bias among health professionals specializing in obesity. *Obesity Research, 11,* 1033–1039.

Schwartz, R. C., Barrett, M. J., & Saba, G. (1985). Family therapy for bulimia. In D. M. Garner & P. E. Garfinkel (Eds.), *Handbook of psychotherapy for anorexia nervosa and bulimia* (pp. 280–310). New York: Guilford Press.

Schwitzer, A., Bergholz, K., Dore, T., & Salimi, L. (1998). Eating disorders among college women: Prevention, education, and treatment responses. *Journal of American College Health, 46*(5), 199–207.

Serfaty, M., Turkington, D., Heap, M., Ledsham, L., & Jolley, E. (1999). Cognitive therapy versus dietary counseling in the outpatient treatment of anorexia nervosa: Effects of the treatment phase. *European Eating Disorders Review, 7*(5), 334–350.

Seidenfeld, M., & Rickert, V. (2001). Impact of anorexia, bulimia and obesity on the gynecologic health of adolescents. *American Family Physician, 64*(3), 445–450.

Seidensticher, J. F., & Tzagournis, M. (1968). Anorexia nervosa: Clinical features and long-term follow-up. *Journal of Chronic Diseases, 21,* 361–367.

Sheehan, H. L., & Summers, V. K. (1949). The syndrome of hypopituitarism. *Quarterly Journal of Medicine, 18,* 319–378.

Shoebridge, P., & Gowers, S. (2000). Parental high concern and adolescent-onset anorexia nervosa: A case–control study to investigate direction of causality. *British Journal of Psychiatry, 176,* 132–137.

Signorini, A., Bellini, O., Pasanisi, F., Contaldo, F., & DeFilippo, E. (2003). Outcome predictors in the short-term treatment of anorexia nervosa: An integrated medical–psychiatric approach. *Eating and Weight Disorders, 8*(2), 168–172.

Silverstone, P. H. (1992). Is chronic low self-esteem the cause of eating disorders? *Medical Hypotheses, 39,* 311–315.

Simmonds, M. (1914). Uber embolische prozesse in der hypophysis. *Archives of Pathology and Anatomy, 217,* 226–239.

Simpson, K. (2002). Anorexia nervosa and culture. *Journal of Psychiatric and Mental Health Nursing, 9*(1), 65–71.

Slupik, R. (1999). Managing adolescents with eating disorders. *International Journal of Fertility and Women's Medicine, 44*(3), 125–130.

Smolak, L., & Murnen, S. (2002). A meta-analytic examination of the relationship between child sexual abuse and eating disorders. *International Journal of Eating Disorders, 31*(2), 136–150.

Sohlberg, S., & Strober, M. (1994). Personality in anorexia nervosa: An update and a theoretical integration. *Acta Psychiatrica Scandinavica, 89*(Suppl. 378), 1–15.

Sokol, M. (2000). Infection-triggered anorexia nervosa in children: Clinical description of four cases. *Journal of Child and Adolescent Psychopharmacology, 10*(2), 133–145.

Sokol, M., Ward, P., Tamiya, H., Kondo, D., Houston, D., & Zabriskie, J. (2002). D8/17 expression on B lymphocytes in anorexia nervosa. *American Journal of Psychiatry, 159*(8), 1430–1432.

Srinivasan, K., Ashok, M., Vaz, M., & Yeragani, V. (2004). Effect of imipramine on linear and nonlinear measures of heart rate variability in children. *Pediatric Cardiology, 25*(1), 20–25.

Steiger, H., Stotland, S., Ghadirian, A. M., & White-head, V. (1995). Controlled study of eating concerns and psychopathological traits in relatives of eating disordered probands: Do familial traits exist? *International Journal of Eating Disorders, 18,* 107–118.

Steiner, H., Kwan, W., Shaffer, T., Walker, S., Miller, S., Sagar, A., et al. (2003). Risk and protective factors for juvenile eating disorders. *European Child and Adolescent Psychiatry, 12*(Suppl. I), I38–I36.

Steiner, H., & Lock, J. (1998). Anorexia nervosa and bulimia nervosa in children and adolescents: A review of the past 10 years. *Journal of the American Academy of Child and Adolescent Psychiatry, 37*(4), 352–359.

Steinhausen, H. C. (1995a). The course and outcome of anorexia nervosa. In K. D. Brownell & C. G. Fairburn (Eds.), *Eating disorders and obesity: A comprehensive handbook* (pp. 234–237). New York: Guilford Press.

Steinhausen, H. C. (1995b). Treatment and outcome of adolescent anorexia nervosa. *Hormone Research, 43,* 168–170.

Steinhausen, H. C. (2002). The outcome of anorexia nervosa in the 20th century. *American Journal of Psychiatry, 159*(8), 1284–1293.

Steinhausen, H., Boyadjieva, S., Grigoroiu-Serbanescu, M., Seidel, R., & Winkler Metzke, C. (2000). A transcultural outcome study of adolescent eating disorders. *Acta Psychiatrica Scandinavica, 101*(1), 60–66.

Stice, E., & Ragan, J. (2002). A preliminary controlled evaluation of an eating disturbance psychoeducational intervention for college students. *International Journal of Eating Disorders, 31*(2), 159–171.

Stice, E., & Shaw, H. (2004). Eating disorder prevention programs: A meta-analytic review. *Psychological Bulletin, 130*(2), 206–277.

Stoving, R., Hangaard, J., Hansen-Nord, M., & Hagen, C. (1999). A review of endocrine changes in anorexia nervosa. *Journal of Psychiatric Research, 33*(2), 139–152.

Strangler, R. S., & Printz, A. M. (1980). DSM-III: Psychiatric diagnosis in a university population. *American Journal of Psychiatry, 137,* 937–940.

Striegel-Moore, R. H. (1993). Etiology of binge eating: A developmental perspective. In C. G. Fairburn & G. T. Wilson (Eds.), *Binge eating: Nature, assessment, and treatment* (pp. 144–172). New York: Guilford Press.

Striegel-Moore, R. H. (1995). A feminist perspective on the etiology of eating. In K. D. Brownell & C. G. Fairburn (Eds.), *Eating disorders and obesity: A comprehensive handbook* (pp. 224–229). New York: Guilford Press.

Striegel-Moore, R., Dohm, F., Kraemer, H., Taylor C., Daniels, S., Crawford, P., et al. (2003). Eating disorders in white and black women. *American Journal of Psychiatry, 160*(7), 1326–1331.

Striegel-Moore, R., & Franko, D. (2003). Epidemiology of binge eating disorder. *International Journal of Eating Disorders, 34,* S19–S29.

Striegel-Moore, R., Leslie, D., Petrill, S., Garvin, V., & Rosenheck, R. (2000). One-year use and cost of inpatient and outpatient services among female and male patients with an eating disorder: Evidence from a national database of health insurance claims. *International Journal of Eating Disorders, 27*(4), 381–389.

Strober, M. (1981). The significance of bulimia in juvenile anorexia nervosa: An exploration of possible etiological factors. *International Journal of Eating Disorders, 1,* 28–43.

Strober, M. (1986). Anorexia nervosa: History and psychological concepts. In K. D. Brownell & J. P. Foreyt (Eds.), *Handbook of eating disorders: Physiology, psychology, and treatment of obesity, anorexia, and bulimia* (pp. 231–246). New York: Basic Books.

Strober, M. (1991). Family-genetic studies of eating disorders. *Journal of Clinical Psychiatry, 52*(10, Suppl.), 9–12.

Strober, M. (1995). Family-genetic perspectives on anorexia and bulimia nervosa. In K. D. Brownell & C. G. Fairburn (Eds.), *Eating disorders and obesity: A comprehensive handbook* (pp. 212–218). New York: Guilford Press.

Strober, M., Freeman, R., Lampert, C., Diamond, J., & Kaye, W. (2000). Controlled family study of anorexia nervosa and bulimia nervosa: Evidence of shared liability and transmission of partial syndromes. *American Journal of Psychiatry, 157*(3), 393–401.

Strober, M., Freeman, R., Lampert, C., Diamond, J., & Kaye, W. (2001). Males with anorexia nervosa: A controlled study of eating disorders in first-degree relatives. *International Journal of Eating Disorders, 29*(3), 263–269.

Strober, M., Lampert, C., Morrell, W., Burroughs, J., & Jacobs, C. (1990). A controlled family study of anorexia nervosa: Evidence of familial aggregation and lack of shared transmission with affective disorders. *International Journal of Eating Disorders, 9*(3), 239–253.

Strober, M., & Yager, J. (1985). A developmental perspective on the treatment of anorexia nervosa in adolescents. In D. M. Garner & P. E. Garfinkel (Eds.), *Handbook of psychotherapy for anorexia nervosa and bulimia* (pp. 363–390). New York: Guilford Press.

Strumia, R., Varotti, E., Manzato, E., & Gualandi, M. (2001). Skin signs in anorexia nervosa. *Dermatology, 203*(4), 314–317.

Studen-Pavlovich, D., & Elliott, M. (2001). Eating disorders in women's oral health. *Dental Clinics of North America, 45* (3), 491–511.

Study Group on Anorexia Nervosa. (1995). Anorexia nervosa: Directions for future research. *International Journal of Eating Disorders, 17,* 235–241.

Stunkard, A. (1993). A history of binge eating. In C. G. Fairburn & G. T. Wilson (Eds.), *Binge eating: Nature, assessment and treatment* (pp. 15–34). New York: Guilford Press.

Stunkard, A., & Allison, K. (2003). Two forms of disordered eating in obesity: Binge eating and night eating.

International Journal of Obesity and Related Metabolic Disorders, 27(1), 1–12.

Sturzenberger, S., Cantwell, P. D., Burroughs, J., Salkin, B., & Green, J. K. (1977). A follow-up study of adolescent psychiatric inpatients with anorexia nervosa. Journal of the American Academy of Child Psychiatry, 16, 703–715.

Swenne, I. (2000). Heart risk associated with weight loss in anorexia nervosa and eating disorders: Electrocardiographic changes during the early phase of refeeding. Acta Paediatrica, 89(4), 447–452.

Swenne, I., & Larsson, P. (1999). Heart risk associated with weight loss in anorexia nervosa and eating disorders: Risk factors for QTc interval prolongation and dispersion. Acta Paediatrica, 88(3), 304–309.

Tasca, G., Flynn, C., & Bissada, H. (2002). Comparison of group climate in an eating disorders partial hospital group and a psychiatric partial hospital group. International Journal of Group Psychotherapy, 52(3), 409–417.

Terre, L. (1993). Developmental trends in health-related behaviors: Implications for preventive interventions. Advances in Medical Psychotherapy, 6, 151–162.

Terre, L., & Burkhart, B. (1996). Problem sexual behaviors in adolescence. In G. Blau & T. Gullotta (Eds.), Adolescent dysfunctional behavior (pp. 139–166). Thousand Oaks: CA: Sage.

Terre, L., & Ghiselli, W. (1997). A developmental perspective on family risk factors in somatization. Journal of Psychosomatic Research, 42(2), 197–208.

Terre, L., Poston, W. S., & Foreyt, J. (2005). Overview and the future of obesity treatment. In D. J. Goldstein (Ed.), The management of eating disorders and obesity (pp. 161–179). Totowa, NJ: Humana Press.

Theander, S. (1970). Anorexia nervosa: A psychiatric investigation of 94 female patients. Acta Psychiatrica Scandinavica, 65(Suppl. 214), 1–194.

Thien, V., Thomas, A., Markin, D., & Birmingham, C. (2000). Pilot study of a graded exercise program for the treatment of anorexia nervosa. International Journal of Eating Disorders, 28(1), 101–106.

Thompson-Brenner, H., Glass, S., & Westen, D. (2003). A multidimensional meta-analysis of psychotherapy for bulimia nervosa. Clinical Psychology Science and Practice, 10(3), 269–287.

Tingelstad, J. (1991).The cardiotoxicity of the tricyclics. Journal of the American Academy of Child and Adolescent Psychiatry, 30, 845–846.

Tobin, D. L., Johnson, C., Steinberg, S, Staats, M., & Baker, D. A. (1991). Multifactorial assessment of bulimia nervosa. Journal of Abnormal Psychology, 100, 14–21.

Treasure, J., & Holland, A. (1995). Genetic factors in eating disorders. In G. I. Szmukler, C. Dare, & J. Treasure (Eds.), Handbook of eating disorders: Theory, treatment and research (pp. 65–81). Chichester, UK: Wiley.

Tuschen, B., & Bents, H. (1995). Intensive brief inpatient treatment of bulimia nervosa. In K. D. Brownell & C. G. Fairburn (Eds.), Eating disorders and obesity: A comprehensive handbook (pp. 354–360). New York: Guilford Press.

Tyrka, A., Waldron, I., Graber, J., & Brooks-Gunn, J. (2002). Prospective predictors of the onset of anorexic and bulimic syndromes. International Journal of Eating Disorders, 32(3), 282–290.

U.S. Food and Drug Administration. (1997). FDA analysis of cardiac valvular dysfunction with use of appetite suppressants, 9/17/97. Retrieved from www.fda.gov/cder/news/slides/index.htm

van Praag, H. M. (1993). "Make-believes" in psychiatry or the perils of progress. New York: Brunner/Mazel.

Vervaet, M., van Heeringen, C., & Audenaert, K. (2004). Personality-related characteristics in restricting versus binging and purging eating disordered patients. Comprehensive Psychiatry, 45(1), 37–43.

Viens, M. J., & Hranchuk, K. (1993). The treatment of bulimia nervosa following a surgery using a stimulus control procedure: A case study. Journal of Behavior Therapy and Experimental Psychiatry, 23, 313–317.

Vitousek, K., & Manke, F. (1994). Personality variables and disorders in anorexia nervosa and bulimia nervosa. Journal of Abnormal Psychology, 103, 137–147.

Vize, C. M., & Cooper, P. J. (1995). Sexual abuse in patients with eating disorders, patients with depression, and normal controls: A comparative study. British Journal of Psychiatry, 167, 80–85.

Vohs, K., Bardone, A., Joiner, T., Abramson, L., & Heatherton, T. (1999). Perfectionism, perceived weight status, and self-esteem interact to predict bulimic symptoms: A model of bulimic symptom development. Journal of Abnormal Psychology, 108(4), 695–700.

Waisberg, J., & Woods, M. (2002). A nutrition and behaviour change group for patients with anorexia nervosa. Canadian Journal of Dietetic Practice and Research, 63(4), 202–205.

Wakeling, A. (1996). Epidemiology of anorexia nervosa. Psychiatry Research, 62, 3–9.

Waller, G. (1998). Perceived control in eating disorders: Relationship with reported sexual abuse. International Journal of Eating Disorders, 23(2), 213–216.

Walsh, B., & Devlin, M. (1998). Eating disorders: Progress and problems. Science, 280, 1387–1390.

Walsh, B. T., Gladis, M., Roose, S. P., Stewart, J. W., Stetner, F., & Glassman, A. H. (1988). Phenelzine vs. placebo in 50 patients with bulimia. Archives of General Psychiatry, 45, 471–475.

Walsh, B. T., Stewart, J. W., Wright, L., Harrison, W., Roose, S. P., & Glassman, A. H. (1982). Treatment of bulimia with monoamine oxidase inhibitors. American Journal of Psychiatry, 139, 1629–1630.

Walsh, B. T., Wilson, G. T., Loeb, K. L., Devlin, M. J., Pike, K. M., Roose, S. P., et al. (1997). Medication and psychotherapy in the treatment of bulimia nervosa. American Journal of Psychiatry, 154, 523–531.

Walsh, J. M., Wheat, M. E., & Freund, K. (2000). Detection, evaluation, and treatment of eating disorders: The role of the primary care physician. *Journal of General Internal Medicine, 15*(8), 577–590.

Ward, A., Ramsay, R., Turnbull, S., Steele, M., Steele, H., & Treasure, J. (2001). Attachment in anorexia nervosa: A transgenerational perspective. *British Journal of Medical Psychology, 74*(Pt. 4), 497–505.

Waters, E., & Kendler, K. (1995). Anorexia nervosa and anorexic-like syndromes in a population-based female twin sample. *American Journal of Psychiatry, 152*(1), 64–71.

Watkins, B., & Lask, B. (2002). Eating disorders in school-aged children. *Child and Adolescent Psychiatric Clinics of North America, 11*(2), 185–199.

Watkins, B., Willoughby, K., Waller, G., Serpell, L., & Lask, B. (2002). Patterns of birth in anorexia nervosa. *International Journal of Eating Disorders, 32*(1), 11–17.

Watson, T., Bowers, W., & Andersen, A. (2000). Involuntary treatment of eating disorders. *American Journal of Psychiatry, 157*(11), 1806–1810.

Webb, W. L., & Gehi, M. (1981). Electrolyte and fluid imbalance: Neuropsychiatric manifestations. *Psychosomatics, 22*, 199–202.

Weiss, T., & Levitz, L. (1976). Diphenylhydantoin treatment of bulimia [Letter to the editor]. *American Journal of Psychiatry, 133*, 1093.

Welch, S. L., & Fairburn, C. G. (1994). Sexual abuse and bulimia nervosa: Three integrated case control comparisons. *American Journal of Psychiatry, 151*, 402–407.

Weltzin, T. E., & Bolton, B. G. (1998). Bulimia nervosa. In V. VanHasselt & M. Hersen (Eds.), *Handbook of psychological treatment protocols for children and adolescents* (pp. 435–465). Mahwah, NJ: Erlbaum.

Weltzin, T. E., Fernstrom, M. H., & Kaye, W. H. (1994). Serotonin and bulimia nervosa. *Nutrition Reviews, 52*, 399–408.

Wentz, E., Gillberg, C., Gillberg, I., & Rastam, M. (2001). Ten-year follow-up of adolescent-onset anorexia nervosa: Psychiatric disorders and overall functioning scales. *Journal of Child Psychology and Psychiatry, 42*(5), 613–622.

Wermuth, B., Davis, K., Hollister, L., & Stunkard, A. (1977). Phenytoin treatment of the binge-eating syndrome. *American Journal of Psychiatry, 134*, 1249–1253.

White, W. C., & Boskind-White, M. (1981). An experiential–behavioral approach to the treatment of bulimarexia. *Psychotherapy: Theory, Research, and Practice, 18*, 501–597.

Wiederman, M., & Pryor, T. (2000). Body dissatisfaction, bulimia, and depression among women: The mediating role of drive for thinness. *International Journal of Eating Disorders, 27*(1), 90–95.

Wildes, J., Emery, R., & Simons, A. (2001). The roles of ethnicity and culture in the development of eating disturbance and body dissatisfaction: A meta-analytic review. *Clinical Psychology Review, 21*(4), 521–551.

Wilfley, D. E., Agras, W. S., Telch, C. F., Rossiter, E. M.,

Schneider, J. A., Cole, A. G., et al. (1993). Group CBT and group interpersonal psychotherapy for nonpurging bulimics: A controlled comparison. *Journal of Consulting and Clinical Psychology, 61*, 296–305.

Wilfley, D. E., & Cohen, L. R. (1997). Psychological treatment of bulimia nervosa and binge eating disorder. *Psychopharmacology Bulletin, 33*(3), 437–454.

Wilfley, D. E., & Rodin, J. (1995). Cultural influences on eating disorders. In K. D. Brownell & C. G. Fairburn (Eds.), *Eating disorders and obesity: A comprehensive handbook* (pp. 78–82). New York: Guilford Press.

Wilfley, D. E., Welch, R., Stein, R., Spurrell, E., Cohen, L., Saelens, B., et al. (2002). A randomized comparison of group cognitive behavioral therapy and group interpersonal psychotherapy for the treatment of overweight individuals with binge-eating disorder. *Archives of General Psychiatry, 59*(8), 713–721.

Willi, J., & Grossman, S. (1983). Epidemiology of anorexia nervosa in a defined region of Switzerland. *American Journal of Psychiatry, 140*, 564–567.

Williamson, D. A., Duchmann, E., Barker, S., & Bruno, R. (1998). Anorexia nervosa. In V. VanHasselt & M. Hersen (Eds.), *Handbook of psychological treatment protocols for children and adolescents* (pp. 413–434). Mahwah, NJ: Erlbaum.

Williamson, D. A., Prather, R. C., Bennett, S. M., Davis, C. J., Watkins, P. C., & Grenier, C. E. (1989). An uncontrolled evaluation of inpatient and outpatient cognitive-behavior therapy for bulimia nervosa. *Behavior Modification, 13*, 340–360.

Williamson, D. A., Zucker, N., Martin, C., & Smeets, M. (2001). Etiology and management of eating disorders. In H. Adams & P. Sutker (Eds.), *Comprehensive handbook of psychopathology* (pp. 641–670). New York: Kluwer.

Williamson, L. (1998). Eating disorders and the cultural forces behind the drive for thinness: Are African-American women really protected? *Social Work in Health Care, 28*(1), 61–73.

Wilson, G. T. (1991). The addiction model of eating disorders: A critical analysis. *Advances in Behaviour Research and Therapy, 13*(1), 27–72.

Wilson, G. T. (1995). Eating disorders and addictive disorders. In K. D. Brownell & C. G. Fairburn (Eds.), *Eating disorders and obesity: A comprehensive handbook* (pp. 165–170). New York: Guilford Press.

Wilson, G. T. (1999). Cognitive behavior therapy for eating disorders: Progress and problems. *Behaviour Research and Therapy, 37*(Suppl. 1), S79–S95.

Wilson, G. T. (2000). Eating disorders and addiction. In W. S. C. Poston & C. Haddock (Eds.), *Food as a drug* (pp. 87–101). New York: Haworth Press.

Wilson, G. T., Eldredge, K. L., Smith, D., & Niles, B. (1991). Cognitive-behavioral treatment with and without response prevention for bulimia. *Behaviour Research and Therapy, 29*, 575–583.

Wilson, G. T., & Fairburn, C. G. (1993). Cognitive treatments for eating disorders. *Journal of Consulting and Clinical Psychology, 61*, 261–269.

Wilson, G. T., & Pike, K. (2001). Eating disorders. In D. H. Barlow (Ed.), *Clinical handbook of psychological disorders* (3rd ed., pp. 332–375). New York: Guilford Press.

Wilson, G. T., Rossiter, E., Kleinfield, E. I., & Lindholm, L. (1986). Cognitive-behavioral treatment of bulimia nervosa: A controlled evaluation. *Behaviour Research and Therapy, 24,* 277–288.

Windauer, U., Lennerts, W., Talbot, P., Touyz, S. W., & Beumont, P. J. V. (1993). How well are 'cured' anorexia nervosa patients?: An investigation of 16 weight-recovered anorexic patients. *British Journal of Psychiatry, 163,* 195–200.

Wiseman, C., Sunday, S., Klapper, F., Harris, W., & Halmi, K. (2001). Changing patterns of hospitalization in eating disorder patients. *International Journal of Eating Disorders, 30*(1), 69–74.

Wiseman, C., Sunday, S., Klapper, F., Klein, M., & Halmi, K. (2002). Short-term group CBT versus psycho-education on an inpatient eating disorder unit. *Eating Disorders: The Journal of Treatment and Prevention, 10*(4), 313–320.

Wolfe, B., Metzger, E., & Jimerson, D. (1997). Research update on serotonin function in bulimia nervosa and anorexia nervosa. *Psychopharmacology Bulletin, 33*(3), 345–354.

Wonderlich, S. A. (1995). Personality and eating disorders. In K. D. Brownell & C. G. Fairburn (Eds.), *Eating disorders and obesity: A comprehensive handbook* (pp. 171–175). New York: Guilford Press.

Wonderlich, S. A., Brewerton, T. D., Jocic, Z., Dansky, B. S., & Abbott, D. W. (1997). Relationship of childhood sexual abuse and eating disorders. *Journal of the American Academy of Child and Adolescent Psychiatry, 36,* 1107–1115.

Wonderlich, S. A., Fullerton, D., Swift, W., & Klein, M. H. (1994). Five-year outcome from eating disorders: Relevance of personality disorders. *International Journal of Eating Disorders, 15,* 233–243.

Woodside, D. B. (1995). The review of anorexia nervosa and bulimia nervosa. *Current Problems in Pediatrics, 25,* 67–89.

Woodside, D., Garfinkel, P., Lin, E., Goering, P., Kaplan, A., Goldbloom, D., et al. (2001). Comparisons of men with full or partial eating disorders, men without eating disorders, and women with eating disorders in the community. *American Journal of Psychiatry, 158*(4), 570–574.

Wooley, S. C. (1995). Feminist influences on the treatment of eating disorders. In K. D. Brownell & C. G. Fairburn (Eds.), *Eating disorders and obesity: A comprehensive handbook* (pp. 294–298). New York: Guilford Press.

Wooley, S. C., & Kearney-Cooke, A. (1986). Intensive treatment of bulimia and body-image disturbance. In K. D. Brownell & J. P. Foreyt (Eds.), *Handbook of eating disorders: Physiology, psychology, and treatment of obesity, anorexia, and bulimia* (pp. 476–502). New York: Basic Books.

Wu, J. C., Hagman, J., Buchsbaum, M. S., Blinder, B., Derrfler, M., Tai, W. Y., et al. (1990). Greater left cerebral hemispheric metabolism in bulimia assessed by positron emission tomography. *American Journal of Psychiatry, 147,* 309–312.

Wurtman, R. J., & Wurtman, J. J. (1984). Nutrients, neurotransmitter synthesis, and the control of food intake. In A. J. Stunkard & E. Stellar (Eds.), *Eating and its disorders* (pp. 77–86). New York: Raven Press.

Yager, J. (1994). Psychosocial treatments for eating disorders. *Psychiatry, 57,* 153–164.

Yager, J. (1995). The management of patients with intractable eating disorders. In K. D. Brownell & C. G. Fairburn (Eds.), *Eating disorders and obesity: A comprehensive handbook* (pp. 374–378). New York: Guilford Press.

Yager, J. (2001). E-mail as a therapeutic adjunct in the outpatient treatment of anorexia nervosa: Illustrative case material and discussion of the issues. *International Journal of Eating Disorders, 29*(2), 125–138.

Zabinski, M., Pung, M., Wilfley, D., Eppstein, D., Winzelberg, A., Celio, A., et al. (2001). Reducing risk factors for eating disorders: Targeting at-risk women with a computerized psychoeducational program. *International Journal of Eating Disorders, 29*(4), 401–408.

Zhu, A., & Walsh, B. (2002). Pharmacologic treatment of eating disorders. *Canadian Journal of Psychiatry, 47*(3), 227–234.

Zipfel, S., Lowe, B., Reas, D., Deter, H., & Herzog, W. (2000). Long-term prognosis in anorexia nervosa: Lessons from a 21–year follow up study. *Lancet, 355,* 721–722.

Zonnevijlle-Bender, M., van Goozen, S., Cohen-Kettenis, P., van Elburg, A., & van Engeland, H. (2002). Do adolescent anorexia nervosa patients have deficits in emotional functioning? *European Child and Adolescent Psychiatry, 11*(1), 38–42.

Author Index

Aarons, G. A., 744
Abbott, D. W., 787
Abbott, R., 209, 218, 227, 561, 563
Abbott, S., 552, 561
Abella, E., 784
Aber, J. L., 607, 631, 689
Abercrombie, H. C., 350
Abidin, R. R., 151, 160
Abikoff, H., 11, 80, 81, 82, 84, 87, 88, 90, 104, 106, 114, 116, 117, 204, 226, 227
Ablon, J. S., 8, 9
Abraham, S. F., 784, 786, 787
Abrahams, N., 651
Abramovitz, A., 6, 281
Abramowitz, A. J., 191, 194
Abramowitz, J. S., 292
Abrams, A., 385
Abrams, D. B., 738, 751
Abramson, L., 340, 341, 342, 350, 354, 685, 686, 787
Abrantes, A. M., 733, 734, 745, 748, 749, 760
Accardo, P. J., 73, 465
Achenbach, T. M., 4, 8, 18, 20, 25, 44, 68, 138, 143, 147, 155, 156, 158, 159, 274, 695, 744
Acker, M. M., 159
Ackerman, D. L., 295
Acton, R., 622, 691
Adam, T., 273, 373
Adams, G., 523, 524, 534, 535
Adams, H. E., 37
Adams, J., 667, 668, 682
Adams, K. D., 548, 555
Adams, M. J., 522, 533
Adams, P., 147, 336, 346, 483, 484
Adams, R. M., 343, 346
Adams, T., 437, 474
Addalli, K. A., 71
Addis, M. E., 31, 299, 376
Addison, O. W., 7
Addy, C., 339, 343
Addy, R., 701
Adelman, H. S., 9, 14, 15
Adler, A. G., 340
Adler, L., 91
Adler, N. A., 678
Adler, R., 145, 202, 217, 218, 219, 227
Administration for Children, Youth and Families, 595, 597, 598, 612
Adrian, C., 351, 354
Advokat, C., 788, 805
Afton, A. D., 221, 222
Ageton, S. S., 157
Aghajanian, G. K., 348
Agras, W. S., 355, 780, 781, 784, 785, 787, 790, 797, 798, 800, 804, 806, 807, 809, 810
Aguar, D., 164, 189, 213
Aguilar, B., 149
Ahia, C. E., 661, 727

Ahlborn, H. H., 180, 219
Ahlsen, G., 461
Ahlsten-Taylor, J., 419
Ahmad, M., 667
Ainsworth, C., 787
Aisemberg, P., 484
Akshoomoff, N., 461, 467
Al Otaiba, S., 537
Al-Shabbout, M., 349
Alain, M., 341
Alanko, L., 461, 462
Alarcon, M., 465
Albano, A. M., 9, 43, 271, 273, 274, 275, 278, 280, 281, 292, 330
Albers, C. A., 10
Albert, M. J., 443
Alberto, P. A., 38
Alberts, E., 72, 73
Albin, J. B., 221, 222
Albin, R. W., 480, 481, 482, 486
Albrecht, R., 342
Albucher, R. C., 701
Aldgate, J., 676
Aldridge, J., 665
Alegria, M., 693
Aleman, A., 652
Alessi, N., 206
Alexander, A. W., 545, 550, 551, 552, 553, 575
Alexander, J. F., 8, 10, 172, 173, 207, 214, 215, 223, 224, 225, 226
Alexander, K. W., 664, 675
Alexander, M. C., 673
Alexander, P. A., 556
Alexander, P. C., 678
Alford, J. D., 436
Alfred, E. D., 77, 81, 444
Algina, J., 165, 166, 212, 225
Alicke, M. D., 16, 17, 28, 29, 38, 41
Alku, P., 461
Allan, R., 783
Allan, W. D., 337, 338
Allard, H. A., 648
Allen, A. J., 91, 94
Allen, D., 457, 472
Allen, D. M., 608
Allen, J., 348, 457, 464, 487
Allen, J. P., 607, 631
Allen, L., 23, 28
Allen, L. B., 302
Allen, S. H., 537
Allessandri, M., 435
Allgood-Merten, B., 342
Allinder, R. M., 574
Allington, R. L., 575
Allison, D. B., 119
Allison, K., 781, 783
Allman, C., 353
Allor, J. H., 537
Alloy, L., 21, 350, 354, 685, 686
Alm, T., 288, 316
Almeida, M. C., 437

Almqvist, F., 415
Alpern, L., 151
Alpert, A., 353, 733
Alpert, J. E., 299, 348
Alpert, J. L., 596
Alterman, A. I., 747
Altham, P., 355
Althause, V., 566
Altmeyer, B. K., 431
Altshuler, J., 687
Alvarado, L., 607
Alvarado, R., 207, 220, 231
Amacher, E., 673
Aman, C. J., 664, 667
Aman, M. G., 93, 95, 205, 207, 226, 414, 415, 416, 436, 439, 441, 442, 443
Amari, A., 425
Amatetti, S., 735
Amato, P. R., 151
Amaya-Jackson, L., 9, 292, 330
Ambrose, S., 611
Ambrosini, P., 205, 338, 347, 349, 386
American Academy of Child and Adolescent Psychiatry, 84
American Academy of Pediatrics, 65, 84, 471
American Association on Mental Retardation, 412, 413, 414, 415, 416
American Association of University Women, 342
American Dietetic Association, 795
American Professional Society on the Abuse of Children, 667, 679
American Psychiatric Association, 20, 25, 65, 67, 68, 69, 70, 137, 138, 139, 146, 147, 152, 157, 274, 336, 337, 412, 415, 416, 421, 433, 456, 457, 458, 459, 463, 489, 681, 736, 779, 780, 781, 782, 783, 784, 785, 790, 791, 792, 794, 795, 796, 797, 809
American Psychological Association, 9, 284, 285, 286, 679
Amianto, F., 785
Amin, T., 465
Amir, R. E., 460
Ammerman, R. T., 4
Amtmann, D., 561, 563
Amundsen, M. J., 6, 28, 284, 285, 286, 287, 295, 298, 489
Anastasi, A., 36.284
Anastopoulos, A. D., 9, 14, 70, 71, 86, 97, 102, 118
Anda, R. F., 648, 650, 651
Anderle, M. J., 350
Anderman, E. M., 355
Anders, P. L., 557
Andersen, A. E., 792, 793, 795, 803, 804, 807
Andersen, P. H., 470
Andershed, H., 142
Anderson, A., 466
Anderson, C. M., 75

Anderson, C. O. L., 731
Anderson, D., 800
Anderson, E., 299, 350
Anderson, G. M., 295
Anderson, J., 152, 422, 427
Anderson, J. C., 271, 339, 648, 649, 650
Anderson, J. W., 74
Anderson, K. A., 734
Anderson, K. G., 736
Anderson, L., 484, 783, 794
Anderson, L. T., 483
Anderson, R. L., 685
Anderson, S., 731
Anderson, S. R., 488
Anderson, V., 484
Andersson, T., 144
Andrade, A., 11, 28, 189, 376
Andreski, P., 76
Andrew, C., 467
Andrews, D., 190
Andrews, D. W., 159, 186, 212, 232
Andrews, J., 7, 353, 378
Andrews, J. A., 70, 339, 345, 347
Andrews, J. N., 99
Andrews, J. S., 733
Andrews, N., 462, 469
Andrews, R., 461
Andrews, V. C., 339
Andrews, W. R., 314
Aneshensel, C. S., 342, 344
Angelini, P. J., 648
Angell, K. E., 340
Angelucci, J., 220
Anglin, T. M., 668, 669
Angold, A., 72, 115, 137, 144, 145, 146,
    189, 216, 271, 280, 298, 339, 650, 693,
    739
Angrist, B., 84
Annis, H. M., 744, 756, 758
Anonymous, 789
Anthony, A., 465, 468
Anthony, B. J., 354
Anthony, J., 695
Anthony, J. C., 210
Anthony, J. L., 533, 542, 543, 550
Antochi, R., 441, 443
Antonello, S., 475
Antshel, K. M., 9, 108, 118
Anzai, N., 795, 796, 797
Aos, S., 166, 174, 178, 185, 188, 212
Appelbaum, P. S., 609
Appelberg, B., 461, 462
Applegate, B., 25, 67, 68, 139, 568
Appleton, A. C., 522, 570, 574
Apter, A., 779, 785
Aragona, J., 606, 610, 611, 613, 616, 617,
    621, 622
Araji, S., 703
Arata, C. M., 656, 658
Arbeile, S., 471
Arbuthnot, J., 146, 173, 174, 214, 215, 219
Archer, J., 146
Arensdorf, A., 6, 28, 284, 285, 286, 287,
    295, 298, 489
Argall, W. J., 787
Argamaso, R. V., 413
Arieti, S., 353
Arin, D. M., 460
Arkinson, M. K., 617
Armenteros, J. L., 206, 226
Armeteros, J. L, 483
Armstrong, F. D., 326
Armstrong, S. C., 439, 441
Armstrong, T. D., 737
Arndt, S., 94, 465
Arnold, C. R., 190
Arnold, D. S., 159
Arnold, J. E., 171, 213
Arnold, K. D., 180, 219
Arnold, L. E., 11, 73, 114, 119, 439, 441
Arnold, L. L., 68
Arnold, M. S., 435
Arnold, S. T., 466
Arnow, B., 797, 798, 800, 804, 806, 807,
    810
Arnsten, A. F. T., 84, 85, 86
Aro, H., 339, 345

Aronson, M., 419
Arrowhead, A., 732
Arthur, J. L., 43
Arthur, M. W., 209, 227
Artner, J., 86
Arvidsson, T., 462
Ary, D. V., 212
Asarnow, J., 13, 24, 37
Asarnow, J. R., 18, 19, 340, 458
Asch, S. E., 569
Asdigian, N., 652, 653, 654
Ash, J. B., 782
Ashok, M., 806
Ashton, V., 662
Ashwin, C., 467
Askeland, E., 172, 229
Asperger, H., 455
Aspland, H., 156, 225, 228, 229
Assemany, A., 679
Association for the Treatment of Sexual
    Abusers, 679
Atabaki, S., 667, 668
Atkeson, B. M., 144, 151, 162, 212
Atkins, M., 625, 629
Atkins, M. S., 105
Atkinson, B. M., 105
Atkinson, L., 9, 621, 622
Attia, E., 805
Attkisson, C., 28
Attwood, T., 475
Atwater, J. D., 187, 215, 227
Audenaert, K., 785
Audrain, J., 733
Aughton, D., 413
Augimeri, L. K., 220
August, G. J., 107
Austin, A. A., 283, 326
Austin, G., 75, 673, 674
Autism Genetic Research Exchange
    Consortium, 465
Avci, A., 806
Avery, D., 330
Avery, I. S., 617
Avison, W. R., 343
Axelrod, S., 431
Axelson, D. A., 295, 350
Ayers, W. A., 28
Ayllon, T., 104, 105, 106, 194, 195, 314,
    611
Aylward, E. H., 75, 552
Ayoub, C., 627, 628, 629
Azar, B., 627
Azar, S. T., 595, 596, 597, 599, 600, 601,
    604, 606, 607, 609, 610, 611, 612, 613,
    614, 615, 616, 617, 618, 619, 620, 621,
    622, 626, 627, 628, 630, 632
Aziz, K., 417
Azqueta, M., 783, 784
Azrin, N. H., 43, 702, 738, 747, 749

Babigian, H. M., 779, 782
Bachanas, P. J., 28
Bachman, J. G., 731, 759
Bachmeyer, M., 428
Bachrach, A. J., 798
Backmund, H., 802
Baden, A. D., 150
Badgley, R. F., 648
Baer, D. M., 6, 7, 10, 40, 44
Baer, J. S., 735
Baer, P. E., 740
Baer, R. A., 107
Baer, S., 67
Bagley, C. C., 650, 651
Baglio, C., 425
Bagner, D. M., 222
Bagwell, C. L., 72, 73, 107
Bahr, C. M., 567
Baieli, S., 461
Bailer, U., 780, 789
Bailet, L. L., 562
Bailey, A., 461, 465
Bailey, J. S., 105, 194, 201, 217
Bailey, K., 299
Bailey, R., 804
Bailey, W. C., 733, 747, 762
Bain, A. M., 561
Baird, G., 443, 457, 461, 462, 463, 483

Bak, S. J., 559
Baker, A. W., 650
Baker, B. L., 25, 160, 435, 436, 484, 485,
    486
Baker, D., 790
Baker, E., 736
Baker, J. A., 602
Baker, J. R., 739
Baker, L., 556, 779, 801
Baker, M., 797
Baker, W. L., 683, 688
Baker-Ward, L., 418
Bakker, D. J., 524, 525
Bal, S., 682, 687
Balach, L., 275
Balachova, T., 9, 615, 616, 617, 621, 623
Balcaltchuk, J., 806
Balderson, B. H., 5
Baldessarini, R. J., 93, 94, 206, 386, 389
Baldry, A. C., 142, 198, 225
Baldwin, B., 797
Baldwin, D. V., 161
Baldwin, M. W., 619
Baldwin, S., 682
Balestracci, K. M., 629
Balge, K. A., 599
Balhorn, M. E., 740
Balise, R., 546
Ball, E. W., 540
Ball, J. D., 72
Ball, L. K., 470
Ball, R., 470
Balla, D., 457
Ballaban-Gil, K., 471
Ballard, R., 736
Ballenger, J. C., 788, 789, 810
Bambara, L., 422
Bamburg, J., 425
Bammer, G., 648, 651
Band, E., 687
Bandura, A., 7, 10, 34, 273, 281, 282, 288,
    290, 314, 318, 351, 739
Banerjee, S., 740
Bank, L., 147, 148, 152, 158, 172, 200,
    214, 224, 226, 340
Barabasz, A. F., 314
Baradaran, L., 665
Barale, F., 467
Baranek, G. T., 457, 465
Baranowska, B., 783
Barbaresi, W. J., 464
Barbarich, N., 806
Barber, M., 462, 658, 659
Barber, N. I., 67
Barberi, A., 789
Barbero, G. J., 340
Barbetta, P. M., 474
Barch, D. M., 350
Barden, N., 348
Bardone, A., 147, 787
Barenz, R., 428, 429
Bargh, J. A., 600
Barker, D., 191
Barker, J., 657, 658, 669
Barker, S., 790, 791, 792, 793, 794
Barkley, R. A., 3, 4, 7, 9, 11, 13, 14, 16,
    25, 26, 27, 30, 34, 36, 39, 43, 65, 67,
    68, 70, 71, 72, 73, 74, 77, 78, 79, 80,
    81, 82, 86, 87, 88, 89, 90, 95, 98, 99,
    101, 102, 103, 104, 105, 109, 110, 111,
    113, 118, 120, 139, 144, 176, 190, 204,
    283, 531, 602, 615, 622, 739
Barlow, D. H., 4, 9, 29, 37, 43, 271, 273,
    274, 275, 276, 277, 278, 279, 280, 281,
    288, 292, 301, 302, 314, 330, 391, 799
Barlow, W. E., 468
Barnby, G., 465
Barnes, G. M., 740, 751, 752
Barnes, H. V., 208, 217, 420
Barnes, K. T., 596, 600, 606, 610, 618
Barnes, M., 513, 516, 517, 518
Barnes, M. C., 28, 513, 520, 524, 531, 555
Barnett, J. Y., 484
Barnett, N. P., 735, 737, 738, 750
Barocas, R., 23
Barocka, A., 350
Baroff, G. S., 416, 430

Baron-Cohen, S., 457, 462, 463, 464, 466, 467, 475
Baron, G., 489
Baron, L., 650
Barr, H. M., 77
Barr, R., 535, 538
Barrera, M., 738, 740
Barrett, K. C., 689
Barrett, M. J., 779
Barrett, P. M., 4, 8, 9, 10, 12, 40, 274, 275, 283, 284, 291, 292, 294, 326, 332
Barrett, R. P., 484
Barrett, S., 14, 30, 80, 102, 111
Barrickman, L. L., 94
Barriga, A. Q., 185
Barrios, B. A., 272, 280, 284
Barrish, H. H., 191, 209
Barron-Quinn, J., 431
Barron, R. W., 522, 523, 547
Barry, C. T., 142, 154, 159
Barry, R. J., 74
Bartelstone, J., 602
Barth, R. P., 198, 201, 617, 619, 620, 622, 652, 676, 677
Barthelemy, C., 467
Bartholomew, T., 793
Bartko, J. J., 203
Bartolucci, G., 459, 471
Barton, C., 173, 223, 224
Barton, S., 487
Bartusch, D. J., 144
Basili, L., 44
Basinger, K. S., 179
Bass, D., 28, 156, 157, 181, 215, 218, 219, 220, 221, 222, 226, 286
Bass, M. P., 465
Basta, J., 682
Bateman, B., 519
Bates, H., III, 566
Bates, J. E., 141, 149, 152
Bates, S., 340
Batterman-Faunce, J. M., 667, 670, 671
Battle, E. K., 811
Battle, R., 568
Baucom, D., 797
Bauer, C. R., 420
Bauer, J., 479, 487
Bauer, L., 77
Baugher, M., 338, 339, 356, 379, 383, 384
Baum, C. G., 164, 213, 214, 226
Baum-Faulkner, D., 612
Bauman, E. D., 733
Bauman, K., 423, 426, 428, 431, 432
Bauman, M. L., 441, 460, 470
Baumann, B. L., 73
Baumeister, A. A., 43, 433
Baumgaerel, A., 70
Bauminger, N., 467, 475
Baumrind, D., 483
Bauserman, R., 680, 681
Bauske, B. W., 171, 229
Bavly, L., 737
Baxter, E. G., 314, 330
Baxter, L. R., 350, 394
Baydar, N., 221
Bayles, K., 149
Bayliss, D. M., 74
Beardslee, W. R., 271, 345, 354, 378, 391
Bearman, S. K., 342, 344
Beattie, D., 488
Beauchaine, T. P., 74, 168, 218, 219, 220, 221, 231
Beauchesne, H., 208
Beaumont, P., 798
Beck, A. T., 160, 273, 277, 279, 350, 351, 362, 379, 381, 753
Beck, J. S., 367
Beck, N. C., 337, 338, 339
Beck, S., 179, 215, 226, 435
Becker, C. B., 299
Becker, D. F., 733, 739
Becker, J. V., 596, 678, 704
Becker, K. D., 143
Becker, O. V., 443
Becker, W. C., 7, 190, 191, 192, 216, 534, 621
Becker-Cottrill, B., 484

Bedway, M., 802
Beebe, T. J., 737
Beede, S. D., 747
Beelmann, A., 107, 179, 215
Beesley, S., 207
Begay, K., 563
Behar, D., 67
Behar, L., 156, 189, 216
Behr, S., 486
Behrens, B. C., 214, 486
Beidel, D. C., 24, 295, 326
Beilke, R. L., 700
Beinfeld, M. C., 789
Beiser, A. S., 667, 668
Belanoff, J., 340
Belchic, J. K., 473
Belin, T. R., 83, 441
Bell, C. C., 391
Bell, D. J., 8, 17
Bell, K., 541
Bell, M., 664
Bell, R. M., 778, 799
Bell, R. Q., 34, 149
Bell, S., 165
Bell-Dolan, D. J., 24, 271, 273, 279, 342
Bellack, A. S., 316
Bellamy, N., 220, 231
Bellinger, D. C., 77, 81, 444
Bellini, O., 807
Bellodi, L., 789
Belmonte, M. K., 467
Belsky, J., 148, 599
Bem, D. J., 278
Bemis, K. M., 798, 800
Bemporad, J. R., 353
Ben, K. R., 482
Ben-Tall, A., 478
Ben-Tovim, D., 778, 788, 804, 808, 809
Bendel, R., 662
Bender, M. E., 86, 106, 109, 110, 111
Bene, E., 695
Benedict, M. A., 676
Bengston, B. S., 682
Benito, N., 483
Benjet, C., 344, 604, 606, 614
Benkelfat, C., 348
Bennett, D. S., 149, 179, 185, 215, 219
Bennett, F. C., 420
Bennett, L. A., 738
Bennett, S. M., 796, 797
Bennett, W. G., 204, 205, 218, 226, 227, 232
Bennett-Johnson, S., 28
Benoit, D., 28
Benoit, M. Z., 299
Benson, B. A., 414
Benson, B. E., 350
Benson, G., 151
Benson, N. J., 522, 523, 547
Bentivoglio, P., 387, 389
Bentler, P. M., 732, 733, 738
Bentovim, A., 650
Bents, H., 795, 799
Bentz, J., 567
Berberich, J. P., 456
Berends, I. E., 525
Berenson, A. B., 667, 668
Beresford, S. A. A., 12
Berg, W., 433
Bergan, J. R., 9
Bergeron, L., 70
Bergh, C., 804
Berghold, K., 787
Bergholz, K., 811
Berglund, P., 3
Bergman, E., 551, 552
Bergman, L., 271, 280
Bergman, T., 468
Berk, L. E., 79, 106
Berkman, M. D., 413
Berkowitz, C., 386
Berkowitz, G., 676
Berkowitz, L., 600, 606
Berliner, L., 595, 657, 658, 659, 663, 683, 691, 692, 693, 694, 702, 703
Berman, J. S., 17, 28
Berman, S. R., 686

Berman, W. H., 351
Bernal, G., 380, 391
Bernal, M. E., 43, 226
Bernard, S., 469
Bernardis, A., 803
Bernbaum, J. C., 420
Bernheimer, L. P., 438
Berninger, V. W., 530, 552, 561, 563
Bernstein, E., 687, 688
Bernstein, G. A., 271, 294
Bernton, D., 628
Berquin, P. C., 75
Berrett, M., 797
Berrick, J. D., 652, 676
Berry, J. M., 443
Berson, N. L., 669
Bertelli, M., 441
Berthiaume, C., 70, 472
Bertrand, J., 462
Bertrand, L., 208
Besalel, V. A., 747
Beschner, G. M., 731
Besharov, D. J., 662, 663
Bessler, A., 71, 739
Bessmer, J., 157, 158
Best, C. L., 658, 668, 685
Betancur, C., 465
Bethke, S., 428
Bettle, N., 782
Bettle, O., 782
Beumont, C. C., 795
Beumont, P. J., 784, 785, 786, 787, 795, 808
Beutler, L., 32, 692, 694, 797
Bezman, R. J., 65, 70
Bhat, P., 568
Bhatti, T., 348
Bhaumik, S., 441
Bialer, I., 84
Bianchi, B., 788
Bianco, E., 468
Bibby, P., 489, 490
Bickerton, W., 379
Bickett, A. D., 623
Bickman, L., 11, 28, 30, 189, 376
Bidwell, R., 795, 796, 797
Biederman, J., 68, 71, 72, 74, 75, 76, 77, 86, 87, 90, 91, 93, 94, 206, 295, 338, 385, 387, 389, 443, 739, 752
Bielecki, J., 425
Bienvenu, T., 465
Bierman, K. L., 147, 155, 179, 186, 211, 232
Bigbee, M. A., 18
Bigelow, K. M., 606, 623, 624
Bigfoot, D. S., 596
Biggs, M., 664
Bigham, M., 469
Biglan, A., 66, 90, 145, 179, 212, 215, 273
Bijou, S., 6, 523
Bilal, R., 752
Billings, A. G., 738
Billington, C., 786
Billstedt, E., 461
Binder, C., 442
Binder, R. L., 655
Binggeli, N. J., 598
Binkoff, J. A., 426, 480
Binstock, T., 469
Binswanger, L., 779
Birch, H. G., 149
Birchler, G. R., 10
Bird, D., 802
Bird, H. R., 271, 733, 739, 745, 752
Bird, S., 704
Birmaher, B., 275, 295, 338, 339, 340, 349, 356, 379, 383, 384, 385, 386, 745
Birmingham, C., 803
Birnbrauer, J. S., 488
Birndorf, S., 784, 792
Birsh, J., 546
Birt, J., 11, 680, 682, 684, 687, 688, 694, 695, 697
Bissada, H., 802
Bitoni, C., 602
Bittle, R., 433
Bjure, J., 783

Blacher, J., 485
Blachman, B. A., 540, 550, 552
Black, C., 468
Black, J., 546
Black, K., 208
Black, R. S., 450
Blackwell, B., 387
Blagys, M. D., 380
Blair, C., 420
Blair, E., 170, 229
Blair, R. J., 142
Blair, S., 786
Blakley, T. L., 683, 688
Blampied, N. M., 200, 202
Blanchard, E. B., 288, 314, 318, 685, 690
Blanco, C., 294
Blane, H., 733
Blankenship, C., 566
Blaske, D. M., 18
Blaskey, L. G., 74
Blattner, J. E., 562
Blaxill, M. F., 470
Blechman, E. A., 12, 43, 143, 161, 184, 202, 225
Bledsoe, Y., 337, 338
Blew, P., 441
Blinder, B., 789
Bliss, C. A., 436
Blitz, C., 732, 738, 743
Block, J., 17, 23, 733, 739, 740
Block, J. H., 17, 23
Block-Pedego, A., 159
Blondis, T. A., 72, 73
Bloomquist, M. L., 107
Blount, R., 72, 652
Blue, J., 597, 601, 618
Blue-Banning, M., 486
Blum, H. M., 147
Blum, R. W., 737
Blumberg, E., 676
Blumberg, E. R., 482, 483
Blume, A. W., 735
Blumenthal, J. D., 72
Blythe, B. J., 617, 619, 620, 622
Boachie, A., 804
Boat, B., 663, 666, 692
Bober, S. L., 595, 596, 606, 607, 613
Bobo, J. K., 745
Bodfish, J. W., 458
Bodin, S. D., 142, 154, 159
Body, G., 353
Boettcher, C., 421
Bogat, G. A., 609
Bogers, W., 350
Boggs, S., 98, 158, 165, 166, 212, 225
Bohlke, K., 469
Boileau, H., 208
Boivin, M., 141, 355
Boland, F., 790
Bolander, F. D., 340
Bolen, R. M., 658, 659, 660, 674, 675
Bolstad, O. D., 190, 213
Bolton, B. G., 790, 792, 793, 795, 796, 797, 801
Bolton, D., 318
Bolton, P., 465
Bonagura, N., 71, 739
Bond, N. W., 272
Bond, S., 471
Bondy, A. S., 290, 316, 332, 476, 479, 490
Bonello-Cintron, C. M., 350
Boney-McCoy, S., 682, 685
Bonner, B., 596, 630, 703
Bonvillian, J., 480
Booij, L., 348
Bookstein, F. L., 77
Boon, F., 441
Boone, C., 683
Boone, R. R., 322
Booth, A. L., 786
Booth, S., 86
Bootzin, R. R., 281, 282, 288, 316
Boppana, V., 204, 226
Bor, B., 160, 169, 212, 225
Bor, W., 97, 100
Borchardt, C. M., 271, 338, 339
Borden, K. A., 107, 109

Borden, S. L., 525, 547, 548, 554, 560
Borduin, C. M., 7, 8, 9, 10, 18, 172, 176, 177, 178, 207, 214, 215, 225, 229, 747
Boren, R., 562
Borger, N., 74
Borgida, E., 670, 673
Borjesson, O., 461
Borkovec, T. S., 279
Borkowski, J. G., 522, 523, 531
Born, C., 350
Born, C. E., 633, 634
Bornstein, P. H., 31, 33, 37, 314
Borowiec, M., 783
Borowitz, S. M., 43
Bos, C. S., 557
Boskind-Lodahl, M., 784, 802
Boskind-White, M., 802
Bostic, J., 386, 387, 389
Boswell, J., 347, 350, 351, 356, 380
Bothwick-Duffy, S. A., 421
Botteron, K. N., 350
Bottoms, B., 664, 666
Botvin, E. M., 736
Botvin, G. J., 732, 733, 736
Boucher, J., 467
Boudewyns, P. A., 701
Boudreau, G., 783, 804
Boulogianni, G., 783, 784
Bouras, N., 442
Bourdeau, P. A., 25
Bousha, D., 606, 607
Bouvard, M., 484
Bove, F., 462
Bow, J., 488, 679
Bowen, G. R., 701
Bower, G. H., 600
Bower, M. E., 596
Bowers, P. G., 524, 525
Bowers, W., 792, 793, 795, 800, 804, 807
Bowlby, J., 351
Bowling, J. B., 436
Bowman, E. S., 688
Bowman, L., 425
Bowyer, C., 801
Box, M. L., 477
Boxer, A. M., 342
Boyadjieva, S., 807
Boyd, A. S., 28
Boyd, R. C., 299
Boyd, S., 488
Boyer, D., 692
Boyko, O. B., 350
Boyle, C., 462, 463
Boyle, F. M., 649
Boyle, M., 84, 87, 102
Boyle, M. C., 18
Boyle, M. H., 70, 72, 73, 145, 147, 648
Braafladt, N., 689
Bradburn, I. S., 804, 809
Bradford, D. C., 18
Bradley, K., 794, 795, 796, 797
Bradley, L., 562
Bradley, R., 512, 514, 572
Bradley, S., 285, 291
Bradley, W., 84
Brady, E. U., 20, 298, 340, 347
Brady, K. T., 739, 745
Brady, M. P., 473, 474
Brady, S. A., 533
Braet, C., 783
Braganza, C., 811
Bragg, R., 561
Braks, K., 795
Brambilla, F., 780, 788, 789
Brambilla, P., 350, 467
Brame, T., 562
Brammer, M., 75, 467
Brandberg, M., 288, 316
Brandner, A. M., 668
Branford, D., 441
Brannan, S. K., 350
Bransford, J. D., 569
Brant, E. F., 685
Brant, R., 656, 657
Brasic, J. R., 484
Brassard, M. R., 598
Braswell, L., 7, 43, 106, 107, 180, 370

Braukmann, C. J., 187, 215, 224, 227
Brauley, J. L., 668
Braun, C. M., 780, 788, 809
Braverman, M., 458
Bray, G. A., 806
Brayden, R. M., 601
Breaux, A. M., 415, 439
Brechman-Toussaint, M., 332
Breen, C., 473, 474
Breen, M., 70, 88
Breer, L., 299
Breese, G. R., 431
Bregman, J., 442, 464
Brehm, K., 195
Breier, J. I., 551, 552
Breiner, J., 435
Breiner, J. L., 164, 214
Breiner, S., 794, 795
Breitholtz, E., 288, 316
Bremmer, R., 98, 102
Bremner, J. D., 348, 350
Bremner, R., 471
Brendgen, M., 154, 200, 208, 209, 217, 221, 227
Brennan, L. C., 489, 490
Brennan, P. A., 145, 354
Brennan-Quattrock, J., 353, 354, 355
Brennen, M., 789
Brent, D., 9, 275, 338, 339, 340, 349, 353, 356, 379, 381, 383, 384, 745
Breslau, N., 76
Brestan, E. V., 9, 615, 616, 617, 621, 623
Bretherton, I., 352
Breton, J., 70
Breton, S. J., 607, 612
Brewer, K. E., 272
Brewerton, T. D., 780, 782, 787, 788, 789, 809, 810
Brewin, C. R., 682, 683
Brezina, T., 152, 153
Bricker, D., 418, 419
Brickman, A., 174, 223, 747
Brickman, J. S., 350
Bridge, J., 338, 339, 356, 379, 383, 384
Briere, J., 657, 658, 660, 675, 679, 680, 688, 692, 700
Briggs-Gowan, M. J., 70
Brightman, A. J., 436
Brinthaupt, V. P., 144
Bristol, M. M., 486
Britcher, J., 653
Britten, K., 435
Broadhurst, D. D., 597, 598
Brocker, E., 783
Brodin, U., 804
Brodkin, E. S., 484
Brodland, G., 807
Brodsky, S. L., 142
Brody, A. L., 350
Brody, C. L., 733
Brody, G. H., 344
Brody, J. L., 747
Brody, M. L., 781
Broks, P., 467
Brome, D., 76
Bromet, E., 685
Brondino, M. J., 66, 157, 177, 178, 221, 224, 226, 747
Brondino, S. J., 9, 21
Bronfenbrenner, U., 10, 353
Bronik, M. D., 367
Bronowski, J., 79
Brook, J., 39, 271, 280, 294, 336, 346, 787
Brookhauser, P. E., 651
Brookman, C., 343
Brookman, L. I., 485
Brooks, A., 561
Brooks, V. B., 276
Brooks-Gunn, J., 340, 342, 344, 347, 420, 787, 809
Brosig, C. L., 662
Broughton, D., 690
Brovedani, P., 484
Browder, D. M., 481
Brown, A., 522, 549, 557
Brown, A. L., 521, 524, 556
Brown, B. S., 747

Brown, C., 23
Brown, C. H., 209, 210
Brown, D., 28, 599, 601
Brown, E., 480
Brown, E. J., 595, 676
Brown, F., 481
Brown, G. G., 76
Brown, G. K., 160
Brown, J., 650, 651
Brown, J. E., 75
Brown, J. H., 734
Brown, K., 387, 389
Brown, K. M., 337, 338
Brown, L., 811
Brown, L. G., 558
Brown, L. K., 692
Brown, M., 601, 618
Brown, M. M., 37, 38, 149
Brown, N., 611
Brown, R. A., 733
Brown, R. D., 328
Brown, R. T., 72, 107, 109
Brown, S., 214, 622, 633, 737
Brown, S. A., 646, 732, 733, 734, 735, 736,
  737, 738, 739, 740, 741, 742, 743, 744,
  745, 746, 747, 748, 749, 750, 751, 752,
  757, 758, 759, 760, 762, 764
Brown, S. E., 608
Brown, T. A., 277, 278, 279
Brown, T. E., 389
Brown, T. L., 177
Brown, V. L., 295
Browne, D., 687
Browne, K., 654, 658, 659
Browne, K. D., 609
Brownell, K. D., 786, 809, 810, 811
Bruce, J., 607
Bruch, H., 779, 793, 794
Bruck, M., 532, 562, 664, 667
Bruder, M. B., 438
Bruna, M. J., 783
Brunk, M., 10, 617, 626
Brunner, J. F., 151
Bruno, M., 698
Bruno, R., 790, 791, 792, 793, 794
Brustolin, A., 804
Bruttini, M., 460
Bryan, J. H., 290, 324
Bryant, B., 682, 687
Bryant, D., 140
Bryant, D. M., 420
Bryant, D. P., 558
Bryant, R., 562
Bryant, S., 547, 685
Bryant-Waugh, R., 778, 782, 783, 792, 793,
  796, 804, 806, 807, 808, 810
Bryson, S. E., 460, 461, 462, 489, 490
Bubl, R., 783
Bucci, J. P., 441, 443
Buch, G. A., 489, 490
Bucholz, K. K., 738, 739
Buchsbaum, M. S., 350, 789
Buck, J. A., 672, 673
Buck, M. J., 633
Buckley, N. K., 192
Buckley, T. C., 685, 690
Budd, K. S., 8
Budrow, M. S., 106, 109, 110, 111
Bueno, G., 606
Buergin, D., 783
Bugental, D., 597, 601, 602, 604, 615, 618,
  633
Buhrmester, D., 204, 217, 226
Buican, B., 439
Buitelaar, J. K., 75, 87, 88, 205, 226, 295,
  484
Buka, S. L., 419
Bukowski, W. M., 355
Bukstein, O., 87, 90
Bukstein, O. G., 87, 90, 203, 204, 207,
  226, 732, 737, 742, 743, 752
Bukstein, O. M., 737
Bulik, C., 780, 781, 785, 786, 788, 789,
  790, 798, 809
Bulkley, J., 666, 669, 670, 671
Bullmore, E. T., 467
Bullock, B. M., 172, 229

Bumbarger, B., 195
Bunch, D. L., 668, 669
Bunke, V., 72
Bunney, W. E., 67
Buntman, A. D., 316
Buntman, S. R., 316
Burack, J. A., 472
Burch, M., 569, 570
Burch, P. R., 182, 183, 215, 218, 220
Burch, S., 484
Burchinal, M. R., 420
Burdick, N. J., 557
Burgard, D., 811
Burge, D., 341, 350, 352, 354
Burgess, E. S., 349, 655
Burgess, R. L., 606
Burke, J., 147, 435
Burke, J. D., 336, 339, 345, 739
Burke, J. E., 522, 523, 531
Burke, K. C., 739
Burke, K. D., 336, 339, 345
Burke, L., 349
Burke, P. M., 338, 387
Burke, R. V., 218, 222
Burkhart, B., 785, 790, 792
Burleson, J. A., 732, 738, 743, 747
Burlingame, G. M., 9
Burnam, M. A., 339, 390
Burns, B., 595, 693
Burns, B. J., 189, 216, 297, 298, 300, 339
Burns, D. D., 757
Burns, G. L., 144, 156, 157, 188
Burns, J. A., 43
Burns, M. S., 522, 532, 534
Burraston, B., 186
Burroughs, J., 807, 809
Burshteyn, D., 119
Burt, S. A., 739
Burton, R., 459, 460, 461, 462, 471
Burton, D. L., 691
Burton, J., 691
Busconi, A., 691
Busemeyer, J. R., 8, 21
Bush, T., 74
Busner, J., 91, 203
Busse, R. T., 159
Bussing, R., 70, 83
Bussey, K., 670
Butler, C., 462
Butler, G., 802
Butler, J., 691
Butler, L., 378
Butler, N., 77
Butter, E. M., 489, 490
Butz, M. R., 436
Buxton, M. E., 752
Bybee, D., 666
Bynner, J., 77
Byrne, J., 413
Byrne, S., 782

Caddell, J., 86
Cadman, D. T., 147
Cady, M. M., 746
Cahill, L. T., 608
Cairney, J., 340
Calderon, R., 345, 346, 353
Caldwell, R. A., 609
Calhoun, K., 37, 797
California Department of Developmental
  Services, 462, 463
Calkins, S., 689
Callaghan, M., 682, 683
Callahan, E. J., 284, 314
Callias, M., 435
Camarata, S. M., 478
Camasso, J. J., 609
Cameron, A. M., 218, 220, 222
Cameron, J., 426
Cameron, M. J., 481, 482
Cameron, S., 665
Camilli, G., 119, 533
Campbell, F. A., 420
Campbell, J., 16
Campbell, K. D., 299
Campbell, K. D. M., 299

Campbell, M., 147, 204, 205, 206, 207,
  218, 226, 227, 232, 483, 484
Campbell, R., 485, 486
Campbell, R. A., 75
Campbell, R. V., 623
Campbell, S., 488, 739
Campbell, S. B., 70, 145, 146, 148, 153,
  204, 205, 218, 226
Campbell, Y., 595
Campione, J., 521, 524
Campis, L. K., 160
Campos, J., 689
Campos, P. E., 28
Campos, R. G., 689
Camras, L. A., 689
Canfield, R. L., 413
Canino, I. A., 44
Cann, W., 170
Cannon, B. O., 488
Cans, C., 463
Canter, W. A., 18
Canterbury, R., 273
Cantor, R. M., 465
Cantos, A. L., 676
Cantwell, D. P., 107, 108, 110, 340, 358
Cantwell, P. D., 807
Capage, L., 165, 213
Capaldi, D. M., 145, 147, 148, 149, 150,
  151, 152
Caporaso, N. E., 733
Capriotti, R., 427
Capuano, F., 294
Caputo, A. A., 142
Caraballo, L., 607
Cardarelli, A., 656, 657, 658, 674, 675,
  676
Cardemil, E. V., 391
Carey, J., 413
Carey, J. C., 443
Carlisle, J., 552
Carlisle, J. F., 556
Carlson, C., 74, 87, 89, 94, 95
Carlson, C. D., 518, 535
Carlson, C. L., 104, 109, 110, 111, 354
Carlson, D. C., 484
Carlson, E., 149
Carlson, E. A., 687, 688
Carlson, E. B., 687, 688
Carlson, G., 18, 19
Carlson, G. A., 24, 37, 337, 338, 339, 340,
  346, 353
Carlson, J., 159
Carlson, J. I., 432, 480, 481
Carlson, P. M., 320
Carmelli, D., 739
Carmichael, D. H., 283, 291, 299, 332
Carnine, D., 66, 90, 523, 524, 534, 535,
  566, 571
Caron, C., 20
Caronna, E. B., 464
Carpenter, E. M., 179
Carpenter, M., 479
Carpentieri, S., 346, 458
Carper, R., 467
Carr, A., 651, 656
Carr, E. G., 20, 43, 422, 426, 427, 432,
  458, 459, 476, 479, 480, 481, 482
Carr, J., 419, 479, 484
Carr, L. G., 733, 739
Carraro, A., 803
Carrera, F., 206
Carrie, A., 465
Carroll, K., 792
Carroll, K. M., 43
Cartelli, L. M., 430
Carter, A. S., 458
Carter, C. M., 477, 479
Carter, F., 798
Carter, J., 797
Carter, M., 658, 659
Cartor, P. G., 214, 221, 486
Cartwright, N., 141
Caruso, D., 784, 792
Carver, C. S., 19
Carver, L., 466
Casat, C., 91, 347, 386, 439
Case, L. P., 523, 531, 568

Caselles, C. E., 597, 599, 601
Casey, B. J., 75
Casey, K., 651
Casey, P. H., 420
Casey, R. J., 17, 28
Casey, S., 481, 482
Cashman, L. A., 292
Cashmore, J., 670, 671
Casiro, O. G., 488
Casper, R. C., 340, 781, 784, 785, 790, 800, 805, 806
Caspi, A., 35, 139, 144, 147, 148, 149, 152, 153, 278, 339, 346, 739
Caspi, C., 147, 153
Cassady, J. C., 73
Cassidy, S., 413
Casson, D. M., 465, 468
Castellanos, F. X., 75, 84, 85, 86
Castillo, E. M., 551, 552
Castro, J., 783, 784
Catalano, R., 141, 145, 209, 218, 227, 599, 733
Cataldo, M. D., 481
Cataldo, M. F., 140, 141, 213
Catanzaro, S. J., 278
Cater, J., 204, 226
Catrambone, R., 569
Catto, S. L., 536
Causey, D. L., 686, 687, 695
Cavallaro, L., 604
Cavallo, F., 804
Cavanaugh, E. R., 747
Cavanaugh, J., 658
Cavell, T. A., 142
Cavins, M. K., 669
Cawley, J. F., 522, 566, 568
Cea-Aravena, J., 119
Ceci, S. J., 664, 667
Cecil, S., 490
Cederblad, M., 75
Celano, M., 686
Celiberti, D. A., 475
Celio, A., 811
Centers for Disease Control and Prevention, 668, 805
Centorrino, F., 443
Ceponiene, R., 461
Cerezo, M. A., 597, 606, 686
Cernichiari, E., 470
Cerny, J. A., 6, 25
Cetta, F., 783
Chacko, A., 9, 11, 97, 98
Chaffin, M., 615, 616, 617, 621, 623, 657, 658, 675, 687, 691, 703
Chakrabarti, S., 462, 469
Challman, T. D., 464
Chamberlain, P., 18, 41, 140, 143, 149, 150, 151, 158, 171, 187, 188, 214, 216, 217, 219, 220, 221, 222, 224, 226, 227, 231, 610, 630
Chamberlin, R., 632
Chambers, W. J., 338
Chambless, D., 284, 295, 378, 421, 797
Chambliss, H., 786
Champion, K., 689, 690
Chan, E., 119
Chan, K. K., 733, 739
Chance, M. W., 660
Chandler, L. K., 437, 473, 476
Chandler, M., 16
Chaney, J. M., 5
Chansky, T. E., 271, 290
Chapman, J. W., 532, 539
Chappell, P. B., 95
Charach, A., 84, 196, 197, 217, 229
Chard, D. J., 527, 553
Chard, K. M., 436
Charitandi, A., 783, 784
Charlop-Christy, M. H., 477
Charlop, M. H., 477
Charman, T., 457, 462, 463
Charney, D., 347, 349
Charney, D. S., 348, 350, 683
Chase, C., 16, 561
Chase-Lansdale, P. L., 634
Chassin, L., 738, 739, 740
Chate, D., 676

Chatoor, I., 109
Chavira, D. A., 299
Chaz, M. G., 466
Cheesman, F. L., 180, 219
Chen, L., 71, 77
Chen, R., 534, 540
Chen, Y. R., 343, 344
Cheney, C. D., 424, 427, 428, 434
Cheng, R., 465
Cheng, Y., 739
Cheong, J., 740
Cherney, M. S., 9
Chernoff, R., 628
Chernyk, B., 792
Chesler, B. E., 780
Chesnick, M., 489
Chess, S., 149
Chess, S., 466
Chez, M., 461
Chhabra, V., 529, 530
Chi, T. C., 73
Chian, D., 470
Childress, D., 465
Childs, G. E., 676
Chiodo, D., 663
Choate, M. L., 302
Chorpita, B. F., 271, 273, 274, 275, 276, 277, 278, 279, 280, 283, 284, 285, 286, 287, 288, 292, 295, 296, 297, 298, 300, 301, 314, 326, 489
Chorzempa, B. F., 561, 562
Choudhury, M., 291
Choudhury, M. S., 9
Chouinard, M. J., 780, 788, 809
Chourmouzi, D., 783, 784
Chowdhry, U., 780, 788
Chrisman, A. K., 295
Christ, A. E., 340
Christ, M. A., 70, 139, 140, 145, 151
Christakis, D. A., 81
Christensen, A., 12, 169, 214
Christensen, C., 561
Christensen, M. J., 601
Christian, R. E., 142, 159, 160
Christiansen, B. A., 738, 740, 744
Christie, D., 780, 788
Christman, A. K., 484
Christophersen, E., 72
Christopherson, B., 691
Christopherson, E. R., 4, 23
Chronis, A., 65, 87, 104, 109, 119
Chronis, A. M., 9, 11, 97, 98
Chropita, B. F., 4, 6, 28, 43, 44
Chrousos, G. P., 348, 349
Chu, B. C., 25, 28, 30, 31, 32
Chu, J. A., 688
Chu, M. P., 77
Chuang, S., 615
Chung, T., 734, 737, 748, 749
Ciancio, D. J., 538
Cicchetti, D., 10, 16, 38, 353, 356, 457, 458, 461, 464, 595, 596, 607, 608, 612, 626, 627, 689, 737, 738
Cicchinelli, L. F., 694
Cifton, A. D., 43
Ciminero, A. R., 36
Cintron, C. B., 350
Cisar, C. L., 473
Claes, M., 148
Claghorn, J. L., 295
Clark, B. S., 462
Clark, C., 348
Clark, D. A., 318
Clark, D. B., 295, 436, 547, 556, 557, 737, 739
Clark, D. L., 119
Clark, D. M., 683
Clark, E., 379
Clark, G. N., 184
Clark, L. A., 277, 278, 279
Clark-Sly, J., 797
Clarke, G., 184, 757
Clarke, G. N., 7, 8, 9, 11, 14, 43, 355, 356, 378, 382, 383
Clarke, J. C., 288, 316
Clarke, R., 442
Clarke, S., 531

Clarke-Stewart, A., 664
Clarkson, S. E., 339
Clarvit, S. R., 295
Clasen, L. S., 75
Clay, M. M., 538
Claycomb, C. D., 75, 76
Clayton, R. R., 739
Clement, P. F., 784
Clement, P. W., 9, 293, 334
Clements, C. B., 142
Clements, C. J., 471
Cleminshaw, H. K., 160
Clevenger, W., 439
Clewes, J., 800, 805
Clingempeel, G. W., 178, 747
Clingerman, S. R., 107
Clingerman, S. T., 109
Clinton, A., 75, 97
Clonan, S., 550, 552
Cloninger, C. R., 739, 787
Clopton, J., 783
Cloutier, P., 686
Clyman, R. B., 630
Cnattingius, S., 789
Coalition for Evidence-Based Policy, 529, 530
Coats, K. I., 379
Coatsworth, J. D., 175, 220, 225, 747, 752
Cobb, J. A., 171
Cober, M., 611
Cobham, V. E., 291, 326
Coe, D., 437
Coe, M. T., 744, 746
Coghill, D., 294, 295, 298
Cognolato, S., 803
Cohen, D., 467, 480
Cohen, D. J., 16, 38, 205, 226, 456, 458, 464, 484
Cohen, H. G., 488
Cohen, I., 489
Cohen, J., 686
Cohen, J. A.293, 326
Cohen, J. A., 698, 700, 701, 702
Cohen, L., 385
Cohen, L. R., 800, 803
Cohen, P., 12, 39, 271, 280, 294, 336, 346, 650, 651, 693, 782, 787
Cohen, R., 8, 14, 175, 214, 220, 226
Cohen, R. M., 75, 350
Cohen, S. J., 733, 747, 762
Cohen-Kettenis, P., 102, 205, 226, 787
Cohn, A. H., 602
Cohn, D. A., 352
Coie, J., 160
Coie, J. C., 231
Coie, J. D., 141, 144, 147, 148, 149, 150, 152, 159, 207, 216
Colby, S. M., 735, 737, 738, 750
Colder, C. R., 740
Cole, C. M., 17
Cole, D. A., 338, 346, 351, 354, 355
Cole, E., 378
Cole, P. M., 689
Cole, R., 208, 212, 226, 632
Coleman, M., 185, 461, 464
Coles, M. E., 292
Colin, V. L., 352
Colineaux, C., 465
Collier, D., 789
Collier-Crespin, A., 443
Colligan, R. C., 464, 747
Collins, F., 465
Colon, S. E., 739
Colt, J. M., 536
Colton, M., 676
Colvin, A., 156
Colvin, G., 158
Comer, D. M., 83, 84
Comi, A. M., 466
Committee for Children, 654
Comparo, L., 665
Compas, B. E., 340, 341, 347, 355, 686
Compton, D. L., 543, 544
Compton, K., 148, 340
Compton, S. N., 3, 9, 295
Condon, S. O., 458

Conduct Problems Prevention Research Group, 8, 23, 143, 144, 160, 186, 210, 211, 220, 221, 227, 230, 232
Cone, J. D., 35
Cone, L. T., 18
Conger, R. D., 340, 341, 344, 606, 610, 611, 623
Conger, R. E., 7
Conger, R. R., 154, 170, 198, 208, 212, 225, 229
Conlon, C. J., 444
Connell, P., 187, 215
Conners, C. K., 67, 115, 116, 119, 274, 386
Conners, K., 443
Conners, S. K., 74, 87, 89, 94, 95
Connolly, A. M., 466
Connolly, B., 419, 420
Connolly, H. M., 805
Connolly, L., 620
Connor, D. F., 84, 85, 86, 87, 88, 95, 109, 203, 204, 205, 217
Connor, R. T., 75, 97
Connor-Smith, J. K., 13, 31, 298
Connors, C. K., 4, 109, 114, 156
Connors, M. D., 214, 622, 633
Connors, M. E., 803
Connors, R. E., 152
Conrad, R., 795
Contaldo, F., 807
Conte,, 657, 658, 663
Conte, E. J., 666
Conte, J., 651, 652, 659, 706
Conte, M., 441
Conway, J., 534, 539
Conway, T., 550, 551, 552, 553, 575
Conyers, C., 428, 429
Cook, C. A., 681
Cook, E. H., 67, 70, 77, 205, 443, 459, 465, 467
Cook, M. D., 649
Cook, R., 472
Cooke, N. L., 437
Coolahan, K., 625, 629
Cooley, M. R., 299
Coolidge, F. L., 74, 76
Coombs-Orme, T., 628
Coon, H., 465
Cooney, G., 692
Cooney, N. L., 751
Coons, P. M., 688
Cooper, G., 569, 619
Cooper, P. J., 782, 788, 798, 799, 809
Cooper, S., 105
Cooper, S. M., 732
Cooper, T., 386, 788
Cooper, Z., 781, 785, 786, 787, 790, 799, 800, 804, 808, 810
Copeland, A. P., 105
Copeland, L. A., 736
Coplan, R. J., 689
Coplin, J. W., 222
Copp, B., 649
Coppel, D. B., 735
Corbett, R., 701
Corcoran, C. M., 339
Cordisco, L. K., 435
Cormier, W. H., 154, 155
Cornell, A. H., 142
Cornwall, E., 281, 314
Corona, R., 471
Cortez, V., 597, 601, 618
Corwin, D. L., 679
Cory-Slechta, D. A., 413
Cosenza, A., 484
Costa, F. M., 740
Costa, J., 789
Costello, A. J., 339, 745
Costello, E. J., 72, 137, 144, 145, 146, 189, 216, 271, 280, 298, 339, 650, 693, 739
Cote, L., 615, 616
Cote, S., 146, 154, 200, 209, 217
Cotler, S., 326
Coulson, T., 488
Coulter, M. L., 669, 674, 675
Coultry, T., 184
Council for Exceptional Children, 417

Courchesne, E., 16, 461, 466, 467
Coury, D. L., 416
Cousins, L., 80, 88, 117
Couvert, P., 465
Cowan, C. P., 352
Cowan, P. A., 10, 352
Cowdery, G. E., 481
Cowell, P. E., 467
Cowen, P. J., 348
Cowie, H., 141
Cox, A., 459, 460, 461, 462, 463, 471
Cox, C., 413
Cox, D. J., 43
Cox, W., 389
Coyne, M. D., 541, 542
Cradock, C., 326
Craig, W. M., 141, 142, 196, 197, 217, 229, 231
Craighead, L. W., 788
Craighead, W. E., 8, 14
Cramond, B., 554
Crandall, K., 441, 442
Cranston, F., 314
Crary, J. L., 805
Craske, M. G., 271
Craver, J. J., 23
Crawford, P., 783
Creamer, V. A., 734, 739, 742, 743, 757, 758, 764
Crick, N. R., 10, 17, 18, 20, 141, 142, 149, 180, 182, 231, 342
Crijnen, A. A. M., 210
Crimmins, D. B., 481, 482
Crimson, M. L., 74, 87, 89, 94, 95, 206, 385, 386
Crisante, L., 229
Crisp, A. H., 779, 781, 787, 792, 799, 801, 807
Criste, T. R., 187, 215
Crits-Christoph, P., 30, 797
Crittenden, P. A., 694
Crittenden, P. M., 600, 612
Crnic, K., 485
Croen, L. A., 463
Croghan, G. G., 747
Croghan, I. T., 747
Crombez, B., 682, 687
Crombez, G., 682, 687
Cronbach, L. J., 36
Crone, D. A., 422, 425, 427
Crook, K., 353
Crooks, C., 9
Crooks, C. V., 616, 634
Crosby, L., 159
Crosby, R., 807
Crosby, R. D., 107
Crosland, K. A., 483
Cross, C. T., 512, 513, 514, 575
Cross Calvert, S., 164, 213
Cross, M., 661
Cross, T. P., 669
Crosse, S. B., 651
Crosswait, C., 14, 30, 80, 102, 111
Crouch, J. L., 178, 608, 686
Crouse-Novak, M. A., 336, 345, 346
Crow, S. J., 800, 806, 807, 808
Crowley, M., 223
Crowley, M. J., 219
Crowley, S. L., 383
Crowley, T. J., 745, 752
Crowson, C., 784
Cruickshank, W. M., 566
Crum, K., 74
Crusto, C., 658
Csernansky, J., 350
Cuccaro, M. L, 343, 345
Cueva, J. E., 206, 226, 483, 484
Cuff, S. P., 343, 345
Cullinan, D., 566
Cully, M., 275
Culp, R. E., 627, 628
Culver, S., 676
Cummings, E. M., 8, 150, 151
Cummings, M., 794, 795, 796, 797
Cummings, S., 795
Cunicelli, E. A., 557
Cunningham, A., 178, 229

Cunningham, A. H., 656, 657, 670, 674, 687, 706
Cunningham, C., 697
Cunningham, C. E., 72, 73, 87, 98, 102, 107
Cunningham, C. J., 806
Cunningham, P. B., 8, 9, 10, 172, 176, 177, 207
Cunningham, P. E., 222, 223
Currier, L. L., 654
Curry, C. J., 413
Curry, J. F., 74, 182, 183, 215, 218, 220, 380
Curtin, G., 563
Curtis, L. J., 150
Curtis, N. M., 7, 178, 229
Curtis, S., 76
Curtiss, K. A., 567
Curwen, T., 704
Cushing, P. J., 141, 213
Cuthbert, M. I., 288, 320
Cutting, L. E., 528, 531, 560
Cyr, M., 678
Cyrd, K., 563
Cyrus, T. A., 667, 669

Daddis, C., 607
Dadds, M. R., 10, 12, 40, 41, 150, 151, 169, 214, 221, 223, 274, 276, 283, 291, 294, 326, 486, 696, 706
Dadson, M., 782, 786, 788, 793, 795
Daga, G., 785, 804
Daggett, J., 437, 473, 474
D'Agostino, J. V., 538
Dahl, M., 789
Dahl, R. E., 349
Dahlem, W. E., 520
Dahlquist, L. M., 326
Dahms, W. T., 806
Dakof, G. A., 731, 747, 748
Daleiden, E., 278, 296, 301, 459
Daleiden, E. L., 4, 6, 43, 44, 273, 300
Dales, L., 469
Daley, D., 19, 30, 97, 98, 102
Daley, S. E., 3, 341
Dalgleish, T., 273, 683
Dalle-Grave, R., 797, 800
Dally, P. D., 787, 807
Dalsgaard, S., 77
Daluiski, A., 782, 783
Daly, D. L., 218, 222
Daly, M., 77
Daly, R. M., 190, 213
Daly, T., 477
Damasio, A. R., 79
D'Amato, M. R., 272
D'Amico, E. J., 646, 734, 735, 738, 747, 748
D'Amico, F., 387
Dammann, J. E., 529
Dancyger, I., 785, 790
Dane, H. A., 142
Danforth, J. S., 67, 68, 72, 73, 86
Dangel, R. F., 37, 187, 229, 602
Daniels, M., 339, 390
Daniels, S., 783
Danielson, A., 350
Danielson, L., 512, 514, 572
Danielsson, B., 462
Danis, B., 150, 159
Dannon, L., 690
Dansky, B. S., 787
Dare, C., 790, 791, 792, 794, 801
Darkes, J., 738
Darling, M., 458
Daro, D. A., 595, 633, 651, 661
Darveaux, D. X., 191
Das, J. P., 525
D'Ateno, P., 472
Datta, P., 431
Davanzo, P. A., 441
Davey, J., 109
David, C. F., 278
David, J., 687
Davidovitch, M., 459
Davidson, H. A., 598
Davidson, J. R. T., 701

Davidson, R. J., 79, 350
Davidson, W. S., 609
Davies, B., 786
Davies, G., 670, 671, 673
Davies, M., 68, 338, 340, 353, 354, 355, 439, 615, 782
Davies, P. T., 10, 150, 151
Davies, S., 468
Davies, S. O., 295
Davies, W. H., 328
Davis, A. F., 318
Davis, B., 353
Davis, C. J., 796, 797
Davis, G. E., 659
Davis, H. T., 204
Davis, J. M., 781, 784, 785, 800
Davis, K., 806
Davis, L., 473
Davis, L. E., 797
Davis, M. A., 43
Davis, M. K., 652, 653
Davis, N., 698
Davis, R., 800, 803, 805
Davis, R. L., 468, 469
Davis, S., 629
Davis, T. E., III, 11
Davis, T. L., 808
Davison, G. C., 277
Daviss, W. B., 387, 389
Dawe, G., 106
Dawson, D. A., 733
Dawson, G., 457, 465, 466, 471, 475, 480, 481, 487
Dawson, V., 669
Day, L. E., 209
De Backer, I., 74
De Bellis, M. D., 349, 707
De Bona, C., 460
De Bortoli, D., 170
De Bourdeauhuij, I., 196, 197, 225
De Haan, E., 295
de Jonge, M., 484
de la Parra, 795
de Leon, G., 752
De Rosier, M. E., 328
de Roux, N., 465
De Troch, C., 442
De Vos, E., 669
Deal, A., 8, 38, 40, 437, 438
Deal, A. G., 439, 482
Deal, T. E., 201, 217
Dean, P., 348
Dean, R. S., 466
Dearing, K. F., 141
Deas, D., 737, 739, 745, 747, 748
Deater-Deckard, K., 152
DeBaryshe, B. D., 740
Deblinger, E., 282, 283, 293, 326, 328, 388, 627, 631, 682, 698, 699, 700, 701
Debourdeaudhuij, I., 682, 687
DeBow, E. F., 686, 687, 695
Decaluwe, V., 783
deCani, J. S., 558
DeCarlo, R., 489
Decoufle, P., 462
Dee, C. C., 108
Deep, A., 668
Deffenbacher, J. L., 314
DeFilippo, E., 807
DeFries, J. C., 532, 567
DeGarmo, D. S., 150, 151, 152, 156, 172, 213, 221, 224, 225
Deitz, S. M., 191, 209
DeJong, A. R., 669
DeJong, S., 386
DeKlyen, M., 149
Del Boca, F. K., 738
del Medico, V., 439
Delaney, M. A., 204, 226
Delaronde, S., 662
DelDotto, J. E., 76
DeLeon, I., 432
Delgado, A. E., 606
Delgado, P. L., 348
Del'Homme, M., 76
Delinsky, S., 785
DeLisi, L. E., 350

DeLoache, J. S., 667
DeLong, G. R., 484
Delprato, D. J., 272, 479
Delquadri, J., 190, 192, 216, 474
Deluty, R. H., 615
Demaray, M. K., 159
Demaree, H. A., 74
DeMaso, D. R., 441
Dembo, R., 752
Demicheli, V., 468
Demler, O., 3
DeModena, A., 348
DeMyer, M. K., 4897
DeMyer, W. E., 487
Denckla, M. B., 75
Denicola, J., 617
Denison, H., 796
Dennis, A., 782, 802
Dennis, M., 458
Deno, S., 573, 574
Denson, R., 76
Denton, C. A., 533, 537, 538, 542, 543, 544, 550, 571
DePalma, M., 525, 547, 548, 555, 560
DePanfilis, D., 609
Department of Public Welfare (PA), 427
dePerczel, M., 531
Derer, K. R., 40
Derivan, A., 205, 206, 226
Derogatis, L., 695
Deroo, L., 735
DeRosier, M. E., 198, 217, 220, 225
deRoss, R., 275
Derrfler, M., 789
Deshler, D. D., 522, 523, 560, 572
Desmond, J. E., 75
Deter, H., 807
Detzer, M. J., 800, 804, 810
Deuel, R. K., 466
Deutch, A. Y., 683
DeVane, C. L., 205
Devany, J., 481
Devine, D., 701
Devinsky, O., 461
Devlin, M. J., 781, 783, 786, 790, 804, 805
Dewey, M. E., 221, 222
deZwaan, M., 780, 783, 787, 788, 789, 790, 800, 805, 806, 807, 809, 810
Diala, C. C., 345
Diamond, A., 67, 70, 75
Diamond, J., 781, 786, 809
Diaz, R. M., 79, 106
Diaz, T., 732, 733
Dicharry, D. C., 631
Dick, T., 656, 657, 670, 674, 687, 692, 706
Dicker, R., 204, 226
Dickson, N., 147, 152, 153
Dickson, S. A., 661, 727
Dickstein, D. P., 75
DiClemente, C., 614
Didonna, F., 807
Dielman, T. E., 736
Dietrich, M. S., 601
Dietz, S. G., 340
DiFilippo, J. M., 341
DiGiuseppe, D. L., 81
DiGiuseppe, R., 28
DiLavore, P. C., 459
Diler, R., 806
Dill, D. L., 688
Dill, P., 809
Dillard, J. P., 620
Dimiceli, S., 465
Ding, Y., 84
Dingemans, A. E., 783
Dinges, K., 187, 215
Dinh, E., 465
Dinkmeyer, D., 165
Dinno, H., 457
DiPietro, E. K., 657
Diseth, T. H, 415, 433, 439
Dissanayake, C., 471
Dittman, R., 804
Dittmann, R., 91

Dittner, C. A., 691
Dix, T. H., 601
Dixon, J., 104, 109, 110, 111
Dobbs, J., 24
Dobson, K., 787
D'Ocon, A., 597, 606
Doctor, R. M., 623, 624
Dodd, J., 179
Dodge, K. A., 10, 20, 37, 38, 107, 141, 142, 144, 147, 149, 152, 159, 180, 182, 186, 207, 220, 230, 232, 689
Doe, T., 651, 661
Doelling, J. L., 676
Doernberg, N., 462, 463
Dohm, F., 781, 783
Doig, T., 652
Dokecki, P., 437
Dolan, L. J., 209
Doleys, D. M., 430
Doll, H. A., 786, 800, 808
Dolz, L., 597, 606
Dombrowski, S. C., 661, 727
Domenech, E., 339
Domingue, D., 489
Domitrovich, C., 195
Donaldson, S. I., 735
Donaldson, S. K., 685
Donenberg, G. R., 5, 16, 30, 298
Dong, M., 648, 650, 651
Donina, W. M., 473
Donkervoet, J. C., 6, 28, 284, 285, 286, 287, 295, 298, 489
Donnellan, A. M., 27, 427
Donnelly, A. C., 595, 633, 661
Donnelly, J. M., 350
Donnelly, K., 548, 554
Donnelly, M., 203
Donnelly, S. L., 465
Donohew, R. L., 739
Donohue, B., 738, 747, 749
Donovan, C., 332
Donovan, C. L., 23, 293
Donovan, D. M., 740
Donovan, J. E., 732, 740
Donovan, M. S., 512, 513, 514, 575
Doolan, M., 156, 225, 228, 229
Dooley, D., 599
Dorado, J. S., 665
Doraiswamy, P. M., 350
Dore, T., 811
Dorer, D. L., 345
Dores, P. A., 479
Dorfmann, S. F., 733, 747, 762
Doris, J., 607
Doris, J. L., 514, 515
Dorn, L. D., 349
Dorn, T. A., 436
Dorsey, M., 423, 426, 428, 431, 432
Dorsey, M. F., 43
Dorta, K. P., 9
DosReis, S., 83, 84, 85, 294, 345
Doss, A. J., 4, 28, 30
Dotemoto, S., 73
Doucette, A., 28
Dougherty, D. D., 295
Douglas, V. I., 67, 96, 106
Doumas, D. M., 10
Downing, J., 8, 662, 663
Doyle, A., 74
Doyle, A. E., 76
Doyle, C., 620
Dozier, M., 612, 630
Dozois, D., 4, 23, 28, 34, 39, 787
Drabman, R., 8, 10, 191
Drach, K. M., 691
Draeger, S., 68
Drain, T., 424
Drake, B., 595, 602
Drake, K. L., 299
Draper, H., 793
Drell, M. J., 681
Drevelengas, A., 783, 784
Drevets, W. C., 349, 350
Drummond, T., 109
du Mazaubrun, C., 463
Dube, S. R., 648, 650, 651
Dubey, D. R., 215

Dubner, A., 675, 682
DuBois, D. L., 356, 383
Dubowitz, H., 623
DuCharme, J., 9, 424, 621, 622
Duchmann, E., 790, 791, 792, 793, 794
Duclos, P., 469
Duesund, L., 803
Duffy, A. L., 40, 291
Dugan, E., 474
Dugan, E. P., 474
Dukes, R. L., 734
Dulcan, M. K., 85, 90, 116, 155, 339, 745, 764
Dumas, J. E., 97, 140, 150, 151, 152, 162, 184, 213, 214, 218, 219, 221, 222, 225, 230, 486, 606
Dumenci, L., 3, 138, 156
Duncan, B. L., 356
Duncan, R. D., 142
Duncan, S. C., 733
Duncan, S. P., 650
Duncan, T., 224
Duncan, T. E., 733
Dunlap, G., 422, 427, 478, 481, 482, 483, 485, 486, 531
Dunlap, G. F. L., 435
Dunlap, K., 6
Dunn, C., 735
Dunn, D., 91
Dunn, M., 457, 472
Dunne, M. P., 649
Dunnington, R. E., 203, 204, 217, 226
Dunson, R. M., 191
Dunst, C. H., 606
Dunst, C. J., 8, 38, 40, 437, 438, 439, 482
DuPaul, G. J., 65, 67, 68, 70, 72, 73, 86, 87, 88, 89, 97, 98, 102, 104, 105, 106, 107, 109, 111, 190
DuPaul, G. L., 29
DuPaul, G. R., 68
Durand, M., 427
Durand, V. M., 428, 459, 480, 481, 482
Durham, T. W., 611
During, S. M., 622
Durlak, J. A., 16, 28, 356, 357, 383
Durning, P., 158
Durston, S., 75
Dusenbury, L., 736
Dush, D. M., 107
Dutka, S., 566, 567, 571
Dutra, R., 660
Duyvesteyn, M. G., 619
Dyer, K., 472
Dykens, E., 459, 471
Dykens, E. M., 444
Dykman, R., 687
Dziuba-Leatherman, J., 651, 652, 653, 654, 655

Eagle, M., 800, 803
Early-Zald, M. B., 787
Easley, M., 197
Eason, L. J., 472
Eastman, C., 273
Eaves, L., 780
Eaves, L. C., 471
Ebert, D., 350
Ebmeier, K. P., 350
Eccles, J. S., 355
Eckenrode, J., 17, 208, 212, 226, 341, 607, 632
Eckert, E. C., 781
Eckert, E. D., 781, 784, 785, 797, 800, 806, 807
Eckert, E. E., 782
Eckert, T. L., 29, 72, 73, 104, 107, 109, 111
Ecton, R. B., 215
Eddy, J. M., 179, 187, 188, 215, 221
Eddy, K., 785
Eddy, M., 480
Edelbrock, C. S., 18, 71, 72, 87, 88, 143, 147, 204, 339, 485, 745
Edell, W. S., 739
Edelson, G., 669, 675
Edelstein, R. S., 657
Edgar-Smith, S., 656, 657

Edwards, A., 462
Edwards, B., 629
Edwards, B. S., 805
Edwards, D., 98, 157, 158
Edwards, G., 7, 9, 67, 71, 72, 73, 74, 103, 118, 176, 432
Edwards, K., 738, 739
Edwards, M., 462
Edwards, M. D., 782
Edwards, W. D., 805
Egan, J., 164, 226
Egan, K., 617, 622, 626
Egel, A. L., 140, 473, 475
Egeland, B., 23, 149, 607, 687, 688
Egolf, B., 602
Egvert, J., 668, 669
Ehlers, A., 682, 683, 687
Ehlert, U., 668
Ehmann, M., 295
Ehrensaft, M. K., 18
Eidem, B., 783
Eifert, G. H., 10
Eigenheer, P., 479
Eigisti, I. M., 464
Eikeseth, S., 488, 489, 490
Eilers, L., 466
Einfeld, S. L., 416
Eisen, A. R., 9, 300, 301
Eisen, M. L., 664
Eisenberg, N., 680, 689
Eisenberg, Z. W., 483
Eisenberger, R., 426
Eisenmajer, R., 459
Eisenstadt, T. H., 156, 157, 158, 165, 190, 213
Eisler, I., 801
Ekdahl, M., 481
Ekman, P., 79
El-Mohandes, A., 611
El-Sayed, E., 74
El-Sheikh, M., 151
Elbaum, B., 538, 539
Elbert, J. C., 28, 489
Elder, G. H., 278, 340, 344, 3412
Eldevik, S., 488
Eldredge, K., 797, 798, 800, 804, 807, 810
Eldredge, R., 607
Elgar, F. J., 150
Eli Lilly & Company, 443
Elkind, G. S., 67
Elkins, I., 739
Elkins, P. D., 322
Ellaway, C., 460
Ellenbogen, M. A., 348
Ellerson, P. C., 633
Elliot, A. J., 8
Elliot-Faust, O., 606
Elliot, R., 32
Elliott, C. E., 221, 222
Elliott, D. M., 657, 658, 675, 679
Elliott, D. S., 157
Elliott, E. J., 202
Elliott, M., 654, 658, 659, 783
Elliott, M. N., 332
Elliott, M. R., 735
Elliott, R. O., 479
Elliott, S. N., 44, 195, 216
Ellis, A., 41
Ellis, B. H., 630
Ellis, D., 473
Ellis, H. D., 461
Ellis, M., 142
Ellis, M. L., 142
Ellis, N., 793, 795
Ellis, P., 611
Ellis, T., 213, 219, 220, 222
Ellis-Macleod, E., 595, 676
Elrod, J. M., 654
Elul, A., 665
Embry, L. H., 161
Emerson, E., 415, 439
Emery, G., 273, 277, 279, 351, 362, 379, 381, 753
Emery, P. C., 441, 443
Emery, R. E., 8, 16, 34, 151
Emmelkamp, P. M. G., 291, 330
Emslie, G. J., 343, 345, 346, 385, 386, 387

Enayati, A., 469
Engelmann, O., 566
Engelmann, S., 523, 534, 566
England, P., 663, 669, 670, 675, 692
Englert, C. S., 522, 526, 527
English, A., 793
English, D. J., 598
Ennett, S. T., 735
Enoch, D., 206
Enron, L. D., 147
Ensign, J., 682
Ensom, R., 682, 685, 686
Entwistle, S. R., 32
Epping, J. E., 686
Epps, J., 156, 180, 220, 226
Epstein, D., 811
Epstein, J. A., 732, 733
Epstein, J. N., 74, 115, 116
Epstein, L. H., 41
Epstein, L. J., 459
Epstein, M. H., 566
Epston, D., 200, 217
Erdley, C. A., 179
Erhardt, D., 72, 107, 203, 204, 217, 226
Erich, S., 676
Erickson, D. B., 156, 160, 166, 225
Erickson, M., 607
Ericsson, M., 788, 789, 790, 810
Erkanli, A., 72, 145, 298, 339, 650, 739
Ernst, M., 75, 484
Erol, N., 44
Erwin, W. J., 798
Esch, B. E., 484
Escobar-Shaves, S., 701
Eso, K., 97
Espinosa, M., 471
Esplin, P. W., 665
Essau, C. A., 146
Estes, A. M., 147, 154, 156, 158, 159, 160
Estroff, T. W., 733
Esveldt-Dawson, K., 14, 181, 215, 225, 226
Etches, P., 417
Etcovitch, J., 80, 81, 88, 117
Eth, S., 698
Evans, I. M., 4, 8, 10, 21, 22, 40, 43
Evans, K., 792, 795, 804, 807
Evans, K. R., 350
Evans, L. D., 430
Evans, M. B., 7, 190, 191, 192, 216
Evans, S., 87, 90
Evans, S. W., 19
Everill, J. T., 787, 802
Everson, M., 663, 666, 669, 674, 675, 692
Ewald, H., 461
Ewigman, B., 604, 620, 633, 651
Ewing, L. J., 145
Exhuthachan, S., 76
Ey, S., 340, 347
Eyberg, S., 616, 623
Eyberg, S. M., 28, 98, 156, 157, 158, 165, 166, 190, 212, 213, 219, 222, 224, 225
Eysenck, H. J., 6, 271
Eyster, C., 666
Ezzell, C. W., 686

Faber, A., 700
Faber, T. L., 75
Fabes, R. A., 186
Fabiano, G. A., 9, 11, 97, 98
Fabsitz, R., 739
Facchini, F., 785
Fagan, J., 739
Fair, C., 662
Fairbank, J. A., 650
Fairbanks, J., 380
Fairbanks, L. A., 350
Fairburn, C. G., 348, 355, 781, 782, 783, 785, 786, 787, 788, 790, 791, 793, 794, 797, 798, 799, 800, 801, 804, 805, 806, 807, 808, 809, 810, 811
Faird, N., 385
Faith, M. S., 119
Falco, R., 523, 524, 571
Falk, J. R., 782
Falk, R., 460
Faller, K. C., 675, 679
Fallon, B., 649

Fallstrom, K., 419
Fals-Stewart, W. S., 10
Famularo, R., 631, 692, 702
Fancis, D. J., 535
Fankhauser, M., 443
Fantuzzo, J., 596, 601, 603, 620, 625, 627, 629
Faraone, S., 71, 72, 74, 76, 77, 86, 87, 90, 206, 389, 739, 752
Faravelli, C., 800
Farber, E. A., 607, 612
Faries, D., 91, 92, 443
Farmer, E., 189, 216, 598, 693
Farnsworth, A., 656, 657, 670, 674, 687, 706
Farquhar, L. C., 631
Farrant, A., 467
Farrell, M. L., 546, 547
Farrell, M. P., 740
Farrell, S. P., 328
Farrington, C. P., 469, 475
Farrington, D. M., 153
Farrington, D. P., 141, 142, 144, 147, 148, 149, 153, 157, 196, 198, 225
Farrington, R., 628
Farris, A. M., 151
Fassbender, L. L., 427
Fassino, S., 785, 804
Fatemi, S. H., 484
Fauber, R. L., 5, 8, 11
Faust, J., 150, 159, 201, 217, 218, 219, 222, 227, 288, 320, 669, 685
Fava, M., 299, 348, 350
Favell, J. E., 43, 485
Favot-Mayaud, I., 469, 475
Feagans, L., 565
Fecteau, S., 472
Federal Bureau of Investigation, 157, 704
Federoff, I., 802
Fee, V., 437
Feehan, C., 379
Feehan, M., 152, 339
Fehlings, D. L., 106
Fehon, D. C., 739
Feil, E., 189
Feil, M., 83, 84
Fein, D., 457, 458, 466, 472, 473, 489, 490
Feinberg, D. T., 107, 108
Feinberg, T. L., 336, 345, 346
Feindler, E. L., 184, 215
Feinfeld, K. A., 160
Feinstein, C., 457, 466, 472, 484
Feiring, C., 682, 686
Feistel, H., 350
Feldlaufer, H., 383
Feldman, H., 415, 439, 484
Feldman, J. F., 76
Feldman, L., 735
Feldman, M. A., 436, 602
Feldman, R. S., 437, 607, 608
Feldmeth, J. R., 691
Felitti, V. J., 648, 650, 651
Feliu, E., 784
Fellbaum, G. A., 190, 213
Fellman, V., 443
Felner, R. D., 13
Felton, D. K., 607
Fendrick, M., 354, 355
Fenichel, G. M., 443
Fennig, S., 796, 797
Fenske, E. C., 476, 488
Fenton, T., 631, 692, 702
Fenton, W. S., 3
Ferdinand, R. F., 146
Ferguson, C., 574
Ferguson, D. L., 437
Ferguson, E., 616
Fergusson, D., 650
Fergusson, D. M., 144, 145, 150, 151, 152, 153, 271, 733
Fermo, J. D., 484
Fernald, G., 545
Fernald, W. B., 481
Fernandez, R. C., 778, 800
Fernandez-Esquer, M., 701
Fernstrom, M. H., 788, 789

Ferrari, M., 8, 14
Ferrel, D. R., 473
Ferron, S., 784
Fetner, H. H., 386
Feurer, I. D., 70
Fewell, R. R., 420
Fichter, M. M., 780, 787, 794, 796, 799, 807
Fiegenbaum, E., 191
Field, K. M., 552
Fier, J., 273
Fierstone, P., 682, 685, 686
Figueroa, J., 179, 215, 226
Fiksenbaum, L., 330
Filipek, P. A., 75, 465
Filliben, T. L., 485
Filstead, W. J., 731
Finch, A. J., Jr., 8, 38, 347, 682
Fincham, F. D., 8
Findling, R. L., 84, 205, 206, 226, 387
Fine, D., 692
Fine, E. M., 84
Fine, M. A., 8, 38
Fine, S., 16
Fineberg, E., 77
Fink, B., 561
Finkel, A. S., 479
Finkel, M. A., 667, 668
Finkelhor, D., 647, 648, 649, 650, 651, 652, 653, 654, 655, 659, 660, 661, 674, 678, 680, 681, 682, 684, 685, 691, 692, 693, 694, 706
Finkelstein, C., 795
Finkelstein, D., 788
Finkelstein, R., 336, 345, 346
Finkenbinder, R., 340
Finlayson, A. J., 459
Finlayson, M. A. J., 565
Finn, S., 792
Fiore, M. C., 733, 747, 762
Firestone, P., 96, 102, 109
First, M., 784
First, M. B., 460
Fischer, C., 203
Fischer, G. J., 650
Fischer, M., 70, 71, 72, 77, 88, 90, 144, 739
Fishbeck, K., 552
Fisher, C., 733
Fisher, C. B., 677
Fisher, J. L., 690, 691
Fisher, L., 142
Fisher, M., 804
Fisher, P., 149, 155, 346, 745, 764
Fisher, P. A., 188, 216, 227, 630
Fisher, W., 432
Fisher, W. W., 425
Fishman, H. C., 103
Fisk, J. L., 524
Fiske, J. A., 704
Fisman, S., 442
Fister, S., 190
Fitzgerald, H. E., 160
Fitzgibbon, M. L., 809
Fitzmaurice, A. M., 566
Fitzpatrick, C., 620
Fiumara, A., 461
Fixsen, D. L., 224
Flagler, S., 23
Flanagan, E., 151
Flanagan, K. D., 141
Flanagan, R., 23
Flannery, K. B., 481
Flannery-Schroeder, E. C., 9, 20, 31, 40, 271, 284, 291, 301, 328, 330
Flavell, J. H., 521, 531
Flay, B., 66, 90
Fleece, E. L., 322
Fleichman, D. H., 193, 216, 225
Fleischman, J., 214, 221, 486
Fleischman, M. J., 43, 171, 212, 213, 218, 219, 222, 229, 624
Fleishner, J. E., 565
Fleiss, K., 80, 81, 88, 117
Fleming, J. E., 147, 648, 651
Fletcher, B. W., 747
Fletcher, J., 28

Fletcher, J. M., 99, 440, 513, 514, 515, 516, 517, 518, 519, 520, 524, 526, 528, 530, 531, 533, 536, 537, 538, 542, 543, 546, 550, 551, 552, 555, 571, 572
Fletcher, K., 9, 14, 30, 67, 71, 72, 73, 74, 80, 90, 102, 103, 111, 118, 144, 176, 739
Fletcher, K. E., 9, 14, 95, 205, 443
Fletcher, K. F., 70, 71
Flewelling, R. L., 734
Flower, L. S., 561
Floyd, E. M., 156
Floyd, F. J., 23
Fluke, J., 662, 663
Flynn, C., 350, 745, 802
Flynn, E., 386
Flynn, J. M., 524, 530
Foa, E. B., 9, 272, 274, 292, 684, 696
Fogarty, L., 666
Fogel, A., 10
Fohr, J., 350
Follette, V. M., 12, 301
Follette, W. C., 20, 298
Follmer, A., 667
Folstein, S. E., 464, 465, 466
Fombonne, E., 462, 463, 464, 469, 489, 782
Fonseca Retana, G., 193, 216, 225, 229
Foorman, B. R., 99, 518, 536, 537, 546, 550, 551, 552, 571
Foote, F., 174, 223, 747
Foote, R., 157, 165, 166, 212, 225
Fora, D. B., 738
Forcier, M., 339, 340, 343, 344, 375
Ford, H., 692
Ford, R. E., 615
Ford, T., 463
Forehan, R., 660
Forehand, R., 7, 9, 23, 43, 44, 98, 105, 113, 139, 140, 141, 143, 144, 150, 154, 155, 157, 158, 160, 162, 163, 164, 165, 166, 189, 202, 207, 212, 213, 214, 219, 220, 221, 222, 225, 231, 283, 353, 435, 602
Forest, M., 437
Foreyt, J. P., 611, 784, 788, 789, 790, 803, 810, 811
Forgatch, M. S., 41, 147, 149, 150, 151, 152, 156, 158, 170, 171, 172, 213, 218, 221, 224, 225, 229, 331, 752
Fornari, V., 785, 790
Forness, S. R., 514, 515, 518
Forrest, P. A., 213
Forsberg, P., 362
Forsell, C., 461
Forsythe, R., 739
Fortin, D., 648
Fossey, M. D., 789
Foster, S., 102, 172, 175, 342
Foster, S. L., 8, 10, 17, 24, 25, 145, 158, 175, 176, 752
Foster-Johnson, L., 733, 752
Fowler, J. S., 84
Fowler, S. A., 476
Fox, J., 18
Fox, J. J., 10, 473, 474
Fox, L., 483, 608
Fox, M. M., 779, 782
Fox, N. A., 17, 689
Fox, T. L., 284, 332
Foxx, R. M., 430, 433, 620
Foy, D., 685
France, K. G., 200, 202
Frances, A., 460, 784
Francis, D. J., 513, 516, 517, 518, 530, 533, 536, 537, 542, 543, 546, 550, 552, 571
Francis, K. L., 477
Francis, S. E., 275, 280, 283, 326
Francke, U., 460
Franco, N., 285
Francoeur, E., 664, 667
Frank, B., 565
Frank, E., 350
Frank, D., 783, 784, 804
Franke, P. J., 675
Frankel, F., 107, 108

Franklin, C. F., 651, 654
Franklin, M., 9
Franklin, M. E., 292
Franklin, R. D., 119
Franko, D., 783, 785
Franks, E. A., 8, 14
Frantz, J., 740, 741
Frary, R. B., 279, 280, 290
Fraser, B., 662, 692
Fraser, J., 356, 378, 379
Fraser, M. W., 595, 602
Fraser, W. I., 462
Frazer, D. R., 142, 159
Frazier, J., 386
Frazier, T. W., 74
Frea, W. D., 475
Fréchette, M., 143
Frederickson, D. D., 657
Freedman, D. X., 467
Freeman, B. J., 471
Freeman, R., 781, 786, 809
Freeman-Longo, R. E., 704
Freidman, M. J., 684
Freire, M., 330
Freissthler, B., 598, 599
Freitag, G., 7, 456
Fremouw, W. J., 606, 784
French, N. H., 14, 181, 215, 225, 226
Freres, D. R., 391
Freud, A., 656
Freud, S., 271
Freudenheim, M., 490
Freund, K., 792
Freund, R. D., 150
Frias, D., 686
Frick, P. J., 67, 70, 139, 140, 142, 145,
  149, 151, 154, 155, 156, 158, 159, 160,
  161, 199, 229, 230, 232
Fried, C. S., 658
Fried, R., 74
Friedlander, R., 442
Friedman, A. G., 23
Friedman, A. S., 731
Friedman, J. L., 72
Friedman, M. A., 354
Friedman, R., 378
Friedrich, W. N., 682, 690, 691, 695, 698,
  700
Friend, A., 353
Friger, M., 736
Frijters, J. C., 524, 525, 547, 548, 555, 560
Frissell, K. C., 734, 736, 744
Frith, U., 458, 460, 462, 467, 480, 562
Fritz, M. S., 462, 464
Frodi, A., 607
Frodl, T., 350
Fromme, K., 734, 735, 738
Froody, R., 606
Frost, H., 797
Frost, L., 476, 479, 490
Frostig, M., 520
Frothingham, T. E., 669
Fry, A. F., 79
Frye, V. H., 466
Fryer, G. E., 653
Fryman, H. M., 670
Fryman, J., 490
Fucci, B. R., 18
Fuchs, D., 421, 512, 514, 522, 527, 528,
  530, 536, 537, 543, 544, 558, 566, 567,
  568, 569, 570, 571, 573, 574
Fuchs, L., 421
Fuchs, L. S., 512, 514, 522, 527, 528, 530,
  536, 537, 543, 544, 558, 566, 567, 568,
  569, 570, 571, 572, 573, 574, 575
Fudge, H., 345
Fuentes, F., 488
Fuhrman, T., 16, 29, 356, 357, 383
Fuhrmann, G., 604
Fulbright, R., 466
Fulbright, R. K., 550
Fulker, D. W., 72
Fulkerson, J. A., 737, 787
Fuller, D., 185, 225
Fuller, T. L., 609
Fullerton, D., 807
Fulmer, D., 541

Funderburk, B., 156, 157, 158, 165, 190,
  213, 615, 616, 617, 621, 623
Funimoto, C., 466
Funkhouser, J. E., 735
Furey, W., 164, 214
Furey, W. A., 164
Furey, W. M., 44
Furr-Holder, C. D. M., 210
Fuster, J. M., 78, 79

Gabardi, L., 195, 227
Gabel, S., 72
Gable, S., 620
Gabrielli, W. F., 441
Gado, M. H., 350
Gadow, K. D., 70, 87, 109, 156, 232, 520
Gaffney, G., 295
Gajzago, C., 487
Galaif, E. R., 732
Gale, J., 378
Gallacher, R., 80, 88, 117
Gallagher, H. M., 328
Gallagher, J. J., 419
Gallimore, R., 438
Gallucci, C., 437
Gamble, W., 352
Gambrill, E. D., 611
Gamby, T. E., 489, 490
Gameroff, M. J., 84, 375
Gammon, G. D., 354, 389
Gammon, P. J., 295
Ganales, D., 204
Ganeles, D., 204
Ganger, W., 676
Gant, D. S., 194, 195
Garan, E., 533
Garbarino, J., 598, 599, 653, 655
Garber, J., 20, 337, 338, 350, 689
Garber, S., 106, 194, 195
Garcia, A., 795
Garcia, J. A., 28
Garcia, M. M., 150
Gardill, M. C., 568
Gardner, D. M., 694
Gardner, J., 83, 84, 85
Gardner, J. F., 91, 294
Gardner, W., 609
Garfinkel, B., 139
Garfinkel, B. G., 349
Garfinkel, P. E., 668, 779, 780, 784,
  785,786, 787, 792, 797, 798, 804, 807
Garfinkel, R., 380
Garfinkle, A. N., 479, 487
Garland, A., 595
Garland, A. F., 676
Garmezy, L. B., 740
Garner, D. M., 785, 787, 797, 798, 800,
  803, 807, 809, 810
Garner, M. V., 800
Garner, R., 556
Garnet, D. M., 780, 798
Garreau, B., 467
Garrison, C. Z., 339, 343, 345
Garvan, C. W., 70
Garvin, V., 796
Gary, F., 70
Gaskill, J., 804
Gaskins, I. W., 557
Gatchel, R. I., 277
Gatley, J. S., 84
Gatsonis, C., 144, 339, 345, 346, 347, 388
Gauber, R., 353
Gauder, N., 70
Gaudin, J. M., 608, 617
Gauld, M., 84, 87
Gauthier, I., 466
Gauvain, M., 438
Gauvin, T. R., 747
Gaylord-Ross, R., 474
Gaynor, S. T., 383
Ge, X., 340, 341, 344
Geddie, L. F., 596
Gee, C., 285
Gee, K., 482
Geen, R., 613
Geer, J. H., 277
Gehi, M., 792

Geier, D. A., 465, 470
Geier, M. R., 465, 470
Geiger, T. C., 142, 231
Geiser, F., 795
Geist, D. E., 389
Geist, R., 803
Gelenberg, A. J., 348
Geller, B., 93, 94, 384, 385, 386
Geller, D. A., 295
Gelles, R., 661
Gemmer, T. C., 182
Gendall, K., 809
Gendreau, P. L., 141
Gendrich, J. G., 194, 195
Gendrich, S. I., 194, 195
Genel, M., 65, 70
Geniesse, R., 107
Genius, M., 657
Genshaft, J. L., 293, 334
Gentile, C. C., 675, 680, 682, 684, 686,
  700
George, C., 354, 607, 615
George, C. W., 787
George, M. S., 350
George, P., 76
Gerber, M. M., 562
Gerdes, A. C., 73
Geretsegger, C., 805
Gerlinghoff, M., 802
Germain, R., 598
German, M., 443
German, V., 143
Germann, G., 573
Germany, E., 355
Gerner, R. H., 350
Gershansky, I. S., 340
Gershater, M., 624
Gershater, R. M., 623, 624
Gershenson, H., 692
Gershon, B., 474
Gersten, R., 193, 216, 225, 229, 523, 524,
  527, 571
Geschwind, D. H., 465
Ghadirian, A. M., 780
Ghaziuddin, M., 461, 466
Ghaziuddin, N., 206, 461, 466, 685
Ghetti, S., 664, 675
Ghiselli, W., 785, 790, 792
Giacin, T. A., 481
Giacobbe-Grieco, T., 481
Giampino, T. L., 71
Gianino, A., 16
Gibbons, F. X., 344
Gibbons, T. A., 179, 185, 215, 219
Gibbs, J. C., 179, 180, 184, 185, 219, 225
Gibson, D., 420
Gibson, L. E., 654, 656
Gidycz, C. A., 652, 653
Giedde, J. N., 75
Gifford-Smith, M., 186, 232
Gil, E., 702
Gil, K. M., 326
Gilbert, B. O., 320
Gilbert, J. R., 465
Gilbert, N., 662, 663
Gilbert, S., 785, 786
Gilchrist, A., 459, 460, 461, 462, 471
Gilchrist, P. N., 795, 796
Giles, W. H., 648, 650, 651
Gill, M. J., 435
Gillberg, C., 72, 457, 459, 461, 462, 464,
  465, 471, 789, 801, 807, 809, 810
Gillberg, I., 461, 465, 783, 807
Giller, H., 138, 230
Gillett, E., 271
Gillham, J. E., 391, 458
Gilliam, J. E., 460
Gilliam, T. C., 465
Gillies, L., 800
Gillin, C., 348
Gillin, J. C., 348
Gillingham, A., 561
Gilliom, M., 149
Gillis, R., 602
Gillispie, E. I., 654
Gillmore, M., 733
Gilmore, S. K., 171, 225

Gilroy, M., 782, 802
Ginsberg, A., 326
Ginsburg, G. S., 271, 283, 285, 291, 292, 299, 332
Gioia, G. A., 67
Giovannoni, J., 663
Girgus, J. S., 17, 338, 340, 341, 686
Giroux, B., 140, 152, 153
Girvin, H., 20
Gither, L. J., 322
Gittelman, R., 104, 386, 739
Gittelman-Klein, R., 71
Gjerde, P. F., 17
Glabe, C., 77
Glabus, M. F., 350
Gladis, M., 805
Gladstone, R., 686
Gladstone, T. R., 273, 354
Glancy, L. J., 752
Glaser, B. A., 213
Glaser, G. H., 612
Glaser, R., 698
Glass, S., 797, 800, 804
Glassberg, M., 485
Glasser, J. W., 468
Glassman, A. H., 805
Glatt, S. J., 86, 88, 204, 217
Glaun, D. E., 787
Gleghorn, A., 739, 748, 752
Glenn, R., 359, 365, 374
Glennon, V. J., 566
Glick, B., 184, 185, 215, 225
Glick, D. R., 631
Glick, L., 459
Glick, M., 459, 471, 569
Glisson, C., 300
Glod, C. A., 67, 75, 386, 683
Glover, D., 141
Glyn, T., 803
Glynn, T., 214
Gnagy, E., 86, 87, 90
Goenjian, A. K., 292, 328
Goering, P., 668, 786
Goetz, D., 349, 353, 354, 355
Goetz, R., 349
Goff, G., 782, 797
Goh, D. S., 658
Goh, H., 481
Goins, C., 620, 627, 629
Gold, E., 686
Gold, M. S., 809
Gold, P. W., 348, 349
Gold, S. R., 687
Gold, V. J., 7, 456
Goldberg, J., 460
Goldberg, R., 747
Goldberg, R. B., 413
Goldberg, S. C., 781, 784, 785, 800
Goldberg-Hamblin, S. E., 484, 485, 486
Goldbloom, D., 668, 786
Golden, N., 783, 784, 794
Golden, O., 663
Golden, R. N., 441, 458
Goldenberg, B., 608
Goldfield, G., 804
Goldfine, P. E., 143
Goldfried, M. R., 5, 22, 32
Golding, J. M., 670, 673
Goldman, J. D. G., 648
Goldman, L. S., 65, 70
Goldman, M. S., 737, 738, 739, 740, 744
Goldsmith, H. H., 78
Goldstein, A. P., 184, 185, 225
Goldstein, D. J., 805, 811
Goldstein, H., 473, 476
Goldstein, J., 656
Goldstein, M. Q., 733, 747, 762
Goldstein, R. B., 336, 346
Goldstein, S., 82, 119, 150, 190
Goldston, D., 339, 346
Golover, G. H., 75
Gomes-Schwartz, B., 656, 657, 658, 674, 675, 676
Gonder-Frederick, L. A., 43
Gonzales-Lopez, A., 473
Gonzalez, L. S., 657
Gonzalez, N., 484

Gonzalez, N. M., 207
Gonzalez, R. E., 299
Good, R. H., III, 573
Goodbloom, D. S., 800, 805
Goode, S., 471
Goodenow, C., 355
Goodlin-Jones, B. L., 459
Goodman, G. S., 657, 663, 664, 665, 666, 667, 669, 670, 671, 673, 674, 675, 692, 698
Goodman, J., 106
Goodman, J. T., 102, 109
Goodman, R., 463
Goodman, S., 150
Goodman, S. H., 25, 693, 733, 739, 745, 752
Goodman-Brown, T., 350, 657
Goodrick, G. K., 803, 809, 811
Goodsitt, A., 794
Goodstein, C., 691
Goodstein, H. A., 566
Goodwin, D. W., 738
Goodwin, F. K., 348
Goodwin, G. M., 350
Goodwin, R., 294
Goodyer, I. M., 353, 355
Gorall, D., 695
Gordan, R. F., 435
Gordis, E. B., 13, 298
Gordon, B., 465
Gordon, B. N., 4, 667
Gordon, C. T., 484
Gordon, D., 351, 354
Gordon, D. A., 43, 173, 174, 180, 214, 215, 219
Gordon, D. S., 657
Gordon, E., 76
Gordon, I., 780, 788
Gordon, J. A., 738, 757
Gordon, J. R., 23
Gordon, M., 105, 160
Gordon, M. A., 650, 671, 672
Gordon, N. J., 438
Gordon, R., 488
Gordon, R. A., 146
Gorey, K., 782
Gorey, K. M., 649
Gorman, B. S., 182, 227
Gorman, J., 806
Gorman-Smith, D., 140, 152, 153
Gosling, A., 439
Gosselin, M., 341
Goteborg, M. J., 462
Gotlib, I., 150
Gotlib, I. H., 25, 336, 341, 346
Gottesman, L., 465
Gottman, J. M., 8, 23, 24, 25, 151
Goudena, P., 652
Goudreau, D., 458
Gough, G., 141
Gough, R., 9, 23
Gould, J., 457, 459, 686
Gould, M. S., 271, 294, 346
Gowers, S., 378, 379, 778, 782, 783, 790, 792, 793, 796, 801, 804, 806, 807, 808, 810
Gowrusankur, J., 355
Graae, F., 11, 13
Grabe, S., 28
Graber, J., 342, 344, 787
Grabowski, L., 220
Graddock, S. G., 747
Grafton, S. T., 75
Graham, D. L., 386
Graham, J. M., 744, 756, 758
Graham, J. W., 735
Graham, L., 783
Graham, P., 23, 415
Graham, S., 180, 232, 512, 522, 523, 531, 561, 562, 563, 564, 565, 568, 572
Grahn, G. L., 151
Gramaglia, C., 785
Grambsch, P., 690
Granada, P., 784
Grandjean, H., 463
Granger, D. A., 16, 17, 28, 29
Granholm, E., 741

Grant, B. F., 733
Grant, K. E., 340, 347
Grant, P. J., 295
Grant, R., 601, 618
Grasley, C., 9, 23, 608, 621, 632
Grattan, J., 379
Graupner, T. D., 471, 489
Graves, A., 564
Graves, K., 173, 174, 214, 219
Graves, M. G., 10
Gravestock, F., 214, 622, 633
Gray, A., 691, 703
Gray, H. M., 808
Gray, J., 628
Gray, J. A., 275, 276, 277, 278, 280
Gray, J. J., 797
Grayson, B., 292
Graziano, A. M., 328
Graziano, W. G., 150
Greden, J., 461
Green, G., 74, 472, 481, 488, 489, 490
Green, J., 459, 460, 461, 462, 471
Green, J. K., 807
Green, K., 164, 189, 213
Green, L., 79
Green, R. S., 806
Green, S., 147
Green, S. M., 70, 144
Green, W. H., 204, 205, 218, 226, 227, 232, 441, 443, 483
Greenbaum, P. E., 733, 738, 752
Greenberg, D. B., 667, 668
Greenberg, G., 109, 110
Greenberg, M. A., 698
Greenberg, M. T., 149, 160, 195, 211, 355
Greenberg, R. L., 273, 277
Greene, B. F., 606, 623, 624
Greene, R. W., 8, 9, 71
Greenfield, B., 80, 88, 117
Greenhill, L., 68, 295
Greenhill, L. L., 74, 84, 85, 87, 89, 90, 94, 95, 203, 204, 205, 439, 615
Greenland, S., 295
Greenley, R. N., 8, 14
Greeno, C., 809
Greenspan, S., 23
Greenstein, D. K., 75
Greenwald, S., 336, 346
Greenway, F. L., 806
Greenwood, C. R., 190, 192, 193, 216, 225
Grega, D. M., 483
Gregg, N., 564
Gregg, V., 179
Greimel, K. V., 805
Greiner, A. R., 86
Greist, D. L., 164, 222
Grella, C. E., 734, 747, 748, 749
Grenier, C. E., 796, 797
Gresham, F. M., 155, 161, 190, 192, 193, 194, 195, 216, 227, 320, 412, 414, 489
Grether, J. K., 463
Greydanus, D., 85, 86, 87, 88, 93, 94, 95, 796
Gries, L. T., 658, 676
Griesler, P. C., 148
Griest, D. L., 141, 158, 160, 162, 164, 213, 214, 216, 221, 222, 225
Griffin, C. C., 568
Griffin, J. C., 431
Griffin, K. W., 732, 733
Griffin, P., 522, 532, 534
Griffin, S. M., 71
Griffioen, D., 288, 316
Griffith, E. M., 466
Griffith, L., 652
Griffiths, D. A., 786
Griffiths, R., 798
Grigoriadis, S., 797
Grigoroiu-Serbanescu, M., 807
Grilo, C. M., 733, 739, 810
Grimes, J. P., 518, 520, 523, 524, 526, 527
Grimme, A. C., 552
Grisso, T., 609
Gritz, E. R., 733, 747, 762
Grizenko, N., 189, 216, 225
Grizzle, K., 748
Groden, G., 489

Groen, A. D., 489
Grolnick, W. S., 355
Grooll, C., 350
Grooms, T., 142
Gross, A. M., 8, 10, 353
Gross, G., 798, 802
Gross, J., 797
Gross, M., 75, 350
Grossman, G., 675
Grossman, J. J., 412
Grossman, P., 191
Grossman, S., 779, 782
Grotpeter, J. K., 142, 342
Grove, W., 807
Grow, C. R., 222
Grusec, J. E., 281, 282, 318
Gualandi, M., 783
Gualtieri, C. T., 13, 386
Guarrera, J., 608
Guelzow, B. T., 13
Guerra, N., 20
Guerra, N. G., 180, 215
Guess, D., 458
Guevremont, D. C., 9, 14, 70, 71, 97, 98, 102, 105, 118
Gugga, S. S., 559
Guidubaldi, J., 160
Guild, J., 190, 192, 216
Guilloud-Bataille, M., 465
Guite, J., 71, 72
Gull, W. W., 779
Gullion, C. M., 345, 386
Gullone, E., 275, 279, 342
Gulotta, C. S., 423, 428
Gunawardene, S., 90, 752
Gundersen, K., 384
Gunderson, D., 173
Gunnar, M. R., 630
Gunsett, R. P., 481
Gunter, H. L., 461
Gunter, P., 190, 474
Gunzerath, L., 733
Guppy, T. E., 562
Gupta, N., 460
Gur, M., 344
Guralnick, M. J., 418, 419
Gurley, D., 271, 280, 294, 336, 346
Gurman, A. S., 10
Gurney, J. G., 462, 464
Gury, E. C., 536
Gusella, J., 802
Gustafson, K. E., 173, 214, 219
Gustafsson, P., 75
Guthrie, D., 24, 37, 438
Guthrie, I., 689
Gutt, S., 795
Guy, S. C., 67
Guzzetta, C., 794, 795, 796, 797

Haapala, D. A., 595
Haarasilta, L., 339, 345
Haas, H., 783
Haas, K., 562
Habib, T., 119
Haddock, C., 809
Hadwin, J., 467, 475
Hafemeister, T. J., 672
Hagan, T. A., 740, 741
Hagberg, B., 460
Hagell, A., 138, 230
Hagen, C., 783
Hagen, R. L., 611
Hagerman, R. J., 415
Haggerty, R., 391
Hagman, J., 789
Hagopian, L. P., 301, 425, 429, 433
Hahn, H., 566
Haines, M., 735
Hains, A. A., 328
Haith, M. M., 468
Hakami, N., 340
Hale, L., 479
Halek, C., 801
Haley, B. E., 470
Halfon, N., 464, 676
Hall, A., 802
Hall, G. A., 479

Hall, J. A., 9, 21, 215, 747
Hall, K., 479
Hall, K. M., 559
Hall, M. L., 425, 430
Hall, R., 620, 629
Hall, R. V., 425, 430
Hall, T., 488
Hallahan, D. P., 512, 514, 515, 519, 521, 522, 523, 526, 546, 562, 564, 566, 572
Halliday-Boykins, C. A., 178, 226, 229
Hallin, A., 483
Hallmayer, J., 464
Hallsten, E. A., 799
Halmi, K. A., 778, 781, 782, 784, 785, 786, 787, 796, 800, 804, 807
Halperin, E., 206
Halperin, J. M., 75, 84, 87, 90, 203
Halpern, R., 419
Halsey, N. A., 466, 469
Halverson, P., 782
Hämäläinen, M., 153
Hamburger, S., 203
Hamburger, S. D., 75, 203, 484
Hamby, D., 438
Hamilton, C. E., 609
Hamilton, D., 283, 735
Hamilton, J., 666
Hamilton, J. D., 5
Hamilton, L., 677
Hamlett, C. L., 522, 566, 567, 568, 569, 570, 571, 573, 574
Hamm, H., 783
Hammen, C., 3, 339, 341, 346, 350, 351, 352, 354, 355, 390
Hammer, M., 607, 608
Hammer, S. J., 469
Hammersley, R., 739
Hammill, D. D., 515, 516, 520
Hammond, M., 108, 156, 158, 168, 207, 213, 218, 221, 222, 225, 231
Hammond, W. A., 778
Han, S. S., 6, 16, 17, 28, 29, 30
Hanashiro, R. Y., 40
Handal, P. J., 340
Handen, B., 415, 427, 430, 439, 442, 484
Handleman, J. S., 435, 471, 472, 487, 488, 489
Hanf, C., 163, 166
Hangaard, J., 783
Hanich, L. B., 568
Hanish, L. D., 186
Hanker, J. P., 668
Hankin, B. L., 25, 340, 341, 342
Hanley, J. H., 66, 214
Hanna, C., 617
Hannah, J. N., 70
Hanner, S., 534
Hansen, C., 285
Hansen, D. J., 611, 657, 658
Hansen, W. B., 735
Hansen-Nord, M., 783
Hanson, C. L., 177, 214, 225
Hanson, K., 151, 811
Hanson, M., 143, 202
Hanson, R. F., 595, 656, 657, 669, 677
Hanson, S. L., 355
Hansson, K., 174, 226, 229
Happaney, K., 602, 618
Happe, F. G. E., 458, 462, 467
Harbin, G. L., 419
Hardan, A., 442, 467, 484
Harden, B. J., 630
Hardesty, V. A., 143
Hardin, M. T., 295
Harding, B., 787, 792, 807
Harding, J., 433
Harding, M., 72, 86, 87
Hardman, R., 797
Hardy, J., 206
Hare, R. D., 159, 232
Hare, V. C., 556
Harenski, K., 350
Hargrave, J., 359, 365, 374
Haring, T., 433, 473, 474
Harman, J. S., 676
Harmon, R., 702
Harmon, R. J., 628

Harn, B., 541, 542
Harnett, P. H., 696, 706
Harnish, J. D., 141
Harper, K., 667
Harper, L. V., 34
Harrell, A. V., 742
Harrington, F. T., 421
Harrington, H., 148, 149, 152, 153
Harrington, K., 75, 97
Harrington, R., 147, 148, 345, 356, 378, 379
Harris, A., 420
Harris, C. A., 568
Harris, K. R., 24, 328, 512, 522, 523, 531, 561, 562, 564, 565, 568, 572
Harris, S. J., 203
Harris, S. L., 8, 10, 14, 435, 436, 471, 472, 473, 475, 477, 485, 487, 488, 489
Harris, S. R., 182
Harris, T. A., 485
Harris, T. R., 650
Harris, W., 796
Harris, W. R., 203
Harrison, C., 72
Harrison, P. A., 737
Harrison, P. J., 781, 782, 783, 786, 787, 788, 790, 791, 797, 800, 805, 806, 807, 809
Harrison, W., 805
Hart, B., 75, 532
Hart, E. L., 67, 68
Hart, S. N., 598
Hartman, R. R., 97, 218, 231
Hartman, V. L., 5
Hartmann, D. P., 18, 29
Hartshorn, J., 792
Hartsough, C. S., 70, 76
Hartung, C. M., 68, 70
Harty, K., 541
Harvey, B., 735
Harvey, E., 72
Harvey, P., 23
Harwood, M., 28, 224
Hasan, N., 204, 226
Hasbrouck, J. E., 584
Hasbury, D., 437
Haskett, M. E., 601, 612, 618
Hassibi, M., 23
Hasting, R. P., 489
Hatch, A., 674, 692
Hatch, M., 91
Hatsukami, D., 781, 797, 806
Hauck, M., 466, 473
Haugaard, J., 668
Hauser, E. R., 465
Hauskamp, B. M., 680, 692
Hawes, R., 322
Hawker, D. M., 781, 799
Hawkins, J. D., 145, 209, 218, 227, 733
Hawkins, R. C., II, 784
Hawkins, R. P., 161, 187
Hawkins, W., 8, 378, 382, 383
Hawley, K. M., 4, 5, 14, 28, 30, 42, 298, 356
Hawley, P. H., 142
Haworth, J., 611
Hay, D., 74, 76
Hay, G. G., 781
Hay, P., 806
Hayek, G., 460
Hayes, J. R., 561
Hayes, M., 687
Hayes, S. C., 12, 20, 37, 68, 96, 290, 301, 322, 330
Haynes, S. N., 8, 20, 37
Hays, B. J., 656
Hays, R. D., 339, 390
Hayward, C., 341, 780, 787, 788, 789, 790, 809, 810
Hazell, P., 95, 347
Hazelrigg, M. D., 30
Hazzard, A., 611, 686
Healy-Farrell, L., 9, 292, 326
Heap, M., 800
Heath, A., 676, 780
Heath, A. C., 350, 739
Heath, G. A., 143

Heathcote, D., 347
Heatherton, T., 787
Heber, R., 412
Hebert, M., 687
Hecht, D., 657
Hechtman, L., 68, 70, 71, 80, 81, 82, 88, 99, 117
Heclos, H. H., 635
Hediger, C., 783
Heerdink, E. R., 439
Heeren, T., 18, 19
Heffelfinger, A. K., 337, 338
Heflin, A. F., 699, 701
Heflin, A. H., 282, 283, 293, 328, 388
Heflinger, C. A., 628
Heger, A., 657
Heggie, D. L., 191, 201, 227
Heiby, E. M., 20, 37
Heide, J. S., 627
Heifetz, L., 436, 485
Heiligenstein, J., 443
Heiligenstein, J. H., 91, 295
Heim, C., 349, 668
Heimberg, R. G., 14, 213, 214, 215, 299
Heinberg, L. J., 786
Heinmaa, M., 800, 803, 805
Heisler, A., 628
Heitler, J. B., 612
Hekimian, E., 597, 618
Heldebrand, T., 337, 338
Heller, T., 158, 204, 217, 225, 226, 232, 455
Heller, W., 467
Hellhammer, D. H., 668
Hellings, J. A., 441, 442, 483
Helmers, K., 349, 688, 695
Helsel, W. J., 279
Hembree-Kigin, T., 165, 213, 623
Hemme, J. M., 9
Hemmelgarn, A., 300
Henderson, C. R., 208, 212, 226, 413, 632
Henderson, J., 800, 804, 810
Henderson, J. Q., 200, 201, 227
Hendren, R. L., 74
Hendricks, A. F. C. J., 143
Henggeler, S. W., 7, 8, 9, 10, 18, 21, 43, 66, 157, 172, 176, 177, 178, 207, 214, 215, 218, 219, 221, 222, 223, 224, 225, 226, 596, 612, 617, 626, 747
Henin, A., 271, 284, 291, 292, 301, 330
Heninger, G. R., 348, 484
Henker, B., 73, 107, 109, 203, 204, 217, 226
Henly, G. A., 741, 742, 743
Hennen, J., 350
Henrich, C. C., 142
Henriksen, T. B., 77
Henry, D., 293, 347, 627, 631, 682, 683
Henry, D. B., 152
Henry, J., 657, 663, 673
Henry, P., 731
Hensrud, D. D., 805
Heo, J., 383
Hepburn, S., 475
Hepinstall, E., 78
Hepps, D., 664
Herbert, J., 353, 355
Herbert, M., 4, 8, 21, 22, 33, 35, 38, 43, 222, 223
Herbison, G. P., 650
Herbison, J., 488
Herman, C. P., 785
Herman, J. L., 684
Herman-Giddens, M. E., 669
Hermecz, D. A., 288, 320
Hermelin, B., 456
Hernandez-Guzman, L., 344
Heron, T. E., 437
Herpertz, S. C., 74
Herpetz-Dahlmann, B., 74
Herrenkohl, E. C., 602
Herrenkohl, R. C., 602
Herrera, V. M., 143
Herreros, B., 783, 784
Herrmann, K. J., 94
Herschell, A. D., 31, 695
Hersen, M., 4, 11, 316

Hershkowitz, I., 665, 666, 673
Hertzig, M. E., 463
Hertzog, C., 23
Hervey, A. S., 74
Hervis, O., 747, 752
Hervis, O. E., 174, 175
Herzberg, D., 341
Herzberger, S. D., 678
Herzing, L. B. K., 465
Herzog, D., 785, 804, 808, 809
Herzog, M., 186
Herzog, W., 807
Hess, R., 13
Hesselbrock, V. M., 738
Hesselink, J. M. K., 805
Hessler, M. J., 337, 338
Hester, C., 809, 810
Hester, R. K., 746, 751
Heston, J., 682, 685
Heubach, K., 554
Heward, W. L., 419, 437, 444
Hewett, F. M., 456
Hewitt, S. K., 690
Hewitt, T., 458
Hexschl, J. E., 682
Heyne, D., 283, 293, 328, 330, 334, 701
Hibbs, E., 9, 203
Hibbs, E. D., 3, 4, 9, 28, 203
Hick, K., 783
Hickling, E., 685, 690
Hickman, C., 458, 480, 481
Hickman, P., 541, 542
Hicks, R., 18
Hiebert, E. H., 522, 536, 539
Higa, C. K., 300
Higgins, A., 180
Higgins, E., 564
Hightower, A. D., 627
Hildebrand, D. G., 490
Hildyard, K., 596
Hill, A., 782
Hill, D. E., 75
Hill, J., 161, 345, 689
Hill, J. H., 320
Hill, J. L., 420
Hill, J. P., 341
Hill, J. W., 221, 222
Hill, K., 467
Hill, K. G., 209, 218, 227
Hill, L. K., 613, 628
Hill, N. L., 142, 159
Hillery, J., 442
Hilliker, D., 459
Hillyard, A., 419
Hilpert, P. L., 290, 320
Hilsenroth, M. J., 380
Hilton, M., 529
Hinds, D., 464
Hinkley, K., 24
Hinojosa Rivera, G., 158, 198, 199, 200, 202, 217, 225
Hinshaw, S. P., 20, 68, 72, 73, 74, 99, 107, 109, 114, 116, 130, 137, 145, 148, 153, 158, 159, 203, 204, 217, 225, 226, 229, 232
Hiralall, A. S., 190
Hirano, H., 783
Hiroto, D., 351, 354
Hirsch, S., 340
Hirschfeld, R. M. A., 348
Hirschman, J. E., 664
Hirt, M. L., 107, 293, 334
Hitzemann, R., 84
Hjalmers, N., 796
Ho, H. H., 471
Ho, M. L., 350
Hoag, M. J., 9
Hoage, C. M., 797
Hoagwood, K., 9, 31, 83, 84, 285, 297, 298, 299, 300
Hobbs, N., 437
Hobbs, S. A., 430
Hoberman, H. M., 345
Hoberman, H. N., 800
Hochgeschwender, U., 789
Hocutt, A. M., 421
Hodapp, R., 412

Hodapp, R. M., 444
Hodes, M., 787, 790, 791
Hodges, E. V. E., 342
Hodges, K., 280, 340
Hodgins, H., 167, 213, 214, 226, 228, 229
Hodgins, S., 147, 148
Hoeber, E. W., 339
Hoehler, F., 431
Hoek, H. W., 781, 782, 783
Hoff, A. L., 5
Hoff, K., 568
Hoffer, D., 552
Hoffman, J. M., 75
Hoffman, K., 619
Hoffman, L., 804
Hoffman, N., 732
Hoffman-Plotkin, D., 607, 615
Hogan, A., 415
Hoge, D. R., 355
Hohmann, A. A., 300
Hoke, J. A., 367
Holahan, J. M., 531
Holcomb, H., 350
Holden, E., 652
Holden, G. W., 21, 218, 220, 222, 633
Holden, J. E., 350
Holder, D., 338, 339, 379, 381, 383, 384
Holder, H. D., 145
Holderness, C. C., 809
Holdrinet, I., 316
Hole, W. T., 484
Hollahan, D. J., 660, 661
Holland, A. J., 780
Holland, C. J., 190, 213
Holland, D., 696, 706
Holland, D. E., 294
Holland, L., 223
Hollander, E., 295, 483
Hollandsworth, J. G., Jr., 10
Holleran, P. A., 150
Hollinsworth, T., 167, 213, 222, 223
Hollister, L., 806
Hollon, S. D., 284, 295, 378, 391
Holman, J., 216
Holmbeck, G. N., 8, 14, 116
Holmberg, J., 459
Holmes, A. S., 470
Holmes, E. A., 682
Holmes, F., 279
Holmes, F. B., 6
Holmes, J. P., 484
Holmes, M. M., 668
Holmes, T., 23
Holmes-Rovner, M., 299
Holowaty, P., 735
Holsboer, F., 348
Holt, G., 442
Holtzman, G., 459
Holtzworth-Munroe, A., 301
Holyoak, K. J., 569
Home, A. M., 197, 217
Honda, H., 462
Honig, A., 348
Hood, K., 166, 213, 219
Hooe, E. S., 278
Hoog, S., 295
Hoogduin, K., 295
Hoogstrate, J., 463
Hook, C. L., 106
Hook, P. E., 520
Hooker, K. A., 23
Hooks, K., 67
Hooven, C., 25
Hoover-Dempsey, K., 437
Hope, R., 798
Hopfer, C., 74
Hopkins, M., 279
Hopmann, M. R., 419
Hops, H., 7, 11, 14, 18, 70, 184, 190, 191, 192, 193, 216, 225, 339, 342, 343, 345, 347, 353, 354, 356, 378, 733, 757
Horgen, K., 809
Horn, W. F., 109, 110
Hornbrook, M., 378
Hornby, H., 676
Horne, A. M., 43, 171, 213
Horner, K. J., 299

Horner, R., 193, 194, 216
Horner, R. H., 422, 425, 427, 480, 481, 482, 485
Hornig, M., 470
Hornstein, N., 688
Horowitz, D., 665, 666, 673
Horowitz, H. A., 352
Horowitz, J., 219, 220, 222, 656,657, 658, 674,675, 676
Horowitz, L. A., 693
Horowitz, M., 682
Horrobin, J. M., 419
Horwitz, A., 629
Horwitz, S. M., 70, 693
Horwood, J., 650
Horwood, L. J., 144, 145, 150, 152, 153, 271, 733
Hoskyn, M., 512, 517, 522, 545, 556, 557, 560
Hosp, J. L., 516
Hotaling, G., 648, 659
Houben, M., 807
Houchens, P., 691
Hough, R., 139, 595
Hough, R. L., 299, 676
Houlihan, M., 432
House, R. F., 747
Houssman, D., 18, 19
Houston, D., 789
Houston, M., 690
Houts, A. C., 34, 43, 222
Houwink-Manville, I., 460
Hovell, M. F., 194, 195
Hoven, C., 85, 90, 116
Hoven, C. W., 693
Howard, B., 9, 12, 43, 281, 282, 290, 291
Howard, B. L., 291, 328
Howard, C., 786
Howard, J., 568
Howard, J. A., 676
Howard, J. K., 537
Howard, J. R., 187, 216, 227
Howard, J. S., 488
Howard, K. I., 340, 375, 376
Howard, M. A., 467
Howard, W., 807
Howe, G. W., 150
Howell, C. T., 4
Howell, J. C., 138
Howell, R., 568
Howes, C., 18, 607
Howing, P. T., 608
Howlin, P., 459, 467, 471, 475, 479
Hoyle, R. H., 739
Hoyson, M., 473
Hoyson, M. H., 488
Hoyt, D. R., 738
Hoza, B., 24, 68, 72, 73, 86, 104, 107, 110
Hranchuk, K., 799
Hrdy, S. B., 635
Hresko, W. P., 526
Hsieh, S. C., 747
Hsu, L. K., 780, 781, 792, 807, 808, 809
Hu, S., 733
Hu, X., 789
Huang, J., 465
Huang, K., 811
Huang-Pollock, C. L., 74
Hubbard, J. A., 107, 141, 231
Hubbard, R. L., 747
Hubble, M. A., 356
Hubert, N., 687
Hudley, C., 180, 232
Hudmon, K. S., 745
Hudson, J., 291
Hudson, J. I., 780, 805
Hudson, J. L., 9, 42
Huesmann, L. R., 147
Huey, S. J., 221
Hughes, M., 685
Hughes, C., 385, 386
Hughes, C. A., 522, 560
Hughes, C. W., 345, 386
Hughes, D. c., 561
Hughes, J., 656
Hughes, J. N., 142, 191
Hughes, M. T., 538, 539

Hughes, P. L., 806
Huizinga, D., 157
Hulley, A., 782
Hultman, C., 789
Humphrey, j., 340
Humphrey, K., 422
Humphrey, L. L., 353
Humphreys, J., 144
Humphreys, L., 164, 213
Humphries, T., 106
Hundleby, J. D., 740
Hundley, M., 150
Hunsley, J., 8, 9, 33, 34, 36, 37
Hunt, R. D., 205, 226
Hunter, M., 669
Hunter, W. M., 674, 675
Huntzinger, R. M., 301
Huon, G., 811
Hupp, S. D. A., 161
Hurlburt, M. S., 299
Hurley, D., 663
Hurley, L. K., 9
Hurley, P., 656, 657, 670, 673, 674, 687, 692, 706
Hurt, R. D., 747
Hurwitz, S. M., 628
Husain, S. A., 353
Hushoff, H. E., 75
Hutcherson, S., 322
Hutching, B., 19
Hutchinson, N. L., 568
Huttenlocher, P. R., 487
Hutton, H. E., 779, 782
Hutton, J., 471
Hviid, A., 469, 470
Hwang, W., 25
Hyer, L., 701
Hyman, C., 148
Hyman, S. L., 465, 466, 469
Hymel, S., 355
Hynd, G., 68
Hynd, G. W., 68, 524
Hyson, M., 687

Iacono, W. G., 739, 789
Ialongo, N., 109, 110, 210, 218, 219, 220
Ialongo, N. S., 210, 218, 227
Iancu, I., 779, 785
Ickowicz, A., 84
Ihnot, C., 554, 584
Ilstrup, D. M., 806
Imber, S. D., 356
Imbierowicz, K., 795
Imuta, F., 462
Imwinkelried, E., 673
Inaba, R., 746
Individuals with Disabilities Education Act Amendments, 150, 152
Ingenmey, R., 477
Ingersoll, B., 82, 119
Ingram, J. L., 465
Ingram, R., 347
Inhelder, B., 526
Inn, A., 738, 744
Insel, T. R., 3
Institute of Medicine, 469, 732
Ireland, J. L., 170, 214
Irvin, L. K., 482, 483
Irvine, A. B., 212
Irvine, J. J., 803
Irwin, L., 415
Irwin, M., 72
Irwin, M. J., 185
Irwin, M. R., 746
Irwin, W., 350
Isacoff, M., 340
Isager, T., 460
Ismond, D. R., 67
Isquith, P. K., 67
Israel, E., 678
Itard, J. M. G., 455
Itin, P., 783
Ito, Y., 67
Ivancic, M. T., 429
Iverson, S., 538
Ivey, J., 350
Iwamasa, G. Y., 8, 44

Iwata, B., 423, 425, 426, 428, 431, 432, 481, 482
Iwata, M., 184
Iwata, N., 343
Iyengar, S., 349
Izard, C. E., 16

Jablensky, A., 25
Jaccard, J., 540, 541
Jack, S., 190
Jackson, B., 288
Jackson, C. T., 473
Jackson, D., 86, 88, 204, 217
Jackson, J. L., 648, 687
Jackson, K. L., 339, 343
Jackson, M. A., 147
Jackson, S., 460
Jackson, T., 785
Jackson, T. W., 191
Jackson, Y., 44
Jacob, R. G., 72
Jacob, T., 151, 160, 740
Jacobi, C., 780, 787, 788, 789, 790, 809, 810
Jacobi, D., 465
Jacobs, B., 156, 225, 228, 229
Jacobs, C., 809
Jacobs, D., 294
Jacobs, G. A., 441
Jacobs, J. R., 158
Jacobs, M. M., 465
Jacobs, M. R., 150, 152
Jacobsen, S. J., 464
Jacobson, J. W., 490
Jacobson, N. S., 12, 301
Jacobson, R. R., 143
Jacobvitz, D., 23
Jacoby, G., 795
Jacquez, F. M., 355
Jadad, A., 469
Jadad, A. R., 84, 87
Jaeger, J. L., 743
Jaenicke, C., 351, 354
Jaffe, P. G., 616, 634
Jaffee, S. R., 149
Jagannathan, R., 609
Jager, M., 350
Jagers, H. D., 187, 229
Jahr, E., 488
Jainchill, N., 752
Jakim, S., 119
Jamain, S., 465
James, B., 702
James, H., 80
James, J. E., 214, 486
James, S., 676
James, S. D., 475
Jameson, P. B., 173
Jamieson, B., 473
Jamieson, E., 353, 355, 649, 650, 656
Jamison, P. J., 520
Janet, P., 779
Janoff-Bulman, R., 682
Janosky, J., 415, 439, 484
Jarecke, R., 205
Jarmon, M., 808
Jarrett, M., 611
Jarry, J. L., 789, 809
Jaselskis, C. A., 443
Jason, L. A., 13, 23, 326
Jasper, S., 475, 476
Jaudes, P. K., 669
Javors, M. A., 203
Javorsky, J., 73
Jaworski, T. M., 682
Jay, M., 783
Jay, S., 687
Jaycox, L. H., 332
Jayson, D., 356, 378, 379
Jeanchild, L., 437
Jeejeebhoy, K., 784
Jeffers, J., 429
Jefferson, T., 468
Jeffrey, J., 548, 555
Jeffries, N. O., 75
Jenike, M. A., 295
Jenkins, J. R., 512, 536, 557

Jennings, K. D., 152
Jennings, S. J., 204, 205, 218, 226, 227, 232
Jenny, C., 667, 668
Jensen, A. L., 4, 6, 28, 30, 31
Jensen, J. B., 349
Jensen, P. S., 3, 4, 9, 13, 20, 28, 68, 72, 84, 85, 90, 116, 273, 294, 336
Jenson, J., 804
Jenson, W., 190, 379
Jerabek, P. A., 350
Jersild, A. T., 279
Jessor, R., 145, 732, 740
Jessor, S. L., 145, 732
Jewell, J., 353
Jick, H., 462, 468, 469
Jilton, R., 28
Jimerson, D., 780, 788, 806
Jin, R., 3
Jitendra, A. K., 568
Joanning, H., 731, 747
Jocelyn, L. J., 488
Jocic, Z., 787
Joe, V. C., 150, 160, 221
Joffe, T., 548, 555
John, K., 354
Johnson, B. R., 678
Johnson, C., 779, 790, 791, 792, 794, 795, 796, 797, 803
Johnson, C. R., 415
Johnson, D., 525
Johnson, D. J., 529, 561
Johnson, D. M., 436, 611
Johnson, E., 489
Johnson, E. M., 735
Johnson, G., 534
Johnson, H. H., 676
Johnson, J., 350, 650, 651, 787
Johnson, J. H., 4
Johnson, M., 141
Johnson, P. G., 608
Johnson, S. B., 13, 320, 489
Johnson, S. M., 190, 192, 213, 216, 429
Johnson, T., 314
Johnson, T. C., 691
Johnson, V., 740
Johnson, W. L., 433
Johnston, C., 8, 70, 72, 102, 150, 151, 160, 161, 163, 222, 604
Johnston, L. D., 731, 732, 759
Johnstone, S. J., 74
Johnson, J. G., 733, 739, 745, 752
Johnson, S., 735
Joiner, T., 278, 343, 354, 686, 787
Jolley, E., 800
Jolly, A. C., 437, 473
Jonas, B. S., 299
Jonas, J. M., 780
Jones, B., 326
Jones, D., 561
Jones, D. J., 779, 782
Jones, D. P. H., 651, 657, 660, 663, 669, 670, 675, 692
Jones, E., 314
Jones, E. D., 574
Jones, F., 203
Jones, G., 473
Jones, J., 77, 91, 682
Jones, J. T., 86, 87, 88
Jones, L. M., 649
Jones, M. C., 6, 271
Jones, R., 798
Jones, R. R., 7, 154, 158, 170, 187, 198, 208, 212, 216, 225, 227, 229
Jones, R. T., 23, 293, 334
Jones, R. W., 631
Jones, S., 520
Jones, S. M., 142
Jones, W., 457, 467, 468, 480, 490
Jones, Y., 185
Jons, P. H., 75
Jonveaux, P., 465
Jordan, D. A., 746
Jordan, N. C., 568
Jorde, L. B., 443
Jorgensen, J. S., 184, 226
Joseph, R. M., 466, 467

Joseph, S., 683
Josephs, A., 314
Josephson, A., 801
Joshi, S., 688
Jou, R. J., 484
Jouriles, E. N., 151
Joyce, P., 798
Joye, N., 668
Joyner, C. D., 612
Juffer, F., 619
Julien, R. M., 203
Jumper, S. A., 680, 692
Junger-Tas, J., 141
Juniper, L., 437
Jurecic, L., 627
Jurgens, M., 428, 429
Jurica, J., 568
Jusko, T. A., 413
Juster, H. R., 14, 213, 214, 215, 299
Juul-Dam, N., 466

Kaczmarek, L., 473
Kaczynski, J., 796
Kaczynski, N. A., 737
Kadden, R. M., 751
Kadesjo, B., 72
Kafantaris, V., 147, 206
Kagan, J., 34, 277, 294
Kahler, C. W., 733
Kahn, J. S., 379
Kahng, S., 431, 432
Kahng, S. W., 425
Kaiser, A. P., 479
Kalas, C., 295
Kalas, R., 745
Kales, S., 340
Kalichman, S. C., 28, 662, 675
Kalin, N. H., 350
Kalsher, M. J., 481
Kaltiala-Heino, R., 142, 782
Kalucy, R. S., 779, 787, 795, 796, 807
Kame'enui, E. J., 523, 541, 542, 573
Kaminer, R. K., 608
Kaminer, U., 743
Kaminer, Y., 732, 733, 737, 738, 742, 743, 747, 752
Kamphaus, K. W., 156
Kamphaus, R., 744, 745
Kamphaus, R. W., 20, 161
Kamps, D., 474
Kamps, D. M., 473, 474
Kamran, M. M., 484
Kandel, D. B., 340, 733, 739, 745, 752
Kandel, E., 19
Kandel, H. J., 314
Kane, M., 9, 43, 281, 282, 290, 291
Kane, M. T., 271, 290, 328
Kane, P., 607
Kanfer, F. H., 4, 7, 8, 13, 21, 22, 33, 35, 37, 38, 40, 41, 42, 282, 290, 328
Kanner, L., 455, 456, 487
Kanwisher, N., 467
Kaplan, A., 786, 787, 797
Kaplan, A. S., 779, 784, 792, 803
Kaplan, D., 484
Kaplan, D. L., 665
Kaplan, H. I., 443
Kaplan, R. M., 330
Kaplan, S., 608, 684
Kaplan, S. J., 608
Kaplan, S. L., 203
Kaprio, J., 339, 345
Kaqtz, A. R., 354
Karajgi, B., 204, 226
Karapurkar, T., 462, 463
Karasoff, P., 482
Karayan, I., 292, 328
Karg, R. S., 9
Karlsson, J., 70
Karns, K., 566, 567, 571
Karoly, P., 42, 282, 290, 328
Karumanchi, S., 443
Karumanchi, V., 443
Karver, M., 28
Karwautz, A., 789
Kasari, C., 467
Kasen, S., 787

Kashani, J. H., 337, 338, 339, 340, 346, 353
Kashdan, T. B., 72
Kashima, K. J., 436
Kasius, M. C., 146
Kaslow, F., 5
Kaslow, N., 685, 686
Kaslow, N. J., 273, 378, 382
Kasorla, I. C., 7
Kassem, L., 674, 675
Kassorla, I. C., 456
Kast, L. C., 23, 653, 654, 655
Kastanaskis, J., 673
Kasten, E. F., 416
Kaster-Bundgaard, J., 8
Kaswan, J., 615
Kataoka, S. H., 332
Kates, K., 482
Katkin, E. S., 74
Katoaka, S. H., 3, 28
Katsovich, L., 95
Katt, J. L., 301
Katusic, S. K., 464
Katz, K. S., 611
Katz, L. F., 8, 25, 151
Katz, R., 797
Katz, R. C., 622
Katz, S. L., 469
Katzaroff, M., 571
Katzir-Cohen, T., 554
Katzman, D., 783, 803
Kauffman, J., 519, 521, 522, 523, 526, 546, 564, 566
Kaufman, A. S., 159
Kaufman, D., 606, 611, 613, 616, 617, 621, 622
Kaufman, J., 275, 340, 347, 349, 608, 745
Kaufman, K., 459, 610, 611, 616, 621, 622, 623, 658, 659
Kaufman, N., 212, 227
Kaufman, N. L., 159
Kaufmann, J. M., 562
Kavale, K. A., 514, 515, 518
Kavanagh, K., 12, 14, 18, 41, 89, 211, 212, 224, 227, 343, 354
Kay, E., 651
Kaye, J. A., 462, 468, 469
Kaye, W., 780, 781, 783, 786, 789, 806, 809
Kaye, W. H., 668, 780, 788, 789, 809
Kayser, A. T., 482, 483
Kazak, S., 465
Kazdin, A. E., 3, 4, 5, 6, 9, 10, 11, 12, 13, 14, 25, 28, 29, 30, 31, 32, 33, 34, 35, 41, 42, 43, 44, 97, 98, 143, 150, 156, 157, 162, 181, 191, 214, 215, 218, 219, 220, 221, 222, 223, 225, 226, 286, 302, 358, 378, 381, 382, 383, 602
Keane, M., 569
Keane, S. P., 472
Keane, T. M., 684
Kearney, C. A., 294, 300
Kearney-Cooke, A., 797, 801, 802
Keel, P. K., 779, 785, 786, 789, 808, 810
Keeler, G., 271, 280, 339
Keeling, B., 561
Keenan, K., 140, 144, 145, 146, 147, 149, 152, 153, 206, 389
Keeney, J. M., 665, 672, 673
Kehle, T. J., 379
Keijsers, G. P. J., 295
Keipe, R., 784, 792
Keith, B., 151
Keith, T., 77
Kellam, S. G., 209, 210, 218, 219, 220, 227
Kelleher, J. P., 443
Kelleher, K. J., 83, 84, 676
Keller, M. B., 271, 345, 804, 808, 809
Keller, M. F., 320
Keller, R. A., 694
Kellet, K., 479
Kelley, J. E., 318
Kelley, L. A., 441
Kelley, S. J., 656, 657
Kelly, B., 566
Kelly, J., 143, 339

Kelly, J. F., 746, 747, 748, 751, 760
Kelly, K. L., 86
Kelly, M., 607
Kelly, M. J., 109
Kelly, M. L., 194
Kelly, P. A., 44
Kelly, R., 657
Kelsey, D., 91, 92
Kem, D. L., 442, 443
Kemmotsu, N., 467
Kemner, C., 484
Kemp, D. C., 480, 481
Kempe, R. S., 628
Kemper, C. C., 314
Kemper, K. J., 119
Kemper, T. L., 460
Kemph, J. P., 205
Kendall, K., 207
Kendall, P. C., 5, 7, 8, 9, 10, 11, 12, 14, 20,
   21, 24, 28, 30, 31, 38, 40, 43, 106, 156,
   180, 213, 214, 215, 220, 226, 271, 273,
   274, 279, 281, 282, 284, 290, 291, 292,
   294, 298, 299, 301, 328, 330, 340, 347,
   358, 370, 373, 381, 382, 383, 429
Kendall-Tackett, K. A., 680, 681, 682, 691,
   692
Kendell, R. E., 25
Kendler, K. S., 780, 789, 790, 809
Kendrick, K., 91, 92
Kennedy, C. H., 433, 481
Kennedy, D. N., 75
Kennedy, F., 787
Kennedy, J. L., 77
Kennedy, N., 442
Kennedy, R. E., 341, 342, 343, 354
Kennedy, S., 668, 783, 798, 805
Kennedy, S. H., 350, 797, 805
Kenny, M., 650
Kent, J., 806
Kent, R., 175, 176
Kenworthy, L., 67
Keogh, B. K., 24
Keown, L. J., 72
Kercher, G., 648
Kerdyck, L., 139
Kermoian, R., 689
Kern, R. A., 439
Kern, T., 602
Kerns, G., 486
Kerns, K. A., 97
Kerr, M., 142
Kerr, M. M., 473
Kerry, I., 782
Kerwin, M. E., 430
Kessel, S. M., 692
Kessler, R., 350, 685, 780
Kessler, R. C., 3
Ketter, T. A., 350, 443
Kettle, L., 85, 90, 116
Key, A., 783
Keyes, S., 17, 23
Keysor, C. S., 203
Khan, L., 484
Khetarpal, S., 275
Kiecolt-Glaser, J. K., 698
Kiely, K., 76
Kiesler, D. J., 301
Kievit, L. W., 656, 657
Kilbane, T., 675
Kilcoyne, J., 654, 658, 659
Kilgore, E., 441
Killalea, A., 468
Killory, E., 805
Kilpatrick, D. G., 649, 656, 657, 658, 668,
   669, 685
Kilts, C. D., 75
Kim, A., 557
Kim, I. J., 344
Kim, R., 271, 290
Kim, T., 76
Kim, Y. S., 95
Kimbrell, T. A., 350
Kinard, E. M., 696
Kinast, C., 612
Kincaid, D., 422
King, A. C., 75
King, B. H., 441, 442, 443

King, C. A., 685
King, G., 662
King, J., 84, 87, 90
King, K. M., 738
King, N., 77
King, N. J., 9, 11, 279, 280, 283, 290, 293,
   314, 328, 330, 334, 701
King, R., 346, 574
King, R. A., 206, 295
King, S., 795
Kingsley, D., 215
Kinlan, J., 294
Kinsbourne, M., 461
Kinscherff, R., 631, 692, 702
Kinzie, J., 811
Kipp, H. I., 73
Kipp, H. L., 86
Kirby, J. R., 524
Kirigin, K. A., 186, 187, 215, 224, 227
Kirigin Ramp, K. A., 227
Kirisci, L., 737, 739, 742, 743
Kirk, S. A., 418, 520, 809
Kirk, W. D., 520
Kirkegaard-Sorensen, L., 19
Kirkley, B. G., 781
Kirkorian, G., 75
Kirschenbaum, D. S., 809
Kiser, L., 297
Kiser, L. J., 682, 685
Kistner, J. A., 278
Kitzman, H., 17, 208, 212, 226, 632
Kitzmann, K. M., 16
Kivlahan, D. R., 735
Kjellgren, G., 462
Klaassen, T., 348
Klajner-Diamond, H., 657
Klancnik, J., 442
Klapper, F., 796, 804
Klaric, J., 115, 116
Klaric, S., 745
Klass, E., 204, 226, 227
Klee, L., 676
Klein, D. N., 336, 346, 685, 733
Klein, H., 784, 792
Klein, M., 804
Klein, M. H., 807
Klein, N. C., 173, 215, 225
Klein, R., 204, 295
Klein, R. D., 216
Klein, R. G., 71, 80, 81, 82, 88, 117, 204,
   205, 226, 227, 739
Kleinfield, E. K., 797
Kleinhans, N., 467
Kleinman, C. S., 206
Kleinman, S., 76, 77
Klevstrand, M., 489
Klin, A., 457, 458, 459, 461, 466, 467,
   468, 480, 490
Kline, R. B., 18
Kling, J., 163
Kling, M. A., 349
Klingman, A., 288, 320
Klingner, J. K., 522, 557, 558, 572
Klinnert, M. D., 226
Klinteberg, B. A., 144
Klorman, R., 290, 320
Klotz, M. L., 16, 17, 28, 29, 38, 41
Kluft, R. P., 688
Klugness, L., 158, 193, 201
Klump, K., 779, 786, 789, 810
Kluszynski, S., 295
Knapp, M., 314
Knapp, P., 615
Kneisz, J., 488
Knight, J., 421
Knight, R. A., 691
Kniskern, D. P., 10
Knitzer, J., 28
Knop, J., 19, 738
Knopik, V. S., 567
Knoster, T. K., 422
Knott, P., 75
Knox, L. S., 9, 43, 281, 292, 330
Knudson, S., 667
Knutson, J. F., 596, 651
Knutson, N. M., 224
Kobak, R., 352

Kochanek, T. T., 419
Kochenderfer, B. J., 141
Koda, V. H., 75
Koedoot, P. J., 439
Koegel, L. K., 435, 476, 477, 478, 479,
   482, 485, 486, 489, 490
Koegel, R. L., 422, 427, 435, 462, 471,
   475, 476, 477, 478, 479, 482, 485, 486,
   487, 489, 490
Koehler, C, 28
Koehly, L. M., 745
Koenig, K., 442
Koepke, T., 801
Koeske, R., 41
Koetting, K., 9
Kogan, E. S., 747
Kogan, S. M., 656, 657, 658
Kohlberg, L., 180
Kohler, F. W., 473
Kohn, A., 426, 443
Kohn, M., 794
Kokotovic, A., 633
Kolko, D., 338, 339, 379, 383, 384
Kolko, D. J., 140, 143, 155, 159, 181, 189,
   201, 203, 204, 216, 217, 218, 219, 222,
   226, 227, 356, 379, 381, 383, 595, 599,
   607, 609, 612, 615, 617, 621, 626, 652,
   656, 676
Kolmen, B., 484
Kologinsky, E., 479, 480
Koloian, B., 72
Kolpacoff, M., 167, 213, 222
Kondas, O., 288, 314
Kondo, D., 789
Kondrick, P. A., 23, 653, 655
Kononen, M., 350
Konstantareas, M. M., 458
Koocher, G. P., 37, 675
Kopeikin, H., 597, 601, 618
Kopet, T., 144, 155
Kopiec, K., 649, 693
Kopp, H. J. P., 141
Kopta, S. M., 375, 376
Korkmaz, B., 471
Korn, Z., 96
Kornhaber, R. C., 288, 290, 320
Kortlander, E., 271, 290
Koselka, M., 283
Kostanski, M., 342
Kosterman, R., 209, 218, 227
Kotchick, B. A., 44, 154, 220, 231, 435
Kotler, J. S., 161, 230
Kotler, L., 782, 783, 804, 805
Kouri, J., 80, 82, 88, 117
Kovacs, M., 144, 336, 337, 338, 339, 340,
   343, 345, 346, 347, 358, 388, 695
Kovalkeski, J., 422
Kovatchev, B., 43
Koverola, C., 606, 617, 629, 657, 685, 690
Kowatch, R. A., 443
Kozak, M. J., 274, 292
Kozloff, M. A., 471
Kraemer, H. C., 114, 350, 355, 780, 783,
   785, 787, 788, 789, 790, 797, 800, 809,
   810
Kraetsch, G. A., 564
Kraizer, S. K., 653
Kramer, J., 738
Kramer, R., 346
Krantz, J. P., 473
Krantz, P. J., 473, 474, 476, 477, 488
Krasnow, A. D., 299, 376
Krasny, L., 465
Kratochvil, C., 91, 443
Kratochwill, T. R., 4, 9, 10
Kratzer, L., 147, 148
Krause, M. S., 375, 376
Krautter, T., 802
Kreft, I. G. G., 734
Krehbiel, G., 216
Kreienkamp, M., 783
Krenz, C., 733
Kresch, L. E., 484
Krieger, R., 608
Krishnamoorthy, J., 442
Kristjanson, A. F., 650
Kristoff, B., 488

Kroeger, K. A., 483
Kroesbergen, E. H., 525
Krohn, M. D., 147
Kroll, J., 299
Kroll, L., 356, 378, 379
Krook, K., 690
Krouse, J. P., 574
Krueger, A. B., 520
Krueger, S., 805
Kruesi, M., 203, 205, 207, 745
Kruger, S., 350
Kruh, I. P., 142
Krystal, J. H., 348, 683
Kuczynski, L., 606
Kuenzel, R., 301
Kuhn, D., 432
Kuhn, J., 667
Kuhn, M. R., 553
Kuhns, J. B., 692
Kuiper, M., 87, 88
Kumar, S., 76
Kumpfer, K. K., 220, 231
Kumpfer, K. L., 658
Kumpulainen, K., 415
Kuntsi, J., 76
Kuperman, S., 94, 738
Kupersmidt, J., 140
Kupfer, D. J., 299
Kupietz, S., 84, 203
Kuroda, J., 281, 285
Kurtines, W. A., 747
Kurtines, W. M., 174, 175, 220, 225, 272,
   281, 282, 283, 285, 291, 292, 299, 330,
   332, 747, 752
Kurtz, P. D., 608
Kusumakar, V., 380
Kutcher, S. P., 349
Kutchins, H., 809
Kutlesic, V., 788, 805
Kuypers, D. S., 192
Kvam, M. H., 657
Kvaternic, M., 651, 654
Kwan, W., 779, 785, 786, 787, 811
Kwasnik, D., 86
Kwok, H. W. M., 483
Kypri, K., 746
Kysela, G., 419

La Malfa, G., 441
Labellarte, M. J., 295
Labori, P. W., 804, 809
Labouvie, E. W., 737, 742
LaBruna, V., 608
Lacerenza, L., 525, 547, 548, 555, 560
Lacey, C., 424
Lacey, J. H., 778, 797, 807
Lachar, D., 439
Lacourse, E., 148, 154, 200, 209, 217
Ladd, G. W., 141
Ladish, C., 156
Lafargue, R. T., 484
Lafer, B., 350
Laffer, P. S., 805
LaFreniere, P. J., 294
LaGana, C., 290, 320
LaGreca, A. M., 292, 686
Lahey, B. B., 25, 67, 68, 70, 73, 139, 140,
   145, 146, 147, 151, 194, 195, 623, 733,
   739, 745, 752
Lahoste, G. J., 77
Lai, C., 465
Lainhart, J. E., 465
Laird, M., 607
Laird, S. B., 742, 743
Lajoy, R., 144
Lakey, J. F., 704
Laliberte, M., 790
Lalli, J. S., 481, 482
LaLonde, C., 16
Lam, A. Y., 465
Lamarch, L., 575
Lamb, J. L., 674, 675
Lamb, M. E., 664, 665, 666, 673
Lamb, S., 656, 657
Lambe, E., 783
Lambert, E. W., 11, 28
Lambert, J., 70

Lambert, J. A., 701
Lambert, M. C., 44
Lambert, M. E., 43
Lambert, M. J., 33
Lambert, N. M., 70, 76
Lambert, S. F., 299
Lambert, W., 214, 221, 376, 486
Lambert, W. E., 189
Lambrecht, L., 459
Lamparski, D., 316
Lampert, C., 345, 346, 786, 809
Lamphear, V., 665
Lampman, C., 16, 29, 356, 357, 383
Lampron, L. B., 20, 182, 183, 215, 218,
   220
Lancioni, G. E., 424
Landaburu, H., 427
Landen, S. J., 436
Landis, H., 348
Lando, H. A., 745
Landsverk, J., 299
Landsverk, J. L., 676
Lane, K. L., 421
Laneri, M., 9, 67, 71, 72, 73, 74, 103, 118,
   176
Lang, A. R., 72, 151
Lang, L. L., 419
Lang, P. J., 79, 273, 689, 798, 799
Lang, R. A., 690
Langdon, N. A., 482
Langenbucher, J. W., 737
Langer, S. N., 481
Langford, S., 84, 87, 90
Langley, A. K., 271, 280
Langlois, A., 608
Langmeyer, D. B., 41
Lanktree, C., 700
Lanphear, B. P., 413
Lansford, J., 186, 232
Lansverk, J., 595
Lantzouni, E., 784
LaPadula, M., 71, 739
LaPerriere, A., 175, 220, 225
LaPierre, A., 747, 752
Laraia, M. T., 788, 789, 810
Larimer, M. E., 735
Larken, S. M., 140
LaRose, L., 43
Larrance, D. L., 601, 618
Larrieu, J. A., 681
Larson, C. L., 350
Larson, R., 792
Larson, S. M., 665
Larsson, H., 76
Larsson, I. O., 74
Larsson, P., 783
Larsson, S., 735
Larzelere, R. E., 187, 215
Laseque, C., 779
Lask, B., 780, 782, 783, 788
Laski, K. E., 477
Last, C. G., 279, 285
Lasure, L. C., 6
Latimer, P., 292
Latimer, W. L., 732
Latimer, W. W., 746, 748
Lau, J., 170, 214, 229
Lauer, K. D., 559
Launay, J., 348, 484
Laundergan, J. C., 731
Launsbury, K., 628
Laurens, K. R., 294
Laurent, J., 278, 347, 350, 351, 356, 380
Lauritsen, M., 461, 470
Lautenschlager, G. J., 150
Lavallee, K. L., 186, 232
LaVeist, T., 345
Lavelle, T., 739
Laver-Bradbury, C., 97, 98
LaVia, M., 804
LaVigna, G. G., 427
Lavigne, V. V., 218, 220, 222
Lavori, P., 271, 299, 345, 808
Law, P. A., 466
Lawendowski, L. A., 735
Lawrence, D., 170, 229

Lawry, W., 686
Lawson, L., 657, 658, 675, 682
Laxer, R. M., 314
Layer, S. A., 423, 428
Lazar, S., 442
Lazarus, A. A., 6, 281
Lazebnik, R., 668, 669
Lazenby, A. L., 458
Le Brocque, R. M., 354
Le Couteur, A., 459, 462, 464
Le Grange, D., 787, 790, 791, 792, 793,
   794, 795, 796, 801
Le, L., 479
Leach, D. J., 488
Leach, J. M., 556
Leaf, P., 70, 345
Leaf, R., 472, 474, 476, 481
Leal, L. L., 314, 330
Learning Disabilities Roundtable, 526
Leatherwood, D., 794, 795, 796, 797
Leavitt, K. L., 633, 634
LeBaron, D., 657
Leblanc, L., 429, 479
LeBlanc, M., 143, 208
Lebnan, V., 202, 217, 218, 219, 227
Lebow, J. L., 5, 44
Lebowitz, B. D., 298
Leboyer, M., 484
Leckman, J. F., 206
LeCouteur, A., 465
Ledbetter, D. H., 465
Ledingham, J., 145, 147
LeDoux, J. M., 517
Ledsham, L., 800
Lee, A., 786
Lee, C., 512, 517, 522, 545, 556, 557, 560
Lee, C. M., 9
Lee, D. S., 557
Lee, F., 71
Lee, M. I., 790
Lee, P. P., 75
Lee, S., 785, 786
Lee, S. S., 20, 73, 137, 145, 148, 153, 229
Lee, T., 7, 8, 176, 177
Lee, V., 273, 616
Lee, Y., 659
Lee-Cavaness, C., 207
Leed-Kelly, A., 745
Leekam, S., 459
Leeman, L. W., 185, 225
Leff, S. S., 220
Lefkowitz, M. M., 147
Lehane, J., 608
Leibowitz, S. F., 780, 798
Leichner, P., 790
Leichtman, M., 664
Leif, P. J., 693
Leifer, M., 674, 675, 676
Leippe, M. R., 670
Leitenberg, H., 284, 314, 654, 656, 659,
   797, 798
Lelio, D. F., 205, 207
Lelon, E., 72
LeMarquand, D., 207
LeMasney, J. W., 661, 727
Lemmon, C., 801
Lenane, M., 203
Lengua, L. J., 160
Lennerts, W., 808
Lenox, M., 350
Lento, J., 737, 738
Leombruni, P., 804
Leon, C. E., 70
Leon, G. E., 792
Leon, G. R., 787
Leon, S. L., 91, 94
Leonard, B., 474
Leonard, B. E., 348
Leonard, B. R., 474
Leonard, H., 292, 295, 460
Leonard, H. L., 388
Leonard, J. C., 781
Leonard, K., 151
Leonard, K. E., 740
Leonard, S., 186
Lepisto, T., 461
Lepore, A. V., 566

Lepore, S. J., 664, 698
Lerer, P., 86
Lerer, R. J., 86
Lerman, C., 733
Lerman, D. C., 481
Lerner, J., 514
Lerner, J. V., 23
Lerner, R. M., 8, 14
Lesch, M., 431
Leschied, A. W., 178, 663
Leske, G., 152, 160
Leslie, A. M., 467
Leslie, D., 796
Leslie, D. R., 649
Leslie, L. K., 299
Letourneau, E., 658, 691, 703
Leufkens, H. G., 439
Leung, A. W., 299
Leung, C., 170, 214, 229
Leung, J., 477
Leung, N., 791, 803
Leung, P., 676
Leung, P. W. L., 44
Leung, S., 170, 214, 229
Lev, J., 279
Leve, L. D., 149, 150, 151, 188, 219, 220, 231
Levene, K. S., 147, 220
Levenson, R. W., 24, 25
Leventhal, B. L., 459, 467
Leventhal, D. L., 77
Leventhal, J. M., 70, 666
Levin, G. M., 205
Levin, L., 474, 475, 480, 481
Levine, A. G., 171, 213
Levine, J., 788
Levine, M., 675
Levine, R., 783
Levis, D. J., 31, 272
Leviton, L., 77, 81, 444
Levitz, L., 806
Levy, B. A., 525, 555
Levy, F., 74, 76
Levy, K. N., 733
Levy, R. L., 28
Lewin, A. B., 425, 431, 432
Lewin, M. L., 413
Lewine, J. D., 461
Lewinsohn, P. M., 7, 8, 9, 11, 14, 43, 70, 184, 336, 339, 342, 344, 345, 346, 347, 355, 356, 378, 383, 733, 737, 739, 745, 757
Lewis, D. O., 612, 691
Lewis, I. A., 648, 659, 660
Lewis, J. C., 597, 601, 618
Lewis, K., 353
Lewis, M., 36, 686
Lewis, M. H., 458
Lewis, R. A., 747
Lewis, S., 281, 282, 288, 314, 320
Lewis-Palmer, T., 194
Lewisohn, P. M., 7, 8, 9, 11, 14, 43, 70
Li, J., 469, 475
Liau, A. K., 185
Liberman,, 520, 533
Liberman, I. Y., 522
Liberzon, I., 701
Licinio, J., 348
Liddle, B., 378
Liddle, H. A., 731, 747, 748
Lidz, C. W., 609
Lie, G., 674
Lieb, R., 166, 174, 178, 185, 188, 212
Lieberman, A. F., 599, 612, 619, 627
Liebert, R. M., 320
Liebowitz, M. R., 295, 805
Liefooghe, A. P. D., 141
Liese, B. S., 753
Lifrak, P. D., 747
Ligezinska, M., 682, 685, 686
Lilenfeld, L., 668, 809
Lilienfeld, S. O., 142, 145, 273
Lilja, J., 735
Limber, S., 609
Lin, E., 668, 786
Lin, E. K., 633
Lin, S. X., 468

Lin, Y., 210, 481
Linan-Thompson, S., 539, 541, 542
Linarello, C., 437
Lincoln, A. J., 461
Lindamood, P., 534, 539, 546, 549, 550
Lindauer, S. E., 483
Lindberg, G., 804
Lindberg, N., 341, 461, 462
Lindemann, M. D., 351
Linden, M., 74, 119
Lindgren, K. A., 350
Lindgren, S., 119
Lindholm, L., 797
Lindsay, D. S., 664
Lindsay, R. C. L., 673
Lindsay, R. L., 443
Lindsey-Dudley, K., 795, 796, 797
Line, G., 443
Linehan, M. M., 12
Ling, W., 340
Lingam, R., 462, 468, 469
Linna, S. L., 415
Linnell, J., 465, 468
Linnet, K. M., 77
Linscott, J., 28
Liotti, M., 74, 350
Lipkin, W. I., 470
Lipovsky, J., 347, 631, 649, 656, 669, 670
Lippke, L. F., 742, 743
Lippmann, J., 293, 700
Lipsey, M. W., 187, 215, 219, 220, 228, 231
Lipsitt, L., 692
Litrownik, A., 480
Littell, J. H., 20
Little, C., 630
Little, S., 288
Little, T. D., 142
Littman, D. C., 150
Liu, J., 465
Livingston, R., 347, 350, 351, 356, 380, 682
Lizardi, H., 685
Lloyd, D. A., 343
Lloyd, J., 519, 521, 522, 523, 526, 546, 564, 566
Loar, L. L., 181, 226
Lobitz, G. K., 190, 213
Lobovits, D. A., 340
Locascio, J. J., 206
Lochman, J. E., 8, 10, 20, 23, 24, 25, 37, 141, 142, 148, 182, 183, 215, 218, 220, 225, 226, 273, 391
Lock, J., 782, 787, 790, 791, 792, 793, 794, 795, 796, 801, 802
Locke, B. L., 436
Lockshin, B., 733
Lockyer, L., 456, 458
Loeb, K., 800
Loeb, K. L., 805
Loeb, M., 479
Loeber, R., 67, 70, 139, 140, 143, 144, 145, 147, 149, 151, 152, 153, 155, 157, 160, 199
Loft, J. D., 25
Logan, G., 67, 87
Logan, J., 84
Logan, T. K., 734
Lombardo, P., 4
London, P., 32
Loney, B. R., 142, 151, 154, 155
Loney, J., 68, 70, 99, 807
Long, E. S., 425
Long, J. S., 487
Long, N., 8, 11, 213, 353
Long, P., 164, 213
Long, P. J., 648, 687
Long, S. H., 608
Lonigan, C. J., 28, 278, 489, 533, 682
Loo, S. K., 74, 119
Lopez, I. D., 86, 88, 204, 217
Lopez, M., 109
Lopreiato, J., 470
Lorber, R., 158, 198, 199, 200, 202, 217, 225, 607
Lorch, E., 350
Lorch, E. P., 67

Lord, C., 459, 464, 471
Lord, K. M., 559
Lorion, R. P., 602
Losel, F., 107
Lösel, F., 179, 215
Losoya, S., 689
Lotspeich, L., 464
Lotspeich, L. J., 465
Lourie, K. J., 692
Lovaas, E. E., 479
Lovaas, O. I., 7, 8, 14, 99, 456, 458, 459, 462, 471, 472, 476, 480, 481, 487, 488, 489
Love, L. C., 687
Love, L. R., 615
Loveland, K. A., 439
Lovett, M., 548, 555
Lovett, M. W., 522, 523, 524, 525, 530, 547, 548, 554, 555, 560
Lovibond, P. F., 272
Lovinger, L., 474
Lovitt, T. C., 523, 562, 566, 567
Low, C., 485
Low, H., 203
Lowe, B., 807
Lowenberg, M., 779
Lubar, J. F., 74
Lubawski, J., 779
Lubbs, H. A., 413
Lubek, R. C., 476
Luborsky, I., 800
Luborsky, L., 743
Luby, E. D., 811
Luby, J. L., 337, 338
Lucas, A., 784
Lucas, C. P., 155, 745, 764
Lucci, D., 458
Luce, S. C., 472, 481
Luckey, D., 17, 208, 212, 226
Lucyshyn, J. M., 481, 482, 483, 486
Luebbert, J. F., 204, 226
Luiselli, J. K., 441, 481, 482
Luk, S., 67
Lukens, E., 353, 354, 355
Lumley, V., 8
Lumpkin, P. W., 283, 291, 299, 330, 332
Lurier, A., 439
Luster, W. C., 187
Luteijn, E., 460
Luteijn, F., 460
Lutzker, J. R., 485, 486, 606, 615, 621, 623, 624
Luus, C. A. E., 670
Lydiard, B., 788, 789
Lydiard, R. B., 789, 810
Lyman, R. D., 160
Lynam, D., 148
Lynam, D. R., 19, 20, 734
Lynch, A., 386
Lynch, D. L., 657, 692
Lynch, F., 378
Lynch, K., 739
Lynch, L., 669
Lynch, M. E., 341
Lynskey, M., 650
Lynskey, M. T., 144, 145, 150, 151, 271, 733
Lyon, G. R., 513, 514, 515, 516, 517, 518, 519, 520, 522, 524, 525, 526, 528, 529, 530, 531, 545, 547, 555, 560, 565
Lyon, R., 28
Lyon, T. D., 663, 664, 665, 674
Lyons, D. M., 348
Lyons-Ruth, K., 28, 151
Lytle, C., 657

Ma, Y., 271, 280, 294, 336, 346
Maas, J. W., 75, 84, 203
Maas, L. C., 75
MacArthur, C., 564
Macaruso, P., 520
MacBrayer, E. K., 150
MacDonald, C., 793
MacDonald, J., 611
MacDonald, J. P., 180, 273
MacDonald, L., 43
MacDonald, R. F., 481

MacDuff, G. S., 476
MacDuff, M. T., 474
Mace, D. E., 184, 226
Mace, F. C., 429, 481
Macedo, C. A., 203
MacFarlane, J., 413
MacFarlane, K., 697
MacIntyre, D., 651, 656
Macintyre, J. C., 206
MacKay, R., 671
Mackay-Soroka, S., 143, 202
MacLean, C., 780
MacLean, W. E., Jr., 415
MacLeod, C., 273
MacLurin, B., 649
MacMillan, A., 652
MacMillan, D. L., 412, 414, 489
MacMillan, H. L., 650
MacMillan, J. H., 652
MacMillan, S., 350
MacMillian, H. L., 648, 649, 652, 656
MacPhee, K., 552
MacPherson, L., 744, 750
MacPherson, T., 652
Madden, P. A. F., 739
Madden, R., 350
Maddox, L. O., 465
Madoki, M. W., 387
Madrid, A., 441, 442, 443
Madsen, C. H., 190, 285
Madsen, K. C., 147
Madsen, K. M., 469, 470
Maestrini, E., 465
Magder, L., 83, 84, 85, 294
Magdol, L., 339, 346
Magee, V., 692
Maggia, G., 788
Magito-McLaughlin, D., 480, 481, 482
Maglieri, K., 429
Magnus, R. D., 387
Magnusson, D., 144, 203
Magnusson, P. K., 465
Magrina, J., 783, 784
Magura, S., 606
Mahaddian, E., 732
Maharg, R., 736
Mahoney, E. M., 804, 809
Mahoney, M. J., 24, 351
Mahoney, W. J., 460
Mahurin, R. K., 350
Main, D., 733
Main, M., 607, 615
Mainprize, E., 805
Maisto, S. A., 737
Mak, A. S., 608
Mak, R., 170, 214, 229
Maki, A., 428, 429
Makin-Byrd, K. N., 596, 600, 610, 614, 618, 620, 627, 630
Makoroff, R. L., 668
Malenfant, L., 23
Malever, M., 85
Malhotra, S., 460
Malik, M., 465, 468
Malina, A., 804
Malkin, A., 349
Malkin, D., 349
Malla, S., 674, 692
Mallick, K., 650, 651
Mallinger, A. G., 350
Mallory, R., 102
Malloy, P., 71, 739
Malone, J., 608
Malone, R. P., 204, 206, 226, 483
Maloney, K., 800
Malson, H., 779
Maltby, N., 466
Mammen, O. K., 599
Manassis, K., 285, 291, 330
Mandel, F., 608, 684
Mandelkern, M. A., 350
Mangiapanello, K., 472
Mangine, S., 628
Manikam, R., 437
Manion, A. P., 670
Manion, I., 620, 629
Manion, I. G., 682, 685, 686

Manjiviona, J., 459, 460
Manke, F., 787
Manly, J. T., 608, 612, 626, 627
Mann, B. J., 18, 215, 747
Mann, E., 612
Mann, J., 288, 290, 314, 316, 320, 322
Mann, L., 519
Mann, R., 480
Mann, T., 811
Mannarino, A. P., 179, 215, 226, 284, 293, 326, 686, 698, 700, 701, 702
Mannheim, G. B., 484
Manning-Courtney, P., 462
Mannucci, E., 800
Mannuzza, S., 71, 739
Manos, M. J., 84
Mantero, M., 788
Manzato, E., 783
Marathe, P., 387
March, J. S., 3, 9, 12, 115, 274, 282, 283, 292, 295, 326, 330, 378, 379, 381, 382, 385, 386, 388, 389
Marchant, R., 661
Marcheschi, M., 441
Marchi, P., 807
Marchione, K. E., 179, 215, 226, 531
Marcotte, D., 341
Marcus, D. J., 466
Marcus, M. D., 793, 794, 798, 799, 800, 801
Marcus, R. N., 387
Marcus, S. C., 84, 294, 375
Mardekian, J., 295
Marholin, D., 104
Mari, J., 806
Maria, K., 557
Mariage, T., 526, 527
Mariani, M. A., 70
Markey, C. N., 779, 785
Markham, C., 701
Markham, K. M., 811
Markham, M. R., 330
Markie-Dadds, C., 97, 100, 160, 168, 169, 170, 200, 202, 207, 212, 214, 225, 228
Markin, D., 803
Markman, H. J., 23
Markowitz, J. S., 484
Markowitz, L. E., 469
Marks, I. M., 271, 279
Marks, R. E., 439, 441
Marlatt, G. A., 734, 735, 738, 740, 750, 757
Marlow, A., 465
Marlow, J. H., 158, 172, 200, 214, 226
Marquard, K., 568
Marquis, J. G., 422, 482
Marrazzi, M. A., 811
Marriott, S. A., 184
Marrs, S., 653
Marrs, S. R., 17, 23
Mars, A., 462
Mars, B. L., 698
Marsh, W. L., 75
Marshall, D. B., 598
Marshall, L., 663
Marsil, D. F., 670, 673
Marsteller, F. A., 343, 386
Marston, D., 527, 573
Martens, B. K., 190, 195, 216
Martens, S. L., 657, 658, 669
Martin, A., 294, 295, 442
Martin, C. L., 186
Martin, C. M., 468
Martin, C. S., 734, 737, 748, 749, 790, 792, 794
Martin, G., 744
Martin, J., 314, 330, 357, 380, 442
Martin, J. L., 481, 648, 649, 650
Martin, J. M., 273
Martin, M. G., 394
Martin, N. G., 739
Martin, N. T., 489, 490
Martin, P. W., 631
Martin, S. E., 663
Martin, S. L., 420
Martinez, C. R., 158, 172

Martinez, M., 465
Martino, S., 689
Martinussen, M., 783
Marton, P., 349
Martone, M., 669
Marttunen, M., 142, 339, 345
Marvin, R., 619
Marx, R. W., 314, 330
Marzillier, J. S., 179, 215, 225, 273
Marzolf, D. P., 667
Mas, C. H., 223
Maschman, T. L., 355
Mash, E. J., 3, 4, 8, 9, 14, 17, 18, 20, 23, 25, 26, 27, 31, 32, 33, 34, 36, 37, 39, 40, 70, 72, 150, 160
Masi, G., 441, 484
Masland, R. H., 413
Mason, D. M., 70
Mason, H., 783
Mason, L., 564, 565
Mason, M., 431
Masse, L. C., 208, 217
Massey, P. S., 416
Masters, K. S., 33
Mastropieri, M. A., 421, 558
Mateer, C. A., 97
Materson, B. J., 784
Mather, N., 573
Mathes, P., 558, 571
Mathes, P. G., 533, 537, 542, 543, 544, 550
Matier, K., 203
Matochik, J. A., 75
Matson, J., 437
Matson, J. L., 279, 322, 425, 436, 477
Matsuishi,, 462
Matt, G. E., 30
Mattes, J. A., 206
Matthews, J., 170
Matthews, L., 74
Matthews, M. A., 634
Matthews, N., 465
Matthys, W., 102
Mattison, R. E., 340
Mattson, A., 203
Matusevich, D., 795
Maudsley, H., 455
Maughan, A., 612, 626, 627
Maughan, B., 77, 147, 161
Maurer, R. G., 490
Mauri, M. C., 788
Maurice, C., 481, 487, 489
Mayberg, H. S., 350
Mayer, L., 805
Mayer, L. S., 209, 210, 218, 219, 220
Mayer, R. G., 428, 429, 430
Mayes, A., 467
Mayfield, J., 166, 174, 178, 185, 188, 212
Mayou, R. A., 682, 687
Mayville, E., 425
Mazaleski, J. L., 481
Mazlish, E., 700
Mazurick, J. L., 157, 218, 219, 220, 221, 222
Mazziotta, J. C., 350
McAfee, J., 437
McAllister, J. A., 339
Mcalpine, D. D., 343
McAtee, M., 422, 482
McAuliffe, S., 415, 439
McBride, C. K., 175, 747
McBride-Chang, C., 680
McBurnett, K., 68, 108, 139, 145, 203
McCabe, K. M., 139
McCabe, M. P., 781, 782, 786
McCallum, M., 320
McCann, J., 682
McCann, S., 350
McCargar, L., 783, 794
McCarthy, D. M., 646, 734, 744, 746, 747, 748, 750
McCarthy, G., 9
McCartney, C., 185
McCartney, K., 81
McCarton, C. M., 420
McCarty, C. A., 81, 143, 144, 338
McCauley, E., 338, 345, 346, 353, 387
McCauley, J. L., 465

McCelland, L., 781
McClannahan, L. E., 473, 474, 476, 477, 488
McClarty, B., 617
McClellan, J. M., 155
McCloskey, L. A., 143
McCloskey, M. S., 328
McClung, T. J., 430
McCombs, A., 353
McConaha, C., 783, 804
McConaughty, S. H., 8
McConaughy, S. H., 155, 744
McConnachie, G., 480, 481
McConnell, S. R., 418, 437, 473, 476
McCool, S., 488
McCord, D., 612
McCord, J., 9, 108, 118, 186, 232, 657
McCormick, M. C., 420
McCormick, M. E., 108
McCormick, N., 648
McCosh, K. C., 432
McCoy, K., 670, 673
McCoy, M. G., 142
McCracken, J., 271, 280
McCracken, J. T., 75, 84
McCrady, B. S., 753, 799
McCrady, F., 459
McCrindle, B., 783
McCurdy, K., 661
McDermott, C., 490
McDermott, J. F., 612
McDermott, P., 743
McDermott, P. A., 147
McDermott, S., 416
McDonald, L., 419
McDonald, T., 676
McDonald, W. M., 350
McDonough, M., 442
McDougle, C. J., 441, 442, 443, 484
McDowell, J. J., 481
McDuff, P., 208, 678
McEachern, A., 650
McEachin, J., 472, 474, 476, 481
McEachin, J. J., 8
McEachran, A., 603, 604, 605, 608, 610
McElroy, L. P., 688
McEvoy, M. A., 473, 474
McEvoy, R., 466
McEwen, B. S., 617
McFarland, J., 484
McFarland, M., 214
McFarlane, A. C., 631, 684, 696, 707, 795, 796
McFarlane, C. M., 795, 796
McGavin, J. K., 790
McGavran, L., 413
McGee, C., 6, 28, 284, 285, 286, 287, 295, 298, 489
McGee, G. G., 437, 477
McGee, R., 72, 152, 339, 340, 345, 608
McGee, R. O., 339
McGhee, D. E., 439
McGilley, B., 785, 792
McGimpsey, B. J., 606
McGinnis, S., 350
McGlashan, T. H., 739
McGloin, J., 608
McGlynn, F. D., 272
McGoey, K., 72, 73, 568
McGoon, M. D., 805
McGough, J. J., 76
McGowan, J., 469
McGrath, E. P., 13, 458
McGrath, P., 102
McGrath, P. J., 150
McGraw, J. M., 663
McGraw-Hill Digital Learning, 573
McGreen, P., 173, 214, 219
McGrew, K., 573
McGue, M., 739, 789
McGuiness, C., 546
McGuiness, D., 546
McGuiness, G., 546
McHale, J. P., 158, 204, 217, 225, 232
McHugh, T. A., 214
McIlvain, H. E., 745
McIntosh, V., 798

McIntyre, A., 628
McIntyre, J., 682, 685, 686
McIntyre, L. L., 485
McIntyre, T. J., 31
McIntyre-Smith, A., 616
McKay, G. D., 165
McKay, K. E., 75
McKeown, R., 343
McKeown, R. E., 339
McKinney, J. D., 565
McKnight, B., 12
McKnight, C. D., 3, 9
McKnight, K. M., 348
McKnight, L., 43
McKnight, P., 523, 560, 735
McLaughlin, D., 422
McLaughlin, F. J., 601
McLaughlin, R. J., 740
McLean, N., 782
McLeer, S., 156, 180, 220, 226
McLeer, S. V., 293, 627, 631, 682, 683
McLellan, A. T., 743
McLeod, B. D., 4, 6, 25, 28, 30, 31
McLoughlin, D., 784
McMahon, P. M., 658
McMahon, R., 164, 213
McMahon, R. J., 7, 8, 9, 14, 43, 44, 98, 113, 139, 140, 143, 144, 147, 154, 155, 156, 157, 158, 159, 160, 161, 163, 164, 165, 166, 189, 200, 202, 207, 208, 211, 212, 213, 214, 218, 219, 221, 222, 225, 228, 229, 230, 283, 602
McMahon, W., 465
McManus, S. M., 159
McMaster, K. L., 543
McMillan, T. M., 631
McMiller, W. P., 299
McMorris, B. J., 738
McMorrow, M., 433
McMorrow, M. J., 620
McMurray, M. B., 86, 87, 88, 204
McMurtry, S. L., 674
McNally, R. J., 272, 273
McNamara, B. H., 676
McNamara, J., 676
McNaughton, N., 276, 277
McNees, M. P., 194, 195
McNeil, C., 165, 213
McNeil, C. B., 31, 156, 157, 158, 161, 165, 190, 213, 612, 615, 616, 623, 695
McNeil, D. W., 31
McNerney, E., 435, 489, 490
McNiel, D. E., 655
McPartland, J., 466, 475, 480, 481
McShane, M., 648
McVey, G., 18
McWatters, M. A., 76
McWilliam, R. A., 419
Meadowcroft, P., 187
Meadows, D., 682
Meals, R., 782, 783
Medenis, R., 109
Medical Research Council, 467, 469
Medland, M. B., 191, 209
Mednick, S. A., 19
Mee-Lee, D., 732
Meesters, C., 330
Megel, M. E., 656
Mehata, P., 546
Mehler, C., 804
Mehler, P. S., 781, 782, 783, 792
Mehta,, 536, 537, 571
Mehta, S., 466
Meichenbaum, D., 7, 24, 106, 372, 523
Meisenzahl, E. M., 350
Melamed, B. G., 285, 288, 320, 322
Melbye, M., 470
Melero-Montes, M. D. M., 462, 469
Meli, C., 461
Meller, W. H., 338, 339
Melloni, R. H., 86, 88, 204, 217
Melnick, G., 752
Melnick, S., 159
Meloni, I., 460
Melton, G. B., 66, 157, 177, 214, 215, 218, 219, 221, 222, 224, 226, 609, 635, 675, 747

Melton, L., 784
Meltzer, H., 463
Meltzoff, A. N., 480
Melzer, A., 654
Mendelson, S., 804
Mendlewicz, L., 787
Mendlowitz, D. R., 44
Mendlowitz, S., 285, 291, 330, 797
Menlove, F. L., 281, 282, 290, 318
Mennen, F. E., 682
Mennin, D., 76
Menold, M. M., 465
Menzies, R. G., 288, 316
Mercer, C. D., 568
Mercer, G. W., 740
Merckelbach, H., 316
Merikangas, K., 354, 809
Merlino, J., 481
Merlo, M., 67, 68
Merrill, L. L., 687
Merriman, U., 205
Merry, S. N., 439, 441
Mers, L., 681
Mervalla, E., 350
Merydith, S. P., 745
Messer, S. C., 353
Metalsky, G. I., 350
Metevia, L., 9, 67, 71, 72, 73, 74, 103, 118, 176
Metrik, J., 744
Metz, B., 489
Metzger, E., 780, 788
Metzler, C. W., 158, 212
Meyer, G., 437
Meyer, J. H., 350
Meyer, K. A., 481
Meyer, L. H., 4, 8, 10, 21, 22, 40, 43, 481, 482
Meyer, R., 285
Meyer, S., 608
Meyers, A. W., 8, 14
Meyers, K., 740, 741, 743
Meyers, R., 625, 629
Meyers, W. C., 206
Meyerson, J., 79
Mezzich, A., 742, 743
Mian, M., 657
Micciolo, R., 807
Michael, J., 479, 481
Michael, K. D., 383
Michael, R., 290, 320
Michelman, J. D., 458
Michelson, D., 91, 92
Michelson, L., 179, 215, 226
Michon, J., 78
Mick, E., 71, 72, 76, 77, 739
Middlebrook, J. L., 150
Midgley, C., 355
Mietzitis, S., 285, 291, 378
Migliaretti, G., 804
Miguel, C., 479
Mihalic, S. F., 187
Mikami, A., 130
Mikhail, C., 790
Mikkelsen, E., 93
Mikulas, W. L., 6
Mikulich, M. S., 91, 94
Mikulich, S. K., 752
Mikulis, D., 783
Milberger, S., 71, 72, 74, 77
Milch, R., 29, 104, 107, 109, 110, 111, 119, 150, 734
Milla, F., 784
Millar, E. A., 340
Miller, B. C., 692
Miller, C., 653
Miller, C. D., 195, 227
Miller, C. M., 179
Miller, D. J., 322
Miller, D. S., 660
Miller, E., 462, 468, 469, 475
Miller, E. T., 750
Miller, G., 195
Miller, G. E., 9, 147, 154, 158, 162, 163, 198, 201, 214, 215, 220, 222, 223, 231
Miller, H., 350
Miller, H. L., 348

Miller, J., 106, 109, 110, 111
Miller, J. H., 522, 568
Miller, J. N., 467
Miller, J. Y., 145, 209
Miller, K., 789
Miller, K. B., 808
Miller, L., 195, 227, 344, 548, 554
Miller, L. J., 75, 76
Miller, L. M., 298
Miller, L. P., 607, 612
Miller, L. R., 601
Miller, L. S., 140
Miller, M., 166, 174, 178, 185, 188, 212, 481
Miller, M. I., 350
Miller, R. L., 205
Miller, S., 779, 785, 786, 787, 811
Miller, S. A., 38
Miller, S. D., 356
Miller, S. L., 8
Miller, S. M., 36
Miller, S. P., 568
Miller, T. L., 146
Miller, W. R., 211, 701, 735, 741, 746, 750, 751
Miller-Perrin, C. L., 17, 23, 651, 652, 653, 655
Miller-Tutzauer, C., 752
Mills, E., 469
Millsap, P. A., 682, 685
Milne, B., 148, 149, 152, 153
Milne, D. C., 293, 334
Milner, J. S., 597, 599, 600, 601, 606, 608, 609, 687
Milstein, V., 688
Miltenberger, R., 8, 427, 428, 429, 655, 790
Milton, D., 92
Minassian, D., 292, 328
M.I.N.D. Institute, 463, 464
Minderaa, R., 75, 205, 226, 460
Mineka, S., 272, 273, 278, 279
Minnich, J., 563
Mintun, M. A., 350
Minuchin, S., 103, 779, 801
Miotto, K., 735
Mirkin, P. K., 574
Mirsky, A. F., 67
Mischel, W., 7, 10
Misumi, K., 462
Mitchell, J., 338, 345, 346, 353, 387
Mitchell, J. E., 781, 782, 784, 792, 797, 800, 805, 806, 807, 808
Mitchell, K. J., 661
Mitchell, S., 665
Miterany, E., 784
Mitrani, V. B., 174
Miyoshi, T., 653
Mizokowa, D. T., 561
Moan, S., 664, 666, 698
Moan-Hardie, S., 665
Moats, L. C., 513, 514, 516, 519, 520, 522, 524, 529, 530, 545, 546, 547, 562
Mock, D., 514, 515, 519, 527
Modan-Moses, D., 784
Moffitt, C., 90, 275, 278, 283, 326
Moffitt, T. E., 19, 35, 139, 144, 147, 148, 149, 152, 153, 339, 346, 739
Moher, D., 84, 87, 90
Mohr, P. J., 798
Mokros, H. B., 340
Moldofsky, H., 785, 798, 807
Molina, B., 72, 73, 87, 90, 107
Molloy, C. A., 462
Molnar, J., 359, 365, 374
Monaco, A. P., 465
Monahan, J., 609
Monastra, V. J., 74
Monk, K., 295
Monroe, A. D., 676
Monson, B. H., 692
Mont, L., 783, 784
Montague, M., 564, 568
Montgomery, S. M., 468, 469
Monti, P. M., 735, 736, 737, 738, 750, 751, 799
Montoya, J., 672

Moody, S. W., 538, 539, 571
Mooney, K. C., 328
Moore, A., 379
Moore, D., 143, 217
Moore, G. J., 350
Moore, K., 188, 216, 630
Moore, K. J., 187, 221
Moore, M. J., 468
Moore, P., 72, 348
Moorehouse, M., 14, 30, 80, 102, 111
Moorer, S. R., 86
Moos, R. H., 738
Moradi, A., 273
Moran, D. J., III, 426
Moran, K., 668
Moran, P., 17
Moran, P. B., 341
Moran, T., 179
Moreau, D., 9, 336, 346, 357, 380
Moreci, P., 349, 745
Moreland, S., 188, 227
Moreno, F. A., 348
Moretti, M. M., 147
Morey, J., 462
Morford, M., 467
Morgan, A., 164, 213
Morgan, C. A., 683
Morgan, D., 190
Morgan, H. G., 807
Morgan, J. C., 108
Morgan, J. J. B., 271
Morgan, P., 527
Morgan, S., 419, 420
Morgan, S. B., 419, 458
Mori, L., 8, 11, 23
Moriarty, D., 202
Morita, Y., 141
Moritsugo, J. N., 13
Moroney, R., 437
Morrell, W., 345, 346, 809
Morren, J., 431
Morrier, M. J., 477
Morris, A. S., 149, 159
Morris, R., 457, 472, 513, 516, 517, 526
Morris, R. D., 529
Morris, R. J., 4
Morris, T. L., 161, 326
Morrison, D., 733
Morrissey-Kane, E., 658
Morrow-Bradley, C., 32
Mortenson, P. B., 470
Mortiz, G., 353
Morton, J., 784
Morton, T., 16, 17, 28, 29
Mortweet, S. I., 4
Moser, J., 656
Moser, R. P., 160
Moses, B. S., 606
Mosher, L., 658, 659
Mosk, M. D., 607
Moskowitz, K. S., 145
Moss, H., 783
Moss, H. B., 737, 739
Moss, S. J., 338, 387
Mostow, A., 16
Mott, D. E. W., 320
Mott, M. A., 732, 734, 737, 739, 740, 741, 748, 750, 752
Motta, R., 675, 682
Mottron, L., 472
Mouridsen, S. E., 460
Mowbray, C., 666
Mowrer, O. H., 6, 272, 683
Mowrer, W. M., 6
Moye, A. W., 801, 802
Mpofu, E., 203, 205
Mrakotsky, C., 337, 338
Mrazek, P., 66, 90, 391
MTA Cooperative Group, 9, 11, 66, 80, 90, 106, 112, 113, 114, 115, 116, 118, 119, 204, 295
Mucci, M., 484
Mudford, O. C., 489, 490
Mueller, B., 74
Mueller, K., 77
Mueller, R. A., 431
Mufson, L., 9, 357, 380, 381, 383

Mukai, L.,, 143, 217
Mulhall, P., 355
Mulick, J. A., 462, 481, 483, 490
Mulle, K., 12, 282, 283, 292, 389
Mullen, P., 648, 649, 650, 651, 701
Mullen, R., 330, 731, 747
Muller, R., 467
Muller, S. D., 285
Mullin, B., 295
Mullins, L. L., 5
Mullins, M., 294
Mullool, J. P., 468
Multisite Violence Prevention Project, 660
Mulvaney, F., 743
Mulvey, E. P., 609
Mumme, D., 689
Mundschenk, N. S., 473
Mundy, P., 466
Munoz, R. F., 391
Munroe-Blum, H., 353, 355
Munt, E. D., 96
Muntaner, C., 345
Murch, S. H., 465, 468
Muris, P., 11, 316, 330
Murnen, S., 788
Murphy, A., 105
Murphy, B., 689
Murphy, C., 462, 463
Murphy, C. M., 151, 281, 282, 288, 316, 608
Murphy, D., 436, 548, 555
Murphy, D. A., 151
Murphy, D. M., 485
Murphy, J. A., 538
Murphy, K. R., 74, 89, 160
Murphy, M., 8, 378, 382, 383
Murphy, W. D., 609
Murray, C., 72, 161, 355
Murray, E., 175, 214, 220, 226
Murray, E. J., 175
Murray, J. C., 465
Murray, M. C., 9, 292, 330
Murray, P. J., 439
Musick, J., 692
Mussell, J. E., 800
Mussen, P. H., 36
Mustill, S., 339
Muthen, B., 733
Muthén, B. O., 210
Myatt, R., 107, 108
Myers, C. A., 545
Myers, D. A., 668
Myers, J. E. B., 673
Myers, K., 345, 346, 353, 743
Myers, L. W., 612
Myers, M. G., 732, 734, 735, 736, 738, 739, 740, 741, 742, 743, 744, 745, 746, 747, 748, 750, 751, 752, 758, 760, 762
Myers, P., 515, 520
Myers, P. A., 668
Myers, R. M., 465
Myers, T., 806
Myerson, N., 330, 701
Myklebust, H., 561
Myles, K. T., 660, 661
Myrtle, A. S., 779

Naar-King, S., 608
Naatanen, R., 461
Nagin, D., 148, 209, 227
Nagin, D. S., 153, 154, 200, 209, 217
Nagle, D. W., 179
Nagle, R. J., 320
Naglieri, J. A., 525
Nagoshi, C. T., 740
Nagoshi, J. T., 193, 216, 225
Nagy, W. E., 552
Naik, B., 441
Najarian, L. M., 292, 328
Najman, J., 649, 736
Nakajima, E., 466
Nakamura, B. J., 6
Nansel, T. R., 141, 142
Nanson, J. L., 76
Narayan, M., 350
Narduzzi, K., 785
Nathanson, R., 658, 665, 670, 698

Natioanl Reading Panel, 520, 533, 535, 539, 546, 553, 557
Nation, M., 658
National Adolescent Perpetrator Network, 704
National Advisory Mental Health Council Workgroup, 298
National Center for Education Statistics, 421, 444, 532
National Center for Prosecution of Child Abuse, 669, 671
National Film Board of Canada, 697
National Institute of Mental Health Autism Research Unit, 424
National Joint Committee on Learning Disabilities, 516
National Research Council, 595
Nauta, M. H., 291, 330
Navarro, A. M., 30
Nay, W. R., 429
Nayak, M. B., 606
Naylor, M., 685
Naylor, S. T., 484
Neal-Barnett, A. M., 8
Neale, M., 780
Needell, B., 676
Needleman, H. L., 444
Needles, D., 144
Neef, N. A., 140, 473
Neeleman, H. L., 77, 81
Neeleman, R., 471
Nef, F., 787
Neft, D., 385
Negri-Shoeltz, N., 427
Neitzert, C. S., 797
Nelki, J. S., 700
Nelson, A., 9
Nelson, B., 338, 349
Nelson, C., 468, 685
Nelson, C. A., 466
Nelson, C. M., 430
Nelson, D. S., 462, 471
Nelson, J. C., 206
Nelson, J. E., 484
Nelson, J. R., 179
Nelson, K. B., 470
Nelson, K. E., 595, 602
Nelson, M. L., 733
Nelson, R. O., 37, 290, 316, 332
Nelson, S., 212, 227
Nelson, S. E., 212
Nelson, W. M., 8, 38, 182, 220
Nelson-Gray, R. O., 301
Nemeroff, C. B., 348, 349
Neshat-Doost, H., 273
Ness, J., 433
Ness, K. K., 462, 464
Neuman, P., 782
Neumann, D. A., 680, 692
Neumann, L., 736
Neumarker, K., 782
Neumarker, U., 782
New, E., 463
New, M., 604
Newberry, A. M., 223
Newby, R., 70, 88
Newby, R. F., 524
Newcomb, A. F., 107
Newcomb, K., 156, 157, 158, 165, 190, 213
Newcomb, M. D., 732, 733
Newcorn, J., 92, 338
Newcorn, J. H., 75
Newdelman, J., 76
Newell, E., 468
Newell, R. M., 173, 223
Newman, A., 282, 290, 328
Newman, C. F., 753
Newman, D. L., 339, 346, 739
Newman, E., 684
Newman, J. E., 179
Newschaffer, C. J., 462, 464
Newsom, C., 458, 462, 472, 480, 481, 483, 487
Newsom, C. D., 426
Newton, J. S., 480
Nezu, A. M., 4, 8, 21

Nezu, C. M., 4, 8, 21
Nezworski, M. T., 24
Ng, S., 229
Ngai, E., 786
Niaura, R. S., 738
Nice, J., 465
Nicholas, E., 664, 666, 698
Nicholas, L., 802
Nickerson, K., 345
Nicoletti, M. A., 350
Niec, L. N., 9
Niederberger, J. M., 659
Niederehe, G., 298
Nielsen, G., 429
Nieminen-von Wendt, T., 461, 462
Nierenberg, A. A., 348
Nietzel, M., 628
Nietzel, M. T., 107
Nigg, J. T., 67, 74, 78, 159
Nihira, K., 438
Niimi, M., 462
Niles, B., 798
Nilsson, D. E., 106, 109, 110, 111
Nilsson, E., 807
Nishi-Strattner, L., 155
Nishimura, C., 465
Nishioka, V., 189
Nitschke, J. B., 350
Nix, R. L., 186, 232, 596, 600, 618, 620, 627, 630
Nixon, R. D. V., 156, 160, 166, 225
Noam, G. G., 16
Nocella, J., 330
Nock, M. K., 42, 218, 223
Noegel, R., 780
Nolan, E. E., 70, 87
Nolen, W. A., 439
Nolen-Hoeksema, S., 17, 338, 340, 341, 343, 686, 811
Noll, J. G., 692, 693
Nomellini, S., 622
Nomura, Y., 380, 381, 383
Norcross, J., 5, 9, 614
Nordahl, T. E., 75, 350
Nordin, V., 461
Norman, D., 74
Norman, P. A., 800, 808
North, J., 43
Northam, E., 202, 217, 218, 219, 227
Northey, K., 170, 229
Norton, J. A., 487
Norton, K., 801
Norton, M. C., 692
Noser, K., 376
Notari-Syverson, N., 537
Nouri, N., 464
Novacenko, H., 349
Novaco, R. W., 182, 602, 622
Novak, S. P., 734
Novikov, I., 784
Nowak-Drabik, K. M., 436, 437
Nowakowska, C., 443
Nudelman, S., 797
Nunez, Z., 672, 673
Nunn, R., 202, 217, 218, 219, 227
Nunn, R. G., 702
Nunno, M., 665, 675
Nurmi, E. L., 465
Nuro, K. F., 43
Nussbaum, B. R., 156
Nussbaum, N., 546
Nye, J., 490
Nyhan, W., 415, 431
NYS Department of Health, 490

Oakes, T. R., 350
Oakland, T., 185, 546
Oates, K., 657
Oates, R. K., 628, 677, 692
Obel, C., 77
Oberklaid, F., 149
Oberlander, L. B., 666
Obermeier, G., 731
Obert, J. L., 735
Obler, M., 280, 284, 316
O'Brien, B., 548, 555
O'Brien, C. P., 743, 747

O'Brien, E. K., 465
O'Brien, J., 437
O'Brien, K., 783
O'Brien, M. L., 109
O'Brien, S., 429, 623
Obrosky, D. S., 338, 345, 346
Obrzut, J. E., 524
O'Connell, D., 347
O'Connell, M. A., 678, 679
O'Conner, P., 19
O'Connor, M. E., 786, 798, 800, 808
O'Connor, N., 456
O'Connor, R. D., 290, 322
O'Connor, R. E., 512, 536, 537, 541, 557
O'Dell, M. C., 476, 477, 478
O'Dell, S. L., 162, 272, 280, 284
Odgers, C. L., 147
Odom, S. L., 437, 473, 474
O'Donnell, D., 72, 86, 87
O'Donnell, J., 1209
Oelwein, P. L., 420
O'Fallon, W., 784
Offer, D., 340
Offord, D. R., 18, 70, 145, 147, 652
Offord, K. P., 747
Oftedal, G., 340
Ogata, J. R., 687, 688
Ogden, T., 172, 178, 226, 229
Ogilvie, D., 648
Ogles, B. M., 33
Ohannessian, C. M., 738
O'Hara, N., 633
O'Hare, F., 564
Ohashi, Y., 462
Öhman, A., 272
Okane, T., 783
Oke, N. J., 474
Okulitch, J. S., 202
Olafson, E., 679
Olafsson, R. F., 141
Oldfield, D., 656
Olds, D., 208, 212, 226, 632
O'Leary, K. D., 6, 7, 38, 151, 175, 176, 190, 191, 192, 216, 608
O'Leary, R. D., 104, 106
O'Leary, S. G., 105, 106, 150, 159, 190, 191, 194
Olfson, M., 294, 375, 380, 381, 383
Olin, S., 298
Oliveri, M. K., 657
Ollendick, T. H., 4, 6, 9, 11, 25, 31, 164, 214, 226, 279, 280, 283, 290, 293, 301, 330, 334, 421, 799
Olley, J., 416
Ollinger, J. M., 350
Olmsted, M. P., 800, 803, 805
Olson, A. E., 159
Olson, D., 695
Olson, E., 685
Olson, J., 608
Olson, L. M., 465
Olson, M., 84
Olson, R., 288, 320, 513, 516, 517, 518, 548, 550
Olson, R. K., 449, 532, 547, 548, 550
Olsson, G. I., 345
Olvera, R. L, 343, 344
Olweus, D., 141, 142, 196, 197, 201, 203, 217, 225, 229
O'Malley, P. M., 731, 732, 759
Omura, R. T., 193, 216, 225
O'Neil, P., 788, 789
O'Neill, R., 158, 435, 480
O'Neill, R. E., 475
Ong, B., 459
Ongur, D., 350
Ontario Ministry of the Attorney General, 673
Open Court Reading, 536
Opland, E., 748, 751
Orbach, I., 18, 19
Orbach, Y., 665, 666, 673
Orcutt, H. K., 670, 671
O'Reilly, M. F., 424
Orelove, F. F., 660, 661
Oren, D. A., 350
Oriol, A., 784

Orlinsky, D. E., 375, 376
Orme, M., 598
Ornitz, E. M., 458
Ornstein, P. A., 667
Orosan, P., 801
Orpinas, P., 197, 217
Orrell-Valente, J., 793, 795
Ort, S. I., 295
Ortega, M., 13
Orts, K., 459
Orvaschel, H., 339, 353, 358, 682, 685, 745
Orwig, D., 299
Osaki, D., 488
Osborne, P., 415, 439
Osgarby, S. M., 696, 706
O'Shaughnessy, M., 785
O'Shea, M., 648, 649
Osman, B. B., 84, 85, 87
Öst, L., 288, 316
Ostensen, E., 783
Oster, J. R., 784
Osterling, J., 457, 466, 471, 480, 487
Ostrander, R., 107
Ostrosky, M., 437, 473
Ostrov, E., 340
Ostuzzi, R., 807
Ota, K. R., 106
O'Toole, B. I., 657, 677, 692
Ott, E. S., 8, 38
Ou, S. R., 420
Ouellette, C., 71
Ouimette, P. C., 685
Oullete, C., 74
Overall, J. E., 206, 226, 483
Overholser, J. C., 341
Overmeyer, S., 75
Overpeck, M., 141, 142
Ovwigho, P. C., 633, 634
Owen, M., 598
Owen, R., 569, 570
Owen, S. M., 156, 188
Owens, J., 655
Owens, J. S., 24
Owens, P., 629
Owens, R. L., 569
Owens, S. M., 156
Oxford, M., 142
Oxman-Martinez, J., 656
Ozonoff, S., 74, 459, 465, 466, 467, 475, 480, 481

Pace, G. M., 432, 481
Packard, D., 472
Packard, T., 109, 110
Padayachi, U. K., 648
Padgett, S., 689
Padron-Gayol, M. V., 206
Pagani, L., 70, 208, 217, 227
Pagani-Kurtz, L., 208, 217
Page, T. J., 429
Pain, K., 417
Paine, M. L., 658
Pajer, K. A., 147
Palinscar, A., 522, 549, 557
Pallonen, U. E., 745
Palmer, A. A., 465
Palmer, D. S., 421
Palmer, P., 465
Palmer, R. L., 779, 784
Palmour, R. M., 348
Palusci, V. J., 667, 669
Pam, A., 789
Panagiotopoulos, C., 783
Pancari, J., 481
Pandina, G. J., 74
Pandina, R. J., 738, 740
Pandit, B. S., 462
Panerai, A., 789
Paniagua, F. A., 96
Panichelli-Mindel, S. M., 271, 284, 291, 301, 330
Panksepp, J., 484
Papa, R., 788
Papanikolaou, K., 465
Papineau, D., 189, 216, 225
Pappadopulos, E. A., 13, 206

Paquette, d., 147
Paradise, J. E., 667, 668
Pardini, D. A., 142
Pare, C., 783, 784
Parham, E. S., 795, 809
Parilla, R., 651
Parish, T. S., 316
Parke, R. D., 599
Parker, A., 739
Parker, C. M., 156
Parker, E. H., 141
Parker, J. D. A., 274
Parker, K. J., 348
Parkman, P. D., 469
Parmar, R. S., 568
Parrila, R. K., 651
Parrish, J. M., 140, 430
Parsons, B. V., 173, 214, 215, 223, 224, 225, 226
Partanen, K., 350
Partington, J. W., 476, 478, 479
Partridge, F., 339
Partridge, S., 676
Pasanisi, F., 807
Pascoe, J. M., 109
Pascual-Marqui, R., 350
Pascualvaca, D., 75
Pate, J. E., 809, 810
Patel, D., 796
Patel, H., 178
Patel, K., 43
Patel, M. R., 423, 428
Paternite, C., 99
Patil, A. A., 461
Patock-Peckham, J. A., 740
Patten, C. A., 747
Patterson, G. R., 7, 10, 14, 33, 34, 35, 41, 96, 99, 140, 143, 146, 147, 148, 149, 150, 151, 152, 153, 154, 156, 157, 158, 160, 161, 170, 171, 172, 186, 195, 198, 200, 208, 212, 213, 214, 218, 219, 221, 222, 224, 225, 226, 228, 229, 232, 482, 610, 740, 752
Patterson, L. J., 350
Paul, R., 456, 458
Paulauskas, S. L., 144, 336, 345, 346, 347, 388
Paulose-Ram, R., 299
Pavlov, I., 271
Pavone, L., 461
Pawl, J. H., 627
Pawluck, D., 782
Pawsey, R., 200
Paxton, S., 793
Pearson, D. A., 439
Pearson, J., 352, 353, 355
Peck, C. A., 437
Peckham-Hardin, K. D., 484, 485, 486
Pecora, P. J., 595, 603, 609
Pedersen, C. B., 470
Pedlow, R., 149
Pedulla, B. M., 37
Peebles, C. D., 681
Peed, S., 164, 212, 225
Peeden, J. N., 466
Peeke, L. A., 273
Pejeau, C., 415
Pelcovitz, D., 608, 684
Peleg, A., 736
Peleg, R., 736
Pelham, W., 19
Pelham, W. E., 68, 70, 72, 73, 86, 87, 88, 90, 104, 106, 107, 109, 110, 111, 115, 141, 151
Pelham, W. E., Jr., 9, 11, 24, 65, 72, 73, 87, 97, 98, 104, 109, 110, 111, 119
Pelios, L., 431
Pelletier-Parker, A., 202
Pelton, G., 484
Pelton, L. H., 598
Penaloza, R. V., 189
Pence, D., 663
Pendleton, V. R., 803
Penick, E. C., 340
Penilla, C., 391
Peniston, E. G., 631
Penn, C., 71

Pennebaker, J. W., 698
Pennington, B. F., 74, 459, 466, 532
Pennington, R., 466, 473
Pennucci, A., 166, 174, 178, 185, 188, 212
Pentz, M. A., 184
Penza, S., 689, 690
Peoples, A., 472
Pepler, D., 142, 147, 167, 196, 197, 213, 214, 217, 220, 226, 228, 229
Pepping, G., 301
Perel, J., 349, 783
Perez, G. A., 223
Perez, J., 467
Perez-Vidal, A., 174, 175, 220, 223, 225, 747, 752
Pericak-Vance, M. A., 465
Perkins, D. N., 569
Perl, E., 204, 226
Perloff, B. F., 456
Perper, J. A., 353
Perry, B. D., 683, 688
Perry, C. L., 787
Perry, D. G., 342
Perry, P. J., 94
Perry, R., 204, 205, 206, 218, 226, 227, 232, 483, 489
Persons, J. B., 301
Persson, H. E., 74
Pestronk, A., 466
Peters, D., 670
Peters, R., 701
Peters, R. D., 8, 14
Peters, T., 784
Petersen, A. C., 340, 341, 342, 343, 347, 354
Peterson, C., 664, 685, 686
Peterson, C. B., 800, 806
Peterson, C. R., 430
Peterson, D., 156
Peterson, G., 688
Peterson, K., 43
Peterson, L., 8, 9, 11, 23, 28, 322, 599, 601, 602, 604, 620, 633, 651
Peterson, L. W., 631
Peterson, R., 682
Peterson, R. A., 273
Peterson, S. L., 485
Peterson, T. R., 747
Petit, L., 632
Petras, H., 210
Petrila, A., 733, 752
Petrill, S., 796
Petropoulos, H., 75
Petropoulos, M. C., 469, 475
Pettinati, H. M., 743
Pettit, G. S., 37, 38, 141, 147, 149, 152, 230
Pettke-Rank, C., 783
Petty, L., 458
Pevalin, D. J., 340
Peveler, R. C., 798, 800
Pevron, A., 678
Pfanner, P., 441
Pfeiffer, S., 185
Pfeiffer, S. I., 187
Pfiffner, L. J., 104, 105, 108, 110, 111, 190, 203
Pfingsten, U., 107
Pham, B., 84, 87, 90
Phelps, L., 109
Phelps, M. E., 350, 394
Philippe, A., 465
Phillips, A., 468
Phillips, A. T., 483
Phillips, E. L., 194, 224
Phillips, J. S., 7
Phillips, N. B., 566, 567
Phillips, P., 667
Phillips, S. D., 595
Phillips, W., 461
Physicians' Desk Reference, 443
Piacentini, J., 11, 13, 271, 280, 295
Piaget, J., 526
Piana, R. C., 355
Piazza, C. C., 423, 425, 428
Piazza, E., 782
Piche, C., 687

Pichichero, M. E., 470
Pick, L., 75
Pickles, A., 147, 148, 345, 465
Pickrel, S. G., 8, 9, 21, 177, 178, 221, 224, 226, 747
Pidgeon, A., 622, 633
Pidgeon, A., 214
Pierce, K., 467, 477
Pierce, L. H., 674
Pierce, R., 674
Pierce, W. D., 424, 427, 428, 434
Piercy, F. P., 747
Piercy, M., 437
Pierloot, R., 807
Pietila, J., 465
Pigott, H. E., 191, 201, 227
Piha, J., 415
Pikas, A., 141
Pike, K., 781, 783, 787, 793, 794, 797, 798, 800, 805
Pilkington, L., 468
Pilkonis, P. A., 298, 356, 599
Pilla, R. S., 141, 142
Pillay, M., 799
Pillay, S. S., 350
Pillow, D. R., 24, 86
Pimentel, S., 9
Pina, A. A., 299
Pincus, D., 156, 157
Pincus, H., 784
Pincus, H. A., 460
Pincus, J. H., 612
Pinderhughes, E., 160
Pine, D., 782
Pine, D. S., 271, 280, 294, 295, 336, 346, 386
Pinker, S., 39
Pinnock, N., 489
Pinsonneault, I., 202
Pintello, D., 674, 675
Pintner, R., 279
Pinto-Martin, J. A., 76
Piquero, A., 152, 153
Piran, N., 805, 811
Pisor, K., 106, 194, 195
Pisterman, S., 102
Pithers, W. D., 691, 703
Pitsavas, G., 783, 784
Pittman, A., 9, 23
Pittman, L. D., 634
Pitts-Conway, V., 474
Piven, J., 465
Pizzagalli, D., 350
Playfair, W. S., 779
Pleak, R., 205
Plen, M., 378
Plesner, A. M., 470
Plienis, A. J., 486
Pliszka, S. R., 74, 75, 84, 87, 88, 89, 93, 94, 95
Plomin, R., 39
Plotkin, R., 618
Plotnicov, K. H., 668, 809
Plummer, B. A., 743
Plummer, C. M., 278
Plunet, M. H., 484
Poduska, J., 210, 218, 227
Pokorni, J. I., 520
Pokorny, A. D., 740
Polaino-Lorente, A., 339
Polcari, A., 75
Polivy, J., 785, 802
Pollack Dorta, K., 380, 381, 383
Pollack, L., 24
Pollack, S., 68, 204
Pollard, R. A., 683, 688
Pollard, S., 70, 109
Pollice, C., 668, 809
Pollock, N., 737
Pollock, V. E., 680, 692
Polloway, E., 414
Polo, A. J., 30, 32
Polster, R. A., 37, 602
Pomeroy, C., 806
Poole, D. A., 664, 673
Pope, H. G., 780, 805
Popkey, C., 604

Poplin, M. S., 526
Poquette, C., 599
Porrino, L. J., 67
Port, L. K., 663, 669, 670, 675, 692
Porter, B., 151
Portnoy, S., 19
Porzelius, L., 786
Posener, J., 350
Posey, D. J., 442, 443, 484
Posten, D., 422
Poston, W. S., 780, 784, 788, 789, 790, 803, 809, 810, 811
Potter, D., 457, 464
Potter, G. B., 185
Potter, H. W., 455
Potter, N., 443
Potter, R. L., 348
Potter, W. Z., 203
Pottle, L. C., 91, 94
Potvin, J. H., 805, 811
Poulin, F., 9, 108, 118, 141, 186, 232
Poulton, L.621, 622
Poulton, L., 9, 143, 202
Pound, J., 657
Povilaitis, T., 599
Powell, B., 619
Powell, J. E., 462
Powell, M. B., 151
Powell, S. B., 458
Powell, S. R., 566, 567
Power, C., 180
Power, T. J., 70, 109
Powers, H. P., 794, 795
Powers, J., 632
Powers, L. E., 485, 486
Powers, M. D., 8
Powers, P. S., 778, 782, 789, 792, 794, 795, 804
Powers, S. W., 164, 214
Poyurovsky, M., 206
Poznanski, E. O., 340
Prather, R. C., 796, 797
Pratt, A., 534, 540
Pratt, H., 796
Pratt, H. D., 85, 86, 87, 88, 93, 94, 95
Pratt, R. D., 470
Premack, D., 425
Prendergast, P., 805
Prentice-Dunn, S., 160
Prentice, K., 569, 570
Prentky, R. A., 691
Presberg, J., 441
Presidential Commission on Law Enforcement and the Administration of Justice, 186
President's Commission on Excellence in Special Education, 513, 514, 578
President's New Freedom Commission on Mental Health, 4
Preskorn, S. H., 387
Presnell, K., 342
Pressley, M., 557
Presson, C. C., 739
Price, D., 468
Price, G. H., 104, 106
Price, J. L., 350
Price, J. M., 737, 738
Price, L. H., 348, 484
Price, R. K., 739
Priel, B., 352
Prien, R., 336
Prieto, S. L., 351
Prince, J., 91, 386
Prinstein, M. J., 686
Printz, A. M., 782
Prinz, R. J., 9, 147, 154, 162, 163, 175, 176, 184, 214, 215, 220, 222, 223, 225, 230, 231
Prior, M., 68, 149, 459, 460, 464, 487
Pritchard, M., 283, 293, 328, 330, 334
Prizmich, L. P., 673
Prochaska, J. O., 9, 20, 614
Prochnow, J. E., 532, 539
Proctor, M. A., 190
Project MATCH Research Group, 748
Prokhorov, A. V., 745
Pronovost, W., 456

Proudfoot, P., 648
Prout, H. T., 436, 437
Provence, S., 458
Provin, M. A., 350
Pruett, R. C., 658
Pruitt, D. B., 682, 685
Prusoff, B. A., 354
Pryor, T., 785, 786, 792
Pugh, K. R., 550
Puig-Antich, J., 206, 338, 349, 353, 354, 355, 358, 386, 745
Pulkkinen, L., 153
Pumariega, A. J., 343, 345, 809, 810
Pung, M., 811
Puntney, J. K., 443
Purdie, D. M., 649
Pure, D. L., 790, 791
Putallaz, M., 38, 147
Putnam, F. W., 681, 687, 688, 689, 692, 693, 695
Pyle, R. L., 781, 782, 784, 797, 800, 806
Pynoos, R. S., 292, 328, 698

Qin, J., 664, 666, 673
Quach, H., 465
Quadflieg, N., 807
Quas, J. A., 664, 666, 667, 669, 670, 671
Quay, H., 4, 78, 139, 156, 415
Querido, J. G., 157, 158, 165
Quinn, P. O., 72
Quinn, W., 731, 747
Quinnell, F. A., 679
Quintero-Howard, C., 807
Quintin, P., 348
Quinton, D., 147, 148
Quitkin, F., 805
Quittner, A. L., 43
Qunaibi, M., 74

Raab, M., 438
Rabe-Hesketh, S., 789
Rabian, B., 273, 285
Rabian, B. A., 328
Rabinovich, H., 338, 349
Rachel, J. V., 747
Rachman, S., 271, 279
Racine, Y. A., 18, 147, 648
Racusin, R., 387, 389
Radojevic, V., 119
Radue, E., 783
Radzikowska, M., 783
Rae, D. S., 336, 339, 345, 739
Raeburn, S. D., 797, 798, 806, 807
Raffaele, L. S., 460
Rafferty, Y., 421
Ragan, J., 804
Raghunathan, T. E., 735
Ragland, E. U., 473
Rahbar, B., 782, 783
Raichle, M. E., 350
Raine, A., 203
Rainey, B., 633
Rains, L. A., 224
Ralveski, E., 797
Ramey, C. T., 418, 420
Ramey, S. L., 420
Ramo, D. E., 746, 750, 751
Rampey, A. H., 805, 811
Ramsay, R., 791
Ramsden, S. R., 141
Ramsey, E., 155, 158, 161, 190, 192, 193, 194, 195, 216, 227, 740
Randall, M., 743
Randall, W., 651
Range, L., 685
Rankin, M. A., 348
Ransby, M., 547, 554
Ransby, M. J., 556
Rantanen, P., 142, 782
Rao, U., 745
Rapee, R. M., 12, 40, 274, 277, 283, 291, 294, 326
Rapin, I., 457, 471, 472
Rapoport, J., 93
Rapoport, J. L., 67, 203, 484
Rapp, N., 473
Rappaport, L., 119

Rappley, M. D., 74, 85, 86, 87, 88, 93, 94, 95
Rapport, M. D., 67, 68, 86, 87, 88, 90, 105
Rasbury, W. C., 4
Rashotte, C. A., 532, 534, 539, 545, 550, 551, 552, 553, 575
Raskind, M., 564
Rasmussen, L. A., 691, 697
Rasmussen, P., 461
Rasmusson, A., 206
Rastam, M., 460, 461, 465, 783, 807
Rathouz, P. J., 147
Ratnofsky, A. C., 651
Ratzan, S., 471
Ratzoni, G., 779, 785
Rau, J. H., 806
Rauch, S. L., 295
Ravan, S. A., 465
Ravitz, A. J., 467
Rawson, R. A., 735
Ray, J., 149
Ray, J. S., 339, 353
Ray, R. S., 7, 171
Rayfield, A., 156, 157
Raymond, N., 805
Rayner, R., 6, 271
Reach, K., 28
Reader, M., 386
Reader, M. J., 75
Realmuto, G. M., 107, 484
Reaney, S., 437, 473
Reas, D., 807
Reaven, J., 475, 488
Reavis, H. K., 190
Reber, M., 156, 180, 220, 226, 416
Rebok, G. W., 209, 210, 218, 219, 220
Recasens, C., 484
Redd, S. C., 469
Reddy, L. A., 187
Reddy, R., 355
Redlich, A. D., 665, 673
Redwood, L., 469
Reece, R., 662
Reed, E., 561
Reed, G., 428
Reed, H. K., 482
Reese, L., 514
Reeve, C. E., 480
Reeve, E. A., 295
Reeves, D., 490
Reeves, J. S., 67
Reeves, R. S., 803
Regier, D. A., 336, 339, 345
Regino, R., 77
Rehm, L. P., 354
Reich, T., 350
Reich, W., 155
Reichler, R. J., 459
Reid, D. K., 526
Reid, J., 108, 150, 607
Reid, J. B., 7, 18, 34, 41, 101, 140, 143, 148, 149, 150, 151, 154, 158, 161, 170, 171, 172, 187, 195, 198, 199, 200, 201, 208, 212, 213, 214, 216, 217, 219, 222, 224, 225, 226, 227, 229, 482, 607, 630
Reid, J. C., 337, 338, 339
Reid, K., 188, 227
Reid, M. J., 166, 167, 168, 185, 192, 207, 212, 213, 218, 219, 220, 221, 223, 225, 228, 231
Reimherr, F. W., 91
Reinecke, M. A., 356, 383
Reinemann, D. H. S., 615
Reiner, S., 184
Reinhart, M., 668
Reinholtz, C., 648
Reis, D., 206
Reiss, A., 386, 414, 415
Reiss, A. L., 75
Reiss, C., 601, 618
Reiss, D., 738
Reiss, S., 273
Reiter, J., 801
Reitman, D., 161
Reitsma, P., 525
Reitzel-Jaffe, D., 9, 23, 609
Reivich, K. J., 391

Rekedal, S., 666
Remer, R., 9, 108, 118
Remy, P., 467
Renner, B. R., 459
Renshaw, P. F., 75, 350
Reppucci, N. D., 658, 668
Reschly, D. J., 516, 518, 520, 523, 524, 526, 527
Rescorla, L., 556
Rescorla, L. A., 3, 4, 138, 155, 156, 158, 159, 274, 458, 695, 744
Resnick, H. S., 656, 657, 658, 668, 669, 685
Resnick, P., 684
Respitz, C., 80, 82, 88, 117
Reul, J. M. H. M., 348
Revilla, J., 667
Reyes, L., 648
Reyna McGlone, C. L., 164, 214, 226
Reynolds, A. J., 420, 632
Reynolds, C., 744, 745
Reynolds, C. R., 20, 156, 274
Reynolds, G. S., 143
Reynolds, V., 9
Reynolds, W. M., 378, 379, 382
Rheinberger, A., 474
Rhodes, J. E., 355
Rhodes, P. H., 468
Rhule, D. M., 161, 208
Ribera, J., 784
Ribordy, S., 689
Ricardi, R. K., 295
Ricca, V., 797, 800
Ricci, L. R., 691
Ricciardelli, L. A., 781, 782, 786
Rice, C., 462, 463
Rice, J. M., 615, 621, 624
Rice, R. E., 739
Rich, B., 460
Rich, B. A., 156
Rich, C. L., 784
Rich, H., 677
Rich, S., 471
Richards, C., 144, 345, 346, 347, 388
Richards, D. A., 631
Richards, M. H., 342
Richards, P., 797
Richards, T. L., 552
Richardson, B., 419
Richardson, J. P., 202
Richardson, M. T., 627
Richdale, A. L., 462
Richman, G., 423, 426, 428, 431, 432
Richmond, B. O., 274
Richter, B., 416
Richter, N. C., 119
Richter, S. S., 740, 748
Richters, J., 72, 273
Richters, J. E., 150, 151
Rick, J., 25
Rickel, A. U., 23, 28
Rickert, V., 782, 783
Riddle, M. A., 294, 295, 345
Riddlesberger, M., 667
Ridge, B., 149
Ridle, M. A., 206
Ridlehuber, H. W., 75
Ridley, M., 39
Ridley-Johnson, R., 322
Riedel, W. J., 348
Rieppi, R., 615
Rieser, J., 569
Rieth, H. J., 567
Rifkin, A., 204, 226
Rigas, C., 807
Riggs, D. S., 696
Riggs, P., 702, 737
Riggs, P. D., 91, 94, 745, 752
Riley, A. W., 146
Riley, J. L., 156
Riley, T., 568
Rimland, B., 487
Rimpela, A., 142
Rimpela, M., 142, 782
Rinaldi, J., 466, 480
Rincover, A., 430, 472, 481
Rind, B., 680, 681

Rindfleisch, N., 675
Ring, H. A., 467
Ring, J., 547, 548, 549, 550
Ring-Kurtz, S., 740, 741
Ringdahl, J., 433
Ringeisen, H., 297
Ringel, J. S., 3, 22
Ringwalt, C. L., 734
Rintelmann, J., 343, 345, 346, 386
Rio, A., 175, 214, 220, 226
Risch, N., 464, 465
Risi, S., 459
Risley, T. R., 7, 456, 532
Risley-Curtiss, C., 628
Riso, L. R., 685
Rispens, J., 652
Rissanen, A., 782
Risucci, D., 525
Ritch, C. R., 484
Ritchie, J., 811
Ritter, B., 281, 282, 288, 314, 316, 318, 322
Ritter, J., 738
Ritterband, L. M., 43
Ritvo, E. R., 471
Rivara, F. P., 735
Rivard, J. C., 595, 602
Rivas-Vazquez, A., 175, 214, 220, 226
Rivera, D., 566
Roache, J., 439
Robb, A., 782, 786, 788, 793, 795
Robbins,, F. R., 486
Robbins, K., 87, 88, 204
Robbins, M. S., 174, 223, 224
Roberts, C. R., 343, 344
Roberts, I., 668
Roberts, M., 164, 212, 213, 225
Roberts, M. C., 4, 8, 9, 10, 23, 292, 322, 601
Roberts, M. D., 611
Roberts, M. W., 150, 158, 160, 221, 430
Roberts, R., 28
Roberts, R. E., 70, 339, 343, 344, 345, 347, 733
Roberts, W., 106
Robertson, C. P., 417
Robertson, D. L., 632
Robertson, J., 347
Robin, A., 18
Robin, A. L., 10, 24, 25, 71, 91, 102, 158, 752, 782, 801, 802
Robin, A. R., 7, 9
Robinette, D., 739
Robins, A. L., 146, 172, 175, 176, 226
Robins, C. J., 24
Robins, L. N., 739
Robinson, C., 601, 618
Robinson, D, 338
Robinson, D. R., 597, 618
Robinson, E., 157, 158
Robinson, E. A., 165, 213, 222
Robinson, G. L., 524
Robinson, J., 208, 217, 413
Robinson, R. O., 461
Robinson, S., 432
Robisnon, G., 461
Robyn, S., 606
Rockert, W., 800, 803, 805
Rodgers, A., 28
Rodick, J. D., 177, 214, 225
Rodier, P. M., 465
Rodin, J., 779, 785
Rodrigue, J. R., 13
Rodriguez, A., 77
Rodriguez, H., 288, 320
Rodriguez, M. C., 484
Roe, D., 796, 797
Roed, I. S., 805
Roehling, P. V., 738, 744
Roerig, J., 800, 805, 806, 807
Roeser, R. W., 355
Rogal, S. S., 702
Rogala, R., 465
Rogan, L., 561
Rogeness, G. A., 203
Roger, H., 469
Roger, J., 442

Rogers, A. I., 784
Rogers, E. S., 152, 160
Rogers, G., 584
Rogers, J., 484
Rogers, R. W., 655
Rogers, S., 466
Rogers, S. J., 457, 459, 466, 471, 487, 488, 489
Rogers, T., 164, 214
Rogers, T. R., 164, 222
Rogers, W., 339, 390
Rogosch, F., 607, 738, 740
Rogosch, F. A., 689, 737, 738
Roguski, K., 783
Rohde, P., 184, 226, 336, 339, 346, 355, 378, 383, 733, 737, 739, 745
Rohrbeck, C. A., 601, 618
Rohsenow, D. J., 701, 735, 737, 738, 750
Roizen, N. J., 72
Rojahn, J., 415, 439
Rolider, A., 432
Roll, D., 424
Rollings, S., 283, 293, 328, 330, 334, 701
Rollnick, S., 211, 735, 741, 746, 750, 751
Roman-Clarkson, S. E., 648
Romancyzk, R. G., 43
Romanczyk, A., 670
Romanczyk, R. G., 481
Romano, E., 70
Romano, J. P., 424
Romans, S. E., 648, 649, 650, 651
Rombough, V., 490
Rome, E., 783
Ronan, K. R., 7, 156, 178, 180, 220, 226, 229, 271, 290
Roncolato, W., 811
Roncoroni, L., 788
Ronit, M., 624
Roodenrys, S., 74
Roosa, M. W., 648
Roose, S. P., 805
Roper, B. L., 18
Roper, M. T., 85, 90, 116
Rorty, M., 787, 808
Rosa, J., 666
Rosario, M., 607, 608
Roscoe, E. M., 425
Rose, E., 534, 539
Rose, J. S., 631, 739
Rose, M., 669
Rosen, C., 651, 652, 659, 706
Rosen, D. S., 782
Rosen, H. S., 201, 217
Rosen, I., 75
Rosen, J. C., 797, 798, 801
Rosen, L. A., 105, 190, 195, 201, 217, 227
Rosen-Sheidley, B., 464, 465, 466
Rosenbaum, A., 104, 106
Rosenbaum, M., 104, 105, 345
Rosenbaum, M. S., 314
Rosenberg, C. R., 206
Rosenberg, D., 692
Rosenberg, M., 652
Rosenberg, R., 19
Rosenberg, T. K., 339
Rosenbinge, J., 783
Rosenblatt, A., 28
Rosenbloom, A., 320
Rosenblum, N. D., 316
Rosenfarb, I., 96, 290, 322, 330
Rosenfield-Schlicter, M. D., 606
Rosenhall, U., 461
Rosenheck, R., 796
Rosenshine, B., 523, 566
Rosenstein, D. S., 352
Rosenthal, N., 350
Rosenthal, R. H., 784
Rosenthal, T. L., 288, 290, 314, 316, 318, 320, 322
Roser, W., 783
Rosman, B. L., 779, 801
Ross, A., 6, 32, 39
Ross, B. H., 569
Ross, C., 469, 688
Ross, C. A., 789
Ross, D. F., 673
Ross, D. M., 70, 119

Ross, R., 202, 217, 218, 219, 227
Ross, S. A., 70, 119
Rossello, J., 380
Rossiter, E. M., 797, 806, 810
Rossotto, E., 787, 808
Rost, B., 783
Rotella, C., 800
Roth, C., 353
Roth, J., 271
Roth, S., 684
Rothbaum, B. O., 43
Rothbaum, B. P., 696
Rothrt, M. L., 299
Rotter, J. C., 288, 293, 316, 334
Rotzien, A., 459
Rounsaville, B. J., 732, 738, 743
Rourke, B. P., 461, 524, 565
Rouse, C. E., 520
Routh, C. P., 221, 222
Rovner, D., 299
Rowan, V. C., 271
Rowe, W. S., 656
Rowe-Hallbert, A., 150, 160, 221
Rowland, C. V., Jr., 787
Rowland, M. D., 8, 9, 10, 172, 176, 177, 207
Roy, A., 799
Royse, D., 628
Ruan, W. J., 141, 142
Rubama, I., 185
Rubenstein, J. L., 18, 19
Rubia, K., 75
Rubin, C., 18, 19
Rubin, K. H., 20, 689
Rubin, R. H., 654
Rubin, R. R., 799
Rubino, K., 692
Rubinstein, M., 691
Ruble, D., 687
Ruble, D. N., 601
Ruch-Ross, H., 692
Rudd, J. M., 678
Rudelli, R., 788
Rudolph, K. D., 3, 341, 350, 352, 355, 390
Rudy, L., 663, 664, 669, 670, 675, 692
Ruef, M., 422
Ruffalo, S. L., 159
Ruggiero, K. J., 657, 685
Ruhl, K. L., 522, 560
Rulliton, W. L., 420
Ruma, P. R., 218, 222
Rumberger, D. T., 28
Rumsey, J., 75
Runtz, M. G., 660, 687, 688
Runyan, D. K., 657, 669, 674, 675
Runyon, M. K., 631, 685
Rusch, F. R., 29
Rush, A. J., 277, 279, 299, 343, 345, 346, 386, 753
Rush, J., 351, 362, 379, 381
Rush, K., 425
Rushton, J. L., 339, 340, 343, 344, 375
Ruskin, E., 471
Russell, D. E., 648, 649, 650, 656, 659, 678
Russell, F. F., 419, 420
Russell, G. F. M., 784, 801, 805, 807
Russell, J., 798
Russell, M., 738
Russell, R., 76
Russo, D. C., 8, 141, 213
Russo, M. F., 145
Rutherford, M., 466
Rutherford, R. B., 430
Rutman, J., 340
Rutter, M., 16, 20, 23, 81, 138, 147, 148, 151, 152, 230, 345, 415, 456, 457, 459, 460, 461, 462, 464, 471, 628
Ryan, E. E., 631
Ryan, J. J., 75, 76
Ryan, N., 340, 349
Ryan, N. D., 93, 94, 336, 338, 349
Ryan, N. E., 356, 383
Ryan, P., 674
Ryan, R. M., 355, 689
Ryan, V., 608
Rydelius, P., 74

Ryding, E., 75
Rynders, J. E., 419
Ryno, L., 796

Saavedra, L. M., 8
Saba, G., 779
Sabol, S. Z., 733
Sacerdote, P., 789
Sachek, J., 78
Sachs, L. A., 119
Sachs, V., 689
Sachsenmaier, T., 670, 671
Sacks, N. R., 808
Sadock, B. J., 443
Saelens, B., 800, 803
Saenz, L., 558
Saez, L., 522, 531
Safer, D. J., 83, 84, 85, 91, 294, 345
Safferman, A., 295
Safford, S., 20, 40, 291
Safir, M. P., 450
Safran, M. A., 299
Safren, S. A., 299
Sagar, A., 779, 785, 786, 787, 811
Saigh, P. H., 316
Sailer, A., 428, 429
Sailor, W., 422, 427, 482
Sainato, D. M., 473
St. Lawrence, J. S., 21
Saitoh, O., 461
Saiz, C. S., 31
Saldana, L., 9, 612, 633, 651
Sale, E., 733
Salimi, L., 811
Salkin, B., 807
Sallee, F. R., 91, 92
Sallows, G. O., 471, 489
Saloman, M. K., 109
Salomon, G., 569
Salomon, R. M., 348
Salt, J., 488
Salter, A., 6
Saltoun, M., 687
Salusso-Deonier, C. J., 810
Salzinger, S., 607, 608, 650, 651
Sambrano, S., 733
Sameroff, A. J., 10, 23
Samit, C., 608
Samoilov, A., 357, 380
Sampson, P. D., 77
Sams, S. E., 111
Samson, Y., 467
Samuel, V. J., 76
Samuelson, H., 345
Sanchez, L. E., 484
Sanchez, R. P., 67
Sandall, S. R., 487
Sander, A. J. B., 355
Sander, J. B., 367
Sanders, M., 631
Sanders, M. R., 12, 41, 97, 100, 150, 160, 168, 169, 170, 200, 202, 207, 212, 214, 221, 223, 225, 228, 229, 485, 486, 622, 633
Sanderson, W. C., 435
Sanderson, W. C., Jr., 105, 277
Sandford, D. A., 612
Sandler, J., 606, 610, 611, 613, 616, 617, 621, 622, 623
Sandman, C. A., 431
Sandnabba, N. K., 690
Sandstrom, M., 461
Sanford, M., 353, 355
Sanger, M., 668, 669
Sanghavi, M., 350
Sanjuan, P., 737
Sansbury, L. E., 150
Sanson, A., 68, 149
Santana, C. A., 782, 789, 792, 804
Santarcangelo, S., 472
Santarelli, G. E., 484, 485, 486
Santhouse, R., 780
Santiago, H., 283
Santisteban, D. A., 174, 175, 220, 223, 225, 747, 752
santor, D. A., 380
Santos, A. B., 8

Santos, C., 439
Santosh, P. J., 443, 483
Santtila, P., 690
Saperstein, L., 651, 652, 659, 706
Sapory, P., 620
Sapyta, J., 28
Sarber, R. E., 606
Sarigiani, P. A., 341, 342, 343, 354
Sas, L. D., 656, 657, 670, 673, 674, 682, 687, 692, 706
Sasher, T. M., 443
Saslawsky, D., 653
Saslow, G., 7
Sass, H., 74
Sassi, R. B., 350
Sasso, G. S., 473
Satterfield, B. T., 110
Satterfield, J. H., 71, 110
Sattler, J. M., 36
Saudargaas, R. A., 7
Saundargas, R. A., 190, 191, 192, 216
Saunders, B. E., 595, 649, 656, 657, 658, 669, 685, 686
Saunders, M., 191, 209
Sauzier, M., 657
Savage, J., 779
Savery, D., 484
Sawyer, J. K., 426
Saxe, R., 467
Saxena, S., 350
Sayegh, L., 189, 216, 225
Sayer, J., 76, 77
Sayger, T. V., 213
Saywitz, K. J., 658, 663, 664, 665, 666, 670, 674, 675, 698
Scahill, L., 95, 294, 295, 442
Scambler, D., 457
Scanlan, J. M., 651
Scanlon, D. M., 519, 533, 534, 540, 541
Scapillato, D., 285, 291, 330
Scarborough, H. S., 556
Scarr, S., 81
Sceery, W., 67
Schachar, R., 67, 84, 87
Schachtel, D., 627, 629
Schachter, H., 84, 87, 90
Schaefer, C. E., 9
Schaefer, S. M., 350
Schaeffer, B., 456, 476, 480
Schaeffer, C. M., 177, 214
Schain, R. J., 456
Schalling, D., 203
Scharzkopf, R. J., 810
Schatschneider, C., 518, 533, 542, 543, 546, 550, 552
Schatzberg, A. F., 348
Schaub-Matt, M., 557
Schaumann, H., 462
Schectman, R. M., 339, 340, 343, 344, 375
Scheeringa, M. S., 681
Schefft, B. K., 4, 8, 13, 21, 22, 33, 35, 37, 38, 40, 41, 42
Scheidt, P. C., 141, 142
Scheier, M. F., 19
Schell, A., 71, 77, 81, 444
Schell, A. M., 110
Schellekens, J., 288, 316
Schendel, D., 469
Scherer, D. G., 66
Schiavo, R. S., 223, 224
Schier, L. M., 733
Schilling, G., 795
Schilling, R. F., 602, 617, 619, 620, 622
Schinke, S. P., 602, 617, 619, 620, 622
Schleifer, D., 93, 94, 387
Schleser, R., 109
Schloredt, K., 345, 346, 353
Schloss, C., 620
Schmaling, K. B., 140, 143, 150, 155, 301
Schmidt, F., 167, 213, 214, 226, 228, 229
Schmidt, K., 343, 354
Schmidt, K. L., 354
Schmidt, M. D., 187, 215
Schmidt, M. E., 203
Schmidt, N. B., 283
Schmidt, S., 345, 346
Schmitz, M., 668

Schmitz, S., 72
Schnack, H. G., 75
Schnakenber-Ott, S. D., 75, 76
Schnedler, R. W., 106, 109, 110, 111
Schneider, A. E., 531
Schneider, J. A., 797, 798, 806
Schneidman, M., 206
Schneiger, A., 212, 227
Schnelle, J. F., 194, 195
Schnoebelen, S., 359, 365, 374
Schnoll, R., 119
Schnurer, A. T., 799
Schoenwald, S. K., 9, 10, 21, 43, 172, 176, 177, 178, 207, 214, 224, 285, 297, 298, 299, 300
Schofield, F., 736
Schoket, D., 752
Scholar, L., 804
Scholing, A., 291, 330
Schonefeld, C., 736
Schonfeld, I. S., 19, 76
Schopler, E., 456, 459, 471, 483
Schothorst, P. F., 76
Schotte, D., 281, 314, 798
Schou, M., 443
Schover, L. R., 462
Schraedley, P. K., 341
Schreck, K. A., 462
Schreibman, D., 151
Schreibman, L., 435, 462, 472, 474, 475, 477, 490
Schreier, H. A., 205
Schrepferman, L., 148, 340
Schroeder, C. S., 4
Schroeder, H. E., 107, 288, 290, 320
Schroeder, S. R., 13, 431, 433, 441, 442
Schroer, R., 416
Schubel, E. A., 84
Schubert, A. B., 75
Schubert, C. J., 668
Schuckit, M. A., 738, 739, 740, 746, 748, 752
Schuele, J. A., 738
Schuhmann, E., 165
Schuhmann, E. M., 165, 166, 212, 225
Schulenberg, J. E., 732
Schuler, R., 342, 344
Schulsinger, F., 738
Schulte, A., 292, 330
Schulte, C., 482
Schulte, D., 301
Schulte, L. E., 651
Schulte, M. T., 736
Schulte-Bahrenberg, T., 301
Schultheis, K., 322
Schultz, J., 678
Schultz, L. A., 226
Schultz, R., 457, 467, 468, 480, 490
Schultz, R. T., 95, 466
Schulze, U., 783, 804
Schumaker, J. B., 184, 195, 522, 523, 560, 567, 572
Schumm, J. S., 571
Schur, S. B., 206
Schwab-Stone, M. E., 70, 155, 346, 745, 764
Schwartz, C. E., 271
Schwartz, D., 787
Schwartz, D. M., 779, 792
Schwartz, E., 782
Schwartz, I. S., 44, 437, 479, 487
Schwartz, J. M., 350, 394
Schwartz, M. B., 786
Schwartz, R. C., 779
Schwartz, R. H., 742
Schwartz, S., 12, 41, 169, 214, 221, 564
Schwartz, S. J., 174, 175, 220, 225, 747, 752
Schwartz, S. T., 203
Schwarzman, A. E., 145, 147
Schwebel, A. I., 8, 38
Schweinhart, L. J., 208, 217, 420
Schweitzer, J. B., 75
Schweitzer, L., 628
Schwitzer, A., 811
Scientific Learning Corporation, 520
Scopetta, M., 175, 214, 220, 226

Scott, K., 608, 609, 621, 632
Scott, K. S., 9
Scott, M. J., 219, 222
Scott, S., 156, 225, 228, 229
Scott, S. S., 601, 618
Scotti, J. R., 161, 481, 482
Scruggs, T. E., 421, 558
Seabaugh, G. O., 567
Seal, B., 480
Sears, M. R., 72
Sebring, D., 608
Secher, S. M., 353, 355
Secord, M., 98
Sedillo, S., 74, 87, 89, 94, 95
Sedlak, A. J., 597, 598
Sedlak, R., 566
Seech, M., 602
Seeley, J. R., 70, 184, 226, 336, 339, 342, 344, 345, 346, 347, 378, 733, 737, 739, 745
Seeley, M. S., 8
Seelig, J., 783
Seese, L., 204, 226, 227
Segal, B., 203
Segev, S., 784
Seguin, J. R., 208, 227
Seidel, R., 807
Seidenfeld, M., 782, 783
Seidensticher, J. F., 807
Seidman, E., 633
Seidman, L. J., 74
Seifer, R., 23, 743
Seifritz, E., 348
Seig, A., 663
Seiverd, K., 74
Selbst, M., 426
Selelyo, J., 676
Seligman, M. E. P., 17, 272, 338, 340, 341, 391, 685, 686
Selin, C. E., 350
Sellars, V., 488
Sells, S. B., 747
Selvin, S., 463
Semple, W. E., 75, 350
Semrud-Clikeman, M., 75, 97
Serafini, L. T., 285
Serbin, L. A., 145, 147
Serfaty, M., 800
Sergeant, J. A., 67, 78
Serketich, W. J., 97, 150, 162, 213, 214, 219, 222
Seroczynski, A. D., 273
Sevcik, B., 574
Severson, H., 159, 189
Sevin, B. M., 423, 428, 477
Sevin, J. A., 477
Sexton, T. L., 8, 10, 172, 173, 207, 223
Seybolt, D., 658
Seymour, F. W., 200, 217
Seymour, R. B., 752
Shadick, R., 279
Shadish, W. R., 30
Shafer, K., 473
Shafer, M. S., 473
Shaffer, D., 19, 139, 155, 745, 764
Shaffer, T., 779, 785, 786, 787, 811
Shafran, C. R., 690
Shafran, R., 785, 786, 787, 790, 799, 800, 804, 810
Shah, M., 204, 226, 227
Shah, P., 350, 441
Shake, M. C., 575
Shalev, A. Y., 684
Shallow, J. R., 687
Sham, P., 789
Shamai, D., 352
Shanahan, T., 533, 535, 538
Shankweiler, D., 522
Shankweiler, D. P., 533
Shannon, M. P., 682
Shanok, S. S., 612
Shapiro, C., 666, 669, 670, 671
Shapiro, C. J., 120
Shapiro, E. G., 462, 464
Shapiro, J. P., 674, 675, 676
Shapiro, R. A., 668
Shapiro, S. T., 430

Shapiro, T., 463, 464
Share, D., 522, 532
Sharma, V., 203
Sharp, S., 196, 197, 229
Sharp, W., 75
Sharpe, M. N., 421
Sharry, J., 620
Shatte, A. J., 391
Shattock, P., 484
Shattuck, R., 455
Shavelson, R., 529
Shaver, P. R., 664, 666
Shaw, B. F., 277, 279
Shaw, B F., 285, 291
Shaw, B. F., 351, 362, 379, 381, 753
Shaw, D. A., 7
Shaw, D. S., 149, 150
Shaw, E. C., 609
Shaw, H., 811
Shaw, J., 783, 794
Shaw, R., 566
Shayne, M., 437
Shaywitz, B., 513, 514, 515, 516, 517, 530, 550, 552, 572
Shaywitz, S. E., 513, 514, 515, 516, 517, 530, 531, 545, 550, 572
Shea, S. H., 733, 739
Shealy, C. N., 628
Shear, M. K., 300
Shedler, J., 733, 739, 740
Sheeber, L., 8, 343, 353, 354, 378, 382, 383
Sheehan, H. L., 779
Sheehan, M., 736
Sheffield, J. K., 23
Sheidow, A. J., 595
Sheils, O., 468
Sheinkopf, S. J., 488
Sheitman, B. B., 484
Sheldrick, R. C., 14, 213, 214, 215
Sheline, Y., 350
Shell, J., 147
Shelton, J. L., 28
Shelton, K. K., 142, 159
Shelton, R. C., 348
Shelton, T. L., 14, 30, 70, 80, 97, 98, 102, 111
Shemilt, J., 488
Shenker, R., 739, 784
Shepard, S., 689
Shepherd, E., 95
Sheppard, K., 210
Sher, K. J., 680, 736
Sherak, D. L., 340
Sherbourne, C. D., 299
Sheridan, S. M., 9, 108
Sherman, D., 598, 599
Sherman, J., 143
Sherman, J. A., 194, 195
Sherman, S. J., 739
Shern, D., 752
Shernoff, E. S., 10
Sherrill, J., 338
Shervette, R. E., III, 72
Sherwin, T., 294
Sherwood, R., 569
Sheslow, D. V., 290, 316, 332
Shestakova, A., 461
Shields, A., 689
Shimizu, Y., 462
Shinn, M. R., 158, 573
Shinnar, S., 471
Shiotsuki, Y., 462
Shipman, K., 689, 690
Shipman, K. L., 607
Shirk, S. R., 28, 31, 350
Shochet, I. M., 696, 706
Shoebridge, P., 790
Shoji, H., 462
Sholomskas, D., 354
Shook, J. E., 810
Shope, J. T., 735, 736
Shore, B. A., 481
Shores, R., 190
Shores, R. E., 473, 474, 629
Short, E. J., 84
Shortt, A. L., 284, 332
Shortt, J., 148, 340

Shortt, L., 735
Shoshan, Y., 435, 489
Shprintzen, R. J., 413
Shure, M. B., 209
Shutty, M. S., 34
Sicotte, N., 780
Siddle, D. A., 272
Sidorenko, E., 568
Sidoti, E. J., 413
Siegal, J. M., 342, 344
Siegel, B., 488
Siegel, G., 479
Siegel, L. J., 4, 322, 340
Siegel, L. S., 73, 107, 522
Siegel, P. T., 801, 802
Siegel, R. M., 668
Siegel, T. C., 156, 157, 181, 215, 218, 226
Siegle, G., 30
Siever, L. J., 203
Sievers, P., 462, 464
Sigafoos, J., 481
Sigman, M., 25, 471
Signorini, A., 807
Sigurdson, E., 652
Sijsenaar, M., 316
Sikand, A., 802
Sikich, L., 206
Silber, T., 793, 795
Silberstein, J., 460
Silbert, J., 523
Silburn, S. R., 170, 229
Sillick, T., 439
Silovsky, J. F., 615, 616, 617, 621, 623, 691, 703
Silva, I., 468
Silva, P., 148
Silva, P. A., 147, 148, 152, 153, 339, 340, 346, 739
Silva, R. R., 147, 207
Silver, R. L., 683, 686
Silverberg, J., 349
Silverman, A. K., 558
Silverman, R., 627
Silverman, W., 686
Silverman, W. K., 8, 271, 272, 273, 281, 282, 283, 285, 291, 292, 294, 299, 300, 301, 330, 332
Silvern, V., 608
Silvernail, D. L., 141
silverstein, J. H., 320
Silverstone, P. H., 787
Silverthorn, P., 142, 154
Silvester, J., 604
Simmel, C., 158, 159
Simmons, A., 75, 462, 467, 468, 469
Simmons, D., 558, 571
Simmons, D. C., 541, 542, 573
Simmons, H., 463
Simmons, J. Q., 487
Simmons-Morton, B., 141, 142
Simms, M., 629
Simms, M. D., 628, 629
Simon, Y., 787
Simonoff, E., 461, 465
Simons, A., 779, 781, 810
Simons, R. F., 231
Simons, R. L., 344
Simos, P. G., 551, 552
Simpkins, C. G., 628
Simpson, D., 470
Simpson, D. D., 747
Simpson, J., 359, 365, 374
Simpson, J. R., 350
Simpson, K., 786
Simpson, T. L., 701
Sims, J. P., 182, 220
Sinclair, B. B., 687
Singer, G., 415
Singer, G. H. S., 484, 485, 486
Singer, H. S., 75
Singh, V. K., 468
Sinha, K., 70
Sintov, N., 736
Sipay, E. R., 534, 540
Siperstein, G. N., 412, 414
Siqueland, L., 9, 24, 43, 281, 282, 290, 291
Sirles, E. A., 675

Siskind, V., 736
Sisson, C., 731
Sisson, L. A., 23
Sisterman Keeney, K., 673
Sivage, C., 105, 109
Skarderud, F., 803
Skare, S. S., 107
Skeels, H., 418
Skeels, H. M., 418
Skiba, R., 574
Skindrud, K., 193, 216, 225
Skinner, B. F., 6, 429, 478, 523
Skinner, H. A., 160
Skinner, M. L., 148, 152, 172
Skinner, W. F., 739
Skodak, M., 418
Skowron, E. A., 615
Skudlarski, P., 550
Skuse, D. H., 465
Slaby, R. G., 180, 215
Slanetz, P. J., 65, 70
Slate, F., 202
Slee, P., 141
Slep, A. M., 150
Slesnick, B., 747
Slifer, K., 423, 426, 428, 431, 432
Slis, V., 676
Sloan, M. A., 85, 86, 87, 88, 93, 94, 95
Sloan, M. T., 85, 90, 116
Slot, N. W., 187, 229
Slotkin, J., 353
Slough, N. M., 211
Slupik, R., 783
Slutske, W. S., 739
Slymen, D. J., 676
Small, A., 484
Small, A. M., 147, 204, 205, 206, 218, 226, 227, 232, 483, 484
Small, M. A., 635
Small, S. G., 534, 540
Smalley, S. L., 76, 465
Smallish, L., 71, 72, 90, 144, 739
Smalls, Y., 425
Smeets, M., 790, 792, 794
Smetana, J., 607
Smied, C. M., 516
Smith, A. C. M., 413
Smith, A. J., 72
Smith, B., 672, 673
Smith, B. H., 87, 90, 120
Smith, C., 648, 659
Smith, C. E., 480, 481, 482
Smith, C. M., 11
Smith Christopher, J., 342
Smith, D., 798
Smith, D. A., 151
Smith, D. D., 566
Smith, D. E., 752
Smith, D. J., 138, 179, 230
Smith, D. K., 188, 219, 227
Smith, D. W., 656, 657, 658, 686
Smith, E. K., 355
Smith, G. T., 738, 739, 740, 744
Smith, H., 678
Smith, I. M., 462
Smith, J., 39
Smith, J. M., Sr., 8
Smith, K., 630
Smith, K. A., 348
Smith, L., 215
Smith, L. A., 177, 214, 218, 219, 221, 222, 226, 747
Smith, M., 461
Smith, N. J., 469
Smith, P., 220, 231
Smith, P. K., 141, 196, 197, 229
Smith, R. G., 481
Smith, S., 676
Smith, S. S., 623
Smith, T., 8, 471, 472, 478, 487, 488, 489, 490
Smith, T. A., 747
Smith-Winberry, C., 110
Smithies, C., 119
Smithmyer, C. M., 141, 231
Smolak, L., 788
Smolen, A., 74

Smolkowski, K., 212
Smyth, J. M., 698
Snarr, J., 74
Snead, B. W., 441
Snow, B., 657
Snow, C., 522, 532, 534
Snow, J., 437
Snow, M. E., 463
Snowling, M. J., 519, 533
Snyder, A. Z., 350
Snyder, H. N., 143
Snyder, J., 8, 10, 148, 150, 152, 195, 340
Snyder, L., 658, 665, 698
Snyder, R., 442
Soares, J. C., 467
Sobesky, W. E., 415
Sobsey, D., 651, 661
Socken, K., 83, 84, 85
Sodersten, P., 804
Soderstrom, H., 461
Soeken, K., 294
Sofronoff, K., 72
Sohlberg, M. M., 97
Sohlberg, S., 787
Sokol, M., 789
Solanto, M. V., 84, 85, 86
Solberg, K. B., 746
Solnick, J. V., 430
Solnit, A. J., 656
Solomon, J., 354
Solomon, M., 205, 459
Somaschini, E., 788
Sondregger, R., 8
Sonnega, A., 685
Sonuga-Barke, E. J. S., 19, 30, 78, 97, 98, 102
Soper, H. V., 479
Sorensen, E., 343, 353, 354
Sorenson, E., 666
Sorenson, T., 657
Sosna, T. D., 156
Sotsky, S. M., 356
Soule, L., 285
Southam-Gerow, M. A., 13, 30, 271, 274, 282, 284, 291, 298, 299, 301, 330, 338
Southwick, S. M., 683
Sowder, B. J., 28
Soydan, H., 220, 231
Soysa, K., 604, 609
Spaccarelli, S., 689
Spadaccini, E., 295
Spagnola, M., 612, 626, 627
Spanier, G. B., 160
Sparen, P., 789
Spargo, E., 784
Sparkman, C. R., 488
Sparks, T., 698
Sparrow, S. S., 457, 458, 459, 461
Spaulding, M., 437
Spear, S. F., 735
Specker, S., 805
Specter, E., 74
Spegg, C., 668
Speier, P. L., 340
Spelke, E. S., 468
Spellman, D. F., 187, 215
Speltz, M. L., 149
Spence, S. H., 23, 179, 215, 225, 274, 275, 281, 291, 293, 314, 332, 336, 378
Spence, S. J., 465
Spencer, T., 76, 91, 92, 295, 389, 443
Spencer, T. J., 72, 73, 86, 87, 91, 93, 94, 387, 739
Spender, Q., 156, 225, 228, 229
Sperber, A. D., 736
Sperling, M. B., 351
Spiker, D., 419, 464, 465
Spillar, R., 320
Spillmann, M. K., 348
Spinner, M., 353, 355
Spirito, A., 687, 735, 737, 738, 750
Spitzer, A., 223
Spitzer, R. L., 68
Spitznagel, E., 350
Spivack, G., 209
Spivak, B., 779, 785
Sponheim, E., 465

Spooner, F., 437, 473
Spracklen, K. M., 186, 232
Spradlin, J. E., 479
Sprafkin, J., 70, 87
Sprague, J., 194
Sprague, J. R., 480, 482
Sprenkle, D. H., 747
Sprich, S., 338
Springer, J. F., 733
Spunt, A. L., 107
Spurlock, J., 44
Spurrell, E., 800, 803
Srinivasan, K., 806
Sroufe, A., 149
Sroufe, L. A., 23, 607, 687, 688
Staats, M., 790
Stachnik, T. J., 191, 209
Stack, C. M., 43
Stack, D. M., 147
Stackhaus, J., 474
Stadolnik, R. F., 202
Stage, S. A., 97, 218, 231
Stagg, V., 152
Staghezza, B. M., 271
Stahl, S. A., 553, 554
Stahmer, A. C., 472, 477
Staib, L. H., 350
Staley, S., 143, 202
Stallard, P., 682
Stallings, P., 274
Stallings, R. R., 676
Stanar, C. R., 43
Stanford, G., 546
Stanger, C., 147
Stangl, D., 693
Stanislaw, H., 488
Staniszewski, D., 197, 217
Stanley, S. M., 23
Stanovich, K., 516, 517, 518, 522, 529, 530, 532
Stanovich, P., 529, 530
Stansbury, R., 299
Stanton, W., 152, 153
Stanton, W. R., 72, 339, 346
Stark, K. D., 9, 43, 273, 343, 347, 350, 351, 353, 354, 356, 359, 365, 367, 373, 374, 378, 380, 382
Stark, L., 687
Stark, M. T., 431
Starling, S. P., 667
Starnes, A. L., 438
Starr, E., 465
State, M. W., 441, 443
State, R. C., 484
Statham, D. J., 739
Statistics Canada, 704
Stattin, H., 142, 144
Staub, D., 437
Staub, S., 179
Staudt, M., 595, 602
Stavrakaki, C., 441, 443
Stechler, G., 18, 19
Stecker, P. M., 567, 573, 574
Steel, H., 628
Steele, B. F., 613
Steele, H., 221, 222, 791
Steele, M., 791
Steele, P., 213, 219, 220, 222
Steele, R., 487
Steele, S., 467
Steenhuis, M. P., 75
Steer, R. A., 160, 293, 326, 698, 700
Steere, J., 798
Stefanatos, G. A., 461
Steffe, M. A., 164
Steffenburg, S., 462, 471
Stehr-Green, P., 470
Steiger, H., 780
Stein, B. D., 332
Stein, D., 809
Stein, D. J., 295
Stein, J. A., 734
Stein, M., 72
Stein, M. A., 68, 70, 72, 73, 77
Stein, M. B., 299, 617
Stein, M. T., 299
Stein, R., 800, 803

Stein, T., 662, 663
Steinbach, K. A., 524, 525, 547, 548, 555, 560
Steinberg, A. M., 292, 328
Steinberg, L. D., 599
Steinberg, S., 790
Steiner, H., 779, 782, 785, 786, 787, 811
Steingard, R., 75, 350, 389, 441
Steinglass, P., 10
Steinhausen, H. C., 798, 804, 807, 808
Steinman, W. M., 104
Steketee, G., 292
Stellfeld, M., 470
Stemmler, M., 340, 347
Stephens, D., 803
Stern, A., 692
Stern, A. E., 657
Stern, C. A., 566
Stern, M., 179, 215, 226
Stern, M. B., 566
Stern, P., 670
Sternberg, K. J., 665, 666, 673
Stetner, F., 805
Stetson, B. A., 739, 742, 743, 764
Stevens, M. C., 457, 472
Stevens, P., 617, 619, 620, 622
Stevens, R., 523, 566
Stevens, V., 196, 197, 225
Stevenson, C. L., 473
Stevenson, H., 625, 629
Stevenson, J., 76
Stevenson, R. E., 413, 416
Stevenson, W. F., 704
Steward, D., 668
Steward, M., 631, 668
Stewart, A., 339, 390
Stewart, D. G., 737, 740, 742, 743
Stewart, J. W., 805
Stewart, M. A., 737, 746, 749
Stewart, S. E., 295
Stewart, S. H., 150
Stewart, S. L., 20
Stewart, S. R., 522
Stewart, T. L., 673
Stice, E., 342, 344, 740, 744, 804, 811
Stichfield, R., 751
Stickeis, A. M., 633
Stickle, T. R., 143, 202, 232
Stigler, K. A., 442
Stillman, B., 561
Stinchfield, R. D., 732, 743, 746, 748
Stocking, S. H., 599
Stodgell, C. J., 465
Stoessel, P. W., 394
Stoewe, J. K., 205
Stoff, D., 24
Stoff, D. M., 207
Stoiber, K. C., 9
Stokes, T. F., 10, 40, 67, 68, 72, 73, 86
Stolke J. J., 439
Stone, V., 466
Stoner, G., 65, 67, 68, 86, 87, 88, 89, 104, 109
Stones, M. H., 683
Stoolmiller, M., 147, 148, 149, 150, 224, 541, 733
Storaasli, R. D., 23
Storey, J., 283
Storey, K., 480
Stormshak, E. A., 9
Storr, C. L., 210
Stotland, S., 780
Stouthamer-Loeber, M., 19, 140, 143, 144, 145, 147, 151, 152, 153, 157, 160, 202
Stovall, A., 627, 629
Stovall, K. C., 612, 630
Stoving, R., 783
Stowe, J., 462, 468, 469
Stowell, R. J., 733
Straatman, A., 608, 621, 632
Stradling, S. G., 219, 222
Strain, G., 795
Strain, P. S., 38, 190, 213, 219, 220, 222, 435, 473, 474, 482, 488, 629
Straka, S. M., 656
Strange, M., 652
Strangler, R. S., 782

Strapko, N., 652
Strassberg, Z., 74
Stratton, H. H., 735
Straus, M. A., 160
Straus, R. B., 677
Strauss, B., 469
Strauss, C. C., 279
Strayhorn, J. M., 97, 98, 159
Strayhorn, J. M., Jr., 8, 39
Street, L. L., 298
Streissguth, A. P., 77
Striegel-Moore, R. H., 781, 783, 785, 786, 796, 802, 809
Strober, M., 345, 346, 779, 780, 781, 785, 786, 787, 789, 792, 801, 809
Stroes, A., 72, 73
Stromme, P., 415, 433, 439
Strosahl, K. D., 9
Stroud, D. D., 657, 658, 669
Stroul, B. A., 188
Strumia, R., 783
Stuart, G. W., 788, 789
Stuart, J. E., 95
Stubbe, D., 294
Stuckey, M. K., 803
Studen-Pavlovich, D., 783
Study Group on Anorexia Nervosa, 810
Stuebing, K. K., 513, 516, 517, 518, 530, 531
Stuetzel, H., 575
Stuewig, J., 143
Stull, S., 349
Stumpf, J., 216
Stunkard, A., 779, 781, 783, 806
Stunkard, J. J., 810
Sturgis, E. T., 164, 189, 213
Sturm, R., 3, 22, 299
Sturmey, P., 480
Sturnick, D., 181, 226
Sturzenberg, S., 807
Suarez, L., 273
Suave, R., 417
Substance Abuse and Mental Health Services Administration, 731
Sudler, N., 352
Sugai, G., 193, 194, 216
Sugrin, I., 318
Sukhodolsky, D. G., 182, 227
Sullivan, K., 274
Sullivan, L., 340
Sullivan, P., 780, 789, 790, 798, 809
Sullivan, P. M., 651
Suls, J., 687
Sultana, C. R., 170
Sulzer-Azaroff, B., 428, 429, 430, 437
Summerfelt, W. T., 376
Summers, V. K., 779
Sumner, G. S., 387
Sunday, S., 787, 796, 804
Sundberg, M. L., 476, 478, 479
Sung, M., 739
Sungum-Paliwal, S. R., 462
Sunohara, G. A., 77
Sunshine, N., 665
Surratt, A., 478
Susman, E. J., 349
Sussman, J., 732, 738, 743
Sussman-Stillman, S., 688
Sutton-Smith, B., 625, 629
Suveg, C., 20
Svedin, C. G., 690
Sveen, O. B., 290, 320
Sverd, J., 87
Swaab-Barneveld, H., 87, 88
Swain, G. E., 739
Swan, G. E., 739
Swank, P. R., 99
Swann, C., 779
Swanson, H. L., 512, 517, 522, 531, 545, 556, 557, 560
Swanson, J., 71, 205, 431
Swanson, J. M., 77, 95, 114, 203, 439
Swanston, H., 677, 692
Swearer, S., 347, 350, 351, 356, 380
Swedo, S. E., 388
Sweeney, L., 156, 160, 166, 225
Sweller, J., 569

Swenne, I., 783
Swenson, C. C., 7, 595, 612, 677
Swettenham, J., 462, 463
Swiderski, R. E., 465
Swift, W., 807
Swim, J., 670, 673
Switzer, E. B., 201, 217
Sylvester, L., 75, 97
Symons, F. J., 484
Syrota, A., 467
Szapocznik, J., 172, 174, 175, 207, 214, 220, 223, 225, 226, 231, 747, 752
Szatmari, P., 70, 353, 355, 459, 471, 490
Szezko, P. R., 350
Szmukler, G. I., 801
Szumowski, E., 72
Szykula, S. A., 171, 213, 229, 624

Tabachnik, N., 21
Tabrizi, M. A., 338
Tagano, D. W., 426
Tager-Flusberg, H., 458, 467
Tageson, C. W., 351
Taghavi, R., 273
Tai, W. Y., 789
Tanaka, J., 466
Tanenbaum, R., 685, 686
Tang, C., 659
Tangel, D. M., 540
Tani, P., 461, 462
Tannenbaum, L. E., 139, 140, 151
Tannock, R., 67, 71, 72, 75, 87
Tapert, S. F., 646, 734, 740, 741, 742, 743, 747, 748, 760
Tapia, M. A., 387
Tapia, M. R., 387
Taplin, P., 607
Taplin, P. S., 212, 222
Taqngel, D. M., 540
Tarbox, J., 427
Tarbox, R., 427
Tarnowski, K. J., 44, 608
Tarter, R. E., 737, 738, 739, 742, 743
Tasca, G., 802
Tashiro, T., 783
Taska, L., 682, 686
Tate, B. G., 430
Tate, S. R., 760
Tatelbaum, R., 632
Taub, E. P., 663, 669, 670, 675, 692
Taubman, M. T., 459
Taussig, C., 208
Taylor, A., 76, 77, 149
Taylor, A. A., 283, 298, 326
Taylor, A. E., 685, 690
Taylor, B., 462, 468, 469, 475
Taylor, B. A., 472, 474, 475, 476, 477
Taylor, C., 77, 783
Taylor, C. M., 682
Taylor, E., 75, 78
Taylor, E. A., 67, 87, 88
Taylor, E. R., 143
Taylor, G. R., 421
Taylor, I. S., 7
Taylor, J., 481
Taylor, J. C., 432
Taylor, L. L., 14, 15
Taylor, M., 190
Taylor, T., 208
Taylor, T. K., 167, 179, 213, 214, 215, 226, 228, 229
Teague, L. A., 484
Teale, P. D., 74
Teasdale, T. W., 738
Tebano-Micci, A., 666
Tebbutt, J., 677, 692
Teicher, M. H., 67, 75, 683
Teitelbaum, O., 490
Teitelbaum, P., 490
Tekell, J. L., 350

Telch, C. F., 797, 798, 800, 804, 806, 807, 810
Temple, J. A., 420
Terdal, L. G., 4, 8, 9, 14, 18, 20, 25, 27, 31, 36, 37, 40
Terr, L., 631
Terr, L. C., 684, 688, 696, 697, 698, 702
Terre, L., 782, 784, 785, 790, 792, 811
Terry, R., 148
Tertinger, D. A., 606
Terwilliger, R. F., 280, 284, 316
Tesch, D., 431
Test, D. W., 437, 473
Testa, M. F., 634
Thakkar-Kolar, R., 631
Thapar, A. J., 76
Tharp, R. G., 7, 10, 37, 44
Theander, S., 785, 787, 807
Thede, L. L., 74, 76
Theisen, F., 804
Thelen, E., 10, 459
Thernlund, G., 75
Thibadeau, S., 441
Thibault, J., 656
Thibodeau, M. G., 477
Thien, V., 803
Thiesse-Duffy, E., 655
Thoennes, N., 679
Thomas, A., 23, 149, 803
Thomas, C., 156, 181, 215, 226
Thomas, D. R., 190
Thomas, F., 731, 747
Thomas, G., 791
Thomas, M., 665
Thomas, S., 671
Thomas, S. E., 747, 748
Thomason, B. T., 28
Thomason, D., 105
Thompsen, W., 462
Thompsom, A. M., 141
Thompson, A., 460, 484, 537
Thompson, J. K., 785, 786
Thompson, K. M., 751
Thompson, L. E., 798
Thompson, L. L., 752
Thompson, M., 19, 30, 97, 98, 102, 787
Thompson, M. G., 779, 792
Thompson, R., 314
Thompson, R. A., 606, 628
Thompson, R. S., 468
Thompson, R. W., 218, 222
Thompson, V. L., 805, 811
Thompson, W. C., 664
Thompson-Brenner, H., 797, 800, 804
Thomsen, C. J., 687
Thomson, J., 97, 552
Thomson, M., 468
Thornberry, T. P., 147
Thornell, A., 76
Thornton, C., 798
Thorsen, P., 469, 470
Thuras, P., 484
Tice, S., 801
Tidwell, R., 669
Tiedemann, G. L., 160, 164, 214, 219
Tiesel, J., 695
Tiet, Q. Q., 140
Tilly, W. D., 422, 518, 520, 523, 524, 526, 527
Timm, M. A., 213, 219, 220, 222, 473, 629
Timnick, L., 650
Tincani, M., 490
Tingelstad, J., 806
Tingstrom, D. H., 191, 216
Tirosh, E., 459
Tisdelle, D. A., 21
Titus, J. B., 466
Tizard, J., 23, 415
Tjaden, P., 679
Tobey, A. E., 671
Tobias, J., 84
Tobin, D. L., 790
Tobin, D. L., 790
Tobler, N. S., 735
Toby, A. E., 670, 671
Todak, G., 353, 354, 355
Todd, A., 194
Todd, A. W., 482

Todd, R. D., 350, 466
Todesco, T., 797, 800
Todhunter, E., 779
Todis, B., 159
Todorov, A., 600
Tolan, P. H., 20, 140, 152, 153
Toledano, A., 784
Tolliver, R. M., 609
Tomblin, J. B., 465
Tomlinson, K. L., 733, 734, 745, 748
Tompson, M., 458
Tompson, M. C., 13
Tomura, N., 783
Tonge, B. J., 279, 283, 293, 328, 330, 334, 701
Torchia, M., 617
Torgesen, J. K., 513, 514, 515, 516, 517, 518, 520, 521, 522, 524, 526, 532, 534, 537, 539, 540, 544, 545, 550, 551, 552, 553, 573, 575
Torre, C., 76
Tortolero, S., 701
Tortu, S., 736
Toth, S. L., 353, 356, 595, 596, 607, 608, 612, 626, 627
Touchette, P. E., 481
Touyz, S. W., 156, 160, 166, 225, 795, 808
Towne, L., 529
Townsend, J., 16, 461, 466
Townsend, M., 437
Tracy, K., 322
Trakowski, J., 283
Tran, C. Q., 460
Tran, T., 75
Trasowech, J. E., 477
Traver, R. E., 746
Treacy, E. C., 677
Treanor, J., 470
Treasure, J., 780, 791
Treatment for Adolescents with Depression Study, 9, 13, 295
Treder, R., 345, 346, 353
Tremblay, C., 687
Tremblay, G., 604, 633, 651
Tremblay, R., 147
Tremblay, R. E., 70, 137, 141, 148, 154, 200, 207, 208, 209, 217, 221, 227
Trentacosta, C., 16
Trepper, T. S., 747
Trickett, P. K., 606, 680, 688, 692, 695
Trivette, C. M., 8, 38, 40, 437, 438, 439, 482
Trocmé, N., 648, 649
Troiani, M., 790
Troisi, A., 441
Tromovitch, P., 680, 681
Tronic, E., 16
Trout, B. A., 187
Troutman, A. C., 38
Tryon, A. S., 472
Tsai, L. Y., 466
Tsuang, M. T., 76
Tu, W., 332
Tubbs, V. K., 456
Tuchman, R., 471
Tuchman, R. F., 459, 462
Tuck, B. F., 561
Tucker, S. B., 67, 68
Tucker, W., 743
Tuff, L., 459
Tufts New England Medical Center, Division of Child Psychiatry, 674
Tuinier, S., 441
Tull, P., 470
Tully, L., 160, 169, 212, 225
Tumner, W., 538
Tumuluru, R., 439
Tune, L. E., 75
Tunmer, W. E., 532, 539
Tupler, L. A., 350
Turbin, M. S., 740
Turbott, S. H., 439, 441
Turco, T. L., 195, 216
Turgay, A., 442
Turkington, D., 800
Turnbull, A. P., 422, 482, 486, 487
Turnbull, H. R., 487

Turnbull, S., 791
Turner, A. P., 750
Turner, C. M., 275
Turner, C. W., 223, 224, 733, 747
Turner, D., 795
Turner, J. E., 338
Turner, J., Jr., 351
Turner, K. M. T., 168, 200, 202, 207, 212, 225, 228
Turner, M., 292, 458, 465
Turner, R. J., 343
Turner, S. M., 24, 295, 326
Turner, T. R., 786
Turovsky, J., 276, 277
Tuschen, B., 795, 799
Tustin, R. D., 612
Tuttle, J. W., 670
Tutty, L. M., 654
Tuynman-Qua, H., 484
Twadell, S., 731
Tweed, D., 693
Twenge, J. M., 340, 343
Twentyman, C. T., 596, 597, 600, 601, 603, 606, 607, 610, 611, 614, 615, 616, 617, 618, 621, 622, 626
Tyler, B., 553
Tyler, K. A., 738
Tyler, L., 142, 159
Tyler, V., 314
Tymchuk, A. J., 602, 606, 623
Tyree, A., 608
Tyrka, A., 787
Tzagournis, M., 807

Ucelli di Nemi, S., 467
Uchigakiuchi, P., 8, 20
Uhlmann, V., 468
Uhry, J. K., 556, 557
Ulaszek, W. R., 72
Ullman, J. B., 734
Ultee, C. A., 288, 316
Umemoto, L. A., 275
Underwood, M. K., 142, 147, 231
Unis, A., 14, 181, 206, 215, 225, 226
Upadhyaya, H. P., 745
Urbain, E. S., 21
Urbina, S., 36, 274
Urdan, T. C., 355
Urey, J. R., 177, 214, 225
Urizar, G., 391
Urquiza, A. J., 612, 615, 616, 623, 700
U.S. Advisory Board on Child Abuse and Neglect, 628
U.S. Department of Health and Human Services, 3, 271, 490, 627, 649, 658, 662, 733
U.S. Food and Drug Administration (FDA), 702, 805
U.S. Public Health Service, 3
Uvebrant, P., 783

Vaccarino, F. J., 789, 809
Vaccaro, D., 151
Vadasy, P., 537
Vaidya, C. J., 75
Vaillant, G. E., 739
Vainio, P., 350
Vaituzis, A. C., 75
Vakalahi, H. F., 740
Vakali, K., 350
Valadez-Meltzer, A., 793, 795
Valdez-Menchaca, M. C., 478
Valdovinos, M. G., 483
Valera, E., 74
Valeri, S. M., 6
Valescu, S., 143
Valkonen-Korhonen, M., 350
Valla, J. P., 70
Vallano, G., 19
Valle, L. A., 609, 615, 616, 617, 621, 623
Valoski, A., 41
Van Bellinghen, M., 442
Van Bourgondien, M. E., 13
van de Wiel, N. M. H., 102
van den Berg, Y. W., 441
van den Broek, P., 67
van den Pol, R. A., 33, 37

Van den Veyver, I. B., 460, 465
Van der Does, A. J. W., 348
Van der Does, W., 348
van der Ende, J., 44, 146
van der Gaag, R. J., 87, 88, 205, 226
van der Hart, O., 696
van der Kolk, B. A., 684, 696, 701
van der Meere, J., 74
van der Meere, J. J., 72, 73
van der Meere, J. P., 67, 78
van der Ploege, H. M., 332
van der Ploege-Stapart, J. D., 332
van der Sar, R. M., 210
Van Dyke, B., 171, 213
van Elburg, A., 787
van Engeland, H., 76, 102, 484, 787
van Furth, E. F., 783
van Goozen, S., 787
Van Hasselt, V. B., 11, 23, 316
van Heeringen, C., 785
van Hoeken, D., 781, 782, 783
Van Hoof, T., 294
Van Horn, Y., 139, 140, 151
Van Houten, R., 23, 432, 477
van IJzendoorn, M. H., 619
Van Kammen, W. B., 140, 144, 145, 152, 153, 157
van Lier, P. A. C., 210
Van Luit, J. E. H., 525
van Melick, M., 330
Van Oost, P., 196, 197, 225, 682, 687
van Praag, H. M., 348, 809, 810
Van Rossem, R., 76
Van Someren, A., 348
Van Voorhis, R., 662, 663
VanBrakle, J., 72, 73
Vance, J. M., 465
Vander Stoep, A., 12
VanDeusen, P., 74
Vanhala, R., 461
Vannier, M., 350
Vara, L. S., 797
Vargas, S., 119, 533
Varotti, E., 783
Vasey, M. W., 273, 276
Vasta, R., 41
Vaughan, K., 561, 563
Vaughn, S., 512, 522, 527, 529, 538, 539, 541, 542, 553, 557, 558, 571, 572, 575
Vaz, M., 806
Veendrik-Meekes, M. J., 441
Veith, V. I., 672
Velez, C. N., 39
Velleman, R., 682
Vellutino, F. R., 519, 520, 533, 534, 540, 541
Velosa, J. F., 294
Venables, P. H., 203
Venning, H. B., 200, 202
Venter, A., 471
Venzke, R., 340
Verduin, T. L., 20, 298
Verhoeven, W. M., 441
Verhulst, F. C., 44, 146, 147
Vernberg, E. M., 292, 686
Vernon, S., 474
Veronen, L., 649, 656
Versage, E. M., 354
Vervaet, M., 785
Vestergaard, M., 469
Vestergren, E., 783
Vickar, D., 417
Victorian Infant Collaborative Study Group, 417
Vieland, V. J., 465
Viens, M. J., 799
Viesselman, J. O., 93
Vigil, J., 75
Vigilante, D., 683, 688
Vik, P. W., 734, 740, 742, 743, 748, 757, 758
Villeponteaux, L., 649, 656
Vincent, J., 206
Vincent, N., 783
Vinet, M. C., 465
Vinke, J., 524, 525
Violatao, C., 657

Virkunen, M., 203
Vitali, A. E., 288, 314
Vitaro, F., 70, 141, 148, 154, 200, 207, 208, 209, 217, 221, 227
Vitelli, F., 460
Vitiello, B., 207, 439
Vitousek, K. M., 787, 798, 800
Vize, C. M., 788
Voeller, K. K. S., 550, 551, 552, 553, 575
Voeltz, L. M., 10
Vogeltanz, N. D., 650
Vohs, K., 787
Volkmar, F. R., 456, 457, 458, 459, 460, 461, 462, 464, 466, 467, 468, 471, 480, 483, 484, 490
Volkow, N. D., 84
Vollmer, T. R., 482
Volpe, A. G., 466
Volpicelli, J. R., 747
von Eye, A., 349
von Knorring, A. L., 345
von Ransom, K. B., 808
von Wendt, L., 461, 462
Voris, J., 682
Vostanis, P., 379
Vuolo, R. D., 348
Vye, N., 569

Wachtel, P. L., 6, 32
Wacker, D., 433
Wade, S. L., 43
Wade, T., 780, 789, 790, 809
Wade, T. J., 340
Wadsworth, S. J., 532
Wagner, B. M., 341, 355
Wagner, E. F., 743
Wagner, E. S., 736
Wagner, H., 595
Wagner, J., 665
Wagner, K., 385, 386
Wagner, K. D., 347, 386, 686
Wagner, R. K., 532, 534, 539, 550, 551, 552, 553, 573, 575
Wahler, R. G., 10, 35, 150, 151, 152, 154, 155, 160, 213, 214, 221, 222, 486, 601, 611
Wahlsten, D., 420
Waibel-Duncan, M. K., 668, 669
Wainwright, A., 490
Wainwright-Sharp, J. A., 461
Waisberg, J., 802
Wakefield, A. J., 465, 468, 469
Wakefield, P. J., 32
Wakeling, A., 781
Wakschlag, L. S., 146, 150, 159
Wakstein, D. J., 456
Wakstein, M. P., 456
Walden, B., 739
Walder, L. O., 147
Waldfogel, J., 420
Waldman, I., 25, 68, 139, 145
Waldron, H. B., 736, 738, 747
Waldron, I., 787
Waldstein, G., 413
Walker, A. M., 143
Walker, C. E., 4, 703
Walker, D., 108
Walker, D. R., 460
Walker, E. F., 38
Walker, H. M., 140, 155, 158, 159, 161, 189, 190, 191, 192, 193, 194, 195, 216, 225, 227, 229
Walker, J. E., 140, 195
Walker, J. L., 145
Walker, K., 314
Walker, L., 43
Walker, M. L., 733
Walker, R. D., 745
Walker, S., 779, 785, 786, 787, 811
Walkup, J. T., 295
Wall, T. L., 733, 739
Wallace, D., 441, 442
Wallace, I. F., 420
Wallace, J. M., Jr., 732
Wallace, M. D., 427
Wallace, S., 465
Wallen, J., 682, 683

Waller, D., 794, 796, 797
Waller, G., 787, 788, 791, 802, 803
Waller, J. L., 343, 345
Waller, N., 687, 688
Waller, P. F., 735
Waller-Perotte, D., 484
Walley, P. B., 164
Wallis, J. M., 337, 338
Walrath, C., 345
Walsh, B. T., 781, 782, 783, 785, 786, 790, 797, 800, 804, 805, 806
Walsh, C., 353, 355
Walsh, C. A., 649, 650, 656
Walsh, J. A., 144, 156, 188
Walsh, J. M., 792
Walsh, M. M., 220
Walsh, S., 808
Walter, H. I., 171, 225
Walter, J. M., 75
Walters, D., 662
Walters, M. S., 3
Walton, L. A., 339
Walton, V. A., 648
Wan, M., 460
Wandersman, A., 658
Wang, G., 84
Wang, L., 350
Wang, P., 350
Wang, P. W., 443
Wang, S., 210
Wannäs, M., 690
Wanzek, J., 557
Ward, A., 791
Ward, B. J., 469
Ward, C. S., 601, 618
Ward, D. M., 178
Ward, E. M., 109
Ward, P., 789
Warman, M., 271, 284, 291, 301, 330
Warner, J. E., 611
Warner, V., 354, 355
Warnke, A., 804
Warren, A. R., 665, 672, 673
Warren, B. L., 674
Warren, M. P., 809
Warren, S. F., 479
Warren-Chaplin, P., 547, 554
Warsh, J. J., 805
Waschbusch, D., 90
Waschbusch, D. A., 141, 144, 150
Wasik, B. H., 420
Wasilewska-Dziubinska, E., 783
Waslick, B., 203, 204
Waslick, B. D., 375
Wassell, J., 181, 215, 223
Wasserman, G. A., 140
Wassermann, E., 203
Wasserstein, J., 461
Wassif, W., 784
Wassink, T. H., 465
Watarai, J., 783
Waterhouse, L., 457, 458, 461, 466, 472, 473
Waterhouse, L. H., 457, 472
Waterman, J., 656, 657
Waters, E., 151, 789
Waters, J., 700
Watkins, B., 650, 780, 782, 788
Watkins, N., 474
Watkins, P. C., 796, 797
Watson, D., 277, 278, 279
Watson, J. B., 6, 271
Watson, S., 159, 177, 201, 214, 217, 218, 219, 222, 225, 227
Watson, T., 793
Watson-Perczel, M., 606
Watt, H., 780, 788
Watthen-Lovaas, N., 479
Weaver, A., 77, 464
Webb, A., 9, 40, 291, 740, 741, 743
Webb, C., 686
Webb, E., 462
Webb, J., 783
Webb, W. L., 784, 792
Weber, J., 6
Webster, C., 147
Webster, I., 102

Webster-Stratton, C., 8, 21, 97, 98, 108, 151, 156, 158, 163, 166, 167, 168, 185, 192, 207, 208, 212, 213, 214, 218, 219, 220, 221, 222, 223, 225, 228, 231, 485, 486, 620, 630
Weckerly, J., 299
Weeks, A., 97, 98
Weeks, G. R., 10
Weeks, K., 437
Weems, C. F., 273, 283, 285, 291, 299, 330, 332
Weersing, V. R., 5, 16, 42, 218, 298, 355, 356, 376, 377, 382, 383
Wehmeyer, M. L., 433
Wehner, E. A., 466
Wehrspann, W., 657
Wei, S., 557
Weidman, C. S., 97, 98, 159
Weiffenbach, B., 77
Weikart, D. P., 208, 217, 420
Weil, J., 220
Weinberg, N. Z., 741
Weinberg, W., 340
Weinberg, W. A., 340, 343, 345, 346, 386
Weincek, L., 674
Weinfield, N. S., 687, 688
Weingart, K. R., 43
Weinrott, M. R., 158, 171, 172, 200, 214, 226, 229
Weinzierl, K. M., 597, 599, 600
Weisman, A., 206
Weisner, T. S., 438
Weiss, A. D., 625, 629
Weiss, B., 16, 17, 28, 29, 30, 38, 41, 149, 298, 337, 338, 689
Weiss, G., 70, 71, 80, 81, 82, 88, 99, 117
Weiss, J. G., 739
Weiss, M. J., 471, 489
Weiss, N. S., 12
Weiss, T., 806
Weissbrod, C. W., 290, 324
Weissman, K., 737, 750
Weissman, M., 380, 381, 383
Weissman, M. M., 9, 294, 336, 346, 354, 355, 357, 380, 733, 739, 745, 752
Weissman, W., 143, 199
Weisz, J. R., 3, 4, 5, 6, 9, 13, 14, 16, 17, 28, 29, 30, 31, 32, 38, 41, 42, 44, 66, 218, 271, 274, 284, 296, 297, 298, 299, 300, 301, 338, 355, 356, 376, 377, 378, 381, 382, 383, 687
Weizman, A., 779, 785
Wekerle, C., 9, 23, 28, 596, 599, 607, 608, 609, 610, 617, 621, 631, 632, 682
Welch, R., 800, 803
Welch, S. L., 786, 788, 800
Wellens, W., 807
Weller, E., 386
Weller, E. B., 93
Weller, R. A., 93
Wells, E., 733
Wells, G. L., 670, 682, 685
Wells, J. K., 23
Wells, J. M., 386
Wells, K. B., 3, 28, 299, 339, 390
Wells, K. C., 10, 11, 23, 115, 116, 141, 162, 164, 182, 183, 189, 213, 214, 215, 218, 221, 222, 225, 226, 228, 273, 430
Wells, L. A., 806
Wells, R. D., 682
Wells, S., 662, 663
Wells, S. J., 609
Welsh, J. D., 17
Welte, J., 752
Weltzin, T. E., 780, 783, 788, 789, 790, 792, 793, 795, 796, 797, 801, 809
Wenning, B., 74
Wentz, E., 460, 461, 783, 807
Werner, E., 457
Werner, J., 457
Werner, N. E., 142
Werner, S. E., 436
Wernicke, J., 91, 92
Werry, J. S., 67, 93, 95, 155, 203, 204, 207
Werthamer, L., 210, 218, 227

Werthamer-Larsson, L., 209
Wesch, D., 624
Wessler, A. E., 24, 271, 273
Wesson, C. L., 574
West, R. W., 43
West, S. A., 91
Westcott, H. L., 651, 660, 670, 671, 673
Westen, D. A., 797, 800, 804
Wetzel, R. J., 7, 10, 37
Wever, W., 74
Wewetzer, C., 783, 804
Whalen, C., 490
Whalen, C. K., 73, 107, 109, 203, 204, 217, 226
Wheat, M. E., 792
Wheeler, J. R., 683
Wheeler, T., 65, 87, 104, 109, 119
Wheelwright, S., 462, 463, 466, 467
Whelan, B. M., 481
Whelan, J. P., 10, 43, 617, 626
Whener, E. A., 457
Wherry, J. N., 687
Whinnery, K., 568
Whisman, M. A., 354
Whitbeck, L. B., 738
Whitcomb, C., 663, 670
Whitcomb, D., 669
White, C., 474
White, D. M., 29
White, G. D., 429
White, H. R., 147, 153, 742
White, J. L., 144
White, J. W., 119
White, M., 200
White, M. A., 190
White, M. J., 472
White, R., 531
White, R. L., 443
White, W. A., 523, 524, 571
White, W. A. T., 524
White, W. C., 784, 802
Whitefield, K., 696, 706
Whitehead, P. C., 663
Whitehead, V., 780
Whitehouse, S., 195
Whitehouse, W., 354, 462
Whiteley, P., 484
Whitley, M. K., 181, 214
Whitman, B. Y., 73
Whitmore, E. A., 752
Whitmore, K., 23, 415
Whittaker, A. H., 76
Whynot, C., 805
Wickramartne, P., 354, 355, 357, 380, 381, 383
Widawski, M. H., 441
Widom, C. S., 608, 628, 676, 692
Wieche, V., 628
Wiederman, M., 785, 786
Wienrott, M. R., 187, 216, 227
Wientzen, J., 691
Wierson, M., 164, 213
Wiesner, M., 144
Wiest, K., 458
Wigal, E., 77
Wigal, S. B., 77
Wigal, T., 77
Wiknertz, A., 796
Wilcox, B. L., 628
Wilcox, D. K., 155
Wilder, A. A., 558
Wildes, J., 779, 781, 810
Wilens, T. E., 72, 76, 86, 87, 90, 91, 93, 94, 385, 386, 387, 389, 739, 752
Wiley, L., 387, 389
Wilfley, D. E., 779, 781, 783, 785, 797, 800, 803, 807, 810, 811
Wilhelmsen, B. U., 735
Wilke, A., 432
Wilkerson, D. S., 466
Willcutt, E. G., 68, 70
Willems, E. P., 10
Willemsen-Swinkels, S. H., 484
Willi, J., 779, 782
Williams, A. A., 170, 229
Williams, A. F., 23
Williams, C., 431, 687

Williams, C. A., 164, 214
Williams, C. E., 293, 334
Williams, D. E., 431
Williams, E., 735
Williams, H., 442, 795
Williams, J. P., 558, 559
Williams, L., 273
Williams, L. M., 649, 680, 681, 682, 691, 692
Williams, M., 203
Williams, P., 668, 669
Williams, R. A., 172, 174, 207, 225, 231
Williams, R. E., 32, 692, 694
Williams, R. L., 479
Williams, S., 152, 339, 345
Williams, S. C. R., 75, 467
Williams, W. L., 427
Williamson, D. A., 790, 791, 792, 793, 794, 796, 797
Williamson, D. E., 340, 349
Williamson, L., 785, 786, 795, 797, 798, 799, 801, 802
Williamson, P., 349
Willis, D., 652
Willis, M. W., 350
Willis, T. J., 99
Willner, A. g., 215, 224
Willoughby, M., 90, 140
Willoughby, M. T., 141
Wills, T. A., 151, 733, 740
Wilsher, C. P., 439, 441
Wilsnack, R. W., 650, 751
Wilsnack, S. C., 650
Wilson, C., 663
Wilson, D., 531
Wilson, D. B., 119, 228
Wilson, E., 779
Wilson, G. T., 6, 38, 301, 355, 781, 785, 787, 793, 794, 797, 798, 799, 800, 801, 805, 809
Wilson, K., 469
Wilson, M. G., 805, 811
Wilson, N. H., 288, 293, 316, 334
Wilson, P. H., 10
Wilson, S. J., 220, 231
Wilton, K., 437
Wiltz, N. A., 171, 225
Windauer, U., 808
Winder, C., 657
Windle, M., 160, 751, 752
Winebarger, A. A., 780
Winett, R. A., 12, 216
Wing, L., 457, 458, 459, 462, 464, 472
Wing, R. R., 41
Wing, W., 74
Winikates, D., 546
Winkler Metzke, C., 807
Winkler, R. C., 12, 216
Winsberg, B. G., 84
Winslow, E. B., 150
Winter, M. G., 18
Winter, M. R., 667, 668
Winterfelt, N., 677
Winters, K., 751
Winters, K. C., 732, 734, 741, 742, 743, 746, 748, 749
Winzelberg, A., 811
Wirth, P. W., 742
Wirtz, P. W., 742
Wise, B., 547, 548, 549, 550
Wiseman, C., 796, 804
Wisniewski, S. R., 299
Witkiewitz, K., 734, 735
Witt, J. c., 44, 195, 216
Wller, C., 748
Wodarski, J. S., 608, 617
Wohlfahrt, J., 469
Wohlfart, J., 470
Wolak, J., 661, 693
Wold, S., 336, 346
Woldorff, M. G., 74
Wolf, J., 473
Wolf, M., 456, 524, 525, 548, 554, 555
Wolf, M. M., 7, 187, 191, 194, 209, 215, 224, 227
Wolfe, B. E., 22, 32, 780, 788

Wolfe, D. A., 4, 9, 23, 25, 28, 43, 595, 596, 599, 603, 604, 605, 606, 607, 608, 609, 610, 611, 613, 616, 617, 620, 621, 622, 623, 629, 631, 632, 634, 652, 673, 674, 675, 680, 682, 686, 700
Wolfe, V. V., 11, 652, 675, 680, 682, 684, 686, 687, 688, 694, 695, 697, 700
Wolfensberger, W., 411
Wolff, L. S., 159
Wolff, S., 458
Wolin, S. J., 738
Wolkow, R., 295
Wolland, J. L., 658
Wolpe, J., 6, 25, 271, 281
Wolpert, C. M., 465
Wolraich, M., 70, 109, 119
Wolter, T. D., 747
Woltzen, M. C., 731
Wonderlich, S. A., 650, 787, 806, 807
Wong, B. L., 24
Wong, B. Y. L., 522, 556
Wong, C., 13
Wong, M., 332, 648
Wong, M. M., 280
Wong, S., 232
Wood, A., 356, 379
Wood, F. B., 513, 514, 515, 516, 517
Wood, J. J., 25
Wood, L. E., 301
Wood, P. A., 139, 299
Wood, W. D., 602
Woodall, C. E., 665
Woodcock, R., 573
Woods, M., 802
Woodside, D. B., 780, 781, 784, 786, 787, 791, 792, 796, 797
Woodward, J., 568
Woodward, A. L., 468
Woodward, L. J., 72, 152
Woody, G. E., 743
Woody, S. R., 298, 435
Woolaway-Bickel, K., 283
Wooley, S. C., 797, 801, 802
Wootton, J. M., 142, 159, 160
World Health Organization, 3, 9, 20, 457, 598
Worling, J., 678, 691, 704
Wornell, G., 203
Worthington, C. K., 520
Wortman, C., 686
Wozniak, J., 71
Wray, L., 620
Wright, A., 811
Wright, F. D., 753
Wright, J., 678
Wright, L., 23, 601, 805
Wright, S., 531
Wright, V., 206, 389
Wruble, L. D., 784
Wu, J., 350
Wu, J. C., 789
Wu, M., 439, 615
Wulfert, E., 96
Wunder, J., 271, 345
Wung, P., 140, 152, 153
Wurtele, S. K., 17, 23, 322, 651, 652, 653, 654, 655
Wurtman, J. J., 780
Wurtman, R. J., 780
Wyatt, G. E., 648, 659, 692
Wymbs, B., 9, 11, 97, 98
Wynn, J. W., 489
Wynne, M. E., 107, 109

Xenakis, S. N., 72

Yaeger, A. M., 733, 740
Yager, J., 787, 792, 793, 797, 801, 804, 808
Yaggi, K. E., 150
Yamashita, F., 462
Yamashita, Y., 466
Yan, W., 568
Yancey, A. K., 342, 344
Yancy, M. G., 367
Yang, H. M., 295
Yang, M. C. K., 43

Yang, N. J., 537
Yang, Y. S., 443
Yang, Z., 141
Yanner, H., 456
Yarbrough, S. C., 482
Yardley, J. K., 739
Yaroslavsky, A., 784
Yaryura-Tobias, J. A., 295
Yates, A., 443
Yaylayan, S., 93
Yazdian, L., 566, 567
Yeager, C. A., 691
Yeargin-Allsopp, M., 462, 463
Yeaton, J., 677
Yeh, C. C., 483
Yeh, M., 5, 139
Yehuda, R., 683, 707
Yeldham, D., 801
Yen, L., 537
Yeo, R. A., 75
Yeragani, V., 806
Yeung-Courchesne, R., 461
Yiannoutsos, C. T., 77
Yih-Ing, H., 747
Yim, L. M., 6, 28, 275, 284, 285, 286, 287,
   295, 298, 489
Yoerger, K. L., 140, 146, 147, 149, 153,
   228, 229
Yokota, A., 471
Yonan, A. L., 465
Yopp, J. M., 9
Yordan, E. A., 668
Yordan, R. A., 668
York, J. L., 421
Yoshikawa, H., 208, 633
Yoshimura, K., 462
Yossi, H., 141
Young, A. D., 350
Young, C., 527
Young, C. C., 219, 220, 222

Young, D., 283, 293, 328, 330, 334
Young, J. E., 351
Young, R., 622, 633
Young, R. W., 214
Young, S. E., 74, 76
Young, S. N., 348
Youngstrom, E. A., 74
Yovanoff, P., 486
Yozwiak, J. A., 670
Yreka, M., 533
Ysseldyke, J. E., 527
Yudell, R. S., 90
Yule, W., 14, 23, 273, 415
Yurcheson, R., 322
Yurgelun-Todd, D., 467, 780
Yuzda, E., 465

Zabinski, M., 811
Zabriskie, J., 789
Zahn, T. P., 203
Zahn-Waxler, C., 17, 18
Zalecki, C. A., 68
Zalenski, S., 488
Zambarano, R. J., 601
Zametkin, A. J., 75
Zanis, D., 740, 741
Zanolli, K., 437, 473
Zappella, M., 460
Zarcone, J. R., 441, 442, 482, 483
Zaroff, M., 679
Zax, M., 23
Zayfert, C., 299
Zeaman, J., 607
Zeanah, C. H., 28, 599, 612, 619, 681
Zeller, R., 189
Zellman, G. L., 662
Zeman, J., 689, 690
Zentall, S. S., 73, 104
Zero to Three, 20
Zettle, R. D., 96

Zetzer, H. A., 692, 694
Zetzsche, T., 350
Zhang, L., 3, 28
Zhang, X., 465
Zhao, J., 789
Zhu, A., 805, 806
Ziegler, S., 196, 197, 217, 229
Zigler, E., 208, 412
Zigmond, N., 514, 516, 529, 571
Zilbovicius, M., 467
Zillman, D., 600
Zima, B. T., 83
Zimet, G. D., 668, 669
Zimmer-Gembeck, M. J., 142, 231
Zimmerman, A. W., 466
Zimmerman, D., 184
Zimmerman, E. G., 458
Zimmerman, F. J., 81
Zimmerman, R., 734, 806
Zimnitzky, B., 441
Zinbarg, R. E., 273
Zingo, J., 437
Zink, M., 8
Zipfel, S., 807
Zipursky, R., 783
Zito, J., 83, 84, 85
Zito, J. M., 84, 91, 294, 345
Zoccolillo, M., 17, 70, 144, 147, 271
Zoghbi, H. Y., 460, 465
Zonana, J., 413
Zonnevijlle-Bender, M., 787
Zubick, S. R., 170, 229
Zucchi, T., 800
Zucker, N., 790, 792, 794
Zucker, R. A., 160
Zupan, B. A., 159, 351
Zuravin, S., 674, 675, 676
Zuravin, S. J., 597, 609
Zwaigenbaum, L., 460, 490

Subject Index

Page numbers followed by an *f* indicate figure, *t* indicate table.

Abecedarian Project, 420
Abuse, emotional, 598. *See also* Maltreatment of children
Abuse, physical
  academic performance and, 608
  conduct problems and, 149
  definition and scope of, 597–598
  depressive disorders and, 353, 382
  overview, 595–596
  sexual abuse and, 651, 675
  by siblings, 678
  See also Maltreatment of children
Academic performance
  atomoxetine and, 92
  behavioral observation and, 158
  classroom behavior management training and, 104
  conduct problems and, 144, 145, 158, 219
  firesetting behaviors and, 143–144
  in maltreated children, 607–608
  New York–Montreal (NYM) multimodal treatment study and, 117–119
  school environment and, 355
  stimulant medication for ADHD and, 86–87
  token reward systems and, 191
Accountability in treatment
  cognitive-behavioral approaches and, 33
  historical developments and, 9
Accuracy in reading, 556
Accurate Reading in Context intervention, 549
Achenbach System of Empirically Based Assessment (ASEBA)
  behavior rating scales in, 156
  conduct problems and, 155, 158
  overview, 744
Achievement Place program, 186–187
Achievement testing, 516
ACTION kits, 374
ACTION treatment program
  implementation of, 360–365, 363t
  overview, 358–360, 390, 393–394
  therapeutic components of, 365–375, 366t, 367f, 368t, 373f, 375f, 376f, 377f
Adaptation difficulties, 4
Adderall, 439. *See* Stimulant medication
Addiction, 736–737. *See also* Substance problems in adolescents
ADHD. *See* Attention-deficit/hyperactivity disorder
Adjustment problems, 675–677, 680
Adolescent Diagnostic Interview (ADI), 743t
Adolescent Transitions Program, 211–212
Adolescents. *See also* Substance problems in adolescents
  autistic spectrum disorders and, 471
  behavioral parent training (BPT) programs and, 102–103

bullying interventions and, 197
conduct problems and, 145–146, 148–149, 152–153
  family-based interventions, 172–178, 214
  lying, 202
  prevention programs and, 211–212
  theft behaviors, 200
depressive disorders and, 338–339, 340, 346
  interpersonal therapy for, 357–358, 380–381
diagnosis of ADHD and, 70–71
disclosure of sexual abuse and, 657
historical developments related to, 7
maltreatment of, 609, 612
oppositional defiant disorder (ODD) and, 139
parent training and, 103
prevalence of depressive disorders in, 339
relational aggression and, 142
sexual abuse and, 648, 659, 678–679, 680
  as sexual abuse offenders, 659–660, 691–692, 704
sexual behavior problems, 690–691, 691–692
structured diagnostic interviews and, 156
Adolescents Drinking Inventory: Drinking and You, 742t
Adoption and Safe Families Act of 1997, 634
Adoption, sexual abuse and, 676
Adrenergic agents, 702
Adrenocorticotropic hormone (ACTH), 348–349
Adulthood
  attention-deficit/hyperactivity disorder in, 71–72
  autistic spectrum disorders and, 471
  conduct problems and, 147, 152
Advocacy groups, 83
Affect
  autistic spectrum disorders and, 471
  cognitive-behavioral interventions and, 24–25
  posttraumatic stress disorder and, 689–690
  self-regulation of, 79
Affect regulation, 684
Affective education, 365–366
Affects, 36
Age
  attention-deficit/hyperactivity disorder and, 68, 70
  autistic spectrum disorders and, 471, 487–488
  conduct problems, 146–147, 219
  depressive disorders, 345
  disclosure of sexual abuse and, 657
  eating disorders and, 781

evaluation of treatment effectiveness, 287t
sexual abuse and, 650
sexual behavior problems, 690–691
stimulant medication for ADHD and, 88
treatment planning and, 16–17
Aggression
  attention-deficit/hyperactivity disorder and, 68, 71
  autism and, 455
  autistic spectrum disorders and, 462
  classification models and, 20
  diagnosis of conduct problems and, 139, 140f, 141
  gender and, 18
  lithium and, 204–205
  in maltreated children, 599–600, 607, 612, 629
  multidisciplinary perspective and, 13
  parent training and, 435
  parental, 151
  prevention and, 23–24
  psychopharmacology and, 203, 206–207, 217, 441, 443
  selective serotonin reuptake inhibitors (SSRIs) and, 385
  sexual abuse prevention programs and, 652
  social skills training and, 107
  stimulant medication for ADHD and, 86
Aggression Replacement Training (ART), 184–185
AIMSweb, 573
Akathisia, 385
Alabama Parenting Questionnaire, 159–160
Alcohol Expectancy Questionnaire (AEQ-A), 744
Alcohol use
  maltreatment of children and, 608
  normative information and, 18
  by parents, 616, 739
  posttraumatic stress disorder and, 685, 701
  in pregnancy, 77, 81, 416, 466
  See also Substance problems in adolescents; Substance use
Allergies, 72
Alpha agonists, 443–444
Amenorrhea, 783
Amygdala
  autistic spectrum disorders and, 467
  depressive disorders and, 350
Analysis–synthesis process, 79
Anatomically correct dolls, 666–667
Angelman syndrome, 465
Anger
  maltreatment of children and, 599, 600
  substance problems in adolescents and, 756
  See also Anger management
Anger Coping intervention, 182–183

Anger management
combined approaches to ADHD
treatment and, 109–110
conduct problems and, 182–183, 215
maltreatment of children and, 602, 606,
622
Anhedonia, 337
Anorexia nervosa
diagnosis and, 784–785
family therapy and, 801–802
group approaches for, 802
historical developments and, 778–780
hospitalization and, 795–796
nature and diagnosis of, 780–785, 780t
overview, 778
personality and, 787
psychoeducation and, 803–804
psychopharmacology and, 804–805
social skills training and, 799
See also Eating disorders
Antecedent–behavior–consequence (A-B-C)
model
assessment and, 35–36
attention-deficit/hyperactivity disorder
and, 96
substance problems in adolescents and,
753–756, 753f
therapeutic decision making and, 22
Antecedent manipulation, 432
Antecedents to a behavior
autistic spectrum disorders and, 481
maltreatment of children and, 622–623
positive behavior support (PBS) and, 424
Anterior cingulate cortex, 350
Anticonvulsants
conduct problems and, 206
eating disorders and, 805, 806
posttraumatic stress disorder and, 702
in pregnancy, 466
Antidepressants
attention-deficit/hyperactivity disorder
and, 92, 93–95
conduct problems and, 206
depressive disorders and, 347, 392
eating disorders and, 788, 804, 805–806,
811
fears and anxieties and, 294–295
mental retardation and, 439, 440t, 441
Antiepileptic medications, 442–443
Antihypertensive agents, 92
Antihypertensive medications, 95
Antipsychotics
autistic spectrum disorders and, 483–484
conduct problems and, 205–206
mental retardation and, 440t, 441–442,
442–443
posttraumatic stress disorder and, 702
Antisocial behavior, parental, 160
Antisocial personality disorder
conduct problems and, 148
parental, 142, 151, 153
Anxiety
attention-deficit/hyperactivity disorder
and, 68, 116
autistic spectrum disorders and, 471
cognitive-behavioral interventions and,
24
conduct problems and, 219
depressive disorders and, 383
developmental information and, 280
gender and, 17–18
overview, 271–280, 275t, 276f, 278f,
297–302, 299f
sexual abuse prevention programs and,
655
stimulant medication for ADHD and, 88
theoretical framework for, 271–274
treatment
cognitive-behavioral interventions and,
326t–333t
components of, 295–297, 296f
exposure interventions, 314t–317t
identifying interventions, 284–285,
286t, 287t, 288
modeling interventions, 318t–325t
other interventions for, 334t–335t
psychopharmacology, 294–295

research on, 288, 289t, 290–295
strategies, 280–284
timing of, 279–280
two-factor theory and, 683
Anxiety disorders
atomoxetine and, 92
attention-deficit/hyperactivity disorder
and, 72
autistic spectrum disorders and, 461
cognitive-behavioral interventions and, 9,
24– 25
comorbidity and, 20
conduct problems and, 144–145
depressive disorders and, 346–347, 349,
387–389
DSM-IV-TR categories of, 27t, 275t
eating disorders and, 783, 784
historical developments related to, 7
multidisciplinary perspective and, 13
Multimodal Treatment Study of ADHD
(MTA) and, 113
overview, 271–280, 275t, 276f, 278f,
297–302, 299f
in parents, 19
posttraumatic stress disorder and, 702
substance problems in adolescents and,
733
treatment
cognitive-behavioral interventions and,
326t–333t
exposure interventions, 314t–317t
modeling interventions, 318t–325t
other interventions for, 334t–335t
psychopharmacology, 294–295
timing of, 279–280
Anxiety management skills, 292
Anxiety sensitivity, 273
Appetite, selective serotonin reuptake
inhibitors (SSRIs) and, 385
Applied behavioral analysis (ABA)
autistic spectrum disorders and, 490
mental retardation and, 421–422
See also Behavior modification
Appraisals, cognitive, 24
Appraisals, self, 600–601
Approach–withdrawal theory, 272–273
Arousability
cognitive-behavioral interventions and,
25
maltreatment of children and, 600
treatment and, 19
Arson. See Firesetting behaviors
Asperger's disorder
comorbidity and, 461
diagnosis of, 459–460, 464
distinguishing from autistic disorder,
458
prevalence rates of, 462–464
sleep problems and, 462
Asperger's Syndrome Diagnostic Interview,
460
Assertiveness, 755–756
Assessment
accountability in treatment and, 33
ACTION treatment program and, 358–
359, 366–367, 366t
anxiety disorders, 274–275
autistic spectrum disorders and, 457–458
cognitive-behavioral systems orientation
and, 35–37
conceptualization of childhood disorders
and, 34
conduct problems and, 154–161, 230–
232
custody disputes and, 679
developmental information and, 16
eating disorders and, 790–792, 7941f
ethnic and cultural factors to consider in,
44–45
functional behavioral assessments and,
422–430, 423f
hospitalization and, 794–795
maltreatment of children and, 603–604,
605t, 606–610
mental retardation and, 414, 433–434,
434f
normative information and, 18–19

prior to sexual abuse prevention
program implementation, 652–653
reading disabilities and, 532
sexual abuse and, 693–696
stimulant medication for ADHD and,
88–89
substance problems in adolescents and,
740–741, 742t–743t, 743–746
systems perspective to, 7
Asthma, 72
Atomoxetine
attention-deficit/hyperactivity disorder
and, 91–93
autistic spectrum disorders and, 484
mental retardation and, 443–444
Attachment
anxiety disorders and, 388
depressive disorders and, 341–342, 354
eating disorders and, 790–791
interventions with maltreating families
and, 629, 630
self-schema development and, 351–353
Attachment status, 221
Attachment theory, 350–353
Attention
depressive disorders and, 337
in Gray's model, 276
substance problems in adolescents and,
761
Attention-deficit/hyperactivity disorder
autistic spectrum disorders and, 484
bupropion and, 386–387
cognitive-behavioral interventions and, 9
comorbidity and, 20–21, 72–73
conceptualization of, 77–80
conduct problems and, 144–146, 157,
218–219, 229–230, 231
depressive disorders and, 346, 389–390
developmental course of, 70–72
diagnosis of, 65, 68, 68t
DSM-IV criteria of, 69t
DSM-IV-TR categories of, 26–27, 26t
etiologies for, 73–76, 81
firesetting behaviors and, 143–144
genetic factors related to, 76–77, 81
historical developments related to, 7
learning disabilities and, 572, 577
mental retardation and, 415
multidisciplinary perspective and, 13
overview, 65, 119–120
in parents, 19, 160, 616
posttraumatic stress disorder and, 683
prevalence and sex ratios of, 70
substance problems in adolescents and,
734, 739, 752
symptoms of, 67–68
treatment of, 65–67, 80–119
assumptions regarding, 81–83
behavioral interventions, 95–108
combined interventions, 109–119
ineffective or unproved, 119
parent training, 435
psychopharmacology, 83–95, 85t,
203–204, 205, 440t, 443
Attention problems
autistic spectrum disorders and, 461–462
DSM-IV criteria of, 69t
posttraumatic stress disorder and, 684
stimulant medication for ADHD and, 86
See also Attention-deficit/hyperactivity
disorder
Attention process training (APT) system, 97
Attention-seeking behavior, 485
Attentional biases, 787
Attributional biases
cognitive-behavioral interventions and,
24, 25
conduct problems and, 149, 220
social functioning and, 38
Attributional processes, 37
Attributional retraining, 282
Attributional styles
anxiety in children and, 273, 279
depressive disorders and, 341
in parents, 19
posttraumatic stress disorder and, 684,
685–686

Attributions
  maltreatment of children and, 617
  regarding child behavior, 604
Atypical antidepressants
  comorbidity and, 386–387
  depressive disorders and, 384t
Atypical antipsychotics, 483–484
Auditory hallucinations, 338
Auditory processing
  assessment and, 520
  treatment and, 519
Authority conflict conduct problems, 153–
    154
Autism Diagnostic Interview—Revised,
    458, 464
Autism Diagnostic Observation Schedule,
    458
Autistic disorder
  behavior modification and, 421
  distinguishing from Asperger's disorder,
    458
  multidisciplinary perspective and, 13
  overview, 416
  prevalence rates of, 462–464
  See also Autistic spectrum disorders
Autistic enterocolitis, 468–469
Autistic psychopathy, 455
Autistic spectrum disorders
  comorbidity and, 461
  etiologies for, 464–471
  historical developments and, 455–456
  nature and diagnosis of, 456–462
  overview, 455, 490–491
  prevalence rates of, 462–464
  treatment
    behavior management and analysis,
      480–483, 482t
    communication skills, 476–480
    early intervention and, 487–490
    family-based interventions, 484–487
    overview, 490–491
    prognosis and, 471–472
    psychopharmacology, 483–484
    social interaction, 472–476
Autoimmune system, 466
Avoidance behavior
  anxiety in children and, 274, 279
  approach–withdrawal theory, 272–273
  eating disorders and, 787
  posttraumatic stress disorder and, 687
  sexual abuse and, 681–682
  trauma-focused psychotherapy and, 697
  two-factor theory and, 272, 683

Baltimore studies, 209–210
Barriers-to-treatment model, 223
Basal ganglia, 350
Baseline data, 433–434, 434f
Behavior
  cognitive-behavioral assessments and, 36
  continuum of programs for, 15f
  on the functional behavior assessment,
    422, 423f
  gender and, 17–18
  See also Conduct problems
Behavior Assessment System for Children,
    Second Edition (BASC)
  conduct problems and, 156
  overview, 744–745
Behavior chain
  interpersonal skills and, 755–756
  substance problems in adolescents and,
    753f
Behavior disorders
  DSM-IV-TR categories of, 26t
  substance problems in adolescents and,
    733
Behavior management
  autistic spectrum disorders and, 480–
    483, 482t
  sexual abuse and, 699, 700
Behavior management, classroom
  attention-deficit/hyperactivity disorder
    and, 103–106
  combining with psychopharmacological
    interventions, 109
  conduct problems and, 159, 190–194

Behavior modification
  mental retardation and, 421– 422
  parent training in, 97–103
  See also Applied behavioral analysis
    (ABA)
Behavior problems
  autistic spectrum disorders and, 462,
    480–483, 482t
  maltreatment of children and, 607, 608,
    612
  puberty and, 342
  sexual abuse and, 680
Behavior rating scales, 156–157
Behavioral analysis
  cognitive-behavioral systems orientation
    and, 35–36
  diagnosis and, 20
  therapeutic decision making and, 22
Behavioral approaches
  attention-deficit/hyperactivity disorder
    and, 95–108
  autistic spectrum disorders and, 484–487
  combining with psychopharmacological
    interventions, 109–119
  comparison studies of, 226
  developmental information and, 14
  eating disorders and, 797–799
  historical developments of, 6–8
  learning disabilities and, 520–521
  maltreatment of children and, 602–603,
    615
  overview, 31, 32–33
Behavioral Coding System, 157–158
Behavioral consultations, 629–630
Behavioral ecology, 10
Behavioral–family systems therapy, 801–
    802
Behavioral generalization
  parent training and, 162
  theft behaviors and, 201
Behavioral inhibition. See Inhibiting
    behavior
Behavioral inhibition system (BIS), 276–
    277, 276f. See also Inhibiting
    behavior
Behavioral model of LDs, 520–521
Behavioral momentum, 424–425
Behavioral observation, 157–159
Behavioral parent training (BPT) programs
  attention-deficit/hyperactivity disorder
    and, 97–103
  autistic spectrum disorders and, 484–485
  New York–Montreal (NYM) multimodal
    treatment study and, 117–119
  See also Parent training
Behavioral problems
  autistic spectrum disorders and, 480–
    483, 482t
  depressive disorders and, 338
  mental retardation and, 415
  reinforcement and, 427–430
Behavioral rehearsals, 102
Behavioral skills training, 653
Beliefs regarding effects of substances, 738,
    753–754
Belonging, sense of, 355
Benzodiazepines
  anxiety disorders and, 388
  eating disorders and, 804
  fears and anxieties and, 294–295
Beta-endorphins, 484
Biases
  eating disorders and, 787
  maltreatment of children and, 610
Binge drinking, 735. See also Substance
    problems in adolescents
Binge-eating disorder
  nature and diagnosis of, 780–785
  overview, 778
  psychoeducation and, 803–804
  treatment and, 800
  See also Eating disorders
Bingeing. See Eating disorders
Biobehavioral model, 737–738, 767
Bioinformational conceptualization of
    anxiety, 273–274
Biological factors

cognitive-behavioral systems orientation
    and, 38–39
  depressive disorders and, 347–349
  eating disorders and, 779–780
  sensitivity to, 7
  substance problems in adolescents and,
    738
Biomedical factors, 412
Bipolar disorder
  attention-deficit/hyperactivity disorder
    and, 71, 72
  depressive disorders and, 339, 346, 389–
    390
  diagnosis and, 336
  psychopharmacology, 442–443
Bipolar subtype of conduct problems, 139
Birth complications
  attention-deficit/hyperactivity disorder
    and, 75–76
  conduct problems and, 149
  eating disorders and, 789
  mental retardation and, 416–417
  premature, 76, 149
Birthweight, 76
Body dissatisfaction
  ethnicity and, 344
  puberty and, 342–343
Body dysmorphic disorder
  body image work and, 801
  eating disorders and, 784
Body image
  eating disorders and, 784, 800–801,
    810
  puberty and, 342–343
Booster sessions
  behavioral parent training (BPT)
    programs and, 102
  depressive disorders and, 392
Borderline personality disorder
  dissociation and, 688
  posttraumatic stress disorder and, 684
Boundaries, depressive disorders and, 353
Boundary conditions, 5t
Breathing retraining, 283
Brief strategic family therapy (BSFT)
  child characteristics and, 220
  comparison studies of, 224–228
  conduct problems and, 174–175
  generalization of, 214
  as prevention, 207
  substance problems in adolescents and,
    747, 752
Broad-based early interventions, 208
Bulimia nervosa
  cognitive-behavioral therapy and, 800
  cultural factors and, 786
  diagnosis and, 784–785
  group approaches for, 802–803
  historical developments and, 778–780
  nature and diagnosis of, 780–785
  overview, 778
  personality and, 787
  psychoeducation and, 803–804
  psychopharmacology, 805–806
  stimulus control strategies and, 799
  See also Eating disorders
Bullying
  comparison studies of interventions,
    225–226
  depressive disorders and, 355
  generalization of treatment and, 216–217
  overview, 141–142
  school-based treatment and, 196–198
Bupropion
  comorbidity and, 386–387, 389
  depressive disorders and, 384–385

Carbamazepine
  conduct problems and, 206
  mental retardation and, 443
Cardiac irregularities with eating disorders,
    783
Caregiver Report Form for Ages 1½–5,
    156
Caretaking system
  foster care and, 674–680
  maltreatment of children and, 597

posttraumatic stress disorder and, 702–703
sexual abuse prevention programs and, 660–661
Case formulation
    ACTION treatment program and, 366–367
    substance problems in adolescents and, 745–746
Case management
    conduct problems and, 188–189, 216
    maltreatment of children and, 603
    in therapeutic foster care, 187
Catapres. *See* Antihypertensive medications
"Catch the Positive" activity, 365, 374
Center at Oregon for Research in the Behavioral Education of the Handicapped (CORBEH)
    comparison studies of, 224–228
    generalization of treatment and, 216
    school-based treatment and, 192–194
Center for Epidemiological Studies Depression Scale (CES-D), 343–344
Central nervous system arousal
    eating disorders and, 788, 805
    in Gray's model, 276
Cerebellum
    attention-deficit/hyperactivity disorder and, 74–75
    autistic spectrum disorders and, 467
Change, commitment for, 22
Change mechanisms, 42
"Change the program" rules, 573–574
Checklist for Autism in Toddlers, 464
Child abduction, prevention and, 23
Child Behavior Checklist
    conduct problems and, 156
    overview, 744
    Sexual Problems scale of, 690
Child-centered therapy, 700
Child characteristics
    conduct problems and, 151, 159, 218–220
    depressive disorders and, 347–353
    disclosure of sexual abuse and, 656–658
    firesetting behaviors and, 143–144
    maltreatment of children and, 612–613
    sexual abuse and, 649–651
Child Dissociative Checklist (CDC), 687–688
Child-focused treatment, 627–631
Child management skills training
    generalization of treatment and, 41
    history of, 7
    overview, 602
Child protection
    prevention of sexual abuse and, 706
    sexual abuse and, 674–680
Child-rearing
    maltreatment of children and, 602, 604
    treatment and, 616
    See also Parenting
Child Sexual Behavior Inventory (CSBI), 690
Child Symptom Inventory—4, 156
Childhood Autism Rating Scale, 458
Childhood disintegrative disorder (CDD)
    diagnosis of, 460
    overview, 455
Childhood disorders
    conceptualization of, 34
    genetic and neurobiological processes and, 38–39
    See also under specific disorders
Children's Social Behavior Questionnaire, 460
Chlorpromazine, 205–206
Chromosome 7, 465
Chromosome 15, 465
Chronic care model of treatment, 13–14, 15f
Cigarette smoking. *See* Tobacco use
Citalopram
    depressive disorders and, 384–385
    eating disorders and, 804
    mental retardation and, 441
Classical conditioning, 271–272

Classification models
    diagnosis and, 20–21
    mental retardation, 411–414
Classroom behavior management
    attention-deficit/hyperactivity disorder and, 103–106
    combining with psychopharmacological interventions, 109
    conduct problems and, 159, 190–194
Classroom environment
    autistic spectrum disorders and, 481
    inclusion and, 420–421
    Individuals with Disabilities Education Act (IDEA), 417
    learning disabilities and, 571
    math disabilities and, 570
    See also School environment
Client-centered therapy
    comparison studies of, 226
    motivation enhancement and, 751
Clinical interviews, 154–156
Clinical therapy, 30–31
Clomipramine
    autistic spectrum disorders and, 484
    obsessive–compulsive disorder and, 295
Clonidine
    conduct problems and, 205
    posttraumatic stress disorder and, 702
    See also Antihypertensive medications
Closed-circuit television in court testimony, 670–672
Clozapine, 442
Coercive punishments
    attention-deficit/hyperactivity disorder and, 9
    conduct problems and, 149–152
Coercive sexual abuse, 650
Cognitions
    autistic spectrum disorders and, 467–468
    cognitive-behavioral assessments and, 36
    learning disabilities and, 521–522
Cognitive approaches, 6–8
Cognitive Assessment System, 525
Cognitive-behavioral approaches
    attention-deficit/hyperactivity disorder and, 106–107
    child characteristics and, 219
    for children, 28–30
    combining with psychopharmacological interventions, 109–119
    comorbidity and, 388, 389
    decision-making approach to, 21–22
    depressive disorders and, 356, 356–358, 378–380, 391, 392–394
        ACTION treatment program, 358–375, 363t, 366t, 367f, 368t, 373f, 375f, 376f, 377f, 390
    developmental information and, 16–19
    diagnosis and, 20–21
    eating disorders and, 797, 799–800, 804, 806–807, 810
    exposure and response prevention (ERP) and, 798
    fears and anxieties and, 273, 288, 290–293, 295–297, 296f, 301–302, 326t–333t
    firesetting behaviors and, 202–203
    individual differences and, 19–20
    interventions with maltreating families and, 626–627
    mathematics instruction and, 566–567
    in the school setting, 104, 106
    sexual abuse and, 700–701
    substance problems in adolescents and, 734–736, 747
    written expression and, 564
    See also Cognitive-behavioral systems orientation
Cognitive-behavioral assessments, 18–19
Cognitive-behavioral models of LDs, 522–523
Cognitive-behavioral skills training
    conduct problems and, 179–183
    substance problems in adolescents and, 749–750, 749t, 750–755, 755–760
Cognitive-behavioral systems orientation
    clinical sensitivity and, 34–35
    combined and multimodal treatments and, 11

conceptualization of childhood disorders, 34
    decision-making processes and, 5t–6
    developmental information and, 14, 16–19
    ethnic and cultural factors to consider in, 44–45
    family involvement in, 37–38
    features of, 31–33
    genetic and neurobiological processes and, 38–39
    historical developments and, 6–9
    operational rules for implementation of treatment, 40
    overview, 9–14, 45
    prototype for, 33–45
    role of assessment in, 35–37
    specialization and, 11
    techniques and technologies used in, 43
    theoretical framework for, 33–34
    treatment generalization and, 40–41
    treatment goals and, 12–13
    treatment processes, 41–42
    See also Cognitive-behavioral approaches
Cognitive-Behavioral Treatment for Sexual Abuse Program (CBT-SAP), 700–701
Cognitive disabilities, 480
Cognitive distortions
    anxiety in children and, 273, 279
    cognitive-behavioral interventions and, 24, 356
    cognitive-behavioral skills training and, 180
    interventions with maltreating families and, 618–620
Cognitive functioning
    attention-deficit/hyperactivity disorder and, 77–78
    autistic disorder and, 458
    in maltreating families, 606
    stress and, 617
Cognitive-interpersonal theory of depression, 350–353
Cognitive models of LDs, 521–522
Cognitive processes
    anxiety in children and, 273
    cognitive-behavioral interventions and, 24–25
    cognitive-behavioral systems orientation and, 38
    generalization of treatment and, 40
Cognitive restructuring
    ACTION treatment program and, 359, 361, 364–365, 371–372
    depressive disorders and, 380–381
    fears and anxieties and, 282
    interventions with maltreating families and, 618–620
    obsessive–compulsive disorder and, 389
Cognitive techniques
    eating disorders and, 799–800
    fears and anxieties and, 282
Cognitive theory
    depressive disorders and, 350–353
    maltreatment of children and, 600
Cognitive triad, 354
Collaboration
    cognitive-behavioral interventions and, 7
    in decision-making processes, 5
    motivation enhancement and, 751
    posttraumatic stress disorder and, 702–703
Collaborative decision-making approaches, 21–22
Collaborative strategic reading, 558
Combined treatments, 11
Communication
    between schools and homes, 105–106
    sexual abuse and, 700
Communication difficulties, 353
Communication disorders, 26t
Communication, functional
    maltreatment of children and, 625
    mental retardation and, 426

Communication skills
  autism and, 416
  autistic spectrum disorders and, 476–480
  investigations of abuse allegations and, 665
  problem-solving communication training (PSCT) and, 175–176
Community-based programs
  conduct problems and, 186–189
  interventions with maltreating families and, 624–625
  mental retardation and, 437–439
  sexual abuse prevention programs and, 661
Community environment, 353
Comorbidity
  anxiety in children and, 298
  attention-deficit/hyperactivity disorder and, 72–73
  autistic spectrum disorders and, 461–462
  conduct problems and, 144–146, 154, 229–230, 231
  depressive disorders and, 338–339, 346–347, 382, 387–390
  diagnosis and, 20–21
  eating disorders and, 783, 784–785
  gender and, 18
  learning disabilities and, 572
  managed care and, 392
  mental retardation and, 414–416
  Multimodal Treatment Study of ADHD (MTA) and, 116
  posttraumatic stress disorder and, 684–685
  stimulant medication for ADHD and, 87, 88
  substance problems in adolescents and, 733–734, 739, 741, 747–748, 761
  treatment and, 83
Comparison studies, 224–228
Compensatory devices to support handwriting and spelling, 563
Compliance training, 163
Compliancy
  attention-deficit/hyperactivity disorder and, 72
  behavioral momentum and, 424–425
  behavioral parent training (BPT) programs and, 100
  diagnosis of conduct problems and, 140–141, 140f
  evaluation of treatment effectiveness, 287t
  maltreatment of children and, 610–611
  parent training and, 435
  school-based treatment and, 195–196
  stimulant medication for ADHD and, 90
  substance problems in adolescents and, 761–762
Comprehension
  autistic spectrum disorders and, 458
  historical developments and, 514
  interventions, 555–560, 572
  learning disabilities and, 517–518
  reading disabilities and, 531
Computer-based instruction, 548–550
Concentration, depressive disorders and, 337
Concerta. See Stimulant medication
Conduct disorder
  assessment and, 154–161
  attention-deficit/hyperactivity disorder and, 68, 71, 72
  comorbidity and, 20–21, 144–146
  depressive disorders and, 389
  developmental processes and, 147–154, 147–154
  diagnosis and, 138–139
  epidemiology of, 146–147
  multidisciplinary perspective and, 13
  Multimodal Treatment Study of ADHD (MTA) and, 113
  overview, 137
  peer relationships and, 73
  social skills training and, 108
  substance problems in adolescents and, 739, 752

Conduct problems
  assessment and, 154–161
  comorbidity and, 144–146, 144–146
  diagnosis and, 138–139
  epidemiology of, 146–147
  future directions in, 229–232
  gender and, 18
  historical developments and, 137–138
  mental retardation and, 415
  overview, 137, 232–233
  risks related to, 41–42
  subtypes of, 139–144, 140f
  treatment/prevention and, 161–212
    community-based programs, 186–189
    for covert CP, 198–203, 199t
    effectiveness of, 212–229
    family-based interventions, 162–178
    prevention and, 207–212
    psychopharmacology, 203–207
    school-based treatment, 189–198
    skills training approaches, 178–186
  See also Behavior
Confidentiality
  depressive disorders and, 391
  maltreatment of children and, 613–614
  mandated reporting laws and, 662
  sexual abuse and, 693
Confirmatory factor analysis, 274–275
Confrontation clause of U.S. constitution, 671
Conjoint family therapy, 747
Conners Rating Scales—Revised, 156
Consequences
  autistic spectrum disorders and, 481–482
  on the functional behavior assessment, 422, 423f
  interventions with maltreating families and, 621
  mental retardation and, 427– 430
  for stealing, 199
  substance problems in adolescents and, 754
Constipation, 462
Constructivist models of LDs, 526–527
Contextual events, 37
Contingencies for Learning Academic and Social Skills (CLASS) program
  comparison studies of, 224–228
  conduct problems and, 192, 193
  generalization of treatment and, 216
Contingency management
  classroom behavior management training and, 104–105, 190–194
  conduct problems and, 232
  eating disorders and, 798
  fears and anxieties and, 283–284, 291
  hospitalization and, 796
Continuing care, 13–14, 15f
Continuity, of conduct problems, 147
Contracting, 611
Control
  in Gray's model, 277
  hospitalization and, 796
Conventional models of treatment, 13–14, 15f
Conversational skills training, 475
Cooperative learning programs
  mental retardation and, 437
  overview, 536–537
  transactional strategies of instruction and, 557
Coping Cat CBT program
  emotional regulation and, 283
  overview, 290–292
  rapport building and, 282
Coping-competence model, 183–184
Coping Course intervention, 226
Coping Koala program, 291
Coping Power intervention
  child characteristics and, 218
  comparison studies of, 226–227
  conduct problems and, 182–183, 215
Coping, ruminative, 341
Coping skills training
  ACTION treatment program and, 367–369
  sexual abuse and, 699
  substance problems in adolescents and, 749–750

Coping strategies
  ACTION treatment program and, 359, 364–365
  autistic spectrum disorders and, 486–487
  depressive disorders and, 352
  developmental information and, 16
  dissociation and, 688
  medical investigation of abuse and, 669
  posttraumatic stress disorder and, 686–687
  relapse prevention and, 757–760
Coping with Depression course, 378
Core Program against Bullying and Antisocial Behavior, 196–197
Corpus callosum, 467
Corrective Reading program, 534
Correspondence training, 96–97
Corticotropin-releasing factor (CRF), 348–349
Cortisol levels, 203
Course of disorder, 70–72, 345. See also under specific disorders
Court cases
  mental retardation and, 417–418
  sexual abuse and, 669–674, 694
Courtroom preparation programs, 673–674
Covert conduct problems
  comparison studies of treatment of, 224–228
  overview, 153–154
  treatment and, 198–203, 199t
  See also Conduct problems
Covert modeling, 281
Criminal behavior
  gender and, 18
  maltreatment of children and, 608
Criminal justice system, 669–674. See also Judicial system
Cue-controlled relaxation, 283
Cultural factors
  anxiety in children and, 299
  brief strategic family therapy and, 174–175
  cognitive-behavioral systems orientation and, 44–45
  conduct problems and, 147, 220, 228–229, 231
  eating disorders and, 785–786
  in maltreating families, 606
  reading disabilities and, 532
  sensitivity to, 7
  sexual abuse and, 650
  substance problems in adolescents and, 732, 733, 751–752
Curriculum-based measurement (CBM), 527–528, 573–575
Custody disputes, sexual abuse and, 679–680, 694
Customary Drinking and Drug Use Record (CDDR), 742t, 743
Cylert
  attention-deficit/hyperactivity disorder and, 91
  mental retardation and, 439

DARE (Drug Abuse Resistance Education) program, 734–735
Data collection stage
  accountability in treatment and, 33
  overview, 22
Day care, 627–630
Day treatment programs
  child characteristics and, 219
  conduct problems and, 189
  interventions with maltreating families and, 627–630
Deceptiveness
  conduct problems and, 142–143
  diagnosis of conduct problems and, 139
Decision-making process
  anxiety in children and, 298–299
  cognitive-behavioral interventions and, 7
  depressive disorders and, 337
  developmental information and, 16
  Individuals with Disabilities Education Act (IDEA), 417
  maltreatment of children and, 603, 609

regarding treatment, 4–5
sexual behavior problems, 692
therapy as, 21–22
Decoding skills
historical developments and, 514
PALS program and, 537
reading disabilities and, 531
Reading Recovery (RR) program and, 538
University of Colorado Studies and, 548–550
Defiance
diagnosis of ADHD and, 71
historical developments related to, 7
Delinquency
aggression and, 141
conduct problems and, 139, 148
gender and, 18
maltreatment of children and, 612
substance problems in adolescents and, 748
Dementia. See Childhood disintegrative disorder (CDD)
Dental abnormalities with eating disorders, 783
Dental care model of treatment, 13–14, 15f
Depression
anxiety in children and, 277–278
attention-deficit/ hyperactivity disorder and, 68, 72
autistic spectrum disorders and, 471
cognitive-behavioral interventions and, 24, 24–25
conduct problems and, 144–145, 148, 219
eating disorders and, 789, 792, 807, 811
etiologies for, 347–353
gender and, 17
historical developments related to, 7
maltreatment of children and, 599, 608
multidisciplinary perspective and, 13
in parents, 19, 72–73, 149–152, 160, 221
posttraumatic stress disorder and, 685–686
substance problems in adolescents and, 739
Depressive disorder not otherwise specified (DDNOS), 336–337
Depressive disorders
comorbidity and, 346–347, 387–390
developmental information and, 337–339
diagnosis of, 336–337
ethnic and cultural factors and, 343–345
gender and, 340–343
onset, course and outcome of, 345–346
overview, 336, 392–394
posttraumatic stress disorder and, 685
prevalence and sex ratios of, 339–340
prevention and, 390–391
substance problems in adolescents and, 734
systems perspective and, 353–355
treatment
ACTION treatment program, 358–375, 363t, 366t, 367f, 368t, 373f, 375f, 376f, 377f, 390
approaches to, 356–358
comorbidity and, 387–390
considering context in, 355–356
ethical and legal considerations, 391–392
managed care, 392
outcome research, 375–383
psychopharmacology, 383–387, 384t, 385f, 440t
vulnerability, 340–341
Dermatological abnormalities with eating disorders, 783
Desipramine
depressive disorders and, 348
eating disorders and, 805, 805–806, 806–807
See also Tricyclic antidepressants
Developmental disorders
DSM-IV-TR categories of, 26t
parent training and, 435–436

Developmental pathway perspective, 229–230
Developmental process
anxiety in children and, 280
assessment and, 154
attention-deficit/hyperactivity disorder and, 458
autistic spectrum disorders and, 458
cognitive-behavioral interventions and, 16–19
conduct problems and, 147–154
depressive disorders and, 337–339
maltreatment of children and, 607–609, 629, 657, 664–665
mental retardation and, 416, 418
regressive autism, 458
sexual behaviors and, 690
social functioning and, 689
substance problems in adolescents and, 737–738
Deviancy training, peer
conduct problems and, 232
overview, 108
skills training approaches and, 186
Dexamethasone suppression test (DST), 348
Dexedrine. See Stimulant medication
Dextroamphetamine
conduct problems and, 203–204
mental retardation and, 439
Diagnosis
anxiety disorders, 274–276, 275t
of attention-deficit/hyperactivity disorder, 65, 69t
autistic spectrum disorders and, 456–462, 490
childhood disorders, 25–27, 26t, 27t
cognitive-behavioral interventions and, 20–21
conduct problems, 137–138, 138–139
of depressive disorders, 336–339
developmental information and, 16
differential, 20–21, 457–458, 461, 784–785
eating disorders and, 780–785, 780t, 781t, 782t, 808–809
mental retardation and, 415
structured diagnostic interviews and, 155
substance problems in adolescents and, 736–737, 741, 744–745
treatment and, 7
See also DSM-IV-TR
Diagnostic and Statistical Manual of Mental Disorders, fourth edition, text revision. See DSM-IV-TR
Diagnostic Interview for Children and Adolescents, 155
Diagnostic Interview Schedule for Children
conduct problems and, 155
overview, 745
Diagnostic overshadowing, 415
Diagnostic–remedial model of LDs, 520
Diarrhea, 462
Diathesis–stress models, 340–341, 347
Dietary interventions, 484
Differential diagnosis
autistic spectrum disorders and, 457–458, 461
eating disorders and, 784–785
importance of, 20–21
Differential reinforcement, 427–428
Direct bullying, 141–142
Direct Instruction
Hospital for Sick Children studies, 547–548
overview, 534–536, 554
reading remediation programs and, 545
task-analytic model of LDs and, 523–524
Direct Observation Form, 156, 158
Disability
maltreatment of children and, 602
sexual abuse and, 651, 657, 659
Discipline
conduct problems and, 149, 153
firesetting behaviors and, 143–144
social functioning and, 38

Disclosure regarding abuse
anatomically correct dolls and, 666–667
child characteristics and, 656–658
maltreatment of children and, 613
mandated reporting laws and, 662
sexual abuse and, 647, 655–656, 706
trauma-focused psychotherapy and, 697
Discontinuation syndrome, 385–386
Discrete-trials teaching, 476–480
Disease model of addiction, 732
Dishonesty. See Deceptiveness
Disinhibition, 385
Disruptive behavior disorders
depressive disorders and, 346–347, 382–383
DSM-IV-TR categories of, 26t
substance problems in adolescents and, 734
Dissemination of a treatment, 228–229
Dissociation
interventions addressing, 702–703
posttraumatic stress disorder and, 687–688
Dissociative Experiences Scale (DES), 687–688
Dissociative identity disorder, 684
Distal events, 35
Distancing behavior, 686–687
DISTAR Arithmetic program, 566
Documentation, 433–435, 434f
Dolls, anatomically correct, 666–667
Domestic violence
maltreatment of children and, 599, 608
sexual abuse and, 651
Donezepil, 484
Dopamine activity
atomoxetine and, 92
attention-deficit/hyperactivity disorder and, 75, 77, 84
autistic spectrum disorders and, 483–484
depressive disorders and, 347–348
Dosage effect, 383
Dose–response effect, 683
Dosing of medication, 88–89
Double-deficit model, 525–526
Down syndrome
differentiating from autistic spectrum disorders, 461
early intervention and, 419–420
Draw-A-Person task, 695
DRD4 (repeater gene), 77
Drug and Alcohol Problem Quick Screen, 742t
Drug Taking Confidence Questionnaire (DTCQ), 744
Drug testing, 762
Drug use
gender and, 17
posttraumatic stress disorder and, 685, 701
in pregnancy, 416
See also Substance problems in adolescents
Drug Use Screening Inventory—Revised (DUSI-R), 742t
DSM-II
attention-deficit/hyperactivity disorder and, 68
conduct problems and, 137
DSM-III
attention-deficit/hyperactivity disorder and, 68
autistic spectrum disorders and, 463–464
conduct problems and, 137–138
DSM-III-R
autistic spectrum disorders and, 463–464
conduct problems and, 137–138
eating disorders and, 780
DSM-IV
attention-deficit/hyperactivity disorder and, 68, 69t
autistic spectrum disorders and, 463
DSM-IV-TR
anxiety disorders, 274–276, 275t
attention-deficit/hyperactivity disorder and, 65, 68
autistic spectrum disorders and, 456–462

DSM-IV-TR *(cont.)*
   childhood disorders, 25–27, 26t, 27t
   cognitive-behavioral interventions and,
      20–21
   conduct problems, 138–139
   depressive disorders, 336–337
   eating disorders and, 779, 780–785,
      780t, 781t, 782t, 784–785
   mental retardation and, 412–413, 415,
      433
   posttraumatic stress disorder and, 681,
      707
   substance problems in adolescents and,
      736–737, 744–745
   See also Diagnosis
Dual-representation theory, 683–684
Duration of treatment
   ACTION treatment program and, 362
   evaluation of treatment effectiveness, 287t
   hospitalization and, 796
   learning disabilities and, 530, 533
Dyadic Parent–Child Interaction Coding
   System II, 157–158
Dynamic Indicators of Basic Early Reading
   Skills, 573
Dysfunction, 5t–6
Dysgraphia, 561
Dyslexia
   definitional issues regarding, 517
   heterogeneity of, 517–518
Dyslexia Training Program, 546
Dysregulation, 142
Dysthymic disorder
   autistic spectrum disorders and, 461
   onset, course and outcome of, 345–346
   prevalence of, 339
Dysthymic disorder (DD), 336

Earlscourt Girls Connection program, 220
Early infantile autism, 455–456
Early intervention
   autistic spectrum disorders and, 471,
      487–490
   conduct problems and, 208, 232
   emphasis on, 7
   fears and anxieties and, 291
   fluency interventions and, 553–554
   learning disabilities and, 576
   maltreatment of children and, 631–633
   mental retardation and, 418–420
   special education and, 575
   substance problems in adolescents and,
      734–736
   See also Prevention
Early Interventions Foster Care model, 630
Early-starter pathway of development,
   147–152
Eating disorders
   assessment and, 790–792, 794f1f
   DSM-IV-TR categories of, 26t
   etiologies of, 785–790
   historical developments and, 778–780
   nature and diagnosis of, 780–785, 780t,
      781t, 782t
   overview, 778, 791f, 808–811
   puberty and, 342
   treatment, 792–808, 793t
      inpatient, 794–797
      multicomponent programs, 797
      outcome predictions, 807–808
      psychopharmacology, 804–807
      psychosocial therapies, 793–794
      psychotherapy, 797–804, 806–807
Ecological model
   autistic spectrum disorders and, 481
   depressive disorders and, 353
   interventions with maltreating families
      and, 625–626
Educable mentally retarded (EMR), 413
Education, completion, 71, 340, 346
Education for All Handicapped Children
   Act, 417. *See also* Individuals with
   Disabilities Education Act (IDEA)
Education of the Handicapped Act
   Amendments, 418. *See also*
   Individuals with Disabilities
   Education Act (IDEA)

Educational factors, 413
Educational functioning, 340
Educational interventions
   attention-deficit/hyperactivity disorder
      and, 83
   firesetting behaviors and, 202–203
   implementation of, 571–576
   lying and, 202
   maltreatment of children and, 632
   mental retardation and, 418–420
   multitiered intervention, 541–544
   operational rules for implementation of,
      40
   reading disabilities and, 532–541
   See also Learning disabilities
Effectiveness of a treatment
   compared to practicality, 66
   conduct problem treatments, 228–229
   fears and anxieties treatment, 284, 285,
      287t, 289t, 297–298
   interventions with maltreating families
      and, 626–627
   learning disabilities and, 529–530
   sexual abuse prevention programs and,
      653–655
Efficacy of a treatment
   compared to practicality, 66
   conduct problem treatments and, 230–
      231
   fears and anxieties treatment, 284, 285,
      286t, 289t
   learning disabilities and, 573
   New York–Montreal (NYM) multimodal
      treatment study and, 118–119
   psychopharmacology, 386
   substance problems in adolescents and,
      746–748
Ego resiliency, 17
Elementary age children
   attention-deficit/hyperactivity disorder
      and, 70–71, 85
   conduct problems and, 162–172, 200,
      202, 214
   FRIENDS program and, 294
   maltreatment of, 607–608, 612, 664–
      665, 667
   mental retardation and, 420–421
   parent training and, 103
   posttraumatic stress disorder and, 682
   prevalence of depressive disorders in,
      339
   schema formation and, 352–353
   sexual abuse and, 657–658, 680
   sexual behavior problems, 690
   structured diagnostic interviews and, 156
   verbal working memory and, 79
Elimination disorders, 26t
Embedded Phonics intervention
   Florida State University study and, 551
   overview, 550
Emotion-focused coping, 687
Emotion regulation
   ACTION treatment program and, 366
   depressive disorders and, 352
   motivation and, 79
   posttraumatic stress disorder and, 689–
      690
   psychoeducation and, 283
   substance problems in adolescents and,
      756–757
   treatment and, 19
Emotional functioning
   anxiety in children and, 274
   cognitive-behavioral interventions and,
      24–25
   substance problems in adolescents and,
      753–754
Emotional processing, 787
Empathy
   autistic spectrum disorders and, 457
   in maltreated children, 607
Empathy training, 475
Empiricism
   cognitive-behavioral approaches and, 33
   substance problems in adolescents and,
      746–748
Empowering interventions, 670

Endocrinological manifestations of eating
   disorders, 783
Energy, loss of, 337
Engagement in treatment
   ACTION treatment program and, 362
   brief strategic family therapy and, 174–
      175
   conduct problems and, 223
   learning disabilities and, 575–576
   maltreatment of children and, 610
Environment
   ACTION treatment program and, 362
   attention-deficit/hyperactivity disorder
      and, 76–77, 81
   autistic spectrum disorders and, 481
   cognitive-behavioral interventions and,
      12, 24
   conduct problems and, 154
   depressive disorders and, 353–355
   eating disorders and, 789–790, 792,
      799–800, 809, 811
   emotional, 25
   inclusion and, 420–421
   maltreatment of children and, 599
   mental retardation and, 419
   parent training and, 435
   positive behavior support (PBS) and, 424
   reading disabilities and, 532
   relapse prevention and, 758–759
   substance problems in adolescents and, 739
   toxins in, 77, 81
Environment, classroom
   autistic spectrum disorders and, 481
   inclusion and, 420–421
   Individuals with Disabilities Education
      Act (IDEA), 417
   learning disabilities and, 571
   math disabilities and, 570
   See also School environment
Environment, family. *See* Family
   environment
Environment, school. *See* School
   environment
Environment, therapeutic, 615– 617
Epilepsy, 462
Epinephrine, 84
EQUIP treatment model, 185
Escitalopram
   depressive disorders and, 384–385
   mental retardation and, 441
Ethical standards
   cognitive-behavioral systems orientation
      and, 42–43
   depressive disorders and, 391–392
Ethnicity
   anxiety in children and, 299
   cognitive-behavioral systems orientation
      and, 44–45
   conduct problems and, 147, 220, 231
   depressive disorders and, 343–345, 375
   evaluation of treatment effectiveness,
      287t
   reading disabilities and, 532
   sensitivity to, 7
   sexual abuse and, 650
   substance problems in adolescents and,
      732, 733, 751–752
Etiological model of LDs
   learning disabilities and, 519f
   overview, 519–520
Etiology
   for ADHD, 73–76, 81
   for autistic spectrum disorders, 464–471,
      490
   for conduct problems, 147–154
   for depressive disorders, 347–353
   eating disorders and, 785–790
   mental retardation, 412–413
   substance problems in adolescents and,
      738–740
Evaluation protocols
   accountability in treatment and, 33
   assessment and, 161
   cognitive-behavioral systems orientation
      and, 37
   stimulant medication for ADHD and,
      88–89

Evidence-based treatments
  clinical sensitivity and, 34–35
  cognitive-behavioral interventions and, 24, 28
  compared to clinical therapy, 30–31
  functional behavioral assessments and, 155
  historical developments and, 9
  interventions with maltreating families and, 625–626
  posttraumatic stress disorder and, 705
  substance problems in adolescents and, 746–748
Evoked response potential (ERP) measures, 74
Evolutionary perspectives, 272
Exclusion, in relational aggression, 142
Executive functioning
  attention-deficit/hyperactivity disorder and, 66, 74, 78–80, 98–99
  autistic spectrum disorders and, 466
  in maltreating families, 606
Exercise, eating disorders and, 810
Exosystem, 353–355
Expectancies, 735–736
Expectancies of parents
  maltreatment of children and, 600–601
  social functioning and, 38
  treatment and, 19
Experiential group therapy, 802–803
Explicit instruction
  comprehension and, 557–558
  learning disabilities and, 531, 577
Exposure and response prevention (ERP)
  comorbidity and, 389
  eating disorders and, 797–798
  in the FOCUS program, 292
Exposure interventions
  eating disorders and, 797–798
  list of, 314t–317t
  overview, 280–281, 295–297, 296f, 301–302
  pairing with modeling techniques, 288
  posttraumatic stress disorder and, 705
  research on, 288, 289t
  sexual abuse and, 696–697, 698, 699–700
Expressive language, 341, 416, 458, 514
Externalizing behavior
  attention-deficit/hyperactivity disorder and, 82
  posttraumatic stress disorder and, 686–687
  sexual abuse and, 680
Externalizing disorders
  mental retardation and, 415
  substance problems in adolescents and, 739
Extinction
  interventions with maltreating families and, 621
  mental retardation and, 428–429
  time outs and, 430
Eyberg Child Behavior Inventory, 156–157
Eye movements, 519

Fact retrieval, math disabilities and, 567–568
Familial risk
  attention-deficit/hyperactivity disorder and, 75, 76–77
  conduct problems and, 149– 152
  See also Genetic factors
Family
  cognitive-behavioral systems orientation and, 37–38
  context of and treatment, 7
  decision-making processes involved in choosing treatment and, 5t
  ethnic and cultural factors to consider in, 44–45
  sexual abuse and, 674–680
  substance problems in adolescents and, 749
Family-based interventions
  autistic spectrum disorders and, 484–487
  child characteristics and, 219
  comparison studies of, 224– 228

conduct problems and, 162–178, 222–224
  effectiveness of, 228–229
  mental retardation and, 419
  substance problems in adolescents and, 747
Family characteristics
  conduct problems and, 220– 222
  eating disorders and, 790–792, 791f
  sexual abuse and, 650
Family conflicts, 71
Family environment
  attention-deficit/hyperactivity disorder and, 76–77
  autistic spectrum disorders and, 481, 482t
  behavioral observation of, 157–158
  cognitive-behavioral systems treatments and, 12
  conduct problems and, 149–152, 159–160
  depressive disorders and, 343, 353–355
  eating disorders and, 790–792
  ethnicity and, 344
  firesetting behaviors and, 143–144
  maltreatment of children and, 595, 598, 599
  self-schema development and, 351–353
  sexual behavior problems in children and, 703
  substance use and, 17, 739–740, 748, 749
  treatment and, 19
Family functioning
  attention-deficit/hyperactivity disorder and, 72
  cognitive-behavioral systems orientation and, 35
  cognitive-behavioral therapy and, 383
  depressive disorders and, 345–346
  firesetting behaviors and, 143–144
  Helping the Noncompliant Child (HNC) parent training program and, 164
  prevention and, 23
  substance problems in adolescents and, 749, 756
Family Management Curriculum (FMC), 211–212
Family therapy
  cognitive-behavioral systems orientation and, 37–38
  conduct problems and, 213–214
  eating disorders and, 801–802
  fears and anxieties and, 291
  generalization of treatment and, 40
  integrating with individual therapy, 7
  interventions with maltreating families and, 626
  research on, 379–380
  systems perspective and, 10
  theft behaviors and, 200
Fast ForWord (FFW) program, 519–520
Fast Track project
  child characteristics and, 220
  conduct problems and, 210–211
Fathering
  depressive disorders and, 343, 354
  maltreatment of children and, 598
  See also Parenting
Fear acquisition theory, 271–272
Fear of stimuli, 272
Fears
  maltreatment of children and, 612
  medical investigation of abuse and, 668–669
  overview, 271, 271–280, 297–302, 299f
  sexual abuse prevention programs and, 655
  theoretical framework for, 271–274
  treatment
    cognitive-behavioral interventions and, 326t–333t
    components of, 295–297, 296f
    exposure interventions, 314t–317t
    identifying interventions, 284–285, 286t, 287t, 288

modeling interventions, 318t–325t
    other interventions for, 334t–335t
    psychopharmacology, 294–295
    research on, 288, 289t, 290–295
    strategies, 280–284
    timing of, 279–280
    two-factor theory and, 683
Feedback
  interventions with maltreating families and, 618
  parent training and, 435
  substance problems in adolescents and, 745–746
Feeding and eating disorders, 26t
Feelings
  acceptance of rather than control of, 12–13
  cognitive-behavioral assessments and, 36
Feminist approaches to treatment, 802
Fernald approach of reading remediation, 545
Fidelity of an intervention, 572–573
Fidelity of Implementation Rating System, 224
Fight–flight system (FFS)
  behavioral inhibition system (BIS) and, 276–277
  depressive disorders and, 348
  sexual abuse and, 683
Financial costs
  maltreatment of children and, 611
  overview, 3
  prevention and, 22–23
Fine motor skills, 460
Fire safety skills, 23
Firesetting behaviors
  comparison studies of interventions, 227
  conduct problems and, 143–144
  generalization of treatment and, 217
  structured diagnostic interviews and, 155
  treatment and, 202–203
Flexibility
  eating disorder treatment and, 794
  fears and anxieties treatment and, 300–301
  in maltreating families, 606
Florida State University study, 551
Fluency
  comprehension and, 556
  Florida State University study and, 551
  interventions, 553–555
  learning disabilities and, 518t
Fluency-oriented reading instruction approach, 554
Fluent speech, 458
Fluoxetine
  autistic spectrum disorders and, 484
  comorbidity and, 388–389
  depressive disorders and, 384–385, 392
  eating disorders and, 805
  mental retardation and, 441
  research on, 379–380
Fluvoxamine
  autistic spectrum disorders and, 484
  mental retardation and, 441
FOCUS program, 292
Food as a reinforcement, 425
Food refusal, 423–424. See also Eating disorders
Format of treatment, 287t
Foster care
  interventions with maltreating families and, 627–630
  multidimensional treatment foster care (MTFC), 187–188, 207, 216, 219, 227, 230–231
  overview, 595
  sexual abuse and, 674–680
  treatment and, 603, 613
Foster care, therapeutic, 187–188
Fragile X syndrome
  comorbidity and, 415–416
  differentiating from autistic spectrum disorders, 461
  mental retardation and, 412

Frequency of treatment
  ACTION treatment program and, 362–363
  evaluation of treatment effectiveness, 287t
Friend to Friend Program, 220
FRIENDS program, 291, 294
Friendship skills training, 475
Frontal cortex, 467
Frontal lobe
  attention-deficit/hyperactivity disorder and, 74–75
  autistic spectrum disorders and, 466
Functional analysis
  autistic spectrum disorders and, 480–481
  cognitive-behavioral systems orientation and, 35–36
  diagnosis and, 20
  overview, 423–424
  substance problems in adolescents and, 753–755, 753f
Functional behavioral assessment
  autistic spectrum disorders and, 482t
  conduct problems and, 155
  mental retardation and, 422–430, 423f
Functional communication, 426–427
Functional family therapy (FFT)
  child characteristics and, 219
  comparison studies of, 224–228
  conduct problems and, 173–174, 223–224
  effectiveness of, 229, 230–231
  generalization of, 214–215
Functionalist perspective, 689
Functioning, child
  DSM-IV criteria of ADHD and, 69t
  treatment goals and, 12
Functioning, family, 12
Functions of a behavior, 422–423, 423f
Funding issues
  maltreatment of children and, 595
  mental retardation and, 444
  Reading Recovery (RR) program and, 539

Garage mechanic approach, 83
Gastrointestinal complaints
  autistic spectrum disorders and, 462
  eating disorders and, 783
Gender
  ACTION treatment program and, 358–359
  attention-deficit/hyperactivity disorder and, 68, 70
  autistic spectrum disorders and, 463, 465
  bullying and, 141
  conduct problems and, 144–145, 146–147, 149, 219, 231
  depressive disorders and, 340, 345–346
  disclosure of sexual abuse and, 657
  eating disorders and, 781, 785–786
  evaluation of treatment effectiveness, 287t
  firesetting behaviors and, 143–144
  maltreatment of children and, 598
  posttraumatic stress disorder and, 685
  relational aggression and, 142
  Rett's disorder and, 460
  sensitivity to, 7
  sexual abuse and, 650, 651
  treatment planning and, 17–18
Generalization of treatment
  cognitive-behavioral systems orientation and, 40–41
  conduct problem treatments, 212–218
  depressive disorders and, 388
  learning disabilities and, 520–521, 530
  maltreatment of children and, 611–612
  parent training and, 162–163
  reading disabilities and, 533
  therapeutic decision making and, 22
Generalized anxiety disorder (GAD)
  cognitive-behavioral therapy and, 290–292
  DSM-IV-TR categories of, 275t

prescriptive treatment approaches and, 300–301
psychopharmacology, 294–295
Genetic factors
  attention-deficit/hyperactivity disorder and, 76–77, 78, 81
  autistic spectrum disorders and, 464–465
  eating disorders and, 788–790
  mental retardation and, 413, 416–417
  Rett's disorder and, 460
  substance problems in adolescents and, 733, 738–739
Genetic processes, 38–39
Gilliam Asperger's Disorder Scale, 460
Gillingham and Stillman approach to handwriting remediation, 561
Goal attainment, 367, 367f
Goal-raising rule, 573–574
Goal setting
  ACTION treatment program and, 364, 366–367, 366t, 367t, 368t
  attention-deficit/hyperactivity disorder and, 96–97
  conduct problems and, 183
  motivation enhancement and, 751
  regarding weight and eating disorders, 795–796
  relapse prevention and, 759–760
  sexual abuse and, 695
  See also Treatment goals
Goals, treatment. See Treatment goals
Good Behavior Game, 209–210
Good Behavior Game Plus Merit, 191
Graduated exposure
  overview, 281
  posttraumatic stress disorder and, 707
  sexual abuse and, 699–700
Gray's model, 276–277, 276f
Grooming behaviors
  adolescents and, 659
  online sexual predators and, 661
Gross motor skills, 460
Group contingencies, 201
Group play therapy, 289t
Group therapy
  ACTION treatment program and, 360–362
  eating disorders and, 802–803
  fears and anxieties and, 291–292
  interventions with maltreating families and, 619, 623, 628
  parent training and, 616
  sexual behavior problems in children and, 703
  skills training approaches and, 186
  Triple P-Positive Parenting Program and, 170
Group token programs, 191
Growth hormone, 349
Growth stunting with eating disorders, 784
Guanfacine. See Antihypertensive medications
Guilt, depressive disorders and, 337
Gynecological complications of eating disorders, 783

Hallucinations, auditory, 338
Haloperidol
  autistic spectrum disorders and, 483–484
  conduct problems and, 205–206, 232
Handwriting
  interventions and, 561–562
  stimulant medication for ADHD and, 86
Head size, autistic spectrum disorders and, 467
Head Start program
  interventions with maltreating families and, 625, 629
  sexual abuse prevention programs and, 654
Headaches, 385
Health care settings, 7–8
Health problems
  eating disorders and, 783–784
  mental retardation and, 416
Healthy Start program, 633
Hearing loss, 461

Hearsay evidence in abuse cases, 672–673
Heller's dementia. See Childhood disintegrative disorder (CDD)
Helping the Noncompliant Child (HNC) parent training program, 163–165
Helplessness, learned. See Learned helplessness
Herpes simplex, 466
Heterogeneity
  conduct problems and, 229–230
  learning disabilities and, 529, 573
Hierarchical behavioral analysis, 36
Hippocampus
  autistic spectrum disorders and, 467
  depressive disorders and, 350
Historical developments
  autistic spectrum disorders and, 455–456
  conduct problems, 137–138
  eating disorders and, 778–780
  learning disabilities and, 514–515, 519–521, 519f
  overview, 6–9
  substance problems in adolescents and, 731–732
Holistic approach, 526–527
Home-based interventions
  autistic spectrum disorders and, 488–490
  maltreatment of children and, 616
Home-based reinforcement programs, 194–195
Home token economy, 100. see also Token reward system
Homework in treatment
  ACTION treatment program and, 364, 365, 371, 374–375, 375f, 376f, 377f
  Helping the Noncompliant Child (HNC) parent training program and, 163
  substance problems in adolescents and, 761–762
Hopelessness
  cognitive-behavioral therapy and, 356
  posttraumatic stress disorder and, 685–686
Hospital for Sick Children studies, 547–548
Hospitalization
  depressive disorders and, 340, 392
  eating disorders and, 792, 794–797, 812n
Hyperactivity
  behavior modification and, 421
  conduct problems and, 149
  DSM-IV criteria of ADHD and, 69t
  firesetting behaviors and, 144
  Multimodal Treatment Study of ADHD (MTA) and, 115
  as a symptom of ADHD, 67–68
Hyperacusis, 461
Hyperarousal, 702
Hypersomnia, 337
Hypervigilance
  attachment style and, 352
  maltreatment of children and, 612
  psychopharmacology and, 702
Hypothalamic–pituitary–adrenal (HPA) axis
  depressive disorders and, 348–349
  sexual abuse and, 668
Hypothesis testing in assessment, 36
Hypothyroidism in pregnancy, 466

Iatrogenic effects
  conduct problems and, 232
  overview, 108
  skills training approaches and, 186
ICD-10, 20–21
Identity formation, 354–355
Idiographic emphasis, 37
Imagery
  fears and anxieties and, 283
  medical investigation of abuse and, 669
  theft behaviors and, 200–201
Imaginary friends, dissociation and, 688
Imipramine, 805. See Tricyclic antidepressants
Immunology, 466

Implementation of interventions
learning disabilities and, 571–576
substance problems in adolescents and, 761–763
Implicit didacticism, 475
Implosion exposure, 281
Impulsivity
attention-deficit/hyperactivity disorder and, 66, 69t, 86, 115
cognitive-behavioral skills training and, 180
cognitive-behavioral therapy and, 106–107
eating disorders and, 789
firesetting behaviors and, 144
historical developments related to, 7
mental retardation and, 416
posttraumatic stress disorder and, 684
substance problems in adolescents and, 739
In vivo strategies
overview, 280–281
sexual abuse prevention programs and, 652–653
Incest
contact with offending relatives and, 677–678
mothers and, 675
by siblings, 678–679
See also Sexual abuse
Incidental training, 477
Inclusion, mental retardation and, 419, 420–421
Incredible Years program
child characteristics and, 219
conduct problems and, 166–168
effectiveness of, 228–229
family characteristics and, 221
as prevention, 207
Indirect bullying, 141–142
Individualized combined treatment (ICT) approach, 200–201
Individuals with Disabilities Education Act (IDEA)
autistic spectrum disorders and, 464
functional behavioral assessments and, 155
learning disabilities and, 515
mental retardation and, 417–418
Independent play, 100
Infancy
conduct problems and, 208
eating disorders and, 789
interventions with maltreating families and, 629–630
Infancy and Early Childhood Visitation Program
comparison studies of, 226
conduct problems and, 208
generalization of treatment and, 217–218
Infant Health and Development Program (IHDP), 420
Inflammatory bowel disease, 468–469
Information processing
learning disabilities and, 521
maltreatment of children and, 600–601
psychoeducational model of LDs and, 520
self-schema and, 351–353
Informed consent, 391
Inhibiting behavior
attention-deficit/hyperactivity disorder and, 66, 74, 78, 80
relational aggression and, 142
See also Behavioral inhibition system (BIS); Impulsivity
Inpatient treatment facilities for addiction, 732
Insecure attachments, 352, 354
Insomnia
autistic spectrum disorders and, 462
depressive disorders and, 337
selective serotonin reuptake inhibitors (SSRIs) and, 385
Instruction
comprehension and, 556–560
direct, 534–536

explicit, 531
in handwriting, 561–562
learning disabilities and, 521–522, 523–524, 526–527, 577
in mathematics, 564–570
in phonics, 533–534
reading remediation programs and, 544–553
Instruction, direct
Hospital for Sick Children studies, 547–548
overview, 534–536, 554
reading remediation programs and, 545
task-analytic model of LDs and, 523–524
Instruction planning, 574–575
Instructional response, 512–513
Insularity, parental, 152
Integration of therapies, 419
Integrative theories
anxiety disorders, 276–279, 276f, 278f
learning disabilities and, 527–528
Intellectual competence. See also Mental retardation
Asperger's disorder and, 459–460
attention-deficit/hyperactivity disorder and, 68, 72
autistic spectrum disorders and, 463, 467, 487–488
depression and, 17
home-based interventions and, 489–490
learning disabilities and, 512–513, 515
substance use and, 17
Interactional context, 154–159
Internal working model, 351–353
Internalizing behavior
attention-deficit/hyperactivity disorder and, 82
conduct problems and, 229–230
posttraumatic stress disorder and, 686–687
puberty and, 342
sexual abuse and, 680
Internalizing disorders
conduct problems and, 144–145
mental retardation and, 415
International Classification of Diseases, 10th revision. See ICD-10
International Dyslexia Association (IDA), 517
Internet
eating disorder treatment and, 811
safety contract regarding, 727
sexual abuse prevention programs and, 661–662
Interpersonal connectedness, 341–342
Interpersonal psychotherapy, 797, 800
Interpersonal skills, 755–756
Interpersonal style
ACTION treatment program and, 361
depressive disorders and, 354
Interpersonal theory, 350–353
Interpersonal therapy for adolescents (IPT-A)
depressive disorders and, 356–358, 392–393
research on, 380–381
Intervention characteristics, 222–224
Intervention in the natural environment, 10
Intervention monitoring, 161
Intervention stage, 22
Interventions
components of in fears and anxiety treatment, 295–297, 296f
conduct problems and, 230–232
continuum of programs for, 15f
decision-making processes and, 5t
gender and, 17–18, 231
identifying for fears and anxiety treatment, 284–285, 286t, 287t, 288
learning disabilities and, 529–531
maltreatment of children and, 610
mental retardation and, 418–420
need for, 27–28
role of assessment in, 35–37
See also Treatment; under specific disorders

Interviews
conduct problems and, 154–156
investigations of abuse allegations and, 663–666
videotaping for use in court, 673
Intraindividual-difference models of LDs, 524–526
Inventory of Drug Taking Situations (IDTS), 744
Investigation of abuse, 662–669
Ipsapirone, 805
IQ
achievement discrepancy, 516, 517
learning disabilities and, 512–513
mental retardation and, 412, 414
testing, 516, 526
Irritability
comorbidity and, 389
depressive disorders and, 337, 339
stimulant medication for ADHD and, 87
Isolation. See Social isolation

Johns Hopkins University Prevention Intervention Research Center Trials, 20910
Judicial system
sexual abuse and, 669–674, 694
trauma-focused psychotherapy and, 697

Kempe Early Education Project, 628
Keystone behaviors, 10
Kinship care, 628. See also Foster care

Labeled praise, 165
Labels
associated with eating disorders, 784
maltreatment of children and, 611
Landau–Kleffner syndrome, 461
Language deficits
autistic spectrum disorders and, 416, 455, 456, 458, 459, 476–480
genetic factors related to, 465
in maltreated children, 607–608
mental retardation and, 415
treatment and, 471
Lapse, 757. See also Relapse prevention
Late-starter pathway of development, 152–153
Lead exposure
attention-deficit/hyperactivity disorder and, 77, 81
mental retardation and, 412, 416
Learned helplessness
posttraumatic stress disorder and, 685–686
sexual abuse and, 683, 684
Learning
continuum of programs for, 15f
historical developments and, 514–515
Learning disabilities
Asperger's disorder and, 459
autistic spectrum disorders and, 480
definitional issues regarding, 515–517
diagnosis of ADHD and, 71
DSM-IV-TR categories of, 26t
heterogeneity of, 517–518, 518t
historical developments and, 514–515
Individuals with Disabilities Education Act (IDEA), 417–418
in maltreated children, 607–608
overview, 512–518, 518t, 576–578
treatment
conceptual approaches to, 518–528, 519f, 521f
mathematics, 565–571
overview, 576–578
putting interventions into practice, 571–576
reading, 531–560
research regarding, 528–531
written language, 560–565
See also Mental retardation
Learning Strategies Curriculum, 560
Legal considerations
depressive disorders and, 391–392
investigations of abuse allegations and, 662–669

Legal considerations (*cont.*)
  maltreatment of children and, 614, 633–635
  mental retardation and, 417–418
  sexual abuse and, 669–674, 694, 706
  time outs and, 430
  trauma-focused psychotherapy and, 697
Legislation, 634–635
Lesch–Nyhan syndrome, 415
Letter knowledge, 533
Life events, 686
Lindamood–Bell Auditory Discrimination in Depth program, 551
Listening comprehension, 517–518
Lithium
  conduct problems and, 204–205, 232
  mental retardation and, 442–443
Live modeling, 281, 288
Loneliness
  autistic spectrum disorders and, 471
  depressive disorders and, 355
Love-bargaining, 659
Lying, 202. *See* Deceptiveness

Maintenance
  substance problems in adolescents and, 760–761
  therapeutic decision making and, 22
Major depressive disorder (MDD)
  autistic spectrum disorders and, 461
  comorbidity and, 387–390
  diagnosis of, 336, 337
  dissociation and, 688
  onset, course and outcome of, 345–346
  posttraumatic stress disorder and, 684, 685
  prevalence of, 339
  prevention and, 391
  selective serotonin reuptake inhibitors (SSRIs) and, 385
Maltreatment of children
  assessment and, 603–604, 605t, 606–610
  conduct problems and, 159
  definition and scope of, 596–598
  depressive disorders and, 353, 382
  overview, 595–596, 635–636
  sexual abuse and, 651
  theoretical–conceptual formulations of, 599–602
  treatment
    considerations for, 610–615
    issues surrounding, 602–603
    legal interventions, 633–635
    methods, 617–631
    overview, 615–617
    prevention and early interventions, 631–633
Managed care, 392
Mandated reporting of abuse
  investigations of abuse allegations and, 662–663
  sexual abuse and, 662
Marijuana Effect Expectancy Questionnaire (MEEQ), 744
Marital conflict of parents
  autistic spectrum disorders and, 486
  child management training and, 41
  cognitive-behavioral systems orientation and, 35
  conduct problems and, 150, 151, 153, 159–160, 221–222
  maltreatment of children and, 616
  parent training and, 436
  treatment and, 19
  Triple P-Positive Parenting Program and, 169
Marital conflicts in adulthood, 340
Maternal depression
  conduct problems and, 149–152
  overview, 72–73
Maternal protection, 674–680, 692
Math disability
  Cognitive Assessment System and, 525
  heterogeneity of, 518t
  overview, 577
  treatment, 565–571
Mathematics calculation, 514

Mathematics problem solving, 568–571
Mathematics reasoning
  historical developments and, 514
  learning disabilities and, 518
Meaning making, 697, 698
Meaning, systems of, 684
Measles–mumps–rebella vaccine, 468–471
Mediated learning, 556–557
Mediational perspective, 356
Mediators of treatment effects
  Multimodal Treatment Study of ADHD (MTA) and, 116–117
  overview, 116
Medical assessment, eating disorders and, 792
Medical investigations of abuse, 667–669
Medical model of LDs
  neuropsychological model and, 524
  overview, 519–520, 519f
Medication. *See* Psychopharmacology
Medication adherence, 386
Memory
  child testimony and, 670
  dual-representation theory and, 683–684
  investigations of abuse allegations and, 664–666
  learning disabilities and, 521
  substance problems in adolescents and, 761
  trauma-focused psychotherapy and, 696–697
Menarche, early
  conduct problems and, 148
  depressive disorders and, 342
Mental defeat, sexual abuse and, 683
Mental retardation
  definition and classification of, 411–414, 444
  DSM-IV-TR categories of, 26t
  future directions in, 444–445
  multidisciplinary perspective and, 13
  overview, 411, 445
  prevention and, 416–417, 445
  psychiatric disorders in addition to, 414–416
  treatment
    behavior problem management, 421–435, 423f, 432f, 434f
    community-based programs, 437–439
    educational services, 417–421
    parent training, 435–436
    psychopharmacology, 439, 440t, 441–444, 445
    psychotherapy, 436–437
    social skills training, 437
Mercury exposure, autistic spectrum disorders and, 469–471
Meta-analysis
  conduct problem treatments, 227–228
  depressive disorders and, 383
  overview, 28
  reviews of treatment for children, 28–30
Metabolism
  attention-deficit/hyperactivity disorder and, 75
  eating disorders and, 788
Metacognition, 521
Methylphenidate
  comparison studies of, 226
  conduct problems and, 203–204
  mental retardation and, 439
  See Stimulant medication
Milieu therapy, 41–42
Mirtazapine, 384–385, 387
MMR vaccine, 468–471
Modeling procedures
  developmental information and, 17
  fears and anxieties and, 281–282
  fluency interventions and, 553
  interventions with maltreating families and, 617–618
  list of, 318t–325t
  mathematics instruction and, 566
  mathematics problem solving and, 568–569
  overview, 295–297, 296f

research on, 288, 289t, 290–293
  transactional strategies of instruction and, 557
Moderational perspective, 356
Moderators of treatment effects
  Multimodal Treatment Study of ADHD (MTA) and, 116–117
  overview, 116
Modular design of psychotherapy
  overview, 301
  sexual abuse and, 695
Monamine hypothesis of depression, 347–348
Monoamine oxidase inhibitors
  depressive disorders and, 384t, 387
  eating disorders and, 805
Montreal Longitudinal–Experimental Study
  conduct problems and, 208–209
  generalization of treatment and, 217–218
Mood disorders
  autistic spectrum disorders and, 461
  DSM-IV-TR categories of, 26t, 27t
  eating disorders and, 783, 784
  posttraumatic stress disorder and, 685
  substance problems in adolescents and, 752
Mood management, 757
Mood stabilizers, 440t, 442–443
Moral reasoning
  Aggression Replacement Training (ART) and, 184–185
  cognitive-behavioral skills training and, 179–180
  conduct problems and, 215
Mortality rates associated with eating disorders, 784
Mothering
  anxiety disorders and, 388
  attention-deficit/hyperactivity disorder and, 72–73
  depressive disorders and, 343, 354
  ethnicity and, 344
  maltreatment of children and, 598
  sexual abuse and, 674–680
  See also Parenting
Motivation
  attention-deficit/hyperactivity disorder and, 83
  disclosure of sexual abuse and, 657
  maltreatment of children and, 610–611
  reinforcement and, 426
  self-regulation of, 79
  substance problems in adolescents and, 761–762
  therapeutic decision making and, 22
Motivation enhancements, 734–735, 749, 750–752
Motivational intervention strategies, 232
Motor impairment
  attention-deficit/hyperactivity disorder and, 75
  depressive disorders and, 337
  in Gray's model, 276
Motor skills disorder, 26t
Multicomponent interventions
  conduct problems and, 232–233
  eating disorders and, 797
  maltreatment of children and, 623–626
  posttraumatic stress disorder and, 705
  sexual abuse and, 699
  skills training and, 184–185
  substance problems in adolescents and, 747
Multidimensional family therapy, 747
Multidimensional treatment foster care (MTFC)
  child characteristics and, 219
  comparison studies of, 227
  conduct problems and, 187–188, 216
  effectiveness of, 230–231
  as prevention, 207
Multidisciplinary perspective
  cognitive-behavioral assessments and, 36
  investigations of abuse allegations and, 663
  overview, 13
Multimodal assessment, 790

Multimodal Treatment Study of ADHD (MTA)
  behavioral parent training (BPT) programs and, 102
  overview, 80, 82, 83, 112–117
  summer treatment program (STP) and, 111
Multimodal treatments
  attention-deficit/hyperactivity disorder and, 80, 110
  comparison studies of, 227–228
  overview, 11
Multiple-gating approaches to screening, 161
Multisensory reading remediation programs, 545–547
Multisite Violence Prevention Project, 660
Multisystemic treatment (MST)
  comparison studies of, 224–228
  conduct problems and, 176–178, 224
  effectiveness of, 230–231
  family characteristics and, 221
  gender and, 18
  generalization of, 214–215
  interventions with maltreating families and, 625–626
  as prevention, 207

Naltrexone, 484
Narrative elaboration, 665
Narrative techniques
  posttraumatic stress disorder and, 705
  sexual abuse and, 698–699
Natural Language Paradigm, 477–478
Nefazodone, 384–385, 387
Negative reinforcement, 426
Neglect
  academic performance and, 608
  antecedents to, 622–623
  assessment and, 606
  definition and scope of, 597–598
  depressive disorders and, 353
  overview, 595–596
  sexual abuse and, 651
  See also Maltreatment of children
Neuroanatomical factors, 349–350
Neurobiological processes
  cognitive-behavioral systems orientation and, 38–39
  eating disorders and, 788–790
Neurochemical stress reaction, 348–349
Neurodevelopmental processes, 38–39
Neurofunctional factors, 349–350
Neuroleptics
  conduct problems and, 205–206
  mental retardation and, 441–442
Neurological factors
  for ADHD, 73–75
  eating disorders and, 783
  learning disabilities and, 519
  sexual abuse and, 707
Neuropeptide modulator alterations, 789
Neuropsychological factors
  autistic spectrum disorders and, 466–467
  conduct problems and, 149
  recent research regarding, 233n
Neuropsychological models of LDs, 524–526
New York–Montreal (NYM) multimodal treatment study
  overview, 80, 82, 117–119
  stimulant medication for ADHD and, 88
No Child Left Behind Act, 573, 576
Noncompliance, treatment
  cognitive-behavioral systems orientation and, 41–42
  maltreatment of children and, 610–611
  parent training and, 435
  parental, 224
Noncompliant child
  parent training and, 163–165
  school-based treatment and, 195–196
Nonverbal learning disability, 461
Nonverbal skills, 458
Nonverbal working memory, 66, 78–79

Norepinephrine
  atomoxetine and, 91–92
  attention-deficit/hyperactivity disorder and, 84
  conduct problems and, 203
  depressive disorders and, 347–348
  eating disorders and, 788
Normalization, autistic spectrum disorders and, 483
Normative information, 18–19
Nortriptyline. See Tricyclic antidepressants

Obesity, eating disorders and, 784
Observation assessments, 694
Observational sessions with maltreating families, 613
Obsessive–compulsive disorder
  atomoxetine and, 92
  autistic spectrum disorders and, 461
  cognitive-behavioral interventions and, 9, 292
  depressive disorders and, 388–389
  DSM-IV-TR categories of, 275t
  eating disorders and, 789, 807
  FOCUS program and, 292
  mental retardation and, 441
  psychoeducation and, 283
  psychopharmacology, 295, 441
Olanzapine
  autistic spectrum disorders and, 484
  eating disorders and, 804
  mental retardation and, 442
Online sexual predators
  safety contract regarding Internet usage, 727
  sexual abuse prevention programs and, 661–662
Onset
  of ADHD, 70–72
  of conduct problems, 139
  of depressive disorders, 345
Ontogenic development, 353
Operant conditioning techniques, 798
Operant speech training, 479–480
Opioids, 484
Oppositional behavior
  behavioral parent training (BPT) programs and, 99
  diagnosis of ADHD and, 71
  diagnosis of conduct problems and, 139, 140f
Oppositional defiant disorder (ODD)
  assessment and, 154–161
  atomoxetine and, 92
  attention-deficit/hyperactivity disorder and, 68, 72
  behavioral parent training (BPT) programs and, 99
  comorbidity and, 144–146
  depressive disorders and, 389
  developmental processes and, 147–154
  diagnosis and, 138–139
  epidemiology of, 146–147
  Multimodal Treatment Study of ADHD (MTA) and, 113
  overview, 137
  peer relationships and, 73
  social skills training and, 108
Oppositionality, 421
Oral language, 532
Organic illness, 39
Orthography. See Spelling skills
Orton–Gillingham approach of reading remediation
  overview, 545–547
  spelling skills and, 562
OSLC parent training program
  adolescents and, 172–173
  effectiveness of, 229, 230–231
  preadolescent children and, 170–172
  theft behaviors, 198–203
Outcome expectancy, anxiety in children and, 273
Outcome, treatment
  assessment and, 161
  attention-deficit/hyperactivity disorder and, 66, 70–72

cognitive-behavioral assessments and, 36
cognitive-behavioral interventions for children, 28–30
cognitive-behavioral systems orientation and, 37
conduct problem treatments, 212–218
decision-making processes and, 5t
depressive disorders and, 340, 375–383
eating disorders and, 807–808, 807–808
foster care and, 628
gender and, 17
indicators to assess, 43–44
interventions with maltreating families and, 631
operational rules for implementation of treatment and, 40
predictors of, 218–224
substance problems in adolescents and, 748–749
therapeutic decision making and, 22
treatment goals and, 12
Overt conduct problems, 153–154
Oxcarbazepine, 443

PALS program
  comprehension and, 558
  implementation of, 571
  multitiered interventions and, 542
  overview, 536–537, 544
  University of Colorado Studies and, 550
Panic disorder
  DSM-IV-TR categories of, 275t
  eating disorders and, 789
Parent–child interaction therapy
  conduct problems and, 165–166
  maltreatment of children and, 612, 616
Parent–child relationship
  atomoxetine and, 92
  behavioral observation of, 157–158
  child temperament and, 39
  conduct problems and, 149–152
  depressive disorders and, 343, 353–354
  eating disorders and, 790–791
  maltreatment of children and, 596, 599, 613, 618
  PCIT and, 623
Parent counseling, 117–119
Parent Daily Report (PDR)
  child characteristics and, 219
  conduct problems and, 158
Parent enhancement training, 214
Parent-focused treatment, 617–622
Parent management training (PMT)
  compared to problem-solving skills training programs, 181–182
  conduct problems and, 215
  family characteristics and, 222
Parent Practice Scale, 159–160
Parent training
  ACTION treatment program and, 390
  anxiety disorders and, 388
  assessing effects of, 159
  attention-deficit/hyperactivity disorder and, 97–103
  autistic spectrum disorders and, 484–487
  child characteristics and, 219
  conduct problems and, 162–178, 223
  family characteristics and, 222
  fears and anxieties and, 283–284
  individual differences and, 19
  maltreatment of children and, 615–617, 620–622
  mental retardation and, 435–436
  problem-solving skills training programs and, 181–182
  research on, 289t
  school-based treatment and, 192
Parental attention, 99–100
Parenting
  Adolescent Transitions Program and, 211–212
  anxiety disorders and, 388
  attention-deficit/hyperactivity disorder and, 72–73, 76–77
  behavioral observation of, 157–158
  cognitive-behavioral systems orientation and, 35

Parenting *(cont.)*
  conduct problems and, 149–152, 159–
    160, 220–222
  depressive disorders and, 353–355
  ethnic and cultural factors to consider in,
    44–45
  firesetting behaviors and, 143–144
  maltreatment of children and, 596, 597,
    604, 606, 614–615, 632
  New York–Montreal (NYM) multimodal
    treatment study and, 117–118
  self-schema development and, 351–353
  sexual behavior problems in children
    and, 691, 703
  substance problems in adolescents and,
    740, 749
  theft behaviors and, 199–200
  See also Child-rearing
Parenting Scale, 159–160
Parents
  ADHD in, 73
  antisocial personality disorder in, 142
  attention-deficit/hyperactivity disorder
    and, 72–73
  decision-making processes involved in
    choosing treatment and, 5*t*
  individual differences in children and, 19
  maltreatment of children and, 610–612,
    615
  psychopathology in, 19, 393
  sexual abuse and, 650, 654, 660–661
  stealing behaviors in children and, 143
  substance use and, 739
  as therapists, 37–38
Paroxetine
  depressive disorders and, 384–385
  discontinuation syndrome and, 385–386
  mental retardation and, 441
Participant modeling, 281
PCIT, 623–624
Peer-assisted learning strategies, 536–537.
  See also Cooperative learning
  programs
Peer attachment, 341–342
Peer Coping Skills (PCS) training program,
  184
Peer deviancy training
  conduct problems and, 232
  overview, 108
  skills training approaches and, 186
Peer groups
  autistic spectrum disorders and, 473–
    474
  conduct problems and, 148, 153, 159,
    232
  school-based treatment and, 192
  skills training approaches and, 186
Peer initiation paradigm
  overview, 473
  social functioning and, 629
Peer mediation, 577
Peer modeling
  fluency interventions and, 553
  relapse prevention and, 759
Peer pressure, 734
Peer rejection, 607
Peer relationships
  atomoxetine and, 92
  attention-deficit/hyperactivity disorder
    and, 73
  conduct problems and, 231
  depressive disorders and, 355
  eating disorders and, 811
  firesetting behaviors and, 143–144
  posttraumatic stress disorder and, 689
  sexual behavior problems in children
    and, 703–704
  social skills training and, 107–108
  substance problems in adolescents and,
    740, 756
Peer-tutoring approaches, 104, 437
Pemoline
  attention-deficit/hyperactivity disorder
    and, 91
  conduct problems and, 203–204
  mental retardation and, 439
Penn Resiliency Program, 391

Perceptual abnormalities
  autistic spectrum disorders and, 461
  posttraumatic stress disorder and, 684
  treatment and, 519
Performance, 82, 96
Perinatal problems
  autistic spectrum disorders and, 466
  cognitive-behavioral systems orientation
    and, 39
  conduct problems and, 149
  eating disorders and, 789
Peritraumatic reactions, 682, 706
Personal Experience Inventory (PEI), 742*t*,
  743
Personal Experience Screening
  Questionnaire (PESQ), 741, 742*t*
Personality
  cognitive-behavioral assessments and, 36
  eating disorders and, 787
  prevention and, 23
  reciprocity and, 34
  sensitivity to, 7
Personality disorders
  autistic spectrum disorders and, 461
  eating disorders and, 783, 784
  individual differences and, 19
  maltreatment of children and, 597
Pervasive developmental disorders
  autistic spectrum disorders and, 456
  DSM-IV-TR categories of, 26*t*
  prevalence rates of, 462–464
Pervasive developmental disorders not
  otherwise specified (PDD NOS),
  460
Pharmacology. *See* Psychopharmacology
PHAST Track Reading Program
  fluency interventions and, 555
  Hospital for Sick Children studies, 547–
    548
  Morris, Lovett, and Wolf studies, 548
Phenylketonuria, 461
Phenytoin sodium, 805, 806
Phobias, 113
Phonics instruction
  effectiveness of, 533–534
  multitiered interventions and, 541–544
  Orton–Gillingham approach of reading
    remediation and, 546–547
  Reading Recovery (RR) program and,
    538, 539
  tutorial studies, 537–541
Phonological Analysis and Blending /Direct
  Instruction (PHAB/DI) program,
  547–548
Phonological awareness
  learning disabilities and, 521
  multitiered interventions and, 542
  Orton–Gillingham approach of reading
    remediation and, 546
  PALS program and, 537
  reading disabilities and, 533
  Reading Recovery (RR) program and,
    539
  University of Colorado Studies and,
    548–550
  University of Washington studies and,
    552
  word reading and, 536
Phrase speech
  autistic spectrum disorders and, 458
  Rett's disorder and, 460
Physical development, 72
Physical examinations in investigations of
  abuse, 667–669
Physical health
  eating disorders and, 783–784
  mental retardation and, 416
Physical impairments, 415
Physical therapy, 803
Physiological hyperarousal, 277–279
Picture Exchange Communication System
  (PECS), 479
Planned ignoring. *See* Extinction
Play
  autistic spectrum disorders and, 458,
    472
  independent, 100

posttraumatic stress disorder and, 681–
  682
sexual behavior problems in children
  and, 703–704
symbolic, 458
trauma-focused psychotherapy and, 697
Population specificity, 25, 33–34
Positive behavior review, 365
Positive behavior support (PBS) model
  autistic spectrum disorders and, 482–
    483, 482*t*
  conduct problems and, 193–194
  generalization of treatment and, 216
  mental retardation and, 422–430, 423*f*
Positive reinforcement
  classroom behavior management training
    and, 105
  extinction, 428
  parent training and, 435
  positive behavior support (PBS) and,
    425–426
Postnatal problems, 149
Posttraumatic stress disorder
  cognitive-behavioral inter- ventions and,
    9, 292–293
  contact with offending relatives and,
    677
  depressive disorders and, 349, 382, 388
  DSM-IV-TR categories of, 275*t*
  interventions with maltreating families
    and, 631
  in maltreated children, 608
  overview, 706–707
  psychoeducation and, 283
  psychopharmacology and, 701–702
  sexual abuse and, 647, 681–690
  tertiary interventions and, 704–705
  treatment and, 695–702
Posttraumatic stress reactions, 680–681
Practicality of a treatment
  compared to efficacy and effectiveness,
    66
  New York–Montreal (NYM) multimodal
    treatment study and, 118–119
Prader–Willi syndrome
  genetic factors related to, 465
  overview, 416
Praise
  home-based reinforcement programs and,
    195
  parent–child interaction therapy and,
    165
  in the school setting, 190
Preadolescent children
  conduct problems and, 162–172, 200,
    202, 214
  eating disorders and, 782
  sexual behavior problems, 690
  structured diagnostic interviews and,
    156
Predictors of a behavior, 422, 423*f*
Prefrontal regions, 74–75
Pregnancy
  maltreatment of children prevention and,
    632
  sexual abuse and, 668
  See also Pregnancy complications;
    Pregnancy, early
Pregnancy complications
  attention-deficit/hyperactivity disorder
    and, 75–76, 77, 81
  autistic spectrum disorders and, 466
  conduct problems and, 149
  eating disorders and, 789
  mental retardation and, 416–417
  See also Prenatal problems
Pregnancy, early
  attention-deficit/hyperactivity disorder
    and, 71
  conduct problems and, 147
  gender and, 18
  maltreatment of children and, 608
  maltreatment of children prevention and,
    632
  sexual abuse and, 668, 692
  See also Pregnancy
Premack principle, 425

Premature birth
attention-deficit/hyperactivity disorder and, 76
conduct problems and, 149
Prenatal/Early Infancy Project, 632
Prenatal problems
attention-deficit/hyperactivity disorder and, 75–76, 77
cognitive-behavioral systems orientation and, 39
conduct problems and, 149
eating disorders and, 789
Prepotent response, 67
Preschool children
anxiety prevention programs and, 294
attention-deficit/hyperactivity disorder and, 70, 84–85
Cognitive-Behavioral Treatment for Sexual Abuse Program (CBT-SAP), 701
conduct problems and, 153, 208
disclosure of sexual abuse and, 657–658
maltreatment of children and, 607, 612, 619, 629–630, 664–665, 667
mental retardation and, 418–420
oppositional defiant disorder (ODD) and, 139
parent training and, 103
posttraumatic stress disorder and, 682
prevalence of depressive disorders in, 339
schema formation and, 352–353
sexual abuse and, 654, 680
sexual behavior problems, 690, 691
structured diagnostic interviews and, 156
verbal working memory and, 79
Preschool participation
autistic spectrum disorders and, 487–488
mental retardation and, 418–420
Prescriptive treatment approaches, 300–301
Preserved speech variant, 460
Prevalence rates
of ADHD, 70
conduct problems, 146
need for interventions and, 28
overview, 3
Prevelance rates
of autistic spectrum disorders, 462–464, 491
of depressive disorders, 339–340
eating disorders and, 781–782
mental retardation and, 415, 416
of sexual abuse, 647–649, 658
of substance use by adolescents, 731
Prevention
of anxiety disorders, 293–294
of attention-deficit/hyperactivity disorder, 81
comparison studies of, 226, 227
conduct problems and, 207–212, 230
continuum of programs for, 15f
of depressive disorders, 390–391
eating disorders and, 810–811
emphasis on, 7, 22–24
fears and anxieties and, 291
intelligence and, 19
learning disabilities and, 575, 578
maltreatment of children and, 595, 596, 631–633
mathematics problem solving and, 569–570
mental retardation and, 416–417, 445
positive behavior support (PBS) and, 424
of reading disabilities, 532–544
sexual abuse, 647, 705–706
substance problems in adolescents and, 734–736
Triple P-Positive Parenting Program component of, 169
See also Early intervention
Primary prevention
eating disorders and, 811
mental retardation and, 416–417
sexual abuse and, 651–662
See also Prevention
Priorities in treatment, 609–610

Proactive aggression
classification models and, 20
contingency management and, 232
diagnosis of conduct problems and, 141
Proactive Reading program, 542
Problem behavior theory, 145–146
Problem-focused interventions, 173–174
Problem formation stage, 22
Problem-solving communication training (PSCT)
for adolescents with ADHD, 102–103
for adolescents with conduct problems, 175–176
comparison studies of, 226
Problem-solving model, 527
Problem-solving skills
ACTION treatment program and, 359, 364–365, 369–371
anxiety in children and, 274, 279
autistic spectrum disorders and, 475
child characteristics and, 220
cognitive-behavioral skills training and, 180
math disabilities and, 568–570
overview, 4–5
posttraumatic stress disorder and, 686–687
problem-solving skills training (PSST) program, 181–182, 215
training in, 14, 284
Problem-solving skills training (PSST) program, 181–182, 215
Procedural math, 567–568
Professional reporting of abuse, 662
Progress monitoring
learning disabilities and, 573–575, 577
substance problems in adolescents and, 760
Progressive muscle relaxation
fears and anxieties and, 283
substance problems in adolescents and, 757
Project for Developmental Disabilities, 436
Project MATH, 566
Project SafeCare, 624
Project 12-Ways, 624
Property destruction
autistic spectrum disorders and, 462
diagnosis of conduct problems and, 139, 140f
Propranolol, 702
Prospective functioning, 79
Protection motivation theory, 655
Protective interventions, 670
Proximal events, 35
Psychoanalytic theory, 271
Psychodynamic theory, 271
Psychoeducation
ACTION treatment program and, 365–366
depressive disorders and, 357
eating disorders and, 803–804
fears and anxieties and, 283
in the FOCUS program, 292
medication adherence and, 386
research on, 289t, 379–380
sexual abuse prevention programs and, 651–662
Psychoeducational model of LDs
compared to cognitive models, 521
overview, 520
Psychological disturbances, 24
Psychological maltreatment, 612
Psychomotor retardation, 337, 339
Psychopathy
maltreatment of children and, 602
in parents, 19
substance problems in adolescents and, 733–734, 745, 752
Psychopharmacology
attention-deficit/hyperactivity disorder and, 83–95, 85t
autistic spectrum disorders and, 483–484
combining with other approaches, 109–119
comparison studies of, 225–226
conduct problems and, 203–207, 230

depressive disorders and, 383–387, 384t, 385f
eating disorders and, 804–807, 811
fears and anxieties and, 294–295
generalization of treatment and, 217
iatrogenic effects and, 232
inpatient facilities' use of, 794
mental retardation and, 439, 440t, 441–444, 445
Multimodal Treatment Study of ADHD (MTA) and, 112–117
posttraumatic stress disorder and, 701–702
in pregnancy, 466
side effects
of antidepressants, 441
of antihypertensive medication, 95
of antipsychotics, 483–484
of mood stabilizers, 443
of neuroleptics, 206, 442
New York–Montreal (NYM) multimodal treatment study and, 119
of selective serotonin reuptake inhibitors (SSRIs), 385
of tricyclic antidepressants, 93–94
substance problems in ado- lescents and, 747–748, 752
See also Medication
Psychosocial influences, 786–788
Psychosocial treatment
attention-deficit/hyperactivity disorder and, 81
conduct problems and, 230
eating disorders and, 793–794
New York–Montreal (NYM) multimodal treatment study and, 117–119
Psychostimulants
comorbidity and, 389
mental retardation and, 439
See also Stimulant medication
Psychotherapy
eating disorders and, 797–804, 806–807
mental retardation and, 436–437
New York–Montreal (NYM) multimodal treatment study and, 117–119
overview, 4
posttraumatic stress disorder and, 696–701
sexual abuse and, 692–696
Puberty
body dissatisfaction during, 342–343
depressive disorders and, 341
eating disorders and, 780
ethnicity and, 344
Pull-out model
mental retardation and, 419
multitiered interventions and, 542–543
Punishment
attention-deficit/hyperactivity disorder and, 9
classroom behavior management training and, 105
coercive, 9, 149–152
conduct problems and, 149
establishing operation and, 424
interventions with maltreating families and, 620
maltreatment of children and, 610
social functioning and, 38
theft behaviors and, 200
Purging. See Eating disorders
Purkinje cells, autistic spectrum disorders and, 467
Purposeful learning, 557

Questioning
interventions with maltreating families and, 619
investigations of abuse allegations and, 663– 666
Quetiapine, 442

Racial factors
disclosure of sexual abuse and, 657
foster care and, 676
sexual abuse and, 650
See also Cultural factors; Ethnicity

Rainbow Game, 697–698
Randomized controlled experiments
    (RCEs), 529
Rapport building
    ACTION treatment program and, 363
    fears and anxieties and, 282
    investigations of abuse allegations and,
        665
RAVE-O program
    fluency interventions and, 554–555
    Hospital for Sick Children studies, 547
    Morris, Lovett, and Wolf studies, 548
Reactive aggression
    classification models and, 20
    diagnosis of conduct problems and, 141
Read Naturally program, 554
Reading comprehension, 517–518, 531
Reading disabilities
    heterogeneity of, 517–518
    instruction planning and, 525–526
    overview, 514, 576–578
    treatment, 531–560
        fluency interventions, 553–555
        prevention and, 532–544
        reading comprehension, 555–560
        reading remediation programs, 544–
            553
    See also Learning disabilities
Reading Recovery (RR) program, 535–536,
    538–539
Reading remediation programs
    fluency interventions and, 553–554
    learning disabilities, 575–576
    overview, 544–553
Rebellious behavior, 153
Receptive language, 514
Recidivism rates
    conduct problem treatments and, 228
    family-based interventions, 214
    functional family therapy and, 173–174
    maltreatment of children and, 613–614,
        623–624
    skills training approaches and, 185, 186
Reciprocal determinism
    depressive disorders and, 351–352
    learning disabilities and, 522–523
Reciprocal inhibition, 281
Reciprocal teaching, 557
Reciprocity
    cognitive-behavioral systems orientation
        and, 34
    systems perspective and, 10
Reconstitution, 79
Refusal skills, 759
Regressive autism
    compared to Landau–Kleffner syndrome,
        461
    overview, 458
    vaccination and, 468–471
Rehearsal
    interventions with maltreating families
        and, 617–618
    learning disabilities and, 521
    relapse prevention and, 758–759
Reinforcement
    ACTION treatment program and, 365
    approach–withdrawal theory, 272–273
    establishing operation and, 424
    hospitalization and, 796
    interventions with maltreating families
        and, 621
    mental retardation and, 427–430
    parent training and, 435
    positive behavior support (PBS) and,
        425–426
    self-injury behaviors and, 431
    social skills training and, 437
    time outs and, 430
    in the Verbal Learning Approach, 478
Reinforcement, positive
    classroom behavior management training
        and, 105
    extinction and, 428
    parent training and, 435
    positive behavior support (PBS) and,
        425–426

Reinforcement programs
    classroom behavior management training
        and, 190–194
    home-based reinforcement programs and,
        194–195
    theft behaviors and, 200–201
    See also Token reward system
Rejection
    depressive disorders and, 342, 353, 354,
        355
    Individuals with Disabilities Education
        Act (IDEA), 417
    internal working model and, 352
    in maltreated children, 607
    sexual abuse and, 659
Relapse prevention
    overview, 749
    substance problems in adolescents and,
        757–760
Relapse recovery plan, 759
Relapse risk
    beliefs regarding effects of substances
        and, 754
    cognitive-behavioral therapy and, 379
    identifying, 757–760
    maintenance of change, 760–761
    substance problems in adolescents and,
        748–749
Relational aggression
    depressive disorders and, 342
    diagnosis of ADHD and, 68
    gender and, 231
    overview, 141, 142
Relationship violence
    cognitive-behavioral interventions and, 9
    conduct problems and, 231
    maltreatment of children and, 608
    prevention and, 23
Relationships
    depressive disorders and, 341–342
    eating disorders and, 792
    posttraumatic stress disorder and, 684
Relationships, peer. See Peer relationships
Relaxation
    fears and anxieties and, 283
    in the FOCUS program, 292
    research on, 379
    substance problems in adolescents and,
        757
    systematic desensitization and, 281
    theft behaviors and, 200–201
Remediation programs
    fluency interventions and, 553–554
    learning disabilities and, 575–576
    overview, 544–553
Reprogramming Environmental
    Contingencies for Effective Social
    Skills (RECESS) program
    comparison studies of, 224–228
    conduct problems and, 192–193
    generalization of treatment and, 216
Research
    behavioral interventions for ADHD, 96–97
    cognitive-behavioral approaches and, 28–
        30, 32–33
    combined approaches to ADHD
        treatment, 109–119
    fears and anxieties treatment, 288, 289t,
        290–295, 314t–335t
    history of, 6–9
    learning disabilities and, 528–531, 577–
        578
    Treatment of Adolescent Depression
        Study (TADS), 378–383
Research-based treatments, 378–381
Research therapy, 30–31
Resiliency
    coping skills and, 368
    maltreatment of children and, 608, 609
Resistance
    cognitive-behavioral systems orientation
        and, 41
    hospitalization and, 796
    maltreatment of children and, 610
    motivation enhancement and, 750–752
    parental, 224

Resourceful Adolescent Program, 696,
    706–707
Resources
    interventions with maltreating families
        and, 620
    neglect and, 606
    support services and, 617
Response cost, 429
Response delay, 798
Response prevention, 797–798
Responsive Reading program, 542–543
Restlessness, 385
Rett's disorder
    diagnosis of, 460, 464
    genetic factors related to, 465
    overview, 416
    prevalence rates of, 463
Revictimization risks, 680–681
Revised Behavior Problems Checklist, 156
Revised Edition of the School Observation
    Coding System, 158
Reward approach
    attention-deficit/hyperactivity disorder
        and, 83
    classroom behavior management training
        and, 104
    fears and anxieties and, 284
    home-based reinforcement programs and,
        194
    home token economy and, 100
Rhesus factor incompatibility, 466
Risk assessment
    investigations of abuse allegations and, 663
    maltreatment of children and, 609
Risk factors
    conduct problems and, 149–152
    eating disorders and, 811
    firesetting behaviors and, 144
    maltreatment of children and, 603–604,
        632
    relapse prevention and, 757–760, 757–
        760
    related to premature termination, 41–42
    sexual abuse and, 651, 668
    substance problems in adolescents and,
        732, 733, 735–736
Risk prediction, 609
Risk-taking behavior, 608
Risperidone
    autistic spectrum disorders and, 484
    conduct problems and, 205–206
    mental retardation and, 442
Ritalin. See Stimulant medication
Rodeo Institute for Teacher Excellence
    (RITE) program, 535
Role playing
    assertiveness and, 755–756
    behavioral parent training (BPT)
        programs and, 102
    maltreatment of children and, 602, 617–
        618
Role structuring, 22
Rubella, 466
Rule adherence
    attention-deficit/hyperactivity disorder
        and, 68
    diagnosis of conduct problems and, 139,
        140f
    sexual abuse and, 678
Rules, classroom, 190
Running away behaviors
    diagnosis of conduct problems and, 139,
        140f
    maltreatment of children and, 612
Rutgers Alcohol Problem Index (RAPI),
    742t

Safer sex practices, 23
Safety of a treatment
    depressive disorders and, 392
    New York–Montreal (NYM) multimodal
        treatment study and, 118–119
Safety, personal
    sexual abuse prevention programs and,
        652–653, 659
    when on the Internet, 661–662, 727

Safety planning, 391–392
Scaffolding
  bullying interventions and, 196
  interventions with maltreating families
    and, 617
  mathematics problem solving and, 569
Scanning, in Gray's model, 276
Schedule for Affective Disorders and
    Schizophrenia for School Age
    Children (K-SADS), 358–359
Schema theory, 569
Schemas
  cognitive-interpersonal theory of
    depression and, 350–353
  depressive disorders and, 352–353
  in Gray's model, 277
  maltreatment of children and, 597, 600
  mathematics problem solving and, 569, 570
Schizoid personality disorder, 458
Schizophrenia
  autistic spectrum disorders and, 455
  dissociation and, 688
  distinguishing from Asperger's disorder,
    458
  eating disorders and, 784
  multidisciplinary perspective and, 13
School adjustment, 15f
School behavior
  atomoxetine and, 92
  behavioral parent training (BPT)
    programs and, 101–102
School dropouts, 71, 340, 346
School environment
  behavioral observation of, 158
  cognitive-behavioral systems treatments
    and, 12
  depressive disorders and, 355
  inclusion and, 420–421
  Individuals with Disabilities Education
    Act (IDEA), 417
  See also Classroom environment
School interventions
  child characteristics and, 220
  classroom behavior management training
    and, 103–106
  conduct problems and, 189–198
  coping-competence model and, 183–184
  generalization of treatment and, 217
  interventions with maltreating families
    and, 625
  meta-analysis of, 29–30
  prevention of sexual abuse and, 651–662
  Seattle Social Development Project, 209
  sexual abuse and, 705
  theft behaviors and, 201
  UCI/OCDE program, 111
School refusal, 300
Seattle Social Development Project, 209
Secondary prevention
  mental retardation and, 416–417
  sexual abuse and, 662–680
  See also Prevention
Secure attachment, 352, 354
Seizure disorders
  autistic spectrum disorders and, 462
  psychopharmacology, 443
Seizures, vaccination and, 468
Selective serotonin reuptake inhibitors
    (SSRIs)
  autistic spectrum disorders and, 484
  cognitive-behavioral therapy and, 393
  comorbidity and, 387–388, 389
  conduct problems and, 206
  depressive disorders and, 348, 384–386,
    384t, 385f, 392
  eating disorders and, 805, 811
  efficacy of, 386
  fears and anxieties and, 294–295
  mental retardation and, 439, 440t, 441
  obsessive–compulsive disorder and, 295
  posttraumatic stress disorder and, 701–
    702
Self-awareness
  ACTION treatment program and, 365–
    366
  autistic spectrum disorders and, 475

Self-control
  attention-deficit/hyperactivity disorder
    and, 78, 109
  cognitive-behavioral skills training and,
    180
  cognitive-behavioral systems orientation
    and, 42
  generalization of treatment and, 40
  interventions with maltreating families
    and, 622
  theft behaviors and, 200–201
Self-control training, 291
Self-directed play, 79
Self-efficacy theory, 273
Self-esteem
  ACTION program and, 373–374, 373f
  attention-deficit/hyperactivity disorder
    and, 73
  comprehension and, 556
  depressive disorders and, 337, 341
  eating disorders and, 787, 810
  in maltreated children, 608
  in parents, 19
  puberty and, 342
  school environment and, 355
  sexual abuse prevention programs and,
    654
  substance problems in adolescents and,
    748
Self-evaluations, 373–374, 373f
Self-help, 811
Self-injury behaviors
  autistic spectrum disorders and, 455,
    462
  mental retardation and, 415, 426, 430–
    433, 432f
  psychopharmacology, 441
  time outs and, 429
Self-instruction, 289t
Self-management
  cognitive-behavioral systems orientation
    and, 42
  fears and anxieties and, 282
Self-map, 373–374, 373f
Self-monitoring
  dissociation and, 687–688
  eating disorders and, 798–799
  fears and anxieties and, 284
Self-perception, 684
Self-regulated strategy development
  learning disabilities and, 523
  written expression and, 564–565
Self-regulation
  attention-deficit/hyperactivity disorder
    and, 78, 79, 96, 98–99
  cognitive-behavioral systems orientation
    and, 42
  learning disabilities and, 572, 577
  math disabilities and, 567–568
  substance problems in adolescents and,
    739
Self-report assessment measures
  conduct problems and, 154–155, 157
  maltreatment of children and, 608
Self-Report Delinquency Scale, 157
Self-schema, 351–353, 354. See also
    Schemas
Self-talk
  fears and anxieties and, 282
  interventions with maltreating families
    and, 620
  medical investigation of abuse and, 669
Semistructured Clinical Interview for
    Children and Adolescents, 155
Sensitivity, clinical, 34–35
Sensory extinction, 432
Sensory impairments, 415, 461
Sentence combining technique, 564
Separation anxiety, 338
Separation anxiety disorder (SAD), 275
Separation, traumatic, 787–788
Sequential assessment, 741
Serotonin neurotransmitter
  autistic spectrum disorders and, 467
  conduct problems and, 203
  depressive disorders and, 347–348

eating disorders and, 783, 788–789
selective serotonin reuptake inhibitors
    (SSRIs) and, 384
Sertraline
  depressive disorders and, 384–385
  mental retardation and, 441
Service utilization, 345
Setting events
  autistic spectrum disorders and, 481
  systems perspective and, 10
Setting generalization, 162
Setting of treatment, 287t
Sexual abuse
  cognitive-behavioral therapy and, 292–
    293
  depressive disorders and, 382
  eating disorders and, 787–788
  overview, 647, 705–707
  posttraumatic stress disorder and, 608,
    681–690
  prevalence and incidence of, 647–649,
    658
  prevention, 23
    child protection and family issues,
      674–680
    disclosure, 651–662
    investigations of abuse allegations,
      662–669
    judicial system involvement and, 669–
      674
    primary, 651–662
    professional reporting, 662
    secondary, 662–680
  psychoeducation and, 283
  treatment, 680–705, 705–707
    dissociative symptoms, 702–703
    offending adolescents, 704
    posttraumatic stress disorder and,
      681–690, 696–702
    psychotherapy for victims and
      families, 692–696
    sexual problems, 690–692, 703–704
  victim characteristics and, 649–651
Sexual behavior
  interventions addressing, 703–704
  maltreatment of children and, 608
  sexual abuse and, 690–692, 705
Sexual problems, 690–692
Sexual Problems scale of the Child
    Behavior Checklist (CBCL), 690
Sexually transmitted diseases, 658, 667,
    668
Shattered assumption theory, 682–683
Shizotypal personality disorder, 458
Short Smoking Consequences
    Questionnaire, 744
Siblings
  autistic spectrum disorders and, 475–476
  generalization among, 164
  incest and, 678–679
  relationships among, 353–354
Side effects
  of antidepressants, 441
  of antihypertensive medication, 95
  of mood stabilizers, 443
  of neuroleptics, 206, 442
  New York–Montreal (NYM) multimodal
    treatment study and, 119
  of selective serotonin reuptake inhibitors
    (SSRIs), 385
  of tricyclic antidepressants, 93–94
  of vaccinations, 468–469
Sign language training, 479
Single-subject designs, 434–435
Situationism
  cognitive-behavioral assessments and, 36
  cognitive-behavioral systems orientation
    and, 37
  systems perspective and, 10
Skills training approaches
  ACTION treatment program and, 364–
    365, 367–369
  compared to pharmacotherapy, 483
  comparison studies of, 227–228
  conduct problems and, 178–186, 215
  fears and anxieties and, 283, 290–292

Skills training approaches *(cont.)*
  firesetting behaviors and, 202–203
  interventions with maltreating families
    and, 620
  motivation enhancement and, 751
  parent training and, 435
Sleep difficulties
  attention-deficit/hyperactivity disorder
    and, 72
  autistic spectrum disorders and, 462
  depressive disorders and, 337
  posttraumatic stress disorder and, 685
Smith–Magenis syndrome
  mental retardation and, 412
  overview, 416
Smoking. *See* Tobacco use
Social anxiety disorder
  cognitive-behavioral therapy and, 290–
    292
  psychopharmacology, 294–295
Social consequences, 96–97
Social functioning
  Asperger's disorder and, 459–460
  atomoxetine and, 92
  autistic spectrum disorders and, 457–
    458, 471, 472–476, 487–488
  cognitive-behavioral systems orientation
    and, 35, 38
  conduct problems and, 149, 153, 159,
    159–160, 215
  depressive disorders and, 341
  maltreatment of children and, 607, 611–
    612, 629
  mental retardation and, 415–416
  prevention and, 23–24
  sexual abuse and, 696
  social skills training and, 106–108
  treatment goals and, 12
Social influences, 785–786
Social information-processing model, 180
Social inhibition, 19
Social initiation peer training, 473–474
Social interaction, 472–476
Social isolation
  maltreatment of children and, 611–612
  in relational aggression, 142
Social learning theory
  anxiety in children, 273
  maltreatment of children and, 602, 624,
    631
  overview, 10
  substance problems in adolescents and,
    738
Social phobia
  autistic spectrum disorders and, 461
  DSM-IV-TR categories of, 275t
  psychopharmacology, 294–295
Social skills deficits, 143–144
Social skills training
  attention-deficit/hyperactivity disorder
    and, 107–108
  autistic spectrum disorders and, 474–
    475
  bullying interventions and, 196
  conduct problems and, 179
  DARE (Drug Abuse Resistance
    Education) program and, 734
  eating disorders and, 799
  mental retardation and, 437
  New York–Montreal (NYM) multimodal
    treatment study and, 117–119
Social support
  autistic spectrum disorders and, 487
  conduct problems and, 152
  continuum of programs for, 15f
  depressive disorders and, 352
  developmental information and, 16
  posttraumatic stress disorder and, 686–
    687
Social support model, 473–474
Social validity
  conduct problem treatments, 212–218
  Helping the Noncompliant Child (HNC)
    parent training program and, 164
  parent training and, 162
Societal-level interventions, 661

Sociocultural models
  eating disorders and, 811
  learning disabilities and, 526–527
Socioeconomic status
  conduct problems and, 149, 150, 152,
    153, 222
  eating disorders and, 807
  firesetting behaviors and, 144
  foster care and, 628, 674
  maltreatment of children and, 596, 598,
    599, 611, 633, 635
  Multimodal Treatment Study of ADHD
    (MTA) and, 113
  parent–child relationship and, 39
  parent training and, 486, 615
  reading disabilities and, 532
  sexual abuse and, 650, 654
  stimulant medication for ADHD and,
    84– 85
Socioemotional problems, 15f
Somatic complaints
  posttraumatic stress disorder and, 684
  sexual abuse and, 668
Somatization disorder, 144
Spanking, Healthy Start program and,
    633
"Spare the rod, spoil the child" belief,
    620
Special education
  autistic spectrum disorders and, 464
  early intervention and, 575
  historical developments and, 514
  mental retardation and, 444
  overview, 578
  prevention and, 578
  See also Learning disabilities
Specific phobia, 275t
Specific skills instruction, 556
Spelling skills
  handwriting and, 561
  interventions and, 562–563
  PALS program and, 537
Stay Safe Program
  disclosure following participation in,
    656
  overview, 651
Stealing. *See* Theft
STEP program, 226
Steps to Independence manual, 436
Stereotypic behavior
  autistic spectrum disorders and, 458–
    459, 471, 480
  mental retardation and, 433, 441
  Rett's disorder and, 460
Stereotyping, 341
Stimulant medication
  adolescents and, 90–91
  attention-deficit/hyperactivity disorder
    and, 84–89, 85t
  combining with other treatments, 109
  conduct problems and, 203–204
  effectiveness of, 90
  generalization of treatment and, 217
  mental retardation and, 440t
Stimuli to a behavior, 481
Stimulus control strategies, 799
Stimulus generalization, 10
Stomach problems, 385
Story grammar, 564
Strategic structural systems engagement
  approach, 223
Strategy instruction
  comprehension and, 556–557, 560
  implementation of, 572
  reading remediation programs and, 545
Strattera
  attention-deficit/hyperactivity disorder
    and, 91–93
  mental retardation and, 443
Stress
  child testimony and, 671–672
  conduct problems and, 151– 152
  depressive disorders and, 341–342, 348–
    349
  external, 35
  maltreatment of children and, 599, 617

medical investigation of abuse and, 668–
    669
  reduction of, 622
  sexual abuse and, 676
Structural behavioral approaches, 747
Structure, 487–488
Structured Clinical Interview for
  Adolescents (SCI), 742t, 743
Structured diagnostic interviews, 154–156
Substance abuse disorders
  atomoxetine and, 92
  pemoline and, 91
  See also Substance use
Substance dependence, 736–737
Substance problems in adolescents
  assessment and, 740–741, 742t–743t,
    743–746
  overview, 731–740, 767
  prevention and, 734–736
  treatment, 746–763
    case example of, 763–767
    clinical course, 748–749
    cognitive-behavioral skills training
      and, 749–750, 749t, 750–755, 755–
      760
    core sessions, 750–755, 753f
    efficacy of, 746–748
    evaluation of treatment effectiveness,
      760
    implementation of, 761–763
    maintenance of change, 760–761
    session structure, 750
  See also Adolescents; Substance use
Substance testing, 762
Substance use
  attention-deficit/hyperactivity disorder
    and, 71
  conduct disorder and, 389
  conduct problems and, 151
  eating disorders and, 783, 784, 789
  gender and, 17
  multisystemic treatment (MST) and, 215
  normative information and, 18
  by parents, 19, 151, 160
  sexual abuse and, 675
  treatment planning and, 745–746
  See also Substance problems in
    adolescents
Substance use disorders, 144
Suicidality
  adolescents and, 338
  comorbidity and, 346
  conduct problems and, 145
  depressive disorders and, 337, 339, 346
  developmental information and, 338
  ethical and legal considerations, 391–392
  ethnicity and, 343
  gender and, 18
  managed care and, 392
  medication adherence and, 386
  normative information and, 18–19
  parent–child relationship and, 353
  research on, 380
  selective serotonin reuptake inhibitors
    (SSRIs) and, 384–385, 702
Summer treatment program (STP), 110–
    111
Support services, 617
Supportive–expressive therapy, 800
Sutter–Eyberg Student Behavior Inventory,
    156–157
Symbolic modeling, 281, 288
Symbolic play, 458
Symptoms
  of attention-deficit/hyperactivity disorder,
    67–68
  of depressive disorders, 336–339
  posttraumatic stress disorder, 681
  stimulant medication for ADHD and, 88
  See also under specific disorders
Syracuse University studies, 550–551
System-induced trauma, 706
Systematic behavioral family therapy, 379
Systematic desensitization
  eating disorders and, 799
  overview, 281

Systems model
  cognitive-behavioral assessments and, 36
  continuum of programs for, 15f
  depressive disorders and, 353–355, 356
  theoretical framework for, 33–34
  See also Cognitive-behavioral systems
    orientation

Tantrums
  autistic spectrum disorders and, 462
  maltreatment of children and, 610
Task-analytic model of LDs
  overview, 520–521
  treatment and, 523–524
Teacher training, 289t
Teachers
  assessment interviews with, 154–155
  classroom behavior management training
    and, 190–194
  depressive disorders and, 355
  fluency interventions and, 553
  home-based reinforcement programs and,
    194–195
  Incredible Years parent tracking program
    and, 167–168
  learning disabilities and, 530
  mental retardation and, 437
  posttraumatic stress disorder and, 702–
    703
Teachers Report Form (TRF), 744
Teaching Family Model (TFM)
  comparison studies of, 227
  conduct problems and, 186–187, 215–
    216, 224
Teasing, peer, 355
Technology
  child testimony and, 670–672
  computer-based instruction, 548–550
  eating disorder treatment and, 811
  interventions with maltreating families
    and, 620
  online sexual predators and, 661–662
  safety contract regarding, 727
  using videotaped testimony in court,
    673
Teen Addiction Severity Index (T-ASI), 743,
    743t
Teen pregnancy
  attention-deficit/hyperactivity disorder
    and, 71
  conduct problems and, 147
  gender and, 18
  maltreatment of children and, 608, 632
  sexual abuse and, 668, 692
  See also Pregnancy
Telephone Interview Report on Stealing
    and Social Aggression (TIROSSA)
  conduct problems and, 158
  as an outcome measure, 199
Temper tantrums, 338
Temperament
  conduct problems and, 149, 159
  eating disorders and, 792
  parent–child relationship and, 39
  substance problems in adolescents and,
    739
  treatment and, 19
Temporal generalization, 214, 216
Temporal myopia, 80, 82–83
Temporary Assistance to Needy Families
    (TANF), 603, 634
Tenex. See Antihypertensive medications
Termination
  premature, 41–42, 223–224
  therapeutic decision making and, 22
Tertiary interventions, 680–705, 704–705
Tertiary prevention, 416–417
Test of Reading Fluency, 573
Test of Word Reading Efficiency, 573
Testimony, child
  hearsay evidence and, 672–673
  psychotherapy and, 694
  sexual abuse and, 669–670
  using videotaped testimony in court,
    673
  via closed circuit television, 670–672

Testing, academic
  coping skills and, 368
  IQ, 516, 526
  learning disabilities and, 512–513
Testosterone, 203
Texas Children's Medication Algorithm,
    385, 385f
Text Structure Program, 559
Theft
  conduct problems and, 139, 140f, 142–
    143
  treatment and, 198–202, 199t, 217,
    231–232
Theme Identification Program, 558–559
Theory of mind, 466, 467–468
Therapeutic alliance
  eating disorders and, 793–794
  interventions with maltreating families
    and, 632
  therapeutic decision making and, 22
  See also Therapeutic relationship
Therapeutic day care, 627–630
Therapeutic foster care, 187–188
Therapeutic milieu, 41–42
Therapeutic relationship
  cognitive-behavioral therapy and, 357
  fears and anxieties and, 282
  maltreatment of children and, 612, 613–
    615, 625–626
  See also Therapeutic alliance
Therapist characteristics, 287t
Thirmerosal, 469–471
Thought disorders, 471
Thoughts
  acceptance of rather than control of, 12–
    13
  cognitive-behavioral assessments and, 36
  learning disabilities and, 521
  substance problems in adolescents and,
    753–754
Thoughts, negative
  ACTION treatment program and, 359,
    361, 366, 371–372
  depressive disorders and, 357
Tic disorders
  atomoxetine and, 92
  DSM-IV-TR categories of, 26t
  stimulant medication for ADHD and,
    87
Tics, problems with, 87
Time out procedure
  Helping the Noncompliant Child (HNC)
    parent training program and, 163
  interventions with maltreating families
    and, 621
  mental retardation and, 429–430
  overview, 100–101
  parent training and, 435
Tobacco use
  in adolescents, 733, 735
  assessment and, 744, 745
  in pregnancy, 77, 81
  psychopharmacology and, 747–748
Token reward system
  conduct problems and, 216
  in the home setting, 100
  mental retardation and, 425
  parent training and, 435
  response cost and, 429
  in the school setting, 104, 191, 192
Toronto Anti-Bullying Intervention, 197
Toxoplasmosis, 466
Toy play, 472
Trainable mentally retarded (TMR), 413
Training, professional
  cognitive-behavioral therapy and, 393
  mental retardation and, 444
Transactional process
  maltreatment of children and, 599
  substance problems in adolescents and,
    738
Transactional strategies of instruction, 557
Transfer of control concept, 291
Transition, mental retardation and, 419
Transportability research, 297–298
Trauma, eating disorders and, 787–788

Trauma-focused cognitive-behavioral
    therapy (TF-CBT), 700
Trauma-focused psychotherapy, 696–701
Trauma symptoms
  eating disorders and, 787–788
  interventions with maltreating families
    and, 630–631
  See also Posttraumatic stress disorder
Traumatic Events Interview, 698
Trazodone, 206
Treatment
  ACTION treatment program, 358–375,
    363t, 366t, 367f, 368t, 373f, 375f,
    376f, 377f
  assessment and, 161
  assumptions regarding, 81–83
  cognitive-behavioral systems orientation
    of, 5t–6
  combined and multimodal, 11
  continuum of programs for, 15f
  decision-making processes involved in
    choosing, 4–5t
  developmental information and, 16–19
  diversity among, 4
  ethnic and cultural factors to consider in,
    44–45
  intelligence and, 19
  maltreatment of children and, 602–603
  managed care and, 392
  operational rules for implementation of,
    40
  processes of, 41–42
  substance use during, 762–763
  See also Interventions; under specific
    disorders
Treatment engagement
  ACTION treatment program and, 362
  brief strategic family therapy and, 174–
    175
  conduct problems and, 223
  learning disabilities and, 575–576
  maltreatment of children and, 610
Treatment, evidence-based. See Evidence-
    based treatments
Treatment generalization. See
    Generalization of treatment
Treatment goals
  ACTION treatment program and, 364
  broadening of, 12–13
  cognitive-behavioral interventions and, 24
  maltreatment of children and, 609–610
  sexual abuse and, 695
  substance problems in adolescents and, 751
  therapeutic decision-making and, 22
  trauma symptoms and, 631
  See also Goal setting
Treatment of Adolescent Depression Study
    (TADS), 378–383, 392–394
Treatment planning
  cognitive-behavioral assessments and, 36
  conduct problems and, 159
  maltreatment of children and, 603
  sexual abuse and, 693–696
  substance problems in adolescents and,
    745–746
  therapeutic decision making and, 22
Tricyclic antidepressants
  attention-deficit/hyperactivity disorder
    and, 93–94
  depressive disorders and, 384, 384t
  eating disorders and, 805–806
  efficacy of, 386
  fears and anxieties and, 294–295
  inefficacy of in treating depressive
    disorders, 347
  mental retardation and, 439, 440t, 441
  posttraumatic stress disorder and, 702
Triggers of disordered eating, 799
Triggers of substance use, 753–755, 753f
Tripartite model, 277–279
Triple P-Positive Parenting Program
  conduct problems and, 168–170
  effectiveness of, 229, 230–231
  interventions with maltreating families
    and, 633
  as prevention, 207

Triple-response system assessment, 10
Truancy, 139, 140*f*
Trust
    eating disorders and, 793–794
    maltreatment of children and, 612
Tryptophan, 348
Tuberous sclerosis, 461
Tutoring
    multitiered interventions and, 541–544
    reading disabilities and, 537– 541
    research on, 289*t*
Twelve-Step programs
    ethnicity and, 752
    family involvement in, 748
    substance problems in adolescents and, 747
Two-factor theory
    anxiety in children, 272
    sexual abuse and, 683

UCI/OCDE program, 111
UMASS/WPS early intervention project, 111–112
University of Colorado studies, 548–550
University of Texas–Houston Intervention Study, 536
University of Texas–Houston study, 551–552
University of Washington studies, 552
Urine screening, 762
Utilization of services, 693

Vaccination, autistic spectrum disorders and, 468–471
Validity of a treatment. *See* Social validity
Valproate, 443
Valproic acid, in pregnancy, 466
Velocardiofacial syndrome, 412
Venlafaxine, 387

Verbal abuse, 608. *See also* Maltreatment of children
Verbal Learning approach, 478–479
Verbal skills
    anatomically correct dolls and, 666–667
    autistic spectrum disorders and, 458, 467
Verbal working memory
    attention-deficit/hyperactivity disorder and, 74, 79
    autistic spectrum disorders and, 466
Vertical behavioral analysis, 36
Vertical prosecution, 670
Videotape use, 620
Vigilance, 276
Vineland Adaptive Behavior Scales
    autistic spectrum disorders and, 457–458
    home-based interventions and, 489
Violence, domestic
    maltreatment of children and, 599, 608
    sexual abuse and, 651
Violence, family
    conduct problems and, 152
    posttraumatic stress disorder and, 685
Violence, maltreatment of children and, 608
Violence, relationship
    cognitive-behavioral interventions and, 9
    conduct problems and, 231
    maltreatment of children and, 608
    prevention and, 23
Visual processing
    assessment and, 520
    treatment and, 519
Voice recognition methods, 563
Vulnerability
    to depressive disorders, 340–341
    ethnicity and, 344

Weight issues
    depressive disorders and, 337
    puberty and, 342–343
What Do I Say Now? video, 654–655
What If Situations Test (WIST), 653
Williams syndrome, 416, 424
Winners group, 696
Word Identification Strategy Training (WIST) program, 547–548
Word prediction software, 563
Word recognition
    Florida State University study and, 551
    historical developments and, 514
    learning disabilities and, 518
    Orton–Gillingham approach of reading remediation and, 546
    reading disabilities and, 532
    University of Colorado Studies and, 548–550
Working memory, 66, 74, 78–79, 82, 96
Worry, 655
Worthlessness, feelings of, 337
Writing interventions, 698–699
Written expression
    historical developments and, 514
    learning disabilities and, 518*t*
    treatment of disabilities in, 560–565, 577
Wyatt v. Stickney (1972), 430

X chromosome, 465

Yearly Progress Pro, 573
Youth Self-Report (YSR), 744

Ziprasidone, 442
Zoloft. *See* Sertraline